SAUNDERS

Q&A REVIEW for the NCLEX-PN® EXAMINATION

SAUNDERS Q&A REVIEW for the NCLEX-PN® EXAMINATION

EDITION 4

LINDA ANNE SILVESTRI, MSN, RN, PhD(c)

Instructor of Nursing
Salve Regina University
Newport, Rhode Island

President
Nursing Reviews, Inc.
and
Professional Nursing Seminars, Inc.
Charlestown, Rhode Island

Instructor
NCLEX-RN® and NCLEX-PN® Review Courses

SAUNDERS
ELSEVIER

SAUNDERS
ELSEVIER

3251 Riverport Lane
St. Louis, Missouri 63043

SAUNDERS Q&A REVIEW FOR THE NCLEX-PN® EXAMINATION ISBN: 978-1-4160-6201-1

Library of Congress Cataloging-in-Publication Data

Silvestri, Linda Anne.
Saunders Q&A review for the NCLEX-PN examination / Linda Anne Silvestri.—4th ed.
p. ; cm.
Includes bibliographical references and index.
ISBN 978-1-4160-6201-1 (pbk. : alk. paper)
1. Practical nursing—Examinations, questions, etc. I. Title. II. Title: Saunders Q&A review for NCLEX-PN. III. Title: Saunders Q and A review for NCLEX-PN. IV. Title: Q&A review for NCLEX-PN.
[DNLM: 1. Nursing, Practical—Examination Questions. WY 18.2 S587sq 2010]
RT62.S532 2010
610.73076—dc22 2009041664

Senior Editor: Kristin Geen
Developmental Editor: Todd McKenzie
Publishing Services Manager: Anne Altepeter
Senior Project Manager: Doug Turner
Multimedia Producer: Keith Jones
Designer: Kim Denando

Printed in the United States of America
Last digit is the print number: 9 8 7 6 5 4 3

To my parents,
To my mother, ***Frances Mary,*** *and in loving memory of my father,* ***Arnold Lawrence,***
who taught me to always love, care, and be the best that I could be.

ABOUT THE AUTHOR

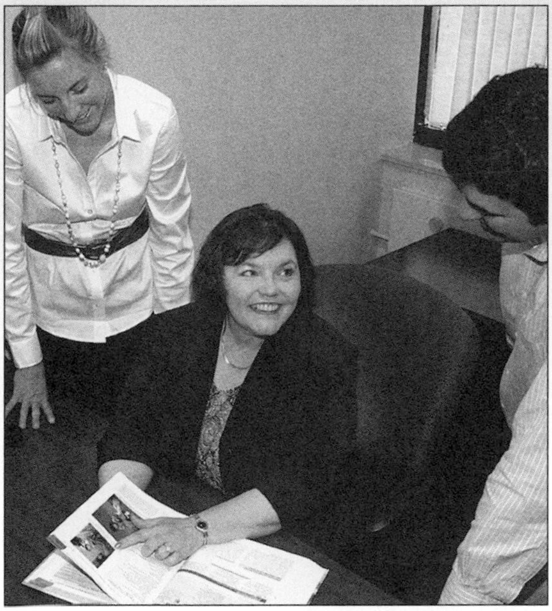

Linda Anne Silvestri

As a child, I always dreamed of becoming either a nurse or teacher. Initially, I chose to become a nurse because I wanted to help others, especially those who were ill. Then I realized that both of my dreams could come true; I could be both a nurse and a teacher. So I pursued my dreams.

I received my diploma in nursing at Cooley Dickinson Hospital School of Nursing in Northampton, Massachusetts. Afterward, I worked at Baystate Medical Center in Springfield, Massachusetts, where I cared for clients in acute medical-surgical units, the intensive care unit, the emergency department, pediatric units, and other acute care units. Later, I received an associate degree from Holyoke Community College in Holyoke, Massachusetts, my BSN from American International College in Springfield, Massachusetts, and my MSN from Anna Maria College in Paxton, Massachusetts, with a dual major in Nursing Management and Patient Education. I have received my PhD candidacy status in Nursing at the University of Nevada, Las Vegas, and I am doing research related to success on the NCLEX exam. I am also a member of the Honor Society of Nursing, Sigma Theta Tau International, Phi Kappa Phi, Golden Key International Honour Society, the Western Institute of Nursing, and the Eastern Nursing Research Society.

As a native of Springfield, Massachusetts, I began my teaching career as an instructor of medical-surgical nursing and leadership-management nursing at Baystate Medical Center School of Nursing in 1981. In 1989 I relocated to Rhode Island and began teaching medical-surgical nursing and psychiatric nursing to RN and LPN students at the Community College of Rhode Island. In 1994 I began teaching nursing at Salve Regina University in Newport, Rhode Island, and remain there as an adjunct faculty member.

My experiences as a student, nursing educator, and item writer for the NCLEX exams aided me as I developed a comprehensive review course to prepare nursing students and graduates for the NCLEX examination. In 1991 I established Professional Nursing Seminars, Inc., and in 2000 I started Nursing Reviews, Inc. Both are companies that conduct review courses for the NCLEX-RN and the NCLEX-PN examinations and assist nursing graduates to achieve their goals of becoming registered nurses or licensed practical/vocational nurses.

Today I conduct review courses for the NCLEX examinations throughout New England and am the author of numerous successful review products. I am so pleased that you have decided to let me join you on your journey to success in testing for nursing school exams and the NCLEX-PN examination!

CONTRIBUTORS

Jill Feranec, LPN
Graduate
Stone Academy
Hamden, Connecticut

Laurent W. Valliere, BS
Vice President
Professional Nursing Seminars, Inc.
Charlestown, Rhode Island

ITEM WRITERS

Patricia Delmoe, RN, MN, ACLS, PALS
Nursing Instructor
Banner Health
Phoenix, Arizona

Marilyn Greer, MS, RN
Associate Professor of Nursing
Rockford College
Rockford, Illinois

Patricia B. Lisk, RN, BSN
Instructor/PCA Coordinator
Augusta Technical College
Aiken, South Carolina

Bruce Austin Scott, MSN, ACNS-BC
Nursing Instructor
San Joaquin Delta College
Stockton, California

Sharon Souter, PhD, RN, CNE
Dean and Associate Professor
College of Nursing
University of Mary Hardin-Baylor
Belton, Texas

Bethany Hawes Sykes, EdD, RN, CEN
Adjunct Faculty
Department of Nursing
Salve Regina University
Newport, Rhode Island

The author and publisher would also like to acknowledge the following individuals for contributions to previous editions of this book:

Nancy Diane Blasdell, MSN, RN
Dartmouth, Massachusetts

Jean DeCoffe, MSN, RN
Lowell, Massachusetts

Kathleen Anne Fiato, RN
Troy, New York

Debbie Jean Fitzgerald, MSN, RN
Norfolk, Virginia

Mary Ann Hogan, MSN, RN, CS
Amherst, Massachusetts

Cathleen J. Massey, LVN
Visalia, California

Yazmin Mojica, RN, MA, MSN/MPH, CNS
Stanton, California

Jo Ann Barnes Mullaney, PhD, RN, CS
Newport, Rhode Island

Roberta P. Ramont, RN, MS
Anaheim, California

Lyndi C. Shadbolt, RN, BSN
Amarillo, Texas

Ruth Sieperman, MN, NNP
Phoenix, Arizona

Deborah W. Toth, MSN, RN
Milan, Ohio

Lucy White RN, MSN
Greencastle, Indiana

CONSULTANT

Nicole Marie Valliere, BSN, RN
Professional Nurse I—Pediatrics
Hasbro Children's Hospital
Providence, Rhode Island

REVIEWERS

Jacqueline B. Arnett, RN, BSN, CPN
Staff Development Coordinator
Life Care Centers of America
Tucson, Arizona

Sally J. Flesch, PhD, RN
Professor of Nursing
Black Hawk College
Moline, Illinois

Anita Garman, RN, BSN, MSN
Staff Nurse
Sutter Gould Medical Foundation
Turlock Medical Clinic
Turlock, California

Dionne Gibbs, RN, BS
Director of Nursing
Centura College
Virginia Beach, Virginia

Melissa Langone, PhD, MSHN, ARNP
Assistant Professor
Health Programs—Nursing
Pasco-Hernando Community College
New Port Richey, Florida

PREFACE

"To know that even one life has breathed easier because you have lived, this is to have succeeded."

—*Ralph Waldo Emerson*

Welcome to *Saunders Pyramid to Success!*
Saunders Q&A Review for the NCLEX-PN® Examination is one in a series of products designed to assist you achieving your goal of becoming a licensed practical/vocational nurse. *Saunders Q&A Review for the NCLEX-PN® Examination* gives you 3200 practice NCLEX-PN test questions based on the 2008 NCLEX-PN test plan developed by the National Council of State Boards of Nursing.

The 2008 test plan for the NCLEX-PN exam identifies a framework based on Client Needs. The Client Needs categories include Safe and Effective Care Environment, Physiological Integrity, Psychosocial Integrity, and Health Promotion and Maintenance. Integrated Processes are also identified as a component of the test plan. These include Caring, Clinical Problem Solving Process (Nursing Process), Communication and Documentation, and Teaching and Learning. This book has been uniquely designed and includes chapters that describe each specific component of the 2008 NCLEX-PN test plan framework and chapters that contain practice questions specific to each component.

NCLEX-PN® TEST PREPARATION

This book begins with information regarding NCLEX-PN preparation. Chapter 1 addresses all of the information related to the 2008 NCLEX-PN test plan and the testing procedures related to the examination. This chapter answers all the questions that you may have about the testing procedures. Chapter 2 discusses the NCLEX-PN from a nonacademic perspective and emphasizes a holistic approach for your individual test preparation. This chapter identifies the components of a structured study plan and pattern, anxiety-reducing techniques, and personal focus issues.

Nursing students want to hear what recent graduates have to say about their experiences with the NCLEX-PN and want to know what it is really like to take this examination. Chapter 3 is written by a nursing graduate who took the NCLEX-PN exam. This chapter addresses the issue of what the NCLEX-PN is all about and includes the graduate's story of success.

Chapter 4, "Test-Taking Strategies," includes all the important strategies that will help you learn how to read a question, how not to read into a question, and how to use the process of elimination and other methods to select the correct response from the options presented.

Client Needs

Chapters 5 through 9 address the 2008 NCLEX-PN test plan component Client Needs. Chapter 5 describes each category of Client Needs as identified by the test plan and lists any associated subcategories, the percentage of test questions for each category, and some of the content included on the NCLEX-PN examination. Chapters 6 through 9 contain practice test questions related specifically to each category of Client Needs. Chapter 6 comprises questions related to Safe and Effective Care Environment; Chapter 7 contains Health Promotion and Maintenance questions; Chapter 8 is made up of Psychosocial Integrity questions; and Chapter 9 contains questions addressing Physiological Integrity.

Integrated Processes

Chapters 10 and 11 address Integrated Processes as identified in the test plan for NCLEX-PN. Chapter 10 describes each Integrated Process. Chapter 11 contains practice test questions related specifically to each Integrated Process, including Caring, Clinical Problem Solving Process (Nursing Process), Communication and Documentation, and Teaching and Learning.

Comprehensive Test

A comprehensive test is included at the end of this book. It consists of 85 practice questions representative of the components of the 2008 test plan framework for NCLEX-PN.

SPECIAL FEATURES OF THE BOOK

Book Design

The book's design uses a unique two-column format. The left column presents the practice questions and options, and the right column provides the corresponding Answers, Rationales, Test-Taking Strategies, Question Categories, Content Areas, and Reference(s). The two-column format makes the review easier because you do not have to flip through pages in search of answers and rationales.

Practice Questions

While you are preparing for the NCLEX-PN examination, it is crucial that you review practice test questions. This book contains 1500 practice questions in NCLEX format, including multiple-choice and alternate item format questions. The accompanying software includes all of the questions from the book, plus an additional 1700 questions, for a total of 3200 test questions.

Alternate Item Format Questions

The alternate item format questions may be presented as fill-in-the-blank, multiple-response, prioritizing (ordered response), image or illustration, or chart/exhibit questions. These questions provide you with practice in prioritizing and decision making and can be found at the end of Chapters 6 through 9 and 11. Additionally, alternate item format questions are integrated throughout the NCLEX-PN review software.

Heart and Lung Sound Questions

Also found on the accompanying software are heart and lung sound questions representative of content addressed in the 2008 NCLEX-PN test plan. Each of these questions is in the NCLEX-style format and presents an audio sound as a component of the question.

Answer Sections for Practice Questions

Each practice question is followed by the correct Answer, Rationale, Test-Taking Strategy, Question Categories, Content Area, and Reference(s). The structure of the answer section is unique and provides the following information for every question:

Rationale: The rationale provides you with significant information about both correct and incorrect options.

Test-Taking Strategy: The test-taking strategy provides you with the logic for selecting the correct option and helps you select an answer to a question on which you must guess. Specific suggestions for review are identified in the test-taking strategy.

Question Categories: Each question is identified based on the categories used by the NCLEX-PN test plan. Additional content area categories are provided with each question to assist you in identifying areas in need of review. The categories identified with each question include Level of Cognitive Ability, Client Needs, Integrated Process, and the specific nursing Content Area. All categories are identified by their full names so that you do not need to memorize codes or abbreviations.

Reference(s): The reference source, including page number, is provided so that you can easily find the information that you need to review in your nursing textbooks.

NCLEX-PN® REVIEW SOFTWARE

You will find an NCLEX-PN review CD packaged in this book. This software contains 3200 questions, 1500 from the book and 1700 additional questions, including multiple-choice, alternate item format, and audio questions. This Windows- and Macintosh-compatible program offers three testing modes for review of the questions.

Study: All questions on Client Needs, Integrated Process, or a specific Content Area. The Answer, Rationale, and Test-Taking Strategy appear after you answer each question.

Quiz: Ten randomly chosen questions on Client Needs, Integrated Process, or a specific Content Area. Results are given and review of the Answer, Rationale, and Test-Taking Strategy is provided after you answer all 10 questions.

Examination: One hundred randomly chosen questions from the entire pool of 3200 questions, chosen according to Client Needs, Integrated Process, or a specific Content Area. Results are given and review is provided after you answer all 100 questions.

The CD allows you to customize your review and determine your areas of strength and weakness. It also provides you with a wealth of practice test questions while simulating the NCLEX-PN experience on your computer.

HOW TO USE THIS BOOK

Saunders Q&A Review for the NCLEX-PN® Examination is especially designed to help you with your successful journey to the peak of the *Pyramid to Success,* becoming a licensed practical/vocational nurse. As you begin your journey through this book, you will be introduced to all of the important points regarding the NCLEX-PN examination, the process of testing, and the unique and special tips regarding how to prepare yourself for this important examination. Read the chapter from the nursing graduate who passed the NCLEX-PN exam, and consider what this graduate has to say about the examination. The test-taking strategy chapter will provide you with important strategies that will guide you in selecting the correct option or assist you in guessing the answer. Read this chapter and practice these strategies as you proceed through your journey with this book.

Once you have completed the introductory components of this book, it is time to begin the practice questions. As you read through each question and select an answer, be sure to read the Rationale and the Test-Taking Strategy. The Rationale provides you with significant information about both the correct and incorrect options, and the Test-Taking Strategy provides you with the logic for selecting the correct option. The strategy also identifies the Content Area that you should review if you had difficulty with the question. Use the reference source provided so that you can easily find the information that you need to review.

As you work your way through *Saunders Q&A Review for the NCLEX-PN® Examination* to identify your areas of strength and weakness, you can return to the companion book, *Saunders Comprehensive Review for the*

NCLEX-PN® Examination, to focus your study on these areas. The companion book and its accompanying software provide you with a comprehensive review of all areas of the nursing content reflected in the 2008 NCLEX-PN test plan, as well as 3700 practice questions that are different from the questions in the book you are holding now.

Another valuable resource for preparing for nursing examinations and the NCLEX-PN examination is *Saunders Strategies for Test Success: Passing Nursing School and the NCLEX® Examination.* This product contains chapters that describe several test-taking strategies and include several sample questions that illustrate how to use the strategy. The sample questions represent all types of question formats, including multiple-choice, fill-in-the-blank, multiple-response, prioritizing (ordered response), chart/texhibit questions, and questions that contain a figure or illustration. In addition to the sample questions in the chapters, 500 practice questions accompany this book. There are 200 practice questions in the book, and the software contains these questions, along with an additional 300 practice questions.

An additional component of the *Saunders Pyramid to Success* is the *Saunders Review Cards for the NCLEX-PN® Examination.* This product provides you with more than 900 practice test questions, including multiple-choice and alternate item format questions such as fill-in-the-blank, multiple response, prioritizing (ordered response), and questions that contain a figure or illustration. The practice question is located on one side of the review card. The reverse side of the review card contains the correct answer, rationale, and question categories for the practice question on the front of the card.

Good luck with your journey through the *Pyramid to Success!* I wish you continued success throughout your new career as a licensed practical/vocational nurse!

Linda Anne Silvestri MSN, RN, PhD(c)

ACKNOWLEDGMENTS

Sincere appreciation and warmest thanks are extended to the many individuals who in their own way have contributed to the publication of this book.

First, I want to acknowledge my parents, who opened my door of opportunity in education. I thank my mother, Frances Mary, for all of her love, support, and assistance as I continuously worked to achieve my professional goals. I thank my father, Arnold Lawrence, who always provided insightful words of encouragement. My memories of his love and support will always remain in my heart. I also thank my best friend and love of my life, Larry; my sister, Dianne Elodia; my brother, Lawrence Peter, and my sister-in-law, Mary; and my nieces and nephews, Gina Marie, Angela, Katie, Nicole, and Nicholas, who were continuously supportive, giving, and helpful during my research and preparation of this publication.

I want to thank all of my nursing students at the Community College of Rhode Island in Warwick who approached me in 1991 and persuaded me to help them prepare to take the NCLEX examination. Their enthusiasm and inspiration led to the commencement of my professional endeavors in conducting NCLEX review courses for nursing students. I also thank the numerous nursing students who have attended my review courses for their willingness to share their needs and ideas. Their input has certainly added a special uniqueness to this publication.

I wish to acknowledge all of the nursing faculty who taught in my NCLEX review courses. Their commitment, dedication, and expertise have certainly assisted nursing students in achieving success with the NCLEX examination. Additionally, a special acknowledgment goes to Laurent W. Valliere for his contribution to this publication, for teaching in my NCLEX review courses, and for his commitment and dedication in assisting my nursing students to prepare for the NCLEX examination from a nonacademic point of view.

I sincerely acknowledge and thank three very important individuals from Elsevier. I thank Nancy O'Brien, my former managing editor, for all of her assistance throughout the preparation of this edition and for her continuous enthusiasm, support, and expert professional guidance, and I thank Kristin Geen, my new managing editor, for all of her assistance in bringing this product to fruition. And I thank Todd McKenzie, my developmental editor, for his extraordinary support. Todd maintains a tremendous role as my developmental editor and definitely has outstanding organizational and prioritizing skills and has maintained order for all of the work that I submitted for manuscript production. I also thank Todd for his dedication to my work, his continuous assistance and support, and for keeping me on schedule with manuscript submission.

A special thank you and acknowledgment goes to four important individuals, Dianne E. Ventrice, Lawrence Fiorentino, Karen Machnacz, and Angela Silvestri. They provided continuous support and dedication to my work in both the NCLEX review courses and in reference support for the fourth edition of this book. Additionally, Angela, who is a senior nursing student at Salve Regina University in Newport, Rhode Island, read the practice questions for this book and has offered feedback based on her nursing student experiences.

I want to acknowledge all of the staff in marketing, especially Bob Boehringer, executive marketing director; Susan Copeland, associate marketing manager; Dan Hughes, Evolve Reach marketing manager; and Kathy Mantz, executive marketing manager, and all of the additional staff at Elsevier for their tremendous assistance throughout the preparation and production of this publication. A special thank you to all of them.

I thank all of the special people in the production department, Anne Altepeter, publishing services manager; Doug Turner, senior project manager; Kim Denando, book designer; and Keith Jones, multimedia producer, all of whom assisted in finalizing this publication.

I would also like to acknowledge Patricia Mieg, former educational sales representative, who encouraged me to submit my ideas and initial work for the first edition of this book to Saunders.

I want to acknowledge all of the contributors, reviewers, and item writers of this publication for their thoughts and ideas. And a special thank you goes to Jill Feranec, LPN, for providing a chapter to this publication regarding her experiences with the NCLEX-PN examination.

I also need to thank Salve Regina University for the opportunity to educate nursing students in the baccalaureate nursing program and for its support during my research and writing of this publication. I would like to especially acknowledge my colleagues, Dr. Peggy Matteson, Dr. JoAnn Mullaney, Dr. Ellen McCarty, and Dr. Bethany Sykes, for all of their support and encouragement.

I wish to acknowledge the Community College of Rhode Island, which provided me the opportunity to educate nursing students in the Associate Degree of Nursing Program, and a special thank you to Patricia

Miller, MSN, RN, and Michelina McClellan, MS, RN, from Baystate Medical Center, School of Nursing, in Springfield, Massachusetts, who were my first mentors in nursing education.

Lastly, a very special thank you to all of my nursing students—past, present, and future. Your love and dedication to the profession of nursing and your commitment to provide health care will bring never-ending rewards!

Linda Anne Silvestri, MSN, RN, PhD(c)

CONTENTS

UNIT

I

NCLEX-PN® Preparation

CHAPTER 1

NCLEX-PN®

THE PYRAMID TO SUCCESS

Welcome to *Saunders Q&A Review for the NCLEX-PN® Examination*, the second component of the Pyramid to Success!

At this time, you have completed the first step in your path toward the peak of the Pyramid with *Saunders Comprehensive Review for the NCLEX-PN® Examination*. Now it is time to continue the journey to becoming a licensed practical or vocational nurse with *Saunders Q&A Review for the NCLEX-PN® Examination!*

As you begin your journey through this book, you will be introduced to all of the important points regarding the NCLEX-PN examination, the process of testing, and the unique and special tips for preparing yourself for this very important examination. You will read what a nursing graduate, who recently passed the NCLEX-PN, has to say about the examination. All of the important test-taking strategies are detailed, which will guide you in selecting the correct option or in making a logical guess when you are unsure about an answer.

Saunders Q&A Review for the NCLEX-PN® Examination contains 3200 NCLEX-PN–style practice questions. The chapters have been developed to provide a description of the components of the NCLEX-PN test plan, including the Client Needs and the Integrated Processes. In addition, chapters have been prepared to contain practice questions specific to each category of the Client Needs and the Integrated Processes. In each chapter that contains practice questions, a rationale, a test-taking strategy, and a reference source that contains a page number are provided with each question. Each question is coded on the basis of the Level of Cognitive Ability, the Client Needs category, the Integrated Process, and the content area being tested. The rationale provides you with significant information regarding both the correct and incorrect options. The test-taking strategy provides you with the logical path to selecting the correct option and identifies the content area to review, if necessary. The reference source and page number provide easy access to the information that you need to review.

Let us continue with our journey up the Pyramid to Success!

THE EXAMINATION PROCESS

An important step in the Pyramid to Success is becoming as familiar as possible with the examination process. The challenge of this examination can arouse significant anxiety. Knowing what the examination is all about and knowing what you will encounter during the process of testing will assist with alleviating your fear and anxiety. The information contained in this chapter addresses the procedures related to the development of the NCLEX-PN test plan, the components of the test plan, and the answers to the questions that are most commonly asked by nursing students and graduates preparing to take the NCLEX-PN. The information in this chapter that relates to the test plan was obtained from the National Council of State Boards of Nursing (NCSBN) Web site (www.ncsbn.org) and the *2008 Detailed Test Plan for the NCLEX-PN® Examination*. Additional information about the test and its development can be obtained by accessing the NCSBN Web site or by writing to the National Council of State Boards of Nursing, 111 East Wacker Drive, Suite 2900, Chicago, Illinois 60601-4277.

CAT NCLEX-PN®

The term *NCLEX-PN* stands for "National Council Licensure Examination for Practical/Vocational Nurses." The term *CAT* stands for "computerized adaptive testing." The CAT NCLEX-PN is a computer-administered examination that the nursing graduate must take and pass to practice as a practical or vocational nurse. This examination measures the competencies required to perform safely and effectively as a newly licensed, entry-level practical or vocational nurse.

CAT AND ANSWERING TEST QUESTIONS

With CAT, the examination is created as you answer each question. All of the test questions are categorized on the basis of the test plan structure and the level of difficulty of the question. As you answer a question, the computer will determine your competency based on the answer that you selected. If you selected the correct answer to a question, the computer scans the question bank and selects a more difficult question. If you selected an incorrect answer, the computer scans the question bank and selects an easier question. This process continues until the test plan requirements are met and a reliable pass-or-fail decision can be made.

When a test question is presented on the computer screen, it must be answered, or the test will not move on. This means that you will not be able to skip questions, go back and review questions, or go back and change answers. Remember, with a CAT examination, after an answer is recorded, all subsequent questions administered depend, to an extent, on the answer selected for that question. Skipping questions and returning to earlier questions are not compatible with the logical methodology of a CAT. The inability to skip questions or to go back and change previous answers will not be a disadvantage to you; rather, you will not fall into the trap of changing a correct answer to an incorrect one with this style of testing.

If you are faced with a question that contains unfamiliar content, you may need to guess the answer. There is no penalty for guessing on this examination. Remember, for the majority of the questions, the answer will be right there in front of you. If you need to guess, use your nursing knowledge to its fullest extent, and think about all of the test-taking strategies that you have practiced in this review program.

You do not need any computer experience to take this examination. A keyboard and question tutorial are provided and administered to all test-takers at the start of the examination. The tutorial will instruct you about the use of the optional on-screen calculator, the use of the mouse, and how to record an answer for the various question types. A proctor is present to explain the use of the computer to ensure your full understanding of how to proceed.

DEVELOPMENT OF THE TEST PLAN

As an initial step in the test-development process, the NCSBN considers the legal scope of nursing practice as governed by state laws and regulations, including the nurse practice act. The NCSBN uses these laws to define the areas on the NCLEX-PN that will assess the competence of candidates for nurse licensure.

The NCSBN also conducts a practice analysis study to determine the framework of the test plan for the NCLEX-PN. The participants in this study include newly licensed practical and vocational nurses. The participants are provided with a list of nursing activities and asked about the frequency of performing these specific activities, their impact on the maintenance of client safety, and the settings in which the activities are performed. Expert analysis of the data obtained from this study guides the development of a framework for entry-level nurse performance that incorporates specific client needs and the processes that are fundamental to the practice of nursing. The NCLEX-PN test plan is derived from this framework. Because nursing practice continues to change, this study is conducted every 3 years. The results of the study that provided the structure for the current test plan were implemented in April 2008.

THE TEST PLAN

The content of the NCLEX-PN reflects the activities that an entry-level practical and vocational nurse must be able to perform to provide clients with safe and effective nursing care. The questions address the Levels of Cognitive Ability, the Client Needs, and the Integrated Processes as identified in the test plan (Box 1-1).

Levels of Cognitive Ability

The NCLEX-PN examination consists of questions that have been written at the cognitive level of application, as well as at higher levels. See Box 1-2 for an example of a question written at the cognitive level of analysis.

Box 1-1 ▲ EXAMINATION QUESTIONS

EACH EXAMINATION QUESTION ADDRESSES:

- A Level of Cognitive Ability
- A Client Needs category
- An Integrated Process

Box 1-2 ▲ LEVEL OF COGNITIVE ABILITY

QUESTION

A nurse is caring for a client who has been diagnosed with tuberculosis. The client is receiving rifampin (Rifadin), 600 mg orally daily. Which laboratory finding would indicate to the nurse that the client is experiencing an adverse reaction?

1. A total bilirubin level of 0.5 mg/dL
2. A white blood cell count of 6000 cells/mm^3
3. A sedimentation rate of 15 mm/hr
4. An alkaline phosphatase level of 25 King-Armstrong units/dL

ANSWER: 4

This question requires you to determine the adverse reactions associated with this medication and to analyze each of the laboratory values identified in the options. Adverse reactions or toxic effects of rifampin include hepatotoxicity, hepatitis, blood dyscrasias, Stevens-Johnson syndrome, and antibiotic-related colitis. The nurse monitors for increased liver function blood test results, bilirubin, blood urea nitrogen, and uric acid levels, because elevations indicate an adverse reaction. The normal alkaline phosphatase level is 4.5 to 13 King-Armstrong units/dL. The normal total bilirubin level is less than 1.5 mg/dL. A normal white blood cell count is 4500 to 11,000 cells/mm^3. The normal sedimentation rate is 0 to 30 mm/hr.

Level of Cognitive Ability: Analysis

Box 1-3 ▲ INTEGRATED PROCESSES OF THE TEST PLAN

Caring
Communication and Documentation
Nursing Process (Clinical Problem-Solving Process)
Teaching and Learning

Client Needs

In the test plan implemented in April 2008, the NCSBN identified a framework based on Client Needs. This framework was selected on the basis of the findings of the practice analysis study. In addition, the Client Needs provide a structure for defining nursing actions and competencies across all settings for all clients and for meeting the requirements of state laws and statutes. The NCSBN identified four major categories of Client Needs. Some categories are further divided into subcategories, and the percentage of test questions in each subcategory is identified. Refer to Chapter 5, "Client Needs and the NCLEX-PN® Test Plan," for a detailed description of these categories and subcategories.

Integrated Processes of the Test Plan

The NCSBN has identified four processes that are fundamental to the practice of nursing. These processes are components of the test plan and are integrated throughout the categories of Client Needs (Box 1-3).

TYPES OF QUESTIONS ON THE EXAMINATION

The types of questions that may be administered on the examination include multiple choice, fill-in-the-blank, multiple response, prioritizing (ordered response), chart/exhibit, and questions that contain a figure or illustration (hot spots). Some questions may require you to use the mouse component of the computer system. For example, you may be presented with a visual that displays the arterial vessels of an adult client. In this visual, you may be asked to "point and click" (using the mouse) on the area where the popliteal pulse can be felt (the hot spot). The NCSBN provides specific directions for you to follow with these questions to guide you in the process of testing. Be sure to read these directions as they appear on the computer screen.

Multiple Choice

Most of the questions that you will be asked to answer will be in the multiple-choice format. These questions will provide you with data about a particular client situation and four answer options.

Box 1-4 ▲ FILL-IN-THE-BLANK QUESTION

QUESTION

A physician's order reads digoxin (Lanoxin), 0.125 mg PO (orally) daily. The medication label reads digoxin (Lanoxin), 0.25 mg/tablet. The nurse prepares how many tablets to administer the dose?

ANSWER: 0.5 Tablet

For this fill-in-the-blank question, you need to focus on the physician's order and the medication dosage that is available. Next, you will use the formula for calculating a medication dose. When you are taking the NCLEX examination, remember to use the on-screen calculator to verify your answer.

FORMULA:

$$\frac{\text{Desired}}{\text{Available}} \times \text{Volume} = \text{tablet}$$

$$\frac{0.125\,\text{mg}}{0.25\,\text{mg}} \times 1\,\text{tablet} = 0.5\,\text{tablet}$$

Fill-in-the-Blank

These types of questions may ask you to perform a medication calculation, to determine an intravenous flow rate, or to calculate an intake and output record for a client. You will need to type in your answer. Read the directions for each question carefully, because you may be asked to round the answer to the nearest whole number or to the nearest tenth. See Box 1-4 for an example of a fill-in-the-blank question.

Multiple Response

For this type of question, you will be asked to select or check all of the options (e.g., nursing interventions) that relate to the information in the question. There is no partial credit given for correct selections. See Box 1-5 for an example of a multiple-response question.

Prioritizing (Ordered Response)

These questions may ask you to number your nursing actions in order of priority. Information will be presented in a question, and, based on the data provided, you will need to determine what you would do first, second, third, and so on. On the NCLEX, you will be asked to use the computer mouse and to "drag and drop" the options in order of priority. See Box 1-6 for an example of a prioritizing (ordered-response) question.

Box 1-5 ▲ MULTIPLE-RESPONSE QUESTION

QUESTION

A nurse is preparing to remove a nasogastric tube from a client. Which of the following actions would the nurse take to perform this procedure? Select all that apply.

1. ☐ Place the client in a supine position.
2. ☑ Assess for the presence of bowel sounds.
3. ☑ Untape the nasogastric tube from the client's nose.
4. ☑ Ask the client to hold his or her breath during the removal of the tube.
5. ☐ Keep the tube attached to the prescribed amount of suction during removal.
6. ☑ Instill 20 mL of air into the nasogastric tube to displace secretions back into the client's stomach.

ANSWER: 2, 3, 4, 6

With a multiple-response question, you will be asked to select or check all of the options (e.g., nursing actions) that relate to the information in the question. To answer this question, visualize the procedure, and think about airway patency, preventing aspiration, and preventing mucosal irritation to identify the correct interventions. After explaining the procedure for tube removal to the client, the nurse assesses for the presence of bowel sounds. The tube is not removed if bowel sounds are absent. The nurse dons clean gloves, places the client in an upright position, and places a towel across the client's chest. The suction is turned off, and the nasogastric tube is disconnected from the suction tube. The nurse instills 20 mL of air into the nasogastric tube to displace secretions back into the client's stomach and to decrease the client's risk of aspiration. The nasogastric tube is then untaped from the client's nose. Finally, the client is instructed to hold the breath during the removal of the tube, and the tube is pulled out in one quick, steady motion.

Figure or Illustration (Hot Spot)

This type of question will provide you with a figure or illustration and ask you to answer the question based on the image. The question could contain a chart, table, figure, or illustration. You may also be asked to use the computer mouse and to "point and click" on a specific area (hot spot) in the visual. A visual or image may appear in any type of question, including a multiple-choice question. See Box 1-7 for an example of a figure or illustration question.

Chart/Exhibit

With this type of question, you will be presented with a problem and a chart or exhibit that you will need to refer to when answering the question. Be sure to read all of the information in the question before deciding on your answer. See Box 1-8 for an example of a chart/exhibit question.

Box 1-6 ▲ PRIORITIZING (ORDERED-RESPONSE) QUESTION

QUESTION

The nurse cares for a client who has arrived to the nursing unit after an appendectomy. List, in order of priority, the actions that the nurse will take. (Number 1 is the first action performed, and number 6 is the last one performed.)

1. Checks for airway patency
4. Checks abdominal dressing
2. Measures the respiratory rate
3. Evaluates heart rate and rhythm
5. Asks the client about any concerns
6. Documents postoperative findings

ANSWER: 1, 4, 2, 3, 5, 6

This question asks you to prioritize nursing actions. Postoperative care begins with the evaluation of the client's ABCs—airway, breathing, and circulation—to assess airway patency to ensure the adequate oxygenation of body organs and tissues. Next, the rate and quality of the client's respirations are determined, and breath sounds are auscultated throughout all lung fields to ensure adequate ventilation. The client's heart rate and rhythm are determined, and the client's blood pressure is checked after respiratory assessment, according to the hierarchy of the ABCs. After the ABCs are complete, the nurse assesses the neurological status and the remaining organ systems and then conducts other assessments (e.g., dressings, drains, tubes, pain) as part of a comprehensive assessment. Finally, the nurse documents the findings.

REGISTERING TO TAKE THE EXAMINATION

The initial step in the registration process is submitting an application to the state board of nursing of the state in which you intend to obtain licensure. You will need to get information from the board of nursing regarding the specific registration process, because the process may vary from state to state. In most states, you may register for the examination online, by mail, or by telephone. The NCLEX candidate Web site is www.vue.com/nclex. Following the registration instructions and completing the registration forms precisely and accurately are important. Registration forms that are not properly completed or not accompanied by the proper fees in the required method of payment will be returned to you and will delay testing. You must pay a fee for taking the examination, and you also may have to pay additional fees to the board of nursing of the state in which you are applying. You will be sent a confirmation letter that

Box 1-7 ▲ FIGURE OR ILLUSTRATION (HOT-SPOT) QUESTION

QUESTION

The nurse notes that this rhythm is being displayed on a client's cardiac monitor. Based on this rhythm, the nurse should take which appropriate action?

1. Contact the physician.
2. Prepare to administer atropine sulfate.
3. Ask the client to perform Valsalva's maneuver.
4. Document the rhythm in the client's medical record.

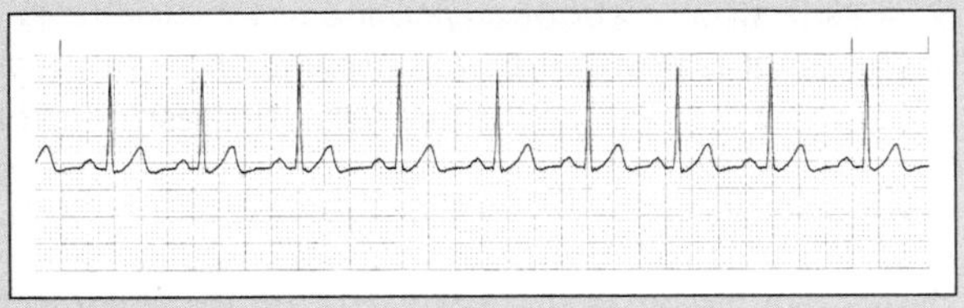

Figure 1-1 (From Ignatavicius, D., & Workman, M. (2006). *Medical-surgical nursing: Critical thinking for collaborative care* (5th ed., p. 716). Philadelphia: Saunders.)

ANSWER: 4

For this question, you are provided with a figure of a rhythm strip and asked about it. Focus on the characteristics of the rhythm. Noting that the rhythm is a normal sinus rhythm will direct you to the correct option. In addition, note that all of the incorrect options identify nursing actions that are performed if the rhythm is abnormal.

Box 1-8 ▲ CHART/EXHIBIT QUESTION

QUESTION

The nurse reviews the laboratory results in a client's chart and determines that which result is abnormal?

1. Sodium 150 mEq/L
2. Potassium 4 mEq/L
3. Fasting glucose 102 mg/dL
4. Blood urea nitrogen 10 mg/dL

CLIENT'S MEDICAL RECORD

Laboratory	Medications	Progress Reports
Sodium 150 mEq/L		
Potassium 4 mEq/L		
Fasting glucose 102 mg/dL		
Blood urea nitrogen 10 mg/dL		

ANSWER: 1

For this question, you are provided with the client's chart and laboratory results. You need to refer to the laboratory results to answer the question. The normal sodium level is 135 to 145 mEq/L. The normal potassium level is 3.5 to 5.1 mEq/L. The normal fasting blood glucose is 70 to 110 mg/dL. The normal blood urea nitrogen is 8 to 25 mg/dL.

indicates that your registration was received. If you do not receive such confirmation within 4 weeks of submitting your registration, you should contact candidate services; this contact information is available on the NCLEX candidate Web site at www.vue.com/nclex.

AUTHORIZATION TO TEST FORM

After your eligibility to test has been determined, your registration form is processed, and an Authorization to Test (ATT) form will be sent to you. You cannot make an appointment for the test until you are declared eligible and until you have received the ATT form. The examination will take place at a Pearson Professional Center, and you can make an appointment online (www.vue.com/nclex) or by telephone. You can schedule an appointment at any Pearson Professional Center. You do not have to take the examination in the same state in which you are seeking licensure. A confirmation of your appointment will be sent to you.

The ATT form contains important information, including your test authorization number, your candidate identification number, and an expiration date. Note the expiration date on the form, because you must complete the test by this date. You also need to take your ATT form to the testing center on the day of your examination; you will not be admitted to the examination if you do not have it.

If, for any reason, you need to cancel or reschedule your appointment to test, you can make the change on the candidate Web site (www.vue.com/nclex) or by calling candidate services. The change needs to be made 1 full business day (24 hours) before your scheduled appointment. If you fail to arrive for the examination or fail to cancel your appointment to test without providing appropriate notice, you will forfeit your examination fee, and your ATT form will be invalidated. This information will be reported to the board of nursing of the state in which you have applied for licensure, and you will be required to register and pay the testing fees again.

It is important that you arrive at the testing center at least 30 minutes before the test is scheduled to begin. If you arrive late for the scheduled testing appointment, you may be required to forfeit your examination appointment. If it is necessary to forfeit your appointment, you will need to reregister for the examination and pay an additional fee, and the board of nursing will be notified that you did not test. A few days before your scheduled date of testing, take the time to drive to the testing center to determine its exact location, the length of time required to arrive at that destination, and any potential obstacles that may delay you (e.g., road construction, traffic, parking).

SPECIAL TESTING CIRCUMSTANCES

If you require special testing accommodations, you should contact the board of nursing before you submit a registration form; the board of nursing will provide you with the procedure for submitting the request. The board of nursing must authorize special testing accommodations. After you receive approval from the state board of nursing, the NCSBN reviews the requested accommodations and also must approve the request. If the request is approved, the testing appointment must be made by an NCLEX program coordinator, whom you can contact by calling NCLEX candidate services 866-469-2539. If it is necessary, you must cancel or reschedule your appointment by contacting an NCLEX program coordinator.

THE TESTING CENTER

The testing center is designed to ensure the complete security of the testing process, and strict candidate identification requirements have been established. To be admitted to the testing center, you must bring the ATT form and two forms of identification. Both forms of identification must be signed and current (nonexpired), and one must contain a recent photograph of you. The name on the piece of identification with the photograph must be the same as the name on the ATT form. A digital fingerprint, signature, and photograph will be taken at the testing center and will accompany the NCLEX examination results to confirm your identity. In addition, if you leave the testing room for any reason, you may be required to have your fingerprint taken again before being readmitted to the room.

Personal belongings are not allowed in the testing room. Secure storage will be provided for you; however, storage space is limited, so you must plan accordingly. The testing center will not assume responsibility for your personal belongings. The testing waiting areas are generally small; therefore, friends or family members who accompany you are not permitted to wait in the testing center while you are taking the examination.

After you have completed the admission process and a brief orientation, the proctor will escort you to your assigned computer. You will be seated at an individual work space area that includes computer equipment, appropriate lighting, an erasable note board, and a marker. No items, including unauthorized scratch paper, are allowed into the testing room. Electronic devices (e.g., watches, beepers, cell phones) are not allowed in the testing room. Eating, drinking, and the use of tobacco are not allowed in the testing room. You will be observed at all times by the test proctor while taking the examination. In addition, video and audio recording of all test sessions occurs. Pearson Professional Centers have no control over the sounds made by others who are typing on the computer. If these sounds are distracting to you, raise your hand to summon the proctor; earplugs are available upon request.

You must follow the directions given by the test center staff, and you must remain seated during the test, except when you have been authorized to leave. If you feel that you have a problem with your computer or that you need an additional note board, a break, or the test proctor, you must raise your hand.

TESTING TIME

The maximum testing time is 5 hours, and this time period includes the tutorial, the sample items, all breaks, and the examination. All breaks are optional, and if you decide to take a break, you must leave the testing room. When you return, you may be required to provide a fingerprint to be readmitted to the testing room.

LENGTH OF THE EXAMINATION

The minimum number of questions that you will need to answer is 85. Of these 85 questions, 60 will be operational (scored) questions, and 25 will be pretest (unscored) questions. The maximum number of questions in the test is 205.

The pretest questions are questions that may be presented as scored questions on future examinations, but they are not identified as such. In other words, you do not know which questions are the unscored questions.

PASS-OR-FAIL DECISIONS

All of the examination questions are categorized by test plan area and level of difficulty. This is an important point to keep in mind when you consider how the computer makes the pass-or-fail decision, because the pass-or-fail decision is not based on a percentage of correctly answered questions.

After the minimum number of questions (85) has been answered, the computer compares the test-taker's ability level with the standard required for passing; this standard required is set based on the expert judgment of several individuals appointed by the NCSBN. If the test-taker is clearly above the passing standard, then he or she passes the examination. If the test-taker is clearly below the passing standard, then he or she fails the examination. If the computer is not able to determine clearly whether the test-taker has passed or failed because the test-taker's ability is close to the passing standard, then the computer continues asking questions. After each question, the computer determines the test-taker's ability. When it becomes clear on which side of the passing standard the test-taker falls, then the examination ends. If the test-taker is administered the maximum number of questions (205 questions), then the computer will make a pass-or-fail decision by recomputing the test-taker's final ability level based on every question answered and comparing it with the passing standard. If the ability level is above the passing standard, then the test-taker passes; if the ability level is not above the passing standard, then the test-taker fails.

If the examination ends because you have run out of time, the computer may not have enough information to make a clear pass-or-fail decision. If this is the situation, the computer will review your performance during testing. If the test-taker's ability was consistently above the passing standard (specifically on the last 60 questions asked), then the test-taker passes. If the test-taker's ability falls below the passing standard, even once, then the test-taker fails.

COMPLETING THE EXAMINATION

After the test has been completed, you will complete a brief computer-delivered questionnaire about your testing experience. When this questionnaire is completed, you need to raise your hand to summon the test proctor, who will collect and inventory all note boards and then permit you to leave.

PROCESSING RESULTS

Every computerized examination is scored twice: once by the computer at the testing center and then again after the examination is transmitted to Pearson Professional Centers. No results are released at the testing center. The board of nursing will mail your results to you approximately 1 month after you have taken the examination. You should not telephone Pearson Professional Centers, the NCSBN, candidate services, or the state board of nursing for results. In some states, results can be obtained via the state Web site or via an NCSBN telephone results service. Information about obtaining NCLEX results by this method can be obtained from the candidate services area of the NCSBN Web site.

CANDIDATE PERFORMANCE REPORT

A candidate performance report is provided to any test-taker who fails the examination. This report provides the test-taker with information about his or her strengths and weaknesses in relation to the test plan and provides a guide for studying and retaking the examination. The test-taker should consult the state board of nursing of the state in which licensure is sought for procedures regarding the time period for retaking the examination.

INTERSTATE ENDORSEMENT

Because the NCLEX-PN examination is a national examination, you can apply to take the examination in any state. After licensure has been received, you can apply for Interstate Endorsement, which involves obtaining another license in another state to practice nursing in that state. The procedures and requirements for Interstate Endorsement may vary from state to state, and these procedures can be obtained from the state board of nursing of the state in which endorsement is sought. You may also be allowed to practice nursing in another state if the state has enacted the Nurse Licensure Compact. The state boards of nursing can be accessed via the NCSBN Web site at www.ncsbn.org.

NURSE LICENSURE COMPACT

It may be possible to hold one license from the state of residency and to practice nursing in another state under the mutual recognition model of nursing licensure if the second state has enacted the Nurse Licensure Compact. To obtain information about the Nurse Licensure Compact and the states that have it, access the NCSBN Web site at www.ncsbn.org.

ADDITIONAL INFORMATION ABOUT THE EXAMINATION

Additional information about the NCLEX-PN examination can be obtained by writing to the National Council of State Boards of Nursing, 111 East Wacker Drive, Suite 2900, Chicago, Illinois 60601-4277. The telephone number for the testing service is 866-293-9600, and the Web site address is www.ncsbn.org.

REFERENCES

Black, J., & Hawks, J. (2009). *Medical-surgical nursing: Clinical management for positive outcomes* (8th ed). St. Louis: Saunders.

Chernecky, C., & Berger, B. (2008). *Laboratory tests and diagnostic procedures* (5th ed). Philadelphia: Saunders.

Christensen, B., & Kockrow, E. (2006). *Foundations of nursing* (5th ed). St. Louis: Mosby.

deWit, S (2009). *Medical-surgical nursing: Concepts & practice*. St. Louis: Saunders.

Hill, S., & Howlett, H. (2009). *Success in practical/vocational nursing: From student to leader* (6th ed). Philadelphia: Saunders.

Hodgson, B., & Kizior, R. (2009). *Saunders nursing drug handbook 2009*. St. Louis: Saunders.

Lilley, L., Harrington, S., & Snyder, J. (2007). *Pharmacology and the nursing process* (5th ed). St. Louis: Mosby.

Linton, A., & Maebius, N. (2007). *Introduction to medical-surgical nursing* (4th ed). Philadelphia: Saunders.

National Council of State Boards of Nursing (Eds.). (2008). *2008 Detailed Test Plan for the NCLEX-PN® Examination*, Chicago: Author.

National Council of State Boards of Nursing, Inc. Web site: www.ncsbn.org. Retrieved on July 25, 2009.

Potter, P., & Perry, A. (2009). *Fundamentals of nursing* (7th ed). St. Louis: Mosby.

Pagana, K., & Pagana, T. (2009). *Mosby's diagnostic and laboratory test reference* (9th ed). St. Louis: Mosby.

CHAPTER 2

Profiles to Success

LAURENT W. VALLIERE, BS

Preparing to take the NCLEX-PN can produce a great deal of anxiety in the nursing graduate. You may be thinking that the NCLEX-PN is the most important examination that you will ever have to take and that it reflects the culmination of everything for which you have worked so hard. The NCLEX-PN is an important exam, because achieving that nursing license defines the beginning of your career as a licensed practical or vocational nurse. A vital ingredient to your success on the NCLEX is avoiding the negative thoughts that allow this examination to seem overwhelming and intimidating. Such thoughts will take full control over your destiny (Box 2-1).

Nursing graduates preparing for the NCLEX must develop a comprehensive plan. The most important component of this plan is identifying the study patterns that helped you to obtain your nursing degree. It is important to begin your planning by reflecting on all of the personal and academic challenges that you experienced during your nursing education. Take time to focus on the thoughts, feelings, and emotions that you experienced before taking an examination while in your nursing program. Examine the methods that you used to prepare for those exams, both academically and psychologically.

Box 2-1 ▲ PROFILES TO SUCCESS

- Avoid negative thoughts that allow the examination to seem overwhelming and intimidating.
- Develop a comprehensive plan to prepare for the examination.
- Examine the study methods and strategies that you used to prepare for exams during nursing school.
- Develop realistic time goals.
- Select a study time period and place that will be most conducive to your success.
- Commit to your own special study methods and strategies.
- Incorporate a balance of exercise, rest, and relaxation into your preparation schedule.
- Maintain healthy eating habits.
- Learn to control anxiety.
- Remember that discipline and perseverance will automatically bring control.
- Remember that this examination is all about you.
- Remember that your self-confidence and your belief in yourself will lead you to success!

These factors are very important considerations when preparing for the NCLEX, because they identify the patterns that worked for you. Think about this for a moment. Your own methods of study must have worked, or you would not be at the point of preparing for the NCLEX-PN.

Each individual requires his or her own methods of preparing for an examination. Graduates who have taken the NCLEX-PN will probably share their experiences and methods of preparing for this challenge with you, and they will provide you with important strategies that they have used. Listen closely to what they have to say, but remember that this examination is all about you. Your identity and what you require in terms of preparation are most important.

Reflect on the methods and strategies that worked for you throughout your nursing program. Do not think that you need to develop new methods and strategies when preparing for the NCLEX. Use what has worked for you. Take some time to reflect on these strategies, write them down on a large blank card, sign your name, and write "LPN" or "LVN" after your name. Post this card in a place where you will see it every morning of every day. Commit to your own special strategies. These strategies reflect your profile and identity and will lead you to success!

A frequent concern of graduates who are preparing for the NCLEX relates to deciding whether they should study alone or become a part of a study group. Examining your profile will help you with this decision. Again, reflect on what has worked for you throughout your nursing program as you prepared for your exams. Remember that your needs are most important. Address your own needs, and do not become pressured by peers who are encouraging you to join a study group if this is not your normal pattern of study. Remember that additional pressure is not what you need at this important time in your life.

Graduates who are preparing for NCLEX frequently inquire about the best method of preparing. First, remember that you are already prepared. In fact, you began preparing for this examination on the first day of your nursing program. The task that you are faced with is to review, in a comprehensive manner, all of the nursing content that you learned as part of your nursing program. It can become totally overwhelming to look at your bookshelf overflowing with the nursing books that you used during nursing school, and your challenge becomes monumental when you look at the boxes of nursing lecture notes that you have accumulated. It is unrealistic to even think that you could read all of those nursing books and lecture notes in preparation for the NCLEX. These books and notes should be used as reference sources, if needed, during your preparation for the NCLEX.

Saunders Comprehensive Review for the NCLEX-PN® Examination has identified for you all of the important nursing content areas relevant to the examination. While you were undertaking this comprehensive review, you should have noted the areas that were unfamiliar or unclear. Be sure that you have taken the necessary time to become familiar with the necessary areas. Now, progress through the Pyramid to Success, and test your knowledge with this book, *Saunders Q&A Review for the NCLEX-PN® Examination*. You may identify nursing content areas that still require further review. Take the time to review these areas as you are guided to do by this book.

Your profile to success requires that you develop realistic time goals for preparing for the NCLEX. It is necessary to take the time to examine your life and all of the commitments that you may have, including family, work, and friends. As you develop your goals, remember to plan time for fun and exercise. To achieve success, you require a balance of both work time and enjoyment time. If you do not plan for some leisure time, you will become frustrated and perhaps even angry. These sorts of feelings will block your ability to focus and concentrate. Remember that you need time for yourself.

Goal development may be a relatively easy process, because you have probably been juggling your life commitments ever since you entered nursing school. Remember that your goal is to identify a daily time frame and time period for you to use when reviewing and preparing for the NCLEX. Open your calendar, and identify the days on which life commitments will not allow you to spend this time preparing. Block those days off, and do not consider them as a part of your review time. Identify the time that is best for you in terms of your ability to concentrate and focus so that you can accomplish the most in your identified time frame. Be sure that you consider a time that is quiet and free of distractions. Many individuals find that the morning hours provide the most productive hours, whereas others may find the afternoon and evening hours to be the most useful. Remember that the NCLEX is all about you; select the time period that will be most conducive to your success.

The place of study is also very important. Select a place that is quiet and comfortable and where you normally do your studying and preparing. Some individuals prefer to study at home in their own environment; if this is your normal pattern, be sure that you are able to free yourself of distractions during your scheduled preparation time. If this is not an option, you may consider spending your preparation time in a library. When selecting your place of study, reflect on what worked best for you during your nursing program.

Selecting the amount of daily preparation time has frequently been a dilemma for many graduates who are preparing for the NCLEX. It is very important to determine a realistic time period that can be adhered to on a daily basis. Set a time frame that will provide you with quality time and that can be realistically achieved. If you do not follow these guidelines, you will become frustrated. This frustration will block your journey toward the peak of the Pyramid to Success.

It is a good idea for you to spend at least 2 hours each day preparing for the NCLEX. This is a realistic time period in terms of both quality and achievability. You may find that, after 2 hours, your ability to focus will diminish. However, you may find on some days that you are able to spend more than the scheduled 2 hours and that your concentration is still present; when these days occur, use them to your advantage.

Discipline and perseverance will automatically bring control. Control will provide you with the momentum that will sweep you to the peak of the Pyramid to Success.

Discipline yourself to spend time preparing for the NCLEX every day. Daily preparation is very important because it maintains a consistent pattern and keeps you in synchrony with the mind flow needed for the day that you are scheduled to take the NCLEX. Some days you may think about skipping your scheduled preparation time because you are not in the mood for study or because you just do not feel like studying. On these days, practice your discipline, and persevere. Stand yourself up, shake off the thoughts of skipping a day, take a deep breath, and get the oxygen flowing throughout your body. Look in the mirror, smile, and say to yourself, "This time is for me, and I can do this!" Look at your card that displays your name with "LPN" or "LVN" after it, and get yourself to that special study place. Remember that discipline and perseverance will bring control!

In the profile to success, academic preparation directs the path to the peak of the Pyramid to Success. However, there are additional factors that will influence your successful achievement, including your ability to control anxiety, physical stamina, rest and relaxation, self-confidence, and your belief that you will achieve success on the NCLEX. You need to take time to think about these important factors and to incorporate them into your daily preparation schedule.

Anxiety is a common concern among students who are preparing to take the NCLEX. Some anxiety is normal and will keep your senses sharp and alert. However, a great deal of anxiety can block your process of thinking and hamper your ability to focus and concentrate. You have already practiced the task of controlling anxiety when you took exams in nursing school. Now you need to continue with this practice and incorporate this control on a daily basis. Each day, before beginning your scheduled preparation time, sit in your quiet special study place, close your eyes, and take a slow, deep breath. Fill your body with oxygen, hold your breath to a count of 4, and then exhale slowly through your mouth. Continue with this exercise, and repeat it four to six times. This exercise will help you to relieve your mind of any unnecessary chatter, and it will deliver oxygen to all of your body tissues and to your brain. On the day that you take the NCLEX, after the necessary pretesting procedures, you will be escorted to your test computer. Practice this breathing exercise before beginning the exam, and use it during the examination if you feel yourself becoming anxious or distracted. Remember that breathing will move oxygen to your brain!

Physical stamina is a necessary component of your readiness for the NCLEX. Plan to incorporate a balance of exercise, rest, and relaxation into your preparation schedule. It is also important that you maintain healthy eating habits. Begin to practice these healthy habits now, if you have not already done so. There are a few points to keep in mind each day as you plan your daily meals. Three balanced meals are important, with snacks such as fruit included between meals. Remember that food items that contain fat will slow you down and that food items that contain caffeine will cause nervousness and sometimes shakiness. These items need to be avoided. Healthy foods that are high in carbohydrates work best to supply you with your energy needs. Remember that your brain can work like a muscle, so it requires those carbohydrates. In addition, be sure that you include necessary fruits and vegetables in your diet (Box 2-2).

If you are the type of individual who does not eat breakfast, work on changing that habit as you are preparing for the NCLEX. Provide your brain with energy in the morning with some form of carbohydrate food; it will make a difference. On the day of the NCLEX, feed your brain and eat a healthy breakfast. In addition, on this very important day, bring a snack such as fruit or a bagel for break time, and feed your brain again so that you will have the energy to concentrate, focus, and complete your examination.

Adequate rest, relaxation, and exercise are important to your preparation process. Many graduates who are preparing for NCLEX have difficulty sleeping, particularly the night before the examination. Begin now to develop methods that will assist you with relaxing your body and mind and that will help you to obtain restful sleep. You may already have a particular method that you use to help you sleep. If not, it may be helpful to try the breathing exercise while you lie in bed to help you to eliminate any mind chatter that is present.

Box 2-2 ▲ HEALTHY EATING HABITS

Eat three balanced meals each day.
Include snacks, such as fruits and vegetables, between meals.
Avoid food items that contain fat.
Avoid food items that contain caffeine.
Consume healthy foods that are high in carbohydrates.

Box 2-3 ▲ CRITICAL WORDS

Believe: Believe in your success every day.
Plan: Plan the study strategies that work for you.
Control: Always maintain command of your emotions, and breathe.
Practice: Review, review, review: practice questions, practice questions, and more practice questions!
Succeed: Believe, plan, control, and practice: "Yes I can!"

It is also helpful to visualize your favorite relaxing place while you do these breathing exercises. Graduates have also stated that listening to quiet music and relaxation tapes have assisted them with relaxing and sleeping. Begin to practice some of these helpful methods now, while you are preparing for the NCLEX, and identify those that work best for you. The night before your scheduled examination is an important one. Spend some time having fun, get to bed early, and incorporate the relaxation methods that you have been using to help you sleep.

Your self-confidence and the belief that you have the ability to achieve success will bring your goals to fruition. Reflect on the profile to success that you maintained during your nursing education. Your confidence and belief in yourself, along with your academic achievements, have brought you to the status of a graduate. Now you are facing one more important challenge (Box 2-3).

Can you meet this challenge successfully? Yes, you can! There is no reason to think otherwise if you have taken all of the necessary steps to ensure that profile to success. Each morning, place your feet on the floor, stand tall, take a deep breath, and smile. With both hands, imagine yourself brushing off any negative feelings. Look at the card that bears your name with the letters "LPN" or "LVN" after it, and tell yourself, "Yes, I can do this successfully!"

Believe in yourself, and you will reach the peak of the Pyramid to Success!

Congratulations, and I wish you continued success in your career as a licensed practical or vocational nurse!

CHAPTER
3

The NCLEX-PN® Examination: From a Graduate's Perspective

JILL FERANEC, LPN

When I made the decision to go to nursing school, I could not believe all that was involved with getting accepted into a program. I had to interview, write an essay, have references, and then take an entrance exam. I knew that all of this would be the very first step in attaining my goal of becoming a licensed practical nurse (LPN). After passing the entrance exam, I decided to go to school part time in the evenings so that I could work full time during the day. I had about a month to prepare myself for school, and I knew that dedication, hard work, and time management lay before me.

I decided very early on that I wanted to learn as much as I could and that I would do my very best to achieve my goal. I knew that study habits were going to be very important to have and maintain throughout the program. I also realized that I would have to give up a lot of my free time for studying.

The first couple of nights attending class were the hardest. The books were piled on, and so were the assignments. I began to look over my new books, and I started to wonder if I would be able to handle all of the work. Although the books were overwhelming at first, I was intrigued by all of the information inside of them. I wanted to learn about everything.

The instructors at my school told us about books to read in addition to the ones we needed for class. After being in school for only 2 months, I went to the bookstore and purchased the book that you are reading right now. This book has thousands of practice questions and answers, rationales for both correct and incorrect options, the test-taking strategies for answering correctly and for taking the NCLEX. I started looking at this question-and-answer book daily. At first I did not know any of the answers—I did not even understand some of the questions—but as time passed, I was able to correlate some of the questions and answers with what I was learning in school. I carried this book with me everywhere. It went into my car in the morning and came out with me at night; it had almost the same mileage as my car! During lunch breaks at work, I tested myself, and I was thrilled when I got a few questions right. I arrived at my clinical sites early and sat in my car to look over this question-and-answer review book. I always read the rationales and the test-taking strategies so that I would understand what each question was really asking. I learned so much, and, by doing this early on in my nursing program, I knew it was going to help prepare me for the NCLEX.

I also used the CDs that accompanied my nursing books and my NCLEX review book. I downloaded as many as I could onto my computer, and then I reviewed the practice questions and answers that related to the course that I was taking at school. This helped me prepare for my nursing school exams and also to prepare for the NCLEX. I found that using the CDs was a good change of pace when studying.

Here is another helpful hint for you: Throughout nursing school, we were given many laboratory values and math formulas to memorize. I wrote them down on small pieces of paper or note cards and put them where I would see them on a daily basis. I posted them on my refrigerator, in my car, and even alongside my bed. After seeing those laboratory values and formulas all the time, I learned them!

I did not participate in study groups, because I knew the study time would turn into a gab session. However, I did turn to fellow students when I felt stressed. Talking to other classmates throughout school was very beneficial, because they understood the pressures that existed. Do not be afraid to seek support from your classmates; they can be so helpful during the trying times!

I was very fortunate to work in a doctor's office as a medical assistant while I was in nursing school. Working there helped me to learn about many aspects of nursing and medicine. I was always asking questions about things I saw or did not understand. I probably seemed like a pest at times, but I was always seeking answers. Never be afraid to ask questions while you are in nursing school or after you graduate.

My study habits never wavered throughout my nursing program. I spent many hours studying every week, but I gave myself one night off each week to do something other than school work. This worked well for me, and I always looked forward to that night.

I thought that I would never get through 23 months of school. There were countless reports, tests, and presentations. Just as you finished one thing, you were given another. Working full time and going to classes at night was exhausting, and I thought the end was never going to come. During all this time, I was thinking about the NCLEX exam, wondering what it was like and if I would pass. During the second year of my nursing program, I started to see the light at the end of the tunnel. It seemed now that time was starting to fly by. I started to wonder if I "knew everything" and if I was really prepared to take the NCLEX exam. Just before school ended, we were given *Saunders Comprehensive Review for the NCLEX-PN® Examination*, which is a companion book to this one that you are reading. This book was my new best friend. I used it to review for my exit exam at school, which I had to pass to graduate, and I passed the exam with no problem! I also used it to prepare for the NCLEX exam, and again I had no problem passing!

After graduation, I did not apply to take the NCLEX right away. I needed time to prepare. I used this book that you are reading and the companion comprehensive review book, and I read each chapter. At the end of each chapter, I completed the practice questions; if I got a question wrong, I was able to go back into the chapter and review the material that I did not understand. Because I knew that the NCLEX was taken on a computer, I made sure that I did 50 to 100 practice test questions every night on the computer using the CD that accompanied these books.

After a few weeks of review, I decided to apply to the state board of nursing. After waiting for more than a month, I finally received an Authorization to Test form. I selected the test center nearest to my home and selected a date to test. (I do not recommend waiting too long to select a date because test dates can fill up quickly.) Now that I had a date to take the NCLEX, I really started to worry. I had all kinds of fears, and I questioned myself repeatedly. I had heard many stories about the NCLEX, including how difficult it was. I was told that some graduates receive only 85 questions to answer and they pass, whereas some receive only 85 questions and fail. I wondered how many questions I would have to answer and how difficult these questions were going to be. With all of these thoughts racing through my head, I took some deep breaths, and then I studied every chance I got.

A week before my test date, I traveled to the test center to make sure that I knew where it was located; I did not want to risk getting lost on the day of the test. I also made sure that I ate healthy and drank plenty of water for the entire week before the exam. Although I was very nervous about the upcoming week, I tried to get plenty of sleep, too.

The day of the exam finally arrived. I felt very confident and was ready to move forward. I arrived at the test center very early. I had allowed myself extra time in case I got caught up in traffic. After being fingerprinted and having my picture taken, I was led into the testing room. I sat down and took some deep breaths. I thought about my 23 months of education and all that I did to reach this moment. I kept telling myself to relax and to stay focused on the questions. After deep breathing and clearing my thoughts, I started the exam.

Of the four options given for multiple-choice questions, two could often be eliminated right away. I found that, if I had difficulty with the last two options, I used test-taking strategies, Maslow's Hierarchy of Needs theory, and the ABCs—airway, breathing, and circulation—to help. After applying one of these test-taking strategies, the correct option usually became obvious. I read each question slowly and carefully and looked at what it was really asking. There was a timer at the bottom of the screen, and, although I knew it was there, I did not pay any attention to it. I took my time with each question.

It seemed as if I had only answered a few questions when the words *Would you like to take a break?* appeared on the screen. Of course I did not want a break; I thought that I was just getting started. After only 10 more questions, the screen went blank. I thought maybe something happened to the computer or that I had failed. I wanted to answer more questions so I could prove that I did know enough. However, I was escorted out of the testing room. It was all over! I felt relieved but exhausted. I looked at the clock in the testing area and saw that I had been in there for about 2 hours. All the way home, I kept thinking about the 85 questions I had answered and all of the choices I had made.

The worst part of the entire NCLEX process is the waiting. After a couple of days, I went to the NCLEX Web site to obtain my results. I decided to pay the small fee to obtain my results early. When the word *PASS* came up on the screen, I could not have been happier!

I look back now, and I do not know why I was so nervous about the NCLEX. I committed myself to studying and learning from the very beginning of my nursing program. I asked a lot of questions and wanted all the answers. If you are determined to work hard, then it is possible to reach your goal. I was in an LPN program 35 years ago and dropped out before graduating. My lifetime goal was to go back into an LPN program and to become the nurse that I always wanted to be. I have reached my goal. Work hard, stay focused, and have confidence in yourself. I wish you the best of luck with taking the NCLEX and in your future nursing career.

CHAPTER

4

Test-Taking Strategies

I. Pyramid to Success (Box 4-1)

II. The "What If...?" Syndrome and How to Avoid Reading Into the Question (Box 4-2)

A. Pyramid points
1. Avoid asking yourself, "Well, what if...?"; this will lead you right into the "forbidden" act of reading into the question.
2. Focus only on the information in the question, read every word, and make a decision about what the question is asking.
3. Look for the strategic words in the question, such as *side effect* or *toxic effect;* strategic words make a difference with regard to what the question is asking about.
4. For multiple-choice questions, multiple-response questions, and questions that require you to number in order of priority, read every option presented before selecting your answers.
5. Always use the process of elimination when options are presented; after you have eliminated some options, reread the question before making your final choice.
6. For fill-in-the-blank questions, focus on the information in the question, and determine what the question is asking; if the question requires you to calculate a medication dose, an intravenous flow rate, or intake and output amounts, recheck your calculations, and always use the on-screen calculator to verify the answer.

Box 4-1 ▲ PYRAMID TO SUCCESS

Avoid asking yourself, "Well, what if...?"; this will lead you right into reading into the question.
Focus only on the information in the question, read every word, and make a decision about what the question is asking.
Look for the strategic words in the question; strategic words make a difference with regard to what the question is asking about.
Always use the process of elimination when options are presented; after you have eliminated some options, reread the question before making your final choice or choices.
Determine if the question contains a positive or negative event query.
Use all of your nursing knowledge, your clinical experiences, and your test-taking skills and strategies to answer the question.

Box 4-2 ▲ PRACTICE QUESTION: AVOIDING THE "WHAT IF...?" SYNDROME AND READING INTO THE QUESTION

QUESTION
A nurse is caring for a hospitalized client with a diagnosis of congestive heart failure who suddenly complains of shortness of breath and dyspnea. The nurse takes which *immediate* nursing action?
1. Calls the physician
2. Administers oxygen to the client
3. Elevates the head of the client's bed
4. Prepares to administer furosemide (Lasix)

ANSWER: 3
Test-Taking Strategy: You may immediately think, what if the client has developed pulmonary edema (a complication of congestive heart failure) and needs a diuretic? However, there is no information in the question that indicates the presence of pulmonary edema. The question simply states that the client suddenly complains of shortness of breath and dyspnea. Read the question carefully. Note the strategic word *immediate,* and focus on the subject—the client's complaints. Although the physician may need to be notified, this is not the immediate action. A physician's order is needed to administer oxygen. Furosemide is a diuretic and may or may not be prescribed for the client. Because there is no data in the question that indicates the presence of pulmonary edema, option 3 is correct. The question is asking you for a nursing action, so that is what you need to look for as you eliminate the incorrect options. Remember to avoid the "What if...?" syndrome!

B. The ingredients of a question (Box 4-3)
   1. The ingredients of a question include the event (a client or clinical situation), the event query, and the options; a fill-in-the blank question will not contain options, and some figure or illustration (hot-spot) questions may or may not contain options.
   2. The client or clinical event provides you with the content that you need to think about when answering the question.
   3. The event query asks something specific about the client or clinical event.
   4. The options are all of the answers provided with the question.
   5. For a multiple-choice question, there will be four options, and you must select one; read every option carefully, and think about the client or clinical event and the event query as you use the process of elimination.
   6. For a multiple-response question, there will be six options, and you must select all options that apply to the event in the question; visualize the event, and use your nursing knowledge and your clinical experience to answer the question.
   7. For a prioritizing (ordered-response) question, you will be required to list, in order of priority (using the computer mouse and dragging and dropping the options), certain nursing interventions or other data; visualize the event, and use your nursing knowledge and clinical experience to answer the question.
   8. A chart/exhibit question will most likely contain options; read the question and all of the information in the chart/exhibit carefully before selecting an answer.

Box 4-3 ▲ MULTIPLE-CHOICE QUESTION: EVENT, EVENT QUERY, AND OPTIONS

QUESTION
Event: A nurse caring for a client with myocardial infarction is helping the client fill out the diet menu request form.

Event Query: The nurse recommends that the client select which of the following beverages from the menu?

Options:
1. Tea
2. Cola
3. Coffee
4. Fruit juice

ANSWER: 4
Test-Taking Strategy: Focus on the client's diagnosis and recall that caffeine needs to be eliminated from the diet because of its stimulating effects. Also, note that options 1, 2, and 3 are comparable or alike in that they are products that contain caffeine; this will direct you to the correct option. Note the ingredients of the question!

III. The Strategic Words (Boxes 4-4 and 4-5)

A. Strategic words focus your attention on a critical point to consider when answering the question; they will assist you with eliminating the incorrect options.
B. Some strategic words may indicate that all of the options are correct and that it will be necessary to prioritize to select the correct option.
C. As you read the question, look for the strategic words; strategic words make a difference with regard to what the question is asking about.

IV. The Subject of the Question (Box 4-6)

A. The subject of the question is the specific topic that the question is asking about.
B. Identifying the subject of the question will assist you with eliminating the incorrect options and direct you to the correct option.

Box 4-4 ▲ COMMON STRATEGIC WORDS

Early or late
Best
First
Initial
Immediately
Most likely or least likely
Most appropriate or least appropriate

Box 4-5 ▲ PRACTICE QUESTION: STRATEGIC WORDS

QUESTION
The nurse is caring for a client receiving digoxin (Lanoxin). The nurse monitors the client for which *early* manifestation of digoxin toxicity?
1. Anorexia
2. Facial pain
3. Photophobia
4. Yellow color perception

ANSWER: 1
Test-Taking Strategy: Focus on the strategic word *early*. The most common early manifestations of toxicity include gastrointestinal disturbances such as anorexia, nausea, and vomiting. Facial pain, personality changes, and ocular disturbances (photophobia, light flashes, halos around bright objects, yellow or green color perception) are also signs of toxicity, but they are not early signs. Remember to look for strategic words!

Box 4-6 ▲ THE SUBJECT OF THE QUESTION

QUESTION

A client who underwent a bronchoscopy was returned to the nursing unit 1 hour ago. The nurse determines that the client is experiencing a complication of the procedure if the nurse notes:

1. An oxygen saturation of 95%
2. A weak gag and cough reflex
3. A respiratory rate of 22 breaths per minute
4. Breath sounds that are greater on the right than on the left

ANSWER: 4

Test-Taking Strategy: Focus on the subject—a complication. Therefore, look for the abnormal piece of data. Begin to answer this question by eliminating options 1 and 3, which are acceptable data. From the remaining options, recall that the client is medicated before this procedure, which would cause a weak gag and cough reflex. Unequal breath sounds are always abnormal. Remember to focus on the subject!

Box 4-7 ▲ PRACTICE QUESTION: POSITIVE EVENT QUERY

QUESTION

A client admitted to the hospital with coronary artery disease complains of dyspnea when at rest. The nurse determines that which of the following items would be *of the most help to the client?*

1. Providing a walker to aid in ambulation
2. Elevating the head of the bed to at least 45 degrees
3. Performing continuous monitoring of oxygen saturation
4. Placing an oxygen cannula at the bedside for use if needed

ANSWER: 2

Test-Taking Strategy: This question is an example of a positive event query. Note the strategic words *of the most help to the client;* these words will direct you to look for the item that is going to have the best immediate effect from the client's perspective. The management of dyspnea is generally directed toward alleviating the cause. Symptom relief may be achieved or at least aided by placing the client at rest with the head of the bed elevated. In severe cases, supplemental oxygen is used. Monitoring the oxygen saturation level detects early complications, but it does not help the client. Likewise, placing an oxygen cannula at the bedside for use would also not help the client. Remember that positive event queries ask you to select an option that is a correct item or statement!

Box 4-8 ▲ PRACTICE QUESTION: NEGATIVE EVENT QUERY

QUESTION

A nurse has reinforced discharge instructions to a client who underwent a right mastectomy with axillary lymph node dissection. Which statement by the client indicates the *need for further instruction* regarding home care measures?

1. "It is alright to use a straight razor to shave under my arms."
2. "I need to be sure that I do not have blood pressures taken or blood drawn from my right arm."
3. "I should inform all of my other health care providers that I have had this surgical procedure."
4. "I need to be sure to wear thick mitt hand covers or to use thick pot holders when I am cooking and touching hot pans."

ANSWER: 1

Test-Taking Strategy: This question identifies an example of a negative event query question. Note the strategic words *need for further instruction;* these words indicate that you need to select an option that identifies an incorrect client statement. Recalling that edema and infection are of concern with this client and that the client needs to be instructed regarding the measures that will avoid trauma to the affected arm will direct you to the correct option. Remember that negative event queries ask you to select an option that is an incorrect item or client statement!

V. Positive and Negative Event Queries
(Boxes 4-7 and 4-8)

A. A positive event query uses strategic words that ask you to select an option that is correct; for example, the event query may read as follows: "Which statement by a client *indicates an understanding* of the side effects of the prescribed medication?"

B. A negative event query uses strategic words that ask you to select an option that is an incorrect item or statement; for example, the event query may read as follows: "Which statement by a client *indicates a need for further teaching* about the side effects of the prescribed medication?"

VI. Questions That Require Prioritizing

A. Questions on the NCLEX may require you to use the skill of prioritizing nursing actions.

B. Look for the strategic words in the question that indicate the need to prioritize (Box 4-9).

C. Remember that when a question requires prioritization, all options may be correct; you may need to determine the correct order of action.

Box 4-9 ▲ COMMON STRATEGIC WORDS THAT INDICATE THE NEED TO PRIORITIZE

Best	Initial
Essential	Most important
First	Next
Highest priority	Primary
Immediate	Vital

Box 4-10 ▲ PRACTICE QUESTION: USE OF THE ABCS

QUESTION

A nurse is caring for a client with Buerger's disease. Which finding would the nurse determine to be a potential complication associated with this disease?

1. Pain with diaphoresis
2. Discomfort in one digit
3. Numbness and tingling in the legs
4. Cramping in the foot while resting

ANSWER: 3

Test-Taking Strategy: Use the ABCs—airway, breathing, and circulation—to answer this question. Buerger's disease (thromboangiitis obliterans) is a recurring inflammation of the small- and medium-sized arteries and veins of the upper and lower extremities that results in thrombus formation and the occlusion of blood vessels. Numbness and tingling in the legs indicate cardiovascular and neurovascular impairment. Remember to use the ABCs—airway, breathing, and circulation—to prioritize.

D. Strategies to use to prioritize include the ABCs—airway, breathing, and circulation; Maslow's Hierarchy of Needs theory; and the steps of the nursing process (clinical problem-solving process).

E. The ABCs (Box 4-10)
   1. Use the ABCs—airway, breathing, and circulation—when selecting an answer or determining the order of priority.
   2. Remember the order of priority: airway, breathing, and circulation.
   3. Airway is always the first priority.

F. Maslow's Hierarchy of Needs theory (Box 4-11; Figure 4-1)
   1. According to Maslow's Hierarchy of Needs theory, physiological needs are the priority, followed by safety and security needs, love and belonging needs, self-esteem needs, and, finally, self-actualization needs; therefore, select the option or determine the order of priority by addressing physiological needs first.
   2. When a physiological need is not addressed in the question or noted in one of the options, continue to use Maslow's Hierarchy of Needs theory as a guide, and look for the option that addresses safety.

Box 4-11 ▲ PRACTICE QUESTION: MASLOW'S HIERARCHY OF NEEDS THEORY

QUESTION

A nurse working in a long-term care facility is assigned to care for four clients on the hospice unit. When planning client rounds, which client would the nurse collect data from *first*?

1. The client who was complaining of severe back pain during the previous shift
2. The client who is being discharged home today and will need assistance packing
3. The client who is bed bound and needs to be turned and repositioned every 2 hours
4. The client who needs assistance applying antiembolic stockings before ambulating to the dining room for breakfast

ANSWER: 1

Test-Taking Strategy: Note the strategic word *first;* this word tells you that you need to prioritize. Use Maslow's Hierarchy of Needs theory. The nurse is working on a hospice unit, which means that he or she is caring for terminally ill clients. These clients need to be comforted, and the nurse needs to maintain a satisfactory lifestyle for these clients throughout the phases of dying. Although all of these clients need the nurse's attention, the client who needs to be seen first would be the client who was in severe pain during the previous shift. The nurse should evaluate this client to see if further pain medication is needed. Alleviating suffering is a priority nursing responsibility. Because pain is often an element of suffering, promoting optimal pain relief is a primary goal. Noting the word *severe* in option 1 will direct you to this option. Remember to use Maslow's Hierarchy of Needs theory to prioritize!

G. Steps of the nursing process (clinical problem-solving process)
   1. Use the steps of the nursing process (clinical problem-solving process) to prioritize.
   2. The steps are data collection, planning, implementation, and evaluation, and they are followed in this order.
   3. Data collection
      a. Data collection questions will address the process of gathering subjective and objective data relative to the client, communicating and documenting information gained during data collection, and contributing to the formulation of nursing diagnoses.
      b. Remember that data collection is the first step in the nursing process (clinical problem-solving process).
      c. When you are asked a question about your initial or first nursing action, look for strategic words in the options that reflect the collection of data relative to the client (Box 4-12).

Nursing Priorities From Maslow's Hierarchy

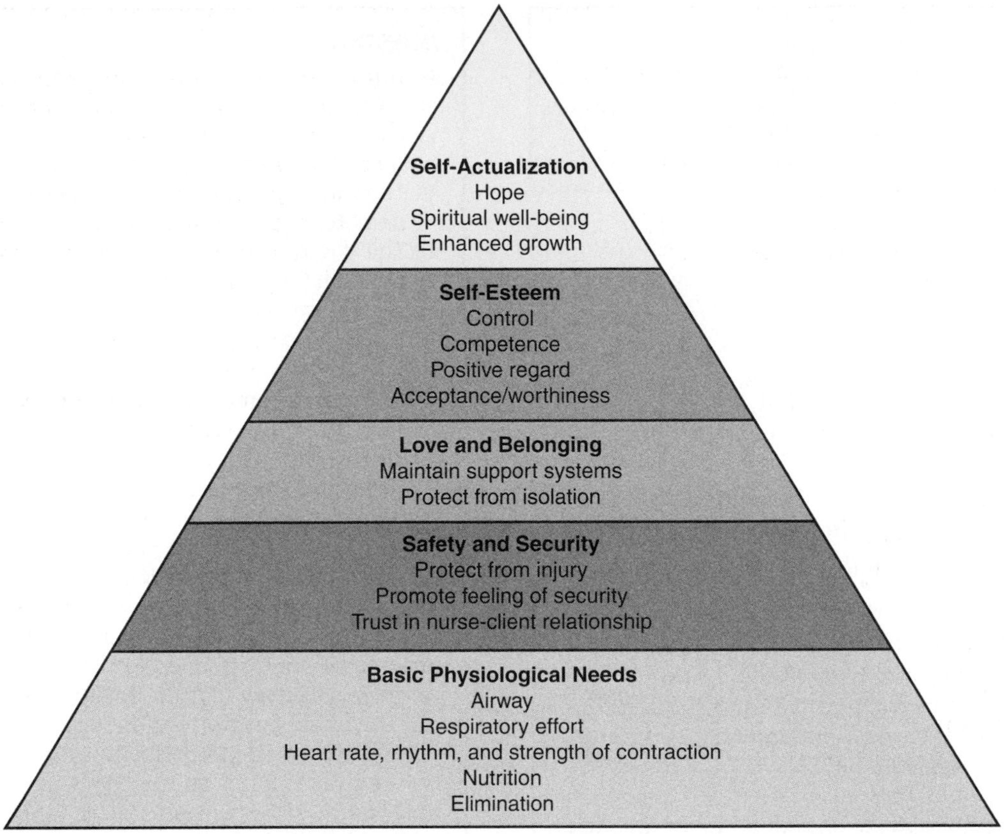

Figure 4-1 Using Maslow's Hierarchy of Needs theory to establish priorities. (From Harkreader, H., Hogan, M., & Thobaben, M. (2007). *Fundamentals of nursing: Caring and clinical judgment* [3rd ed., p. 209]. Philadelphia: Saunders.)

Box 4-12 ▲ DATA COLLECTION: STRATEGIC WORDS

Check	Identify
Collect	Monitor
Determine	Observe
Find out	Obtain information
Gather	Recognize

d. If an option contains the concept of the collection of client data, it is best to select that option (Box 4-13).
e. If a data collection action is not one of the options, follow the steps of the nursing process (clinical problem-solving process) as your guide to select your initial or first action.
f. *Possible exception to the guideline:* If the question presents an emergency situation, read carefully; in an emergency situation, an intervention may be the priority.

4. Planning: Planning questions will require providing input into plan development, assisting with the formulation of the goals of care, and assisting with the development of a plan of care (Box 4-14).
5. Implementation (Box 4-15)
   a. Implementation questions address the process of assisting with organizing and managing care, providing care to achieve established goals, and communicating and documenting nursing interventions thoroughly and accurately.
   b. Focus on a nursing action rather than a medical action when you are answering a question, unless the question is asking you what prescribed medical action is anticipated.
   c. On the NCLEX-PN, the only client that you need to be concerned about is the client in the question that you are answering; remember that the client in the question on the computer screen is your only assigned client.
   d. Answer the question from a textbook and ideal perspective, and remember that the nurse has all the time and resources needed and readily available at the client's bedside; for example, within the context of the question, you do not need to run to the treatment room to obtain sterile gauze, because the sterile gauze will be at the client's bedside.
   e. Remember to avoid the "What if...?" syndrome.

Box 4-13 ▲ PRACTICE QUESTION: THE NURSING PROCESS/DATA COLLECTION

QUESTION

A nurse enters a client's room and finds the client slumped down in a chair. The client's breathing is shallow, and a pulse is present. Based on this data, the nurse determines that the priority would be to:

1. Call the doctor immediately.
2. Have the secretary call a code blue.
3. Check the vital signs and level of consciousness.
4. Ask the unit clerk to call the family immediately.

ANSWER: 3

Test-Taking Strategy: Focus on the data in the question, and note the strategic word *priority.* Use the steps of the nursing process. Option 3 is the only option that addresses data collection. In addition, the use of the ABCs—airway, breathing, and circulation—will direct you to option 3. The client is breathing and has a pulse; therefore, additional data is needed before any other action is performed. The vital signs and level of consciousness should be checked. After those assessments are made, the physician is notified and will then contact the family. A code blue is not indicated at the present time. Remember that data collection is the first step of the nursing process.

Box 4-14 ▲ PRACTICE QUESTION: THE NURSING PROCESS/PLANNING

QUESTION

A client is admitted to the hospital with a diagnosis of acute pancreatitis. The nurse plans care knowing that which problem occurs with this disorder?

1. Alteration in comfort related to abdominal pain
2. Excess fluid volume related to sodium retention
3. Alteration in fluid and electrolyte balance related to hyperkalemia
4. Potential for hypoglycemia related to a low blood glucose level secondary to increased insulin secretion

ANSWER: 1

Test-Taking Strategy: This question relates to planning nursing care and asks you to identify the problem that occurs with acute pancreatitis. Note the word *acute,* and use your medical terminology skills. Remember that *-itis* indicates inflammation; this will direct you to option 1. Remember that planning is the second step of the nursing process!

Box 4-15 ▲ PRACTICE QUESTION: THE NURSING PROCESS/IMPLEMENTATION

QUESTION

A visitor brings a suicidal client a brightly packaged gift. The nurse accompanies the visitor to the client's room and takes which action?

1. Suggests that the client open the gift
2. Reinforces the safety policies with the client
3. Tells the client what a beautiful package this is
4. Lets the visitor spend time alone with the client

ANSWER: 1

Test-Taking Strategy: Implementation questions address the process of organizing and managing care. The nurse must be concerned with the safety of the client. The visitor may or may not be aware of the client's suicidal thoughts or of the hospital's safety policies. The client should open the gift in the presence of the nurse so that sharp or unsafe objects can be locked in the client's safety box. Leaving the package unattended in the room with the client is hazardous. Options 2, 3, and 4 are incorrect and unsafe. Remember that implementation is the third step of the nursing process!

Box 4-16 ▲ PRACTICE QUESTION: THE NURSING PROCESS/EVALUATION

QUESTION

A nurse provides instructions to a pregnant woman about food items to consume that contain folic acid. Which statement made by the client *indicates an adequate understanding* of these food items?

1. "I will eat yogurt every day."
2. "I will eat a banana every day."
3. "A glass of milk each day will be sufficient."
4. "Green leafy vegetables, whole grains, and fruits are important to eat."

ANSWER: 4

Test-Taking Strategy: Note the strategic words *indicates an adequate understanding.* These words indicate that this is an evaluation-type question. Options 1 and 3 can be eliminated first because they are comparable or alike in that both yogurt and milk are dairy products and are high in calcium. To select from the remaining options, remember that bananas are high in potassium. Remember that evaluation is the fourth step of the nursing process!

6. Evaluation (Box 4-16)
   a. Evaluation questions address the comparing of actual outcomes of care with the expected outcomes and on communicating and documenting findings.
   b. These questions focus on assisting with determining the client's response to care and identifying factors that may interfere with achieving expected outcomes.
   c. With an evaluation question, watch for negative event queries; they are frequently used in evaluation-type questions.

Box 4-17 ▲ PRACTICE QUESTION: COMMUNICATION

QUESTION

A client who is scheduled for surgery to be placed in skeletal traction says to the nurse, "I'm not sure if I want to have this skeletal traction or if the skin traction would be best to stabilize my fracture." Based on the client's statement, the nurse should make which response?

1. "There is no reason to be concerned. I have seen lots of these procedures."
2. "Skeletal traction is much more effective than skin traction in your situation."
3. "You have concerns about skeletal versus skin traction for your type of fracture?"
4. "Your fracture is very unstable. You will die if you do not have this surgery performed."

ANSWER: 3

Test-Taking Strategy: Use therapeutic communication techniques. Select the option that enhances communication and addresses the client's feelings and concerns; this will direct you to option 3. Remember to use therapeutic communication techniques and to focus on the client's feelings!

VII. Client Needs

A. Safe and Effective Care Environment
   1. These questions address the concepts of the nurse providing nursing care; collaborating with other health care team members to facilitate effective client care; and protecting clients, significant others, and health care personnel from environmental hazards.
   2. Focus on safety with these types of questions, and remember the importance of handwashing, call bells, bed positioning, and the appropriate use of side rails.

B. Physiological Integrity
   1. These questions address the concepts of the nurse providing comfort and assistance during the performance of activities of daily living; providing care related to the administration of medications; and monitoring clients receiving parenteral therapies.
   2. These questions also address the nurse's ability to reduce the client's potential for developing complications or health problems related to treatments, procedures, or existing conditions, as well as the nurse's role in providing care to clients with acute, chronic, or life-threatening physical health conditions.
   3. Focus on Maslow's Hierarchy of Needs theory with these types of questions, and remember that physiological needs are a priority and are addressed first.
   4. Use the ABCs—airway, breathing, and circulation—and the steps of the nursing process (clinical problem-solving process) when selecting an option that addresses physiological integrity.

C. Psychosocial Integrity
   1. These questions address the concepts of the nurse providing nursing care that promotes and supports the emotional, mental, and social well-being of the client and significant others.
   2. Content addressed in these questions relates to supporting and promoting the client or significant others' ability to cope, adapt, or solve problems in situations such as illnesses, disabilities, and stressful events (e.g., abuse, neglect, violence).
   3. You may be asked communication-type questions that relate to how you would respond to a client, a client's family member or significant other, or to other health care team members.
   4. Use therapeutic communication techniques to answer communication questions because of their effectiveness in the communication process.
   5. Remember to select the option that focuses on the client's, the client's family members', or the significant others' thoughts, feelings, concerns, anxieties, or fears (Box 4-17).

D. Health Promotion and Maintenance
   1. These questions address the concepts of the nurse providing and assisting with the direction of nursing care to promote and maintain health.
   2. Content addressed in these questions relates to assisting the client and significant others during the normal, expected stages of growth and development from conception through advanced old age and providing client care related to the prevention and early detection of health problems.
   3. Use teaching and learning theory if the question addresses client teaching; remember that client willingness, desire, and readiness to learn are the first priorities.
   4. Watch for negative event queries, which are frequently found in questions that address health promotion and maintenance and client education.

VIII. Eliminating Comparable or Alike Options (Box 4-18)

A. When reading the options, look for options that are comparable or alike; these options will include a similar concept or nursing action.

B. Comparable or alike options can be eliminated as possible answers.

Box 4-18 ▲ PRACTICE QUESTION: ELIMINATE COMPARABLE OR ALIKE OPTIONS

QUESTION

A nurse is caring for a client who has bipolar disorder with aggressive social behavior. Which of the following activities would initially be most appropriate for this client?

1. Chess
2. Writing
3. Ping-Pong
4. Basketball

ANSWER: 2

Test-Taking Strategy: Options 1, 3, and 4 are comparable or alike in that they are activities that the client cannot do alone and that are competitive. Solitary activities that require a short attention span with mild physical exertion are the most appropriate initial activities for a client who is aggressive. Competitive games (options 1, 3, and 4) should be avoided because they can stimulate aggression and increase psychomotor activity. Remember to eliminate options that are comparable or alike!

Box 4-19 ▲ PRACTICE QUESTION: ELIMINATE OPTIONS THAT CONTAIN CLOSE-ENDED WORDS

QUESTION

A nurse reinforces instructions to the parents of an infant with hip dysplasia regarding the care of the Pavlik harness. Which instruction provided by the nurse is accurate?

1. The harness must be worn 8 hours a day.
2. The harness is removed to check the skin and for bathing.
3. The infant should never be moved when out of the harness.
4. The harness must be removed for feedings and diaper changes.

ANSWER: 2

Test-Taking Strategy: Visualize the Pavlik harness; this will assist you with eliminating options 3 and 4. Select option 2 over option 1 because the time frame in option 1 is rather short. In addition, note the close-ended words *must* in options 1 and 4 and *never* in option 3. Remember to avoid options that contain close-ended words!

IX. Eliminate Options That Contain Close-Ended Words (Box 4-19)

A. Close-ended words include *all, always, every, must, none, never,* and *only.*

B. Eliminate options that contain close-ended words; these words infer a fixed or extreme meaning, and thus these types of options are usually incorrect.

C. Options that contain open-ended words such as *may, usually,* or *generally* should be considered as possible correct options.

X. Look for the Umbrella Option (Box 4-20)

A. When answering a question, look for the umbrella option.

B. The umbrella option is one that is a broad or universal statement and that usually contains the concepts of the other options within it.

C. The umbrella option will be the correct answer.

Box 4-20 ▲ PRACTICE QUESTION: LOOK FOR THE UMBRELLA OPTION

QUESTION

A nurse is developing a plan of care for a client with Ménière's disease. The priority nursing interventions should focus on which of the following?

1. Safety measures
2. Dietary restrictions
3. Activity limitations
4. Knowledge about medication therapy

ANSWER: 1

Test-Taking Strategy: Focus on the client's disorder—Ménière's disease—and recall the pathophysiology associated with this disease. All of the options identify a component of the plan of care for this client, but remember that safety is a priority. In addition, note that option 1 is the umbrella option in that it is a broad statement or intervention. Remember to look for the umbrella option!

XI. Use the Guidelines for Delegating and Making Assignments (Box 4-21)

A. You may be asked a question that will require you to decide how you will delegate a task or assign clients to other health care providers.

B. Focus on the information in the question and the task or assignment that is to be delegated.

C. After you have determined what task or assignment is to be delegated, consider the client's needs; match the client's needs with the scope of practice of the health care providers identified in the question.

D. The nurse practice act and any practice limitations define the aspects of care that can be delegated and those that must be performed by a nursing assistant, a licensed practical or vocational nurse, or a registered nurse.

E. Noninvasive interventions (e.g., skin care, range-of-motion exercises, ambulation, grooming, hygiene) can generally be assigned to a nursing assistant.

Box 4-21 ▲ PRACTICE QUESTION: USE THE GUIDELINES FOR DELEGATING AND MAKING ASSIGNMENTS

QUESTION

A nurse in charge of a long-term care unit is planning the client assignments for the day. A licensed practical nurse (LPN) and a nursing assistant are on the nursing team. Which client would the nurse *most appropriately* assign to the LPN?

1. The client who is scheduled for an electrocardiogram and a chest x-ray
2. The client with stable congestive heart failure who has early-stage Alzheimer's disease
3. The client who was treated for dehydration who is weak and needs assistance with bathing
4. The client with emphysema who is receiving oxygen (2 L via nasal cannula) and who becomes dyspneic on exertion

ANSWER: 4

Test-Taking Strategy: The nurse would most appropriately assign the client with emphysema to the LPN. This client has an airway problem and has the highest-priority needs of the clients presented in the options. The clients described in options 1, 2, and 3 can be cared for appropriately by the nursing assistant. Remember to match the client's needs with the scope of practice of the health care provider!

Box 4-22 ▲ PRACTICE QUESTION: ANSWERING PHARMACOLOGY QUESTIONS

QUESTION

An iodine solution is prescribed for a client. The client calls the nurse at the clinic and complains of a brassy taste and burning sensations in the mouth. The nurse tells the client to:

1. Contact the physician.
2. Continue the medication.
3. Take half of the prescribed dose for the next 24 hours.
4. Stop the medication for the next 24 hours and then continue to take it as prescribed.

ANSWER: 1

Test-Taking Strategy: Use medication guidelines to help you answer this question. Eliminate options 3 and 4 first because the nurse cannot legally alter medication prescriptions without a physician's order. Considering the client symptoms presented in the question, eliminate option 2 as a reasonable choice. The chronic ingestion of iodine can produce iodism. The client needs to be instructed about the symptoms of iodism, which includes a brassy taste, burning sensations in the mouth, soreness of gums and teeth, frontal headache, coryza, salivation, and skin eruptions. The client needs to notify the physician if these symptoms occur. Remember to use medication guidelines to answer pharmacology questions!

F. A licensed practical or vocational nurse can perform the tasks that a nursing assistant can perform; in addition, he or she can perform certain invasive tasks, such as applying dressings; suctioning; urinary catheterization; and administering oral, subcutaneous, and intramuscular injections, as well as some intravenous piggyback medications.

G. A registered nurse can perform the tasks that a licensed practical or vocational nurse can perform and is responsible for assessment, planning care, supervising care, and initiating teaching.

XII. Answering Pharmacology Questions (Box 4-22)

A. If you are familiar with the medication, use your nursing knowledge to answer the question.

B. Remember that the question will identify both the generic name and the trade name of the medication.

C. If the question identifies a medical diagnosis, then try to make a relationship between the medication and the diagnosis; for example, you can determine that cyclophosphamide (Cytoxan) is an antineoplastic medication if the question refers to a client with breast cancer who is taking this medication.

D. Try to determine the classification of the medication being addressed to assist you with answering the question; identifying the classification will assist with determining the medication's action and/or side effects; for example, diltiazem (*Card*izem) is a cardiac medication.

E. Recognize the common side effects associated with each medication classification, and then relate the appropriate nursing interventions to each side effect; for example, if the side effect is hypertension, then the associated nursing intervention would be to monitor the blood pressure.

F. Learn the medications that belong to a classification by looking for commonalities in their names; for example, medications that are xanthine bronchodilators end with *-line* (e.g., theophyl*line*).

G. Look at the medication name and use medical terminology to assist with determining the medication action; for example, Lopressor lowers *(lo)* the blood pressure *(pressor)*.

H. If the question requires a medication calculation, remember that an on-screen calculator is available on the computer; talk yourself through each step to be sure that the answer makes sense, and recheck the calculation before answering the question, particularly if the answer seems like an unusual dosage.

I. Pyramid points to remember
   1. The client should generally not take an antacid with medication because the antacid will affect the absorption of the medication.
   2. Capsules should not be opened, and enteric-coated and sustained-release tablets should not be crushed.
   3. The client should never adjust or change a medication dose or abruptly stop taking a medication.
   4. The nurse never adjusts or changes the client's medication dosage or discontinues a medication.
   5. The client needs to avoid taking any over-the-counter medications or other medications (e.g., herbal preparations) unless they are approved for use by the health care provider.
   6. The client needs to avoid alcohol and smoking.
   7. Medications are never administered if the order is difficult to read or unclear or if it identifies an unusual dose.

REFERENCES

deWit, S. (2005). *Fundamental concepts and skills for nursing* (2nd ed.). Philadelphia: Saunders.

Harkreader, H., Hogan, M. A., & Thobaben, M. (2007). *Fundamentals of nursing: Caring and clinical judgment* (3rd ed.). Philadelphia: Saunders.

Hill, S., & Howlett, H. (2009). *Success in practical/vocational nursing: From student to leader* (6th ed.). Philadelphia: Saunders.

Hockenberry, M., & Wilson, D. (2007). *Wong's nursing care of infants and children* (8th ed.). St. Louis: Mosby.

Hodgson, B., & Kizior, R. (2009). *Saunders nursing drug handbook 2009.* St. Louis: Saunders.

Huber, D. (2006). *Leadership and nursing care management* (3rd ed.). Philadelphia: Saunders.

Lehne, R. (2007). *Pharmacology for nursing care* (6th ed.). St. Louis: Saunders.

Leifer, G. (2005). *Maternity nursing* (9th ed.). Philadelphia: Saunders.

Meiner, S., & Leuckenotte, A. (2006). *Gerontologic nursing* (3rd ed.). St. Louis: Mosby.

Morrison-Valfre, M. (2005). *Foundations of mental health care* (3rd ed.). St. Louis: Mosby.

National Council of State Boards of Nursing (Eds.). (2008). *2008 Detailed Test Plan for the NCLEX-PN® Examination.* Chicago: Author.

National Council of State Boards of Nursing, Inc. Web site: http://www.ncsbn.org/. Retrieved July 25, 2009.

Potter, P., & Perry, A. (2009). *Fundamentals of nursing* (7th ed.). St. Louis: Mosby.

Price, D., & Gwin, J. (2005). *Thompson's pediatric nursing* (9th ed.). Philadelphia: Saunders.

Skidmore-Roth, L. (2008). *2008 Mosby's nursing drug reference* (21st ed.). St. Louis: Mosby.

UNIT
II

Client Needs

CHAPTER 5

Client Needs and the NCLEX-PN® Test Plan

CLIENT NEEDS

In the new test plan implemented in April 2008, the National Council of State Boards of Nursing (NCSBN) identified a framework based on Client Needs. This framework was selected on the basis of an analysis of the findings of a practice analysis study of newly licensed practical and vocational nurses in the United States. The study identified the nursing activities performed by these entry-level nurses. In addition, according to the NCSBN, the Client Needs categories provide a structure for defining nursing actions and competencies across all settings for all clients. The NCSBN identifies four major categories of Client Needs. Some categories are further divided into subcategories, and the percentage of test questions in each subcategory is identified (Table 5-1).

Safe and Effective Care Environment

The Safe and Effective Care Environment category addresses content related to the nurse's roles in providing nursing care and collaborating with other health care team members to promote the achievement of client outcomes and to protect clients, family members, significant others, and other health care personnel from environmental hazards. The Safe and Effective Care Environment category includes two subcategories: Coordinated Care and Safety and Infection Control. The NCSBN identifies nursing content related to the subcategories of this Client Needs category (Box 5-1); refer

TABLE 5-1 ▲ CLIENT NEEDS AND PERCENTAGE OF TEST QUESTIONS

CLIENT NEEDS CATEGORY	QUESTIONS (%)
SAFE AND EFFECTIVE CARE ENVIRONMENT	
Coordinated Care	12-18
Safety and Infection Control	8-14
HEALTH PROMOTION AND MAINTENANCE	7-13
PSYCHOSOCIAL INTEGRITY	8-14
PHYSIOLOGICAL INTEGRITY	
Basic Care and Comfort	11-17
Pharmacological Therapies	9-15
Reduction of Risk Potential	10-16
Physiological Adaptation	11-17

From the National Council of State Boards of Nursing (Eds.). (2008). *Detailed Test Plan for the NCLEX-PN® Examination.* Chicago: Author.

Box 5-1 ▲ NCLEX-PN® CONTENT: SAFE AND EFFECTIVE CARE ENVIRONMENT

COORDINATED CARE

- Advance directives
- Advocacy
- Client-care assignments
- Client rights
- Concepts of management and supervision
- Confidentiality and information security
- Consultation with members of the health care team
- Continuity of care
- Establishing priorities
- Ethical practice
- Information technology
- Informed consent
- Legal responsibilities
- Performance improvement
- Referral processes
- Resource management
- Staff education

SAFETY AND INFECTION CONTROL

- Accident and error prevention
- Incident, event, irregular occurrence, and variance reports
- Disaster and security planning
- Ergonomic principles
- Handling hazardous and infectious materials
- Injury prevention and safety, including home safety
- Medical and surgical asepsis
- Safe use of equipment
- Standard and other precautions
- Use of restraints and safety devices

From the National Council of State Boards of Nursing (Eds.). (2008). *Detailed Test Plan for the National Council Licensure Examination for Practical/Vocational Nurses.* Chicago: Author. Refer to the National Council of State Boards of Nursing Web site for more information about the test plan: www.ncsbn.org.

Box 5-2 ▲ SAFE AND EFFECTIVE CARE ENVIRONMENT QUESTIONS

COORDINATED CARE

A nurse is planning the client assignments for the day. Which of the following is the most appropriate assignment for the nursing assistant?

1. The client who requires colostomy irrigation
2. The client receiving continuous tube feedings
3. The client who requires stool specimen collections
4. The client who has difficulty swallowing food and fluids

ANSWER: 3

Rationale: This question addresses the subcategory Coordinated Care in the Client Needs category of Safe and Effective Care Environment, and it specifically addresses content related to client care assignments. Delegation tasks must be consistent with the individual's level of expertise and licensure or lack of licensure. In this situation, the most appropriate assignment for the nursing assistant would be to care for the client who requires stool specimen collections, which is a noninvasive task. The client with difficulty swallowing food and fluids is at risk for aspiration, and colostomy irrigations and tube feedings are not performed by unlicensed personnel. Remember that the health care provider needs to be competent and skilled at performing the task or activity that has been assigned.

SAFETY AND INFECTION CONTROL

A client with tuberculosis (TB) is scheduled to go to the radiology department for a chest x-ray. Which nursing intervention would be appropriate when preparing to transport the client?

1. Apply a mask to the client.
2. Apply a mask and gown to the client.
3. Apply a mask, gown, and gloves to the client.
4. Notify the x-ray department so that personnel can be sure to wear masks when the client arrives.

ANSWER: 1

Rationale: This question addresses the subcategory Safety and Infection Control in the Client Needs category of Safe and Effective Care Environment, and it specifically addresses content that is related to airborne precautions. Clients who have or are suspected of having TB should wear a mask when out of the hospital room to prevent the spread of the infection to others. A gown and gloves are not necessary.

to the NCSBN Web site at www.ncsbn.org for information about the NCLEX test plan. The Coordinated Care subcategory (12% to 18%) addresses content related to facilitating effective client care through collaboration with other health care team members. The Safety and Infection Control subcategory (8% to 14%) addresses content that tests the knowledge, skills, and abilities required to protect clients and health care personnel from health and environmental hazards. Box 5-2 presents examples of questions that address these two subcategories. Refer to Chapter 6, "Safe and Effective Care Environment," for practice questions that reflect this Client Needs category.

Health Promotion and Maintenance

The Health Promotion and Maintenance category (7% to 13%) addresses the principles that are related to growth, development, and the aging process. This Client Needs category also addresses content that tests the knowledge, skills, and abilities required to assist the client, family members, and significant others with preventing health problems, recognizing alterations in health, and developing health practices that promote and support wellness. The NCSBN identifies nursing content that is related to this Client Needs category (Boxes 5-3 and 5-4); refer to the NCSBN Web site at www.ncsbn.org for information about the NCLEX test plan. Refer to Chapter 7, "Health Promotion and Maintenance," for practice questions that reflect this Client Needs category.

Box 5-3 ▲ NCLEX-PN® CONTENT: HEALTH PROMOTION AND MAINTENANCE

Aging process
Antepartum, intrapartum, and postpartum periods and newborn care
Data collection techniques
Developmental stages and transitions
Expected body-image changes
Family planning
Health promotion and screening programs
High-risk behaviors
Human sexuality
Immunizations
Lifestyle choices
Preventing disease
Self-care

From the National Council of State Boards of Nursing (Eds.). (2008). *Detailed Test Plan for the National Council Licensure Examination for Practical/Vocational Nurses.* Chicago: Author. Refer to the National Council of State Boards of Nursing Web site for information about the test plan: www.ncsbn.org.

Psychosocial Integrity

The Psychosocial Integrity category (8% to 14%) addresses content that tests the knowledge, skills, and abilities required to promote and support the emotional, mental, and social well-being of the client, family members, and significant others. The NCSBN identifies nursing content related to this Client Needs category (Boxes 5-5 and 5-6); refer to the NCSBN Web site at www.ncsbn.org for information about the NCLEX test plan. Refer to Chapter 8, "Psychosocial Integrity," for practice questions that reflect this Client Needs category.

Box 5-4 ▲ HEALTH PROMOTION AND MAINTENANCE QUESTIONS

A postpartum nurse has instructed a new mother regarding how to bathe her newborn infant. The nurse demonstrates the procedure to the mother, and, on the following day, asks the mother to perform the procedure. Which observation by the nurse indicates that the mother is performing the procedure correctly?

1. The mother cleans the ears and then moves to the eyes and the face.
2. The mother begins to wash the newborn infant by starting with the eyes and face.
3. The mother washes the arms, chest, and back, followed by the neck, arms, and face.
4. The mother washes the newborn infant's entire body and then washes the eyes, face, and scalp.

ANSWER: 2

Rationale: This question addresses the Client Needs category of Health Promotion and Maintenance, and it specifically addresses the postpartum period. The bathing of a newborn should start with the eyes and face and with the cleanest area first. Next, the external ears and behind the ears are cleaned. The newborn infant's neck should be washed, because formula, lint, and breast milk will often accumulate in the folds of the neck. The hands and arms are then washed. The infant's legs are washed next, with the diaper area washed last. Remember to always start with the cleanest area of the body and to proceed to the dirtiest area.

A client with atherosclerosis asks a nurse about dietary modifications to lower the risk of heart disease. The nurse encourages the client to eat which of the following foods to lower this risk?

1. Fresh cantaloupe
2. Broiled cheeseburger
3. Baked chicken with skin
4. Mashed potato with gravy

ANSWER: 1

Rationale: This question addresses the Client Needs category of Health Promotion and Maintenance, and it specifically addresses health and wellness. To lower the risk of heart disease, the diet should be low in saturated fat, with the appropriate number of total calories. The diet should be low in red meat and include more white meat with the skin removed. Dairy products should be low in fat, and foods with high amounts of empty calories should be avoided. Fresh fruits and vegetables are naturally low in fat.

Box 5-5 ▲ NCLEX-PN® CONTENT: PSYCHOSOCIAL INTEGRITY

Abuse and neglect
Behavior interventions and management
Coping mechanisms
Crisis intervention
Cultural awareness
End-of-life issues
Grief and loss
Mental health and mental illness concepts
Religious and spiritual influences on health
Sensory and perceptual alterations
Situational role changes
Stress management
Substance abuse disorders
Suicide precautions
Support systems
Therapeutic communication
Therapeutic environment
Unexpected body-image changes
Violence precautions

From the National Council of State Boards of Nursing (Eds.). (2008). *Detailed Test Plan for the National Council Licensure Examination for Practical/Vocational Nurses.* Chicago: Author. Refer to the National Council of State Boards of Nursing Web site for information about the test plan: www.ncsbn.org.

Physiological Integrity

The Physiological Integrity category includes four subcategories: Basic Care and Comfort, Pharmacological Therapies, Reduction of Risk Potential, and Physiological Adaptation. The NCSBN identifies nursing content related to the subcategories of this Client Needs category (Box 5-7); refer to the NCSBN Web site at www.ncsbn.org for information about the NCLEX test plan. The Basic Care and Comfort subcategory (11% to 17%) addresses content that tests the knowledge, skills, and abilities required to provide comfort and assistance with the performance of activities of daily living. The Pharmacological Therapies subcategory (9% to

Box 5-6 ▲ PSYCHOSOCIAL INTEGRITY QUESTIONS

The nurse is planning care for a client who is experiencing anxiety after a myocardial infarction. Which priority nursing intervention should be included in the plan of care?

1. Answer questions with factual information.
2. Provide detailed explanations of all procedures.
3. Limit family involvement during the acute phase.
4. Administer an antianxiety medication to promote relaxation.

ANSWER: 1

Rationale: This question addresses the Client Needs category of Psychosocial Integrity, and it specifically addresses content related to fear and anxiety. Accurate information reduces fear, strengthens the nurse–client relationship, and assists the client with dealing realistically with the situation. Providing detailed information may increase the client's anxiety, so information should be provided simply and clearly. Limiting family involvement may or may not be helpful, because the client's family may be a source of support for the client. Medication should not be used unless necessary.

A nurse in the mental health clinic is assisting with collecting data from a family with a diagnosis of domestic violence. Which of the following factors would the nurse initially want to include during data collection?

1. The coping style of each family member
2. The family's anger toward the intrusiveness of the nurse
3. The family's current ability to use community resources
4. The family's denial of the violent nature of their behavior

ANSWER: 1

Rationale: This question addresses the Client Needs category of Psychosocial Integrity, and it specifically addresses domestic violence. Note the strategic word *initially.* At the beginning, data collection includes a careful history of each family member. Options 2, 3, and 4 address the family as a whole; option 1 addresses each family member.

Box 5-7 ▲ NCLEX-PN® CONTENT: PHYSIOLOGICAL INTEGRITY

BASIC CARE AND COMFORT
Assistive devices
Elimination
Mobility and immobility
Nonpharmacological pain interventions
Nutrition and oral hydration
Palliative and comfort care
Personal hygiene
Rest and sleep

REDUCTION OF RISK POTENTIAL
Diagnostic tests
Laboratory values
Potential for alterations in body systems
Potential for complications of diagnostic tests, procedures, surgery, and health alterations
Therapeutic procedures
Vital signs

PHARMACOLOGICAL THERAPIES
Adverse and toxic effects
Contraindications and compatibilities
Dosage calculations
Intended effects
Medication administration
Pharmacological actions
Pharmacological agents
Side effects

PHYSIOLOGICAL ADAPTATION
Alterations in body systems
Basic pathophysiology
Fluid and electrolyte imbalances
Medical emergencies
Radiation therapy
Unexpected responses to therapies

From the National Council of State Boards of Nursing (Eds.). (2008). *Detailed Test Plan for the National Council Licensure Examination for Practical/Vocational Nurses.* Chicago: Author. Refer to the National Council of State Boards of Nursing Web site for information about the test plan: www.ncsbn.org.

15%) addresses content that tests the knowledge, skills, and abilities required to provide care related to the administration of medications and to the monitoring of clients receiving parenteral therapies. The Reduction of Risk Potential subcategory (10% to 16%) addresses content that tests the knowledge, skills, and abilities required to reduce the client's potential for developing complications or health problems related to existing conditions, treatments, and procedures. The Physiological Adaptation subcategory (11% to 17%) addresses content that tests the knowledge, skills, and abilities required to participate in providing care to clients with acute, chronic, or life-threatening physical health conditions. Box 5-8 provides practice questions that address these subcategories. Refer to Chapter 9, "Physiological Integrity," for practice questions that reflect this Client Needs category.

Box 5-8 ▲ PHYSIOLOGICAL INTEGRITY QUESTIONS

BASIC CARE AND COMFORT

A client with right-sided weakness needs to learn how to use a cane for home maintenance of mobility. The nurse plans to teach the client to position the cane by holding it in which of the following ways?

1. With the left hand and 6 inches lateral to the left foot
2. With the right hand and 6 inches lateral to the right foot
3. With the left hand, with the cane placed in front of the left foot
4. With the right hand, with the cane placed in front of the right foot

ANSWER: 1
Rationale: This question addresses the subcategory Basic Care and Comfort in the Client Needs category of Physiological Integrity, and it specifically addresses content related to the use of an assistive device. The client is taught to hold the cane on the opposite side of the weakness because, with normal walking, the opposite arm and leg move together (called *reciprocal motion*). The cane is placed 6 inches lateral to the fifth toe.

PHARMACOLOGICAL THERAPIES

A nurse is caring for a client with hypertension who is receiving torsemide (Demadex) 5 mg orally daily. Which of the following would indicate to the nurse that the client may be experiencing an adverse reaction related to the medication?

1. A chloride level of 98 mEq/L
2. A sodium level of 135 mEq/L
3. A potassium level of 3.1 mEq/L
4. A blood urea nitrogen (BUN) level of 15 mg/dL

ANSWER: 3
Rationale: This question addresses the subcategory Pharmacological Therapies in the Client Needs category of Physiological Integrity, and it specifically addresses content related to the adverse effect of a medication. Torsemide is a loop diuretic that can produce acute, profound water loss; volume and electrolyte depletion; dehydration; decreased blood volume; and circulatory collapse. Option 3 is the only option that indicates an electrolyte depletion, because the normal potassium level is 3.5 to 5.1 mEq/L. The normal sodium level is 135 to 145 mEq/L, the normal chloride level is 98 to 107 mEq/L, and the normal BUN level is 5 to 20 mg/dL.

REDUCTION OF RISK POTENTIAL

The nurse is caring for a client scheduled to undergo a renal biopsy. To minimize the risk of postprocedure complications, the nurse reports which of the following laboratory results to the physician before the procedure?

1. Potassium: 3.8 mEq/L
2. Serum creatinine: 1.2 mg/dL
3. Prothrombin time: 15 seconds
4. Blood urea nitrogen (BUN): 18 mg/dL

ANSWER: 3
Rationale: This question addresses the subcategory Reduction of Risk Potential in the Client Needs category of Physiological Integrity, and it specifically addresses a potential postprocedure complication of a diagnostic test. Postprocedure hemorrhage is a complication after renal biopsy. Because of this, the prothrombin time is assessed before the procedure. The normal prothrombin time range is 11 to 12.5 seconds. The nurse ensures that these results are available and reports abnormalities promptly. The normal BUN level is 5 to 20 mg/dL, the normal serum creatinine level is 0.6 to 1.3 mg/dL, and the normal potassium level is 3.5 to 5.1 mEq/L.

PHYSIOLOGICAL ADAPTATION

A pregnant client tells a nurse that she felt wetness on her peripad and that she found some clear fluid. The nurse immediately inspects the perineum and notes the presence of the umbilical cord. Which action should the nurse take first?

1. Monitor the fetal heart rate.
2. Notify the registered nurse.
3. Transfer the client to the delivery room.
4. Place the client in Trendelenburg's position.

ANSWER: 4
Rationale: This question addresses the subcategory Physiological Adaptation in the Client Needs category of Physiological Integrity, and it specifically addresses an acute and life-threatening physical health condition. On inspection of the perineum, if the umbilical cord is noted, the nurse immediately places the client into Trendelenburg's position to relieve cord compression. The registered nurse is notified, who then contacts the health care provider. The nurse monitors the fetal heart rate, and the client is transferred to the delivery room as prescribed by the health care provider.

REFERENCES

Black, J., & Hawks, J. (2009). *Medical-surgical nursing: Clinical management for positive outcomes* (8th ed.). St. Louis: Saunders.

Chernecky, C., & Berger, B. (2008). *Laboratory tests and diagnostic procedures* (5th ed.). Philadelphia: Saunders.

Christensen, B., & Kockrow, E. (2006). *Foundations of nursing* (5th ed.). St. Louis: Mosby.

deWit, S. (2009). *Medical-surgical nursing: Concepts & practice*. St. Louis: Saunders.

Hill, S., & Howlett, H. (2009). *Success in practical/vocational nursing: From student to leader* (6th ed.). Philadelphia: Saunders.

Hodgson, B., & Kizior, R. (2009). *Saunders nursing drug handbook 2009*. St. Louis: Saunders.

Lilley, L., Harrington, S., & Snyder, J. (2007). *Pharmacology and the nursing process* (5th ed.). St. Louis: Mosby.

Linton, A., & Maebius, N. (2007). *Introduction to medical-surgical nursing* (4th ed.). Philadelphia: Saunders.

National Council of State Boards of Nursing (Eds.). (2008). *Detailed Test Plan for the NCLEX-PN® Examination*. Chicago: Author.

National Council of State Boards of Nursing, Inc. Web site: http://www.ncsbn.org/. Retrieved July 25, 2009.

Potter, P., & Perry, A. (2009). *Fundamentals of nursing* (7th ed.). St. Louis: Mosby.

CHAPTER

6

Safe and Effective Care Environment

1. A nurse is preparing to transfer an average-sized client with right-sided hemiplegia from the bed to the wheelchair. The client is able to support weight on the unaffected side, and the nurse plans to use the hemiplegic transfer technique. The client is sitting upright in bed with the legs dangling over the side. For the safest transfer, where should the wheelchair be positioned?

1 Next to either leg
2 Near the client's left leg
3 Near the client's right leg
4 As space in the room permits

Level of Cognitive Ability: Application
Client Needs: Safe and Effective Care Environment
Integrated Process: Nursing Process/Implementation
Content Area: Fundamental Skills

Answer: 2

Rationale: Although the space in the room is an important consideration for the placement of a wheelchair for a transfer, when the client has an affected lower extremity, movement should always occur toward the client's unaffected (strong) side. For example, if the client's right leg is affected and the client is sitting on the edge of the bed, then the wheelchair is positioned next to the client's left side; this wheelchair position allows the client to use the unaffected leg effectively and safely.

Test-Taking Strategy: Use the process of elimination, and focus on the subject: the safest transfer for the client. Although option 4 is a consideration for wheelchair positioning, it is not the safest answer. Option 2 will provide the safest transfer, because positioning the wheelchair next to the client's unaffected leg allows the client to use the stronger leg more effectively for a safe transfer. Review transfer techniques if you had difficulty with this question.

References

Christensen, B., & Kockrow, E. (2006). *Foundations of nursing* (5th ed., p. 391). St. Louis: Mosby.
Potter, P., & Perry, A. (2009). *Fundamentals of nursing* (7th ed., p. 1261). St. Louis: Mosby.

---

2. A nurse is preparing to leave the room of a client with a tracheostomy. The nurse ensures that the client has which of the following means of communication readily available before leaving the room?

1 Call bell
2 Letter board
3 Picture board
4 Pen and paper

Level of Cognitive Ability: Application
Client Needs: Safe and Effective Care Environment
Integrated Process: Communication and Documentation
Content Area: Adult Health/Respiratory

Answer: 1

Rationale: Before leaving the room, the nurse ensures that the call bell is readily available. A client who cannot speak must have a means of contacting a nurse who is not in the room. The other options facilitate communication when the nurse is already present in the client's room.

Test-Taking Strategy: Use the process of elimination and your knowledge of basic principles of communication to answer this question. Note the strategic words *tracheostomy* and *leaving the room*. Remember that options that are comparable or alike are often incorrect; with this in mind, eliminate options 2, 3, and 4. Review these methods of communication if you had difficulty with this question.

Reference

Christensen, B., & Kockrow, E. (2006). *Foundations of nursing* (5th ed., pp. 361, 442). St. Louis: Mosby.

---

3. A licensed practical nurse (LPN) is asked to prepare a room for a child who will be admitted to the pediatric unit with a diagnosis of tonic-clonic seizures. The LPN prepares the room and plans to place which of the following items at the bedside?
   1 A suction apparatus and oxygen
   2 A tracheotomy set and oxygen
   3 An endotracheal tube and an airway
   4 An emergency cart and padded side rails

Level of Cognitive Ability: Application
Client Needs: Safe and Effective Care Environment
Integrated Process: Nursing Process/Planning
Content Area: Child Health

Answer: 1
Rationale: Tonic-clonic seizures cause a tightening of all of the body's muscles that is followed by tremors. An obstructed airway and increased oral secretions are the major complications during and after a seizure. A suction apparatus, oxygen, and an airway are helpful to prevent choking and cyanosis in these clients. Options 2, 3, and 4 are incorrect. Inserting a tracheostomy or endotracheal tube is not done in this situation. It is not necessary to have an emergency cart at the bedside, but a cart should be available in the treatment room or on the nursing unit.

Test-Taking Strategy: Use the process of elimination. Recalling that tonic-clonic seizures produce excessive oral secretions and airway obstruction will assist you with selecting the correct option. Review the plan of care associated with seizure precautions if you had difficulty with this question.

Reference
Price, D., & Gwin, J. (2008). *Pediatric nursing: An introductory text* (10th ed., p. 254). St. Louis: Saunders.

---

4. A child is admitted to the hospital with an undiagnosed exanthema (rash) that covers the trunk profusely and that is sparse on the extremities. During data collection, the nurse discovers that the child was exposed to varicella 2 weeks ago. The appropriate and immediate nursing intervention will be to:
   1 Immediately place the child in any available bed.
   2 Place the child in a private room on strict isolation.
   3 Check the progression of the exanthema, and report it to physician.
   4 Allow the child to play in the playroom until orders are received from the physician.

Level of Cognitive Ability: Application
Client Needs: Safe and Effective Care Environment
Integrated Process: Nursing Process/Implementation
Content Area: Child Health

Answer: 2
Rationale: A child with undiagnosed exanthema should be placed on strict isolation in a private room. Varicella causes a profuse rash on the trunk with a sparse rash on the extremities. It is important to prevent the spread of this communicable disease by placing the child in isolation until further diagnosis and treatment can be made. Options 1, 3, and 4 are incorrect.

Test-Taking Strategy: Use the process of elimination. Option 2 prevents the child from exposing other children and keeps staff, visitors, and others at minimal risk. Option 4 unnecessarily exposes other children and the environment to varicella. Admitting the child to "any" room is inappropriate. Checking the progression of the exanthema is correct, but it is not the immediate intervention. Review the care of the child with exanthema if you had difficulty with this question.

References
Hockenberry, M., & Wilson, D. (2007). *Nursing care of infants and children* (7th ed., pp. 668-669). St. Louis: Mosby.
Hockenberry, M., & Wilson, D. (2009). *Wong's essentials of pediatric nursing* (8th ed., pp. 462, 707). St. Louis: Mosby.

---

5. A rehabilitation center nurse is planning the client assignments for the day. Which of the following clients should the nurse assign to the nursing assistant?
   1 A client who had a below-the-knee amputation

Answer: 2
Rationale: The nurse is legally responsible for client assignments and must assign tasks based on the guidelines of nurse practice acts and the job description of the employing agency. Clients who have had below-the-knee amputations, who are scheduled for invasive diagnostic procedures, or who are scheduled to be transferred to a hospital for coronary artery bypass surgery have

2 A client on strict bedrest who is undergoing a 24-hour urine collection
3 A client who is scheduled for transfer to the hospital for coronary artery bypass surgery
4 A client who is scheduled for transfer to the hospital for an invasive diagnostic procedure

Level of Cognitive Ability: Application
Client Needs: Safe and Effective Care Environment
Integrated Process: Nursing Process/ Implementation
Content Area: Delegating/Prioritizing

both physiological and psychosocial needs. The nursing assistant has been trained to care for clients who are on bedrest and who require urine collections. The nurse will provide instructions, but the tasks required for these duties are within the role description of a nursing assistant.

Test-Taking Strategy: Note that the question asks for the assignment that can be delegated to the nursing assistant. When you are asked questions that relate to delegation, think about the role description of the employee and the needs of the client. The process of elimination easily directs you to option 2. Review the responsibilities related to delegation if you had difficulty with this question.

Reference

deWit, S. (2009). *Medical-surgical nursing: Concepts & practice* (pp. 3-4). St. Louis: Saunders.

---

6. A nurse is preparing to administer a continuous tube feeding via a feeding pump and notes that the electrical cord for the pump has only two prongs. Which of the following is the appropriate action?
1 Use the pump anyway.
2 Contact the physician.
3 Run the pump on the battery.
4 Obtain a three-prong grounded plug.

Level of Cognitive Ability: Application
Client Needs: Safe and Effective Care Environment
Integrated Process: Nursing Process/ Implementation
Content Area: Fundamental Skills

Answer: 4

Rationale: Electrical equipment must be maintained in good working order and should be grounded. (The third, longer prong in an electrical plug is the ground prong.) Theoretically, the ground prong carries any stray electrical current back to the ground, whereas the other two prongs carry the power to the piece of electrical equipment. There is no reason to contact the physician. Running the pump on the battery is not the most appropriate nursing action because the battery will run out, especially with the feeding being continuous.

Test-Taking Strategy: Use the process of elimination, and note the strategic words *only two prongs*. Principles of basic electrical safety should assist with directing you to the correct option. Review these principles if you had difficulty with this question.

Reference

Potter, P., & Perry, A. (2009). *Fundamentals of nursing* (7th ed., pp. 819, 842). St. Louis: Mosby.

---

7. A nurse is questioning a client about potential hazards in the home environment. Which of the following items, if identified by the client, is an indication that the client needs further instruction about home safety?
1 Carpeted stairs secured with carpet tacks
2 Clothes hamper at the end of the hallway
3 Wet spots on the ceramic-tiled bathroom floor
4 Skid-resistant, small area rugs in the living room

Answer: 3

Rationale: Injuries in the home frequently result from wet spots on the floor (regardless of the type of flooring); small rugs on the stairs and floor; and clutter on bedside tables, closet shelves, the top of the refrigerator, and bookshelves. Area rugs and runners should not be used on or near stairs. Any carpeting on the stairs should be secured with carpet tacks. Care should also be taken to ensure that end tables are secure and have stable straight legs. Nonessential items should be placed in drawers to eliminate clutter.

Test-Taking Strategy: Use the process of elimination, and note the strategic words *needs further instruction*. These words indicate a negative event query and ask you to select an option that is an unsafe situation. Recalling the principles related to home safety will assist with directing you to the correct option. Review these principles if you had difficulty with this question.

Level of Cognitive Ability: Comprehension
Client Needs: Safe and Effective Care Environment
Integrated Process: Teaching and Learning
Content Area: Fundamental Skills

References
deWit, S. (2009). *Medical-surgical nursing: Concepts & practice* (p. 197). St. Louis: Saunders.
Potter, P., & Perry, A. (2009). *Fundamentals of nursing* (7th ed., p. 813). St. Louis: Mosby.

---

8. A hospitalized client with a history of alcohol abuse tells the nurse, "I am leaving now. I have to go. I don't want any more treatment. I have things that I have to do right away." The client has not been discharged. In fact, the client is scheduled for an important diagnostic test in 1 hour. After the nurse discusses the client's concerns with the client, the client dresses and begins to walk out of the hospital room. Which of the following is the appropriate nursing action?

1 Notify the registered nurse (RN).
2 Call security to block all of the exit areas.
3 Restrain the client until the physician can be reached.
4 Tell the client that he or she cannot return to the hospital if he or she leaves now.

Answer: 1
Rationale: A nurse can be charged with false imprisonment if a client is made to wrongfully believe that he or she cannot leave the hospital. Most health care facilities have documents that the client is asked to sign that relate to the client's responsibilities when the client leaves against medical advice. The licensed practical nurse should notify the RN, who will ask the client to sign these documents before he or she leaves. The RN should request that the client wait to speak to the physician before leaving, but, if the client refuses to do so, the nurse cannot hold the client against his or her will. Restraining the client and calling security to block the exits constitutes false imprisonment. All clients have a right to health care at any time and cannot be told otherwise.

Test-Taking Strategy: Use the process of elimination. Keeping the concept of false imprisonment in mind, eliminate options 2 and 3, because they are comparable or alike. Eliminate option 4, because all clients have a right to health care. Review the points related to false imprisonment if you had difficulty with this question.

Level of Cognitive Ability: Application
Client Needs: Safe and Effective Care Environment
Integrated Process: Nursing Process/Implementation
Content Area: Fundamental Skills

Reference
Christensen, B., & Kockrow, E. (2006). *Foundations of nursing* (5th ed., p. 231). St. Louis: Mosby.

---

9. Two nurses are in the cafeteria having lunch in a quiet, secluded area. A physical therapist from the physical therapy department joins the nurses. During lunch, the nurses discuss a client who was physically abused. After lunch, the physical therapist provides therapy to the abused client and asks the client questions about the physical abuse. The client discovers that the nurses told the therapist about the abuse event and is emotionally harmed. The consequences associated with the nurses' discussion about the client are associated with which of the following?

1 They can be charged with libel.
2 They can be charged with slander.
3 There are no consequences, because they had their discussion in a secluded area.

Answer: 2
Rationale: Defamation is false communication or careless disregard for the truth that causes damage to someone's reputation, either in writing (libel) or verbally (slander). The most common examples are giving out inaccurate or inappropriate information from the medical record; discussing clients, families, or visitors in public areas; or speaking negatively about co-workers. The event described could cause emotional harm to the client, and the nurses could be charged with slander. This event also violates the client's right to confidentiality.

Test-Taking Strategy: When answering the question, use the process of elimination and your knowledge about the law and the legal responsibilities of the nurse to protect the client. Eliminate options 3 and 4 first. From the remaining options, it is necessary to know that slander involves a verbal discussion about a client. Review the nurse's legal responsibilities if you had difficulty with this question.

4 There are no consequences, because the physical therapist is involved in the client's care.

Level of Cognitive Ability: Comprehension
Client Needs: Safe and Effective Care Environment
Integrated Process: Nursing Process/ Implementation
Content Area: Fundamental Skills

Reference

Christensen, B., & Kockrow, E. (2006). *Foundations of nursing* (5th ed., p. 22). St. Louis: Mosby.

---

10. A nurse has administered a dose of diazepam (Valium) to the client. The nurse should take which most important action before leaving the client's room?
1 Close the shades.
2 Turn off the overhead light.
3 Put up the side rails on the bed.
4 Turn down the volume of the television.

Level of Cognitive Ability: Application
Client Needs: Safe and Effective Care Environment
Integrated Process: Nursing Process/ Implementation
Content Area: Pharmacology

Answer: 3
Rationale: Diazepam is a sedative/hypnotic medication with anticonvulsant and skeletal muscle relaxant properties. The nurse should institute safety measures before leaving the client's room to ensure that the client does not injure himself or herself. The most frequent side effects of this medication are dizziness, drowsiness, and lethargy. Therefore the nurse puts the side rails up on the client's bed before leaving the room to prevent falls. Options 1, 2, and 4 may be helpful measures that provide a comfortable, restful environment; however, option 3 is the one that provides for the client's safety.

Test-Taking Strategy: Note the strategic words *most important*, and use Maslow's Hierarchy of Needs theory. Remember that if a physiological need is not present, safety takes priority. Recalling that this medication is a sedative/hypnotic drug directs you to option 3. Review diazepam if you had difficulty with this question.

References

Christensen, B., & Kockrow, E. (2006). *Foundations of nursing* (5th ed., p. 371). St. Louis: Mosby.
Hodgson, B., & Kizior, R. (2009). *Saunders nursing drug handbook 2009* (pp. 345-347). St. Louis: Saunders.

---

11. A client has cognitive-perceptual difficulties and problems with fine motor coordination. The client's nurse should read the progress notes from which of the following health care team members to obtain suggestions for working with this client?
1 Social worker
2 Speech pathologist
3 Recreational therapist
4 Occupational therapist

Level of Cognitive Ability: Application
Client Needs: Safe and Effective Care Environment
Integrated Process: Nursing Process/ Implementation
Content Area: Adult Health/Neurological

Answer: 4
Rationale: The occupational therapist focuses on the development or relearning of fine motor skills. Social workers, speech pathologists, and recreational therapists do not address these types of client problems.

Test-Taking Strategy: Focus on the subject of the question: cognitive-perceptual difficulties and problems with fine motor coordination. Each of the incorrect options names a health team member who is not involved with fine motor skills, retraining, or cognitive-perceptual skill development. Review this information if you are unfamiliar with the roles of the health care members identified in the options.

Reference

Christensen, B., & Kockrow, E. (2006). *Foundations of nursing* (5th ed., p. 230). St. Louis: Mosby.

12. A postpartum client has been diagnosed with endometritis. The nurse who is reinforcing teaching about how to prevent the spread of infection to the newborn should tell the mother to:

1 Keep the newborn in the Isolette.
2 Ask visitors to not hold the newborn.
3 Wear a mask to prevent the spread of airborne droplets.
4 Wash the hands carefully before picking up the newborn.

Level of Cognitive Ability: Application
Client Needs: Safe and Effective Care Environment
Integrated Process: Teaching and Learning
Content Area: Maternity/Postpartum

Answer: 4

Rationale: Infection can be transmitted through contaminated items (e.g., hands, bed linens) of clients with endometritis. Handwashing is one of the most effective methods for preventing the transmission of this infectious disease, because it breaks the chain of infection. Options 2 and 3 are not related to the route of transmission of this infection, and option 1 is unnecessary.

Test-Taking Strategy: Use the process of elimination. Eliminate options 2 and 3 first because they are not related to the route of transmission. Choose correctly from the remaining options by using concepts related to the spread of infectious disease and maternal-infant bonding. Review endometritis if you had difficulty with this question.

Reference

Leifer, G. (2008). *Maternity nursing: An introductory text* (10th ed., pp. 344, 409). Philadelphia: Saunders.

---

13. A 2-month-old infant is admitted to the hospital. The nurse should perform which of the following actions to maintain the infant's safety and to reduce the risk of sudden infant death syndrome (SIDS)?

1 Make sure that only plastic bottles and toys are used.
2 Place the infant in a supine position in preparation for sleep.
3 Take the pacifier out of the infant's mouth before the infant falls asleep.
4 Cover the crib with netting when the child is not being directly observed.

Level of Cognitive Ability: Application
Client Needs: Safe and Effective Care Environment
Integrated Process: Nursing Process/Implementation
Content Area: Child Health

Answer: 2

Rationale: The American Academy of Pediatrics recommends the supine position for sleep to reduce the risk of SIDS. Plastic bottles and toys are not needed yet, because a 2-month-old cannot hold them. Pacifiers are considered safe and appropriate at this age. Safety netting is not necessary at this age, because the infant cannot roll over or stand alone.

Test-Taking Strategy: Use the process of elimination. The subject of the question is a nursing action that is appropriate to ensure infant safety. Eliminate option 1 because of the close-ended word *only*. Your knowledge of age-appropriate care and techniques to reduce the risk of SIDS will assist you with selecting the correct option from those that remain. Review the prevention of SIDS if you had difficulty with this question.

Reference

Christensen, B., & Kockrow, E. (2006). *Foundations of nursing* (5th ed., p. 1013). St. Louis: Mosby.

---

14. Sertraline (Zoloft) is prescribed to treat depression. The nurse reviews the client's record and consults the physician if which of the following is noted?

1 A history of diabetes mellitus
2 A history of myocardial infarction
3 The use of phenelzine sulfate (Nardil)
4 A history of irritable bowel syndrome

Level of Cognitive Ability: Analysis
Client Needs: Safe and Effective Care Environment

Answer: 3

Rationale: Sertraline (Zoloft) is a serotonin reuptake inhibitor and an antidepressant medication. Potentially fatal reactions may occur if sertraline is administered concurrently with a monoamine oxidase inhibitor (MAOI), such as phenelzine sulfate. MAOIs should be stopped at least 14 days before sertraline therapy is started. Conversely, sertraline should be stopped at least 14 days before MAOI therapy begins. Options 1, 2, and 4 are not of concern with this medication.

Integrated Process: Nursing Process/Data Collection
Content Area: Pharmacology

Test-Taking Strategy: Knowledge about the interactions and contraindications associated with the use of sertraline is necessary to answer this question. Remember that potentially fatal reactions may occur if sertraline is administered concurrently with an MAOI. Review MAOI interactions if you had difficulty with this question.

Reference

Hodgson, B., & Kizior, R. (2009). *Saunders nursing drug handbook 2009* (p. 1051). St. Louis: Saunders.

---

15. A nurse prepares to give an injection to a client. The nurse does which of the following after giving the injection?

1 Breaks the needle and discards it
2 Recaps the needle and discards the syringe in the disposal unit
3 Places the uncapped needle and syringe in a labeled cardboard box
4 Places the uncapped needle and syringe in a labeled, rigid plastic container

Level of Cognitive Ability: Application
Client Needs: Safe and Effective Care Environment
Integrated Process: Nursing Process/Implementation
Content Area: Fundamental Skills

Answer: 4
Rationale: Standard precautions include specific guidelines for the handling of sharps and needles. Needles should not be recapped, bent, broken, or cut after use; rather, they should be disposed of in a labeled, impermeable container specifically used for this purpose. Needles should not be discarded in cardboard boxes, because they could puncture the cardboard and cause a needle stick injury. Needles should never be left lying around after use.

Test-Taking Strategy: Use the process of elimination. Recalling that needles should never be broken or recapped assists with eliminating options 1 and 2. Noting that option 3 identifies a container that could be punctured assists with its elimination. Review standard precautions if you had difficulty with this question.

Reference

deWit, S. (2009). *Medical-surgical nursing: Concepts & practice* (p. 120). St. Louis: Saunders.

---

16. A licensed practical nurse (LPN) is assisting a registered nurse (RN) with developing a plan of care for a client who will be hospitalized for the insertion of an internal cervical radiation implant. Which of the following does the LPN suggest be included in the client's plan of care?

1 Limiting visitors' time to 60-minute visits
2 Placing the client in a private room close to the nurses' station
3 Placing a lead container and long-handled forceps in the client's room
4 Reinserting the implant into the vagina immediately if it becomes dislodged

Level of Cognitive Ability: Comprehension
Client Needs: Safe and Effective Care Environment
Integrated Process: Nursing Process/Planning
Content Area: Adult Health/Oncology

Answer: 3
Rationale: The client's room should be marked with appropriate signs that state the presence of radiation. Visitors are limited to 30-minute visits. The client should be placed in a private room at the end of the hall, because this location provides less of a chance of others being exposed to radiation. A lead container and long-handled forceps should be kept in the client's room at all times during internal radiation therapy. If the implant becomes dislodged, the nurse should pick it up with long-handled forceps and place it in the lead container; it would not be reinserted by the nurse.

Test-Taking Strategy: Use the process of elimination and your knowledge about the precautions and care for a client with a radiation implant to answer the question. Eliminate option 1 because of the lengthy time frame for visits. Eliminate option 2 because of the words *close to the nurses' station.* Knowing that it is not within the scope of nursing practice to reinsert the implant assists with the elimination of option 4. Review the precautions for internal radiation therapy if you had difficulty with this question.

Reference

Christensen, B., & Kockrow, E. (2006). *Adult health nursing* (5th ed., p. 829). St. Louis: Mosby.

---

17. A nurse is assigned to care for a 4-week-old infant who is scheduled for a pyloromyotomy. The nurse plans to do which of the following when caring for the infant?

1 Restrain the infant in a high chair.
2 Elevate the head of the infant's bed.
3 Feed the infant 1 oz of formula every hour.
4 Place the infant in a lying-down position for feedings.

Level of Cognitive Ability: Application
Client Needs: Safe and Effective Care Environment
Integrated Process: Nursing Process/Planning
Content Area: Child Health

Answer: 2

Rationale: Preoperatively, the infant's status is nothing by mouth (NPO), and the infant is stabilized with intravenous fluids and electrolytes. The head of the bed is elevated to reduce the risk of aspiration. The physician may also prescribe a prone position. Options 3 and 4 are not accurate during the preoperative period, because the infant is kept NPO. An infant is not restrained in a high chair.

Test-Taking Strategy: Use the process of elimination. Eliminate options 3 and 4 first. The infant is not fed lying down and is NPO. Next, eliminate option 1 because you would not restrain an infant in a high chair. Review the preoperative positioning of an infant who is scheduled for pyloromyotomy if you had difficulty with this question.

Reference

Leifer, G. (2007). *Introduction to maternity and pediatric nursing* (5th ed., p. 636). Philadelphia: Saunders.

---

18. A nurse who is employed in a long-term care facility has planned a get-together for clients and their families to celebrate the birthday of a client who is turning 100 years old. During the party, the nurse takes pictures of some of the clients and plans to submit the pictures to the local newspaper. Which client right has the nurse violated?

1 Assault
2 Battery
3 Invasion of privacy
4 False imprisonment

Level of Cognitive Ability: Comprehension
Client Needs: Safe and Effective Care Environment
Integrated Process: Nursing Process/Implementation
Content Area: Fundamental Skills

Answer: 3

Rationale: Invasion of privacy takes place when an individual's private affairs are unreasonably invaded. Taking photographs of a client is an example of such a violation. Telling the client that he or she cannot leave the hospital constitutes an example of false imprisonment. Threatening to place a client in restraints is an example of an assault. Performing a procedure without consent is an example of battery.

Test-Taking Strategy: Use the process of elimination. Note the strategic words *takes pictures*. Focus on the event identified in the question to assist with directing you to the correct option. Review the events that constitute an invasion of privacy if you had difficulty with this question.

Reference

Christensen, B., & Kockrow, E. (2006). *Foundations of nursing* (5th ed., p. 25). St. Louis: Mosby.

---

19. A nurse overhears a client asking the physician if the results of a biopsy indicated cancer. The physician tells the client that the results have not been returned when in fact the physician is aware that the results of the biopsy indicated the presence of malignancy. The nurse is upset that the physician has not shared the results with the client and

Answer: 3

Rationale: Defamation is false communication or careless disregard for the truth that causes damage to someone's reputation, either in writing (libel) or verbally (slander). An assault occurs when a person puts another person in fear of a harmful or offensive contact. Negligence involves the actions of professionals that fall below the standard of care for a specific professional group. Although the physician may be aware of the client's biopsy results, the physician decides when it is best to share such a diagnosis with the client.

tells another nurse that the physician has lied to the client and that this physician probably lies to all of the clients. Which legal tort has the nurse violated with this statement?
1 Libel
2 Assault
3 Slander
4 Negligence

Level of Cognitive Ability: Comprehension
Client Needs: Safe and Effective Care Environment
Integrated Process: Nursing Process/ Implementation
Content Area: Fundamental Skills

Test-Taking Strategy: Use the process of elimination. You should eliminate options 2 and 4 first by recalling the definitions of these items. Recalling that slander constitutes verbal defamation will direct you to option 3. Review the torts identified in each option if you had difficulty with this question.

Reference
Christensen, B., & Kockrow, E. (2006). *Foundations of nursing* (5th ed., p. 22). St. Louis: Mosby.

---

20. A nurse employed in a long-term care facility is preparing to administer medication to a client and notes that the order for furosemide (Lasix) is higher than the recommended dosage. The nurse calls the physician to clarify the order and asks the physician to prescribe a dosage within the recommended range. The physician refuses to change the order and instructs the nurse to administer the dose as prescribed. Which of the following actions should the nurse take?
1 Discontinue the order.
2 Contact the nursing supervisor.
3 Administer the dose as prescribed.
4 Call the state medical board, and report the physician.

Level of Cognitive Ability: Application
Client Needs: Safe and Effective Care Environment
Integrated Process: Nursing Process/ Implementation
Content Area: Fundamental Skills

Answer: 2
Rationale: If the physician writes an order that requires clarification, it is the nurse's responsibility to contact the physician for clarification. If there is no resolution regarding the order because the order remains as it was written after the nurse talked with the physician or because the physician cannot be located, then the nurse should contact the nurse manager or supervisor for further clarification regarding what the next step should be. Under no circumstances should the nurse proceed to carry out the order until clarification is obtained. Option 1 is not within the scope of nursing practice, and option 4 is a premature action.

Test-Taking Strategy: Use the process of elimination. Eliminate option 3 first because this is an unsafe action. Eliminate option 1 next because this action is outside of the scope of nursing practice. Option 4 is premature and should be eliminated. In addition, the nurse should follow the organizational chain of command and seek assistance from the nursing supervisor. Review the nursing responsibilities related to a physician's orders if you had difficulty with this question.

References
Christensen, B., & Kockrow, E. (2006). *Foundations of nursing* (5th ed., p. 705). St. Louis: Mosby.
Linton, A. (2007). *Introduction to medical-surgical nursing* (4th ed., p. 33). Philadelphia: Saunders.

---

21. The nurse is administering medications to a client and administers a 250-mg oral dose of methyldopa (Aldomet) instead of the prescribed 125 mg dose. The nurse discovers the error when documenting that the medication has been administered. Which of the following is an inappropriate nursing action regarding the incident?

Answer: 3
Rationale: An incident report needs to be completed whenever an unusual incident occurs. The incident report is confidential and privileged information; it should not be copied, placed in the chart, or have any reference made to it in the client's record. A complete entry in the client's record should be made concerning the incident; the incident report is not a substitute for such an entry. The client's blood pressure should be monitored because this medication is an antihypertensive. The physician should be notified.

1 Complete an incident report.
2 Monitor the client's blood pressure.
3 Make a copy of the incident report for the physician.
4 Document a complete entry in the client's record concerning the incident.

Level of Cognitive Ability: Application
Client Needs: Safe and Effective Care Environment
Integrated Process: Nursing Process/ Implementation
Content Area: Fundamental Skills

Test-Taking Strategy: Use the process of elimination, and note the strategic word *inappropriate*. This word indicates a negative event query and asks you to select an option that is an incorrect nursing action. Knowing that methyldopa is an antihypertensive medication will assist you with eliminating option 2, and knowing that an incident report needs to be completed when a medication error occurs will assist you with eliminating option 1. Recalling that incident reports should not be copied will direct you to option 3 from the remaining options. Review the nursing responsibilities related to incident reports if you had difficulty with this question.

Reference
Christensen, B., & Kockrow, E. (2006). *Foundations of nursing* (5th ed., pp. 112, 115). St. Louis: Mosby.

---

22. A nurse who has recently graduated asks another licensed practical nurse (LPN) about the need to obtain professional liability insurance. Which of the following is the appropriate response for the LPN to make?

1 "The hospital insurance covers your actions."
2 "Nurses should have their own malpractice insurance."
3 "Lawsuits are filed against physicians and the hospital, so you are safe without it."
4 "It is very expensive, and you really don't need it, because the hospital covers you."

Level of Cognitive Ability: Application
Client Needs: Safe and Effective Care Environment
Integrated Process: Nursing Process/ Implementation
Content Area: Fundamental Skills

Answer: 2
Rationale: Nurses need their own liability insurance for protection against malpractice lawsuits. Nurses erroneously assume that they are protected by an agency's professional liability policies. Usually, when a nurse is sued, the employer is also sued for the nurse's actions or inactions. Although this is the norm, nurses are encouraged to have their own malpractice insurance.

Test-Taking Strategy: Note the subject of the question—the need to obtain professional liability insurance. This should easily direct you to option 2. Also note that options 1, 3, and 4 are comparable or alike in that they all refer to not obtaining the malpractice insurance. Review liability related to malpractice insurance if you had difficulty with this question.

Reference
Christensen, B., & Kockrow, E. (2006). *Foundations of nursing* (5th ed., pp. 13, 24, 1267, 1269). St. Louis: Mosby.

---

23. A licensed practical nurse witnesses an accident in which a victim was hit by a car. The nurse stops at the scene of the accident and administers safe care to the victim, who sustained a compound fracture of the femur. The victim is hospitalized and later develops sepsis as a result of the fractured femur. The victim files suit against the nurse who provided care at the scene of the accident. Which of the following most accurately describes the nurse's immunity from this suit?

Answer: 3
Rationale: A Good Samaritan law is passed by the state legislature to encourage nurses and other health care providers to provide care to a person when an accident, emergency, or injury occurs, without fear of being sued for the care provided. Called *immunity from suit,* this protection usually applies only if all of the conditions of the law are met, such as the heath care provider receives no compensation for the care provided and the care given is not willfully and wantonly negligent.

1 The Good Samaritan Law will not protect the nurse.
2 The Good Samaritan Law protects lay persons and not professional health care providers.
3 The Good Samaritan Law will protect the nurse if the care given at the scene was not negligent.
4 The Good Samaritan Law always provides immunity from suit, even if the nurse accepted compensation for the care provided.

Level of Cognitive Ability: Comprehension
Client Needs: Safe and Effective Care Environment
Integrated Process: Nursing Process/ Implementation
Content Area: Fundamental Skills

Test-Taking Strategy: Focus on the information in the question, and use the process of elimination. Options 1 and 2 are comparable or alike and are incorrect statements that can be eliminated first. Eliminate option 4 next because it is incorrect, and there is no evidence in the question that the nurse accepted compensation for the care provided. Review the Good Samaritan Law if you had difficulty with this question.

Reference

Christensen, B., & Kockrow, E. (2006). *Foundations of nursing* (5th ed., pp. 27-28, 744). St. Louis: Mosby.

---

24. A nurse who is working in a long-term care facility responds after hearing someone calling, "Help, the bed is on fire!" Upon entering the room, the nurse finds an older client slapping at the flames on the bedspread with a pillow. Both of the client's hands have been burned. Which action should the nurse take first?
1 Pull the nearest fire alarm.
2 Close the door of the room.
3 Remove the client from the room.
4 Run to get the nearest fire extinguisher.

Level of Cognitive Ability: Application
Client Needs: Safe and Effective Care Environment
Integrated Process: Nursing Process/ Implementation
Content Area: Fundamental Skills

Answer: 3
Rationale: During a fire emergency, the steps to follow are summed up with the acronym *RACE:* **R**emove the victim; **A**ctivate the alarm; **C**ontain the fire; and **E**xtinguish as needed. This is a universal standard that may be applied to any type of fire emergency. Option 3 is correct, because the client is removed from the area. Option 1 would be the next step (activate the alarm), followed by option 2 (contain the fire) and then option 4 (extinguish as needed).

Test-Taking Strategy: Note the strategic word *first.* With this in mind, sequence the activities with the use of the RACE acronym; this will direct you to option 3. Review fire safety if you had difficulty with this question.

Reference

Christensen, B., & Kockrow, E. (2006). *Foundations of nursing* (5th ed., p. 365). St. Louis: Mosby.

---

25. An adult client is brought to the emergency department by ambulance after being hit by a car. The client is unconscious and in shock. A perforated spleen is suspected, and emergency surgery is required immediately to save the client's life. There are no family members present. With regard to informed consent for the surgical procedure, the nurse understands that which of the following is the best nursing action?
1 Ask the hospital chaplain to sign the consent form.

Answer: 2
Rationale: Generally, there are only two instances in which the informed consent of an adult client is not needed. One instance is when an emergency is present and delaying treatment for the purpose of obtaining informed consent would result in injury or death; the second instance is when the client waives the right to give informed consent. It is inappropriate to ask the hospital chaplain to sign the consent form. Requesting that the nursing supervisor initiate a court order for the surgical procedure delays necessary life-saving interventions. Although the client's family needs to be notified, calling a family member to obtain telephone consent before the surgical procedure also delays necessary life-saving interventions.

2 Transport the client to the operating room immediately.
3 Call the nursing supervisor to initiate a court order for the surgical procedure.
4 Call a family member to obtain telephone consent before the surgical procedure.

Level of Cognitive Ability: Application
Client Needs: Safe and Effective Care Environment
Integrated Process: Nursing Process/ Implementation
Content Area: Fundamental Skills

Test-Taking Strategy: Use the process of elimination. Option 1 can be eliminated first. Next, note the strategic words *surgery is required immediately*. Options 3 and 4 would delay treatment and should be eliminated. Review the issues surrounding informed consent if you had difficulty with this question.

References
Black, J., & Hawks, J. (2009). *Medical-surgical nursing: Clinical management for positive outcomes* (8th edition, p. 2191). St. Louis: Saunders.
Potter, P., & Perry, A. (2009). *Fundamentals of nursing* (7th ed., pp. 332-333). St. Louis: Mosby.

---

26. A nurse is asked to check the corneal reflex of an unconscious client. The nurse should use which of the following as the safest stimulus when touching the client's cornea?
1 Sterile glove
2 Wisp of cotton
3 Sterile drop of saline
4 Tip of a 1-mL syringe

Level of Cognitive Ability: Application
Client Needs: Safe and Effective Care Environment
Integrated Process: Nursing Process/ Implementation
Content Area: Adult Health/Neurological

Answer: 3
Rationale: The client who is unconscious is at great risk for corneal abrasion. The safest way to test the corneal reflex is by using a drop of sterile saline. Options 1, 2, and 4 can cause injury to the cornea.

Test-Taking Strategy: Use the process of elimination. Remember that options that are comparable or alike are not likely to be correct. In this case, each of the incorrect options is a solid substance, and the correct option is a liquid. Review the method for checking the corneal reflex if you had difficulty with this question.

References
Black, J., & Hawks, J. (2009). *Medical-surgical nursing: Clinical management for positive outcomes* (8th edition, p. 1685). St. Louis: Saunders.
Perry, A., & Potter, P. (2010). *Clinical nursing skills & techniques* (7th ed., p. 490). St. Louis: Mosby.

---

27. A client tells the nurse that she has seen many articles in the health care section of the newspaper about case management and asks the nurse what this means. To provide accurate information, the nurse tells the client which of the following?
1 "It represents an interdisciplinary health care delivery system."
2 "One nurse takes care of one client and is responsible for that client."
3 "One nurse supervises all of the other employees when they care for clients."
4 "A single case manager plans the care for all of the clients in the nursing unit."

Level of Cognitive Ability: Application
Client Needs: Safe and Effective Care Environment
Integrated Process: Nursing Process/ Implementation
Content Area: Fundamental Skills

Answer: 1
Rationale: Case management represents an interdisciplinary health care delivery system to promote the appropriate use of hospital personnel and material resources to maximize hospital revenues while providing for optimal outcomes of care. Case management involves managing client care by managing the client care environment. Options 2, 3, and 4 are incorrect descriptions.

Test-Taking Strategy: Use the process of elimination. Note that options 2, 3, and 4 are comparable or alike in that they all address a single individual managing the client care environment. Review the basic characteristics of case management if you had difficulty with this question.

Reference
Christensen, B., & Kockrow, E. (2006). *Foundations of nursing* (5th ed., pp. 13, 93). St. Louis: Mosby.

28. A client is scheduled for a bone marrow aspiration. The nurse plans to use which of the following skin cleansing agents before this procedure to prevent infection as a result of the procedure?
1 Alcohol swabs
2 Soap and water
3 Povidone-iodine
4 Hydrogen peroxide

Level of Cognitive Ability: Application
Client Needs: Safe and Effective Care Environment
Integrated Process: Nursing Process/Planning
Content Area: Fundamental Skills

Answer: 3
Rationale: Before a bone marrow aspiration procedure, the needle insertion site is cleansed with an antiseptic solution such as povidone-iodine. This helps reduce the number of bacteria on the skin and decreases the risk of infection after the procedure. The other options are incorrect because they would not produce this effect.

Test-Taking Strategy: Use the process of elimination and your knowledge of general asepsis and topical cleansing agents to answer this question. Recalling that a bone marrow aspiration procedure is invasive will assist with directing you to the correct option. Review bone marrow aspiration if you had difficulty with this question.

References
Chernecky, C., & Berger, B. (2008). *Laboratory tests and diagnostic procedures* (5th ed., p. 243). Philadelphia: Saunders.
Monahan, F., Sands, J., Marek, J., Neighbors, M., & Green, C. (2007). *Phipps' medical-surgical nursing: Health and illness perspectives* (8th ed., p. 906). St. Louis: Mosby.

---

29. A nurse arrives to work the day shift and is assigned to care for a client with terminal cancer. The nurse notes that the client has been receiving an opioid analgesic every 3 hours for pain. When the nurse enters the client's room, the client states, "I'm so glad you're here. The medicine never works when the nurse who cared for me last night gives it to me." The nurse has previously observed this same occurrence with both this client and other clients and suspects that the night nurse is substance impaired. Which of the following actions will the nurse take?
1 Report the information to the police.
2 Report the information to a supervisor.
3 Call the impaired nurse organization, and report the nurse.
4 Call the night nurse who gave the medication and discuss the event with that nurse.

Level of Cognitive Ability: Application
Client Needs: Safe and Effective Care Environment
Integrated Process: Nursing Process/Implementation
Content Area: Fundamental Skills

Answer: 2
Rationale: Nurse practice acts require reporting any suspicion of substance-impaired nurses. The board of nursing has jurisdiction over the practice of nursing and may develop plans for treatment and supervision. The situation described should be reported to the nursing supervisor, who will then report it to the board of nursing. Option 4 is incorrect and may cause a conflict, and options 1 and 3 are premature actions.

Test-Taking Strategy: Use the process of elimination. Remember to follow the channel of organizational structure to report events such as this one. By reporting the information, the nurse alerts the institution about the potential problem and sets the stage for further investigation and appropriate action. Review the appropriate nursing actions when substance abuse in the workplace is suspected if you had difficulty with this question.

References
deWit, S. (2009). *Medical-surgical nursing: Concepts & practice* (p. 1134). St. Louis: Saunders.
Ignatavicius, D., & Workman, M. (2010). *Medical-surgical nursing: Patient-centered collaborative care* (6th ed., p. 82). St. Louis: Saunders.

---

30. A nurse is assisting with providing emergency treatment for a client who is experiencing ventricular tachycardia. The licensed practical nurse understands that

Answer: 2
Rationale: Safety during defibrillation is essential for preventing injury to the client and to the personnel assisting with the procedure. The person performing the defibrillation ensures that all

which action by the registered nurse provides the safest environment during a defibrillation attempt?

1 Placing no lubricant on the paddles
2 Performing a visual and verbal check of "all clear"
3 Holding the client's upper torso stable while the defibrillation is performed
4 Handing the charged paddles separately to the person who is performing the defibrillation

Level of Cognitive Ability: Application
Client Needs: Safe and Effective Care Environment
Integrated Process: Nursing Process/Implementation
Content Area: Adult Health/Cardiovascular

personnel are standing clear of the bed with a verbal and visual check of "all clear." Charged paddles should never be handed to other personnel. For the shock to be effective, some type of conductive medium (e.g., lubricant, gel) must be placed between the paddles and the skin. The client is not touched during the defibrillation procedure.

Test-Taking Strategy: Use the process of elimination, and focus on the subject: safe principles of defibrillation. Option 2 involves a verbal and visual check of "all clear," which provides for the safety of all involved. Review the principles related to safety and defibrillation if you had difficulty with this question.

Reference

Proehl, J. (2009). *Emergency nursing procedures* (4th ed., p. 399). St. Louis: Saunders.

---

31. A nurse is in the process of giving a client a bed bath. During the procedure, the unit secretary calls the nurse on the intercom to ask the nurse to answer an emergency phone call. What is the appropriate nursing action?

1 Finish the bath before answering the phone call.
2 Walk out of the room and answer the phone call.
3 Put the call light within the client's reach, and answer the phone call.
4 Leave the door open so that the client can be monitored, and answer the phone call.

Level of Cognitive Ability: Application
Client Needs: Safe and Effective Care Environment
Integrated Process: Nursing Process/Implementation
Content Area: Fundamental Skills

Answer: 3

Rationale: When an emergency phone call must be answered, one appropriate action is to ask another nurse to accept the call; however, this is not one of the options. If it is necessary for the nurse to answer the call and to leave the room temporarily, the door should be closed or the room curtains pulled around the bathing area to provide privacy. The client should be covered with a blanket, and, to maintain safety, the call light should be placed within the client's reach.

Test-Taking Strategy: Use the process of elimination. Note the strategic words *emergency phone call;* this should assist with the elimination of option 1. From the remaining options, the only option that addresses client safety and comfort is option 3. Review these safety measures if you had difficulty with this question.

References

Christensen, B., & Kockrow, E. (2006). *Foundations of nursing* (5th ed., p. 449). St. Louis: Mosby.
Potter, P., & Perry, A. (2009) *Fundamentals of nursing* (7th ed., p. 868). St. Louis: Mosby.

---

32. An adolescent asks a nurse about the procedure for becoming an organ donor. The nurse most accurately tells the adolescent that:

1 Written consent is never required to become a donor.
2 A donor must be 18 years old or older to provide consent.
3 An individual who is at least 16 years old can sign papers to become a donor.
4 The family is responsible for making

Answer: 2

Rationale: Any person 18 years old or older may become an organ donor by indicating his or her consent in writing. In the absence of appropriate documentation, a family member or legal guardian may authorize the donation of the decedent's organs.

Test-Taking Strategy: Use the process of elimination. Noting that two of the options address an age provides a clue that one of these options may be correct. In this case, it is best to select the higher age. Review the procedure for organ donation if you had difficulty with this question.

the decision about organ donation at the time of death.

Level of Cognitive Ability: Application
Client Needs: Safe and Effective Care Environment
Integrated Process: Nursing Process/ Implementation
Content Area: Fundamental Skills

Reference

Marriner-Tomey, A. (2009). *Guide to nursing management and leadership* (8th ed., pp. 498-499). St. Louis: Mosby.

---

33. A nurse who is employed in the medical unit of a local hospital arrives at work and is told to report (float) to the pediatric unit for the day. Several pediatric admissions occurred during the night, and the pediatric unit needs assistance with caring for the children. The nurse has never worked in the pediatric unit and is anxious about floating to this area. Which of the following is the appropriate nursing action?

1 Call the nursing supervisor.
2 Refuse to float to the pediatric unit.
3 Ask another nurse to float to the pediatric unit.
4 Report to the pediatric unit, and identify tasks that can be safely performed.

Level of Cognitive Ability: Application
Client Needs: Safe and Effective Care Environment
Integrated Process: Nursing Process/ Implementation
Content Area: Fundamental Skills

Answer: 4

Rationale: Floating is an acceptable legal practice used by hospitals to solve their understaffing problems. Legally, a nurse cannot refuse to float unless a union contract guarantees that nurses can work only in specified areas or the nurse can prove a lack of knowledge for the performance of assigned tasks. When this situation occurs, the nurse should set priorities and identify potential areas of harm to the client. A nurse cannot refuse an assignment and should not ask another nurse to perform an assignment. The supervisor would be called if the nurse is asked to perform a task that could not be safely performed.

Test-Taking Strategy: Use the process of elimination. Note the strategic word *appropriate.* Options 2 and 3 can be eliminated first because a nurse cannot refuse an assignment or ask someone else to perform an assignment. From the remaining options, it is premature to call the nursing supervisor. Therefore option 4 is the appropriate action. Review nursing responsibilities related to floating if you had difficulty with this question.

Reference

Linton, A. (2007). *Introduction to medical-surgical nursing* (4th ed., pp. 33-34). Philadelphia: Saunders.

---

34. A nurse is orienting a nursing assistant to the clinical nursing unit. The nurse should intervene if the nursing assistant does which of the following during a routine handwashing procedure?

1 Keeps the hands lower than the elbows
2 Washes continuously for 10 to 15 seconds
3 Uses 3 to 5 mL of soap from the dispenser
4 Dries the hands from the forearm down to the fingers

Level of Cognitive Ability: Application
Client Needs: Safe and Effective Care Environment

Answer: 4

Rationale: Proper handwashing procedure involves wetting the hands and wrists and keeping the hands lower than the forearms so that water flows toward the fingertips. The nurse uses 3 to 5 mL of soap and scrubs for 10 to 15 seconds using a rubbing and circular motion. The hands are rinsed and then dried from the fingers to the forearms. The paper towel is discarded, and a second paper towel is used to turn off the faucet to avoid hand contamination.

Test-Taking Strategy: Use the process of elimination, and note the strategic word *intervene.* This word indicates a negative event query and asks you to select an option that is an incorrect action performed by the nursing assistant. Visualize each option, and use basic principles of asepsis to answer this question. Review the handwashing procedure if you had difficulty with this question.

Integrated Process: Nursing Process/ Implementation
Content Area: Leadership/Management

Reference

Christensen, B., & Kockrow, E. (2006). *Foundations of nursing* (5th ed., p. 281). St. Louis: Mosby.

---

35. A 22-year-old client who was struck by a car while jogging is brought to the emergency department by the ambulance team. Emergency measures are instituted but are unsuccessful. The client's fiancée is with the client and tells the nurse that the client is an organ donor. In anticipation that the client's eyes will be donated, which of the following should the nurse do first?

1 Ask the fiancée to obtain the client's will from the lawyer.
2 Call the National Eye Bank Center to confirm that the client is a donor.
3 Position the deceased client supine, and place dry sterile dressings over the eyes.
4 Elevate the head of the bed, close the deceased client's eyes, and place a small ice pack on the eyes.

Level of Cognitive Ability: Application
Client Needs: Safe and Effective Care Environment
Integrated Process: Nursing Process/ Implementation
Content Area: Fundamental Skills

Answer: 4
Rationale: When a corneal donation is anticipated, the head of the bed is elevated, the deceased client's eyes are closed, and a small ice pack is placed on the client's eyes. Within 2 to 4 hours, the eyes are enucleated, and the cornea is usually transplanted within 24 to 48 hours. Options 1 and 3 are incorrect actions, and option 2 is not an initial action.

Test-Taking Strategy: Note the strategic word *first.* Note that the subject of the question is the donation of the eyes; this should assist you with eliminating options 1 and 2. Knowing how to care for the eyes of a deceased organ donor will lead you to option 4. Review this procedure if you had difficulty with the question.

Reference

Ignatavicius, D., & Workman, M. (2010). *Medical-surgical nursing: Patient-centered collaborative care* (6th ed., p. 1091). St. Louis: Saunders.

---

36. A client with metastatic bladder cancer is admitted to the hospital for chemotherapy. During data collection, the client tells the nurse that a living will was prepared 2 years ago and asks if the will needs to be updated. Which of the following is the appropriate nursing response?

1 "Living wills are valid for 6 months."
2 "The will can't be changed after it is written."
3 "You will have to discuss the issue with your lawyer."
4 "A living will should be reviewed yearly with your physician."

Level of Cognitive Ability: Application
Client Needs: Safe and Effective Care Environment
Integrated Process: Nursing Process/ Implementation
Content Area: Fundamental Skills

Answer: 4
Rationale: The client should discuss the living will with a physician, and it should be reviewed annually to ensure that it contains the client's current wishes and desires. Options 1 and 2 include inaccurate information. Option 3 is not an appropriate response and places the client's question on hold.

Test-Taking Strategy: Use the process of elimination. Options 1 and 2 include inaccurate information and can be eliminated first. Although changing a living will would require consultation with a lawyer, the appropriate and accurate nursing response would be to inform the client that the living will should be reviewed annually. Review the procedures related to living wills if you had difficulty with this question.

Reference

Christensen, B., & Kockrow, E. (2006). *Foundations of nursing* (5th ed., p. 205). St. Louis: Mosby.

---

37. A licensed practical nurse (LPN) is preparing to suction a client with a diagnosis of acquired immunodeficiency syndrome. The LPN should gather which of the following supplies to perform this procedure safely?

1 Gloves, gown, and mask
2 Gown, mask, and protective eyewear
3 Gloves, mask, and protective eyewear
4 Gloves, gown, and protective eyewear

Level of Cognitive Ability: Application
Client Needs: Safe and Effective Care Environment
Integrated Process: Nursing Process/Implementation
Content Area: Fundamental Skills

Answer: 3

Rationale: Standard precautions include the use of gloves whenever there is actual or potential contact with blood or body fluids. During suctioning, the nurse wears gloves, a mask, and protective eyewear or a face shield. Impervious gowns are worn in those instances when it is anticipated that there will be contact with a large amount of body fluids or blood.

Test-Taking Strategy: Use the process of elimination. Note that the subject of the question is suctioning, so expect airborne secretions with this procedure. Basic knowledge of standard precautions would direct you to an option that includes a mask, protective eyewear, and gloves; the only option that contains these three items is option 3. Review standard precautions if you had difficulty with this question.

Reference

deWit, S. (2009). *Medical-surgical nursing: Concepts & practice* (pp. 120, 1189-1190). St. Louis: Saunders.

---

38. A licensed practical nurse (LPN) who is employed in a long-term care facility is observing a nursing assistant ambulating a client with right-sided weakness. The LPN determines that the nursing assistant was performing the procedure safely if the LPN observed the nursing assistant:

1 Standing behind the client
2 Standing in front of the client
3 Standing on the left side of the client
4 Standing on the right side of the client

Level of Cognitive Ability: Comprehension
Client Needs: Safe and Effective Care Environment
Integrated Process: Nursing Process/Evaluation
Content Area: Leadership/Management

Answer: 4

Rationale: When walking with a client, the nurse should stand on the client's affected side. The nurse should position the free hand on the client's shoulder so that the client can be pulled toward the nurse in the event that the client falls forward. The client should be instructed to look up and outward rather than at his or her feet. Options 1, 2, and 3 are incorrect.

Test-Taking Strategy: Use the process of elimination. Note the strategic words *right-sided weakness;* this will assist you with eliminating option 3. Eliminate options 1 and 2, because neither of these places the nurse in a strategic position should the client lose balance and begin to fall forward or backward. Recalling that support is needed on a client's affected side will direct you to option 4. Review the procedures for ambulating clients if you had difficulty with this question.

Reference

deWit, S. (2009). *Medical-surgical nursing: Concepts & practice* (p. 779). St. Louis: Saunders.

---

39. A nurse is caring for a client who is receiving a dose of an intramuscular antibiotic. The nurse enters the client's room to administer the prescribed antibiotic, and the client tells the nurse that the medication burns and that he does not want the medication to be given. The nurse tells the client that the medication is necessary and administers the medication. Which of the following can the client legally charge as a result of the nursing action?

1 Assault
2 Battery

Answer: 2

Rationale: An assault occurs when a person puts another person in fear of a harmful or offensive contact. For this intentional tort to be actionable, the victim must be aware of the threat of harmful or offensive contact. Battery is actual contact with one's body. Negligence involves actions below the standards of care. Invasion of privacy occurs when the individual's private affairs are unreasonably invaded. In the event described, the nurse can be charged with battery, because the nurse administers a medication that the client has refused.

3 Negligence
4 Invasion of privacy

Level of Cognitive Ability: Comprehension
Client Needs: Safe and Effective Care Environment
Integrated Process: Nursing Process/ Implementation
Content Area: Fundamental Skills

Test-Taking Strategy: Use the process of elimination. Note that the client refuses the medication but that the nurse administers the medication anyway; this should direct you to option 2. Review the descriptions associated with the terms in each option if you had difficulty with this question.

Reference
Christensen, B., & Kockrow, E. (2006). *Foundations of nursing* (5th ed., p. 22). St. Louis: Mosby.

---

40. A licensed practical nurse (LPN) is reinforcing teaching given by a registered nurse to the parents of a child with celiac disease. The LPN reminds the parents to do which of the following to ensure that the diet is safe based on the child's physical needs?

1 Restrict corn and rice in the diet.
2 Serve pasta dishes instead of cereals with grain.
3 Keep the intake of fresh starchy vegetables to a minimum.
4 Read food labels carefully to avoid hidden sources of gluten.

Level of Cognitive Ability: Application
Client Needs: Safe and Effective Care Environment
Integrated Process: Teaching and Learning
Content Area: Child Health

Answer: 4
Rationale: Gluten is added to many foods, such as hydrolyzed vegetable protein derived from cereal grains. Grains are also frequently added to processed foods as thickening or fillers. Because of this, it is important to read food labels. Gluten is found primarily in the grains of wheat and rye; rice, corn, and other vegetables are acceptable in a gluten-free diet. Many pasta products contain gluten and should be avoided.

Test-Taking Strategy: Use the process of elimination. Begin to answer this question by recalling that a gluten-free diet is indicated for the management of celiac disease, and remember which foods are high in gluten. Choose correctly by selecting the umbrella option. Review celiac disease and the gluten-free diet if you had difficulty with this question.

Reference
Price, D., & Gwin, J. (2008). *Pediatric nursing: An introductory text* (10th ed., p. 250). St. Louis: Saunders.

---

41. A nurse notes that a child who has been diagnosed with intussusception has a formed, brown bowel movement. The nurse should take which initial action to ensure that a safe plan of care is implemented for the child?

1 Prepare the child for hydrostatic reduction.
2 Ask the child about any increase in abdominal pain.
3 Warn the child and her parents that surgery is imminent.
4 Report the passage of the normal stool to the registered nurse (RN).

Level of Cognitive Ability: Application
Client Needs: Safe and Effective Care Environment
Integrated Process: Nursing Process/ Implementation
Content Area: Child Health

Answer: 4
Rationale: The passage of a formed, brown bowel movement usually indicates that an intussusception has reduced itself. The nurse immediately reports this data to the RN, who will in turn report it to the physician. This finding may change the course of the plan of care. Increased abdominal pain is not expected, because the child's gastrointestinal tract is likely to be more functional. The finding does not indicate the need for immediate surgery.

Test-Taking Strategy: Use the process of elimination. Recalling that the passage of a normal stool may indicate that an intussusception is resolving or has resolved will direct you to option 4. Review the care of the child with intussusception if you had difficulty with this question.

Reference
Price, D., & Gwin, J. (2008). *Pediatric nursing: An introductory text* (10th ed., pp. 160-162). St. Louis: Saunders.

42. A psychotic client is belligerent and agitated, making aggressive gestures, and pacing in the hallway. To ensure a safe environment, which of the following is the nurse's highest priority?

1. Assisting other staff with restraining the client
2. Providing safety for the client and for other clients on the unit
3. Providing comfort and consolation to the other clients on the unit
4. Politely asking the client to calm down and to regain control over his or her behavior

Level of Cognitive Ability: Application
Client Needs: Safe and Effective Care Environment
Integrated Process: Nursing Process/Implementation
Content Area: Mental Health

Answer: 2

Rationale: A psychotic client who is out of control may require seclusion to ensure the safety of the client and of the other clients on the unit. The correct option is the only one that addresses the safety needs of both the client and others. Options 1 and 3 do not provide for the client's safety needs or rights. In addition, there are specific policies and guidelines that must be followed with regard to restraining a client. Option 4 may be ineffective, and it does not address the safety needs of others in the unit.

Test-Taking Strategy: The subject of the question is safety; note the strategic words *belligerent, agitated,* and *aggressive.* Use the process of elimination and Maslow's Hierarchy of Needs theory to prioritize the nursing actions. Option 2 is the umbrella option and addresses the safety of all. Review the care of the psychotic client if you had difficulty with this question.

Reference

Varcarolis, E., & Halter, M. (2009). *Essentials of psychiatric mental health nursing: A communication approach to evidence-based care* (pp. 286, 1291-1292). St. Louis: Saunders.

---

43. A client with Bell's palsy is scheduled for magnetic resonance imaging (MRI). The nurse should implement which of the following to ensure a safe environment in preparation for this test?

1. Apply metal-tipped electrodes to the client's chest.
2. Remove all objects that contain metal from the client.
3. Shave the client's groin for the insertion of a femoral catheter.
4. Ensure that the client maintains nothing-by-mouth (NPO) status for 24 hours before the procedure.

Level of Cognitive Ability: Application
Client Needs: Safe and Effective Care Environment
Integrated Process: Nursing Process/Implementation
Content Area: Adult Health/Neurological

Answer: 2

Rationale: An MRI uses magnetic fields to produce a diagnostic image. All metal objects (e.g., rings, bracelets, hairpins, watches) should be removed from the client. The client's history should also be reviewed to determine if the client has any internal metallic devices (e.g., orthopedic hardware, pacemakers, shrapnel). A femoral catheter is not inserted for this procedure. For an abdominal MRI, the client is usually NPO, but this is not necessary for an MRI of the head. In addition, maintaining NPO status for 24 hours is unnecessary and may be harmful to the client. Metal-tipped electrodes are not used for this test.

Test-Taking Strategy: Use the process of elimination. Note the physiological location as it relates to the client's diagnosis. Recalling that metallic objects cannot be in place during an MRI and focusing on the client's diagnosis will direct you to option 2. Review client preparation for an MRI if you had difficulty with this question.

Reference

Chernecky, C., & Berger, B. (2008). *Laboratory tests and diagnostic procedures* (5th ed., p. 750). Philadelphia: Saunders.

---

44. A nurse who is assisting with the care of a client who has been in a coma for more than 1 year is told by the physician to stop the tube feeding that is providing sustenance to the client. The nurse, who is aware of the legal basis needed for carrying out the order, first determines whether which of the following requirements has been met?

Answer: 4

Rationale: The client's family or legal guardian can make treatment decisions, generally in collaboration with physicians, other health care workers, and other trusted advisors. The nurse first checks for family authorization before discontinuing the treatment. After doing this, option 3 would be appropriate. Although options 1 and 2 may be necessary in some events, these options are not the first actions to take in this situation.

1 Institutional ethics committee approval
2 A court order to discontinue the treatment
3 A written order by the physician to remove the tube
4 Authorization by the family to discontinue the treatment

Level of Cognitive Ability: Application
Client Needs: Safe and Effective Care Environment
Integrated Process: Nursing Process/Implementation
Content Area: Fundamental Skills

Test-Taking Strategy: Note the strategic word *first;* this tells you that the correct option is determined according to a proper sequence of action. Recalling that the family or legal guardian can make decisions about discontinuing treatment will direct you to option 4. Review the legal principles surrounding end-of-life decisions if you had difficulty with this question.

Reference

deWit, S. (2009). *Medical-surgical nursing: Concepts & practice* (pp. 186-187). St. Louis: Saunders.

---

45. A nurse who is assisting a physician with the insertion of a Miller-Abbott tube should do which of the following to ensure a safe environment and to decrease the client's risk of aspiration?
1 Place the client in a high-Fowler's position.
2 Assist with inserting the tube with the balloon inflated.
3 Instruct the client to bear down if there is an urge to gag.
4 Ask the client to cough when the tube reaches the nasopharynx.

Level of Cognitive Ability: Application
Client Needs: Safe and Effective Care Environment
Integrated Process: Nursing Process/Implementation
Content Area: Adult Health/Gastrointestinal

Answer: 1
Rationale: A Miller-Abbott tube is a nasoenteric tube used to correct a bowel obstruction and to decompress the intestine. A high-Fowler's position decreases the risk of aspiration if vomiting occurs. The physician inserts the tube with the balloon deflated in a manner similar to that used with a nasogastric tube. The client usually sips water to facilitate the passage of the tube through the nasopharynx and the esophagus. Options 2, 3, and 4 are incorrect actions.

Test-Taking Strategy: Use the process of elimination. The subject of the question is decreasing the risk of aspiration during the insertion of a Miller-Abbott tube. Eliminate option 2 first, because the tube could not be inserted with the balloon inflated. Next, eliminate options 3 and 4, because coughing and bearing down will not facilitate the passage of the tube. Review the procedure for the insertion of nasoenteric tubes if you had difficulty with this question.

Reference

deWit, S. (2009). *Medical-surgical nursing: Concepts & practice* (p. 705). St. Louis: Saunders.

---

46. A nurse who is assisting with the care of a client with cancer is following medication orders to manage the cancer pain. Which of the following strategies should the nurse follow to ensure adequate and safe pain control?
1 Try multiple simultaneous medications for maximum pain relief.
2 Rely entirely on prescription and over-the-counter medications for pain relief.
3 Ensure that the client is kept at a low baseline pain level to avoid sedation or addiction.
4 Start with low medication doses and gradually increase to a dose that

Answer: 4
Rationale: The most appropriate approach is to begin with low doses and to increase the dose as needed to maintain a dose that relieves the pain. Option 2 ignores the benefits of other options that may relieve pain, such as massage, therapeutic touch, and music. Keeping the client at a baseline level of pain is an inappropriate practice. Multiple medication interventions do not guarantee effectiveness and can also be unsafe.

Test-Taking Strategy: Use the process of elimination. Begin to answer this question by eliminating options 1 and 2 because of the words *multiple* and *entirely*. Choose correctly between the remaining options by remembering the basic principles of pain management. Review these principles if you had difficulty with this question.

relieves the pain without exceeding the maximal daily dose.

Level of Cognitive Ability: Application
Client Needs: Safe and Effective Care Environment
Integrated Process: Nursing Process/Implementation
Content Area: Adult Health/Oncology

Reference

Christensen, B., & Kockrow, E. (2006). *Adult health nursing* (5th ed., pp. 840-841). St. Louis: Mosby.

---

47. A licensed practical nurse (LPN) is reinforcing instructions given by a registered nurse to a client regarding how to take medications after discharge from the hospital. The LPN should use which of the following approaches to best ensure the safe administration of medication in the home?

1 Show the client the proper way to take the prescribed medications.
2 Tell the client to double up on the medications if a dose has been missed.
3 Count the number of pills remaining in the prescription bottle once a week.
4 Allow the client to verbalize and demonstrate the correct administration procedure.

Level of Cognitive Ability: Application
Client Needs: Safe and Effective Care Environment
Integrated Process: Teaching and Learning
Content Area: Fundamental Skills

Answer: 4

Rationale: The most effective method of teaching to ensure the safe self-administration of medications in the home setting is to have the client verbalize and demonstrate how to take medications. This ensures that the client has both the knowledge and the physical ability to comply with medication therapy. Option 1 is useful early in the teaching or learning process, but it is not the best method, because it does not allow the client to demonstrate his or her own ability. Option 2 is incorrect, because it is a dangerous and incorrect statement. Option 3 is unrealistic and does not enhance self-care.

Test-Taking Strategy: Use the process of elimination. Eliminate options 2 and 3 first by remembering the general guidelines for safe medication administration and teaching and learning principles. From the remaining options, select the one that most universally addresses the full abilities needed by the client after discharge. Review teaching and learning principles if you had difficulty with this question.

Reference

Potter, P., & Perry, A. (2009). *Fundamentals of nursing* (7th ed., p. 712). St. Louis: Mosby.

---

48. A client with thrombophlebitis is being treated with heparin sodium therapy. The registered nurse asks the licensed practical nurse to check the medication supply to ensure that the antidote for this therapy is available. The nurse checks the medication supply for which medication?

1 Protamine sulfate
2 Streptokinase (Streptase)
3 Phytonadione (vitamin K)
4 Aminocaproic acid (Amicar)

Level of Cognitive Ability: Application
Client Needs: Safe and Effective Care Environment
Integrated Process: Nursing Process/Implementation
Content Area: Pharmacology

Answer: 1

Rationale: Protamine sulfate is the antidote for heparin sodium. Streptokinase is a thrombolytic agent used to dissolve blood clots. Vitamin K is the antidote for warfarin (Coumadin). Amicar is an antifibrinolytic used to prevent the breakdown of clots that have already been formed.

Test-Taking Strategy: Specific knowledge of the antidote to heparin sodium is needed to answer this question correctly. Remember that protamine sulfate is the antidote for heparin sodium. Review common antidotes if you had difficulty with this question.

Reference

Kee, J., Hayes, E., & McCuistion, L. (2009). *Pharmacology: A nursing process approach* (6th ed., p. 678). St. Louis: Saunders.

49. A nurse who is assisting with the care of a client with cardiomyopathy should give priority attention to which of the following to ensure client safety?

1 Administering vasodilator medications
2 Conducting a thorough pain assessment
3 Taking measures to prevent orthostatic changes when the client stands
4 Telling the client about the importance of avoiding over-the-counter medications

Level of Cognitive Ability: Application
Client Needs: Safe and Effective Care Environment
Integrated Process: Nursing Process/Implementation
Content Area: Adult Health/Cardiovascular

Answer: 3

Rationale: Orthostatic changes can occur in the client with cardiomyopathy as a result of impaired venous return; these changes could lead to dizziness and falls. Vasodilators should not be administered. There is no mention of pain in the question, and pain may not directly affect safety in this event. Option 4 is an accurate statement, but it is not directly related to the subject of the question.

Test-Taking Strategy: The subject of the question is a nursing measure that will protect the safety of a client with cardiomyopathy. The only logical option is the one that deals with the prevention of the orthostatic changes that can occur with cardiomyopathy. Review the care of the client with cardiomyopathy if you had difficulty with this question.

References

deWit, S. (2009). *Medical-surgical nursing: Concepts & practice* (pp. 480-481). St. Louis: Saunders.
Linton, A. (2007). *Introduction to medical-surgical nursing* (4th ed., pp. 667-668). Philadelphia: Saunders.

---

50. A licensed practical nurse (LPN) is reinforcing teaching given by the registered nurse to a client who has been diagnosed with endocarditis. The LPN explains that it is important for this client to use an electric razor rather than a straight razor for shaving for which of the following reasons?

1 An electric razor can be sanitized more easily.
2 Straight razors harbor too many microorganisms.
3 The client is at higher risk for infection from any nick or cut.
4 Any cuts or skin injuries should be avoided while taking anticoagulants.

Level of Cognitive Ability: Application
Client Needs: Safe and Effective Care Environment
Integrated Process: Teaching and Learning
Content Area: Adult Health/Cardiovascular

Answer: 4

Rationale: Clients with endocarditis are at risk for developing thrombi along the walls of the heart, which could become emboli that may lead to a brain attack (stroke). For this reason, clients with endocarditis are treated with anticoagulant therapy to prevent thrombus formation. Clients who are taking anticoagulants should implement measures to prevent injury and subsequent bleeding. The other options are incorrect, because they emphasize infection rather than bleeding.

Test-Taking Strategy: Use the process of elimination, and recall that the client with endocarditis is receiving anticoagulant therapy. Remember that comparable or alike options are not likely to be correct. With this in mind, eliminate each of the incorrect options, because they deal with infection rather than bleeding. Review the care of the client with endocarditis if you had difficulty with this question.

Reference

Ignatavicius, D., & Workman, M. (2010). *Medical-surgical nursing: Patient-centered collaborative care* (6th ed., p. 785). St. Louis: Saunders.

---

51. A licensed practical nurse (LPN) is assisting a registered nurse (RN) with caring for a client who just underwent cardiac catheterization via the femoral artery approach. The nurse should avoid taking which of the following actions when caring for this client because it would be unsafe?

1 Resuming prescribed medications
2 Having the client sit upright for a meal
3 Encouraging the client to drink extra fluids

Answer: 2

Rationale: For 6 hours after cardiac catheterization via the femoral approach (or per physician's orders), the client should not bend or hyperextend the affected leg to avoid blood vessel occlusion or hemorrhage. This means that having the client sit upright would be contraindicated. Precatheterization medications are generally resumed after the procedure. Asking the client to wiggle the toes to determine neurovascular status is acceptable and should be done, because vascular status could be impaired if a hematoma or thrombus were developing. Fluids should be increased to help with eliminating the contrast medium through the kidneys.

4 Asking the client to wiggle the toes when collecting data about the neurovascular status

Level of Cognitive Ability: Application
Client Needs: Safe and Effective Care Environment
Integrated Process: Nursing Process/Implementation
Content Area: Adult Health/Cardiovascular

Test-Taking Strategy: Use the process of elimination. Note the strategic words *avoid* and *unsafe*. These words indicate a negative event query and ask you to select an option that is an incorrect action. Use your knowledge of postcatheterization care, and keep in mind that the femoral access site was used; this will direct you to option 2. Review postcardiac catheterization care if you had difficulty with this question.

Reference

Chernecky, C., & Berger, B. (2008). *Laboratory tests and diagnostic procedures* (5th ed., p. 297). Philadelphia: Saunders.

---

52. A nurse is delivering a meal tray to a client with heart failure. The nurse should remove which item from the tray before bringing it to the client's bedside because the food item would be unsafe for the client to consume?

1 Sherbet
2 Green beans
3 Baked chicken
4 Saltine crackers

Level of Cognitive Ability: Application
Client Needs: Safe and Effective Care Environment
Integrated Process: Nursing Process/Implementation
Content Area: Adult Health/Cardiovascular

Answer: 4
Rationale: Clients with heart failure should monitor and restrict their sodium intake. Saltine crackers are high in sodium and should be avoided. Green beans and sherbet are low in sodium. Baked chicken would contain only physiologic saline because it is an animal product and thus would not have to be avoided by the client.

Test-Taking Strategy: The subject of the question is knowing that a client with heart failure should eat a low-sodium diet. Note the strategic word *unsafe;* this word indicates a negative event query and asks you to select an option that is an incorrect food item. Use the process of elimination to select the food that is highest in sodium. Review foods that are high in sodium if you had difficulty with this question.

Reference

Linton, A. (2007). *Introduction to medical-surgical nursing* (4th ed., pp. 660, 664). Philadelphia: Saunders.

---

53. An older client with diabetes mellitus is vomiting because of gastroenteritis. The nurse should do which of the following to maintain oral intake to safely minimize the risk of dehydration?

1 Give only sips of water until the client is able to tolerate solid foods.
2 Withhold all food and fluids until vomiting has ceased for at least 8 hours.
3 Restrict the client to clear liquids for at least 3 days to allow for bowel rest.
4 Encourage the client to drink up to 8 to 12 ounces of fluid every hour while awake.

Level of Cognitive Ability: Application
Client Needs: Safe and Effective Care Environment
Integrated Process: Nursing Process/Implementation
Content Area: Adult Health/Gastrointestinal

Answer: 4
Rationale: Small amounts of fluid may be tolerated even when vomiting is present. The client should be offered up to 8 to 12 ounces of liquid that contains both glucose and electrolytes hourly. The diet should be advanced to a regular diet as soon as it is tolerated and should include a minimum of 100 to 150 grams of carbohydrates daily. Options 1, 2, and 3 are incorrect actions because they will not maintain adequate oral intake.

Test-Taking Strategy: Use the process of elimination. Begin to answer this question by eliminating options 1 and 2 because of the close-ended words *only* and *all*. Choose correctly from the remaining options, knowing that a 3-day time frame is excessive. Review measures to minimize dehydration if you had difficulty with this question.

Reference

deWit, S. (2009). *Medical-surgical nursing: Concepts & practice* (p. 927). St. Louis: Saunders.

54. A client who does not have an artificial airway has a new order for a sputum culture. The nurse should avoid doing which of the following to obtain a suitable specimen?
 1 Obtain the specimen early in the morning.
 2 Have the client take deep breaths before coughing.
 3 Ask the client to rinse the mouth before expectoration.
 4 Place the culture container lid facedown on the bedside table.

Level of Cognitive Ability: Application
Client Needs: Safe and Effective Care Environment
Integrated Process: Nursing Process/Implementation
Content Area: Fundamental Skills

Answer: 4
Rationale: The lid would be contaminated if it is placed facedown on the bedside table; this could lead to inaccurate test results. The client should rinse the mouth or brush the teeth before specimen collection to avoid contaminating the specimen. The client should take deep breaths before expectoration for best sputum production. The specimen is optimally obtained early in the morning, because sputum has a longer amount of time to collect in the airways during sleep.

Test-Taking Strategy: Use the process of elimination, and note the strategic word *avoid*. This word indicates a negative event query and asks you to select an option that is an incorrect nursing action. Use your knowledge of the principles of aseptic technique to choose correctly. Review these principles if you had difficulty with this question.

References
Chernecky, C., & Berger, B. (2008). *Laboratory tests and diagnostic procedures* (5th ed., pp. 1034-1035). Philadelphia: Saunders.
deWit, S. (2009). *Medical-surgical nursing: Concepts & practice* (p. 287). St. Louis: Saunders.

---

55. A nurse is implementing measures to prevent the spread of infection to other clients. The nurse understands that which of the following is the best way to prevent the spread of infection?
 1 Use proper handwashing techniques.
 2 Use sterile technique with all procedures.
 3 Never stop in the middle of performing a procedure.
 4 Read the policy and procedure manual before performing treatments.

Level of Cognitive Ability: Comprehension
Client Needs: Safe and Effective Care Environment
Integrated Process: Nursing Process/Implementation
Content Area: Fundamental Skills

Answer: 1
Rationale: Proper handwashing is the best way to prevent the spread of infection. All procedures do not require sterile technique. Reading the policy and procedure manual does not guarantee that infection will not spread. It may be necessary in some situations to stop in the middle of a procedure, but option 3 is not the best way to prevent the spread of infection.

Test-Taking Strategy: Focus on the subject of the question—the best way to prevent the spread of infection—and use the process of elimination. Recalling the basic principles of infection prevention will direct you to option 1. Review these basic principles if you had difficulty with this question.

Reference
deWit, S. (2009). *Medical-surgical nursing: Concepts & practice* (pp. 119-120). St. Louis: Saunders.

---

56. A nurse is carrying out an order to obtain a sputum sample, which must be obtained via the saline inhalation method. The nurse helps the client to use the nebulizer safely and effectively by encouraging the client to do which of the following?
 1 Hold the nebulizer under the nose.
 2 Keep the lips closed lightly over the seal.
 3 Keep the lips closed tightly over the seal.
 4 Alternate one vapor breath with one breath from room air.

Answer: 2
Rationale: Inhaling vaporized saline is an effective means of helping a client to cough productively. The vapor condenses on the respiratory mucosa, thus stimulating the cough reflex and the expectoration of secretions. The nurse tells the client to close the mouth lightly over the mouthpiece; it is not necessary to form a tight seal. The client inhales vaporized saline with each breath until coughing results. The nebulizer is not held under the nose.

Test-Taking Strategy: Focus on the subject—using the saline inhalation method to obtain a sputum specimen. Visualizing this procedure will direct you to option 2. Review this procedure if you had difficulty with this question.

Level of Cognitive Ability: Application
Client Needs: Safe and Effective Care Environment
Integrated Process: Nursing Process/Implementation
Content Area: Adult Health/Respiratory

References
Chernecky, C., & Berger, B. (2008). *Laboratory tests and diagnostic procedures* (5th ed., p. 1035). Philadelphia: Saunders.
Potter, P., & Perry, A. (2009). *Fundamentals of nursing* (7th ed., p. 1437). St. Louis: Mosby.

---

57. A client has a tracheostomy with a nondisposable inner cannula. After completing tracheostomy care, the nurse reinserts the inner cannula into the tracheostomy tube immediately after doing which of the following?

1 Suctioning the airway
2 Rinsing it in sterile water
3 Drying it with a sterile cotton ball
4 Lightly tapping it dry against a sterile surface

Level of Cognitive Ability: Application
Client Needs: Safe and Effective Care Environment
Integrated Process: Nursing Process/Implementation
Content Area: Adult Health/Respiratory

Answer: 4
Rationale: The nurse reinserts the inner cannula immediately after tapping it dry against a sterile surface. After it has been inserted, it is turned clockwise to lock it into place. It should not be dried with a cotton ball, which could leave cotton particles on the cannula. The client's airway is suctioned before tracheostomy care is performed. The cannula is rinsed in sterile water before it is tapped dry.

Test-Taking Strategy: The wording of the question tells you that there is a particular sequence that must be followed to complete the steps of the procedure. Use the process of elimination to determine that the step that would be performed immediately before reinsertion would be related to drying the tube. Review the procedure for tracheostomy care if you had difficulty with this question.

Reference
Christensen, B., & Kockrow, E. (2006). *Foundations of nursing* (5th ed., pp. 566-567). St. Louis: Mosby.

---

58. A nurse is assisting with the care of a client with a nasogastric (NG) tube. The nurse understands that which of the following would be the most potentially hazardous method for checking tube placement when caring for the client?

1 Measuring the pH of the gastric aspirate
2 Submerging the NG tube in water to check for bubbling
3 Aspirating the NG tube with a 50-mL syringe for gastric contents
4 Instilling 10 to 20 mL of air into the NG tube while auscultating over the stomach

Level of Cognitive Ability: Comprehension
Client Needs: Safe and Effective Care Environment
Integrated Process: Nursing Process/Implementation
Content Area: Adult Health/Respiratory

Answer: 2
Rationale: The most potentially hazardous method of checking NG tube placement is to submerge the end of the tube in water to observe for bubbling. This could put the client at risk for aspiration if the client breathed in fluid while the tube was in the lungs. Each of the other methods described is acceptable. The best method of determining tube placement is to verify it by x-ray.

Test-Taking Strategy: Use the process of elimination, and note the strategic words *most potentially hazardous.* This tells you that the correct answer is an option that puts the client at risk for possible injury. Evaluate each of the options, noting that, in this case, the correct option puts the client at risk for aspiration. Review the procedure for confirming NG tube placement if you had difficulty with this question.

Reference
Christensen, B., & Kockrow, E. (2006). *Foundations of nursing* (5th ed., p. 592). St. Louis: Mosby.

---

59. An older client who has not been hospitalized previously is extremely anxious after hospital admission. To provide a safe environment for the client and minimize

Answer: 4
Rationale: Several general interventions will reduce the hospitalized client's level of stress. These include acknowledging the client's feelings, offering information, providing social support, and

the stress of hospitalization, the nurse should do which of the following?
1 Keep visitors to the minimum number possible.
2 Keep the door open and the room lights on at all times.
3 Admit the client to a room far away from the nurse's station.
4 Allow the client to have as many choices related to care as possible.

Level of Cognitive Ability: Application
Client Needs: Safe and Effective Care Environment
Integrated Process: Nursing Process/Implementation
Content Area: Fundamental Skills

letting the client have control over choices related to care. Options 1 and 3 could increase anxiety, whereas option 2 could add to the disruption created by the hospitalization and interfere with the client's sleep pattern.

Test-Taking Strategy: Use the process of elimination, and note the strategic words *safe* and *minimize the stress.* This tells you that the correct option is one that calms the client's feelings of fear and anxiety after being placed in a foreign environment. Use general principles related to safety and stress reduction to answer the question. Review these principles if you had difficulty with this question.

Reference
Wold, G. (2008). *Basic geriatric nursing* (4th ed., pp. 164, 323). St. Louis: Mosby.

---

60. A client with pulmonary tuberculosis (TB) asks the nurse how this disease was contracted. The nurse replies that TB is commonly spread by which of the following methods?
1 Sneezing
2 Shaking hands
3 Contact with stool
4 Contact with urine

Level of Cognitive Ability: Comprehension
Client Needs: Safe and Effective Care Environment
Integrated Process: Nursing Process/Implementation
Content Area: Adult Health/Respiratory

Answer: 1
Rationale: TB is spread by droplet nuclei, which become airborne when the infected client laughs, sings, sneezes, or coughs. An individual must inhale the droplet nuclei for the chain of infection to continue. TB is not spread by shaking hands or by contact with stool or urine.

Test-Taking Strategy: The subject of the question is the method of TB transmission. Recalling that TB is a respiratory disorder and spread by droplet nuclei will direct you to the correct option. Review TB, infection control measures, and respiratory isolation technique if you had difficulty with this question.

Reference
Linton, A. (2007). *Introduction to medical-surgical nursing* (4th ed., p. 564). Philadelphia: Saunders.

---

61. A nurse is collecting data about a client's risk of committing suicide. Which of the following is the best question for the nurse to ask the client?
1 "Do you have a death wish?"
2 "Do you wish your life was over?"
3 "Do you ever think about ending it all?"
4 "Have you ever thought of killing yourself?"

Level of Cognitive Ability: Application
Client Needs: Safe and Effective Care Environment
Integrated Process: Nursing Process/Data Collection
Content Area: Mental Health

Answer: 4
Rationale: A suicide risk assessment requires direct communication between the client and the nurse. It is important to provide a question that is directly related to the risk for suicide. Options 1, 2, and 3 do not directly address the subject of the question. Option 4 is the most direct option.

Test-Taking Strategy: Use the process of elimination. Note the strategic word *best.* Also, note the word *killing*. Option 4 directly addresses the subject of suicide. Review the assessment of suicide risk if you had difficulty with this question.

Reference
deWit, S. (2009). *Medical-surgical nursing: Concepts & practice.* (p. 1113). St. Louis: Saunders.

---

62. A physical assessment of a suicidal client was performed on admission to the inpatient unit. The nurse reviews the findings and recognizes that this is an important part of the admission process because it alerts the nurse to:
1 Baseline data
2 Abnormalities
3 Existing medical problems
4 Evidence of physical self-harm

Level of Cognitive Ability: Comprehension
Client Needs: Safe and Effective Care Environment
Integrated Process: Nursing Process/Data Collection
Content Area: Mental Health

Answer: 4
Rationale: The physical assessment of a suicidal client should be thorough and should focus on the evidence of self-harm and the formulation of a plan for the suicide attempt. Although all of the options are correct, option 4 is most appropriate for the suicidal client. Clients with a history or evidence of self-harm are greater suicide risks.

Test-Taking Strategy: Use the process of elimination, and focus on the subject of the question. Remember that physical evidence of self-harm is an important component of the assessment process of a suicidal client. Review the characteristics of the client at risk for suicide if you had difficulty with this question.

References
deWit, S. (2009). *Medical-surgical nursing: Concepts & practice* (pp. 1113-1114). St. Louis: Saunders.
Linton, A. (2007). *Introduction to medical-surgical nursing* (4th ed., p. 1262). Philadelphia: Saunders.

---

63. A nurse who is assisting with the care of suicidal clients in a psychiatric nursing unit should plan to implement special precautions at which of the following times of increased risk?
1 Day shift
2 Weekdays
3 Shift change
4 8 AM to 2 PM

Level of Cognitive Ability: Application
Client Needs: Safe and Effective Care Environment
Integrated Process: Nursing Process/Planning
Content Area: Mental Health

Answer: 3
Rationale: During shift changes, fewer staff members may be available to observe clients. The staff in a psychiatric nursing unit should increase precautions during shift changes for clients identified as suicidal. Other times of increased risk for suicides are weekends (not weekdays) and night shifts (not day shifts).

Test-Taking Strategy: Use the process of elimination. Remember that options that are comparable or alike are not likely to be correct, so eliminate options 1 and 4 first. Choose between the remaining options by selecting the time when fewer staff members would be available to observe clients. Review the care of the client at risk for suicide if you had difficulty with this question.

Reference
Fortinash, K., & Holoday-Worret, P. (2008). *Psychiatric mental health nursing* (4th ed., p. 476). St. Louis: Mosby.

---

64. A nurse is assisting with the admission of a postoperative client from the postanesthesia care unit to the surgical nursing unit. The nurse should do which of the following for the safety of the client?
1 Ask the client to slide from the stretcher to the bed.
2 Move the client rapidly from the stretcher to the bed.
3 Put the side rails up after moving the client from the stretcher.
4 Uncover the client before transferring him or her from the stretcher to the bed.

Level of Cognitive Ability: Application
Client Needs: Safe and Effective Care Environment

Answer: 3
Rationale: Because the client may still be experiencing residual effects of anesthesia, the nurse should raise the side rails after transferring the client from the stretcher to the bed. It is not realistic to ask the client to slide from the stretcher to the bed because of the effects of anesthesia and postoperative pain. Hurried movements and rapid changes in position should be avoided because these predispose the client to hypotension. During the transfer of the client after surgery, the nurse should avoid exposing the client because of potential heat loss, respiratory infection, and shock.

Test-Taking Strategy: Use the process of elimination. Begin to answer this question by eliminating options 2 and 4 first because they are not standard nursing interventions. Choose between the remaining options, knowing that the subject of the question is client safety and that the only option that addresses safety is option 3. Review the care of the postoperative client if you had difficulty with this question.

Integrated Process: Nursing Process/ Implementation
Content Area: Fundamental Skills

Reference
Linton, A. (2007). *Introduction to medical-surgical nursing* (4th ed., p. 266). Philadelphia: Saunders.

---

65. A nurse is caring for a child with a fever. The nurse implements which safe action when giving this child a tepid tub bath?
1 Add isopropyl alcohol to the bath water.
2 Let the child soak in the tub for 10 minutes.
3 Slowly add cool water to the warmer bath water.
4 Warm the water to the same body temperature of the child.

Level of Cognitive Ability: Application
Client Needs: Safe and Effective Care Environment
Integrated Process: Nursing Process/ Implementation
Content Area: Child Health

Answer: 3
Rationale: Cool water should be added to an already warm bath, because this will cause the water temperature to slowly drop. The child will be able to gradually adjust to the changing water temperature and will not experience chilling. The child should be kept in a tepid tub bath for 20 to 30 minutes to achieve maximum results. Alcohol is toxic and contraindicated for tepid sponge or tub baths. To achieve the best cooling results for the child with a fever, the water temperature should be at least 2 degrees lower than the child's body temperature.

Test-Taking Strategy: Use the process of elimination. Begin to answer this question by eliminating option 4 because this would not lower the child's temperature. Eliminate option 1 next, knowing that isopropyl alcohol should not be used. To choose correctly between the remaining options, you must be familiar with either the time frames indicated to lower a temperature with a tepid bath or the proper methods for cooling the bath water. Review measures to treat hyperthermia if you had difficulty with this question.

References
Leifer, G. (2007). *Introduction to maternity and pediatric nursing* (5th ed., p. 491). Philadelphia: Saunders.
Price, D., & Gwin, J. (2008). *Pediatric nursing: An introductory text* (10th ed., pp. 35, 373). St. Louis: Saunders.

---

66. A nurse is assisting with the care of a child who underwent the surgical repair of a cleft lip the previous day. The nurse should implement which safe nursing intervention when caring for the surgical incision?
1 Clean the incision only if serous exudate forms.
2 Remove the Logan bar carefully to clean the incision.
3 Rub the incision gently with a sterile cotton-tipped swab.
4 Rinse the incision with sterile water after using diluted hydrogen peroxide, if prescribed.

Level of Cognitive Ability: Application
Client Needs: Safe and Effective Care Environment
Integrated Process: Nursing Process/ Implementation
Content Area: Child Health

Answer: 4
Rationale: The incision should be rinsed with sterile water when it is cleaned with a solution other than water or saline. The Logan bar is intended to maintain the integrity of the suture line; removing the Logan bar on the first postoperative day is incorrect because removal would increase tension on the surgical incision. The incision is cleaned after every feeding and when serous exudate forms. The incision should be dabbed and not rubbed to maintain its integrity.

Test-Taking Strategy: Use the process of elimination. Eliminate option 2 first, recalling that the Logan bar maintains the integrity of the suture line. Eliminate option 1 because of the word *only* and option 3 because of the word *rub.* Review the care of a child after the surgical repair of a cleft lip if you had difficulty with this question.

Reference
Price, D., & Gwin, J. (2008). *Pediatric nursing: An introductory text* (10th ed., p. 102). St. Louis: Saunders.

---

67. A nurse is assigned to care for an older client who has been identified as a victim of physical abuse. When planning care for this client, the nurse's priority is focused toward:

1 Adhering to the mandatory abuse reporting laws
2 Removing the client from any immediate danger
3 Referring the abusing family member for treatment
4 Encouraging the client to file charges against the abuser

Level of Cognitive Ability: Application
Client Needs: Safe and Effective Care Environment
Integrated Process: Nursing Process/Planning
Content Area: Mental Health

Answer: 2
Rationale: Whenever the abused client remains in the abusive environment, priority must be placed on determining whether the person is in any immediate danger. If so, emergency action must be taken to remove the client from the abusive situation. Options 1 and 3 may be appropriate interventions but are not the priority. Option 4 is not an appropriate intervention at this time and may produce increased fear and anxiety in the client.

Test-Taking Strategy: Use the process of elimination. Eliminate option 4 first because this action may produce increased fear and anxiety in the client. Use Maslow's Hierarchy of Needs theory to select from the remaining options. Remember that if a physiological need is not present, then safety is the priority; this should direct you to option 2, which is the only option that directly addresses client safety. Review the care of the victim of abuse if you had difficulty with this question.

References
Fortinash, K., & Holoday-Worret, P. (2008). *Psychiatric mental health nursing* (4th ed., p. 504). St. Louis: Mosby.
Wold, G. (2008). *Basic geriatric nursing* (4th ed., pp. 23-25). St. Louis: Mosby.

---

68. When planning safe activities for the depressed client during the early stages of hospitalization, the nurse should:

1 Plan nothing until the client asks to participate in milieu activities.
2 Offer the client a menu of daily activities and insist that the client participate in all of them.
3 Provide a structured daily program of activities and encourage the client to participate in them.
4 Provide an activity that is quiet and solitary in nature to avoid increased fatigue, such as working on a puzzle or reading a book.

Level of Cognitive Ability: Application
Client Needs: Safe and Effective Care Environment
Integrated Process: Nursing Process/Implementation
Content Area: Mental Health

Answer: 3
Rationale: A depressed person is often withdrawn. In addition, the person experiences difficulty concentrating, loss of interest or pleasure, low energy, fatigue, feelings of worthlessness, and poor self-esteem. The plan of care should provide successful experiences in a stimulating yet structured environment. Options 1 and 4 are restrictive, and option 2 is demanding.

Test-Taking Strategy: Use the process of elimination. Remember that the depressed client requires a structured and stimulating program. Options 1 and 4 are too restrictive and offer little or no structure or stimulation. Option 2 is eliminated because of the high demands placed on the client. Review the care of the client with depression if you had difficulty with this question.

Reference
Fortinash, K., & Holoday-Worret, P. (2008). *Psychiatric mental health nursing* (4th ed., pp. 521-522). St. Louis: Mosby.

---

69. A nurse is caring for a client under contact isolation. After the nursing care has been performed, which protective item worn during client care should the nurse remove first when leaving the room?

1 Mask
2 Gown

Answer: 3
Rationale: The nurse should remove his or her gloves first because these are the items that are the most contaminated. The nurse then carefully removes the mask by touching only the elastic or mask strings; ungloved hands will not become contaminated by touching only these areas. The nurse then unties the neck strings and the back strings of the gown and allows the gown to fall from his or her shoulders. The nurse removes his or her hands from the

3 Gloves
4 Eyewear

Level of Cognitive Ability: Application
Client Needs: Safe and Effective Care Environment
Integrated Process: Nursing Process/Implementation
Content Area: Fundamental Skills

sleeves without touching the outside of the gown, holds the gown inside at the shoulder seams, folds it inside out, and discards it in the appropriate trash receptacle or laundry bag. The nurse removes eyewear or goggles and then washes his or her hands.

Test-Taking Strategy: Use your knowledge of standard precautions and of the methods used to prevent contamination. Visualize the correct process of removing contaminated clothing and items after caring for a client. Remember that the gloves are the items that are the most contaminated. Review these precautions and procedures if you had difficulty with this question.

References

Christensen, B., & Kockrow, E. (2006). *Foundations of nursing* (5th ed., p. 285). St. Louis: Mosby.
Linton, A. (2007). *Introduction to medical-surgical nursing* (4th ed., p. 172). Philadelphia: Saunders.

---

70. Ultraviolet light (UVL) therapy is prescribed in the treatment plan of a client with psoriasis. The nurse reinforces instructions to the client regarding safety measures related to the therapy. Which statement made by the client indicates the need for further instruction?
1 "Each treatment will last 30 minutes."
2 "I should wear eye goggles during the treatment."
3 "I will expose only the area that requires treatment."
4 "I will cover my face with a loosely applied covering."

Level of Cognitive Ability: Comprehension
Client Needs: Safe and Effective Care Environment
Integrated Process: Teaching and Learning
Content Area: Adult Health/Integumentary

Answer: 1

Rationale: Safety precautions are required during UVL therapy. Most UVL treatments require the person to stand in a light-treatment chamber for up to 15 minutes. It is best to expose only those areas that require treatment to the UVL. Wearing protective wraparound goggles prevents the exposure of the eyes to UVL. If it does not require treatment, the face should be shielded with a loosely applied cloth. Direct contact with the light bulbs of the treatment unit should be avoided to prevent the burning of the skin.

Test-Taking Strategy: Note the strategic words *indicates the need for further instruction.* These words indicate a negative event query and ask you to select an option that is an incorrect client statement. Note that option 1 refers to a time frame of 30 minutes, which is an extensive time period for exposure to UVL. Review client instructions for UVL treatments if you had difficulty with this question.

Reference

Ignatavicius, D., & Workman, M. (2010). *Medical-surgical nursing: Patient-centered collaborative care* (6th ed., pp. 507-508). St. Louis: Saunders.

---

71. A nurse is assigned to care for a client who sustained a burn injury. The nurse reviews the physician's orders and should question the registered nurse about which order?
1 Monitor the weight daily.
2 Monitor the urine output hourly.
3 Maintain the nasogastric tube with intermittent suction.
4 Administer morphine sulfate intramuscularly every 3 hours as needed for pain.

Level of Cognitive Ability: Application
Client Needs: Safe and Effective Care Environment

Answer: 4

Rationale: Oral, subcutaneous, and intramuscular routes for administering medications are contraindicated in a client with a burn because of the poor absorption factor. When the fluid balance is stabilized, oral opioid agents can be used. Options 1, 2, and 3 are all appropriate interventions for a client with a burn.

Test-Taking Strategy: Use the process of elimination, and note that the subject of the question relates to the order that should be questioned. Read each option carefully, and think about the physiology that occurs in the client with a burn. Recalling that poor absorption will occur with medications administered by the oral, subcutaneous, or intramuscular routes will direct you to option 4. Review pain management for the client with a burn if you had difficulty with this question.

Integrated Process: Nursing Process/Implementation
Content Area: Adult Health/Integumentary

References
Black, J., & Hawks, J. (2009). *Medical-surgical nursing: Clinical management for positive outcomes* (8th ed., p. 1251). St. Louis: Saunders.
Christensen, B., & Kockrow, E. (2006). *Adult health nursing* (5th ed., pp. 107, 109). St. Louis: Mosby.

---

72. A nurse is caring for an older client who had a hip pinned after it was fractured. When planning nursing care, the nurse should avoid which of the following to minimize the chance of further injury?
1 Leaving the side rails down
2 Answering the call bell promptly
3 Keeping the call bell within reach
4 Ensuring that the nightlight is working

Level of Cognitive Ability: Application
Client Needs: Safe and Effective Care Environment
Integrated Process: Nursing Process/Implementation
Content Area: Adult Health/Musculoskeletal

Answer: 1
Rationale: Safe nursing actions for preventing injury to the client include keeping the side rails up, keeping the bed in a low position, and providing a call bell that is within the client's reach. Responding promptly to the client's use of the call light minimizes the chance that the client will try to get up alone, which could result in a fall. Nightlights are built into the lighting systems of most facilities, and the bulbs in these lights should be routinely checked to ensure that they are working.

Test-Taking Strategy: Use the process of elimination. Note the strategic word *avoid;* this word indicates a negative event query and asks you to select an option that is an incorrect action. Because options 2 and 3 are standard safety measures, they are eliminated first. The use of a nightlight would help prevent falls; this is also helpful and so can be eliminated. Review common safety measures if you had difficulty with this question.

References
Christensen, B., & Kockrow, E. (2006). *Foundations of nursing* (5th ed., p. 351). St. Louis: Mosby.
deWit, S. (2009). *Medical-surgical nursing: Concepts & practice* (p. 193). St. Louis: Saunders.

---

73. A nurse has reinforced instructions to a parent regarding safe methods of preventing Lyme disease. Which statement made by the parent would indicate the need for additional instruction?
1 "We should wear hats when we go on our hiking trip."
2 "Wearing long-sleeved tops and long pants is important."
3 "We should wear closed shoes and socks that can be pulled up over our pants."
4 "We should avoid the use of insect repellents because they will attract the ticks."

Level of Cognitive Ability: Comprehension
Client Needs: Safe and Effective Care Environment
Integrated Process: Teaching and Learning
Content Area: Adult Health/Immune

Answer: 4
Rationale: To prevent Lyme disease, individuals should be instructed to use an insect repellent on the skin and clothes when the individuals are in areas in which ticks are likely to be found. Long-sleeved tops, long pants, closed shoes, and a hat or cap should be worn. If possible, heavily wooded areas or areas with thick underbrush should be avoided. Socks can be pulled up and over pant legs to prevent ticks from entering under the clothing.

Test-Taking Strategy: Note the strategic words *need for additional instruction.* These words indicate a negative event query and ask you to select an option that is an incorrect client statement. Use the process of elimination, and note that option 4 uses the word *avoid.* Reading carefully will assist with directing you to this option. Review measures to prevent contact with ticks if you had difficulty with this question.

Reference
Ignatavicius, D., & Workman, M. (2010). *Medical-surgical nursing: Patient-centered collaborative care* (6th ed., p. 356). St. Louis: Saunders

---

74. A client with paraplegia has a risk for injury related to the spasticity of the leg muscles. The nurse avoids which action when caring for this client?

1 Using restraints to immobilize the limbs
2 Administering a prn order for a muscle relaxant
3 Removing potentially harmful objects placed near the client
4 Performing range-of-motion exercises with the affected limbs

Level of Cognitive Ability: Application
Client Needs: Safe and Effective Care Environment
Integrated Process: Nursing Process/Implementation
Content Area: Adult Health/Neurological

Answer: 1

Rationale: Using limb restraints will not alleviate spasticity and could harm the client so should be avoided. The use of muscle relaxants may be helpful if the spasms cause discomfort to the client or pose a risk to the client's safety. Removing potentially harmful objects is a good basic safety measure. Range-of-motion exercises are beneficial for stretching muscles, which may diminish spasticity.

Test-Taking Strategy: Use the process of elimination. Note the strategic word *avoids;* this word indicates a negative event query and asks you to select an option that is an incorrect action and one that is potentially harmful to the client. This will direct you to option 1. Review the care of the client with limb spasticity if you had difficulty with this question.

References

Christensen, B., & Kockrow, E. (2006). *Adult health nursing* (5th ed., pp. 744-745). St. Louis: Mosby.
Linton, A. (2007). *Introduction to medical-surgical nursing* (4th ed., pp. 491, 495). Philadelphia: Saunders.

---

75. A client is admitted to the hospital with severe hypoparathyroidism. The nurse should do which of the following activities to promote client safety?

1 Keep the room slightly cool.
2 Institute seizure precautions.
3 Keep the head of the bed lowered.
4 Use a waist restraint continuously.

Level of Cognitive Ability: Application
Client Needs: Safe and Effective Care Environment
Integrated Process: Nursing Process/Implementation
Content Area: Adult Health/Endocrine

Answer: 2

Rationale: Hypoparathyroidism results from insufficient parathyroid hormone, which leads to low serum calcium levels. Hypocalcemia can cause tetany, which, if untreated, can lead to seizures. The nurse should institute seizure precautions to maintain a safe environment. The other options do nothing to help this health problem or to promote a safe environment for this client.

Test-Taking Strategy: Use the process of elimination, and note the strategic words *hypoparathyroidism* and *client safety.* Answer this question by recalling the complications of low calcium levels, which are tetany and ultimately seizures. With these in mind, eliminate each of the incorrect options. Review the complications associated with hypoparathyroidism if you had difficulty with this question.

References

Christensen, B., & Kockrow, E. (2006). *Adult health nursing* (5th ed., p. 537). St. Louis: Mosby.
Linton, A. (2007). *Introduction to medical-surgical nursing* (4th ed., p. 999). Philadelphia: Saunders.

---

76. A nurse is assisting with preparing a plan of care for a client being admitted to the hospital for the insertion of a cervical radiation implant. Which safe activity should the nurse suggest for this client after the implant has been inserted?

1 Maintain bedrest.
2 Sit in a chair when out of bed.

Answer: 1

Rationale: The client with a cervical radiation implant should be maintained on bedrest in the dorsal position to prevent the movement of the radiation source. The head of the bed is elevated to a maximum of 10 to 15 degrees for comfort. Turning the client on the side is avoided. If turning is absolutely necessary, a pillow is placed between the client's knees; with the body in straight alignment, the client is logrolled.

3 Maintain a side-lying position.
4 Elevate the head of the bed 45 degrees.

Level of Cognitive Ability: Application
Client Needs: Safe and Effective Care Environment
Integrated Process: Nursing Process/Planning
Content Area: Adult Health/Oncology

Test-Taking Strategy: Consider the anatomical location of the implant and the risk of dislodgement. Options 2, 3, and 4 can cause dislodgement of the implant. Review the care of the client with a radiation implant if you had difficulty with this question.

Reference

Christensen, B., & Kockrow, E. (2006). *Adult health nursing* (5th ed., p. 829). St. Louis: Mosby.

---

77. A nurse is assigned to care for a client who has returned to the nursing unit after an oral cholecystogram. At this point in time, the nurse should question which of the following physician's orders in the medical record?

1 Monitor for nausea and vomiting.
2 Monitor the client's hydration status.
3 Maintain a clear liquid status for 72 hours.
4 Monitor the client for abdominal discomfort.

Level of Cognitive Ability: Application
Client Needs: Safe and Effective Care Environment
Integrated Process: Nursing Process/Implementation
Content Area: Adult Health/Gastrointestinal

Answer: 3

Rationale: The client should be able to resume a normal diet after the nurse has ensured that the client's gastrointestinal (GI) function is normal. It is not necessary to keep the client on clear liquids for 72 hours after the procedure. The nurse would monitor the client for complaints of GI discomfort, nausea, and vomiting. The nurse would also assess the hydration status as part of routine care for the client undergoing a GI diagnostic test.

Test-Taking Strategy: Use the process of elimination. Note the strategic words *at this point* and *question*. This tells you that the correct option is one that would have been needed before the procedure but that is no longer necessary. Note that options 1, 2, and 4 are assessments that are appropriate after this procedure; option 3 is an intervention that is not necessary at this time. Review care after an oral cholecystogram if you had difficulty with this question.

Reference

deWit, S. (2009). *Medical-surgical nursing: Concepts & practice* (p. 744). St. Louis: Saunders.

---

78. A nurse employed in a physician's office is asked to check a client who is at low risk for contracting tuberculosis (TB) for the results of the purified protein derivative (PPD) test implanted 72 hours previously. The nurse determines that the PPD induration has a diameter of 11 mm. What action should the nurse take next?

1 Notify the physician.
2 Ask the client for permission to repeat the test.
3 Document the normal finding in the client's record.
4 Tell the client to make an appointment with a pulmonologist.

Level of Cognitive Ability: Application
Client Needs: Safe and Effective Care Environment
Integrated Process: Nursing Process/Implementation
Content Area: Adult Health/Respiratory

Answer: 1

Rationale: An area of induration that measures 10 mm or more is considered a positive reading and indicates exposure to tuberculosis. The nurse who observes a positive PPD reading notifies the physician immediately. The physician would then order a chest x-ray to determine whether the client has clinically active TB or old, healed TB lesions. A sputum culture would then be performed to confirm a diagnosis of active TB. Option 3 is incorrect because the reading is not a normal finding. Option 2 is incorrect because the test results are positive. A physician rather than a nurse would request a consultation with a pulmonologist.

Test-Taking Strategy: Note the strategic word *next*. Begin to answer this question by eliminating option 2 as incorrect. Option 4 is eliminated because it is not a nursing responsibility to obtain physician consultations. Knowing that the results indicate a positive test will direct you to option 1. Review the PPD test if you had difficulty with this question.

Reference

Chernecky, C., & Berger, B. (2008). *Laboratory tests and diagnostic procedures* (5th ed., pp. 758-759). Philadelphia: Saunders.

79. A nurse reinforces information about tuberculosis (TB) disease and recuperation to a client diagnosed with TB. The nurse determines that the client understands the information presented if the client states that it is possible to return to work when:

1 Five sputum cultures are negative
2 Three sputum cultures are negative
3 The purified protein derivative test and chest x-ray are negative
4 The sputum culture and purified protein derivative test are negative

Level of Cognitive Ability: Comprehension
Client Needs: Safe and Effective Care Environment
Integrated Process: Nursing Process/Evaluation
Content Area: Adult Health/Respiratory

Answer: 2
Rationale: The client must have sputum cultures performed every 2 to 4 weeks after the initiation of anti-TB medication therapy. The client may return to work when the results of three sputum cultures are negative, because the client is considered noninfectious at that point. One negative sputum culture is not sufficient, and five negative cultures are unnecessary.

Test-Taking Strategy: Use the process of elimination. Knowing that a positive purified protein derivative test never reverts to negative helps you to eliminate options 3 and 4. From the remaining options, it is necessary to know that three negative sputum cultures are required. Review the teaching points related to TB if you had difficulty with this question.

Reference
deWit, S. (2009). *Medical-surgical nursing: Concepts & practice* (p. 327). St. Louis: Saunders.

---

80. A registered nurse tells a licensed practical nurse (LPN) that a client who is suspected of having tuberculosis (TB) is being admitted to the hospital and asks the LPN to prepare a room for the client. The LPN prepares the room, knowing that this client's room needs to provide which of the following?

1 Venting to the roof and ultraviolet light
2 Ultraviolet light and three room air exchanges per hour
3 Ten room air exchanges per hour and venting to the roof
4 Venting to the outside, six room air exchanges per hour, and ultraviolet light

Level of Cognitive Ability: Application
Client Needs: Safe and Effective Care Environment
Integrated Process: Nursing Process/Planning
Content Area: Adult Health/Respiratory

Answer: 4
Rationale: The client with TB must be admitted to a private room that provides at least six air exchanges per hour. The room should provide venting to the outside and have ultraviolet lights installed. Options 1, 2, and 3 are inaccurate and would not provide adequate protection for preventing the transmission of the infection.

Test-Taking Strategy: Begin to answer this question by recalling the specific requirements of physical facilities that are used when caring for clients with TB. Knowing that ultraviolet light is required helps you to eliminate option 3. From the remaining options, note that the correct option is the only one that addresses all of the room requirements. Review these protective requirements if you had difficulty with this question.

Reference
Christensen, B., & Kockrow, E. (2006). *Foundations of nursing* (5th ed., p. 292). St. Louis: Mosby.

---

81. A client diagnosed with tuberculosis (TB) is scheduled for an x-ray. Which nursing intervention is appropriate for the nurse to perform when sending the client to the x-ray department?

1 Apply a mask to the client.
2 Apply a mask and gown to the client.
3 Apply a mask, gown, and gloves to the client.
4 Notify the x-ray department so that the personnel will know to wear masks when the client arrives.

Answer: 1
Rationale: Clients who have or who are suspected of having TB should wear a mask when they are out of their rooms. A high-efficiency particulate air respirator (mask) is worn by the nurse when caring for the client with TB. A gown and gloves are not needed for the client.

Test-Taking Strategy: Use the process of elimination. The subject of the question relates to the times that the client is out of his or her room. It would be impossible for everyone outside of the client's room to wear a mask, so option 4 can be eliminated. Remember that TB is transmitted via the airborne route; this will help you to eliminate options 2 and 3. Review the transmission of TB if you had difficulty with this question.

Level of Cognitive Ability: Application
Client Needs: Safe and Effective Care Environment
Integrated Process: Nursing Process/Implementation
Content Area: Adult Health/Respiratory

References

Christensen, B., & Kockrow, E. (2006). *Foundations of nursing* (5th ed., p. 280). St. Louis: Mosby.
deWit, S. (2009). *Medical-surgical nursing: Concepts & practice.* (p. 327). St. Louis: Saunders.

---

82. An extremely angry and aggressive client on the mental health inpatient unit has been placed in restraints. When working with this client, the nurse should suggest removal of the restraints when the client:

1 Divulges all of the reasons for the aggressive behavior
2 Has been sedated and is still experiencing sedative effects
3 Apologizes and tells the nurse that it will not happen again
4 Initiates no aggressive acts for an hour after the release of two leg restraints

Level of Cognitive Ability: Application
Client Needs: Safe and Effective Care Environment
Integrated Process: Nursing Process/Implementation
Content Area: Mental Health

Answer: 4
Rationale: The best indicator that the client's behavior is under control is when the client refrains from aggression after being partially released from the restraints. Restraints are initially placed around the waist, wrists, and ankles. The ankle restraints are removed first, one at a time, at regular intervals. The wrist and waist restraints are removed together when the client continues to exhibit nonaggressive behavior.

Test-Taking Strategy: To answer this question accurately, you must be familiar with the legal and ethical issues involving restraints as they are used for patients with aggressive mental illness. Remember that the best indicator that the client's behavior is under control is when the client refrains from aggression after being partially released from the restraints. Review these protocols and procedures if you had difficulty with this question.

Reference

Varcarolis, E., & Halter, M. (2009). *Essentials of psychiatric mental health nursing: A communication approach to evidence-based care* (pp. 434, 524). St. Louis: Saunders.

---

83. A client who has been admitted to the mental health unit with obsessive-compulsive disorder repeatedly cleans the bathroom fixtures. The client has become enraged and has started to bite and kick a roommate for occupying the bathroom. Which of the following actions should the nurse take first?

1 Physically restrain the client.
2 Notify the risk-management department.
3 Provide a safe environment for both clients.
4 Administer a medication to provide chemical restraint.

Level of Cognitive Ability: Application
Client Needs: Safe and Effective Care Environment
Integrated Process: Nursing Process/Implementation
Content Area: Mental Health

Answer: 3
Rationale: The first action of the nurse is to provide an environment that is safe for both clients. This may take a variety of forms, depending on individual circumstances, agency protocols, and written physician orders. Seclusion, chemical restraint, and physical restraint are only used when alternative and less-restrictive measures are not effective for controlling the client's behavior.

Test-Taking Strategy: Use Maslow's Hierarchy of Needs theory to answer this question. Physiological and safety needs come first. In this situation, the correct answer is the option that is the most global and that meets the needs of both clients identified in the question. Review the care of the client who is physically aggressive if you had difficulty with this question.

Reference

Varcarolis, E., & Halter, M. (2009). *Essentials of psychiatric mental health nursing: A communication approach to evidence-based care* (p. 428). St. Louis: Saunders.

---

84. A physician orders a 12-lead electrocardiogram (ECG) to be performed on a client. The client is concerned about the safety of the test, and the nurse provides information to the client. Which of the following would indicate that the client understands the test?

1 "I cannot breathe while the ECG is running."
2 "I should lie still while the ECG is being done."
3 "When the ECG begins, I must take a deep breath."
4 "If I move when the ECG begins, I will be shocked."

Level of Cognitive Ability: Comprehension
Client Needs: Safe and Effective Care Environment
Integrated Process: Nursing Process/Evaluation
Content Area: Adult Health/Cardiovascular

Answer: 2
Rationale: Good contact between the skin and electrodes is necessary to obtain a clear 12-lead ECG printout. Therefore the electrodes are placed on the flat surfaces of the skin just above the ankles and wrists. Movement may cause a disruption in that contact and artifact, which makes the ECG printout difficult to read. The client does not have to hold the breath or take a deep breath during the procedure. The client should be reassured that the procedure will not produce a shock.

Test-Taking Strategy: Use the process of elimination. While a 12-lead ECG is being performed, it is best if the client does not move the extremities; this will help a clear ECG reading to be obtained. Options 1, 3, and 4 are inappropriate statements. Review the procedure for obtaining an ECG if you had difficulty with this question.

Reference
Chernecky, C., & Berger, B. (2008). *Laboratory tests and diagnostic procedures* (5th ed., pp. 461-462). Philadelphia: Saunders.

---

85. A nurse is assisting with planning the discharge of a client with chronic anxiety and assists with selecting the goals that will promote a safe environment at home. The appropriate maintenance goal should focus on which of the following?

1 Ignoring feelings of anxiety
2 Identifying anxiety-producing events
3 Continuing contact with a crisis counselor
4 Eliminating all anxiety from the daily events

Level of Cognitive Ability: Application
Client Needs: Safe and Effective Care Environment
Integrated Process: Nursing Process/Planning
Content Area: Mental Health

Answer: 2
Rationale: Recognizing events that produce anxiety allows the client to prepare to cope with anxiety or to avoid a specific stimulus. Counselors will not be available for all anxiety-producing events, and this option does not encourage the development of internal strengths. Ignoring feelings will not resolve anxiety. It is impossible to eliminate all anxiety from daily events.

Test-Taking Strategy: Use the process of elimination. Eliminate option 4 first because of the close-ended word *all*. Eliminate option 1 next because feelings should not be ignored. From the remaining options, select option 2; it is more client centered, and it provides preparation for the client to deal with anxiety when it occurs. Review the goals for the client with chronic anxiety if you had difficulty with this question.

Reference
Stuart, G. (2009) *Principles and practices of psychiatric nursing* (9th ed., p. 570). St. Louis: Mosby.

---

86. A nurse is planning to reinforce instructions to a client with chronic vertigo about safety measures to prevent the worsening of symptoms or injury. Which safety instruction should the nurse provide to the client?

1 Remove clutter in the home.
2 Turn the head slowly when spoken to.
3 Drive at times when you do not feel dizzy.

Answer: 1
Rationale: The client with chronic vertigo should avoid driving and using public transportation; the sudden movements involved in each could precipitate an attack. To further prevent vertigo attacks, the client should change position slowly and should turn the entire body (not just the head) when spoken to. If vertigo does occur, the client should immediately sit down or grasp the nearest piece of stable furniture. The client should maintain a clutter-free home with throw rugs removed, because the effort of regaining balance after slipping could trigger vertigo.

4 Go to the bedroom and lie down when vertigo is experienced.

Level of Cognitive Ability: Application
Client Needs: Safe and Effective Care Environment
Integrated Process: Teaching and Learning
Content Area: Adult Health/Neurological

Test-Taking Strategy: Use the process of elimination. Begin to answer this question by eliminating options 3 and 4 first because they put the client at greatest risk of injury as a result of vertigo. From the remaining options, note that option 1 is a safer intervention than option 2. Review safety measures for the client with chronic vertigo if you had difficulty with this question.

References

Christensen, B., & Kockrow, E. (2006). *Adult health nursing* (5th ed., p. 675). St. Louis: Mosby.
Ignatavicius, D., & Workman, M. (2010). *Medical-surgical nursing: Patient-centered collaborative care* (6th ed., p. 1127). St. Louis: Saunders.

---

87. A nurse is assigned to care for a client with Parkinson's disease who has recently begun taking levadopa (L-dopa). Which of the following is most important to check before ambulating the client?

1 The client's history of falls
2 Assistive devices used by the client
3 The client's postural (orthostatic) vital signs
4 The degree of intention tremors exhibited by the client

Level of Cognitive Ability: Comprehension
Client Needs: Safe and Effective Care Environment
Integrated Process: Nursing Process/Data Collection
Content Area: Pharmacology

Answer: 3
Rationale: Clients with Parkinson's disease are at risk for postural (orthostatic) hypotension from the disease. This problem worsens when L-dopa is introduced, because the medication can also cause postural hypotension, thus increasing the client's risk for falls. Although knowledge of the client's use of assistive devices and history of falls is helpful, it is not the most important piece of data based on the information in this question. Clients with Parkinson's disease generally have resting rather than intention tremors.

Test-Taking Strategy: Use the process of elimination, and focus on the subject of the question—the most important piece of data before ambulating a client taking L-dopa. Postural hypotension presents the greatest safety risk to the client. Review safety measures for the client with Parkinson's disease if you had difficulty with this question.

Reference

Kee, J., Hayes, E., & McCuistion, L. (2009). *Pharmacology: A nursing process approach* (6th ed., pp. 335-336). St. Louis: Saunders.

---

88. A nurse is giving a bed bath to a client who is on strict bedrest. To safely increase venous return, the nurse bathes the client's extremities by using:

1 Long, firm strokes from distal to proximal areas
2 Short, patting strokes from distal to proximal areas
3 Firm, circular strokes from proximal to distal areas
4 Smooth, light strokes back and forth from proximal to distal areas

Level of Cognitive Ability: Application
Client Needs: Safe and Effective Care Environment
Integrated Process: Nursing Process/Implementation
Content Area: Fundamental Skills

Answer: 1
Rationale: Long, firm strokes in the direction of venous flow promote venous return when the extremities are bathed. Circular strokes are used on the face. Short, patting strokes and light strokes are not as comfortable for the client and do not promote venous return.

Test-Taking Strategy: Use the process of elimination. Eliminate options 3 and 4 first because a stroke from proximal to distal will not promote venous return. From the remaining options, select option 1 because long, firm strokes will promote venous return and client comfort. Review the bed bathing procedure if you had difficulty with this question.

References

Christensen, B., & Kockrow, E. (2006). *Foundations of nursing* (5th ed., p. 447). St. Louis: Mosby.
Perry, A., & Potter, P. (2010). *Clinical nursing skills & techniques* (7th ed., p. 431). St. Louis: Mosby.

89. A nurse is preparing to give an intramuscular (IM) injection that is irritating to the subcutaneous tissues. The drug reference recommends that it be given using the Z-track technique. Which of the following procedural steps would cause the tracking of the medication through the subcutaneous tissues?

1 Massaging the site after injecting the medication
2 Retracting the skin to the side before piercing the skin with the needle
3 Preparing a 0.2-mL air lock in the syringe after drawing up the medication
4 Attaching a new sterile needle to the syringe after drawing up the medication

Level of Cognitive Ability: Application
Client Needs: Safe and Effective Care Environment
Integrated Process: Nursing Process/Implementation
Content Area: Fundamental Skills

Answer: 1
Rationale: The Z-track variation of the standard IM technique is used to administer IM medications that are highly irritating to subcutaneous and skin tissues. Attaching a new sterile needle is done so that the new needle will not have any medication adhering to the outside that could be irritating to the tissues. Preparing an air lock keeps the needle clean of medication on insertion, and, as the air is injected behind the medication, it will provide a seal at the point of insertion to prevent tracking of the medication. Retracting the skin provides a seal over the injected medication to prevent tracking through the subcutaneous tissues. The site should not be massaged because this can lead to tissue irritation.

Test-Taking Strategy: Use the process of elimination, and focus on the subject of the question—tracking of the medication. Options 2, 3, and 4 are procedural steps for Z-track injection. Option 1 is incorrect; Z-track injections are not massaged because this could lead to tracking and tissue irritation. Review the procedure for administering Z-track injections if you had difficulty with this question.

Reference
Christensen, B., & Kockrow, E. (2006). *Foundations of nursing* (5th ed., p. 731). St. Louis: Mosby.

---

90. A nurse is preparing to suction a client's tracheostomy. In which position should the client be safely placed to ideally promote deep breathing and coughing?

1 Supine position
2 Lateral position
3 High-Fowler's position
4 Semi-Fowler's position

Level of Cognitive Ability: Application
Client Needs: Safe and Effective Care Environment
Integrated Process: Nursing Process/Implementation
Content Area: Fundamental Skills

Answer: 4
Rationale: If it is not contraindicated, before suctioning a tracheostomy, the client is placed in semi-Fowler's position to promote deep breathing, maximum lung expansion, and productive coughing. With the client in this position, gravity pulls downward on the diaphragm, which allows greater chest expansion and lung volume. Options 1 and 2 would not provide maximum lung expansion. The high-Fowler's position would not allow for easy visualization of the tracheotomy or easy access of the suction catheter.

Test-Taking Strategy: Use the process of elimination. You can eliminate options 1 and 2 first because they are comparable or alike options. From the remaining options, eliminate option 3 because the high-Fowler's position would not allow for easy visualization of the tracheostomy or easy access of the suction catheter. Review the procedure for suctioning a tracheostomy if you had difficulty with this question.

Reference
Christensen, B., & Kockrow, E. (2006). *Foundations of nursing* (5th ed., p. 565). St. Louis: Mosby.

---

91. The pregnant client is at full term. The fetal heart rate (FHR) is being monitored for a baseline rate. The nurse is satisfied with the results and tells the client that the baby is safe and that the baby's heart

Answer: 3
Rationale: The average FHR for a baby at term is 140 beats per minute. The normal range is 120 to 160 beats per minute; therefore option 3 is the only correct option.

rate is within normal limits. The nurse bases this interpretation on which of the following data?
1 FHR of 80 beats per minute
2 FHR of 90 beats per minute
3 FHR of 140 beats per minute
4 FHR of 170 beats per minute

Level of Cognitive Ability: Comprehension
Client Needs: Safe and Effective Care Environment
Integrated Process: Nursing Process/Data Collection
Content Area: Maternity/Antepartum

Test-Taking Strategy: Knowledge of the normal FHR is required to answer this question. Remember that the normal range is 120 to 160 beats per minute. Review the FHR if you had difficulty with this question.

Reference
Leifer, G. (2008). *Maternity nursing: An introductory text* (10th ed., p. 114). Philadelphia: Saunders.

---

92. A nurse is caring for a client who is dying and is a potential organ donor. The nurse reviews the client's medical record and identifies a contraindication to organ donation if which of the following is documented in the client's record?
1 Age of 38 years
2 Hepatitis B infection
3 Allergy to penicillin-type antibiotics
4 Negative rapid plasma reagin laboratory result

Level of Cognitive Ability: Comprehension
Client Needs: Safe and Effective Care Environment
Integrated Process: Nursing Process/Data Collection
Content Area: Fundamental Skills

Answer: 2
Rationale: A potential organ donor must meet age eligibility requirements, which vary by organ; for example, donors must be less than 65 years old for kidney donation, less than 55 years old for pancreas and liver donation, and less than 40 years old for heart donation. The donor should be free of communicable disease (e.g., human immunodeficiency virus, hepatitis), and the involved organ may not be diseased. Another contraindication to transplant is malignancy, with the exceptions of noninvolved skin or corneas.

Test-Taking Strategy: Use the process of elimination, and note the strategic word *contraindication.* With this in mind, eliminate option 1 first. Because allergies are not part of the decision-making criteria, eliminate option 3 next. Option 4 indicates an absence of syphilis (a communicable disease), which leaves option 2 (hepatitis B) as the correct option. Review the contraindications to organ donation if you had difficulty with this question.

Reference
deWit, S. (2009). *Medical-surgical nursing: Concepts & practice* (p. 860). St. Louis: Saunders.

---

93. A client with chronic renal failure has an indwelling catheter in the abdomen that is used for peritoneal dialysis. While bathing, the client spills water on the dressing that covers the catheter. The licensed practical nurse reports the occurrence to the registered nurse (RN) and plans to immediately assist with which of the following?
1 Changing the dressing
2 Removing the catheter
3 Flushing the peritoneal dialysis catheter
4 Scrubbing the catheter with povidone-iodine

Level of Cognitive Ability: Application
Client Needs: Safe and Effective Care Environment

Answer: 1
Rationale: Clients with peritoneal dialysis catheters are at high risk for infection. Because bacteria can reach the catheter insertion site more easily through a wet dressing, the nurse ensures that the dressing is kept dry at all times. The catheter is not removed; it is placed surgically by the physician, and it is needed for further dialysis treatments. Flushing the catheter is not indicated. Scrubbing the catheter with povidone-iodine is done at the time of connection or disconnection of peritoneal dialysis by the RN.

Test-Taking Strategy: Use the process of elimination. The subject of the question is that the dressing is wet. The correct option would focus on the dressing rather than the catheter; this eliminates options 2, 3, and 4. Review the principles of asepsis if you had difficulty with this question.

Integrated Process: Nursing Process/Planning
Content Area: Adult Health/Renal

References

Christensen, B., & Kockrow, E. (2006). *Foundations of nursing* (5th ed., pp. 270-271). St. Louis: Mosby.
Linton, A. (2007). *Introduction to medical-surgical nursing* (4th ed., p. 875). Philadelphia: Saunders.

---

94. A client who suffered a severe head injury has had vigorous treatment to control cerebral edema. Brain death has now been determined. The nurse assigned to assist with caring for the client prepares to carry out which of the following orders that will maintain the viability of the kidneys before organ donation?

1 Checking the respirations
2 Monitoring the temperature
3 Administering intravenous (IV) fluids
4 Performing frequent range-of-motion exercises with the extremities

Level of Cognitive Ability: Application
Client Needs: Safe and Effective Care Environment
Integrated Process: Nursing Process/Implementation
Content Area: Fundamental Skills

Answer: 3
Rationale: Perfusion to the kidney is affected by blood pressure, which is in turn affected by blood vessel tone and fluid volume. Therefore the client who was previously dehydrated to control intracranial pressure is now in need of rehydration to maintain perfusion to the kidneys. The nurse prepares to infuse IV fluids as ordered and to continue monitoring the urine output. Checking the respirations and temperature and performing frequent range-of-motion exercises with extremities will not maintain the viability of the kidneys.

Test-Taking Strategy: Use the process of elimination. Note the subject of the question—maintaining the viability of the kidneys. This implies an action orientation, which guides you to look for options that involve intervention rather than data collection. With this in mind, eliminate options 1 and 2 first. You would choose the correct of the remaining two options by comparing their benefits to the kidneys. Review the interventions related to the care of the potential kidney donor if you had difficulty with this question.

Reference

Ignatavicius, D., & Workman, M. (2010). *Medical-surgical nursing: Patient centered collaborative care* (6th ed., p. 1631). St. Louis: Saunders.

---

95. A nurse is assisting in the emergency department of a small local hospital when a client with multiple gunshot wounds arrives by ambulance. The nurse is asked to care for the client's personal belongings, which may be needed as legal evidence. Which of the following actions by the nurse is contraindicated in the proper handling of legal evidence?

1 Give the clothing and wallet to the family.
2 Cut the clothing along seams, avoiding bullet holes.
3 Place the personal belongings into a labeled, sealed paper bag.
4 Initiate a log (custody log) that provides tracking information regarding the handling of items needed for evidence.

Level of Cognitive Ability: Application
Client Needs: Safe and Effective Care Environment
Integrated Process: Nursing Process/Implementation
Content Area: Fundamental Skills

Answer: 1
Rationale: Basic rules for handling evidence include limiting the number of people with access to the evidence, initiating a chain-of-custody log to track the handling and movement of evidence, and carefully removing clothing to avoid destroying evidence. This usually includes cutting clothes along seams and avoiding areas where there are obvious holes or tears. Potential evidence is never released to the family to take home.

Test-Taking Strategy: Use the process of elimination. Note the strategic word *contraindicated;* this word indicates a negative event query and asks you to select the option that is an incorrect action. You should be directed to option 1 because giving the belongings to the family may be jeopardizing evidence. Review the proper handling of legal evidence if you had difficulty with this question.

Reference

Proehl, J. (2009). *Emergency nursing procedures* (4th ed., pp. 889-893). St. Louis: Saunders.

96. A nurse working on a medical nursing unit during an external disaster is called to assist with the care of clients coming into the emergency department and asked to assist the triage nurse. Using principles of prioritizing, the nurse initiates care for a client with which of the following injuries first?

1 Fractured tibia
2 Penetrating abdominal injury
3 Bright red bleeding from a neck wound
4 Open severe head injury and a deep coma

Level of Cognitive Ability: Application
Client Needs: Safe and Effective Care Environment
Integrated Process: Nursing Process/Implementation
Content Area: Delegating/Prioritizing

Answer: 3

Rationale: The client with arterial bleeding from a neck wound is in immediate need of treatment to save the client's life. According to the triage process, the client in this classification would be issued a red tag. The client with a penetrating abdominal injury would be tagged yellow and classified as "delayed," requiring intervention within 30 to 60 minutes. A green or "minimal" designation would be given to the client with a fractured tibia; this client requires intervention but can provide self-care, if needed. A designation of "expectant" and a color code of black would be applied to the client with massive injuries and a minimal chance of survival; these clients are given supportive care and pain management but are given definitive treatment last.

Test-Taking Strategy: Use the process of elimination. To answer this question accurately, you must be able to apply principles of prioritizing to the clients identified in the options. Eliminate options 1 and 2 first because they are less in need of immediate care. Select between options 3 and 4 by determining which client has the better chance of a positive outcome after intervention. Review the principles of prioritizing if you had difficulty with this question.

Reference

Ignatavicius, D., & Workman, M. (2010). *Medical-surgical nursing: Patient-centered collaborative care* (6th ed., pp. 163-164). St. Louis: Saunders.

---

97. A nurse is collecting data about home safety from an older client who is at risk for falls. The nurse determines that which of the following items in the home poses a potential risk for the client?

1 Scatter rugs
2 Shower seat
3 Bathroom handrails
4 Railings on the staircase

Level of Cognitive Ability: Comprehension
Client Needs: Safe and Effective Care Environment
Integrated Process: Nursing Process/Data Collection
Content Area: Adult Health/Musculoskeletal

Answer: 1

Rationale: The incidence of falls by older clients can be reduced with the use of bathroom safety equipment such as a shower seat and handrails. In addition, the home should have railings on all staircases and ample lighting. Scatter rugs could potentially cause the older client to fall and should be removed or at least secured with a nonskid backing.

Test-Taking Strategy: Use the process of elimination. The subject of the question is a factor in the home that poses a risk to the client. Begin to answer by eliminating options 3 and 4, which provide physical support to the client and pose no risk. Using this same line of reasoning, eliminate option 2. Review measures to prevent falls if you had difficulty with this question.

Reference

Wold, G. (2008). *Basic geriatric nursing* (4th ed., pp. 154-155). St. Louis: Mosby.

---

98. A client who received a dose of chemotherapy 12 hours ago is incontinent of urine while in bed. The nurse safely wears which of the following when cleaning the client?

1 Mask and gloves
2 Gown and gloves
3 Mask, gown, and gloves
4 Gown, gloves, and eyewear

Answer: 2

Rationale: The client who has received chemotherapy will have antineoplastic agents or their metabolites in body fluids and excreta for 48 hours. For this reason, the nurse should wear protection when dealing with likely sources of contamination. In this instance, the nurse should wear gloves and a gown to protect the hands and uniform from contamination.

Level of Cognitive Ability: Application
Client Needs: Safe and Effective Care Environment
Integrated Process: Nursing Process/Implementation
Content Area: Adult Health/Oncology

Test-Taking Strategy: Use the process of elimination. Begin to answer this question by reasoning that the potential source of contamination in this event is the client's urine. Because urine present on the hospital gown and bedclothes is not likely to splash, you can eliminate the options that identify a mask or eyewear. This leaves option 2 as the correct answer. Review chemotherapy contamination guidelines if you had difficulty with this question.

Reference
Ignatavicius, D., & Workman, M. (2010). *Medical-surgical nursing: Patient-centered collaborative care.* (6th ed., p. 423). St. Louis: Saunders.

---

99. A clinic nurse is providing instructions to the mother of a child who was diagnosed with mumps. The mother is concerned about her other children and asks the nurse how the infection is transmitted. The nurse informs the mother that mumps is transmitted by:

1 Airborne droplets
2 Contact with tears
3 The fecal-oral route
4 Contact with body sweat

Level of Cognitive Ability: Application
Client Needs: Safe and Effective Care Environment
Integrated Process: Teaching and Learning
Content Area: Child Health

Answer: 1
Rationale: Mumps is transmitted via airborne droplets, salivary secretions, and possibly the urine. Options 2, 3, and 4 are incorrect.

Test-Taking Strategy: Use the process of elimination, and focus on the subject of the question—the method of transmission of mumps. Remember that mumps is transmitted via airborne droplets, salivary secretions, and possibly the urine. Review the transmission route of mumps if you had difficulty with this question.

Reference
Price, D., & Gwin, J. (2008). *Pediatric nursing: An introductory text* (10th ed., p. 267). St. Louis: Saunders.

---

100. A nurse is assisting with preparing a client scheduled for a bone marrow aspiration. The client asks the nurse if the procedure will be painful. To provide the client with accurate information, the nurse should incorporate which of the following into a response to the client?

1 There is no pain from the procedure at all.
2 The procedure is painful, but the client will be under anesthesia.
3 A local anesthetic is used, but there is some pain during aspiration.
4 The procedure is very painful, but the client will be heavily medicated beforehand.

Level of Cognitive Ability: Application
Client Needs: Safe and Effective Care Environment
Integrated Process: Nursing Process/Implementation
Content Area: Fundamental Skills

Answer: 3
Rationale: A local anesthetic is used to anesthetize the skin and subcutaneous tissue to minimize tissue discomfort with needle insertion. The client will feel some pain briefly when the sample is aspirated out of the marrow. Options 1, 2, and 4 are not true statements.

Test-Taking Strategy: Use the process of elimination. Recalling that the procedure may be performed at the bedside will assist you with eliminating options 2 and 4. Knowing that the procedure is invasive will help you to eliminate option 1. Review bone marrow aspiration if you had difficulty with this question.

Reference
Chernecky, C., & Berger, B. (2008). *Laboratory tests and diagnostic procedures* (5th ed., p. 243). Philadelphia: Saunders.

---

101. A nurse is preparing to assist a client from the bed to a chair with the use of a hydraulic lift. The nurse should do which of the following to move the client safely with this device?

1 Position the client in the center of the sling.
2 Have three staff members available to assist.
3 Have the client grasp the chains that attach the sling to the lift.
4 Lower the client rapidly after he or she is positioned over the chair.

Level of Cognitive Ability: Application
Client Needs: Safe and Effective Care Environment
Integrated Process: Nursing Process/ Implementation
Content Area: Fundamental Skills

Answer: 1

Rationale: One person may operate a hydraulic lift. The client is positioned in the center of the sling, which is then attached to chains or straps that connect the sling to the lift. The client's hands and arms are crossed over the chest, and the client is raised from the bed into a sitting position. The lift raises the client off of the mattress and lowers the client slowly after the sling is positioned over the chair.

Test-Taking Strategy: Use the process of elimination, and focus on the subject—safe transfer. Visualizing this procedure will assist with directing you to option 1. Review the safe transfer procedure if you had difficulty with this question.

References

Christensen, B., & Kockrow, E. (2006). *Foundations of nursing* (5th ed., p. 396). St. Louis: Mosby.
Perry, A., & Potter, P. (2010). *Clinical nursing skills & techniques* (7th ed., p. 213). St. Louis: Mosby.

---

102. An older client in a long-term care facility is at risk for injury because of confusion. Because the client's gait is stable, which method of restraint, if prescribed, would be best used by the nurse to prevent injury to the client?

1 Vest restraint
2 Waist restraint
3 Alarm-activating bracelet
4 Chair with a locking lap tray

Level of Cognitive Ability: Application
Client Needs: Safe and Effective Care Environment
Integrated Process: Nursing Process/ Implementation
Content Area: Fundamental Skills

Answer: 3

Rationale: If the client is confused and has a stable gait, the least intrusive method of restraint is the use of an alarm-activating bracelet or "wandering bracelet." This allows the client to move about the residence freely while preventing him or her from leaving the premises. A vest or waist restraint or a chair with a locking lap tray is more intrusive than an alarm-activating bracelet.

Test-Taking Strategy: Use the process of elimination, your knowledge of the various restraint methods, and the ethical and legal consequences of restraint to eliminate each of the incorrect options. The words *stable gait* will also guide your selection. Review the guidelines related to the use of restraints if you had difficulty with this question.

Reference

Perry, A., & Potter, P. (2010). *Clinical nursing skills & techniques* (7th ed., p. 334). St. Louis: Mosby.

---

103. A nurse is suctioning the airway of a client with a tracheostomy. To safely perform the procedure, the nurse should do which of the following?

1 Turn on wall suction to 190 mm Hg.
2 Withdraw the catheter while continuously suctioning.
3 Insert the catheter until the client coughs or resistance is felt.
4 Reenter the catheter into the tracheostomy after suctioning the client's mouth.

Level of Cognitive Ability: Application
Client Needs: Safe and Effective Care Environment

Answer: 3

Rationale: The wall suction unit is maintained between 120 and 180 mm Hg of pressure; this allows for the adequate removal of secretions while protecting the airway from trauma. The nurse inserts the catheter until resistance is felt and then withdraws it 1 cm to move away from the mucosa. The nurse suctions intermittently and does not reenter the tracheostomy after suctioning the client's mouth.

Test-Taking Strategy: Use the process of elimination. Remembering that mucosal trauma can occur during suctioning will assist you with eliminating options 1 and 2. From the remaining options, visualizing this procedure will direct you to option 3. Review the tracheostomy suctioning procedure if you had difficulty with this question.

Integrated Process: Nursing Process/ Implementation
Content Area: Adult Health/Respiratory

Reference

Potter, P., & Perry, A. (2009). *Fundamentals of nursing* (7th ed., pp. 935-936). St. Louis: Mosby.

---

104. Furosemide (Lasix) 40 mg orally has been prescribed for a client. The nurse administers furosemide 80 mg to the client at 10:00 AM. After discovering the error, the nurse completes an incident report. Which of the following should the nurse document on this report?

1. "Lasix 80 mg was administered at 10:00 AM."
2. "Lasix 80 mg was given to the client instead of 40 mg."
3. "The wrong dose of medication was given to the client at 10:00 AM."
4. "I meant to give 40 mg of Lasix but I was rushed to get to another client who needed me and I gave the wrong dose."

Level of Cognitive Ability: Application
Client Needs: Safe and Effective Care Environment
Integrated Process: Communication and Documentation
Content Area: Fundamental Skills

Answer: 1

Rationale: When filing an incident report, the nurse should state the facts clearly. The nurse would not record assumptions, opinions, judgments, or conclusions about what occurred. Option 1 is the only statement that states the facts clearly.

Test-Taking Strategy: Read the occurrence as stated in the question. Using the process of elimination, select the option that clearly and most directly states what has occurred. Option 4 is eliminated first because it contains unnecessary information. Option 2 provides a judgment. Option 3 is incorrect because it assigns blame to the nurse. Option 1 clearly and simply states the occurrence. Review the documentation guidelines associated with completing incident reports if you had difficulty with this question.

Reference

Christensen, B., & Kockrow, E. (2006). *Foundations of nursing* (5th ed., p. 112). St. Louis: Mosby.

---

105. A nurse employed in a long-term care facility assists a nursing assistant with completing an incident report for a client who was found sitting on the floor. After completing the report, which of the following should the nurse avoid?

1. Notifying the nursing supervisor
2. Asking the unit secretary to call the physician
3. Forwarding the incident report to the nursing director's office
4. Documenting in the nurses' notes that an incident report was filed

Level of Cognitive Ability: Application
Client Needs: Safe and Effective Care Environment
Integrated Process: Nursing Process/ Implementation
Content Area: Fundamental Skills

Answer: 4

Rationale: Nurses are advised not to document the filing of an incident report in the nurses' notes. Information in the medical record can be considered evidence, and the record can be obtained by subpoena if a lawsuit is filed. Incident reports inform the facility's administration of the incident so that risk-management personnel can consider changes to prevent similar occurrences in the future. Incident reports also alert the facility's insurance company to a potential claim and to the need for further investigation. Options 1, 2, and 3 are accurate interventions.

Test-Taking Strategy: Use the process of elimination. Note the strategic word *avoid;* this word indicates a negative event query and asks you to select an option that is an incorrect action. Options 1, 2, and 3 all relate to the notification of individuals or departments. Option 4 relates to inappropriate documentation. Review the guidelines for the completion of incident reports if you had difficulty with this question.

Reference

Christensen, B., & Kockrow, E. (2006). *Foundations of nursing* (5th ed., p. 112). St. Louis: Mosby.

---

106. A physician is visiting a client in the nursing unit and is called to another nursing unit to assess a client in extreme pain. The physician tells the nurse, "I'm in a hurry. Can you write the order to decrease the atenolol (Tenormin) to 25 mg daily?" Which of the following is the appropriate nursing action?

1 Write the order as stated.
2 Call the nursing supervisor to write the order.
3 Inform the client of the change of medication.
4 Ask the physician to return to the nursing unit to write the order.

Level of Cognitive Ability: Application
Client Needs: Safe and Effective Care Environment
Integrated Process: Nursing Process/Implementation
Content Area: Fundamental Skills

Answer: 4
Rationale: Nurses are not to accept verbal orders from physicians because of the risk of errors. Although the client will be informed about the change in the treatment plan, this is not the most appropriate action at this time. The physician should write the new order.

Test-Taking Strategy: Use the process of elimination. Recalling that verbal orders are not acceptable will assist you with selecting the correct option. Options 1 and 2 are comparable or alike, so they can be eliminated. Option 3 is appropriate for a later time. Option 4 clearly identifies the nurse's responsibility in this event. Review the nurse's responsibilities related to implementing the physician's orders if you had difficulty with this question.

Reference
Christensen, B., & Kockrow, E. (2006). *Foundations of nursing* (5th ed., p. 703). St. Louis: Mosby.

---

107. A nurse has prepared a client for an intravenous pyelogram. The nurse determines that the client is knowledgeable about the procedure if the client states the need to report which of the following sensations immediately?

1 Nausea
2 Difficulty breathing
3 Salty taste in the mouth
4 Warm, flushed feeling in the body

Level of Cognitive Ability: Comprehension
Client Needs: Safe and Effective Care Environment
Integrated Process: Nursing Process/Evaluation
Content Area: Adult Health/Renal

Answer: 2
Rationale: Intravenous pyelography is a contrast study of the kidneys that determines the presence of a variety of disorders of the kidneys, ureters, and bladder. Normal sensations during the injection of the iodine-based radiopaque dye include a warm, flushed feeling; a salty taste in the mouth; and transient nausea. Difficulty breathing, wheezing, hives, and itching signal an allergic response and should be reported immediately. This response is prevented by asking the client about allergies to iodine or shellfish before the procedure.

Test-Taking Strategy: Use the ABCs—airway, breathing, and circulation; this will direct you to option 2. Review intravenous pyelography if you had difficulty with this question.

Reference
Chernecky, C., & Berger, B. (2008). *Laboratory tests and diagnostic procedures* (5th ed., p. 682). Philadelphia: Saunders.

---

108. Which activity by the family of an infant with respiratory syncytial virus who is receiving ribavirin (Virazole) indicates a knowledge deficit regarding the management of the disease process?

1 The infant's pregnant aunt visits the infant.
2 The infant's grandfather, who has asthma, is told that he may not visit.
3 Before leaving the infant's room, all family members wash their hands.

Answer: 1
Rationale: Whenever anyone is receiving ribavirin, there are precautions taken to prevent exposure to the medication. Everyone who enters the room while the client is receiving ribavirin should wear gowns, masks, gloves, and hair coverings. Anyone who is pregnant or considering pregnancy and anyone with a history of respiratory problems or reactive airway disease should not care for or visit anyone who is receiving ribavirin. Good handwashing is necessary before leaving the room, because handwashing prevents the spread of germs.

4 The family members wear gowns, gloves, masks, and hair coverings when they visit the infant.

Level of Cognitive Ability: Comprehension
Client Needs: Safe and Effective Care Environment
Integrated Process: Teaching and Learning
Content Area: Child Health

Test-Taking Strategy: Note the strategic words *indicates a knowledge deficit;* these words indicate a negative event query and ask you to select an option that is an incorrect activity by a family member. This will assist with directing you to option 1. Review ribavirin and the associated precautions if you had difficulty with this question.

Reference
McKinney, E., James, S., Murray, S., & Ashwill, J. (2009). *Maternal-child nursing* (3rd ed., p. 1193). St. Louis: Mosby.

---

109. A client in the nursing unit has an order for dextroamphetamine sulfate (Dexedrine) 25 mg orally daily. The nurse plans to collaborate with the dietician to limit the amount of which item on the client's dietary trays?

1 Fat
2 Starch
3 Protein
4 Caffeine

Level of Cognitive Ability: Application
Client Needs: Safe and Effective Care Environment
Integrated Process: Nursing Process/Implementation
Content Area: Pharmacology

Answer: 4
Rationale: Dextroamphetamine sulfate is a central nervous system (CNS) stimulant. Caffeine is also a stimulant and should be limited for the client taking this medication. In addition, the client should be taught to limit his or her own caffeine intake. Fat, starch, and protein do not need to be limited while taking this medication.

Test-Taking Strategy: Use the process of elimination, and recall that this medication is a CNS stimulant. Next, evaluate each of the options to determine the additive stimulation that each provides. Knowing that caffeine is a stimulant will direct you to option 4. Review dextroamphetamine sulfate if you had difficulty with this question.

Reference
Kee, J., Hayes, E., & McCuistion, L. (2009). *Pharmacology: A nursing process approach* (6th ed., p. 302). St. Louis: Saunders.

---

110. A hospitalized client with hypertension is receiving captopril (Capoten). To ensure client safety, the nurse should be sure that the client does which of the following?

1 Drinks plenty of water
2 Sits up and stands slowly
3 Eats foods that are high in potassium
4 Takes in sufficient amounts of high-fiber foods

Level of Cognitive Ability: Application
Client Needs: Safe and Effective Care Environment
Integrated Process: Teaching and Learning
Content Area: Adult Health/Cardiovascular

Answer: 2
Rationale: Orthostatic hypotension is a concern for clients taking antihypertensive medications. Clients are advised to avoid standing in one position for significant amounts of time, to change positions slowly, and to avoid extreme warmth (e.g., showers, bath, hot tubs, weather). Clients are also taught to recognize the symptoms of orthostatic hypotension, including dizziness, lightheadedness, weakness, and syncope. The use of this medication does not require the eating of foods that are high in potassium or fiber or the drinking of plenty of water.

Test-Taking Strategy: Use the process of elimination, and note the client's diagnosis. Recalling that captopril is an antihypertensive will assist with directing you to option 2. Remember that orthostatic hypotension is a potential concern with all types of antihypertensives. Review captopril if you had difficulty with this question.

Reference
Mosby. (2008). *2008 Mosby's nursing drug reference* (21st ed., p. 220). St. Louis: Mosby.

111. A nurse is assisting with planning care for the client who is scheduled for admission to the nursing unit after femoral–popliteal bypass grafting. The nurse understands that which of the following would be unsafe for use because it would impair circulation to the affected extremity?

1 Sheepskin
2 Bed cradle
3 Elastic wraps
4 Lightweight blanket

Level of Cognitive Ability: Comprehension
Client Needs: Safe and Effective Care Environment
Integrated Process: Nursing Process/Planning
Content Area: Adult Health/Cardiovascular

Answer: 3

Rationale: The use of sheepskin, a bed cradle, and lightweight blankets can promote warmth to the extremity and protect it from harm. Elastic wraps, if ordered, would be used when the client is out of bed to reduce edema, but they could impair circulation and wound healing. Frequently the limb that has been operated on is left unwrapped for monitoring and is not covered by elastic wraps or pneumatic boots. However, these devices may be placed on the alternate extremity.

Test-Taking Strategy: Use the process of elimination, and note the strategic word *unsafe.* Recall that the limb that has been operated on needs frequent monitoring, warmth, and protection; this will direct you to option 3. Review the care of the client after femoral–popliteal bypass grafting if you had difficulty with this question.

Reference

deWit, S. (2009). *Medical-surgical nursing: Concepts & practice* (p. 445). St. Louis: Saunders.

---

112. A nurse is changing a dressing on a venous stasis ulcer that is clean and that has a growing bed of granulation tissue. The nurse should safeguard wound integrity by avoiding the use of which of the following dressing materials?

1 Hydrocolloid dressing
2 Vaseline gauze dressing
3 Wet-to-dry saline dressing
4 Wet-to-wet saline dressing

Level of Cognitive Ability: Application
Client Needs: Safe and Effective Care Environment
Integrated Process: Nursing Process/Implementation
Content Area: Fundamental Skills

Answer: 3

Rationale: The use of wet-to-dry saline dressings provides a mechanical debridement whereby both devitalized and viable tissue are removed; this method should not be used on a clean, granulating wound. Granulation tissue in a venous stasis ulcer is protected with the use of wet-to-wet saline dressings, Vaseline gauze, or moist occlusive dressings such as hydrocolloid dressings, as prescribed.

Test-Taking Strategy: Use the process of elimination. Note the strategic word *avoiding;* this word indicates a negative event query and asks you to select an option that is an incorrect type of dressing. Note that the wound is clean with granulation tissue, which needs protection. Note that options 1, 2, and 4 all have one thing in common—continuous moisture; this will direct you to option 3 because it is the only dressing that could disrupt this healing tissue. Review the principles related to wound care if you had difficulty with this question.

References

Christensen, B., & Kockrow, E. (2006). *Adult health nursing* (5th ed., pp. 393-394). St. Louis: Mosby.

Ignatavicius, D., & Workman, M. (2010). *Medical-surgical nursing: Patient-centered collaborative care* (6th ed., p. 493). St. Louis: Saunders.

---

113. A licensed practical nurse (LPN) is assisting with caring for an older client being admitted to the nursing unit with severe digoxin toxicity from the accidental ingestion of a week's supply of the medication. The registered nurse asks the LPN to check the

Answer: 4

Rationale: Digoxin immune Fab is an antidote for severe digoxin toxicity. It contains an antibody produced in sheep that antigenically binds any unbound digoxin in the serum and removes it. It also binds the digoxin that is reentering the bloodstream from the tissues, which is then excreted by the kidneys. Potassium chloride and furosemide are other medications that are commonly used in

medication supply to see if the antidote for digoxin toxicity is available. The LPN checks the medication supply for which medication?

1 Protamine sulfate
2 Furosemide (Lasix)
3 Potassium chloride (K-Dur)
4 Digoxin immune Fab (Digibind)

Level of Cognitive Ability: Application
Client Needs: Safe and Effective Care Environment
Integrated Process: Nursing Process/ Implementation
Content Area: Pharmacology

conjunction with digoxin for cardiac conditions. Protamine sulfate is the antidote for heparin.

Test-Taking Strategy: Use the process of elimination. Note the relationship between the name of the medication in the question and the correct option. Review digoxin immune Fab if you had difficulty with this question.

Reference

Hodgson, B., & Kizior, R. (2009). *Saunders nursing drug handbook 2009* (pp. 357-358). St. Louis: Saunders.

---

114. A client receiving lisinopril (Prinivil) has a white blood cell (WBC) count of 3800 cells/mm^3. The nurse should plan to do which of the following when caring for this client?

1 Follow aseptic technique diligently.
2 Place the client on respiratory isolation.
3 Use antibacterial soap when bathing the client.
4 Request prophylactic antibiotics from the physician.

Level of Cognitive Ability: Application
Client Needs: Safe and Effective Care Environment
Integrated Process: Nursing Process/Planning
Content Area: Pharmacology

Answer: 1

Rationale: Clients taking angiotensin-converting enzyme inhibitors such as lisinopril are at risk for the development of neutropenia. These clients require the use of strict aseptic technique by the nurse, and they should also be taught to report signs and symptoms of infection (e.g., sore throat, fever) to the physician. The WBC count with differential may be monitored monthly for up to 6 months in clients deemed at risk. Options 2, 3, and 4 are unrelated to the information in the question.

Test-Taking Strategy: Use the process of elimination. Noting that the WBC count is low and that a low count places the client at risk for infection will direct you to option 1. Review lisinopril and the associated nursing interventions if you had difficulty with this question.

References

Mosby. (2008). *2008 Mosby's nursing drug reference* (21st ed., p. 620). St. Louis: Mosby.
Lehne, R. (2007). *Pharmacology for nursing care* (6th ed., p. 472). Philadelphia: Saunders.

---

115. A client with obsessive-compulsive disorder spends many hours during the day and night washing his or her hands. When initially planning a safe environment, the nurse allows the client to continue this behavior because:

1 It increases self-esteem.
2 It relieves the client's anxiety.
3 It decreases the chance of infection.
4 It gives the client a feeling of self-control.

Level of Cognitive Ability: Comprehension
Client Needs: Safe and Effective Care Environment
Integrated Process: Nursing Process/Planning
Content Area: Mental Health

Answer: 2

Rationale: The compulsive act provides immediate relief from anxiety and is used to cope with stress, conflict, or pain. Although the client may feel the need to increase self-esteem, that is not the primary goal. Options 1, 3, and 4 are not reasons for allowing the client to continue the compulsive act.

Test-Taking Strategy: Use the process of elimination. Recalling that the behavior associated with compulsive disorders relieves anxiety will direct you to option 2. Review obsessive-compulsive disorder if you had difficulty with this question.

Reference

Varcarolis, E., & Halter, M. (2009). *Essentials of psychiatric mental health nursing: A communication approach to evidence-based care* (pp. 148, 184). St. Louis: Saunders.

---

116. A client is scheduled to undergo cardiac catheterization for the first time. Which of the following points should the nurse plan to include in the preprocedure teaching to provide the client with accurate information?

1 The procedure is performed in the operating room.
2 The initial catheter insertion is quite painful; after that, there is little or no pain.
3 The client may feel fatigue and have various aches because it is necessary to lie quietly on a hard x-ray table for approximately 4 hours.
4 The client may feel certain sensations at various points during the procedure, such as skipped heart beats; a flushed, warm feeling; a desire to cough; and palpitations.

Level of Cognitive Ability: Application
Client Needs: Safe and Effective Care Environment
Integrated Process: Nursing Process/Planning
Content Area: Adult Health/Cardiovascular

Answer: 4
Rationale: During the preprocedure teaching, the client should be told that the procedure is performed in a darkened cardiac catheterization room and that electrocardiogram leads are attached to the limbs. A local anesthetic is used, so there is little to no pain with catheter insertion. The x-ray table is hard and may be tilted periodically. The procedure may take up to 2 hours, and the client may feel various sensations with catheter passage and dye injection.

Test-Taking Strategy: Use the process of elimination. Eliminate option 1 because this procedure is not performed in the operating room. Eliminate option 3 because 4 hours is too long of a time frame and option 2 because the procedure is not *quite painful*. Review client preparation for cardiac catheterization if you had difficulty with this question.

Reference
Chernecky, C., & Berger, B. (2008). *Laboratory tests and diagnostic procedures* (5th ed., p. 297). Philadelphia: Saunders.

---

117. A nurse is inserting an indwelling Foley catheter. When the nurse inflates the balloon, the client immediately complains of pain. The appropriate nursing action is to:

1 Call the physician.
2 Tell the client that the discomfort will pass.
3 Withdraw 1 mL from the balloon of the catheter.
4 Deflate the balloon and insert it further into the bladder.

Level of Cognitive Ability: Application
Client Needs: Safe and Effective Care Environment
Integrated Process: Nursing Process/Implementation
Content Area: Fundamental Skills

Answer: 4
Rationale: The appropriate procedure if the client complains of pain after the balloon is inflated is to deflate the balloon and insert it further into the bladder. If the client complains of pain, the balloon is most likely positioned in the urethra. Options 2 and 3 are incorrect actions. It is not necessary to call the physician.

Test-Taking Strategy: Focus on the data in the question. Visualizing this procedure and thinking about the anatomy of the urinary system will direct you to option 4. Review the insertion of a Foley catheter if you had difficulty with this question.

Reference
Potter, P., & Perry, A. (2009). *Fundamentals of nursing* (7th ed., p. 1159). St. Louis: Mosby.

---

118. A nurse is caring for a client who is scheduled to have an arthrogram using a contrast dye. Which of the following pieces of data collected by the nurse has the highest priority?

1 Allergy to contrast dye
2 Whether the client wishes to void before the procedure

Answer: 1
Rationale: Because of the risk of allergy, the nurse places highest priority on determining whether the client has an allergy to contrast dye, iodine, or shellfish. The nurse also reinforces information about the test, tells the client about the need to remain still during the procedure, and encourages the client to void before the procedure for comfort.

3 The ability of the client to remain still during the procedure
4 Whether the client has any remaining questions about the procedure

Level of Cognitive Ability: Comprehension
Client Needs: Safe and Effective Care Environment
Integrated Process: Nursing Process/Data Collection
Content Area: Fundamental Skills

Test-Taking Strategy: Use the process of elimination. Note the strategic words *highest priority;* these words tell you that more than one or all of the options are correct. Although options 2, 3, and 4 are all important, only option 1 is related to a medical risk. The consequence of a possible allergic reaction makes this the correct option. Review the procedure for an arthrogram if you had difficulty with this question.

Reference
Chernecky, C., & Berger, B. (2008). *Laboratory tests and diagnostic procedures* (5th ed., p. 169). Philadelphia: Saunders.

---

119. A nurse is reinforcing discharge instructions for a client with a spinal cord injury. To provide a safe home-care environment, which of the following should be the priority?
1 Follow-up laboratory and diagnostic tests
2 What the physician has indicated needs to be taught
3 Including the significant others in the teaching session
4 Assisting the client with dealing with long-term care placement

Level of Cognitive Ability: Application
Client Needs: Safe and Effective Care Environment
Integrated Process: Teaching and Learning
Content Area: Adult Health/Neurological

Answer: 3
Rationale: Involving the client's significant others in discharge teaching is a priority for the client with a spinal cord injury, because the client will need the support of the significant others. Knowledge and understanding of what to expect will help both the client and the significant others deal with the limitations. A physician's order is not necessary for providing instructions; this is an independent nursing action. Laboratory and diagnostic testing are inappropriate discharge instructions for this client. Long-term placement is not the only option for clients with spinal cord injuries.

Test-Taking Strategy: Use the process of elimination. Eliminate option 4 first because long-term placement is not the only discharge option. Eliminate option 2 next; although the physician's orders should be addressed, teaching is an independent nursing action. From the remaining options, consider the client's diagnosis. Home care and support will be needed, which will direct you to option 3. Review the care of the client with a spinal cord injury and the teaching and learning principles if you had difficulty with this question.

Reference
Linton, A. (2007). *Introduction to medical-surgical nursing* (4th ed., p. 504). Philadelphia: Saunders.

---

120. A nurse is asked to assist with applying electrocardiogram (ECG) electrodes to a diaphoretic client. The nurse should do which of the following to keep the electrodes from coming loose?
1 Secure the electrodes with adhesive tape.
2 Place clear, transparent dressings over the electrodes.
3 Apply lanolin to the skin before applying the electrodes.
4 Apply tincture of benzoin to the skin before applying the electrodes.

Level of Cognitive Ability: Application
Client Needs: Safe and Effective Care Environment

Answer: 4
Rationale: Tincture of benzoin is commonly used with a diaphoretic client to help the electrodes adhere to the skin. Placing adhesive tape or a clear dressing over the electrodes will not help the adhesive gel of the actual electrode make better contact with the diaphoretic skin. Lanolin or any other lotion makes the skin slippery and prevents good initial adherence.

Test-Taking Strategy: Use the process of elimination, and focus on the subject—keeping the electrodes from coming loose; this will assist you with eliminating option 3. Note that options 1 and 2 are comparable or alike in that they both provide an external form of providing security for the electrodes. Only option 4 addresses direct contact with the skin. Review the application of ECG electrodes to a diaphoretic client if you had difficulty with this question.

Integrated Process: Nursing Process/Implementation
Content Area: Adult Health/Cardiovascular

References
Pagana, K., & Pagana, T. (2009). *Mosby's diagnostic laboratory test reference* (9th ed., p. 36). St. Louis: Mosby.
Perry, P., & Potter, P. (2010). *Clinical nursing skills and techniques* (7th ed., p. 1192). St. Louis: Mosby.

---

121. A nurse observes a client wringing his hands and looking frightened. The client reports that he is feeling out of control. Which approach by the nurse will maintain a safe environment?

1 Isolate the client in a "time-out" room.
2 Move the client to a quiet room and talk about his feelings.
3 Observe the client in an ongoing manner but do not intervene.
4 Administer the ordered as-needed anxiety medication immediately.

Level of Cognitive Ability: Application
Client Needs: Safe and Effective Care Environment
Integrated Process: Nursing Process/Implementation
Content Area: Mental Health

Answer: 2
Rationale: The anxiety symptoms demonstrated by this client require some form of intervention. Moving the client decreases environmental stimulus, and talking gives the nurse an opportunity to identify the cause of the client's feelings and to identify appropriate interventions. Isolation is appropriate if the client is a danger to himself or others. There is no indication in the question that the client poses a threat to others. Medication is used only when other noninvasive approaches have been unsuccessful.

Test-Taking Strategy: Use the process of elimination, and note the strategic word *frightened.* Eliminate options 3 and 4 first, recalling that an intervention is necessary and that medication is used only when other noninvasive approaches have been unsuccessful. From the remaining options, select option 2 because it addresses the client's feelings. Review the care of the client with anxiety if you had difficulty with this question.

Reference
Varcarolis, E., & Halter, M. (2009). *Essentials of psychiatric mental health nursing: A communication approach to evidence-based care* (p. 132). St. Louis: Saunders.

---

122. A client has Buck's extension traction applied to the right leg. The nurse should perform which safe intervention to prevent complications of the device?

1 Provide pin care once per shift.
2 Inspect the skin of the right leg frequently.
3 Massage the skin of the right leg with lotion every 8 hours.
4 Release the weights on the right leg for range-of-motion exercises daily.

Level of Cognitive Ability: Application
Client Needs: Safe and Effective Care Environment
Integrated Process: Nursing Process/Implementation
Content Area: Adult Health/Musculoskeletal

Answer: 2
Rationale: Buck's extension traction is a type of skin traction. The nurse inspects the skin of the limb in traction frequently for irritation or inflammation. Massaging the skin with lotion is not indicated. The nurse never releases the weights of traction unless specifically ordered to do so by the physician. There are no pins to care for with skin traction.

Test-Taking Strategy: Use the process of elimination. Knowledge of Buck's extension traction allows you to eliminate options 1 and 4. There are no pins, and the nurse never removes weights without a specific order to do so. Because the apparatus and traction would have to be removed to apply lotion, the correct answer is to inspect the skin. Also note that option 2 addresses the first step of the nursing process, data collection. Review the care of the client in Buck's extension traction if you had difficulty with this question.

Reference
Ignatavicius, D., & Workman, M. (2010). *Medical-surgical nursing: Patient-centered collaborative care* (6th ed., p. 1190). St. Louis: Saunders.

123. A nurse is assisting during a code, and the physician is preparing to defibrillate the client. Which item can safely remain in contact with the client while the client is defibrillated?

1 Oxygen
2 Ventilator
3 Backboard
4 Nitroglycerin patch

Level of Cognitive Ability: Application
Client Needs: Safe and Effective Care Environment
Integrated Process: Nursing Process/Implementation
Content Area: Adult Health/Cardiovascular

Answer: 3

Rationale: Flammable materials such as oxygen, metal devices, and liquids that are capable of carrying electricity are removed from the client and bed before defibrillation. The nitroglycerin patch may have a metal backing and should be removed. A ventilator delivers oxygen to the client. The backboard is needed to immediately resume cardiopulmonary resuscitation (CPR) if defibrillation is unsuccessful.

Test-Taking Strategy: Use the process of elimination. Options 1 and 2 are comparable or alike and so are eliminated first. From the remaining options, remember that the nitroglycerin patch may have a metallic backing and should be removed. Review the principles of CPR if you had difficulty with this question.

References

Ignatavicius, D., & Workman, M. (2010). *Medical-surgical nursing: Patient-centered collaborative care* (6th ed., pp. 756-757). Philadelphia: Saunders.

Perry, A., & Potter, P. (2010). *Clinical nursing skills & techniques* (7th ed., pp. 725-727). St. Louis: Mosby.

---

124. A licensed practical nurse (LPN) is reinforcing the discharge instructions provided by the registered nurse to an adult client who is a victim of family violence. The LPN plans to include:

1 Specific information about self-defense classes
2 Instructions to call the police the next time the abuse occurs
3 Exploration of the pros and cons of remaining with the abusive family member
4 Specific information regarding safe havens and shelters in the client's neighborhood

Level of Cognitive Ability: Application
Client Needs: Safe and Effective Care Environment
Integrated Process: Nursing Process/Planning
Content Area: Mental Health

Answer: 4

Rationale: Assisting the victim of family violence with a specific plan for removing himself or herself from the abuser (e.g., safe havens, hotlines) is essential. An abused person is usually reluctant to call the police. Teaching the victim to fight back (e.g., self-defense classes) is not appropriate when dealing with a violent person. An exploration of the pros and cons of remaining with the abusive family member is an inappropriate and unhelpful intervention.

Test-Taking Strategy: Use Maslow's Hierarchy of Needs theory to recall that safety is the priority when a physiological condition is not present. Option 4 addresses safety. Review the care of the client who is a victim of abuse if you had difficulty with this question.

Reference

Varcarolis, E., & Halter, M. (2009). *Essentials of psychiatric mental health nursing: A communication approach to evidence-based care* (p. 390). St. Louis: Saunders.

---

125. A nurse is caring for a client who has recently has a plaster leg cast applied. The nurse should take which safe action to prevent the development of compartment syndrome?

1 Elevate the limb and apply ice to it.
2 Elevate the limb and cover it with bath blankets.
3 Keep the affected leg horizontal and apply heat to it.
4 Place the leg in a slightly dependent position and apply ice to it.

Answer: 1

Rationale: Compartment syndrome is prevented by controlling edema; elevation and the application of ice optimally achieve this. Therefore, options 2, 3, and 4 are incorrect.

Test-Taking Strategy: Use the process of elimination. Knowing that edema is controlled or prevented with limb elevation helps you to eliminate options 3 and 4. From the remaining options, think about the effects of ice as compared with bath blankets. Ice further controls edema, whereas bath blankets produce heat and prevent the air circulation needed for the cast to dry. This will direct you to option 1. Review the measures that prevent compartment syndrome if you had difficulty with this question.

Level of Cognitive Ability: Application
Client Needs: Safe and Effective Care Environment
Integrated Process: Nursing Process/Implementation
Content Area: Adult Health/Musculoskeletal

References

Black, J., & Hawks, J. (2009). *Medical-surgical nursing: Clinical management for positive outcomes* (8th ed., p. 516). St. Louis: Saunders.
Ignatavicius, D., & Workman, M. (2006). *Medical-surgical nursing: Critical thinking for collaborative care* (5th ed., p. 1198). St. Louis: Saunders.
Linton, A. (2007). *Introduction to medical-surgical nursing* (4th ed., p. 921). Philadelphia: Saunders.

---

126. An 8-year-old child admitted to the hospital has a recent history of sexual abuse by an adult family member. The licensed practical nurse assigned to assist with caring for the child notes that the child is withdrawn and appears frightened. Which of the following describes the best plan for the initial nursing encounter to convey concern and support?

1 Introduce yourself and explain to the child that he or she is safe in the hospital.
2 Introduce yourself and tell the child that the nurse would like to sit with him or her for awhile.
3 Introduce yourself and then ask the child to express how he or she feels about the events that led up to this admission.
4 Introduce yourself, explain your role, and ask the child to act out the sexual encounter with the abuser with the use of art therapy.

Level of Cognitive Ability: Application
Client Needs: Safe and Effective Care Environment
Integrated Process: Nursing Process/Implementation
Content Area: Child Health

Answer: 2
Rationale: The initial role of the nurse working with an abused victim is to establish trust. This is accomplished by providing a nonthreatening, stable, and safe environment. Establishing trust takes time. Victims of sexual abuse may exhibit fear and anxiety because of the recent incident. In addition, they may fear further abuse. When initiating contact with a child victim of sexual abuse who demonstrates a fear of others, it is best to convey a willingness to spend time and to move slowly to initiate activities that may be perceived as threatening. After a rapport has been established, the nurse may explore the child's feelings or use various therapeutic modalities to encourage a recounting of the offensive experience.

Test-Taking Strategy: Note the strategic word *initial,* and focus on the subject—conveying concern and support. Option 2 explains how to establish trust during an initial encounter by spending time with the child in a nonthreatening atmosphere. Options 3 and 4 may be implemented after trust and rapport are established. Option 1 may be appropriate but does not convey concern and support on the part of the nurse. Review the care of the child who is a victim of abuse if you had difficulty with this question.

References

Leifer, G. (2007). *Introduction to maternity and pediatric nursing* (5th ed., p. 568). Philadelphia: Saunders.
Price, D., & Gwin, J. (2008). *Pediatric nursing: An introductory text* (10th ed., p. 174). St. Louis: Saunders.

---

127. A physician is about to defibrillate a client with ventricular fibrillation and says, in a loud voice, "CLEAR!" The nurse immediately does which of the following?

1 Removes the backboard
2 Steps away from the bed
3 Shuts off the intravenous (IV) infusion going into the client's arm
4 Places the conductive gel pads for defibrillation on the client's chest

Level of Cognitive Ability: Application
Client Needs: Safe and Effective Care Environment

Answer: 2
Rationale: For the safety of all personnel, everyone must stand back and be clear of all contact with the client and the client's bed when the defibrillator paddles are being discharged. It is the primary responsibility of the person using the defibrillator paddles to communicate the "clear" message loudly enough for all to hear and to ensure everyone's compliance. All personnel must immediately comply with this command. The gel pads should have been placed on the client's chest before the defibrillator paddles were applied. The backboard is left in place for resuming cardiopulmonary resuscitation, if necessary. Shutting off the IV infusion has no useful purpose.

Integrated Process: Nursing Process/Implementation
Content Area: Adult Health/Cardiovascular

Test-Taking Strategy: Use the process of elimination, and focus on the subject of the question—safety during defibrillation. Stepping back from the bed prevents the nurse from being defibrillated along with the client. Review safety measures related to defibrillation if you had difficulty with this question.

Reference

Black, J., & Hawks, J. (2009). *Medical-surgical nursing: Clinical management for positive outcomes* (8th ed., pp. 1470-1471). St. Louis: Saunders.

---

128. A nurse receives a telephone call from the laboratory and is told that an initial report of a urine culture identifies the presence of several different organisms. The nurse evaluates that this most likely means which of the following?

1. The specimen was contaminated.
2. The client has a kidney infection.
3. The client has a bladder infection.
4. The specimen was mishandled in the laboratory.

Level of Cognitive Ability: Comprehension
Client Needs: Safe and Effective Care Environment
Integrated Process: Nursing Process/Evaluation
Content Area: Fundamental Skills

Answer: 1
Rationale: The presence of several different organisms in a urine culture usually indicates that contamination has occurred. The urinary tract is normally sterile, and infection, if it occurs, is usually with one organism. A repeat of the urine culture is indicated.

Test-Taking Strategy: Use the process of elimination, and note the strategic words *most likely*. There is no information in the question that indicates that the laboratory personnel mishandled the specimen. A urine culture will not discriminate between bladder or kidney infection; the clinical picture would help to differentiate this. Remember that specimen contamination is the most frequent reason that several different organisms are cultured; most urinary tract infections are caused by a single organism, such as *Escherichia coli*. Review the causes of specimen contamination if you had difficulty with this question.

References

Chernecky, C., & Berger, B. (2008). *Laboratory tests and diagnostic procedures* (5th ed., pp. 232-233). Philadelphia: Saunders.
Christensen, B., & Kockrow, E. (2006). *Foundations of nursing* (5th ed., p. 502). St. Louis: Mosby.

---

129. A nurse is evaluating the client's safe use of a cane for left-sided weakness. The nurse should intervene and correct the client if the nurse observes the client doing which of the following?

1. Holding the cane on the right side
2. Moving the cane when the right leg is moved
3. Leaning on the cane when the right leg swings through
4. Keeping the cane 6 inches out to the side of the right foot

Level of Cognitive Ability: Comprehension
Client Needs: Safe and Effective Care Environment
Integrated Process: Teaching and Learning
Content Area: Adult Health/Musculoskeletal

Answer: 2
Rationale: The cane is held on the stronger side to minimize stress on the affected extremity and provide a wide base of support. The cane is held 6 inches lateral to the fifth toe and moved forward with the affected leg. The client leans on the cane for added support while the stronger side swings through.

Test-Taking Strategy: Focus on the strategic words *should intervene and correct the client*. Knowing that the cane is held on the stronger side helps you eliminate options 1 and 4 first. To select between the remaining options, recall that the client moves the cane with the weaker leg and leans on it for support when the stronger leg swings through. Review the correct use of a cane if you had difficulty with this question.

Reference

deWit, S. (2009). *Medical-surgical nursing: Concepts & practice* (p. 779). St. Louis: Saunders.

---

130. A nurse instructs a mother caring for an infant with acute infectious diarrhea about measures to prevent the spread of pathogens. Which action by the mother indicates a need for further teaching?

1 Washes the infant's hands after changing the diaper
2 Restrains the infant's hands when changing the diaper
3 Places the soiled diaper in a sealed, double plastic bag
4 Applies a cloth diaper snugly after cleaning the perineum

Level of Cognitive Ability: Comprehension
Client Needs: Safe and Effective Care Environment
Integrated Process: Teaching and Learning
Content Area: Child Health

Answer: 4
Rationale: Cloth diapers do not have elastic in the legs; this could allow for seepage of the infectious stool and cause the spread of pathogens. Also, liquid stool makes the diaper wet, which also promotes the spread of disease. Disposable plastic diapers have elastic in the legs, high absorbency, and plastic on the outside; these features decrease the transmission of pathogens. Option 1 prevents the spread of pathogens through handwashing. Option 2 prevents the infant from coming into contact with the infectious material. Option 3 identifies the appropriate disposal of infectious waste.

Test-Taking Strategy: Note the strategic words *need for further teaching.* These words indicate a negative event query and ask you to select an option that is an incorrect action by the mother. Use the principles of standard precautions, which include handwashing, the proper disposal of body fluids and waste, and avoiding contact with body fluid. The only option that does not accurately reflect these precautions is option 4. Review standard precautions if you had difficulty with this question.

Reference
Leifer, G. (2007). *Introduction to maternity and pediatric nursing* (5th ed., pp. 297, 302, 678). Philadelphia: Saunders.

---

131. A nurse administers medications to the wrong client. During the investigation of the incident, it was determined that the nurse failed to check the client's identification bracelet before administering the medications. In this event, negligence has occurred because negligence is:

1 Strictly prohibited by the institution's own policies
2 Strictly prohibited by the state's nurse practice act
3 Defined as a crime that results in the injury of a client
4 Defined as the failure to meet established standards of care

Level of Cognitive Ability: Comprehension
Client Needs: Safe and Effective Care Environment
Integrated Process: Nursing Process/Evaluation
Content Area: Fundamental Skills

Answer: 4
Rationale: The legal definition of negligence is the failure to meet accepted standards of care. Option 3 is an incorrect definition of negligence, although injury may have come to the client as a result of the error. Both the institution and the nurse practice act have provisions that identify and discourage acts of negligence.

Test-Taking Strategy: Use the process of elimination. Options 1 and 2 are true in that the purpose of the nurse practice act and of the institutional policies and procedures is to protect the public from harm; however, they identify and discourage acts of negligence rather than "strictly prohibit" negligence. From the remaining options, select option 4 because it is the umbrella option. Review the concepts related to negligence if you had difficulty with this question.

Reference
Christensen, B., & Kockrow, E. (2006). *Foundations of nursing* (5th ed., pp. 22, 24). St. Louis: Mosby.

---

132. A nurse is told that an assigned client has acquired methicillin-resistant *Staphylococcus aureus* (MRSA). In addition to standard precautions, the nurse places the client on which type of transmission-based precautions?

Answer: 2
Rationale: Contact precautions are precautions that include standard precautions and the use of barrier precautions such as gloves and impermeable gowns. Contact precautions are used for clients with diarrhea, antibiotic-resistant infections, or draining wounds that are not contained by sterile dressings. The goal of these precautions is to eliminate disease transmission from direct

1 Enteric precautions
2 Contact precautions
3 Airborne precautions
4 Respiratory precautions

Level of Cognitive Ability: Application
Client Needs: Safe and Effective Care Environment
Integrated Process: Nursing Process/ Implementation
Content Area: Fundamental Skills

contact with the client or from indirect contact through an intermediary infected object or surface that has been in contact with the client (e.g., instruments, linens, dressing materials). Enteric precautions, airborne precautions, and respiratory precautions are not necessary.

Test-Taking Strategy: Focus on the client's diagnosis, and think about the method of transmission of the infection to others. Eliminate options 3 and 4 first because they are comparable or alike. Recalling that MRSA can be transmitted by contact with the infecting organism will assist with directing you to option 2. Review contact precautions if you had difficulty with this question.

Reference

Christensen, B., & Kockrow, E. (2006). *Foundations of nursing* (5th ed., p. 293). St. Louis: Mosby.

---

133. A prenatal client who has acquired the sexually transmitted virus *Condyloma acuminatum* (human papillomavirus) asks the nurse to again explain the treatment of the infection. The nurse should reinforce additional information about which of the following safe treatments with this client?
1 Laser therapy
2 Interferon therapy
3 Cytotoxic medications
4 No therapy is available for this condition.

Level of Cognitive Ability: Application
Client Needs: Safe and Effective Care Environment
Integrated Process: Nursing Process/ Implementation
Content Area: Maternity/Antepartum

Answer: 1
Rationale: For the pregnant client, laser therapy is the most effective method of destroying human papillomavirus. This therapy is localized, whereas medications (which are considered toxic to the fetus) would have a systemic effect. The primary neonatal effect of the virus is respiratory or laryngeal papillomatosis, although the exact route of perinatal transmission is unknown. Options 2, 3, and 4 are incorrect.

Test-Taking Strategy: Use the process of elimination, and begin by eliminating option 4. Remember that options that are comparable or alike are not likely to be correct. With this in mind, eliminate options 2 and 3 next because they are both medications. Review the care of the prenatal client with a *Condyloma acuminatum* infection if you had difficulty with this question.

Reference

Leifer, G. (2008). *Maternity nursing: An introductory text* (10th ed., p. 393). Philadelphia: Saunders.

---

134. A licensed practical nurse (LPN) has been instructed to move a client from the bed to a chair 1 day after a total knee replacement. The LPN reviews the physician's orders and should expect to note which of the following orders to protect the knee joint?
1 Obtain a walker to minimize weight bearing by the client on the affected leg.
2 Lift the client to the bedside chair, leaving the continuous passive motion (CPM) machine in place.
3 Apply a compression bandage around the dressing, and put ice on the knee while the client is seated.

Answer: 4
Rationale: On the first postoperative day, the nurse assists the client with getting out of bed after stabilizing the affected joint with a knee immobilizer. The surgeon orders weight-bearing limits on the affected leg. The leg is elevated while the client is sitting in the chair to minimize edema. A compression dressing should already be in place on the wound. The CPM machine is used only while the client is in bed. Ambulation is not started until the second postoperative day.

Test-Taking Strategy: Use the process of elimination. Focus on the subject—the protection of the knee joint. This will direct you to option 4 because a knee immobilizer will protect the joint. Review postoperative care after a total knee replacement if you had difficulty with this question.

4 Apply a knee immobilizer before moving the client, and elevate the leg that has been operated on while the client is seated.

Level of Cognitive Ability: Comprehension
Client Needs: Safe and Effective Care Environment
Integrated Process: Nursing Process/Implementation
Content Area: Adult Health/Musculoskeletal

References

Christensen, B., & Kockrow, E. (2006). *Adult health nursing* (5th ed., p. 146). St. Louis: Mosby.

Ignatavicius, D., & Workman, M. (2010). *Medical-surgical nursing: Patient-centered collaborative care* (6th ed., pp. 333-334). St. Louis: Saunders.

---

135. A nurse is collecting information from a client about the client's suicide potential. The nurse should ask the client which significant question?

1 "Why do you want to hurt yourself?"
2 "Do you have a plan to commit suicide?"
3 "Has anyone in your family committed suicide?"
4 "Can you describe how you are feeling right now?"

Level of Cognitive Ability: Application
Client Needs: Safe and Effective Care Environment
Integrated Process: Nursing Process/Data Collection
Content Area: Mental Health

Answer: 2

Rationale: When collecting information about suicide risk, the nurse must determine if the client has a suicide plan. Clients who have a definitive plan pose a greater risk for suicide. Options 1, 3, and 4 do not directly provide this information.

Test-Taking Strategy: Use the process of elimination, and note the strategic word *significant.* Option 2 directly determines the presence of a suicide plan. Review the risks for suicide potential if you had difficulty with this question.

References

deWit, S. (2009). *Medical-surgical nursing: Concepts & practice* (pp. 1113-1114). St. Louis: Saunders.

Varcarolis, E., & Halter, M. (2009). *Essentials of psychiatric mental health nursing: A communication approach to evidence-based care* (pp. 416-417). St. Louis: Saunders.

---

136. A client is admitted to a long-term care facility with a diagnosis of Parkinson's disease. The nurse gives information about the client's condition to a visitor assumed to be a family member. The nurse has violated which legal concept of the nurse–client relationship?

1 Incompetency
2 Invasion of privacy
3 Communication techniques
4 Teaching and learning principles

Level of Cognitive Ability: Comprehension
Client Needs: Safe and Effective Care Environment
Integrated Process: Nursing Process/Implementation
Content Area: Fundamental Skills

Answer: 2

Rationale: Discussing a client's condition without the client's permission violates the client's rights and places the nurse in legal jeopardy. This action is an invasion of privacy and affects the client's confidentiality. Incompetence could lead to negligence, but this legal concept is not related to the subject identified in the question. Communication techniques relate to the nurse–client relationship. Teaching and learning principles are considered concepts of standards of practice.

Test-Taking Strategy: Use the process of elimination. Focus on the subject of the question—the sharing of information—to direct you to option 2. Review client rights if you had difficulty with this question.

Reference

Christensen, B., & Kockrow, E. (2006). *Foundations of nursing* (5th ed., p. 25). St. Louis: Mosby.

---

137. A client has an order for valproic acid (Depakene) 250 mg once daily. To maximize the client's safety, the nurse plans to schedule the medication:

1 With lunch
2 At bedtime

Answer: 2

Rationale: Valproic acid is an anticonvulsant that causes central nervous system (CNS) depression. Its side effects include sedation, dizziness, ataxia, and confusion. When the client is taking this medication as a single daily dose, administering it at bedtime negates the risk of injury from sedation and enhances client safety.

3 After breakfast
4 Before breakfast

Level of Cognitive Ability: Application
Client Needs: Safe and Effective Care Environment
Integrated Process: Nursing Process/Implementation
Content Area: Pharmacology

Test-Taking Strategy: Use the process of elimination. Note the strategic words *maximize the client's safety.* Recalling that this medication is an anticonvulsant with CNS depressant properties leads you to think of sedation as a side effect. Select option 2 because it allows the sedative effects of the medication to occur at a time when the client is sleeping and therefore the client is less likely to become injured. Review the side effects of valproic acid if you had difficulty with this question.

Reference

Kee, J., Hayes, E., & McCuistion, L. (2009). *Pharmacology: A nursing process approach* (6th ed., p. 329). St. Louis: Saunders.

---

138. A client who had a synthetic cast placed on the right arm 24 hours ago to treat a fractured ulna tells the nurse that he wants to take a shower. Based on the review of the data related to the injury and the type of cast, which of the following is the best response to ensure a safe environment?

1 "The cast padding will never dry."
2 "It may lead to a serious infection."
3 "Hot water may soften the synthetic cast."
4 "It is not safe for you to shower at this time."

Level of Cognitive Ability: Application
Client Needs: Safe and Effective Care Environment
Integrated Process: Nursing Process/Implementation
Content Area: Adult Health/Musculoskeletal

Answer: 4
Rationale: It may be unsafe for the client to shower with a cast on the arm because the client could slip and fall. Water does not damage the synthetic cast; however, the cast padding could get wet, and wet padding traps moisture that may lead to skin maceration and breakdown. Water may soften a plaster cast, but it has no effect on a synthetic cast. A shower will not cause an infection.

Test-Taking Strategy: Note the strategic words *synthetic* and *best response.* Also note the close-ended word *never* in option 1. Use Maslow's Hierarchy of Needs theory. Option 4 specifically addresses safety. Review the care of the client with a synthetic cast if you had difficulty with this question.

Reference

Linton, A. (2007). *Introduction to medical-surgical nursing* (4th ed., p. 922). Philadelphia: Saunders.

---

139. A client is prepared to receive elective cardioversion to treat atrial fibrillation. Which of the following is an unsafe preprocedure observation?

1 The client's digoxin has been withheld for the last 48 hours.
2 The defibrillator has the synchronizer turned on and is set at 50 joules.
3 The client has received an intravenous (IV) dose of midazolam (Versed).
4 The client is wearing a nasal cannula that is delivering oxygen at 2 L/min.

Level of Cognitive Ability: Comprehension
Client Needs: Safe and Effective Care Environment
Integrated Process: Nursing Process/Data Collection
Content Area: Adult Health/Cardiovascular

Answer: 4
Rationale: Digoxin may be withheld for up to 48 hours before cardioversion because it increases ventricular irritability and may cause ventricular dysrhythmias after countershock. The client typically receives an IV dose of a sedative or antianxiety agent. The defibrillator is switched to synchronizer mode to time the delivery of the electrical impulse to coincide with the QRS wave and to avoid the T wave, which could cause ventricular fibrillation; the energy level is typically set at 50 to 100 joules. During the procedure, any oxygen is removed temporarily because oxygen supports combustion, and a fire could result from electrical arcing.

Test-Taking Strategy: Note the strategic words *unsafe preprocedure observation.* Recalling the concepts related to oxygen combustion will direct you to option 4. Review the procedures related to defibrillation and cardioversion if you had difficulty with this question.

Reference

Ignatavicius, D., & Workman, M. (2010). *Medical-surgical nursing: Patient-centered collaborative care* (6th ed., p. 756). St. Louis: Saunders.

---

140. A nurse administers an incorrect dose of digoxin (Lanoxin) to a client. During the subsequent investigation of the error, it is determined that the nurse did not note the client's heart rate of 45 beats per minute before administering the medication. Failure to adequately collect data in this event is addressed under which function of the nurse practice act?

1. Defining the specific educational requirements for licensure in the state
2. Describing the scope of practice of licensed and unlicensed care providers
3. Identifying the process for disciplinary action if standards of care are not met
4. Recommending specific terms of incarceration for nurses who violate the law

Level of Cognitive Ability: Comprehension
Client Needs: Safe and Effective Care Environment
Integrated Process: Nursing Process/Data Collection
Content Area: Fundamental Skills

Answer: 3
Rationale: In this scenario, acceptable standards of care were not met (i.e., the nurse failed to adequately assess the client before administering a medication). Option 3 refers specifically to the event described in the question, whereas options 1, 2, and 4 do not.

Test-Taking Strategy: Focus on the information provided in the question, and use the process of elimination to direct you to option 3, which refers specifically to the event described in the question. Review information related to the nurse practice act if you had difficulty with this question.

References

deWit, S. (2009). *Medical-surgical nursing: Concepts & practice.* (pp. 2, 17). St. Louis: Saunders.

Potter, P., & Perry, A. (2009). *Fundamentals of nursing* (7th ed., p. 705). St. Louis: Mosby.

---

141. A nurse is observing a nursing assistant talking to a client who is hearing impaired. The nurse should intervene if the nursing assistant does which of the following while communicating with the client?

1. Speaks in a normal tone
2. Speaks clearly to the client
3. Faces the client when speaking
4. Speaks directly into the impaired ear

Level of Cognitive Ability: Application
Client Needs: Safe and Effective Care Environment
Integrated Process: Nursing Process/Implementation
Content Area: Leadership/Management

Answer: 4
Rationale: When communicating with a hearing-impaired client, the nurse should speak in a normal tone to the client and should not shout. The nurse should talk directly to the client while facing him or her and speak clearly. If the client does not seem to understand what is said, the nurse should express the statement differently. Moving closer to the client and toward the better ear may facilitate communication, but the nurse should avoid talking directly into the impaired ear.

Test-Taking Strategy: Use the process of elimination. Note the strategic words *the nurse should intervene* and *directly into the impaired ear;* this will direct you to option 4. Review communication techniques to use when dealing with hearing-impaired clients if you had difficulty with this question.

Reference

deWit, S. (2009). *Medical-surgical nursing: Concepts & practice* (p. 630). St. Louis: Saunders.

---

142. Which statement made by a nursing student indicates an understanding of the concepts associated with suicide and suicidal intentions?

1. "Only psychotic individuals commit suicide."
2. "Suicide attempts are just attention-seeking behaviors."

Answer: 4
Rationale: Most people who commit suicide have given definite clues or warnings about their intentions. The individual who is suicidal is not necessarily psychotic or even mentally ill. A suicide attempt is not an attention-seeking behavior, and each act should be taken very seriously. Suicide is not an inherited condition; it is an individual condition.

3 "Suicide runs in the family, so there is nothing that health care personnel can do about it."
4 "Many individuals who really do kill themselves have talked about their suicidal intentions to others."

Level of Cognitive Ability: Comprehension
Client Needs: Safe and Effective Care Environment
Integrated Process: Nursing Process/Evaluation
Content Area: Mental Health

Test-Taking Strategy: Use the process of elimination. Eliminate option 1 because of the word *only.* Eliminate option 2 because of the words *just attention-seeking behaviors.* Eliminate option 3 because of the words *there is nothing that health care personnel can do about it.* Review concepts related to suicide if you had difficulty with this question.

Reference
Fortinash, K., & Holoday-Worret, P. (2008). *Psychiatric mental health nursing* (4th ed., p. 469). St. Louis: Mosby.

---

143. A nurse working in a crisis center receives a telephone call from a client who states that he wants to kill himself and has a loaded gun on the table. Which of the following is the best initial nursing intervention?
1 Try to contact the physician.
2 Ask the client why he wants to kill himself.
3 Keep the client talking and ask for consent to send medical assistance to help him.
4 Insist that the client give you his name and address so that you can send the police immediately.

Level of Cognitive Ability: Application
Client Needs: Safe and Effective Care Environment
Integrated Process: Nursing Process/Implementation
Content Area: Mental Health

Answer: 3
Rationale: During a crisis, the nurse must take an authoritative, active role to promote the client's safety. When a client verbalizes that he has a loaded gun in his home and wants to kill himself, the client's safety is the primary concern. Keeping the client on the phone and asking the client for consent to send medical assistance is the best intervention. Insisting may anger the client and cause him to hang up. Asking the client why he wants to kill himself is not the initial intervention. Likewise, contacting the physician is not the appropriate intervention at this time.

Test-Taking Strategy: Use the process of elimination, keeping the focus of the client's safety in mind. Option 3 is the umbrella option and encompasses the necessary actions. Review emergency measures during a suicide-related crisis if you had difficulty with this question.

Reference
Varcarolis, E., & Halter, M. (2009). *Essentials of psychiatric mental health nursing: A communication approach to evidence-based care* (pp. 417-418). St. Louis: Saunders.

---

144. A nurse in a long-term care facility determines the need to place a vest restraint on a client, but the client does not want a vest restraint applied. The best nursing action is to:
1 Contact the physician.
2 Apply the restraint anyway.
3 Compromise with the client and use wrist restraints.
4 Medicate the client with a sedative and then apply the restraint.

Level of Cognitive Ability: Application
Client Needs: Safe and Effective Care Environment
Integrated Process: Nursing Process/Implementation
Content Area: Fundamental Skills

Answer: 1
Rationale: The use of restraints should be avoided if possible. If the nurse determines that a restraint is necessary, the procedure should be discussed with the client's family, and an order should be obtained from the physician. The physician's order protects the nurse from liability. The nurse should carefully explain to the client and the client's family the reasons that the restraint is necessary, the type of restraint selected, and the anticipated duration of restraint.

Test-Taking Strategy: Use the process of elimination. Eliminate option 2 first; if the nurse applied the restraint to a client who was refusing the procedure, then the nurse could be charged with battery. Options 2 and 4 are comparable or alike, so option 4 can be eliminated next. Option 3 could be an unsafe and ineffective procedure if the vest restraint was initially considered necessary. Review the issues surrounding the use of restraints if you had difficulty with this question.

Reference
deWit, S. (2009). *Medical-surgical nursing: Concepts & practice* (p. 198). St. Louis: Saunders.

145. A client is being discharged from the hospital and will receive oxygen therapy at home. The nurse is reinforcing instructions with the client and family about oxygen safety measures in the home. Which statement indicates that the client requires further instruction?

1 "I will call the physician if I experience any shortness of breath."
2 "I will keep my scented candles within 5 feet of my oxygen tank."
3 "I will not sit in front of my wood-burning fireplace with my oxygen on."
4 "I realize that I should check the oxygen level of the portable tank frequently."

Level of Cognitive Ability: Comprehension
Client Needs: Safe and Effective Care Environment
Integrated Process: Teaching and Learning
Content Area: Fundamental Skills

Answer: 2
Rationale: Oxygen is a highly combustible gas. Although it will not spontaneously burn or cause an explosion, oxygen can easily cause a fire to ignite in a client's room if it comes in contact with a spark from a cigarette, a candle, or electrical equipment. Oxygen in high concentrations is highly combustible and causes fire to spread quickly. The client should contact the physician if shortness of breath occurs.

Test-Taking Strategy: Use the process of elimination. Note the strategic words *requires instruction.* These words indicate a negative event query and ask you to select an option that is an incorrect client statement. Remembering that oxygen is a highly combustible gas will direct you to option 2. Review teaching points related to home care and oxygen if you had difficulty with this question.

Reference
deWit, S. (2009). *Medical-surgical nursing: Concepts & practice* (p. 352). St. Louis: Saunders.

---

146. A nurse is assisting with planning care for a client diagnosed with deep vein thrombosis (DVT) of the left leg. Which intervention should the nurse plan to avoid?

1 Elevating the client's left leg
2 Applying moist heat to the client's left leg
3 Ambulating the client in the hall once per shift
4 Administering acetaminophen (Tylenol) to the client, as prescribed

Level of Cognitive Ability: Application
Client Needs: Safe and Effective Care Environment
Integrated Process: Nursing Process/Planning
Content Area: Adult Health/Cardiovascular

Answer: 3
Rationale: Standard management of the client with DVT includes bedrest for the length of time prescribed; limb elevation; relief of discomfort with warm, moist heat and analgesics, as needed; anticoagulant therapy; and monitoring for signs of pulmonary embolism. Ambulation is contraindicated because it increases the likelihood of dislodgement of the thrombus, which could travel to the lungs and become a pulmonary embolism.

Test-Taking Strategy: Use the process of elimination. Note the strategic word *avoid;* this word indicates a negative event query and asks you to select an option that is an incorrect action. The application of heat and limb elevation are indicated to reduce inflammation and edema, so options 1 and 2 are eliminated. Tylenol relieves discomfort and is also indicated. This leaves ambulation, which could lead to pulmonary embolism. Review the care of the client with DVT if you had difficulty with this question.

Reference
Linton, A. (2007). *Introduction to medical-surgical nursing* (4th ed., pp. 710-711). Philadelphia: Saunders.

---

147. A nurse is assisting with the care of a client in labor who has a history of sickle cell anemia. Knowing that the client has a high risk for sickling crisis during labor, the nurse should give priority to implementing which safe nursing action to prevent a crisis from occurring?

1 Reassure and encourage the client.
2 Maintain strict handwashing technique.

Answer: 3
Rationale: Administering oxygen as needed is an effective intervention to prevent sickle cell crisis during labor. The client is at high risk for being unable to meet the oxygen demands of labor and thus unable to prevent sickling. Option 1 is a generally helpful nursing measure, but it is not related to the prevention of sickling crisis. Option 2 is a safe nursing action, but it does nothing to prevent sickling crisis. Option 4 is not realistic and would not prevent sickling crisis.

3 Ensure that the client uses oxygen during labor.
4 Remind the client to not bear down for more than 3 seconds

Level of Cognitive Ability: Application
Client Needs: Safe and Effective Care Environment
Integrated Process: Nursing Process/Implementation
Content Area: Maternity/Intrapartum

Test-Taking Strategy: Focus on the subject of the question—a safe nursing action that will help prevent sickling crisis. Note that the question contains the strategic word *priority*, and use the ABCs—airway, breathing, and circulation. Select the option that addresses the subject of the question and that supports the client's airway. Review measures to prevent sickle cell crisis if you had difficulty with this question.

Reference

Leifer, G. (2008). *Maternity nursing: An introductory text* (10th ed., p. 265). Philadelphia: Saunders.

---

148. A client who is admitted to the labor and delivery unit in labor has active genital herpes lesions present in the genital tract. The licensed practical nurse should reinforce the teaching given by the registered nurse about which of the following immediate plans for the client?
1 Placement on protective isolation
2 Preparation for a cesarean delivery
3 Preparation for spontaneous vaginal delivery
4 Imminent artificial rupture of the membranes

Level of Cognitive Ability: Application
Client Needs: Safe and Effective Care Environment
Integrated Process: Teaching and Learning
Content Area: Maternity/Intrapartum

Answer: 2
Rationale: Cesarean delivery reduces the risk of neonatal infection from a mother in labor who has either herpetic genital tract lesions or ruptured membranes. Options 3 and 4 would expose the fetus to the virus. Standard precautions are necessary, but protective isolation is not.

Test-Taking Strategy: Use the process of elimination, and note the strategic words *lesions present in the genital tract.* Use your knowledge of the labor process and disease transmission to reason that the infant should not be born vaginally; this would help you to eliminate option 3. Eliminate option 4 next, knowing that this could also expose the fetus to the virus. Eliminate option 1 because standard precautions are needed but protective isolation is not. Review the care of the client with active genital herpes lesions if you had difficulty with this question.

Reference

Leifer, G. (2008). *Maternity nursing: An introductory text* (10th ed., p. 270). Philadelphia: Saunders.

---

149. A client with possible renal disease is scheduled to undergo diagnostic testing by intravenous pyelogram (IVP). To ensure client safety, the nurse should be certain to collect data from this client about a history of which of the following?
1 Allergy to shellfish or iodine
2 Family incidence of renal disease
3 Frequent and chronic antibiotic use
4 Long-term use of diuretic medications

Level of Cognitive Ability: Application
Client Needs: Safe and Effective Care Environment
Integrated Process: Nursing Process/Data Collection
Content Area: Adult Health/Renal

Answer: 1
Rationale: A client undergoing diagnostic testing that involves the use of a contrast medium (e.g., IVP) should be questioned about allergy to shellfish, seafood, or iodine; this would identify a potential allergic reaction to the contrast dye that may be used in such a test. The other items are useful as part of the general health history, but they are not as critical as the allergy determination.

Test-Taking Strategy: Use the process of elimination. Note the strategic words *to ensure client safety.* These words imply that more than one or all of the options may be correct but that one of them is most important for the client's safety. Eliminate options 3 and 4 first because they both involve collecting data about prior medication therapy. Choose correctly between the remaining options by using your knowledge of the IVP procedure. Review preprocedure care for an IVP if you had difficulty with this question.

Reference

Chernecky, C., & Berger, B. (2008). *Laboratory tests and diagnostic procedures* (5th ed., p. 682). Philadelphia: Saunders.

---

150. A nurse is carrying out an order for a 24-hour urine collection for a client with a suspected renal disorder. Which of the following actions should the nurse avoid to ensure proper collection technique?

1 Refrigerate the container or place it on ice.
2 Save all voidings after the first one during the 24-hour period.
3 Ask the client to void at the end time, and add this specimen to the container.
4 Ask the client to void at the start time, and place this specimen in the container.

Level of Cognitive Ability: Application
Client Needs: Safe and Effective Care Environment
Integrated Process: Nursing Process/Implementation
Content Area: Adult Health/Renal

Answer: 4

Rationale: To collect a 24-hour urine specimen, the nurse should ask the client to void at the beginning of the collection period and then discard the urine sample. This is done because the urine in that voiding has been in the bladder for an unknown period of time. All subsequent voided urine is saved in a container, which is placed on ice or refrigerated. The nurse should ask the client to void at the finish time and then add this sample to the collection. The nurse labels the container, places it on fresh ice, and sends it to the laboratory immediately.

Test-Taking Strategy: Note the strategic word *avoid;* this word indicates a negative event query and asks you to select an option that is an incorrect nursing action. Focus on the subject of the question—proper collection technique for a 24-hour urine specimen. Visualize the procedure, and use your knowledge of this basic procedure to answer the question. Review the procedure for a 24-hour urine collection if you had difficulty with this question.

Reference

deWit, S. (2009). *Medical-surgical nursing: Concepts & practice* (p. 821). St. Louis: Saunders.

---

151. A licensed practical nurse assisting a registered nurse with caring for a client in active labor should do which of the following to best prevent fetal heart rate decelerations?

1 Begin preparations for a cesarean delivery.
2 Encourage upright or side-lying maternal positions.
3 Measure maternal and fetal vital signs every 30 minutes.
4 Suggest asking the physician about the advisability of an oxytocin (Pitocin) drip.

Level of Cognitive Ability: Application
Client Needs: Safe and Effective Care Environment
Integrated Process: Nursing Process/Implementation
Content Area: Maternity/Intrapartum

Answer: 2

Rationale: Side-lying and upright positions (e.g., walking, standing, squatting) can improve venous return and encourage effective uterine activity, which in turn will reduce the likelihood of fetal heart rate decelerations. Cesarean delivery will not prevent decelerations. Measuring the vital signs every 30 minutes will do nothing to prevent decelerations. Oxytocin could aggravate fetal heart rate decelerations because of increased uterine activity and decreased uteroplacental perfusion.

Test-Taking Strategy: Use the process of elimination, and note the strategic words *prevent fetal heart rate decelerations.* Eliminate each of the incorrect options because they do not have an immediate effect on the physiological status of the mother or the fetus. Remember that side-lying and upright positions will encourage effective uterine activity and provide a safe environment. Review measures to prevent fetal heart rate decelerations if you had difficulty with this question.

Reference

Leifer, G. (2008). *Maternity nursing: An introductory text* (10th ed., p. 116). Philadelphia: Saunders.

---

152. A nurse employed in a clinic is assisting with the care of a client with diabetes mellitus who is 36 weeks pregnant. The results of three previous weekly nonstress tests have been reactive, but this week the test was nonreactive after 40 minutes. The nurse should expect that

Answer: 1

Rationale: A nonreactive test requires further evaluation, thus indicating the need for a contraction stress test. To send the client home for 3 days could place the fetus in jeopardy. Hospitalizing the client for either induction of labor or continuous fetal monitoring is premature without further diagnostic test data.

the physician will prescribe which of the following to safely monitor this client?
1 A contraction stress test
2 Admission to the hospital for continuous fetal monitoring
3 Admission to the hospital for immediate induction of labor
4 A follow-up appointment in 3 days to repeat the nonstress test

Level of Cognitive Ability: Analysis
Client Needs: Safe and Effective Care Environment
Integrated Process: Nursing Process/Planning
Content Area: Maternity/Antepartum

Test-Taking Strategy: Use the process of elimination. Begin to answer this question by eliminating options 2 and 3 because they are unnecessary at this time. Choose correctly between the remaining options by selecting the one that provides further evaluation. Review the meanings of nonstress test results if you had difficulty with this question.

Reference
Leifer, G. (2008). *Maternity nursing: An introductory text* (10th ed., p. 65). Philadelphia: Saunders.

---

153. A nurse who begins to administer medications to a client via a nasogastric feeding tube suspects that the tube has become clogged. Which of the following safe actions should the nurse take first?
1 Aspirate the tube.
2 Flush the tube with warm water.
3 Prepare to remove and replace the tube.
4 Flush the tube with a carbonated liquid such as cola.

Level of Cognitive Ability: Application
Client Needs: Safe and Effective Care Environment
Integrated Process: Nursing Process/Implementation
Content Area: Fundamental Skills

Answer: 1
Rationale: The nurse should first attempt to unclog the feeding tube by aspirating it. If this does not work, the nurse should try to flush the tube with warm water. Carbonated liquids such as cola may also be used, but only if agency policy identifies this practice as acceptable. The replacement of the tube is the last step if others are unsuccessful.

Test-Taking Strategy: Use the process of elimination, and note the strategic word *first*. Focusing on this word and noting the word *clogged* will direct you to option 1. Review interventions for a clogged nasogastric feeding tube if you had difficulty with this question.

Reference
deWit, S. (2009). *Medical-surgical nursing: Concepts & practice* (p. 705). St. Louis: Saunders.

---

154. A client with depression who was admitted to the psychiatric unit the previous day suddenly begins smiling and stating that the current episode of depression has lifted. The client continues to be talkative and engages in conversation with other clients on the unit. The licensed practical nurse consults with the registered nurse, knowing that which of the following changes should be made to the client's treatment plan?
1 Allow increased in-room activities.
2 Increase the level of suicide precautions.
3 Allow the client to spend time off of the unit.

Answer: 2
Rationale: A depressed client who has been hospitalized for only 1 day is unlikely to have a dramatic cure. A sudden elevation in mood probably indicates that the client has decided to harm himself or herself, so an increase in the level of suicide precautions is indicated to keep the client safe. Option 1 is not indicated, and options 3 and 4 could place the client at increased risk.

Test-Taking Strategy: Use the process of elimination. Each of the incorrect options supports the client's idea that the depression has resolved. Keeping in mind that safety is of the utmost importance, eliminate each of the incorrect options. Review the care of the depressed client if you had difficulty with this question.

4 Reduce the dosage of antidepressant medication.

Level of Cognitive Ability: Analysis
Client Needs: Safe and Effective Care Environment
Integrated Process: Nursing Process/Planning
Content Area: Mental Health

Reference

Fortinash, K., & Holoday-Worret, P. (2008). *Psychiatric mental health nursing* (4th ed., p. 471). St. Louis: Mosby.

---

155. A child is seen in the health care clinic, and initial testing for human immunodeficiency virus (HIV) is performed because of the child's exposure to HIV infection. Which of the following home-care instructions should the nurse provide to the parents of the child?

1 Avoid sharing toothbrushes.
2 Avoid all immunizations until the diagnosis is established.
3 Wipe up any blood spills with soap and water and allow them to air dry.
4 Wash the hands with half-strength bleach if they come in contact with the child's blood.

Level of Cognitive Ability: Application
Client Needs: Safe and Effective Care Environment
Integrated Process: Teaching and Learning
Content Area: Child Health

Answer: 1

Rationale: Immunizations must be kept up to date (no live virus vaccines are administered if the child has HIV infection). Blood spills are wiped up with a paper towel; the area is then washed with soap and water, rinsed with bleach and water, and allowed to air dry. The hands are washed with soap and water if they come in contact with blood. Parents are instructed that toothbrushes are not to be shared because of the risk of others contracting HIV infection.

Test-Taking Strategy: Use the process of elimination. Eliminate option 2 first because of the close-ended word *all.* Eliminate option 3 next based on the knowledge that blood spills should be cleaned with a bleach solution. Eliminate option 4 because bleach would be very irritating and caustic to the skin. Review the home-care instructions for the child exposed to HIV infection if you had difficulty with this question.

References

Price, D., & Gwin, J. (2008). *Pediatric nursing: An introductory text* (10th ed., p. 88). St. Louis: Saunders.
McKinney, E., James, S., Murray, S., & Ashwill, J. (2009). *Maternal-child nursing* (3rd ed., p. 1054). St. Louis: Mosby.

---

156. The physician tells the nurse that a client admitted with a neurological problem will be scheduled for magnetic resonance imaging (MRI). The nurse questions the physician about this procedure based on a client history of which of the following?

1 Heart failure
2 Cardiac dysrhythmias
3 Chronic airflow limitation
4 Prosthetic valve replacement

Level of Cognitive Ability: Application
Client Needs: Safe and Effective Care Environment
Integrated Process: Nursing Process/Data Collection
Content Area: Adult Health/Neurological

Answer: 4

Rationale: The client scheduled for MRI removes all metallic objects because of the magnetic field generated by the device. A careful history is done to determine if any metal objects have been implanted in the client, such as orthopedic hardware, pacemakers, artificial heart valves, aneurysm clips, or intrauterine devices. These may heat up, become dislodged, or malfunction during the procedure, and the client may be ineligible for the procedure if there is a significant risk. The remaining options pose no risk to the client scheduled for MRI.

Test-Taking Strategy: Use the process of elimination, and focus on the subject—contraindications to MRI. Noting the word *magnetic* in the name of the test will direct you to option 4. Review MRI if you had difficulty with this question.

Reference

Chernecky, C., & Berger, B. (2008). *Laboratory tests and diagnostic procedures* (5th ed., pp. 750-751). Philadelphia: Saunders.

---

157. A clinic nurse is providing instructions to a mother whose child was diagnosed with rubeola (red measles). To prevent the infection from spreading to her other children, the mother asks the nurse how the measles are transmitted. The nurse informs the mother that rubeola is transmitted by which the following?

1 Saliva
2 Fecal–oral route
3 Airborne particles
4 Contact with sweat

Level of Cognitive Ability: Application
Client Needs: Safe and Effective Care Environment
Integrated Process: Teaching and Learning
Content Area: Child Health

Answer: 3
Rationale: Rubeola is transmitted via airborne particles or by direct contact with infectious droplets. Options 1, 2, and 4 are incorrect.

Test-Taking Strategy: Knowledge regarding the route of transmission of rubeola is required to answer this question. Remember that rubeola is transmitted via airborne particles or by direct contact with infectious droplets. Review the route of transmission of rubeola if you had difficulty with this question.

Reference

Price, D., & Gwin, J. (2008). *Pediatric nursing: An introductory text* (10th ed., p. 266). St. Louis: Saunders.

---

158. A nurse is called to a client's room by another nurse. When the second nurse arrives at the room, he sees that a fire has occurred in the client's waste basket. The first nurse has removed the client from the room. What is the second nurse's next action?

1 Confine the fire.
2 Evacuate the unit.
3 Extinguish the fire.
4 Activate the fire alarm.

Level of Cognitive Ability: Application
Client Needs: Safe and Effective Care Environment
Integrated Process: Nursing Process/ Implementation
Content Area: Fundamental Skills

Answer: 4
Rationale: Remember the acronym *RACE* to set priorities when a fire occurs: **R**emove the victim; **A**ctivate the alarm; **C**ontain the fire; and **E**xtinguish as needed. In this event, the client has already been rescued from the immediate vicinity of the fire. The next action is to activate the fire alarm.

Test-Taking Strategy: Remember the order of the *RACE* acronym to set priorities to answer the question. Review fire safety if you had difficulty with this question.

References

Christensen, B., & Kockrow, E. (2006). *Foundations of nursing* (5th ed., pp. 364-365). St. Louis: Mosby.

---

159. A licensed practical nurse (LPN) employed in a long-term care facility is making the assignments for the day. When delegating a task, the LPN gives authority and responsibility to a team member by:

1 Suggesting how to complete the task
2 Checking to be sure the task is complete
3 Completing the task for the team member
4 Waiting for the team member to report the results of the completed task

Answer: 4
Rationale: Authority for task completion is not given to the team member by directing or participating but by allowing the team member to be responsible for completing the task on his or her own. Options 1, 2, and 3 do not delegate authority and responsibility to the person performing the task.

Test-Taking Strategy: Use the process of elimination, and focus on the subject—giving authority and responsibility to a team member. Note that options 1, 2, and 3 are comparable or alike in that they all have the LPN involved in task completion. Review the principles related to delegation if you had difficulty with this question.

Level of Cognitive Ability: Application
Client Needs: Safe and Effective Care Environment
Integrated Process: Nursing Process/ Implementation
Content Area: Delegating/Prioritizing

Reference

deWit, S. (2009). *Medical-surgical nursing: Concepts & practice* (pp. 3-4). St. Louis: Saunders.

---

160. Which action is unsafe when inserting an indwelling bladder catheter?

1 Coiling the tubing of the collection bag
2 Lubricating the catheter tip with water-soluble jelly
3 Inflating the balloon after the catheter is in the bladder
4 Stopping catheter advancement just as urine appears in the catheter tubing

Level of Cognitive Ability: Application
Client Needs: Safe and Effective Care Environment
Integrated Process: Nursing Process/ Implementation
Content Area: Fundamental Skills

Answer: 4

Rationale: The catheter should be advanced 1 to 2 inches beyond the point where the flow of urine is first noted; this ensures that the balloon is fully in the bladder before it is inflated. Each of the other options represents correct procedure. The catheter tip is lubricated for easier insertion. The balloon is inflated after the catheter is in the bladder. The tubing should be coiled (not kinked), and the collection bag should be placed lower than the level of the bladder.

Test-Taking Strategy: Note the strategic word *unsafe;* this word indicates a negative event query and asks you to select the option that is an incorrect nursing action. Visualizing this procedure and recalling that the catheter is advanced 1 to 2 inches after urine is seen will direct you to option 4. Review the insertion of an indwelling bladder catheter if you had difficulty with this question.

Reference

Christensen, B., & Kockrow, E. (2006). *Foundations of nursing* (5th ed., p. 577). St. Louis: Mosby.

---

161. An emergency department nurse asks a licensed practical nurse (LPN) to assist with preparing a client who has sustained a gunshot wound for surgery. The LPN removes the client's clothing and places a hospital gown on the client. Which of the following indicates the appropriate nursing action regarding the client's clothing, which is stained with blood?

1 Discard the clothing.
2 Place the clothing in a paper bag.
3 Place the clothing in a plastic bag.
4 Give the clothing to a family member or significant other.

Level of Cognitive Ability: Application
Client Needs: Safe and Effective Care Environment
Integrated Process: Nursing Process/ Implementation
Content Area: Fundamental Skills

Answer: 2

Rationale: Any evidence of crime discovered during an examination is saved and recorded. The clothing is not given to a family member or significant other. The documentation of evidence includes the bodily location from which the evidence was obtained and when or to whom it was delivered. Evidence should be maintained in its original condition. Clothing is stored in a paper bag instead of plastic to prevent decomposition. If clothing must be cut off of the client, special attention is taken to not inadvertently destroy evidence.

Test-Taking Strategy: Use the process of elimination. Note the strategic words *gunshot wound,* and identify the subject of the question—the legal consideration of evidence related to a crime. Options 1 and 4 can be eliminated first. From the remaining options, recalling that articles can decompose in a plastic bag will direct you to option 2. Review the emergency care of a client involved in a crime if you had difficulty with this question.

Reference

Proehl, J. (2009). *Emergency nursing procedures* (4th ed., pp. 889-893). St. Louis: Saunders.

162. At the beginning of the shift, a client reports severe pain to the nurse, even though pain medication was administered several times during the night. The nurse notes that the client has been complaining of this severe pain every morning for the last 3 days and that the same nurse has cared for this client for the last 3 nights. The nurse suspects that the night nurse is not administering the pain medication to the client as prescribed. According to the nurse practice act, which of the following should the nurse who discovered this situation do?

1 Call the police.
2 Notify the impaired nurse organization.
3 Report the information to the nursing supervisor.
4 Wait until the next morning and talk to the night nurse.

Level of Cognitive Ability: Application
Client Needs: Safe and Effective Care Environment
Integrated Process: Nursing Process/Implementation
Content Area: Fundamental Skills

Answer: 3
Rationale: The nurse practice acts require reporting the suspicion of impaired nurses. The board of nursing has jurisdiction over the practice of nursing and may develop plans for treatment and supervision. The suspicion should be reported to the nursing supervisor, who then notifies the board of nursing. Option 4 can cause further injury to the client. Options 1 and 2 will not alert the health care agency to the problem.

Test-Taking Strategy: Use the process of elimination. Option 4 can be eliminated first because this action can cause further injury to this client. Use principles of prioritizing, and focus on the subject—ethical and legal responsibilities. The nurse should report the information and alert the health care agency to the potential problem, which will lead to further investigation and action. Review the ethical and legal issues related to the suspicion of impaired nurses if you had difficulty with this question.

References
deWit, S. (2009). *Medical-surgical nursing: Concepts & practice* (p. 17). St. Louis: Saunders.
Potter, P., & Perry, A. (2009). *Fundamentals of nursing* (7th ed., pp. 326-327). St. Louis: Mosby.

---

163. A client with an infection is receiving antibiotics by intramuscular (IM) injection. Because this client is also on anticoagulant therapy, the nurse knows that safety for this client should include which of the following?

1 Decreasing the IM needle size
2 Doubling the dose of the anticoagulant
3 Prolonging the pressure applied to the IM site after each injection
4 Applying a pressure bandage to the injection site after each IM injection

Level of Cognitive Ability: Application
Client Needs: Safe and Effective Care Environment
Integrated Process: Nursing Process/Implementation
Content Area: Pharmacology

Answer: 3
Rationale: Anticoagulants place the client at risk for bleeding. Prolonged pressure over the site of an IM injection will assist with preventing bleeding into the tissues that surround the injection site. Doubling the dose of the anticoagulant is incorrect, and a pressure bandage is unnecessary. Decreasing the IM needle size may be helpful, but it is not the most appropriate action.

Test-Taking Strategy: Use the process of elimination. Option 2 can be eliminated because the dose of an anticoagulant would not be doubled. From the remaining options, select option 3, recalling that bleeding is a concern when the client is taking an anticoagulant and because this action is necessary after every IM injection. Review the safety measures for a client receiving anticoagulants if you had difficulty with this question.

Reference
Ignatavicius, D., & Workman, M. (2010). *Medical-surgical nursing: Patient-centered collaborative care* (6th ed., p. 819). St. Louis: Saunders.

---

164. When a medication is being administered, which of the following is the safest and most accurate way for the nurse to verify the identity of the client?

Answer: 1
Rationale: One of the six rights of medication administration is the right client, which can only be accurately verified by checking the identity band. The client may also be asked his or her

1 Check the identity band.
2 Call out the client's name.
3 Ask the client to state his or her name.
4 Ask another nurse to verify the client's identity.

Level of Cognitive Ability: Comprehension
Client Needs: Safe and Effective Care Environment
Integrated Process: Nursing Process/Implementation
Content Area: Fundamental Skills

name, but this action may not be reliable, particularly if the client has periods of confusion. Options 2 and 4 can result in medication errors.

Test-Taking Strategy: Use the process of elimination and your knowledge of the six rights of medication administration. Remember that the safest and most accurate way for the nurse to verify the identity of a client is by checking the identity band. Review the six rights of medication administration if you had difficulty with this question.

Reference
Christensen, B., & Kockrow, E. (2006). *Foundations of nursing* (5th ed., p. 704). St. Louis: Mosby.

---

165. A nurse has developed a plan of care for a client diagnosed with a brain attack (stroke). The nurse should be most concerned with which of the following aspects of care when this client begins to ambulate?
1 Safety
2 Hygiene
3 Hydration
4 Elimination

Level of Cognitive Ability: Comprehension
Client Needs: Safe and Effective Care Environment
Integrated Process: Nursing Process/Planning
Content Area: Fundamental Skills

Answer: 1
Rationale: Safety is the primary concern when the client is ambulating. Although hydration, hygiene, and elimination are also concerns in the plan of care, safety is the priority.

Test-Taking Strategy: Use the process of elimination. Noting the strategic words *begins to ambulate* will direct you to option 1. Review the care of the client with a stroke who is beginning to ambulate if you had difficulty with this question.

Reference
Christensen, B., & Kockrow, E. (2006). *Adult health nursing* (5th ed., p. 733). St. Louis: Mosby.

---

166. A nurse demonstrates awareness of the single most important infection control technique when doing which of the following?
1 Using gloves when giving a bed bath
2 Using sterile gloves when providing perineal care
3 Washing hands before and after every client contact
4 Using sterile technique for an abdominal dressing change

Level of Cognitive Ability: Application
Client Needs: Safe and Effective Care Environment
Integrated Process: Nursing Process/Implementation
Content Area: Fundamental Skills

Answer: 3
Rationale: The most important infection control measure is the prevention of the spread of infection, which is accomplished by frequent handwashing. Options 1 and 4 are correct techniques, but they are not the most important infection control technique. Using sterile gloves for perineal care is not necessary and is costly; clean gloves are sufficient for this procedure.

Test-Taking Strategy: Use the process of elimination, and note the strategic words *single most important.* Recalling the basics of infection control will direct you to option 3. Review the importance of handwashing if you had difficulty with this question.

Reference
deWit, S. (2009). *Medical-surgical nursing: Concepts & practice* (pp. 119-120). St. Louis: Saunders.

---

167. A client has been placed on contact precautions. To prevent the spread of infection, the nurse should do which of the following?

Answer: 2
Rationale: When the client is on contact precautions, a mask is not necessary. However, a mask is necessary for respiratory precautions. Sterile gloves are not required for all client contacts, although

1 Restrict all visitors.
2 Perform meticulous handwashing frequently.
3 Wear a mask and a gown with all client contacts.
4 Wear sterile gloves for all contacts with the client.

Level of Cognitive Ability: Application
Client Needs: Safe and Effective Care Environment
Integrated Process: Nursing Process/Implementation
Content Area: Fundamental Skills

clean gloves may be worn. All visitors need not be restricted from visiting if they are instructed in the measures that prevent infection. Meticulous and frequent handwashing is necessary.

Test-Taking Strategy: Use the process of elimination, and focus on the strategic words *contact precautions*. Eliminate options 1, 3, and 4 because of the close-ended word *all*. Review the measures for contact precautions if you had difficulty with this question.

Reference

deWit, S. (2009). *Medical-surgical nursing: Concepts & practice* (p. 121). St. Louis: Saunders.

---

168. A nurse is assisting with the care of a client with hyperparathyroidism. The nurse does which of the following to help safely minimize the effects of the disease process?
1 Restrict fluids to 1000 mL per day.
2 Explain the benefits of a diet that is high in milk products.
3 Encourage the liberal use of calcium carbonate antacids (Tums).
4 Assist the client to ambulate in the hall three times a day for 15 minutes.

Level of Cognitive Ability: Application
Client Needs: Safe and Effective Care Environment
Integrated Process: Nursing Process/Implementation
Content Area: Adult Health/Endocrine

Answer: 4
Rationale: The client with hyperparathyroidism is predisposed to hypercalcemia and to renal calculi formation; therefore ambulation is important. A diet that is high in milk products would add to the client's calcium load. Calcium carbonate contains calcium and is therefore not the best choice as an antacid. Fluids should not be restricted because fluids aid in the excretion of calcium via the kidneys and prevent the formation of calcium-containing renal stones.

Test-Taking Strategy: Use the process of elimination. Recalling that the client is predisposed to hypercalcemia will help you to eliminate options 2 and 3 first. Recalling that fluid will help reduce the likelihood of the development of renal stones will direct you to option 4 from the remaining options. Review the care of the client with hyperparathyroidism if you had difficulty with this question.

References

Christensen, B., & Kockrow, E. (2006). *Adult health nursing* (5th ed., p. 536). St. Louis: Mosby.
Ignatavicius, D., & Workman, M. (2010). *Medical-surgical nursing: Patient-centered collaborative care* (6th ed., p. 1462). St. Louis: Saunders.

---

169. A nurse is evaluating a client's readiness for discharge and is performing a home safety assessment to determine if there are any environmental hazards in the home. Which statement made by the client should the nurse further investigate?
1 "I live in a one-story house."
2 "I use smoke detectors in my home."
3 "I don't have any nightlights in the house."
4 "I have removed the scatter rugs from the house."

Level of Cognitive Ability: Comprehension
Client Needs: Safe and Effective Care Environment
Integrated Process: Nursing Process/Evaluation
Content Area: Fundamental Skills

Answer: 3
Rationale: If the client tells the nurse that there are no nightlights in the home, the nurse should investigate further. Nightlights assist with preventing falls among clients who may need to get up during the night. Options 1, 2, and 4 do not pose environmental hazards in the home.

Test-Taking Strategy: Use the process of elimination, and focus on the strategic words *further investigate*. Look for the option that identifies an environmental hazard to the client; this will direct you to option 3. Review environmental hazards in the home if you had difficulty with this question.

Reference

Linton, A. (2007). *Introduction to medical-surgical nursing* (4th ed., p. 307). Philadelphia: Saunders.

---

170. A nurse is caring for a client with a hiatal hernia. To prevent tracheal aspiration, the nurse should do which of the following?
1 Administer antacids as needed.
2 Instruct the client to not smoke.
3 Instruct the client to lose weight.
4 Elevate the head of the bed on 4- to 6-inch blocks.

Level of Cognitive Ability: Application
Client Needs: Safe and Effective Care Environment
Integrated Process: Nursing Process/Implementation
Content Area: Adult Health/Gastrointestinal

Answer: 4
Rationale: Regurgitation with tracheal aspiration is a major complication of a hiatal hernia. Although antacids, the avoidance of smoking, and losing weight will assist with alleviating the discomfort that can occur, these measures will not prevent aspiration.

Test-Taking Strategy: Use the process of elimination, and note the subject of the question—preventing tracheal aspiration. Options 1, 2, and 3 are all interventions that may be used with the client with a hiatal hernia, but they do not prevent regurgitation and aspiration; option 4 is the only option that will help prevent this from occurring. Review the care of the client with a hiatal hernia if you had difficulty with this question.

Reference
Linton, A. (2007). *Introduction to medical-surgical nursing* (4th ed., p. 762). Philadelphia: Saunders.

---

171. A nurse is discussing the home environment with a client preparing for discharge to determine if there are any fire hazards in the home. Which of the following statements by the client should the nurse further explore?
1 "I don't burn candles in my house."
2 "I should plan and practice escape routes in case of a fire."
3 "I use smoke detectors and check the batteries faithfully every 2 years."
4 "My space heaters are located at least 3 feet from any items or furniture."

Level of Cognitive Ability: Comprehension
Client Needs: Safe and Effective Care Environment
Integrated Process: Nursing Process/Evaluation
Content Area: Fundamental Skills

Answer: 3
Rationale: Smoke detectors should be used; however, clients need to be instructed to test the batteries monthly and to change the batteries every 6 months. The client should also be instructed to keep a multipurpose fire extinguisher on hand in case of fire. Options 1, 2, and 4 identify correct actions regarding fire safety in the home.

Test-Taking Strategy: Note the strategic words *further explore;* these words indicate a negative event query and ask you to select an option that is an incorrect client statement. Recalling that smoke detector batteries need to be checked monthly and changed every 6 months will direct you to option 3. Review fire safety measures if you had difficulty with this question.

Reference
Christensen, B., & Kockrow, E. (2006). *Foundations of nursing* (5th ed., p. 365). St. Louis: Mosby.

---

172. Spironolactone (Aldactone) is prescribed for a client with hypertension. To ensure safety, the licensed practical nurse should consult with the registered nurse before giving which medication that has already been prescribed for the client?
1 Digoxin (Lanoxin)
2 Docusate sodium (Colace)
3 Potassium chloride (Slow-K)
4 Warfarin sodium (Coumadin)

Level of Cognitive Ability: Application
Client Needs: Safe and Effective Care Environment
Integrated Process: Nursing Process/Implementation
Content Area: Pharmacology

Answer: 3
Rationale: Spironolactone is a potassium-sparing diuretic that places the client at risk for hyperkalemia. If a potassium supplement were prescribed, the nurse would question the order. Docusate sodium is a stool softener, and warfarin sodium is an anticoagulant. Digoxin is a cardiac glycoside.

Test-Taking Strategy: Use the process of elimination and your knowledge of the medication classification of spironolactone. Recalling that this medication is a potassium-sparing diuretic will direct you to option 3. Review spironolactone if you had difficulty with this question.

Reference
Hodgson, B., & Kizior, R. (2009). *Saunders nursing drug handbook 2009* (p. 1076). Philadelphia: Saunders.

---

173. A nurse administers digoxin (Lanoxin) 0.25 mg instead of the prescribed order of 0.125 mg. The nurse discovers the error while charting the medication. The nurse completes an incident report and notifies the physician of the incident. Which of the following is the next appropriate nursing action?

1 Document the incident in the client's record.
2 Place the incident report in the client's record.
3 Send the incident report to the risk-management department.
4 Make a copy of the incident report and send it to the physician's office.

Level of Cognitive Ability: Application
Client Needs: Safe and Effective Care Environment
Integrated Process: Nursing Process/Implementation
Content Area: Fundamental Skills

Answer: 1
Rationale: The incident report is confidential and privileged information. It should not be copied, placed in the client's record, or have any reference made to it in the client's record. It is the physician's responsibility to sign the incident report before it is sent to the risk-management department. A copy should not be made or sent to the physician's office. The incident report is not a substitute for a complete entry in the client's record regarding the incident.

Test-Taking Strategy: Use the process of elimination, and note the strategic word *next.* Recalling the purpose of an incident report and the nurse's responsibilities regarding the report and documentation will direct you to option 1. Review the nurse's responsibilities regarding incident reports if you had difficulty with this question.

Reference
Christensen, B., & Kockrow, E. (2006). *Foundations of nursing* (5th ed., p. 112). St. Louis: Mosby.

---

174. A clinic nurse is caring for a pregnant woman with acquired immunodeficiency syndrome (AIDS) who is exhibiting signs of fever, weight loss, and candidiasis. The nurse should place highest priority on which intervention?

1 Providing emotional support to the mother
2 Assessing the mother's history for AIDS risk factors
3 Using disposable gloves when in contact with nonintact skin
4 Providing clear information about the consequences of AIDS on the unborn child

Level of Cognitive Ability: Application
Client Needs: Safe and Effective Care Environment
Integrated Process: Nursing Process/Implementation
Content Area: Maternity/Antepartum

Answer: 3
Rationale: Standard precautions should be used when caring for a pregnant client with AIDS. Options 1 and 4 are part of the plan of care, but, according to Maslow's Hierarchy of Needs theory, they have a lesser priority. Option 2 is not a timely intervention because the client has already acquired the virus.

Test-Taking Strategy: Use the process of elimination, and note the strategic words *highest priority.* Use Maslow's Hierarchy of Needs theory to eliminate options 1 and 4. From the remaining options, noting that the client has AIDS will eliminate option 2. Review the care of the client with AIDS if you had difficulty with this question.

Reference
Leifer, G. (2008). *Maternity nursing: An introductory text* (10th ed., pp. 393, 409). Philadelphia: Saunders.

---

175. A nurse should put on gloves to perform which of the following nursing interventions when working with a neonate?

1 Feeding the infant
2 Providing cord care

Answer: 2
Rationale: Standard precautions indicate that unsterile, clean gloves should be worn when touching nonintact skin. The nurse wears gloves when changing the baby's diaper and providing cord care. Gloves are not necessary for the activities in options 1, 3, and 4.

3 Discharging the infant
4 Changing the infant's clothes

Level of Cognitive Ability: Application
Client Needs: Safe and Effective Care Environment
Integrated Process: Nursing Process/Implementation
Content Area: Maternity/Postpartum

Test-Taking Strategy: Use the process of elimination. Recalling that wearing gloves is necessary when in contact with nonintact skin will direct you to option 2. Review standard precautions if you had difficulty with this question.

Reference

Leifer, G. (2008). *Maternity nursing: An introductory text* (10th ed., pp. 185, 409). Philadelphia: Saunders.

---

176. A nurse is assigned to care for a hospitalized client. Which of the following interventions in the general plan of care specifically upholds an item listed in the Patient's Bill of Rights?
1 Maintain accurate and current client information.
2 Act in a manner that reinforces the client's dignity.
3 Incorporate available and appropriate teaching reference materials.
4 Consult with other health care team members about discharge planning.

Level of Cognitive Ability: Comprehension
Client Needs: Safe and Effective Care Environment
Integrated Process: Nursing Process/Implementation
Content Area: Fundamental Skills

Answer: 2
Rationale: Option 2 reflects the items identified in the client's bill of rights. The other nursing interventions reflect competent care but are not directly mentioned in this document.

Test-Taking Strategy: Use the process of elimination, and focus on the subject of the question—the client's bill of rights. Recalling these rights will direct you to option 2. Review the client's rights if you had difficulty with this question.

Reference

Christensen, B., & Kockrow, E. (2006). *Foundations of nursing* (5th ed., pp. 15, 24-25). St. Louis: Mosby.

---

177. A nurse is assigned to care for a client with hypoparathyroidism. Which of the following interventions should the nurse focus on if the priority of care is to maintain a safe environment for this client?
1 Implementing seizure precautions
2 Keeping the client comfortably cool
3 Keeping the bed in a modified Trendelenburg's position
4 Applying chest and ankle restraints after raising the side rails

Level of Cognitive Ability: Application
Client Needs: Safe and Effective Care Environment
Integrated Process: Nursing Process/Implementation
Content Area: Adult Health/Endocrine

Answer: 1
Rationale: Hypoparathyroidism causes a deficiency of parathyroid hormone that leads to low serum calcium levels. Untreated hypocalcemia can cause tetany and seizure activity. The nurse should anticipate such a complication and institute seizure precautions to maintain a safe environment. The client's temperature does not elevate with this disorder. In addition, this disorder does not cause hypotension and does not require the modified Trendelenburg's position. Option 4 could cause injury to the client if seizure activity occurred.

Test-Taking Strategy: Use the process of elimination, and recall the pathophysiology associated with hypoparathyroidism. Focus on the strategic words *safe environment;* this direct you to option 1. Review hypoparathyroidism if you had difficulty with this question.

Reference

Linton, A. (2007). *Introduction to medical-surgical nursing* (4th ed., p. 999). Philadelphia: Saunders.

---

178. A nurse is beginning an intermittent enteral tube feeding. Which of the following nursing actions has the highest priority?

Answer: 2
Rationale: The highest priority is determining tube placement. Initiating a tube feeding without checking tube placement places the client at risk for aspiration, which can lead to pneumonia.

1 Weighing the client beforehand
2 Determining proper tube placement
3 Measuring intake and output each shift
4 Preparing the amount of formula needed

Level of Cognitive Ability: Application
Client Needs: Safe and Effective Care Environment
Integrated Process: Nursing Process/Implementation
Content Area: Fundamental Skills

Options 1, 3, and 4 are routine care items for a client receiving enteral feedings, but they are not the highest priority.

Test-Taking Strategy: Note the strategic words *highest priority*, and use the ABCs—airway, breathing, and circulation. This will direct you to option 2. Remember that initiating a tube feeding without checking tube placement places the client at risk for aspiration. Review enteral feedings if you had difficulty with this question.

Reference

deWit, S. (2009). *Medical-surgical nursing: Concepts & practice* (pp. 704-705). St. Louis: Saunders.

---

179. A client is being discharged to return home after a spinal fusion. The nurse should suggest a consultation with the continuing-care nurse regarding the need for follow-up modification of the home environment if the client states which of the following?

1 The bathroom has hand railings in the shower.
2 There are three steps to get up to the front door.
3 The family has rented a commode for use by the client.
4 The bedroom and bathroom are on the second floor of the home.

Level of Cognitive Ability: Comprehension
Client Needs: Safe and Effective Care Environment
Integrated Process: Nursing Process/Planning
Content Area: Adult Health/Musculoskeletal

Answer: 4

Rationale: Stair-climbing may be restricted or limited for several weeks after spinal fusion. Options 1 and 3 are useful to the client. Option 2 would not cause as many problems as option 4.

Test-Taking Strategy: Use the process of elimination. Options 1 and 3 are useful to the client and can be eliminated first. To select between options 2 and 4 (both of which involve stairs), you should determine that option 2 is least problematic, whereas option 4 poses a significant problem to the client who is restricted from stair-climbing. Review the activity restrictions required after spinal fusion if you had difficulty with this question.

Reference

Christensen, B., & Kockrow, E. (2006). *Adult health nursing* (5th ed., p. 185). St. Louis: Mosby.

---

180. A nurse caring for a client at home notes the presence of multiple straight and wavy threadlike lines beneath the client's skin and suspects the presence of scabies. Which of the following precautions will the nurse institute until the physician is contacted?

1 Putting on a pair of gloves
2 Donning a mask and gloves
3 Putting on a gown and gloves
4 Avoiding sitting on the client's furniture

Level of Cognitive Ability: Application
Client Needs: Safe and Effective Care Environment
Integrated Process: Nursing Process/Implementation
Content Area: Adult Health/Integumentary

Answer: 3

Rationale: The nurse should wear a gown and gloves during close contact with a person infested with scabies. Masks are not necessary. Transmission via clothing and other inanimate objects is uncommon. Scabies is usually transmitted from person to person by direct skin contact. All contacts that the client has had should be treated at the same time.

Test-Taking Strategy: Consider the mode of transmission of scabies, and use the process of elimination. Because scabies is transmitted by direct skin contact, eliminate options 1, 2, and 4. Review standard precautions and the transmission mode of scabies if you had difficulty with this question.

Reference

Linton, A. (2007). *Introduction to medical-surgical nursing* (4th ed., pp. 172, 1142). Philadelphia: Saunders.

---

181. A nurse administers the morning dose of digoxin (Lanoxin) to a client. When charting the medication, the nurse discovers that a dose of 0.25 mg was administered rather than the prescribed dose of 0.125 mg. Which of the following actions will the nurse take?

1 Complete an incident report.
2 Administer an additional 0.125 mg.
3 Tell the client that too much medication was administered and that an error was made.
4 Tell the client that the dose administered was not the total amount and administer the additional dose.

Level of Cognitive Ability: Application
Client Needs: Safe and Effective Care Environment
Integrated Process: Nursing Process/Implementation
Content Area: Fundamental Skills

Answer: 1
Rationale: In accordance with the agency's policies, nurses are required to file incident reports when an event arises that could or did cause client harm. If a dose of 0.125 mg was prescribed and a dose of 0.25 mg was administered, then the client received too much medication; additional medication is not required and in fact could be detrimental. The client should be informed when an error has occurred but in a professional manner so as not to cause fear and concern. In many situations, the physician will discuss these issues with the client.

Test-Taking Strategy: Use the process of elimination. Simple math calculation will assist you with eliminating both options 2 and 4. From the remaining options, select option 1 because it is the nurse's responsibility to complete an incident report form. Review nursing responsibilities related to medication errors if you had difficulty with this question.

Reference
Christensen, B., & Kockrow, E. (2006). *Foundations of nursing* (5th ed., p. 112). St. Louis: Mosby.

---

182. A nursing assistant is caring for a client who has an indwelling urinary catheter. The nurse determines that the nursing assistant needs instructions about the care of the client if the nursing assistant:

1 Keeps kinks out of the tubing
2 Uses soap and water to cleanse the perineal area
3 Lets the drainage tubing rest under the client's leg
4 Keeps the drainage bag below the level of the bladder

Level of Cognitive Ability: Application
Client Needs: Safe and Effective Care Environment
Integrated Process: Nursing Process/Implementation
Content Area: Leadership/Management

Answer: 3
Rationale: Proper care of an indwelling catheter is especially important to prevent infection. The nurse and all caregivers must use strict aseptic technique when emptying the drainage bag or obtaining urine specimens. The perineal area is cleansed thoroughly with mild soap and water at least twice a day and after a bowel movement. The drainage bag is kept below the level of the bladder to prevent urine from being trapped in the bladder, and, for the same reason, the drainage tubing is not placed under the client's leg. The tubing must be allowed to drain freely at all times.

Test-Taking Strategy: Use the process of elimination. Note the strategic words *needs instructions;* this indicates a negative event query and asks you to select an option that is an incorrect action. Eliminate option 2 first because this is a basic standard of care for the client with an indwelling catheter. Option 1 is consistent with principles of care and will assist with the promotion of drainage. From the remaining options, recall that option 4 promotes drainage and that option 3 could impede drainage; thus the answer to the question is option 3. Review the care of the client with an indwelling urinary catheter if you had difficulty with this question.

References
Christensen, B., & Kockrow, E. (2006). *Adult health nursing* (5th ed., p. 479). St. Louis: Mosby.
deWit, S. (2009). *Medical-surgical nursing: Concepts & practice* (p. 829). St. Louis: Saunders.

---

183. A client is scheduled for bronchoscopy. The priority is to ensure which of the following?

1 Asking the client about allergies to shellfish

Answer: 3
Rationale: Bronchoscopy requires that an informed consent be obtained from the client before the procedure. The client receives nothing by mouth for at least 6 hours before the procedure. It is unnecessary to inquire about allergies to shellfish

2 Restricting the diet to clear liquids on the day of the test
3 Checking that an informed consent for the procedure is signed
4 Checking for an order for preprocedure prophylactic antibiotics

Level of Cognitive Ability: Application
Client Needs: Safe and Effective Care Environment
Integrated Process: Nursing Process/Implementation
Content Area: Adult Health/Respiratory

before this procedure because no contrast dye is injected. There is also no need for prophylactic antibiotics.

Test-Taking Strategy: Focus on the name of the procedure. Recalling that bronchoscopy is an invasive procedure and thus requires an informed consent will direct you to the correct option. Review bronchoscopy if you had difficulty with this question.

Reference

Chernecky, C., & Berger, B. (2008). *Laboratory tests and diagnostic procedures* (5th ed., p. 262). Philadelphia: Saunders.

---

184. A client with acquired immunodeficiency syndrome who has cytomegalovirus retinitis is receiving ganciclovir sodium (Cytovene). The nurse should plan to do which of the following while the client is taking this medication?
1 Monitor blood glucose levels for elevation.
2 Administer the medication on an empty stomach only.
3 Apply pressure to venipuncture sites for at least 2 minutes.
4 Provide the client with a soft toothbrush and an electric razor.

Level of Cognitive Ability: Application
Client Needs: Safe and Effective Care Environment
Integrated Process: Nursing Process/Planning
Content Area: Pharmacology

Answer: 4
Rationale: Ganciclovir sodium causes neutropenia and thrombocytopenia as the most frequent side effects. For this reason, the nurse monitors the client for signs and symptoms of bleeding and implements the same precautions that are used for a client receiving anticoagulant therapy. These include providing a soft toothbrush and an electric razor to minimize the risk of trauma that could result in bleeding. The medication may cause hypoglycemia but not hyperglycemia, and it does not have to be taken on an empty stomach. Venipuncture sites should be held for approximately 10 minutes.

Test-Taking Strategy: Use the process of elimination. Eliminate option 2 because of the close-ended word *only* and option 3 because of the words *2 minutes*. Recalling that ganciclovir causes neutropenia and thrombocytopenia directs you to option 4 from the remaining options. Review ganciclovir if you had difficulty with this question.

Reference

Hodgson, B., & Kizior, R. (2009). *Saunders nursing drug handbook 2009* (pp. 528-530). St. Louis: Saunders.

---

185. A client is scheduled to have an inferior vena cava (IVC) filter inserted. The nurse should place highest priority on determining whether the surgeon wants which of the following medications held during the preoperative period?
1 Furosemide (Lasix)
2 Famotidine (Pepcid)
3 Multivitamin with minerals
4 Warfarin sodium (Coumadin)

Level of Cognitive Ability: Analysis
Client Needs: Safe and Effective Care Environment
Integrated Process: Nursing Process/Data Collection
Content Area: Adult Health/Cardiovascular

Answer: 4
Rationale: The nurse is careful to question the surgeon about whether warfarin sodium should be administered during the preoperative period before the insertion of an IVC filter. This medication is often withheld during the preoperative period to minimize the risk of hemorrhage during surgery. The other medications may also be withheld if specifically ordered, but usually they are discontinued as part of an order for nothing by mouth after midnight.

Test-Taking Strategy: Note that the question contains the strategic words *highest priority;* to choose the correct option, you must recall the action of an anticoagulant. Remember that when a client is taking an anticoagulant, a risk for bleeding exists. Review the adverse effects of warfarin sodium if you had difficulty with this question.

Reference

Ignatavicius, D., & Workman, M. (2010). *Medical-surgical nursing: Patient-centered collaborative care* (6th ed., pp. 682, 820). St. Louis: Saunders.

---

186. A nurse aspirates 40 mL of undigested formula from a client's nasogastric tube. Before administering the tube feeding, the nurse does which of the following with the 40 mL of gastric aspirate?

1 Pours it into the nasogastric tube through a syringe with the plunger removed
2 Discards it properly and records it as output on the client's intake and output record
3 Dilutes it with water and injects it into the nasogastric tube by putting pressure on the plunger
4 Mixes it with the formula and pours it into the nasogastric tube through a syringe without a plunger

Level of Cognitive Ability: Application
Client Needs: Safe and Effective Care Environment
Integrated Process: Nursing Process/Implementation
Content Area: Fundamental Skills

Answer: 1
Rationale: After checking residual feeding contents, gastric contents are reinstilled into the stomach by removing the syringe bulb or plunger and pouring the gastric contents via the syringe into the nasogastric tube. Gastric contents should be reinstilled to maintain the client's electrolyte balance. The gastric aspirate does not need to be mixed with water or formula, and it should not be discarded or injected by putting pressure on the plunger.

Test-Taking Strategy: Use the process of elimination. Remembering that the removal of the gastric contents could disturb the client's electrolyte balance will assist you with eliminating option 2. Eliminate option 3 because of the word *pressure.* Recalling that aspirated gastric contents should be immediately replaced will direct you to the correct option. Review the procedure for administering tube feedings if you had difficulty with this question.

Reference
Christensen, B., & Kockrow, E. (2006). *Foundations of nursing* (5th ed., p. 654). St. Louis: Mosby.

---

187. A nurse has an order to obtain a urinalysis from a client with an indwelling urinary catheter. To prevent the contamination of the specimen, the nurse should avoid which of the following?

1 Clamping the tubing of the drainage bag
2 Obtaining the specimen from the urinary drainage bag
3 Aspirating a sample from the port on the drainage system
4 Wiping the port on the drainage system with an alcohol swab before inserting the syringe

Level of Cognitive Ability: Application
Client Needs: Safe and Effective Care Environment
Integrated Process: Nursing Process/Implementation
Content Area: Fundamental Skills

Answer: 2
Rationale: A urine specimen is not taken from the urinary drainage bag. Because it undergoes chemical changes, the urine that is sitting in the bag does not necessarily reflect the client's current status. In addition, it may become contaminated with bacteria from the opening of the system.

Test-Taking Strategy: Note the strategic word *avoid;* this word indicates a negative event query and asks you to select an option that is an incorrect action. Use the process of elimination, and focus on the subject—preventing contamination; this should direct you to the correct option. Review the procedure for obtaining a urine specimen from an indwelling urinary catheter if you had difficulty with this question.

Reference
Christensen, B., & Kockrow, E. (2006). *Foundations of nursing* (5th ed., p. 578). St. Louis: Mosby.

---

188. A client requests pain medication from the nurse. After administering the intramuscular (IM) injection, what should the nurse do next?

1 Recap the needle.
2 Place the syringe on the overbed table.
3 Assist the client to ambulate to aid in absorption.

Answer: 4
Rationale: After administering an IM injection, the nurse should next apply gentle pressure to the site with an alcohol swab to prevent bleeding and to assist with medication absorption. The needle is not recapped or placed on the overbed table; rather, the needle and syringe are placed in the appropriate puncture-resistant receptacle. The client who is in pain should not be ambulated to aid in medication absorption.

4 Apply gentle pressure to the site with an alcohol swab.

Level of Cognitive Ability: Application
Client Needs: Safe and Effective Care Environment
Integrated Process: Nursing Process/ Implementation
Content Area: Fundamental Skills

Test-Taking Strategy: Use the process of elimination, and note the strategic word *next*. Visualize this procedure, and use your knowledge of the principles related to the safe administration of IM medication to direct you to option 4. Review the procedure for administering an IM injection if you had difficulty with this question.

References

Christensen, B., & Kockrow, E. (2006). *Foundations of nursing* (5th ed., p. 730). St. Louis: Mosby.
Perry, A., & Potter, P. (2010). *Clinical nursing skills & techniques* (7th ed., pp. 602-603). St. Louis: Mosby.

---

189. A nurse in a well-baby clinic is providing safety instructions to a mother of a 1-month-old infant. Which safety instruction is most appropriate at this age?

1 Lock up all poisons.
2 Cover all electrical outlets.
3 Do not shake the infant's head.
4 Remove hazardous objects from low places.

Level of Cognitive Ability: Comprehension
Client Needs: Safe and Effective Care Environment
Integrated Process: Teaching and Learning
Content Area: Child Health

Answer: 3
Rationale: The most important age-appropriate instruction is to not shake or vigorously jiggle the infant's head. Options 1, 2, and 4 become important instructions to provide to the mother as the child reaches the age of 6 months and begins to explore the environment.

Test-Taking Strategy: Use the process of elimination. Focus on the age of the infant to direct you to the correct option. A 1-month-old is not at the developmental level of exploring the environment; this will help you to eliminate options 1, 2, and 4. Review age-appropriate safety measures if you had difficulty with this question.

Reference

Leifer, G. (2007). *Introduction to maternity and pediatric nursing* (5th ed., p. 543). Philadelphia: Saunders.

---

190. A 17-year-old female client is about to be discharged with her new baby. Which of the following statements, if made by the client, indicates the need for further teaching regarding safety measures for her baby?

1 "I keep all my pots and pans in my lower cabinets."
2 " I will not use the microwave to heat my baby's formula."
3 "I have locks on all of the cabinets that hold my cleaning supplies."
4 "I have a car seat that I will put in the front seat to keep my baby safe."

Level of Cognitive Ability: Comprehension
Client Needs: Safe and Effective Care Environment
Integrated Process: Teaching and Learning
Content Area: Maternity/Postpartum

Answer: 4
Rationale: A baby car seat should never be placed in the front seat because of the potential for injury on impact. Any cabinets that contain dangerous items that the baby could swallow should be locked. Microwaves should never be used to heat bottle formula because the formula could burn or even scald the baby's mouth. Although the bottle may only feel warm, it could contain hot spots that could severely damage the baby's mouth. It is perfectly safe to leave pots and pans in the lower cabinets for the baby to investigate when he or she begins to explore the environment, as long as they are not made of glass; glass items, if broken, could harm the baby.

Test-Taking Strategy: Note the strategic words *need for further teaching;* these words indicate a negative event query and ask you to select an option that is an incorrect client statement. Use the process of elimination to identify the option that would cause injury to the baby. Review infant safety measures if you had difficulty with this question.

Reference

Price, D., & Gwin, J. (2008). *Pediatric nursing: An introductory text* (10th ed., pp. 189, 192). St. Louis: Saunders.

---

191. A nurse is caring for a 9-month-old child after cleft palate repair. The nurse has applied elbow restraints to the child. The mother visits the child and asks the nurse to remove the restraints. Which of the following is the appropriate nursing action?

1 Remove both restraints.
2 Remove a restraint from one extremity.
3 Tell the mother that the restraints cannot be removed.
4 Loosen the restraints but tell the mother that they cannot be removed.

Level of Cognitive Ability: Application
Client Needs: Safe and Effective Care Environment
Integrated Process: Nursing Process/ Implementation
Content Area: Child Health

Answer: 2

Rationale: Elbow restraints are used after cleft palate repair to prevent the child from touching the repair site, which could cause accidental rupture and tearing of the sutures. The restraints can be removed one at a time only if a parent or nurse is in constant attendance. Options 1, 3, and 4 are inaccurate nursing actions.

Test-Taking Strategy: Use the process of elimination. Eliminate options 3 and 4 first because they are comparable or alike. From the remaining options, recall the purpose of the restraints after this surgical procedure; this will direct you to option 2, which is the safest nursing action. Review postoperative nursing interventions after cleft palate repair if you had difficulty with this question.

Reference

Price, D., & Gwin, J. (2008). *Pediatric nursing: An introductory text* (10th ed., p. 103). St. Louis: Saunders.

---

192. A nurse is caring for a hospitalized child with rubella (German measles). Which of the following precautions should the nurse institute while caring for this child?

1 Enteric precautions
2 Protective isolation
3 Contact precautions
4 Reverse isolation procedures

Level of Cognitive Ability: Application
Client Needs: Safe and Effective Care Environment
Integrated Process: Nursing Process/ Implementation
Content Area: Child Health

Answer: 3

Rationale: The care of a child with rubella involves airborne precautions and contact isolation. Airborne precautions require the use of masks. Contact precaution requires the use of gowns and gloves for contact with any infectious material. Contaminated articles must be bagged and labeled before reprocessing. Options 1, 2, and 4 are not specific to the care of a child with rubella.

Test-Taking Strategy: Use the process of elimination. Eliminate options 2 and 4 because they are comparable or alike. From the remaining options, recalling that the transmission of rubella is by direct contact with infectious droplets will direct you to option 3. Review the method of transmission of rubella if you had difficulty with this question.

Reference

Hockenberry, M., & Wilson, D. (2009). *Wong's essentials of pediatric care* (8th ed., p. 461). St. Louis: Mosby.

---

193. A nurse is caring for a child who was diagnosed with erythema infectiosum (fifth disease). The child's mother asks the nurse how this disease is transmitted. The nurse informs the mother that fifth disease is transmitted by which of the following routes?

1 Saliva
2 Fecal–oral route
3 Airborne particles
4 Contact with sweat

Answer: 3

Rationale: Fifth disease is transmitted via airborne particles, respiratory droplets, blood, blood products, or transplacental means. Options 1, 2, and 4 are incorrect regarding the mode of transmission of fifth disease.

Test-Taking Strategy: Knowledge regarding the mode of transmission of fifth disease is required to answer this question. Remember that fifth disease is transmitted via airborne particles, respiratory droplets, blood, blood products, and transplacental means. Review fifth disease if you had difficulty with this question.

Level of Cognitive Ability: Application
Client Needs: Safe and Effective Care Environment
Integrated Process: Teaching and Learning
Content Area: Child Health

Reference

McKinney, E., James, S., Murray, S., & Ashwill, J. (2009). *Maternal-child nursing* (3rd ed., p. 1018). St. Louis: Mosby.

---

194. A nurse is giving a bed bath to a client and notes the need for another towel. Which nursing action will the nurse take?

1 Using a bath blanket as a towel
2 Borrowing the roommate's towel
3 Going to the linen room to get the towel
4 Washing the hands and obtaining a towel from the linen room

Answer: 4

Rationale: To avoid spreading the client's germs, the nurse's hands must be washed before leaving the client's room. It is never appropriate to borrow other clients' supplies because this will spread germs. It is not appropriate to use a bath blanket as a towel.

Test-Taking Strategy: Use your knowledge regarding the basic principles related to bathing a client and visualize the event to direct you to option 4. Review the basic principles for administering a bed bath if you had difficulty with this question.

Level of Cognitive Ability: Application
Client Needs: Safe and Effective Care Environment
Integrated Process: Nursing Process/Implementation
Content Area: Fundamental Skills

Reference

Potter, P., & Perry, A. (2009). *Fundamentals of nursing* (7th ed., pp. 869-876). St. Louis: Mosby.

---

195. A nurse is determining a family member's ability to use sterile gloves to perform a dressing change. Which statement indicates to the nurse that the family member requires further teaching?

1 "Whichever glove I decide to put on first is up to me."
2 "I know that I can use the inner wrapper as a sterile field."
3 "If I touch the glove on the counter, I should open another pair."
4 "I don't have to worry about washing my hands because I have sterile gloves."

Answer: 4

Rationale: The hands must always be washed—even when sterile gloves are used—to keep germs from spreading. The inner wrapper makes an excellent area for use because it is sterile. If the gloves touch anything unsterile, they must be considered contaminated, and a new package of sterile gloves must be used. Which glove is put on first is up to the individual as long as sterile technique is not compromised.

Test-Taking Strategy: Note the strategic words *requires further teaching;* these words indicate a negative event query and ask you to select an option that is an incorrect statement. Recalling the principles of sterile technique will direct you to option 4. Review sterile technique if you had difficulty with this question.

Level of Cognitive Ability: Comprehension
Client Needs: Safe and Effective Care Environment
Integrated Process: Teaching and Learning
Content Area: Fundamental Skills

References

deWit, S. (2009). *Medical-surgical nursing: Concepts & practice* (pp. 119-120). St. Louis: Saunders.
Potter, P., & Perry, A. (2009). *Fundamentals of nursing* (7th ed., p. 667). St. Louis: Mosby.

---

196. A nurse is preparing to leave a client's room and must remove a gown, a mask, and gloves before leaving the room. Which of the following interventions could lead to the spread of infection?

1 Taking the gloves off first before removing the gown

Answer: 2

Rationale: The gown must be rolled from inside out to prevent the organisms on the outside of the gown from contaminating other areas. Gloves are considered the most contaminated protective items that the nurse wears and therefore must be removed first. The hands should be washed after removing the protective items to eliminate any germs that are still present. Ungloved hands

2 While removing the gown, avoiding rolling it from inside out
3 Washing the hands after the entire procedure has been completed
4 Using ungloved hands, removing the gown using the neck ties

Level of Cognitive Ability: Application
Client Needs: Safe and Effective Care Environment
Integrated Process: Nursing Process/ Implementation
Content Area: Fundamental Skills

should be used to remove the gown to prevent contaminating the back of the gown with germs from the gloves.

Test-Taking Strategy: Note the strategic words *lead to the spread of infection.* Visualize this procedure, and use the process of elimination with this focus in mind to direct you to the correct option. Review the procedure for removing protective clothing when leaving a client's room to prevent infection if you had difficulty with this question.

Reference
deWit, S. (2009). *Medical-surgical nursing: Concepts & practice* (p. 123). St. Louis: Saunders.

---

197. A nurse is caring for a hospitalized child with rubeola (red measles). Which of the following precautions should the nurse institute when caring for the child?
1 Wearing gloves
2 Wearing a gown
3 Wearing a mask
4 Wearing goggles

Level of Cognitive Ability: Application
Client Needs: Safe and Effective Care Environment
Integrated Process: Nursing Process/ Implementation
Content Area: Child Health

Answer: 3
Rationale: Rubeola is transmitted via airborne particles or direct contact with infectious droplets. The treatment of rubeola is symptomatic, whether the child is hospitalized or remains at home. If hospitalized, however, airborne isolation precautions are required. During the febrile period, the child should be restricted to quiet activities and bedrest. Respiratory isolation for a child with rubeola requires masks for those who are in close contact with the child. Gowns, gloves, or goggles are not specifically indicated. Strict handwashing is advised after touching the child or contaminated objects and before caring for another child. Articles that are contaminated should be bagged and labeled before reprocessing.

Test-Taking Strategy: Note the strategic word *hospitalized.* Recalling that rubeola is transmitted via airborne particles or direct contact with infectious droplets will direct you to option 3. Review the procedures for caring for a hospitalized child with rubeola if you had difficulty with this question.

Reference
Price, D., & Gwin, J. (2008). *Pediatric nursing: An introductory text* (10th ed., pp. 41, 266). St. Louis: Saunders.

---

198. A nurse has checked a client's vision and is addressing safety needs related to deficits experienced as a result of normal age-related changes. Which statement by the client indicates the need for further discussion about safety?
1 "I should avoid nighttime driving."
2 "I should have bright orange strips of tape installed at the edge of stairs."
3 "I should keep the lights turned on in the stairways and hallways at night."
4 "I should have a high-gloss paint put on the walls to increase light reflection."

Level of Cognitive Ability: Comprehension
Client Needs: Safe and Effective Care Environment

Answer: 4
Rationale: Age-related changes in the eye (e.g., diminished or absent pupillary response, decreased retinal blood supply) can cause night blindness, the inability to see as a result of glare, and deficits of depth and color perception. Using high-gloss paint on the walls will increase glare and make it more difficult for the client to see. All of the other options are appropriate safety measures.

Test-Taking Strategy: Note the strategic words *need for further discussion.* These words indicate a negative event query and ask you to select an option that is an incorrect intervention. Recalling that high-gloss paint will cause a glare will easily direct you to option 4. Review the safety measures for normal age-related vision changes if you had difficulty with this question.

Integrated Process: Teaching and Learning
Content Area: Fundamental Skills

Reference
Perry, A., & Potter, P. (2006). *Clinical nursing skills & techniques* (6th ed., p. 1338). St. Louis: Mosby.

---

199. A nurse is caring for an 8-month-old infant with a diagnosis of febrile seizures. When planning this infant's care, the nurse should anticipate the need for which of the following items?
1 Restraints
2 Padded sides on the crib
3 A code cart at the bedside
4 A padded tongue blade taped to the head of the bed

Level of Cognitive Ability: Application
Client Needs: Safe and Effective Care Environment
Integrated Process: Nursing Process/Planning
Content Area: Child Health

Answer: 2
Rationale: Padded crib sides will protect the child from injury during seizure activity. A padded tongue blade should never be used. During a seizure, nothing should be placed in a child's mouth; the child should be placed in a side-lying position but should not be restrained. A code cart should be available but need not be placed at the bedside.

Test-Taking Strategy: Use the process of elimination. Recalling that safety is an issue during seizure activity will direct you to option 2. Review the precautions to take when seizure activity is a risk if you had difficulty with this question.

Reference
Price, D., & Gwin, J. (2008). *Pediatric nursing: An introductory text* (10th ed., p. 254). St. Louis: Saunders.

---

200. A licensed practical nurse has been asked to do a safety survey at a children's day care center. All of the children cared for at the center are between the ages of 1 and 3 years. Of the following safety hazards, which presents the greatest hazard to a toddler at the center?
1 A hot water heater set above 120° F
2 Toys with small, loose parts in the playroom
3 A swimming pool in the neighbor's gated yard
4 Toxic plants located in the front yard of the center

Level of Cognitive Ability: Analysis
Client Needs: Safe and Effective Care Environment
Integrated Process: Nursing Process/Data Collection
Content Area: Child Health

Answer: 2
Rationale: Toys in the playroom should be the first concern because the toddlers will play in this area. Options 3 and 4 identify safety hazards that are not in the toddlers' play area and would not be the first priority. Water temperature should be a priority in a toddler's home, where scalding could occur during bathing; this would be a secondary consideration in a day care setting.

Test-Taking Strategy: Note the strategic words *greatest hazard to a toddler,* and focus on the setting—a day care center. This focus and the process of elimination will direct you to option 2. Review safety in a day care center if you had difficulty with this question.

Reference
Price, D., & Gwin, J. (2008). *Pediatric nursing: An introductory text* (10th ed., pp. 188, 192). St. Louis: Saunders.

---

201. A nurse is reinforcing instructions to the mother of a preschool child with hemophilia. The nurse instructs the mother to do which of the following to promote a safe but normal environment?
1 Examine toys and the play area for sharp objects.
2 Restrict the child from playing in an outdoor playground.

Answer: 1
Rationale: Examining toys and equipment in the play area will prevent potential injuries. Protective equipment may be necessary when the child first becomes mobile, but, by preschool age, this equipment should only be needed during bike riding and other activities that present a risk of injury. Outdoor playgrounds can present hazards, and activities in these areas should be supervised rather than restricted. The child is overprotected if allowed to play only when directly supervised by a family member. Parents should reduce their anxiety and give the child some independence.

3 Insist that the child wear a helmet and elbow pads during all waking hours.
4 Allow the child to use play equipment only when a parent or older sibling is present.

Level of Cognitive Ability: Application
Client Needs: Safe and Effective Care Environment
Integrated Process: Teaching and Learning
Content Area: Child Health

Test-Taking Strategy: Use the process of elimination. Eliminate options 2, 3, and 4 because of the close-ended words *restrict, all,* and *only.* Review the safety measures for a child with hemophilia if you had difficulty with this question.

Reference

Price, D., & Gwin, J. (2008). *Pediatric nursing: An introductory text* (10th ed., pp. 192, 247). St. Louis: Saunders.

---

202. Seizure precautions have been ordered for a client. The nurse should avoid doing which of the following when planning care for the client?

1 Turning on the lights in the room at night
2 Maintaining the bed in the lowest position
3 Assisting the client to ambulate in the hallway
4 Monitoring the client closely while the client is showering

Level of Cognitive Ability: Application
Client Needs: Safe and Effective Care Environment
Integrated Process: Nursing Process/Planning
Content Area: Adult Health/Neurological

Answer: 1

Rationale: A quiet, restful environment is provided as part of seizure precautions. This includes undisturbed times for sleep and a nightlight for safety. The client should be accompanied during activities such as bathing and walking so that assistance is readily available and injury is minimized if a seizure begins. The bed is maintained in the low position for safety.

Test-Taking Strategy: Use the process of elimination. Note the strategic word *avoid.* This word indicates a negative event query and asks you to select an option that is an incorrect nursing action. Eliminate options 3 and 4 because they indicate safe planning. Eliminate option 2 next because it also represents an item that addresses client safety. Review the care of the client with orders for seizure precautions if you had difficulty with this question.

References

Ignatavicius, D., & Workman, M. (2010). *Medical-surgical nursing: Patient-centered collaborative care* (6th ed., p. 959). St. Louis: Saunders.
Potter, P., & Perry, A. (2009). *Fundamentals of nursing* (7th ed., p. 844). St. Louis: Mosby.

---

203. A client with active tuberculosis is admitted to the medical-surgical unit. When planning a bed assignment, the nurse follows proper acid-fast bacteria isolation precautions when he or she does which of the following?

1 Transfers the client to the intensive care unit
2 Places the client in a private, well-ventilated room
3 Assigns the client to a double room because intravenous antibiotics will be administered
4 Assigns the client to a double room and places a "Strict Handwashing" sign outside the door

Answer: 2

Rationale: According to category-specific (respiratory) isolation precautions, acid-fast bacteria isolation always requires a private room. The room used should be well ventilated and should provide at least 6 exchanges of air per hour; it should also be ventilated to the outside, if possible. Option 2 is the only appropriate option.

Test-Taking Strategy: Note that the question states *active tuberculosis.* Eliminate options 3 and 4 because they are comparable or alike in that they both involve a double room. Eliminate option 1 by focusing on the client's diagnosis. Review the care of the client with active tuberculosis if you had difficulty with this question.

Reference

Christensen, B., & Kockrow, E. (2006). *Adult health nursing* (5th ed., p. 429). St. Louis: Mosby.

Level of Cognitive Ability: Application
Client Needs: Safe and Effective Care Environment
Integrated Process: Nursing Process/Planning
Content Area: Adult Health/Respiratory

---

204. A nurse is caring for a client in pelvic traction. To ensure safety, which physician order requires clarification?
1 Keep the client in good alignment.
2 Raise the head of the bed 30 degrees.
3 Observe for pressure points over the iliac crest.
4 Apply the pelvic girdle snugly over the client's pelvis and iliac crest.

Level of Cognitive Ability: Application
Client Needs: Safe and Effective Care Environment
Integrated Process: Nursing Process/Implementation
Content Area: Adult Health/Musculoskeletal

Answer: 2
Rationale: The foot of the bed is raised to prevent the client from being pulled down in bed by the traction. The head of the bed is usually kept flat, and good body alignment is maintained. The girdle should be applied snugly so that it does not slip off. The skin should be checked for pressure sores.

Test-Taking Strategy: Use the process of elimination, and note the strategic words *requires clarification*. Options 1 and 3 are fundamental principles and are eliminated first. From the remaining options, visualizing the procedure will direct you to option 2. Review the procedure for pelvic traction if you had difficulty with this question.

Reference
Christensen, B., & Kockrow, E. (2006). *Adult health nursing* (5th ed., p. 175). St. Louis: Mosby.

---

205. A client is admitted to the long-term care facility with a diagnosis of Parkinson's disease. The nurse gives information about the client's condition to a visitor who is assumed to be a family member. The nurse has violated which legal concept of the nurse–client relationship?
1 Assault
2 Invasion of privacy
3 Battery
4 Negligence

Level of Cognitive Ability: Comprehension
Client Needs: Safe and Effective Care Environment
Integrated Process: Nursing Process/Implementation
Content Area: Fundamental Skills

Answer: 2
Rationale: Discussing a client's condition without the client's permission violates the client's rights and places the nurse in legal jeopardy. This action by the nurse invades privacy and affects the confidentiality issue of client rights. Assault occurs when one person puts another person in fear of a harmful contact. Negligence is conduct that falls below the standard of care. Battery is an intentional touching of another's body without consent to do so.

Test-Taking Strategy: Use the process of elimination. Focusing on the subject of the question—sharing information and what constitutes an invasion of privacy—will direct you to the correct option. Review client rights if you had difficulty with this question.

Reference
Christensen, B., & Kockrow, E. (2006). *Foundations of nursing* (5th ed., p. 25). St. Louis: Mosby.

---

206. A nurse is collecting data about the client's risk for falls. The nurse recognizes that which of the following factors promotes safety?
1 Cataracts
2 Use of nitroglycerin
3 Episodes of dizziness
4 Use of orthopedic shoes

Answer: 4
Rationale: Several factors can increase the client's risk for falls: impaired vision, medications that cause dizziness or orthostatic hypotension, and problems with balance and coordination. Cataracts represent a vision impairment, which could increase the client's risk. Dizziness obviously increases the likelihood of a fall. Nitroglycerin could cause orthostatic hypotension, which is also a potential risk. Orthopedic shoes are specially fitted for the client and are generally sturdy and safe.

Level of Cognitive Ability: Comprehension
Client Needs: Safe and Effective Care Environment
Integrated Process: Nursing Process/Data Collection
Content Area: Fundamental Skills

Test-Taking Strategy: Use the process of elimination, and note the strategic words *promotes safety*. To select the correct option, evaluate each of the items in terms of the potential of that item to make the client fall. Orthopedic shoes are beneficial to the client and provide stability; this should direct you to option 4. Review the risk factors for falls if you had difficulty with this question.

References

Christensen, B., & Kockrow, E. (2006). *Foundations of nursing* (5th ed., p. 1119). St. Louis: Mosby.
Wold, G. (2008). *Basic geriatric nursing* (4th ed., p. 154). St. Louis: Mosby.

---

207. A nurse enters the laundry room to empty a bag of dirty linens and discovers a fire. The nurse activates the alarm, closes the laundry room door, and obtains the fire extinguisher to extinguish the fire. To prepare to use the fire extinguisher, the nurse first:

1 Pulls the pin on the fire extinguisher
2 Squeezes the handle on the extinguisher
3 Puts on a mask before using the extinguisher
4 Puts on a pair of gloves before touching the extinguisher

Level of Cognitive Ability: Application
Client Needs: Safe and Effective Care Environment
Integrated Process: Nursing Process/Implementation
Content Area: Fundamental Skills

Answer: 1

Rationale: A fire can be extinguished by using a fire extinguisher. To use the extinguisher, the pin is pulled first. The extinguisher should then be aimed at the base of the fire. The handle of the extinguisher is squeezed, and the fire is extinguished by sweeping the extinguisher from side to side to coat the area evenly. Although the nurse should be cautious when using a fire extinguisher, it is not necessary to don gloves or a mask; these actions would delay the process of extinguishing the fire.

Test-Taking Strategy: Use the process of elimination. Eliminate options 3 and 4 first because these actions would delay the process of extinguishing the fire. Remember the acronym *PASS* to prioritize in the use of a fire extinguisher: **P**ull the pin; **A**im at the base of the fire; **S**queeze the handle; and **S**weep from side to side to coat the area evenly. Review the appropriate use of a fire extinguisher if you had difficulty with this question.

Reference

Christensen, B., & Kockrow, E. (2006). *Foundations of nursing* (5th ed., p. 365). St. Louis: Mosby.

---

208. A nurse is caring for a client receiving chemotherapy. On review of the morning laboratory results, the nurse notes that the white blood cell count is extremely low, and the client is immediately placed on neutropenic precautions. The client's breakfast tray arrives, and the nurse inspects the meal and prepares to bring the tray into the client's room. Which of the following actions should the nurse take before bringing the meal to the client?

1 Removing the coffee from the breakfast tray
2 Asking the client if he or she feels like eating at this time
3 Calling the dietary department to ask for disposable utensils
4 Removing the fresh-squeezed orange juice from the breakfast tray

Answer: 4

Rationale: For the immunocompromised client, a low-bacteria diet is implemented; this includes avoiding fresh fruits and vegetables and ensuring that food is thoroughly cooked. It is not necessary to remove the coffee from the tray. Disposable utensils are used for clients who are infectious and who present a risk of transmitting an infection to others. It is best to encourage the client to eat because nutrition is very important for a client receiving chemotherapy who is immunocompromised.

Test-Taking Strategy: Use the process of elimination, and focus on the subject of the question—neutropenic precautions. Eliminate option 2 because this is not the best measure for the client who requires nutrition. Eliminate option 1 because there is no reason for it. Knowing that fresh fruits and vegetables present a threat to this client or that disposable utensils are used for the client who is infectious will direct you to option 4. Review the interventions for the client with hematological toxicity if you had difficulty with this question.

Level of Cognitive Ability: Application
Client Needs: Safe and Effective Care Environment
Integrated Process: Nursing Process/Implementation
Content Area: Adult Health/Oncology

Reference

Christensen, B., & Kockrow, E. (2006). *Adult health nursing* (5th ed., p. 833). St. Louis: Mosby.

---

209. A nurse is assigned to care for a client on contact precautions. When reviewing the client's record, the nurse notes that the client has a health care–associated (nosocomial) infection caused by methicillin-resistant *Staphylococcus aureus*. The client has an abdominal wound that requires irrigation and a tracheostomy attached to a mechanical ventilator that requires frequent suctioning. The nurse gathers supplies before entering the client's room. Which of the following protective items will the nurse need when caring for this client?

1 Gloves and a gown
2 Gloves and goggles
3 Gloves, a gown, and goggles
4 Gloves, a gown, and shoe protectors

Answer: 3

Rationale: Goggles are worn to protect the mucous membranes of the eye during interventions that may produce splashes of blood, body fluids, secretions, and excretions. In addition, contact precautions require that gloves be used and a gown worn if direct client contact is anticipated. Shoe protectors are not necessary.

Test-Taking Strategy: Use the process of elimination. Note the strategic words *contact precautions, irrigation,* and *frequent suctioning*. Visualizing the nursing care required to perform these procedures will direct you to option 3. Review transmission-based precautions if you had difficulty with this question.

References

deWit, S. (2009). *Medical-surgical nursing: Concepts & practice* (pp. 1189-1190). St. Louis: Saunders.
Linton, A. (2007). *Introduction to medical-surgical nursing* (4th ed., p. 172). Philadelphia: Saunders.

Level of Cognitive Ability: Application
Client Needs: Safe and Effective Care Environment
Integrated Process: Nursing Process/Implementation
Content Area: Fundamental Skills

---

210. A nurse who is assigned to work with a hospitalized client should do which of the following to maintain standard precautions?

1 Conduct handwashing only before donning gloves.
2 Dispose of sharps, needles, and syringes in a labeled plastic bag.
3 Use protective equipment, such as a mask and gloves, when collecting data from the client.
4 Institute protective measures when the potential for exposure to blood or body fluids exists.

Answer: 4

Rationale: Protective measures are necessary when exposure is likely or anticipated, but they are not necessary for all client contacts or for data collection. Sharps, needles, and syringes must be disposed of in puncture-resistant containers. Handwashing must be performed before and after all procedures and client contacts, regardless of the use of gloves.

Test-Taking Strategy: Use the process of elimination. Eliminate option 1 first because of the close-ended word *only*. Eliminate option 2 next because of the words *plastic bag*. From the remaining options, recalling that protective measures are necessary when exposure is likely or anticipated will direct you to option 4. Review standard precautions if you had difficulty with this question.

Reference

deWit, S. (2009). *Medical-surgical nursing: Concepts & practice* (pp. 1189-1190). St. Louis: Saunders.

Level of Cognitive Ability: Application
Client Needs: Safe and Effective Care Environment
Integrated Process: Nursing Process/Implementation
Content Area: Fundamental Skills

211. A nurse has administered an injection to a client. After the injection, the nurse accidentally drops the syringe on the floor. Which of the following actions by the nurse is appropriate?

1 Call the housekeeping department to pick up the syringe.
2 Recap the needle and then use forceps to discard the syringe.
3 Carefully pick up the syringe from the floor and gently recap the needle.
4 Carefully pick up the syringe from the floor and dispose of it in a sharps container.

Level of Cognitive Ability: Application
Client Needs: Safe and Effective Care Environment
Integrated Process: Nursing Process/Implementation
Content Area: Fundamental Skills

Answer: 4

Rationale: Syringes should never be recapped in any circumstances to prevent being stuck by a contaminated needle. Syringes should always be placed in sharps containers immediately after use to prevent injury from a needle stick. It is not appropriate to ask housekeeping to pick up the syringe.

Test-Taking Strategy: Use the process of elimination. Eliminate options 2 and 3 because they are comparable or alike. Use principles related to standard precautions to direct you to option 4. Review the procedure for discarding needles if you had difficulty with this question.

References

Christensen, B., & Kockrow, E. (2006). *Foundations of nursing* (5th ed., p. 353). St. Louis: Mosby.

Potter, P., & Perry, A. (2009). *Fundamentals of nursing* (7th ed., p. 660). St. Louis: Mosby.

---

212. After discussing the use of restraints with a client and family, a physician has written an order for wrist restraints to be applied to the client. The nurse instructs the nursing assistant to apply the restraints. When checking the client, which of the following observations indicates that the nursing assistant performed unsafe care and needs teaching about the safe use of restraints?

1 The restraints were released every 2 hours.
2 The restraints were applied snugly and tightly.
3 A safety knot was used to secure the restraints.
4 The call light was placed within reach of the client's hand.

Level of Cognitive Ability: Comprehension
Client Needs: Safe and Effective Care Environment
Integrated Process: Teaching and Learning
Content Area: Leadership/Management

Answer: 2

Rationale: Restraints should never be applied tightly because they could impair circulation. A safety knot should be used because it can easily be released in an emergency. Restraints must be released every 2 hours for inspection of the skin, assessment of circulation, and range-of-motion exercises. The call light must always be placed within the client's reach so that the client can use it to obtain assistance.

Test-Taking Strategy: Note the strategic words *performed unsafe care;* these words indicate a negative event query and ask you to select an option that is an incorrect action. Using the process of elimination and noting the word *tightly* in option 2 will direct you to this option. Review the care of the client with restraints if you had difficulty with this question.

Reference

deWit, S. (2009). *Medical-surgical nursing: Concepts & practice* (p. 1149). St. Louis: Saunders.

---

213. A nurse is caring for a child with bronchiolitis caused by respiratory syncytial virus (RSV). Which of the following precautions will the nurse institute when caring for the child to decrease the spread of organisms?

Answer: 1

Rationale: RSV can live on paper or skin for up to 1 hour and on cribs or other nonporous surfaces for up to 6 hours. Although RSV is not airborne, it is highly communicable, and it is usually transferred by the hands. Meticulous handwashing

1 Contact isolation
2 Enteric precautions
3 Protective isolation
4 Respiratory isolation

Level of Cognitive Ability: Application
Client Needs: Safe and Effective Care Environment
Integrated Process: Nursing Process/ Implementation
Content Area: Child Health

decreases the spread of organisms. Personnel who care for children with RSV should maintain contact isolation, which includes wearing gloves and gowns and practicing good handwashing.

Test-Taking Strategy: Knowledge regarding the method of transmission of RSV is required to answer this question. Remember that RSV is highly communicable and that it is usually transferred by the hands. Review RSV and its mode of transmission if you had difficulty with this question.

Reference

Leifer, G. (2007). *Introduction to maternity and pediatric nursing* (5th ed., p. 577). Philadelphia: Saunders.

---

214. Which of the following items would be appropriate for the nurse to wear if there is the potential for body fluid to splatter into the mouth or nose while caring for the client?
1 Cap
2 Mask
3 Gown
4 Goggles

Level of Cognitive Ability: Application
Client Needs: Safe and Effective Care Environment
Integrated Process: Nursing Process/ Implementation
Content Area: Fundamental Skills

Answer: 2
Rationale: A mask would offer full protection of the nose and mouth. Goggles would protect the eyes from getting injured. A gown would protect the nurse's uniform. A cap would protect the nurse's hair.

Test-Taking Strategy: Note the strategic words *mouth or nose;* the only item that would protect these areas is a mask. Review standard precautions if you had difficulty with this question.

Reference

Christensen, B., & Kockrow, E. (2006). *Foundations of nursing* (5th ed., p. 280). St. Louis: Mosby.

---

215. A nurse is assigned to care for four clients. The nurse implements which of the following to prevent the spread of infection from client to client?
1 Using clean technique with all procedures
2 Performing sterile technique with all procedures
3 Using proper handwashing techniques when necessary
4 Reading about performing treatments in the policy and procedure manual

Level of Cognitive Ability: Application
Client Needs: Safe and Effective Care Environment
Integrated Process: Teaching and Learning
Content Area: Fundamental Skills

Answer: 3
Rationale: Proper handwashing is the best way to prevent the spread of infection. Reading the policy and procedure manual does not guarantee that infection will not spread. All procedures do not require sterile technique, and clean technique alone is not always appropriate.

Test-Taking Strategy: Focus on the subject of the question—preventing the spread of infection. Recalling the importance of handwashing will direct you to option 3. Review the importance of handwashing if you had difficulty with this question.

References

Christensen, B., & Kockrow, E. (2006). *Foundations of nursing* (5th ed., pp. 281-282). St. Louis: Mosby.
deWit, S. (2009). *Medical-surgical nursing: Concepts & practice* (pp. 119-120, 126). St. Louis: Saunders.

---

216. A nurse needs to collect a midstream urine specimen from a female client. Which of the following indicates that the nurse understands the principles of using proper technique to collect the specimen?

1. Cleansing the meatus with antiseptic pads using upward strokes
2. Making sure that the fingers do not touch the inside of the collection container
3. Letting go of the labia after it is cleansed and asking the client to urinate
4. Instructing the client to urinate in the container after the labia have been cleansed

Level of Cognitive Ability: Application
Client Needs: Safe and Effective Care Environment
Integrated Process: Nursing Process/Implementation
Content Area: Fundamental Skills

Answer: 2
Rationale: The inside of the container is sterile, and sterility must be maintained. Fingers touching the inside would contaminate the container. The meatus should be cleansed from front to back (toward the anus); upward strokes would carry bacteria from the anal region. The labia should remain open during the procedure. The client should urinate a small amount into the toilet before urinating into the specimen container to allow some of the organisms near the meatus to leave the area.

Test-Taking Strategy: Use the process of elimination, and identify the option that would prevent contamination. This will direct you to option 2. Review the procedure for collecting a midstream urine specimen if you had difficulty with this question.

Reference

Christensen, B., & Kockrow, E. (2006). *Foundations of nursing* (5th ed., p. 503). St. Louis: Mosby.

ALTERNATE ITEM FORMAT QUESTIONS

Prioritizing (Ordered Response)

217. List in order of priority the steps for correctly performing handwashing. Number 1 is the first step, and number 6 is the last step.

___ Turn on the water.
___ Dry the hands with a paper towel.
___ Allow the warm water to wet the hands.
___ Turn the water faucet off with the paper towel.
___ Apply soap to the hands and rub them vigorously.
___ Keep the hands pointed downward and then rinse them.

Level of Cognitive Ability: Application
Client Needs: Safe and Effective Care Environment
Integrated Process: Nursing Process/Implementation
Content Area: Delegating/Prioritizing

Answer: 1, 5, 2, 6, 3, 4
Rationale: The water is turned on first. The hands are then wet with warm water, soap is applied, and the hands are rubbed vigorously to cleanse them of germs. The hands are pointed downward so that the germs flow into the sink rather than backward up the hands and arms when they are rinsed. The hands are dried and the faucet is turned off with the use of paper towels to prevent the hands from becoming recontaminated.

Test-Taking Strategy: Visualize the procedure. Thinking about the principles related to asepsis and avoiding contamination will help you to determine the correct order of action. Review the procedure for handwashing if you had difficulty with this question.

Reference

Christensen, B., & Kockrow, E. (2006). *Foundations of nursing* (5th ed., pp. 281-282). St. Louis: Mosby.

Multiple Response

218. A client was brought to the emergency department after an episode of acute anginal pain. The client was hospitalized, and diagnostic studies were performed.

Answer: 1, 2, 3, 5
Rationale: Copies of a living will should be kept with the medical record, at the physician's office, and in the client's home. A copy will also be retained in the client's lawyer's office. These

After treatment, the client was discharged. The client is readmitted to the hospital and tells the nurse that a living will was prepared during the last hospital admission. The nurse understands that a copy of this document can be obtained from which locations? Select all that apply.

- ❒ 1 The client's home
- ❒ 2 The physician's office
- ❒ 3 The client's lawyer's office
- ❒ 4 The client's daughter's home
- ❒ 5 The medical record at the hospital
- ❒ 6 The hospital emergency department files

Level of Cognitive Ability: Comprehension
Client Needs: Safe and Effective Care Environment
Integrated Process: Nursing Process/Implementation
Content Area: Fundamental Skills

documents are not maintained in emergency department files or in the home of another person other than the client.

Test-Taking Strategy: Focus on the subject—maintaining a copy of the client's living will. It would seem reasonable that the physician would keep a copy of this document in the medical files. The client would certainly have a copy in his or her home, because this document identifies the client's wishes. It would also seem reasonable that a copy would be maintained in the client's medical record to provide guidance to care providers if an event arose during hospitalization that required referral to this document. It is not realistic for an emergency department to maintain such documents in their files. In addition, this document would not be kept in another person's home, because this would violate the client's right to privacy. Review the procedures related to living wills if you had difficulty with this question.

Reference
Christensen, B., & Kockrow, E. (2006). *Foundations of nursing* (5th ed., p. 205). St. Louis: Mosby.

Fill-in-the-Blank

219. A client is to receive 1000 mL of 5% dextrose at 125 mL per hour. The drop factor is 10 drops (gtt) per mL. To administer the infusion safely, the nurse adjusts the flow rate at how many drops per minute? (Round answer to the nearest whole number.)

Answer: _____ gtt per minute

Level of Cognitive Ability: Application
Client Needs: Safe and Effective Care Environment
Integrated Process: Nursing Process/Implementation
Content Area: Fundamental Skills

Answer: 21 gtt per minute
Rationale: The first step is to determine how many hours the intravenous (IV) solution will last. This requires the simple division of the total volume of mL to be infused (1000 mL) by the total mL per hour (125 mL), which results in 8 hours. Convert the hours to minutes (8 hours = 480 minutes), and then use the formula to calculate the flow rate.
Formula:

$$\frac{\text{Total volume in mL} \times \text{drop factor}}{\text{Time in minutes}} = \text{Flow rate in drops per minute}$$

$$\frac{1000\text{ mL} \times 10\text{ gtt}}{480\text{ minutes}} = \frac{10{,}000}{480} = 20.8 \text{ or } 21 \text{ gtt per minute}$$

Test-Taking Strategy: Use the formula for calculating an IV flow rate. Remember that you need to convert hours to minutes. Recheck your work, and verify the answer with a calculator. Review the formula for IV flow rates if you had difficulty with this question.

Reference
Potter, P., & Perry, A. (2009). *Fundamentals of nursing* (7th ed., pp. 1007-1010). St. Louis: Mosby.

Multiple Response

220. A nurse is caring for a client with leukemia who is receiving chemotherapy. The nurse reviews the client's laboratory results and notes that the client's neutrophil count is less than 1000 cells/mm^3.

Answer: 3, 5, 6
Rationale: A client who has a low neutrophil count is at risk for infection, so interventions are aimed at preventing this occurrence. Individuals with a cold or respiratory infection should not be in contact with the client. Because clients with low white blood

Choose the nursing interventions that specifically apply to the care of the client. Select all that apply.

❒ 1 Pad the side rails.
❒ 2 Place the client in a semiprivate room.
❒ 3 Restrict visitors with colds or respiratory infections.
❒ 4 Remove all hazards and sharp objects from the environment.
❒ 5 Implement a low-bacteria diet that excludes fresh fruits, vegetables, and milk products.
❒ 6 Place a clean mask on the client if the client needs to leave the room for a diagnostic test.

Level of Cognitive Ability: Application
Client Needs: Safe and Effective Care Environment
Integrated Process: Nursing Process/Implementation
Content Area: Adult Health/Oncology

cell counts often become infected with their own microorganisms through their gastrointestinal tracts, a low-bacteria diet is prescribed. The client should wear a clean mask when outside of his or her room, especially in heavily traveled public areas such as corridors, elevators, and waiting rooms. Invasive procedures are avoided as much as possible to prevent the entrance of microorganisms into the client's body, and the client's temperature is monitored frequently to detect any early signs of infection. The client should be encouraged to shower daily to remove bacteria from the skin and perianal area. The client should be placed in a private room. Padding the side rails and removing all hazards and sharp objects from the environment would be implemented if the client had thrombocytopenia and was at risk for bleeding.

Test-Taking Strategy: Note that the client has a low neutrophil count. Recalling that this low count places a client at risk for infection will help you to identify the appropriate interventions. Review the interventions for the client at risk for infection if you had difficulty with this question.

Reference

Linton, A. (2007). *Introduction to medical-surgical nursing* (4th ed., pp. 604-605). Philadelphia: Saunders.

Figure/Illustration

221. The physician's order is to administer 5 mg of enalapril maleate (Vasotec) orally twice daily. The nurse reads the label on the medication bottle and safely prepares how many tablets to administer one dose?

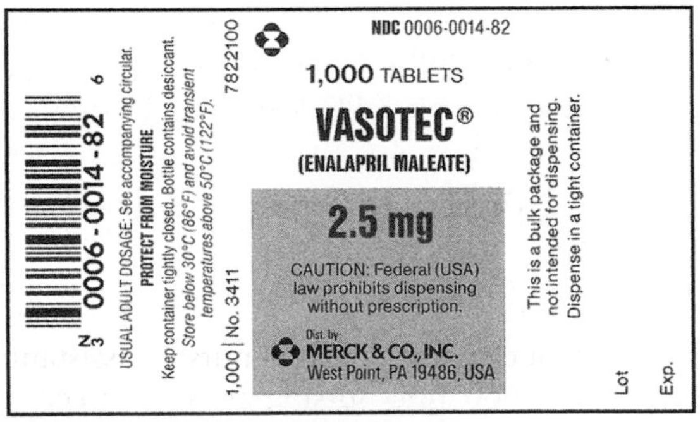

Figure 6-1 Vasotec medication label. (From Kee, J., & Marshall, S. [2009]. *Clinical calculations: With applications to general and specialty areas* [6th ed., p. 141]. Philadelphia: Saunders.)

Answer: _____ tablets

Level of Cognitive Ability: Application
Client Needs: Safe and Effective Care Environment
Integrated Process: Nursing Process/Implementation
Content Area: Fundamental Skills

Answer: 2 tablets
Rationale: Use the formula for calculating medication doses.
Formula

$$\frac{\text{Desired}}{\text{Available}} \times \text{Quantity} = \text{Dose}$$

$$\frac{5\text{ mg}}{2.5\text{ mg}} \times 1\text{ tablet} = 2\text{ tablets}$$

Test-Taking Strategy: Perform the calculation on a piece of paper, and follow the formula for the calculation of the correct dose. Use a calculator to recheck your work, and make sure that the answer makes sense. Review the medication calculation formula if you had difficulty with this question.

Reference

Kee, J., & Marshall, S. (2009). *Clinical calculations: With applications to general and specialty areas* (6th ed., pp. 86, 141). Philadelphia: Saunders.

Multiple Response

222. The nurse understands that a transparent film wound-care product can be safely used for which types of wounds? Select all that apply.

- ❒ 1 Infected wounds
- ❒ 2 Superficial wounds
- ❒ 3 Partial-thickness wounds
- ❒ 4 Wounds with little or no exudates
- ❒ 5 Wounds with sloughing or necrosis
- ❒ 6 Wounds with tunneling or sinus tracts

Level of Cognitive Ability: Comprehension
Client Needs: Safe and Effective Care Environment
Integrated Process: Nursing Process/Planning
Content Area: Adult Health/Integumentary

Answer: 2, 3, 4, 5

Rationale: A transparent film wound-care product allows for the visualization of the wound and provides a moist environment that promotes granulation tissue and the autolysis of necrotic tissue. It allows oxygen and water vapor to escape while remaining impermeable to bacteria and contaminants. This type of product is used for superficial wounds, partial-thickness wounds, wounds with little or no exudates, and wounds with sloughing or necrosis. It is not recommended for wounds that are infected, those with heavy exudates, or those with tunneling or sinus tracts; gauze dressings would be used for these types of wounds.

Test-Taking Strategy: Focus on the subject—a transparent film wound-care product. Visualize this type of wound-care product. Recalling that it allows for the visualization of the wound and that it retains moisture will direct you to the correct options. Review the characteristics of a transparent film dressing if you had difficulty with this question.

References

Black, J., & Hawks, J. (2009). *Medical-surgical nursing: Clinical management for positive outcomes* (8th ed., p. 316). St. Louis: Saunders.

Perry, A., & Potter, P. (2010). *Clinical nursing skills and techniques* (7th ed., pp. 1015-1016). St. Louis: Mosby.

Multiple Response

223. Which of the following clients have needs that can be safely cared for by a nursing assistant? Select all that apply.

- ❒ 1 A client on strict bedrest
- ❒ 2 A client who requires nasogastric tube feedings every 4 hours
- ❒ 3 A client who requires abdominal wound dressing changes every 8 hours
- ❒ 4 A client who requires transport via stretcher to the radiology department for a chest x-ray
- ❒ 5 A client who requires bladder scanning to check for the amount of residual after every voiding
- ❒ 6 A client who requires stool collection and the testing of the stool for blood with blood-testing strips

Level of Cognitive Ability: Application
Client Needs: Safe and Effective Care Environment
Integrated Process: Nursing Process/Implementation
Content Area: Delegating/Prioritizing

Answer: 1, 4, 5, 6

Rationale: Delegation is an activity that involves assigning responsibility for certain tasks to other people. The nurse needs to know each staff member's capabilities as well as the constraints dictated by licensure and education level. A nursing assistant is an unlicensed person and lacks the education needed to provide care to clients who require invasive treatments or clients with complex needs. Administering a tube feeding is an invasive procedure that needs to be performed by a licensed health care provider. Changing an abdominal dressing is an invasive procedure that requires the use of aseptic technique and that also needs to be performed by a licensed health care provider. The clients described in options 1, 4, 5, and 6 have needs that can be met by the nursing assistant; these needs are noninvasive, and the nursing assistant receives training in performing the tasks required.

Test-Taking Strategy: Note that the question asks about the clients that can be cared for by the nursing assistant. Remembering that the nursing assistant is unlicensed and that he or she can perform tasks that are noninvasive will direct you to the correct options. Review the principles related to delegating and the role of the nursing assistant if you had difficulty with this question.

Reference

Marriner-Tomey, A. (2009). *Guide to nursing management and leadership* (8th ed., pp. 52-56). St. Louis: Mosby.

Chart/Exhibit

224. Which documentation entry is incomplete?

Client's Medical Record Nursing Notes			
Date	Time	Note	Signature
1. 2/9/11	1530	Awake and oriented to time, place, and person.	Jane Doe, LPN
2. 2/9/11	1600	Abdominal dressing changed.	Jane Doe, LPN
3. 2/9/11	1630	To radiology via wheelchair for chest x-ray.	Jane Doe, LPN
4. 2/9/11	1730	Returned from radiology. Assisted from wheelchair to bedside chair per client's request. Daughter visiting client.	Jane Doe, LPN

Answer: _____

Level of Cognitive Ability: Comprehension
Client Needs: Safe and Effective Care Environment
Integrated Process: Communication and Documentation
Content Area: Fundamental Skills

Answer: 2
Rationale: The principles of documentation imply rules for legibility, correct use of terminology and abbreviations, brevity, sequence of occurrence, completeness, confidentiality, and the signing of notes made in the client's medical record. Notations about dressings need to include the location of the dressing, the nature of the secure attachment of the dressing to the client, and the amount as well as the description of any drainage observed. If a dressing is removed, the condition of the skin and the wound under it should be described. The notations in options 1, 3, and 4 are complete.

Test-Taking Strategy: Focus on the subject—the incomplete documentation note. Remember that when the client has a dressing and the dressing is changed, it is necessary to document a complete description of the wound. Review the principles related to documentation if you had difficulty with this question.

Reference

Harkreader, H., Hogan, M.A., & Thobaben, M. (2007). *Fundamentals of nursing: Caring and clinical judgement* (3rd ed., pp. 232, 239, 241). Philadelphia: Saunders.

Fill-in-the-Blank

225. A physician prescribes 1000 mL of normal saline to be infused over 12 hours. The drop factor is 15 drops (gtt) per mL. To administer the infusion safely, the nurse adjusts the flow rate at how many drops per minute? (Round answer to the nearest whole number.)

Answer: _____ gtt per minute

Level of Cognitive Ability: Application
Client Needs: Safe and Effective Care Environment
Integrated Process: Nursing Process/Implementation
Content Area: Fundamental Skills

Answer: 21 gtt per minute
Rationale: Use the formula for calculating intravenous (IV) drip rates.
Formula:

$$\frac{\text{Total volume in mL} \times \text{drop factor}}{\text{Time in minutes}} = \text{Flow rate in drops per minute}$$

$$\frac{1000\text{ mL} \times 15\text{ drops}}{720\text{ minutes}} = \frac{15000}{720} = 20.8, \text{ or } 21\text{ gtt per minute}$$

Test-Taking Strategy: Use the formula for calculating an IV flow rate. Remember that you need to convert hours to minutes. Recheck your work, and verify the answer with a calculator. Review the formula for IV flow rates if you had difficulty with this question.

Reference

Potter, P., & Perry, A. (2009). *Fundamentals of nursing* (7th ed., pp. 1007-1010). St. Louis: Mosby.

Fill-in-the-Blank

226. A nurse takes the temperature of a client and obtains a reading of 37.5° C. The reading needs to be converted to degrees Fahrenheit before it is documented. The nurse would document what as the final measurement?

Answer: _____° F

Level of Cognitive Ability: Application
Client Needs: Safe and Effective Care Environment
Integrated Process: Nursing Process/ Implementation
Content Area: Fundamental Skills

Answer: 99.5° F
Rationale: Use the formula for converting degrees Celsius to degrees Fahrenheit: take the Celsius measurement, multiply it by 1.8, and add 32.
Formula:

$$F = (1.8 \times C) + 32$$
$$F = (1.8 \times 37.5) + 32$$
$$F = 99.5°$$

Test-Taking Strategy: Note that the question asks you to convert degrees Celsius to degrees Fahrenheit. Use the formula for this conversion, and verify the answer with a calculator. Review this formula and how to use it to convert temperature measurements if you had difficulty with this question.

Reference
Harkreader, H., Hogan, M.A., & Thobaben, M. (2007). *Fundamentals of nursing: Caring and clinical judgement* (3rd ed., p. 117). Philadelphia: Saunders.

Multiple Response

227. Which of the following conditions require airborne precautions? Select all that apply.

- ❐ 1 Chickenpox
- ❐ 2 Acute diarrhea
- ❐ 3 Wound infection
- ❐ 4 Respiratory tuberculosis
- ❐ 5 Respiratory syncytial virus
- ❐ 6 Severe acute respiratory syndrome (SARS)

Level of Cognitive Ability: Application
Client Needs: Safe and Effective Care Environment
Integrated Process: Nursing Process/ Implementation
Content Area: Fundamental Skills

Answer: 1, 4, 6
Rationale: Airborne precautions are used to prevent infection when the infectious organism is capable of remaining in the air for prolonged periods of time and of being transported in the air for distances of more than 3 feet; therefore these precautions are necessary for chickenpox, tuberculosis, and SARS. Contact precautions are used when working with clients who have infections that are spread by direct or indirect contact. The conditions noted in options 1, 2, and 5 are spread by contact with the organism.

Test-Taking Strategy: Focus on the subject—conditions that require the use of airborne precautions. Think about the pathophysiology and nursing care associated with each condition identified in the options to answer correctly. Review these conditions and airborne and contact precautions if you had difficulty with this question.

Reference
Potter, P., & Perry, A. (2009). *Fundamentals of nursing* (7th ed., p. 645). St. Louis: Mosby.

Multiple Response

228. Which of the following statements are appropriate to document on an incident report for a client who experienced a fall? Select all that apply.

- ❐ 1 The client fell out of bed.
- ❐ 2 The client was found lying on the floor.
- ❐ 3 No bruises or injuries are noted on the client.
- ❐ 4 The client's physician was called and notified.

Answer: 2, 3, 4, 5
Rationale: An incident or adverse-occurrence report is a tool used by health care facilities to document situations that have caused harm or that have the potential to cause harm to clients, employees, or visitors. Common situations that require the completion of an incident report include medication errors, falls, and accidental needle sticks. When completing documentation on an incident report, the same principles used when documenting in a client's medical record are followed. Only facts are documented; the nurse would not document interpretations of the situation (options 1 and 6 are interpretations).

❒ 5 The client is alert and oriented to date, time, and place.

❒ 6 The client apparently failed to call the nurse for assistance with getting out of bed.

Level of Cognitive Ability: Application
Client Needs: Safe and Effective Care Environment
Integrated Process: Communication and Documentation
Content Area: Fundamental Skills

Test-Taking Strategy: Focus on the subject—accurate documentation notes in an incident report. Recalling the principles related to documentation and that the nurse would document facts rather than interpretations will direct you to the correct options. Review the principles related to documentation if you had difficulty with this question.

Reference:
Potter, P., & Perry, A. (2009). *Fundamentals of nursing* (7th ed., pp. 336, 403). St. Louis: Mosby.

REFERENCES

Black, J., & Hawks, J. (2009). *Medical-surgical nursing: Clinical management for positive outcomes* (8th ed.). St. Louis: Saunders.

Chernecky, C., & Berger, B. (2008). *Laboratory tests and diagnostic procedures* (5th ed.). Philadelphia: Saunders.

Christensen, B., & Kockrow, E. (2006). *Adult health nursing* (5th ed.). St. Louis: Mosby.

Christensen, B., & Kockrow, E. (2006). *Foundations of nursing* (5th ed.). St. Louis: Mosby.

deWit, S (2009). *Medical-surgical nursing: Concepts & practice*. St. Louis: Saunders.

Fortinash, K., & Holoday-Worret, P. (2008). *Psychiatric mental health nursing* (4th ed.). St. Louis: Mosby.

Harkreader, H., Hogan, M. A., & Thobaben, M. (2007). *Fundamentals of nursing: Caring and clinical judgement* (3rd ed.). Philadelphia: Saunders.

Hockenberry, M., & Wilson, D. (2007). *Nursing care of infants and children* (7th ed.). St. Louis: Mosby.

Hockenberry, M., & Wilson, D. (2009). *Wong's essentials of pediatric care* (8th ed.). St. Louis: Mosby.

Hodgson, B., & Kizior, R. (2009). *Saunders nursing drug handbook 2009*. Philadelphia: Saunders.

Ignatavicius, D., & Workman, M. (2010). *Medical-surgical nursing: Patient-centered collaborative care*. (6th ed.). St. Louis: Saunders.

Kee, J., Hayes, E., & McCuistion, L. (2009). *Pharmacology: A nursing process approach* (6th ed.). St. Louis: Saunders.

Kee, J., & Marshall, S. (2009). *Clinical calculations: With applications to general and specialty areas* (6th ed.). Philadelphia: Saunders.

Leifer, G. (2007). *Introduction to maternity and pediatric nursing* (5th ed.). Philadelphia: Saunders.

Leifer, G. (2008). *Maternity nursing: An introductory text* (10th ed.). Philadelphia: Saunders.

Lilley, L., Harrington, S., & Snyder, J. (2007). *Pharmacology and the nursing process* (5th ed.). St. Louis: Mosby.

Linton, A. (2007). *Introduction to medical-surgical nursing* (4th ed.). Philadelphia: Saunders.

Marriner-Tomey, A. (2009). *Guide to nursing management and leadership* (8th ed.). St. Louis: Mosby.

McKenry, L., Tessier, E., & Hogan, M. (2006). *Mosby's pharmacology in nursing* (22nd ed.). St. Louis: Mosby.

McKinney, E., James, S., Murray S., & Ashwill, J. (2009). *Maternal-child nursing* (3rd ed.). St. Louis: Mosby.

Monahan, F., Sands, J., Marek, J., Neighbors, M., & Green, C. (2007). *Phipps' medical-surgical nursing: Health and illness perspectives* (8th ed.). St. Louis: Mosby.

Mosby. (2008). *2008 Mosby's nursing drug reference* (21st ed.). St. Louis: Mosby.

Pagana, K., & Pagana, T. (2009). *Mosby's diagnostic laboratory test reference* (9th ed.). St. Louis: Mosby.

Perry, A., & Potter, P. (2010). *Clinical nursing skills & techniques* (7th ed.). St. Louis: Mosby.

Potter, P., & Perry, A. (2009). *Fundamentals of nursing* (7th ed.). St. Louis: Mosby.

Price, D., & Gwin, J. (2008). *Pediatric nursing: An introductory text* (10th ed.). St. Louis: Saunders.

Proehl, J. (2009). *Emergency nursing procedures* (4th ed.). St. Louis: Saunders.

Stuart, G. (2009). *Principles and practices of psychiatric nursing* (9th ed.). St. Louis: Mosby.

Varcarolis, E., & Halter, M. (2009). *Essentials of psychiatric mental health nursing: A communication approach to evidence-based care*. St. Louis: Saunders.

Wold, G. (2008). *Basic geriatric nursing* (4th ed.). St. Louis: Mosby.

CHAPTER

7

Health Promotion and Maintenance

229. A nurse is performing a neurovascular check on a client. Which of the following is the best method to use when checking a client's pupillary reaction to light?

1 Turn the light on directly in front of the eye and watch for a response.
2 Ask the client to follow the light through the six cardinal positions of gaze.
3 Check the pupil size and then have the client alternate between watching the light and watching the examiner's finger.
4 Instruct the client to look straight ahead and then shine the light on the client, moving it from the temporal area to the eye.

Level of Cognitive Ability: Application
Client Needs: Health Promotion and Maintenance
Integrated Process: Nursing Process/Data Collection
Content Area: Adult Health/Neurological

Answer: 4
Rationale: Option 4 identifies the correct procedure for checking a client's pupillary reaction to light. Option 1 relates to the pupillary response to light, but shining the light directly into the client's eye without asking the client to focus on a distant object is not an appropriate technique. Option 2 assesses for eye movement related to cranial nerves III, IV, and VI. Option 3 assesses the accommodation of the eye rather than the eye's response to light.

Test-Taking Strategy: Use the process of elimination, and focus on the subject—pupillary assessment. Visualize this technique and each description given in the options to answer the question. Review basic neurological checks if you had difficulty with this question.

Reference

Perry, A., & Potter, P. (2010). *Clinical nursing skills & techniques* (7th ed., p. 124). St. Louis: Mosby.

---

230. When a client is asked to describe how she performs a breast self-examination (BSE), she describes the appropriate monthly palpation of the breasts and nipples. The nurse determines that the client requires instruction regarding which important component of the BSE?

1 Inspection
2 Percussion
3 Auscultation
4 Mammography

Level of Cognitive Ability: Comprehension
Client Needs: Health Promotion and Maintenance
Integrated Process: Teaching and Learning
Content Area: Adult Health/Oncology

Answer: 1
Rationale: Standing before a mirror to inspect the breasts for puckering, dimpling, or changes in contour is an important component of the BSE. Percussion and auscultation are not components of the BSE. Although mammography is a test for breast cancer, it is not a component of the BSE.

Test-Taking Strategy: Focus on the subject—the correct procedure for a BSE. Note the strategic words *the client requires instruction*. These words indicate a negative event query and ask you to select the item that needs to be taught to the client. Although percussion and auscultation are components of a physical examination, they are not components of a BSE. In addition, although mammography is another test for breast cancer, it is not a part of a BSE. Remember that inspection is the first step of the BSE. Review the BSE if you had difficulty with this question.

Reference

Linton, A. (2007). *Introduction to medical-surgical nursing* (4th ed., pp. 1038-1039). Philadelphia: Saunders.

---

231. A nurse is reviewing the record of a client suspected of having malignant melanoma. Which finding, if documented in the client's record, should the nurse recognize as a warning sign for malignant melanoma?

1 Genital warts
2 Dimpling of the skin
3 A mole that has turned blue
4 A mole with round, smooth borders

Level of Cognitive Ability: Comprehension
Client Needs: Health Promotion and Maintenance
Integrated Process: Nursing Process/Data Collection
Content Area: Adult Health/Oncology

Answer: 3
Rationale: Shades of blue in a mole are considered ominous for malignant melanoma. Genital warts are associated with cancer of the cervix. The dimpling of the skin of the breast is associated with breast cancer. A mole with round, smooth borders would be a normal finding.

Test-Taking Strategy: Focus on the subject of the question—malignant melanoma. Recalling the characteristics of malignant melanoma will direct you to option 3. Review the signs of malignant melanoma if you had difficulty with this question.

Reference
Linton, A. (2007). *Introduction to medical-surgical nursing* (4th ed., pp. 1143-1144). Philadelphia: Saunders.

---

232. A nurse is auscultating the breath sounds of a client. The nurse avoids which data collection technique because it is incorrect?

1 Using the bell of the stethoscope
2 Asking the client to sit straight up
3 Placing the stethoscope directly on the client's skin
4 Having the client breathe slowly and deeply through the mouth

Level of Cognitive Ability: Application
Client Needs: Health Promotion and Maintenance
Integrated Process: Nursing Process/Data Collection
Content Area: Adult Health/Respiratory

Answer: 1
Rationale: The bell of the stethoscope is not used to auscultate breath sounds. The client should ideally sit up and breathe slowly and deeply through the mouth. The diaphragm of the stethoscope, which is warmed before use, is placed directly on the client's skin rather than over a gown or clothing.

Test-Taking Strategy: Use the process of elimination. Noting the strategic word *incorrect* and recalling this fundamental technique directs you to option 1. Review auscultation as a basic physical examination data collection technique if you had difficulty with this question.

References
Jarvis, C. (2008) *Physical examination and health assessment* (5th ed., p. 454). Philadelphia: Saunders.
Potter, P., & Perry, A. (2009) *Fundamentals of nursing* (7th ed., p. 595). St. Louis: Mosby.

---

233. A nurse in a health screening clinic is caring for a 39-year-old white female client. The client has a blood pressure of 152/92 mm Hg at rest, a total cholesterol level of 190 mg/dL, and fasting blood glucose level of 114 mg/dL. The nurse should focus attention on which risk factor for coronary artery disease (CAD) noted in this client?

1 Age
2 Hypertension
3 Hyperlipidemia
4 Glucose intolerance

Level of Cognitive Ability: Comprehension
Client Needs: Health Promotion and Maintenance

Answer: 2
Rationale: Hypertension, cigarette smoking, and hyperlipidemia are major risk factors of CAD. Glucose intolerance, obesity, and response to stress are also contributing factors. Age is a nonmodifiable risk factor. The client's total cholesterol and blood glucose levels fall just within the normal range.

Test-Taking Strategy: Identifying the abnormal finding in the question will assist you with selecting the correct option. Option 1 can be eliminated first because age is a nonmodifiable risk factor. From the remaining options, note that the blood pressure is the only abnormal finding. Review the risk factors associated with CAD if you had difficulty with this question.

Reference
deWit, S. (2009). *Medical-surgical nursing: Concepts & practice* (p. 435). St. Louis: Saunders.

Integrated Process: Nursing Process/Data Collection
Content Area: Adult Health/Cardiovascular

---

234. A nurse is reviewing the health records of the prenatal clients scheduled to be seen in the health care clinic. The nurse determines that which of the following clients is at least risk for gestational hypertensive disorder?

1 A client with a history of gestational hypertension
2 A client who has been diagnosed with a hydatidiform mole
3 A client who is 20 years old, gravida 2, weighing 115 pounds
4 A client who was diagnosed with diabetes mellitus 10 years previously

Level of Cognitive Ability: Analysis
Client Needs: Health Promotion and Maintenance
Integrated Process: Nursing Process/Data Collection
Content Area: Maternity/Antepartum

Answer: 3
Rationale: Gestational hypertension is the development of mild hypertension during pregnancy in a previously normotensive client without proteinuria or pathologic edema. The clients in options 1, 2, and 4 are at high risk for the development of gestational hypertension. With regard to option 3, if the client had been younger than 18 or older than 35 years old and underweight or overweight, then she would have been at risk; however, she falls within normal age and weight criteria.

Test-Taking Strategy: Note the strategic words *least risk*. These words indicate a negative event query and ask you to select the client that is not at risk for gestational hypertension. Note that option 3 is the only option that identifies a client who does not have a preexisting health problem. Review the risks associated with gestational hypertension if you had difficulty with this question.

Reference
Leifer, G. (2007). *Introduction to maternity and pediatric nursing* (5th ed., p. 91). Philadelphia: Saunders.

---

235. A child is to receive a measles, mumps, and rubella (MMR) vaccine. During data collection, the nurse notes that the child is allergic to eggs. Which of the following should the nurse anticipate being prescribed for this child?

1 Administration of a killed measles vaccine
2 Elimination of this vaccine from the immunization schedule
3 Administration of epinephrine (Adrenalin) before the administration of the MMR vaccine
4 Administration of diphenhydramine (Benadryl) and acetaminophen (Tylenol) before the administration of the MMR vaccine

Level of Cognitive Ability: Analysis
Client Needs: Health Promotion and Maintenance
Integrated Process: Nursing Process/Planning
Content Area: Child Health

Answer: 1
Rationale: Live measles vaccine is produced from chick embryo cell culture, so the possibility of anaphylactic hypersensitivity in children with egg allergies should be considered. If there is a question of sensitivity, children should be tested before the administration of the MMR vaccine. If a child tests positive for sensitivity, the killed measles vaccine may be given as an alternative. The use of medications before the administration of a vaccine is not a normal procedure. A vaccine would not be eliminated from the immunization schedule.

Test-Taking Strategy: Use the process of elimination. Option 2 can be eliminated first because a vaccine would not be eliminated from the immunization schedule. Eliminate options 3 and 4 next because they are comparable or alike and because the use of medications before a vaccine is not normal procedure. Recalling that live measles vaccine is produced from chick embryo cell culture will direct you to option 1. Review the procedures related to the administration of vaccines if you had difficulty with this question.

References
Leifer, G. (2007). *Introduction to maternity and pediatric nursing* (5th ed., p. 720). Philadelphia: Saunders.
Price, D., & Gwin, J. (2008). *Pediatric nursing: An introductory text* (10th ed., p. 130). St. Louis: Saunders.

236. A nursing instructor asks a nursing student about killed or inactivated vaccines. The student responds by describing these vaccines as:

1. Bacterial toxins that have been made inactive by either chemicals or heat
2. Vaccines that contain pathogens that have been made inactive by either chemicals or heat
3. Vaccines that have their virulence (potency) diminished so that they do not produce a full-blown clinical illness
4. Vaccines that have been obtained from the pooled blood of many people and that provide antibodies to a variety of diseases

Level of Cognitive Ability: Comprehension
Client Needs: Health Promotion and Maintenance
Integrated Process: Teaching and Learning
Content Area: Child Health

Answer: 2

Rationale: Killed or inactivated vaccines are vaccines that contain pathogens that have been made inactive by either chemicals or heat. These vaccines, which are noninfectious, cause the body to produce antibodies. Their disadvantage is that they elicit a limited immune response from the body, so several doses are necessary. Examples of this type of vaccine include the Salk polio vaccine, the rabies vaccine, and the pertussis vaccine. Option 1 identifies toxoids. Option 3 identifies live (attenuated) vaccines. Option 4 identifies human immunoglobulin.

Test-Taking Strategy: Use the process of elimination. Note the relationship between inactivated vaccines in the question and option 2. Review inactivated vaccines if you had difficulty with this question.

References

Potter, A., & Perry, P. (2010). *Clinical nursing skills & techniques* (7th ed., p. 813). St. Louis: Mosby.
Price, D., & Gwin, J. (2008). *Pediatric nursing: An introductory text* (10th ed., p. 129). St. Louis: Saunders.

---

237. The nurse is asked to monitor a client with cardiac disease for the presence of cyanosis. Which body area is the best site for checking for this condition?

1. The nailbeds
2. In the sclerae
3. Over the palms of the hands
4. At the junction of the hard and soft portions of the palate

Level of Cognitive Ability: Application
Client Needs: Health Promotion and Maintenance
Integrated Process: Nursing Process/Data Collection
Content Area: Adult Health/Cardiovascular

Answer: 1

Rationale: The presence of cyanosis can best be seen in the nailbeds, the conjunctivae, and the oral mucosa. Pallor is best seen in the buccal mucosa or the conjunctivae, particularly in dark-skinned clients. Jaundice can be best assessed in the sclera, near the limbus at the junction of the hard and soft portions of the palate, and over the palms.

Test-Taking Strategy: Focus on the subject—cyanosis. Use your knowledge of data collection techniques related to the presence of cyanosis to answer this question to direct you to option 1. Review these techniques if you had difficulty with this question.

References

deWit, S. (2009). *Medical-surgical nursing: Concepts & practice* (p. 369). St. Louis: Saunders.
Ignatavicius, D., & Workman, M. (2010). *Medical-surgical nursing: Patient-centered collaborative care* (6th ed., pp. 474-475). St. Louis: Saunders.

---

238. A nurse is assisting with monitoring a client who has undergone shoulder arthroplasty for brachial plexus compromise by checking the status of the musculocutaneous nerve. Which data collection technique should the nurse implement?

1. Ask the client to spread all of the fingers wide and to resist pressure.
2. Ask the client to raise the forearm, and then assess for the flexion of the biceps.

Answer: 2

Rationale: To assess musculocutaneous nerve status, the nurse checks for the flexion of the biceps by having the client raise the forearm. Poor biceps flexion may indicate compromise of the musculocutaneous nerve. Options 1, 3, and 4 are incorrect techniques.

Test-Taking Strategy: Use the process of elimination, and focus on the subject—the data collection technique used to determine the status of the musculocutaneous nerve. Recalling the anatomical location of the nerve and visualizing each of the techniques described in the options will direct you to option 2. Review this data collection technique if you had difficulty with this question.

3 Ask the client to move the thumb toward the palm and then back to the neutral position.
4 Ask the client to grasp the nurse's hand, and then note the strength of the client's first and second fingers.

Level of Cognitive Ability: Application
Client Needs: Health Promotion and Maintenance
Integrated Process: Nursing Process/Data Collection
Content Area: Adult Health/Musculoskeletal

References

Ignatavicius, D., & Workman, M. (2010). *Medical-surgical nursing: Patient-centered collaborative care* (6th ed., pp. 281-282). St. Louis: Saunders.
Lewis, S., Heitkemper, M., Dirksen, S., & Bucher, L. (2007). *Medical-surgical nursing: Assessment and management of clinical problems* (7th ed., p. 1665). St. Louis: Mosby.
Monahan, F., Sands, J., Marek, J., Neighbors, M., & Green, C. (2007). *Phipps' medical-surgical nursing: Health and illness perspectives* (8th ed., pp. 1634-1635, 1637). St. Louis: Mosby.

---

239. A client is diagnosed with pernicious anemia. The nurse understands that which of the following risk factors is associated with the development of this type of anemia?
1 Gastric resection
2 Inadequate iron in the diet
3 Musculoskeletal disorders
4 Central nervous system disorders

Level of Cognitive Ability: Comprehension
Client Needs: Health Promotion and Maintenance
Integrated Process: Nursing Process/Data Collection
Content Area: Adult Health/Gastrointestinal

Answer: 1
Rationale: One major risk factor for the development of pernicious anemia is gastric resection. Inadequate iron in the diet is not specifically associated with this type of anemia; however, it is associated with iron-deficiency anemia. Central nervous system and musculoskeletal manifestations may occur as a result of pernicious anemia.

Test-Taking Strategy: Use the process of elimination. Recalling that the parietal cells of the stomach secrete the intrinsic factor necessary for vitamin B_{12} absorption and that pernicious anemia is caused by a deficiency of the intrinsic factor will direct you to option 1. Review pernicious anemia if you had difficulty with this question.

Reference

Linton, A. (2007). *Introduction to medical-surgical nursing* (4th ed., pp. 583, 763-764). Philadelphia: Saunders.

---

240. A nurse is planning to assist with testing the function of a client's vestibulocochlear nerve (cranial nerve VIII). The nurse should gather which items to assist with the performance of the test?
1 Tuning fork and audiometer
2 Snellen chart and ophthalmoscope
3 Flashlight and pupil size chart or millimeter ruler
4 Safety pin, hot and cold water in test tubes, and cotton wisp

Level of Cognitive Ability: Application
Client Needs: Health Promotion and Maintenance
Integrated Process: Nursing Process/Implementation
Content Area: Adult Health/Neurological

Answer: 1
Rationale: The vestibulocochlear nerve (cranial nerve VIII) is responsible for auditory acuity as well as bone and air conduction. The audiometer assesses the client's hearing, and the tuning fork tests bone and air conduction. The supplies noted in options 2, 3, and 4 are used for testing cranial nerves II, III, and V, respectively.

Test-Taking Strategy: Focus on the subject—the vestibulocochlear nerve. Recalling the function of this nerve will direct you to option 1. Review the technique for testing cranial nerve VIII if you had difficulty with this question.

References

Jarvis, C. (2008) *Physical examination and health assessment* (5th ed., p. 669). Philadelphia: Saunders.
Linton, A. (2007). *Introduction to medical-surgical nursing* (4th ed., pp. 1192-1193). Philadelphia: Saunders.

---

241. A nurse is assisting with evaluating the deep tendon reflexes of a pregnant client. The nurse exposes the woman's lower leg, places one hand under the woman's knee to raise it slightly off the bed, and uses the percussion hammer to strike the patellar tendon just below the patella. The nurse documents the response as 4+. This response is interpreted as:

1 Normal
2 Diminished
3 Very brisk or hyperactive
4 Increased or brisker than average

Level of Cognitive Ability: Analysis
Client Needs: Health Promotion and Maintenance
Integrated Process: Nursing Process/Evaluation
Content Area: Maternity/Antepartum

Answer: 3

Rationale: The normal response is extension and forward thrusting of the foot. A 1+ response indicates a diminished response, 2+ indicates a normal response, 3+ indicates an increased or brisker-than-average response, and 4+ indicates a very brisk or hyperactive response.

Test-Taking Strategy: Use the process of elimination and your knowledge of data collection techniques and the evaluation of deep tendon reflexes to answer this question. Noting the strategic words *response as 4+* will direct you to option 3. Review the data collection technique for the deep tendon reflexes if you had difficulty with this question.

Reference

Leifer, G. (2008). *Maternity nursing: An introductory text* (10th ed., p. 260). Philadelphia: Saunders.

---

242. To maintain a child's developmental skills while the child is hospitalized, the nurse should encourage a 1-year-old child who was born 2 months early to:

1 Sit independently
2 Walk independently
3 Build a tower of three blocks
4 Indicate wants by pointing or grunting

Level of Cognitive Ability: Application
Client Needs: Health Promotion and Maintenance
Integrated Process: Nursing Process/Implementation
Content Area: Child Health

Answer: 1

Rationale: For premature infants, a nurse needs to calculate the developmental age by deducting the time of prematurity from the age of the child until the child reaches the age of 2 years. In this case, subtracting 2 months from 1 year results in an adjusted age of 10 months. A 10-month-old infant can sit independently. By the age of 15 months, a child should walk independently and indicate wants by pointing and grunting. By the age of 18 months, a child should be able to build a tower of three blocks.

Test-Taking Strategy: Use the process of elimination. Note the strategic words *1-year-old child who was born 2 months early.* Apply your knowledge of the psychomotor skills that would be present in a 10-month-old child to answer the question. Review growth and development concepts if you had difficulty with this question.

Reference

Price, D., & Gwin, J. (2008). *Pediatric nursing: An introductory text* (10th ed., pp. 126-127). St. Louis: Saunders.

---

243. A client has been newly diagnosed with hypertension. The nurse plans to do which of the following as the first step in teaching the client about the disorder?

1 Decide on the teaching approach
2 Plan for the evaluation of the session
3 Gather all available resource materials
4 Identify the client's knowledge and needs

Level of Cognitive Ability: Application
Client Needs: Health Promotion and Maintenance

Answer: 4

Rationale: Determining what to teach a client begins with an assessment of the client's own knowledge and learning needs. After these have been determined, the nurse can effectively plan a teaching approach and determine the actual content and resource materials that may be needed. The evaluation is performed after teaching is completed.

Test-Taking Strategy: Note the strategic word *first.* Use the steps of the nursing process (clinical problem-solving process), and remember that data collection is the first step. Review teaching and learning principles if you had difficulty with this question.

Integrated Process: Teaching and Learning
Content Area: Fundamental Skills

Reference

Christensen, B., & Kockrow, E. (2006). *Adult health nursing* (5th ed., p. 381). St. Louis: Mosby.

---

244. A nurse is reinforcing discharge instructions to a client after elbow arthroplasty. Which instruction should the nurse provide to the client?

1. Do not lift anything that weighs more than 10 pounds.
2. Playing sports with the operative arm should be avoided.
3. Triceps and biceps strengthening exercises can be started in 6 weeks.
4. Elbow flexion and extension exercises are avoided for at least 2 weeks.

Level of Cognitive Ability: Application
Client Needs: Health Promotion and Maintenance
Integrated Process: Teaching and Learning
Content Area: Adult Health/Musculoskeletal

Answer: 2
Rationale: After elbow arthroplasty, elbow flexion and extension exercises are allowed as tolerated. Clients should not lift more than 5 pounds, and they should not begin triceps and biceps strengthening exercises for 3 months. The client will not be able to use the operative arm to play sports.

Test-Taking Strategy: Use the process of elimination. Considering the involvement of this surgical procedure and the anatomical location will direct you to option 2. Review client teaching points after elbow arthroplasty if you had difficulty with this question.

Reference

Ignatavicius, D., & Workman, M. (2010). *Medical-surgical nursing: Patient-centered collaborative care* (6th ed., pp. 335-336). St. Louis: Saunders.

---

245. During a difficult vaginal delivery, a large-for-gestational-age (LGA) infant suffers a fracture of the left clavicle. The infant is being discharged to home with an immobilizing sling, and the nurse reinforces home-care instructions to the parents. Which parent statement would indicate that further instruction is necessary?

1. "Will my baby's arm always be paralyzed?"
2. "The primary purpose of the immobilization is to provide comfort."
3. "We understand that the final diagnosis was made by x-ray study and physical examination."
4. "Our doctor explained that this is a complication associated with the delivery of a large infant."

Level of Cognitive Ability: Comprehension
Client Needs: Health Promotion and Maintenance
Integrated Process: Teaching and Learning
Content Area: Maternity/Postpartum

Answer: 1
Rationale: The complications of a vaginal LGA birth are associated with the need to assist the process with forceps, vacuum extraction, or both. Even without mechanical assistance, the clavicles may fracture during delivery if the infant is LGA. The diagnosis is made by physical examination of the infant and by x-ray study. Immobilization will provide comfort. The infant's arm will not be paralyzed.

Test-Taking Strategy: Note the strategic words *further instruction is necessary.* These words indicate a negative event query and ask you to select an option that is an incorrect statement. Recalling that the injury is temporary and treatable will direct you to option 1. Review clavicle fracture in an LGA infant if you had difficulty with this question.

Reference

Leifer, G. (2008). *Maternity nursing: An introductory text* (10th ed., p. 300). Philadelphia: Saunders.

---

246. A nurse provides home-care instructions to parents about their postmature infant's nutritional needs. Which parent statement indicates an understanding of the necessary care of the infant?

Answer: 4
Rationale: A postmature infant is poorly nourished and has wasting and growth restriction as a result of placental dysfunction. These infants need early and more frequent feedings to help compensate for the period of poor nutrition in utero. They are at

1 "Our baby is at risk for high blood sugars."
2 "Cold stress is not likely to occur in our baby."
3 "Letting our baby sleep through feedings is OK."
4 "We should anticipate that our baby may require more frequent feedings."

Level of Cognitive Ability: Comprehension
Client Needs: Health Promotion and Maintenance
Integrated Process: Nursing Process/Evaluation
Content Area: Maternity/Postpartum

risk for hypoglycemia and cold stress. It is best to not allow the infant to sleep through the scheduled feeding times because of the risk for hypoglycemia.

Test-Taking Strategy: Knowledge of the nutritional needs of a postmature infant is necessary to answer this question. Noting that option 4 directly relates to feeding and nutritional needs will direct you to this option. Review the care of the postmature infant if you had difficulty with this question.

Reference

Leifer, G. (2008). *Maternity nursing: An introductory text* (10th ed., p. 309). Philadelphia: Saunders.

---

247. A nurse is caring for an infant classified as small for gestational age (SGA). When gathering data about the maternal history, the nurse checks for which major risk factor that may result in an SGA infant?
1 Smoking
2 Maternal age
3 Marital status
4 Maternal blood type

Level of Cognitive Ability: Analysis
Client Needs: Health Promotion and Maintenance
Integrated Process: Nursing Process/Data Collection
Content Area: Maternity/Antepartum

Answer: 1
Rationale: Maternal smoking interferes with placental flow and oxygenation; this in turn impairs fetal growth and may result in an SGA infant. Options 2, 3, and 4 are not factors that contribute to an SGA infant.

Test-Taking Strategy: Use the process of elimination and your knowledge of the risk factors associated with an SGA infant to answer this question. Recalling the effects of smoking on the fetus will direct you to option 1. Review the risk factors associated with SGA infants if you had difficulty with this question.

Reference

Leifer, G. (2008). *Maternity nursing: An introductory text* (10th ed., p. 302). Philadelphia: Saunders.

---

248. A nurse is teaching a client who has been placed on a low-cholesterol diet about appropriate dessert items. The nurse teaches the client that which item is acceptable to eat?
1 Sherbet
2 Ice cream
3 Pound cake
4 Frosted slice of cake

Level of Cognitive Ability: Application
Client Needs: Health Promotion and Maintenance
Integrated Process: Teaching and Learning
Content Area: Fundamental Skills

Answer: 1
Rationale: Desserts that are higher in cholesterol include high-fat frozen desserts (e.g., ice cream) and high-fat cakes (e.g., frosted and pound cakes). Most store-bought pies and cookies are also high in fat. The best low-fat dessert choices include angel food cake; frozen desserts such as sorbet, sherbet, Italian ice, and frozen yogurt; and other desserts that are specifically labeled "low fat."

Test-Taking Strategy: Focus on the subject—a low-cholesterol diet. Review each option while keeping this subject in mind to direct you to option 1. Review food items that are high in cholesterol if you had difficulty with this question.

References

Nix, S. (2009). *Williams' basic nutrition and diet therapy* (13th ed., pp. 38, 478). St. Louis: Mosby.
Linton, A. (2007). *Introduction to medical-surgical nursing* (4th ed., p. 96). Philadelphia: Saunders.

249. A preschool child is in the preoperational phase of cognitive development. The nurse understands that if 5 ounces of juice were poured into a short glass and the same amount was poured into a tall skinny glass, the child will think there is more juice in the tall glass. The nurse knows that the child has not yet developed an understanding of:

1 Centering
2 Artificialism
3 Egocentricism
4 Symbolic functioning

Level of Cognitive Ability: Comprehension
Client Needs: Health Promotion and Maintenance
Integrated Process: Nursing Process/Data Collection
Content Area: Child Health

Answer: 1
Rationale: Centering is the tendency to concentrate on a single outstanding characteristic of an object while excluding its other features. Egocentricism is a type of thinking in which children have difficulty seeing a point of view other than their own. Artificialism is the idea that the world and everything in it are created by people. Symbolic functioning is the creation of a mental image to stand for something that is not there.

Test-Taking Strategy: Knowledge of characteristics of the preoperational phase of cognitive development is necessary to answer this question. Remember that centering is the tendency to concentrate on a single outstanding characteristic of an object while excluding its other features. Review the preoperational phase of development if you had difficulty with this question.

Reference
Price, D., & Gwin, J. (2008). *Pediatric nursing: An introductory text* (10th ed., p. 222). St. Louis: Saunders.

---

250. A nurse in a well-baby clinic is collecting data about the language and communication developmental milestones of a 7-month-old infant. The nurse understands that which of the following begins to occur in the infant at this developmental age?

1 Cooing sounds
2 Use of gestures
3 Babbling sounds
4 Increased interest in sounds

Level of Cognitive Ability: Comprehension
Client Needs: Health Promotion and Maintenance
Integrated Process: Nursing Process/Data Collection
Content Area: Child Health

Answer: 4
Rationale: An increased interest in sounds occurs between the ages of 6 and 8 months. Babbling sounds begin between the ages of 3 and 4 months. Between the ages of 1 and 3 months, the infant will produce cooing sounds. The use of gestures and the imitation of sounds occur between the ages of 9 and 12 months.

Test-Taking Strategy: Use the process of elimination. Noting the age of the infant will help you to eliminate options 1 and 3 because the developmental milestones cited in these options occur at an earlier age. From the remaining options, focus on the age of the child to direct you to option 4, remembering that the use of gestures occurs later in infants. Review these developmental milestones if you had difficulty with this question.

Reference
Price, D., & Gwin, J. (2008). *Pediatric nursing: An introductory text* (10th ed., p. 126). St. Louis: Saunders.

---

251. A nurse obtains an older client's height and weight on admission to a long-term care facility. The nurse describes normal age-related changes in height and in the musculoskeletal system to the client. The client demonstrates an understanding of these changes if which client statement is made?

1 "I must have osteoporosis."
2 "I'm shorter because my cartilage is overgrown."
3 "We will use these results to determine my ideal body weight."

Answer: 4
Rationale: Age-related changes in the musculoskeletal system include decreased bone density, increased bony prominence, a kyphotic posture, cartilage degeneration, decreased range of motion, muscle atrophy, decreased strength, and slowed movement. Option 4 identifies correct information. Only a physician can give a diagnosis of osteoporosis. Although height and weight are used to determine ideal body weight, this is unrelated to age-related changes.

Test-Taking Strategy: Use the process of elimination. Note the strategic words *demonstrates an understanding.* Focus on the subject—changes related to height—to direct you to option 4. Review these age-related changes if you had difficulty with this question.

4 "I'm shorter because I don't have as much bone density as I used to."

Level of Cognitive Ability: Comprehension
Client Needs: Health Promotion and Maintenance
Integrated Process: Nursing Process/Evaluation
Content Area: Fundamental Skills

References

deWit, S. (2009). *Medical-surgical nursing: Concepts & practice* (p. 767). St. Louis: Saunders.
Wold, G. (2008). *Basic geriatric nursing* (4th ed., pp. 36-37). St. Louis: Mosby.

---

252. A nurse is assisting with the development of a teaching plan for an older client with hypertension. The client will be discharged to home and must learn to manage diet and medications. To facilitate the client's learning process, the nurse will first:

1 Set priorities for the client.
2 Use only one teaching method.
3 Determine the client's readiness to learn.
4 Plan 30-minute teaching sessions only in the evening after visiting hours are over.

Level of Cognitive Ability: Application
Client Needs: Health Promotion and Maintenance
Integrated Process: Teaching and Learning
Content Area: Fundamental Skills

Answer: 3
Rationale: Until the client is ready to learn, teaching sessions will be ineffective. Teaching should be performed in short sessions early in the day, when the client is well rested. It is important to include the client in the development of the teaching plan and to set priorities with the client. Varied teaching methods (e.g., verbal instruction) are best. Visual aids and written material should be provided for later reference.

Test-Taking Strategy: Use the process of elimination to assist you with answering the question. Remember that data collection is the first step in the nursing process; option 3 addresses the process of data collection. Review teaching and learning principles if you had difficulty with this question.

References

deWit, S. (2009). *Medical-surgical nursing: Concepts & practice* (p. 441). St. Louis: Saunders.
Wold, G. (2008). *Basic geriatric nursing* (4th ed., pp. 210-211). St. Louis: Mosby.

---

253. The nurse has been teaching an older client about influenza vaccine. The nurse determines that the client needs more instruction when the client states:

1 "I'll get the flu vaccine this fall."
2 "I should get the vaccine every year."
3 "I should get a flu vaccine even though I'm healthy."
4 "I don't need the vaccine this year because I had one last year."

Level of Cognitive Ability: Comprehension
Client Needs: Health Promotion and Maintenance
Integrated Process: Teaching and Learning
Content Area: Fundamental Skills

Answer: 4
Rationale: New influenza vaccines are developed every year based on predictions of which strains of the virus will be active. Clients should be advised to get the vaccine every year. Options 1, 2, and 3 are correct statements about the influenza vaccine.

Test-Taking Strategy: Note the strategic words *needs more instruction*. These words indicate a negative event query and ask you to select an option that is an incorrect statement. Use the process of elimination and your knowledge of this vaccine to answer the question. Recalling that the vaccine is administered yearly will direct you to option 4. Review the influenza vaccine if you had difficulty with this question.

Reference

Wold, G. (2008). *Basic geriatric nursing* (4th ed., p. 41). St. Louis: Mosby.

---

254. A client tells the nurse, "I did not take my heart medication today because I did not want to get that terrible headache again." The nurse should make which appropriate response to this client?

Answer: 4
Rationale: Some cardiac medications, particularly the nitrates, dilate the body's arteries; this can increase blood flow to the brain and cause headaches. These headaches are usually transient and treatable with over-the-counter pain relievers (e.g.,

1 "If you are getting a headache, it is best to stand up when taking your heart medication."
2 "You were correct to not take your heart medication. Headaches are a sign of an allergic reaction."
3 "Headaches are just something you'll have to get used to if you don't want to have another heart attack."
4 "The side effect of headaches will probably decrease in a few days. In the meantime, we can ask your physician about the use of acetaminophen (Tylenol) to relieve the discomfort."

Level of Cognitive Ability: Application
Client Needs: Health Promotion and Maintenance
Integrated Process: Teaching and Learning
Content Area: Pharmacology

acetaminophen). Standing can result in orthostatic hypotension. The client should not stop taking medication without advice from a physician.

Test-Taking Strategy: Use the process of elimination. Eliminate option 2 because the client should always take medication as prescribed. Option 1 will not relieve the headache and may result in orthostatic hypotension. Option 3 is a nontherapeutic response. Review client teaching related to nitrates if you had difficulty with this question.

References

Kee, J., Hayes, E., & McCuistion, L. (2009). *Pharmacology: A Nursing process approach* (6th ed., p. 634). St. Louis: Saunders.
Lehne, R. (2007). *Pharmacology for nursing care* (6th ed., p. 575). Philadelphia: Saunders.

---

255. A nurse is collecting information about weight loss from an obese client. What data collection method should the nurse use to most accurately determine the effectiveness of a weight-loss program?
1 Monitor the weight.
2 Review calorie counts.
3 Review laboratory results.
4 Monitor intake and output daily.

Level of Cognitive Ability: Application
Client Needs: Health Promotion and Maintenance
Integrated Process: Nursing Process/Data Collection
Content Area: Fundamental Skills

Answer: 1
Rationale: The most accurate weight-loss measurement entails weighing the client at the same time of day, while he or she is wearing the same clothes, on the same scale. Some physicians recommend weekly weighing rather than daily weighing. Options 2, 3, and 4 help measure nutrition and hydration status.

Test-Taking Strategy: Use the process of elimination. Note the similarity between the words *weight loss* in the question and *weight* in the correct option. Review the most accurate method for determining weight loss if you had difficulty with this question.

References

Ignatavicius, D., & Workman, M. (2010). *Medical-surgical nursing: Patient-centered collaborative care* (6th ed., pp. 1389-1390) St. Louis: Saunders.
Linton, A. (2007). *Introduction to medical-surgical nursing* (4th ed., pp. 775-776). Philadelphia: Saunders.

---

256. Which of the following items, if identified during data collection, is most important for a client to modify to lessen the risk for coronary artery disease (CAD)?
1 Elevated triglyceride levels
2 Elevated serum lipase levels
3 Elevated low-density lipoproteins (LDL) levels
4 Elevated high-density lipoproteins (HDL) levels

Level of Cognitive Ability: Analysis
Client Needs: Health Promotion and Maintenance

Answer: 3
Rationale: LDLs are more directly associated with CAD than other lipoproteins. LDL levels, along with cholesterol levels, have a higher associative and predictive value for CAD than triglyceride levels. In addition, HDLs are inversely associated with the risk of CAD. Lipase is a digestive enzyme that breaks down ingested fats in the gastrointestinal tract.

Test-Taking Strategy: Note the strategic words *most important*, and focus on the subject—lessening the risk of CAD. Remember that LDLs are more directly associated with CAD than other lipoproteins. Review the risk factors for CAD if you had difficulty with this question.

Integrated Process: Nursing Process/Data Collection
Content Area: Adult Health/Cardiovascular

Reference
deWit, S. (2009). *Medical-surgical nursing: Concepts & practice* (p. 489). St. Louis: Saunders.

---

257. The mother of an adolescent tells the nurse that her child refuses to eat meat and is concerned that the child will get sick from poor nutrition. Which response to the mother is most helpful for dealing with an adolescent vegetarian?

1 "You should take your child to the doctor because eating this way causes health problems."
2 "This is just a phase. Keep preparing meals as you always have, and your child will come around."
3 "People follow vegetarian diets for many reasons. A vegetarian diet can provide needed nutrients if it is planned carefully."
4 "Your child will not eat meat, but I assume she is a lacto-ovo vegetarian. She will get adequate protein from dairy products."

Level of Cognitive Ability: Application
Client Needs: Health Promotion and Maintenance
Integrated Process: Teaching and Learning
Content Area: Child Health

Answer: 3
Rationale: A vegetarian diet can provide needed nutrients if it is planned carefully; the nurse should provide nutritional information about this type of diet to the mother. Option 3 provides the most helpful information. Option 1 will cause unnecessary alarm in the mother. Option 2 may not be accurate and is an assumption on the nurse's part. Option 4 makes an assumption that may not be accurate.

Test-Taking Strategy: Note the strategic words *most helpful,* and recall therapeutic communication techniques to direct you to option 3. Review vegetarian diets if you had difficulty with this question.

Reference
Leifer, G. (2007). *Introduction to maternity and pediatric nursing* (5th ed., p. 457). Philadelphia: Saunders.

---

258. Preschool-age children are at risk for accidents. The nurse teaches parents that these children have the developmental skills to be responsible for:

1 Staying away from strange dogs
2 Knowing what is and is not harmful
3 Wearing a helmet when riding a bike
4 Making decisions about joining a gang

Level of Cognitive Ability: Comprehension
Client Needs: Health Promotion and Maintenance
Integrated Process: Teaching and Learning
Content Area: Child Health

Answer: 3
Rationale: Preschool-age children are at risk for accidents because their judgment is overruled by curiosity. A preschooler has the developmental skills to be responsible for wearing a helmet when riding a bike. In addition, wearing a helmet can become a habit very quickly with parental insistence and behavior training. Although these children may know safety rules, a strange dog may attract their attention. A preschool-age child may not have the developmental skill of knowing what is and is not harmful, and he or she cannot be expected to make sound decisions.

Test-Taking Strategy: Note the age group of the child. Use your knowledge of safety issues and the psychosocial development of this age group to answer the question. Review safety issues and the preschooler if you had difficulty with this question.

Reference
Price, D., & Gwin, J. (2008). *Pediatric nursing: An introductory text* (10th ed., p. 286). St. Louis: Saunders.

---

259. A nurse is reinforcing dietary home-care instructions to a client with coronary artery disease (CAD). Which statement by the client indicates an understanding of the recommended dietary practices?

1 "I should become a strict vegetarian."
2 "I should eliminate all cholesterol and fat from my diet."
3 "I should use polyunsaturated oils, eat low-fat cheese, and drink skim milk."
4 "I should substitute eggs and whole milk for meat to get adequate dietary protein."

Level of Cognitive Ability: Comprehension
Client Needs: Health Promotion and Maintenance
Integrated Process: Nursing Process/Evaluation
Content Area: Fundamental Skills

Answer: 3

Rationale: A client with CAD needs to avoid foods that are high in saturated fat and cholesterol (e.g., eggs, whole milk, red meat) because they contribute to increases in low-density lipoproteins. The use of polyunsaturated oils, skim milk, and complex carbohydrates is recommended to control hypercholesterolemia. The client does not have to become a strict vegetarian or eliminate all cholesterol and fat from the diet to control the disorder.

Test-Taking Strategy: Use the process of elimination to eliminate options 1 and 2 because of the close-ended words *strict* and *all*. Eliminate option 4 next because these items are high in cholesterol. Review the dietary measures for the client with CAD and foods that are high in cholesterol if you had difficulty with this question.

Reference

Christensen, B., & Kockrow, E. (2006). *Adult health nursing* (5th ed., p. 359). St. Louis: Mosby.

---

260. A nurse is collecting data from a client who has been diagnosed with coronary artery disease (CAD). Which of the following data are modifiable risk factors for the development of CAD?

1 Age and obesity
2 Gender and ethnicity
3 Family history and stress
4 Hypertension and cigarette smoking

Level of Cognitive Ability: Comprehension
Client Needs: Health Promotion and Maintenance
Integrated Process: Nursing Process/Data Collection
Content Area: Adult Health/Cardiovascular

Answer: 4

Rationale: Nonmodifiable risk factors for CAD cannot be controlled; they include age, gender, family history, and ethnicity. Modifiable risk factors can be controlled; they include the cholesterol level, hypertension, cigarette smoking, and obesity.

Test-Taking Strategy: Note the strategic word *modifiable*. Use the process of elimination, and note that only option 4 contains factors that can be controlled or changed. Review modifiable risk factors if you had difficulty with this question.

Reference

Christensen, B., & Kockrow, E. (2006). *Adult health nursing* (5th ed., pp. 335, 359, 378). St. Louis: Mosby.

---

261. A nurse has reinforced home-care instructions with a client with pulmonary embolism regarding measures to prevent recurrence after discharge from the hospital. The nurse determines that the instructions have been effective if the client states an intention to:

1 Limit fluid intake.
2 Sit down whenever possible.
3 Continue to wear supportive hose.
4 Cross the legs only at the ankle and not at the knee.

Level of Cognitive Ability: Comprehension
Client Needs: Health Promotion and Maintenance

Answer: 3

Rationale: Recurrence of pulmonary embolism can be minimized by the wearing of elastic or supportive hose to enhance venous return. The client can also enhance venous return by avoiding crossing the legs at the knee or ankle, interspersing periods of sitting with walking, and doing active foot and ankle exercises. The client should also take in sufficient fluids to prevent hemoconcentration and hypercoagulability.

Test-Taking Strategy: Use the process of elimination, and focus on the subject—measures to prevent the recurrence of pulmonary embolism. Recalling that prolonged immobilization and hypercoagulability can lead to pulmonary embolism will direct you to option 3. Review the measures for preventing the recurrence of pulmonary embolism if you had difficulty with this question.

Integrated Process: Nursing Process/Evaluation
Content Area: Adult Health/Respiratory

References

Ignatavicius, D., & Workman, M. (2010). *Medical-surgical nursing: Patient-centered collaborative care* (6th ed., p. 678). St. Louis: Saunders.
Linton, A. (2007). *Introduction to medical-surgical nursing* (4th ed., p. 547). Philadelphia: Saunders.

---

262. A nurse is reinforcing home-care instructions regarding the need to begin long-term anticoagulant therapy for a client who has atrial fibrillation. Which explanation describes the reasoning for this therapy?

1 "This dysrhythmia decreases the amount of blood flow from the heart, which can lead to blood clots forming in the brain."
2 "The antidysrhythmic medications you are taking cause blood clots as a side effect, so you need this medication to prevent them."
3 "Because of this dysrhythmia, blood backs up in the legs and puts you at risk for blood clots; this is also called 'deep vein thrombosis.'"
4 "Because the atria are 'quivering,' blood flows sluggishly through them. Clots can form along the heart wall, which could then loosen and travel to the lungs or brain."

Level of Cognitive Ability: Application
Client Needs: Health Promotion and Maintenance
Integrated Process: Teaching and Learning
Content Area: Adult Health/Cardiovascular

Answer: 4

Rationale: A severe complication of atrial fibrillation is the development of thrombi. The blood stagnates in the "quivering" atria because of the loss of organized atrial muscle contraction and "atrial kick," which can account for up to 30% of the cardiac output. The blood that pools in the atria can then clot, which increases the risk for pulmonary and cerebral emboli. Options 1, 2, and 3 are incorrect descriptions.

Test-Taking Strategy: Use the process of elimination, and focus on the client's diagnosis. Note the relationship of the words *fibrillation* in the question and *quivering* in the correct option. Review atrial fibrillation and the development of thrombi if you had difficulty with this question.

References

Christensen, B., & Kockrow, E. (2006). *Adult health nursing* (5th ed., p. 391). St. Louis: Mosby.
Kee, J., Hayes, E., & McCuistion, L. (2009). *Pharmacology: A nursing process approach* (6th ed., pp. 679-680). St. Louis: Saunders.

---

263. A client with prostatitis asks the nurse, "Why do I need to take a stool softener? The problem is with my urine, not my bowels!" The nurse should provide which explanation to the client?

1 "This is a standard medication order for anyone with an abdominal problem."
2 "This will keep the bowel free of feces, which will decrease the swelling inside."
3 "Being constipated puts you at more risk for developing complications of prostatitis."
4 "This will help you to avoid constipation, because straining is painful with prostatitis."

Answer: 4

Rationale: Prostatitis is an inflammation of the prostate gland. Stool softeners are prescribed for the client with prostatitis to prevent constipation, which can be painful. Stool softeners are not a standard medication order for anyone with an abdominal problem. Stool softeners have no direct effect on decreasing swelling, and they do not prevent complications (e.g., chronic prostatitis).

Test-Taking Strategy: Use the process of elimination. The response in option 1 may be eliminated first because it is nonspecific and nonhelpful. The bowel is never "free of feces," so option 2 can be eliminated next. From the remaining options, recalling the action and purpose of stool softeners directs you to option 4. Review the care measures for the client with prostatitis if you had difficulty with this question.

Level of Cognitive Ability: Application
Client Needs: Health Promotion and Maintenance
Integrated Process: Nursing Process/Implementation
Content Area: Adult Health/Renal

References

Christensen, B., & Kockrow, E. (2006). *Adult health nursing* (5th ed., p. 487). St. Louis: Mosby.

Ignatavicius, D., & Workman, M. (2006). *Medical-surgical nursing: Patient-centered collaborative care* (6th ed., p. 1733). St. Louis: Saunders.

---

264. A client with Parkinson's disease has begun therapy with levodopa. The nurse provides home-care instructions about the medication and determines that the client understands the action of the medication if the client verbalizes that results may not be apparent for:

1 1 week
2 24 hours
3 2 to 3 days
4 2 to 3 weeks

Level of Cognitive Ability: Analysis
Client Needs: Health Promotion and Maintenance
Integrated Process: Nursing Process/Evaluation
Content Area: Pharmacology

Answer: 4

Rationale: Parkinson's disease is a debilitating disease that affects motor ability and that is characterized by tremor, rigidity, akinesia (slow movement), and postural instability. Signs and symptoms of Parkinson's disease usually begin to resolve within 2 to 3 weeks of starting therapy, although marked improvement may not be seen for up to 6 months in some clients. Clients should understand this concept to help them to comply with medication therapy.

Test-Taking Strategy: Focus on the client's diagnosis and the characteristics associated with this medication. Remember that the effects of levodopa begin within 2 to 3 weeks of starting therapy, although marked improvement may not be seen for up to 6 months in some clients. Review the effects of levodopa if you had difficulty with this question.

Reference

Kee. J., Hayes, E., & McCuistion, L. (2009). *Pharmacology: A nursing process approach* (6th ed., p. 336). St Louis: Saunders.

---

265. A nurse is participating in a prostate screening clinic and determines that a client understands the shared educational information if the client tells another participant that:

1 A daily supplement of vitamin E prevents benign prostatic hypertrophy (BPH).
2 Cigarette smoking triples the chance of developing BPH.
3 Increased intake of green leafy vegetables prevents BPH.
4 An annual digital rectal examination beginning at age 50 should be performed for early detection.

Level of Cognitive Ability: Comprehension
Client Needs: Health Promotion and Maintenance
Integrated Process: Nursing Process/Evaluation
Content Area: Adult Health/Renal

Answer: 4

Rationale: BPH is thought to result from an alteration in the client's androgen levels, although the exact cause is still unknown. Increasing age is a risk factor for developing BPH, and an annual digital rectal examination and a prostate-specific antigen test should be performed beginning at age 50. Increased intake of green leafy vegetables does not prevent BPH. Vitamin E and cigarette smoking have no known relationship with BPH.

Test-Taking Strategy: Use the process of elimination. Recalling that advancing age is a primary risk factor assists you with eliminating options 1, 2, and 3. Also, the setting of the question is a prostate screening clinic, and so the focus should be on detection; this will guide you to option 4. Review the concepts related to BPH if you had difficulty with this question.

Reference

deWit, S. (2009). *Medical-surgical nursing: Concepts & practice* (p. 166). St. Louis: Saunders.

---

266. A client is being discharged home after a prostatectomy. The nurse reinforces home-care instructions and instructs the client to:

1 Wait 1 week before mowing the lawn.
2 Avoid lifting more than 50 pounds for 4 to 6 weeks after surgery.

Answer: 4

Rationale: A prostatectomy is the surgical removal of part of the prostate gland. Postoperatively, the client should notify the physician if there are any signs of infection, pain, bleeding, or urinary obstruction. Lifting more than 20 pounds is prohibited for 4 to 6 weeks after surgery. Other strenuous activities that could increase intraabdominal tension are also restricted (e.g., mowing the

3 Drink at least 15 glasses of water a day to minimize clot formation.
4 Notify the physician if fever, increased pain, or inability to void occurs.

Level of Cognitive Ability: Application
Client Needs: Health Promotion and Maintenance
Integrated Process: Teaching and Learning
Content Area: Adult Health/Renal

lawn). The client should take in 6 to 8 glasses of water or nonalcoholic beverages per day to minimize the risk of clot formation. Drinking 15 glasses of water per day is excessive.

Test-Taking Strategy: Use the process of elimination. Eliminate option 3 as excess fluid intake. Eliminate options 1 and 2 next because their activities are also excessive. This leaves option 4 as being correct. The client should notify the physician if signs of infection or obstruction occur. Review postoperative prostatectomy home-care instructions if you had difficulty with this question.

Reference

Linton, A. (2007). *Introduction to medical-surgical nursing* (4th ed., pp. 1092-1093). Philadelphia: Saunders.

---

267. A nurse is teaching a client with acute renal failure to include high-quality proteins in the diet. The nurse tells the client to avoid which food item because it is a low-quality protein source?
1 Fish
2 Eggs
3 Chicken
4 Broccoli

Level of Cognitive Ability: Application
Client Needs: Health Promotion and Maintenance
Integrated Process: Teaching and Learning
Content Area: Adult Health/Renal

Answer: 4
Rationale: High-quality proteins come from animal sources and include such foods as eggs, meat, and fish. Low-quality proteins are derived from plant sources and include vegetables and foods made from grains. The renal diet is limited with regard to the amount of protein consumed; therefore it is important that high-quality proteins be ingested.

Test-Taking Strategy: Use the process of elimination. Note that chicken, eggs, and fish are all derived from animal sources, whereas broccoli is a plant. Review high-quality protein foods if you had difficulty with this question.

Reference

deWit, S. (2009). *Medical-surgical nursing: Concepts & practice* (p. 100). St. Louis: Saunders.

---

268. A client is ready to be discharged from the hospital and will be changing a wound dressing at home. The nurse assists with determining the client's ability to care for the dressing site. The best way to evaluate the client's ability is to:
1 Ask the client to verbalize wound site care.
2 Ask the client to change the wound dressing.
3 Review the entire discharge plan with the client again.
4 Demonstrate the dressing change for the client one last time before discharge.

Level of Cognitive Ability: Comprehension
Client Needs: Health Promotion and Maintenance
Integrated Process: Teaching and Learning
Content Area: Fundamental Skills

Answer: 2
Rationale: The acquisition of psychomotor skills is best evaluated by observing how a client carries out a procedure. The client may be able to verbalize how to do the procedure but may not be able to actually perform the psychomotor functions required. Reviewing the entire plan and demonstrating it again will not evaluate the client's ability.

Test-Taking Strategy: Use the process of elimination. Note the strategic words *evaluate* and *client's ability*. The correct option should involve some type of active client participation. Having the client actively demonstrate a procedure is always the best method of evaluating a psychomotor skill. Remember this concept of the teaching and learning process if you had difficulty with this question.

Reference

Christensen, B., & Kockrow, E. (2006). *Foundations of nursing* (5th ed., pp. 344-345). St. Louis: Mosby.

---

269. A nurse is reinforcing home-care instructions to a client being discharged with a peripheral intravenous (IV) line in place. The nurse plans to teach the client which most important concept for preventing peripheral IV infections when receiving home IV therapy?

1 Change the IV tubing and fluid containers daily.
2 Redress the IV site daily and cleanse it with alcohol.
3 Check the IV site carefully every day for redness and edema.
4 Carefully wash your hands with antibacterial soap before working with the IV site or equipment.

Level of Cognitive Ability: Application
Client Needs: Health Promotion and Maintenance
Integrated Process: Teaching and Learning
Content Area: Fundamental Skills

Answer: 4

Rationale: It is important for the client to realize the necessity of handwashing before working with IV fluids. Although the assessment of the IV site is important, it does not actively prevent infection. The IV site does not need to be redressed daily unless the dressing becomes wet, soiled, or loose. The IV containers should be changed daily, and the tubing should be changed every 48 to 72 hours, depending on the home-care agency policies.

Test-Taking Strategy: Note the strategic words *most important.* Read the question carefully and note that infection prevention is the concept that should be taught to the client. Remember that the number one priority of infection prevention always includes proper handwashing technique. Review measures to prevent infection if you had difficulty with this question.

References

Christensen, B., & Kockrow, E. (2006). *Foundations of nursing* (5th ed., p. 283). St. Louis: Mosby.

deWit, S. (2009). *Medical-surgical nursing: Concepts & practice* (p. 64). St. Louis: Saunders.

---

270. A client who is scheduled for the implantation of an automatic internal cardioverter-defibrillator (AICD) asks the nurse why there is a need to keep a diary after insertion and what should be written in the diary. The nurse teaches the client that the primary purpose of the diary is to:

1 Determine which activities to avoid.
2 Document events that precipitate a countershock.
3 Provide a count of the number of shocks delivered.
4 Record a variety of data that are useful for the physician as part of medical management.

Level of Cognitive Ability: Application
Client Needs: Health Promotion and Maintenance
Integrated Process: Teaching and Learning
Content Area: Adult Health/Cardiovascular

Answer: 4

Rationale: The client with an AICD maintains a log or diary that includes the date and time of the shock, activity that occurred before the shock, any symptoms that were experienced, the number of shocks delivered, and how the client felt after the shock. The information is used by the physician to adjust the medical regimen (especially medication therapy), which must be maintained after AICD insertion.

Test-Taking Strategy: Focus on the subject—the primary purpose of the log or diary; this implies a comprehensive response. Each of the incorrect options lists one of the items that should be logged in the diary, but the correct option is the only one that can be considered a primary purpose. Option 4 is the umbrella option. Review home-care instructions for a client with an AICD if you had difficulty with this question.

Reference

Ignatavicius, D., & Workman, M. (2010). *Medical-surgical nursing: Patient-centered collaborative care* (6th ed., p. 761). St. Louis: Saunders.

---

271. A nurse is determining a hypertensive client's understanding of dietary modifications to control the disease process. The nurse evaluates the client's understanding as satisfactory if the client makes which of the following meal selections?

Answer: 3

Rationale: A client with hypertension should avoid food products that are high in sodium content. Foods from the meat group that are higher in sodium include bacon, luncheon meat, chipped or corned beef, kosher meat, smoked or salted meat or shellfish, peanut butter, and a variety of shellfish.

1 Corned beef, fresh carrots, and boiled potatoes
2 Hot dog on a bun, sauerkraut, and baked beans
3 Turkey, baked potato, and salad with oil and vinegar
4 Scallops, French fries, and salad with bleu cheese dressing

Level of Cognitive Ability: Comprehension
Client Needs: Health Promotion and Maintenance
Integrated Process: Nursing Process/Evaluation
Content Area: Adult Health/Cardiovascular

Test-Taking Strategy: Use the process of elimination. Eliminate options 1 and 2 first because these are highly processed meats that are high in sodium. (The sauerkraut in option 2 is also high in sodium.) The shellfish and commercial dressing help you to eliminate option 4 next. Review foods that are high in sodium if you had difficulty with this question.

Reference

Linton, A. (2007). *Introduction to medical-surgical nursing* (4th ed., pp. 107, 719, 724-725). Philadelphia: Saunders.

---

272. A nurse reinforces home-care instructions for a client who will be taking warfarin sodium (Coumadin) indefinitely. The nurse determines that the client needs further instructions if the client states the need to:
1 Use a soft toothbrush.
2 Use only a straight razor for shaving.
3 Avoid drinking alcohol while taking warfarin sodium.
4 Carry identification about the medication being taken.

Level of Cognitive Ability: Analysis
Client Needs: Health Promotion and Maintenance
Integrated Process: Teaching and Learning
Content Area: Pharmacology

Answer: 2

Rationale: Warfarin sodium (Coumadin) is an oral anticoagulant. Client instructions for oral anticoagulant therapy include taking the medication only as prescribed and at the same time each day. The client should not take other medications (including over-the-counter medications) without physician approval and should avoid alcohol. The client should notify all caregivers about the medication and carry a Medic-Alert identification card. The client is instructed to report any signs of bleeding (and to prevent them whenever possible) and to adhere to the schedule for follow-up blood work. The client should use a soft toothbrush to prevent bleeding from the gums during toothbrushing and an electric razor rather than a straight razor because a straight razor can cause nicks and resultant bleeding.

Test-Taking Strategy: Note the strategic words *needs further instructions.* These words indicate a negative event query and ask you to select an option that is an incorrect statement. Measures to teach clients on anticoagulant therapy generally deal with the prevention of bleeding and the interference of medication effects. Only option 2 represents a danger in one of these areas; therefore it is the option to select. Also note the close-ended word *only* in option 2. Review warfarin sodium if you had difficulty with this question.

Reference

Hodgson, B., & Kizior, R. (2009). *Saunders nursing drug handbook 2009* (p. 219). St. Louis: Saunders.

---

273. A nurse has reinforced home-care instructions to a client being discharged from the hospital with an arterial ischemic leg ulcer. The nurse determines that further instruction is needed if the client makes which statement?
1 "I should wear shoes and socks."
2 "I should apply lotion to my feet."

Answer: 4

Rationale: Foot-care instructions for the client with peripheral arterial ischemia are the same as those given to the client with diabetes mellitus. However, to enhance blood flow, the client with arterial disease should avoid raising the legs above the level of the heart unless instructed to do so as part of an exercise program (e.g., Buerger-Allen exercises) or unless venous stasis is present as well.

3 "I should cut my toenails straight across."
4 "I should raise my legs above the level of my heart periodically."

Level of Cognitive Ability: Comprehension
Client Needs: Health Promotion and Maintenance
Integrated Process: Teaching and Learning
Content Area: Adult Health/Cardiovascular

Test-Taking Strategy: Note the strategic words *further instruction is needed.* These words indicate a negative event query and ask you to select an option that is an incorrect client statement. Use the process of elimination, and focus on the subject—arterial ischemic leg ulcer. The word *ischemia* suggests that you should enlist the aid of gravity to enhance blood flow. Recalling the principles related to an arterial problem directs you to option 4. Review the care of the client with peripheral arterial disease if you had difficulty with this question.

Reference
Linton, A. (2007). *Introduction to medical-surgical nursing* (4th ed., p. 711). Philadelphia: Saunders.

---

274. A nurse is providing home-care instructions to a pregnant diabetic client regarding nutrition and insulin needs during pregnancy. The nurse determines that the client understands dietary and insulin needs if the client states that she may require which of the following during the second half of the pregnancy?
1 Increased insulin
2 Decreased insulin
3 Increased caloric intake
4 Decreased caloric intake

Level of Cognitive Ability: Comprehension
Client Needs: Health Promotion and Maintenance
Integrated Process: Nursing Process/Evaluation
Content Area: Maternity/Antepartum

Answer: 1
Rationale: Glucose crosses the placenta, but insulin does not. High fetal demands for glucose in combination with the insulin resistance caused by hormonal changes during the last half of pregnancy can result in an elevation of maternal blood glucose levels. This increases the mother's demand for insulin and is referred to as the diabetogenic effect of pregnancy. Caloric intake is not affected by diabetes.

Test-Taking Strategy: Use the process of elimination and your knowledge of the pathophysiology associated with diabetes to help you answer the question. Eliminate options 3 and 4 first because diabetes does not change caloric needs. Recalling that the need for insulin may decrease during the first half of pregnancy and increase during the second half will direct you to option 1. Review the effects of diabetes on pregnancy and insulin needs if you had difficulty with this question.

Reference
Leifer, G. (2008). *Maternity nursing: An introductory text* (10th ed., pp. 266-267). Philadelphia: Saunders.

---

275. A nurse is monitoring a pregnant woman for the presence of pitting edema. Which of the following methods should the nurse implement to check the edema level?
1 The nurse uses the fingertips of the index and middle finger and presses into the ankles for a period of 3 to 5 seconds.
2 The nurse presses the fingertips of the index and middle finger against the shin and holds pressure for 2 to 3 seconds.
3 The nurse uses the fingertips of the index and middle finger, presses against the abdomen, and holds pressure for 2 to 3 seconds.

Answer: 2
Rationale: To evaluate for the presence of pitting edema, the nurse uncovers the woman's lower leg, presses the fingertips of the index and middle fingers against the shin, and holds the pressure for 2 to 3 seconds. Options 1, 3, and 4 are inaccurate techniques for assessing the presence of pitting edema.

Test-Taking Strategy: Use the process of elimination. Visualize each technique described in the options to assist with selecting the correct option. Review ways to evaluate for pitting edema if you had difficulty with this question.

Reference
McKinney, E., James, S., Murray, S., & Ashwill, J. (2009). *Maternal-child nursing* (3rd ed., pp. 623-624). St. Louis: Mosby.

4 The nurse uses the fingertips of the index and middle finger, presses against the upper arm, and holds pressure for 3 to 5 seconds.

Level of Cognitive Ability: Application
Client Needs: Health Promotion and Maintenance
Integrated Process: Nursing Process/Data Collection
Content Area: Maternity/Antepartum

---

276. A nurse reinforces home-care instructions to a pregnant woman regarding measures for relieving low back pain. Which statement by the client indicates an understanding of these measures?
1 "I will do the pelvic tilt exercises."
2 "I will wear an abdominal support."
3 "I should wear shoes with a higher heel."
4 "I should work at relaxing my abdominal muscles when I stand."

Level of Cognitive Ability: Comprehension
Client Needs: Health Promotion and Maintenance
Integrated Process: Nursing Process/Evaluation
Content Area: Maternity/Antepartum

Answer: 1
Rationale: Pelvic tilt exercises decrease strain on the muscles of the abdomen and lower back; this strain is caused by the added weight of the abdomen and the shift in the center of gravity. An abdominal support should only be worn if recommended by the physician. Relaxing the abdominal muscles adds to the problem. Wearing higher-heeled shoes adds to the muscle strain and exaggerates the shift in the center of gravity.

Test-Taking Strategy: Use the process of elimination, and visualize each option. Eliminate option 2 because an abdominal support needs to be prescribed by a physician. Eliminate option 3 because higher-heeled shoes can cause an unsafe condition. Eliminate option 4 because relaxing the abdominal muscles while standing can increase back discomfort. Review the measures to relieve back discomfort if you had difficulty with this question.

Reference
Leifer, G. (2007). *Introduction to maternity and pediatric nursing* (5th ed., pp. 64, 66). Philadelphia: Saunders.

---

277. The mother of a 5-year-old child who has been newly diagnosed with diabetes mellitus is very concerned about her child going to school and participating in social events. The nurse assists with developing a plan of care and suggests formulating which of the following goals?
1 The child's normal growth and development will be maintained.
2 The child will use effective coping mechanisms to manage anxiety.
3 The child and family will discuss all aspects of the illness and its treatments.
4 The child and family will integrate diabetes care into patterns of daily living.

Level of Cognitive Ability: Analysis
Client Needs: Health Promotion and Maintenance
Integrated Process: Nursing Process/Planning
Content Area: Child Health

Answer: 4
Rationale: The family and the child should integrate the care and management of diabetes into their daily living to effectively manage social events in the child's life. The other options are all goals for the family; however, they do not deal with social issues.

Test-Taking Strategy: Use the process of elimination, and focus on the subject—participation in social events. Integrating diabetes into the patterns of daily living is the only one of the options presented that deals with social issues. Review growth and development concepts and psychosocial issues related to diabetes care in a child if you had difficulty with this question.

Reference
Price, D., & Gwin, J. (2008). *Pediatric nursing: An introductory text* (10th ed., p. 301). St. Louis: Saunders.

---

278. A nurse is obtaining a health history from a client and is collecting data regarding the risk factors associated with osteoporosis. Which piece of data reported by the client places the client at low risk for osteoporosis?

1. History of a chronic illness
2. Cigarette smoking for 40 years
3. Consumption of a high-calcium diet
4. Excessive alcohol intake for 40 years

Level of Cognitive Ability: Analysis
Client Needs: Health Promotion and Maintenance
Integrated Process: Nursing Process/Data Collection
Content Area: Adult Health/Musculoskeletal

Answer: 3

Rationale: Risk factors associated with osteoporosis include a diet that is deficient in calcium. Options 1, 2, and 4 include risk factors that are associated with osteoporosis. Additional risk factors include postmenopausal age, long-term used of corticosteroids, family history of osteoporosis, sedentary lifestyle, and long-term use of anticonvulsants and furosemide.

Test-Taking Strategy: Note the strategic words *low risk.* Recalling the causes and risk factors associated with osteoporosis directs you to option 3. Review these risk factors if you had difficulty with this question.

Reference

Linton, A. (2007). *Introduction to medical-surgical nursing* (4th ed., p. 906). Philadelphia: Saunders.

---

279. A postpartum nurse is caring for a client who delivered a viable baby 2 hours previously. The nurse palpates the fundus and notes the character of the lochia. Which characteristic of the lochia does the nurse expect to note at this time?

1. Pink-colored lochia
2. White-colored lochia
3. Serosanguineous lochia
4. Dark red-colored lochia

Level of Cognitive Ability: Comprehension
Client Needs: Health Promotion and Maintenance
Integrated Process: Nursing Process/Data Collection
Content Area: Maternity/Postpartum

Answer: 4

Rationale: When checking the perineum, the lochia is monitored for amount, color, and the presence of clots. The color of the lochia during the fourth stage of labor (the first 1 to 4 hours after birth) is a dark red color. Options 1, 2, and 3 are not expected characteristics of the lochia at this time.

Test-Taking Strategy: Use the process of elimination. Note that the question refers to a client who delivered 2 hours previously; this should direct you to option 4. Review the expected findings of a perineal assessment during the immediate postpartum period if you had difficulty with this question.

Reference

Leifer, G. (2008). *Maternity nursing: An introductory text* (10th ed., pp. 227-228). Philadelphia: Saunders.

---

280. A nurse reinforces home-care instructions to a client with systemic lupus erythematosus (SLE). Which statement by the client indicates the need for further instruction regarding the measures to use to manage fatigue?

1. "I should sit whenever possible."
2. "I should avoid long periods of rest."
3. "I should take a hot bath in the evening."
4. "I should engage in moderate low-impact exercise when not fatigued."

Level of Cognitive Ability: Comprehension
Client Needs: Health Promotion and Maintenance
Integrated Process: Teaching and Learning
Content Area: Adult Health/Musculoskeletal

Answer: 3

Rationale: To help reduce fatigue in the client with SLE, the nurse should instruct the client to sit whenever possible, avoid hot baths, schedule moderate low-impact exercises when not fatigued, and maintain a balanced diet. The client is not instructed to rest for long periods because this promotes joint stiffness.

Test-Taking Strategy: Note the strategic words *need for further instruction.* These words indicate a negative event query and ask you to select an option that is an incorrect client statement. Focus on the subject—the management of fatigue. The process of elimination should direct you to option 3. Review the measures to prevent fatigue in the client with SLE if you had difficulty with this question.

References

Christensen, B., & Kockrow, E. (2006). *Adult health nursing* (5th ed., pp. 95-96). St. Louis: Mosby.
Swearingen, P. (2008). *All-in-one care planning resource: Medical-surgical, pediatric, maternity, & psychiatric nursing care plans* (2nd ed., p.508). St. Louis: Mosby.

---

281. A nursing student is assigned to care for a postpartum client. The nursing instructor reviews the nursing care plan developed by the student and asks the student to describe the process of involution. Which of the following is an accurate description of this process?

1 "Involution refers to the inverted uterus that is beginning to return to normal."
2 "Involution refers to the gradual reversal of the uterine muscle into the abdominal cavity."
3 "Involution refers to the descent of the uterus into the pelvic cavity occurring at a rate of 2 cm daily."
4 "Involution is the progressive descent of the uterus into the pelvic cavity occurring at a rate of approximately 1 cm per day."

Level of Cognitive Ability: Comprehension
Client Needs: Health Promotion and Maintenance
Integrated Process: Teaching and Learning
Content Area: Maternity/Postpartum

Answer: 4

Rationale: Involution is the progressive descent of the uterus into the pelvic cavity. After birth, descent occurs at a rate of approximately 1 fingerbreadth or 1 cm per day. Options 1, 2, and 3 are incorrect descriptions.

Test-Taking Strategy: Knowledge of the definition and process of involution is necessary to answer this question. Use medical terminology to assist you with defining the term and selecting the correct option. Remember that involution is a progressive descent of the uterus into the pelvic cavity at a rate of approximately 1 fingerbreadth or 1 cm per day. Review involution if you had difficulty with this question.

Reference

Leifer, G. (2008). *Maternity nursing: An introductory text* (10th ed., p. 226). Philadelphia: Saunders.

---

282. A nursing instructor asks the student assigned to work in the labor and delivery department about the purpose of the placenta. Which of the following is a correct response?

1 "It cushions and protects the fetus."
2 "It maintains the body temperature of the fetus."
3 "It prevents antibodies and viruses from passing to the fetus."
4 "It provides an exchange of nutrients and waste products between the mother and the fetus."

Level of Cognitive Ability: Comprehension
Client Needs: Health Promotion and Maintenance
Integrated Process: Teaching and Learning
Content Area: Maternity/Intrapartum

Answer: 4

Rationale: The placenta provides an exchange of nutrients and waste products between the mother and the fetus. The amniotic fluid surrounds, cushions, protects, and maintains the body temperature of the fetus. Nutrients, medications, antibodies, and viruses can pass through the placenta.

Test-Taking Strategy: Knowledge of the purpose of the placenta and the amniotic fluid is necessary to answer this question. Remember that the placenta provides nutrients. Review the structure and function of the placenta and the amniotic fluid if you had difficulty with this question.

Reference

Leifer, G. (2008). *Maternity nursing: An introductory text* (10th ed., pp. 31-32). Philadelphia: Saunders.

---

283. A nurse is preparing to check the fetal heartbeat of a pregnant woman who is at 20 weeks' gestation. Which piece of equipment is most appropriate for the nurse to use?

1 A fetoscope
2 A fetal heart monitor

Answer: 1

Rationale: The fetal heartbeat can first be heard with a fetoscope at 18 to 20 weeks' gestation. If a Doppler ultrasound device is used, the fetal heart rate (FHR) can be detected as early as 10 weeks' gestation. Options 3 and 4 do not adequately assess the fetal heartbeat. A fetal heart monitor is used during labor or in other situations when the FHR requires continuous monitoring.

3 An adult stethoscope
4 The bell of a stethoscope

Level of Cognitive Ability: Application
Client Needs: Health Promotion and Maintenance
Integrated Process: Nursing Process/Data Collection
Content Area: Maternity/Intrapartum

Test-Taking Strategy: Use the process of elimination. Eliminate options 3 and 4 first because they are comparable or alike. Knowing that a fetal heart monitor is used for continuous monitoring directs you to option 1. Review the data collection techniques associated with fetal heart monitoring if you had difficulty with this question.

Reference

Leifer, G. (2007). *Introduction to maternity and pediatric nursing* (5th ed., p. 132). Philadelphia: Saunders.

---

284. A client arrives at the prenatal clinic for her first prenatal assessment. The client tells the nurse that the first day of her last menstrual period was August 19, 2011. Using Nägele's rule, the nurse determines that which of the following is the estimated date of delivery?

1 May 26, 2012
2 June 12, 2012
3 June 26, 2012
4 May 12, 2012

Level of Cognitive Ability: Comprehension
Client Needs: Health Promotion and Maintenance
Integrated Process: Nursing Process/Data Collection
Content Area: Maternity/Antepartum

Answer: 1

Rationale: The accurate use of Nägele's rule requires that the woman it is being applied to have a regular 28-day menstrual cycle. Add 7 days to the first day of the last menstrual period (LMP), subtract 3 months, and then add 1 year to that date to obtain the estimated date of delivery. In this case, the first day of the LMP was August 19, 2011; add 7 days to get August 26, 2011; subtract 3 months to get May 26, 2011; and then add 1 year to get May 26, 2012.

Test-Taking Strategy: Use caution when following the steps of Nägele's rule to determine the estimated date of delivery. Read all of the options carefully, and note the dates and years before selecting an option. Review Nägele's rule if you had difficulty with this question.

Reference

Leifer, G. (2008). *Maternity nursing: An introductory text* (10th ed., p. 42). Philadelphia: Saunders.

---

285. A nurse reinforces home-care instructions to a client taking diazepam (Valium) 5 mg orally three times daily. Which statement by the client indicates the need for additional instruction?

1 "A glass of wine every day with dinner helps me to relax."
2 "When do you think I'll be able to start tapering off the medication?"
3 "I was very drowsy when I began to take this medication, but now I feel all right."
4 "I think I am coming down with the flu. What can I take that will not interfere with this medication?"

Level of Cognitive Ability: Comprehension
Client Needs: Health Promotion and Maintenance
Integrated Process: Teaching and Learning
Content Area: Pharmacology

Answer: 1

Rationale: Diazepam (Valium) is a benzodiazepine. If a central nervous system depressant (e.g., alcohol) is taken with a benzodiazepine, additive effects can occur that may cause respiratory depression or even be lethal. Diazepam may cause initial drowsiness. It should not be discontinued abruptly because the client may develop withdrawal symptoms. Many over-the-counter medications that are used to treat the flu contain ingredients that interact with diazepam.

Test-Taking Strategy: Note the strategic words *need for additional instruction*. These words indicate a negative event query and ask you to select an option that is an incorrect statement. Recalling that alcohol needs to be avoided with the administration of medication directs you to option 1. Review client teaching points related to the use of benzodiazepines if you had difficulty with this question.

Reference

Hodgson, B., & Kizior, R. (2009). *Saunders nursing drug handbook 2009* (p. 347). Philadelphia: Saunders.

---

286. A client with thromboangiitis obliterans (Buerger's disease) asks the nurse what home-care measures can be implemented to alleviate the symptoms. The nurse tells the client which of the following about this disorder and symptom control?

1. "There is no current treatment."
2. "Surgery is the most successful therapy."
3. "Warmth, exercise, and smoking cessation are most helpful."
4. "Analgesics are primarily used to control the symptom of pain."

Level of Cognitive Ability: Application
Client Needs: Health Promotion and Maintenance
Integrated Process: Teaching and Learning
Content Area: Adult Health/Cardiovascular

Answer: 3
Rationale: The main goals of treatment for thromboangiitis obliterans are the same as for peripheral arterial insufficiency. Thus the client is taught measures to increase circulation, which include enhancing vasodilatation through warmth, exercise, and smoking cessation. Options 1, 2, and 4 are incorrect.

Test-Taking Strategy: Use the process of elimination. Option 1 is unrealistic. Surgery is not a likely choice because this disorder has both arterial and venous involvement, which eliminates option 2. Option 4 is of limited use because the pain is caused by ischemia. Review the therapeutic management of Buerger's disease if you had difficulty with this question.

Reference
Christensen, B., & Kockrow, E. (2006). *Adult health nursing* (5th ed., p. 388). St. Louis: Mosby.

---

287. A client is being discharged with a peripheral intravenous (IV) site for continued home IV therapy. When planning for the discharge, the nurse reinforces which home-care measure to help prevent phlebitis and infiltration?

1. Cleanse the site daily with alcohol.
2. Gently massage the area around the site daily.
3. Immobilize the extremity until the IV is discontinued.
4. Keep the cannula stabilized or anchored properly with tape.

Level of Cognitive Ability: Application
Client Needs: Health Promotion and Maintenance
Integrated Process: Teaching and Learning
Content Area: Fundamental Skills

Answer: 4
Rationale: The principles of maintaining IV therapy at home are the same as in the hospital. It is important to ensure that the IV site is anchored properly to reduce the risk of phlebitis and infiltration. Massaging the site may actually contribute to catheter movement and tissue damage. Dressings that surround peripheral IV sites are changed and cleansed at various times (usually every 2 to 5 days), depending on facility protocols. Most dressings are to remain intact unless they become wet, soiled, or loose. Immobilizing the extremity is not routinely necessary for peripheral IV sites. Armboards for immobilization are only used if a site is near a joint and the IV is positional.

Test-Taking Strategy: Use the process of elimination. Focus on the subject—preventing phlebitis and infiltration. Option 4 is the only action that will prevent these complications. Review the interventions related to phlebitis and infiltration if you had difficulty with this question.

Reference
deWit, S. (2009). *Medical-surgical nursing: Concepts & practice* (p. 61). St. Louis: Saunders.

---

288. Diltiazem hydrochloride (Cardizem) is prescribed for the client with Prinzmetal's angina. The nurse reinforces home-care instructions to the client regarding this medication. Which statement made by the client indicates the need for further instruction?

1. "I will take the medication after meals."
2. "I will call the physician if shortness of breath occurs."
3. "I will rise slowly when getting out of bed in the morning."
4. "I will avoid activities that require alertness until my body gets used to the medication."

Answer: 1
Rationale: Diltiazem hydrochloride is a calcium-channel blocker. It is administered before meals and at bedtime, as prescribed. Hypotension can occur, and the client is instructed to rise slowly. The client should avoid tasks that require alertness until a response to the medication is established. The client should call the physician if an irregular heartbeat, shortness of breath, pronounced dizziness, nausea, or constipation occurs.

Test-Taking Strategy: Use the process of elimination, and note the strategic words *need for further instruction.* These words indicate a negative event query and ask you to select an option that is an incorrect statement. Recalling that this medication is used for angina may assist you with eliminating options 2, 3, and 4 because many of the cardiac medications lower blood pressure. Review diltiazem hydrochloride if you had difficulty with this question.

Level of Cognitive Ability: Analysis
Client Needs: Health Promotion and Maintenance
Integrated Process: Teaching and Learning
Content Area: Pharmacology

Reference

Hodgson, B., & Kizior, R. (2009). *Saunders nursing drug handbook 2009* (p. 360). Philadelphia: Saunders.

---

289. A nurse explains the risk factors associated with breast cancer to a client. The nurse determines that the client requires further explanation if the client states that which of the following is a risk factor?

1 Nulliparity
2 Late age of menarche
3 A history of breast cancer
4 A family history of breast cancer

Level of Cognitive Ability: Comprehension
Client Needs: Health Promotion and Maintenance
Integrated Process: Teaching and Learning
Content Area: Adult Health/Oncology

Answer: 2

Rationale: Factors that increase the risk for breast cancer include an early age of menarche (especially younger than 12 years), a late age of menopause or more than 40 years of menses, and a first full-term pregnancy after the age of 30 to 35 years. Options 1, 3, and 4 are also risk factors.

Test-Taking Strategy: Use the process of elimination, and note the strategic words *requires further explanation*. These words indicate a negative event query and ask you to select an option that is an incorrect statement. You should be able to easily eliminate options 3 and 4 because they are risk factors for breast cancer. From the remaining options, remembering that a greater number of years of menses increases the risk directs you to option 2. Review the risk factors for breast cancer if you had difficulty with this question.

References

Christensen, B., & Kockrow, E. (2006). *Adult health nursing* (5th ed., p. 604). St. Louis: Mosby.
deWit, S. (2009). *Medical-surgical nursing: Concepts & practice* (p. 963). St. Louis: Saunders.

---

290. When caring for the client with thromboangiitis obliterans (Buerger's disease), the nurse incorporates measures to help the client cope with the lifestyle changes that are required to control the disease process. The nurse initiates a referral to which of the following resources to best help the client achieve this goal?

1 Occupational therapist
2 Medical social worker
3 Pain management clinic
4 Smoking cessation program

Level of Cognitive Ability: Application
Client Needs: Health Promotion and Maintenance
Integrated Process: Nursing Process/Implementation
Content Area: Adult Health/Cardiovascular

Answer: 4

Rationale: Smoking is highly detrimental to clients with Buerger's disease, and they are advised to stop smoking completely. Given that smoking is a form of chemical dependency, referral to a smoking cessation program may be helpful for many clients. For many clients, symptoms are relieved or alleviated after they stop smoking. The other resources listed are unnecessary for this client based on the information presented in the question.

Test-Taking Strategy: Use the process of elimination. Recalling that this disorder is characterized by the inflammation and thrombosis of the smaller arteries and veins directs you to option 4. Review the treatment goals for the client with Buerger's disease if you had difficulty with this question.

Reference

Christensen, B., & Kockrow, E. (2006). *Adult health nursing* (5th ed., p. 388). St. Louis: Mosby.

---

291. A nurse has reinforced home-care instructions to a client being discharged to home after an abdominal aortic

Answer: 4

Rationale: The client can walk as tolerated after the repair or resection of an AAA, including walking outdoors. Walking is a

aneurysm (AAA) resection. The nurse determines that the client understands the instructions if the client states that an appropriate activity is to:
1 Mow the lawn.
2 Play 18 holes of golf.
3 Lift objects up to 30 pounds in weight.
4 Walk as tolerated, including out of doors.

Level of Cognitive Ability: Comprehension
Client Needs: Health Promotion and Maintenance
Integrated Process: Nursing Process/Evaluation
Content Area: Adult Health/Cardiovascular

healthy and beneficial activity during the postoperative period. The client should not lift objects that weigh more than 15 to 20 pounds for 6 to 12 weeks or engage in any activities that involve pushing, pulling, or straining. Driving is also prohibited for several weeks.

Test-Taking Strategy: Use the process of elimination. To answer this question, evaluate each option in terms of the strain it could put on the sutured graft; this directs you to option 4. Review the discharge instructions after an AAA repair if you had difficulty with this question.

Reference
Swearingen, P. (2008). *All-in-one planning resource: Medical-sugical, pediatric, maternity, & psychiatric nursing care plans* (2nd ed., p. 150). St. Louis: Mosby.

---

292. A nurse is reinforcing home-care dietary instructions with a client taking triamterene (Dyrenium). The nurse plans to include which of the following in a list of acceptable foods?
1 Oranges
2 Bananas
3 Baked potatoes
4 Pears canned in water

Level of Cognitive Ability: Application
Client Needs: Health Promotion and Maintenance
Integrated Process: Nursing Process/Planning
Content Area: Pharmacology

Answer: 4
Rationale: Triamterene is a potassium-sparing diuretic, and clients taking this medication should be cautioned against eating foods that are high in potassium unless they are taking a potassium-losing diuretic with it. Many foods are high in potassium, especially unprocessed foods and many vegetables, fruits, potatoes, and fresh meats. Because potassium is very water soluble, foods that are prepared in water are often lower in potassium. Of the options provided, pears canned in water provide the lowest source of potassium.

Test-Taking Strategy: Focus on the name of the medication, and recall that triamterene is a potassium-sparing diuretic. Next, determine which food item is lowest in potassium and thus acceptable for the client to consume; this will direct you to option 4. Review triamterene and the foods that are high in potassium if you had difficulty with this question.

References
deWit, S. (2009). *Medical-surgical nursing: Concepts & practice* (p. 48). St. Louis: Saunders.
Hodgson, B., & Kizior, R. (2009). *Saunders nursing drug handbook 2009* (pp. 1171-1172). Philadelphia: Saunders.

---

293. A nurse has reinforced home-care instructions to the parents of a child after heart surgery. Which parent statement indicates the need for further instruction?
1 "My child can return to school for full days 1 week after discharge."
2 "My child should avoid crowds and people for 1 week after discharge."
3 "My child should be allowed to play inside but not outside at this time."

Answer: 1
Rationale: The child who had undergone heart surgery can usually return to school the third week after hospital discharge but should only go for half days for the first week (depending on physician preference). Returning to school for full days 1 week after discharge will be too strenuous for the child and will place the child at risk for infection. Outdoor play should be omitted for several weeks, and indoor play should be allowed as tolerated. The child should avoid crowds for 1 week after discharge, including crowds at day care centers and churches. The parents should notify the physician if any difficulty with breathing occurs.

4 "I should call the physician if my child develops faster or harder breathing than normal."

Level of Cognitive Ability: Comprehension
Client Needs: Health Promotion and Maintenance
Integrated Process: Teaching and Learning
Content Area: Child Health

Test-Taking Strategy: Note the strategic words *indicates the need for further instruction*. These words indicate a negative event query and ask you to select an option that is an incorrect statement. Recalling the principles related to the prevention of infection and the complications of surgery directs you to option 1. Review the home-care instructions for the child after heart surgery if you had difficulty with this question.

Reference

McKinney, E., James, S., Murray, S., & Ashwill, J. (2009). *Maternal-child nursing* (3rd ed., p. 1260). St. Louis: Mosby.

---

294. A nurse assisting with teaching female clients how to prevent pelvic inflammatory disease (PID) should tell the clients which of the following?

1 Douche monthly.
2 Avoid unprotected intercourse.
3 Single sexual partners should be avoided.
4 Consult with a gynecologist regarding the placement of an intrauterine device (IUD).

Level of Cognitive Ability: Application
Client Needs: Health Promotion and Maintenance
Integrated Process: Teaching and Learning
Content Area: Fundamental Skills

Answer: 2

Rationale: PID is any inflammatory condition of the female pelvic organs, especially one caused by a bacterial infection. The primary prevention of PID includes avoiding the following: unprotected intercourse, multiple sexual partners, the use of an IUD, and douching.

Test-Taking Strategy: Use the principle of exposure of the pelvic area as a cause of infection. With this concept in mind, you should be able to eliminate options 1, 3, and 4. Review preventive measures for PID if you had difficulty with this question.

Reference

Linton, A. (2007). *Introduction to medical-surgical nursing* (4th ed., p. 1051). Philadelphia: Saunders.

---

295. A nurse in a well-baby clinic is collecting data about the motor development of an 18-month-old child. Which of the following is the highest level of development that the nurse would expect to note in this child?

1 The child snaps large snaps.
2 The child builds a tower of two blocks.
3 The child builds a tower of four to five blocks.
4 The child puts on simple clothes independently.

Level of Cognitive Ability: Comprehension
Client Needs: Health Promotion and Maintenance
Integrated Process: Nursing Process/Data Collection
Content Area: Child Health

Answer: 3

Rationale: A child is expected to be able to build a tower of four to five blocks at the age of 18 months. A child should be able to build a tower of two blocks at the age of 15 months. A child is expected to be able to snap large snaps and put on simple clothes independently at the age of 30 months.

Test-Taking Strategy: Visualize each of the fine motor skills presented in the options to help you select the correct option. Note that options 2 and 3 are comparable or alike in that they address a similar task but with different developmental levels; this may indicate that one of these options is correct. Noting the age of the child directs you to option 3. Review these developmental milestones if you had difficulty with this question.

Reference

Price, D., & Gwin, J. (2008). *Pediatric nursing: An introductory text* (10th ed., p. 177). St. Louis: Saunders.

---

296. A nurse reinforces instructions to a new mother who is about to breast-feed her newborn infant. Which statement by the mother indicates the need for further instruction?

1 "I should turn my newborn infant on his side facing me."
2 "When my newborn opens his mouth, I should draw him the rest of the way onto my breast."
3 "I should tilt my nipple upward or squeeze the areola and push it into my newborn infant's mouth."
4 "I should place a clean finger in the side of my newborn infant's mouth to break the suction before removing my baby from my breast."

Level of Cognitive Ability: Comprehension
Client Needs: Health Promotion and Maintenance
Integrated Process: Teaching and Learning
Content Area: Maternity/Antepartum

Answer: 3
Rationale: The mother is instructed to avoid tilting the nipple upward or squeezing the areola and pushing it into the baby's mouth. Options 1, 2, and 4 are correct procedures for breast-feeding.

Test-Taking Strategy: Note the strategic words *need for further instruction*. These words indicate a negative event query and ask you to select an option that is an incorrect statement. Visualize the descriptions given in each of the options; this will help you to eliminate options 1, 2, and 4. Reading option 3 carefully and noting that the word *pushing* suggests force or resistance should direct you to this option. Review breast-feeding instructions if you had difficulty with this question.

Reference
Leifer, G. (2008). *Maternity nursing: An introductory text* (10th ed., pp. 210-212). Philadelphia: Saunders.

---

297. The parents of a male newborn who is not circumcised request information about how to clean the newborn's penis. The nurse should provide the parents with which information?

1 "Retract the foreskin and cleanse the glans with every diaper change."
2 "Retract the foreskin and cleanse the glans when bathing your newborn."
3 "Do not retract the foreskin during cleaning because this may cause adhesions."
4 "Retract the foreskin no farther than it will easily go, and replace it over the glans after cleaning."

Level of Cognitive Ability: Application
Client Needs: Health Promotion and Maintenance
Integrated Process: Teaching and Learning
Content Area: Child Health

Answer: 3
Rationale: In newborn boys, the prepuce is continuous with the epidermis of the glans and is nonretractable. Forced retraction may cause adhesions to develop. It is best to allow separation to occur naturally, which takes place between 3 years of age and puberty. Most foreskins are retractable by 3 years of age and should be pushed back gently for cleaning once a week.

Test-Taking Strategy: Use the process of elimination. Note that options 1, 2, and 4 are comparable or alike in that they indicate the need to retract the foreskin; retracting the foreskin is not recommended in an uncircumcised newborn boy. Option 3 is the only selection that states that the foreskin should not be retracted. Review parent teaching points related to the care of an uncircumcised newborn if you had difficulty with this question.

Reference
Leifer, G. (2007). *Introduction to maternity and pediatric nursing* (5th ed., p. 290). Philadelphia: Saunders.

---

298. A nurse is teaching a client with thromboangiitis obliterans (Buerger's disease) about interventions to use to control the disease process. The nurse tells the client that which measure should be avoided?

1 Keep the extremities cool.

Answer: 1
Rationale: Buerger's disease is an occlusive disease that affects the small and medium arteries and veins. Interventions are directed at preventing progression of Buerger's disease. The client should maintain warmth in the extremities, especially by avoiding exposure to cold. Other interventions include conveying the need for immediate smoking cessation and providing the medications

2 Inspect the extremities for signs of infection.
3 Take nifedipine (Procardia) as directed.
4 Inspect the extremities for signs of ulceration.

Level of Cognitive Ability: Application
Client Needs: Health Promotion and Maintenance
Integrated Process: Teaching and Learning
Content Area: Adult Health/Cardiovascular

prescribed for vasodilation (e.g., the calcium-channel blocker nifedipine [Procardia], the α-adrenergic blocker prazosin [Minipress]). The client should inspect the extremities and report signs of infection or ulceration.

Test-Taking Strategy: Note the strategic word *avoided*. This word indicates a negative event query and asks you to select an option that is an incorrect measure. Recalling that the client with Buerger's disease should maintain warmth in the extremities directs you to option 1. Review the home-care measures for the client with Buerger's disease if you had difficulty with this question.

Reference

Christensen, B., & Kockrow, E. (2006). *Adult health nursing* (5th ed., p. 388). St. Louis: Mosby.

---

299. A nurse is reinforcing teaching to a client about the self-administration of betamethasone dipropionate (Qvar; an inhaled corticosteroid) and albuterol (Proventil; an inhaled bronchodilator) for the treatment of asthma. The nurse determines that teaching has been effective when the client states:

1 "I'll keep the inhalers in the refrigerator."
2 "I can use an inhaler for a week past the expiration date."
3 "I will take the bronchodilator first, then the corticosteroid."
4 "I will take the corticosteroid first, wait a few minutes, and then take the bronchodilator."

Level of Cognitive Ability: Analysis
Client Needs: Health Promotion and Maintenance
Integrated Process: Teaching and Learning
Content Area: Pharmacology

Answer: 3

Rationale: When betamethasone dipropionate and albuterol are taken together, the bronchodilator should be taken first to open the airways. This allows for better penetration of the corticosteroid into the bronchial tree. In addition, the client should wait 5 minutes after administering the bronchodilator before administering the corticosteroid. Inhalers do not need to be refrigerated, and medication should not be taken after the expiration date.

Test-Taking Strategy: Use the process of elimination. Option 2 is eliminated first because medication should not be taken past the expiration date. From the remaining options, recalling that the airways should be dilated first will direct you to option 3. Review the procedure for administering these respiratory medications if you had difficulty with this question.

Reference

Kee, J., Hayes, E., & McCuistion, L. (2009). *Pharmacology: A nursing process approach.* (6th ed., pp. 607-610). St. Louis: Saunders.

---

300. A nurse reinforces instructions to a mother about measures to reduce the incidence of gastroesophageal reflux disease (GERD) in her child. Which statement by the mother indicates the need for further instruction?

1 "I should buy bottle nipples that have smaller holes."
2 "I will give my child small feedings often throughout the day."
3 "I should add a small amount of cereal to my child's formula."

Answer: 1

Rationale: In GERD, the transfer of gastric contents into the esophagus occurs. With regard to feeding the child with this disorder, the bottle nipple holes should be larger to allow for the easy flow of thicker formula. This child's formula will most likely be thickened with cereal to increase the consistency and decrease the incidence of regurgitation. The child should receive smaller feedings throughout the day. Sucking on a pacifier in an upright position facilitates the flow of food through the esophagus.

4 "I will give my child a pacifier and maintain him in an upright position after meals."

Level of Cognitive Ability: Comprehension
Client Needs: Health Promotion and Maintenance
Integrated Process: Teaching and Learning
Content Area: Child Health

Test-Taking Strategy: Use the process of elimination, and note the strategic words *need for further instruction*. These words indicate a negative event query and ask you to select an option that is an incorrect statement. Noting the words *small feedings, add a small amount of cereal*, and *maintain him in an upright position* in options 2, 3, and 4, respectively, will assist you with eliminating these options. Review the feeding procedures for a child with GERD if you had difficulty with this question.

Reference

Leifer, G. (2007). *Introduction to maternity and pediatric nursing* (5th ed., p. 642). Philadelphia: Saunders.

---

301. A licensed practical nurse is assisting a registered nurse at a health screening clinic. Which client behavior is significant and indicates the need for the reinforcement of brain attack (stroke) prevention education?

1 Eats two bowls of high-fiber grain cereal with skim milk for breakfast
2 Has a blood pressure of 126/80 mm Hg and has lost 10 pounds recently
3 Uses oral contraceptives and condoms for pregnancy and disease prevention
4 Works as the manager of a busy medical-surgical unit and jogs 2 miles each day

Level of Cognitive Ability: Comprehension
Client Needs: Health Promotion and Maintenance
Integrated Process: Teaching and Learning
Content Area: Adult Health/Neurological

Answer: 3
Rationale: Obesity, hypertension, hyperlipidemia, smoking, and the use of oral contraceptives are all modifiable risk factors associated with brain attack (stroke). Oral contraceptive use may be discouraged because of the side effect of clot formation. In option 1, the client eats a fairly low-fat meal. In option 2, the client has borderline elevated blood pressure but has made a change in lifestyle. In option 4, the client has a stressful job but uses a stress-reduction method.

Test-Taking Strategy: Note the strategic words *need for the reinforcement*. These words indicate a negative event query and ask you to select an option that is a high-risk behavior. Recalling that the use of oral contraceptives is a modifiable risk factor for brain attack (stroke) will direct you to the correct option. Review the risk factors related to brain attack (stroke) if you had difficulty with this question.

Reference

Ignatavicius, D., & Workman, M. (2010). *Medical-surgical nursing: Patient-centered collaborative care* (6th ed., p. 1033). St. Louis: Saunders.

---

302. A nurse caring for an adult client who had a brain attack (stroke) plans to check the plantar reflex. What is the best way to elicit this reflex?

1 Tap the Achilles' tendon with a reflex hammer.
2 Gently prick the client's skin on the dorsum of the foot in two places.
3 Firmly stroke the lateral sole of the foot and under the toes with a blunt instrument.
4 Hold the sides of the client's great toe, and, while moving it, ask the client what position it is in.

Level of Cognitive Ability: Application
Client Needs: Health Promotion and Maintenance

Answer: 3
Rationale: The plantar reflex is elicited by firmly stroking the lateral sole of the foot and under the toes with a blunt instrument. The toes plantarflex normally, but they dorsiflex and fan out when an abnormal response is present. Option 1 assesses gastrocnemius muscle contraction, option 2 assesses two-point discrimination, and option 4 assesses proprioception.

Test-Taking Strategy: Focus on the subject—checking the plantar reflex. Note the relationship between the subject and option 3. Review this data collection technique if you had difficulty with this question.

Reference

Christensen, B., & Kockrow, E. (2006). *Adult health nursing* (5th ed., p. 125). St. Louis: Mosby.

Integrated Process: Nursing Process/Data Collection
Content Area: Adult Health/Neurological

---

303. A nurse is assigned to reinforce dietary measures to a client with coronary artery disease. The nurse should plan to take which action first if the client expresses frustration about the dietary regimen?
1 Notify the registered nurse (RN).
2 Leave the client alone for a while.
3 Continue with the dietary teaching.
4 Identify the cause of the frustration.

Level of Cognitive Ability: Application
Client Needs: Health Promotion and Maintenance
Integrated Process: Nursing Process/Data Collection
Content Area: Adult Health/Endocrine

Answer: 4
Rationale: The first action by the nurse should be to determine the cause of the frustration. Continuing to teach and leaving the client alone may block the communication and learning processes. The RN may need to be notified of the client's frustration, but the first action is to determine the cause.

Test-Taking Strategy: Note the strategic word *first*, and use the steps of the nursing process; remember that data collection is the first step. Options 1, 2, and 3 represent the implementation phases of the nursing process. The only data collection choice is option 4. Review teaching and learning principles if you had difficulty with this question.

Reference
deWit, S. (2009). *Medical-surgical nursing: Concepts & practice* (pp. 495, 499). St. Louis: Saunders.

---

304. A nurse is trying to determine the client's adjustment to a new diagnosis of coronary heart disease. Which of the following questions should the nurse ask to elicit the most useful response from the client?
1 "Do you understand the use of your new medications?"
2 "Are you going to schedule your follow-up physician visit?"
3 "Do you have anyone at home to help with housework and shopping?"
4 "How do you feel about the lifestyle changes you are planning to make?"

Level of Cognitive Ability: Application
Client Needs: Health Promotion and Maintenance
Integrated Process: Communication and Documentation
Content Area: Adult Health/Cardiovascular

Answer: 4
Rationale: Open-ended questions are needed to explore a client's reactions or feelings in response to an identified situation. Close-ended questions generally elicit a "yes" or "no" response exclusively. Option 4 is the only question that is open-ended and that explores the client's feelings about the disease.

Test-Taking Strategy: Use the process of elimination and therapeutic communication techniques. All of the incorrect options are closed-ended questions. Avoid close-ended questions, and always select the option that addresses client feelings. Review therapeutic communication techniques if you had difficulty with this question.

Reference
deWit, S. (2009). *Medical-surgical nursing: Concepts & practice* (pp. 9, 359). St. Louis: Saunders.

---

305. A licensed practical nurse (LPN) is assisting a school nurse with the routine health assessment of 11-year-old children. The LPN expects to assist with screening for:
1 Scoliosis
2 Meningitis

Answer: 1
Rationale: Scoliosis is a common deformity that affects children who have some degree of spinal curvature. Screening for the disorder generally begins in the fifth grade. There is no routine screening test for meningitis. Congenital hip disorder and PKU are screened for in newborns.

3 Phenylketonuria (PKU)
4 Congenital hip disorder

Level of Cognitive Ability: Comprehension
Client Needs: Health Promotion and Maintenance
Integrated Process: Nursing Process/Data Collection
Content Area: Child Health

Test-Taking Strategy: Knowledge of disorders common to school-age children and of routine screenings is needed to select the correct option. Rely on your clinical experience to eliminate the incorrect options if you are unfamiliar with this information. PKU is screened for in newborns, and the word *congenital* in option 4 suggests that it is screened for in infancy. Review screening procedures for these disorders if you had difficulty with this question.

Reference

Price, D., & Gwin, J. (2008). *Pediatric nursing: An introductory text* (10th ed., pp. 347, 349). St. Louis: Saunders.

---

306. A nurse is assisting with taking a history from a client suspected of having testicular cancer. Which data is most helpful for determining the client's risk factors?

1 Age
2 Number of sexual partners
3 Geographic location of residence
4 Marital status and number of children

Answer: 1

Rationale: Age is a basic but important risk factor for testicular cancer. The disease is the most common malignancy in males between the ages of approximately 18 and 34 years. Other risk factors include a history of undescended testis and a family history of testicular cancer. Options 2 and 4 are unrelated risk factors. The geographic location of residence is not a major risk factor.

Level of Cognitive Ability: Comprehension
Client Needs: Health Promotion and Maintenance
Integrated Process: Nursing Process/Data Collection
Content Area: Adult Health/Oncology

Test-Taking Strategy: Knowledge of the risk factors for testicular cancer assists you with answering the question correctly. Remember that the disease is the most common malignancy in males between the ages of approximately 18 and 34 years. Review the risk factors related to testicular cancer if you had difficulty with this question.

Reference

Linton, A. (2007). *Introduction to medical-surgical nursing* (4th ed., p. 1099). Philadelphia: Saunders.

---

307. A nurse is assisting at a health screening clinic and collecting data from clients about environmental risk factors for neurological disorders. Which factor places the client at least risk for a neurological disorder?

1 Exposure to pesticides
2 Ventilation in the work area
3 Adequate lighting in the work area
4 Exposure to fumes from things such as paints or bonding agents (glues)

Answer: 2

Rationale: The nurse assesses the risk of exposure to neurotoxic fumes and chemicals, including paint, bonding agents, and pesticides. The nurse also inquires about the adequacy of ventilation in the home and work area. The adequacy of lighting in the work area is unrelated to an environmental risk factor for a neurological disorder.

Level of Cognitive Ability: Analysis
Client Needs: Health Promotion and Maintenance
Integrated Process: Nursing Process/Data Collection
Content Area: Adult Health/Neurological

Test-Taking Strategy: Use the process of elimination. Note the strategic words *places the client at least risk;* this should direct you to option 2. Review environmental risk factors related to neurological disorders if you had difficulty with this question.

References

Christensen, B., & Kockrow, E. (2006). *Foundations of nursing* (5th ed., p. 55). St. Louis: Mosby.
deWit, S. (2009). *Medical-surgical nursing: Concepts & practice* (p. 164). St. Louis: Saunders.

---

308. A nurse is assisting with testing the reflexes of a client. The nurse tests the pharyngeal reflex by:

1 Stroking the skin on an abdominal quadrant
2 Stimulating the back of the throat with a tongue depressor
3 Stroking the outer plantar surface of the foot from heel to toe
4 Stimulating the perianal skin or gently inserting a gloved finger into the rectum

Level of Cognitive Ability: Application
Client Needs: Health Promotion and Maintenance
Integrated Process: Nursing Process/Data Collection
Content Area: Adult Health/Neurological

Answer: 2

Rationale: The pharyngeal (gag) reflex is tested by touching the back of the throat with an object such as a tongue depressor. The abdominal reflex, the plantar reflex, and the anal reflex are described in options 1, 3, and 4, respectively. A positive response to each of these reflexes is considered normal.

Test-Taking Strategy: Focus on the subject—the pharyngeal reflex. Recalling that the word *pharyngeal* refers to the pharynx or the back of the throat directs you to option 2. Review the testing of the pharyngeal reflex if you had difficulty with this question.

Reference

Potter, P., & Perry, A. (2009). *Fundamentals of nursing* (7th ed., p. 588). St. Louis: Mosby.

---

309. A nurse caring for a client with atrial fibrillation checks for a pulse deficit by:

1 Palpating the radial pulse for quality while auscultating the apical pulse volume
2 Auscultating the apical pulse for an irregular rate while palpating the radial pulse rate
3 Auscultating the apical pulse for a regular pulse while palpating the radial pulse for quality
4 Palpating the radial pulse for quality while auscultating the apical pulse for an irregular rate

Level of Cognitive Ability: Application
Client Needs: Health Promotion and Maintenance
Integrated Process: Nursing Process/Data Collection
Content Area: Adult Health/Cardiovascular

Answer: 2

Rationale: In clients with atrial fibrillation, the pulse is irregular. Pulse deficit is a condition in which the peripheral pulse rate is less than the ventricular contraction rate and is a characteristic of atrial fibrillation. When a pulse rate is irregular, the apical pulse should be auscultated for the irregularity and the radial pulse should be palpated for the pulse deficit. The descriptions in options 1, 3, and 4 are inaccurate.

Test-Taking Strategy: Use the process of elimination, and consider the nature of atrial fibrillation. Pulse deficit determines irregularity and rate. Option 2 is the only option that addresses the assessment of both the apical and radial rates. Review the procedure for checking the pulse deficit if you had difficulty with this question.

Reference

Linton, A. (2007). *Introduction to medical-surgical nursing* (4th ed., p. 633). Philadelphia: Saunders.

---

310. A client is seen in the health care clinic 2 weeks after a segmental resection of the upper lobe of the left lung. The nurse is assisting with collecting information from the client and notes that the client is sitting stiffly in the examining room chair with the right arm held close to the chest. The nurse determines that it is most important to ask the client about:

Answer: 3

Rationale: Failure of the client to perform active range-of-motion exercises as prescribed after lung surgery allows for the formation of adhesions of the incised muscle layer and leads to dysfunction syndrome. Only option 3 relates to the information in the question.

1 The client's ability to ambulate
2 Dietary habits and the effectiveness of support services
3 Compliance with the prescribed arm and shoulder exercises
4 The physical characteristics of the client's house and the number of steps

Level of Cognitive Ability: Application
Client Needs: Health Promotion and Maintenance
Integrated Process: Nursing Process/Data Collection
Content Area: Adult Health/Respiratory

Test-Taking Strategy: Note the strategic words *sitting stiffly.* Focus on the client data in the question to direct you to the correct option. Only option 3 relates to the nurse's observations. Review postoperative measures associated with lung surgery if you had difficulty with this question.

Reference

Black, J., & Hawks, J. (2009). *Medical-surgical nursing: Clinical management for positive outcomes* (8th ed., p. 1261). St. Louis: Saunders.

---

311. A nurse is evaluating a client's understanding of health measures to prevent coronary artery disease (CAD). Which client statement indicates a need for teaching?
1 "I should restrict my intake of fried foods."
2 "I could bring on a heart attack if I exercise."
3 "I should take my medicines at the same times each day."
4 "If I quit smoking, I will eventually lose my risk for heart disease caused by smoking."

Level of Cognitive Ability: Comprehension
Client Needs: Health Promotion and Maintenance
Integrated Process: Teaching and Learning
Content Area: Adult Health/Cardiovascular

Answer: 2
Rationale: CAD affects the arteries that provide blood, oxygen, and nutrients to the myocardium. A sedentary lifestyle is a major risk factor for the development of CAD. Exercise may reduce the risk of CAD by decreasing weight, reducing blood pressure, and elevating the high-density lipoprotein level. All of the other options are health measures to prevent CAD.

Test-Taking Strategy: Use the process of elimination. Note the strategic words *need for teaching.* These words indicate a negative event query and ask you to select an option that is an incorrect statement. Remember that exercise is a key component of preventing this disease. Review the prevention measures associated with CAD if you had difficulty with this question.

Reference

Linton, A. (2007). *Introduction to medical-surgical nursing* (4th ed., p. 653). Philadelphia: Saunders.

---

312. A nurse is providing dietary instructions to a client with a uric acid renal stone. Which dietary instruction should the nurse provide to the client?
1 Seafood is allowed in the diet.
2 Increase your intake of legumes.
3 Organ-meat–type foods can be included in the diet.
4 Increase your intake of cranberries and citrus fruits.

Level of Cognitive Ability: Application
Client Needs: Health Promotion and Maintenance
Integrated Process: Nursing Process/Implementation
Content Area: Adult Health/Renal

Answer: 2
Rationale: Dietary intervention may be important for the management of renal stones. Dietary instructions to the client with a uric acid stone include increasing the intake of legumes, green vegetables, and fruits (except prunes, grapes, cranberries, and citrus fruits) to increase the alkalinity of the urine. The client should also be instructed to decrease purine sources, which include organ meats, gravies, red wines, goose, venison, and seafood.

Test-Taking Strategy: Use the process of elimination and your knowledge of the dietary instructions for a client with uric acid stones. Recalling that the goal is to increase the alkalinity of the urine will direct you to option 2. Review the dietary instructions associated with uric acid renal stones if you had difficulty with this question.

References
Ignatavicius, D., & Workman, M. (2010). *Medical-surgical nursing: Patient-centered collaborative care* (6th ed., p. 1574). St. Louis: Saunders.
Nix, S. (2009). *Williams' basic nutrition and diet therapy* (13th ed., p. 430). St. Louis: Mosby.

---

313. A nurse reinforces home-care instructions to a client with Bell's palsy about treatment measures for the disorder. Which statement by the client indicates a need for further instruction?

1 "I should eat small meals and soft foods frequently."
2 "I should place ice packs to the affected side of my face."
3 "I should protect my affected eye by using an eye patch."
4 "I should place artificial tears into my affected eye four times daily."

Level of Cognitive Ability: Comprehension
Client Needs: Health Promotion and Maintenance
Integrated Process: Teaching and Learning
Content Area: Adult Health/Neurological

Answer: 2
Rationale: Bell's palsy is an acute and temporary paralysis of cranial nerve VII (facial nerve). Therapeutic management for the client with this condition includes providing moist heat packs to the affected area. The client is instructed to eat small amounts of soft foods frequently and to protect the affected eye by using an eye patch. The client is also instructed to use artificial tears four times daily and to manually close the affected eye from time to time.

Test-Taking Strategy: Use the process of elimination, and note the strategic words *need for further instruction.* These words indicate a negative event query and ask you to select an option that is an incorrect statement. Read each option carefully and consider the anatomical area that is affected to assist you with answering the question; this should direct you to option 2. Review the treatment of Bell's palsy if you had difficulty with this question.

Reference
Christensen, B., & Kockrow, E. (2006). *Adult health nursing* (5th ed., p. 735). St. Louis: Mosby.

---

314. While reviewing the nursing care plan of a hospitalized child who is immobilized because of skeletal traction, a licensed practical nurse notes that the registered nurse has documented a nursing diagnosis of *Delayed growth and development* related to immobilization and hospitalization. Which of the following evaluative statements indicates a positive outcome for this child?

1 The fracture heals without complications.
2 The caregivers verbalize safe and effective home care.
3 The child maintains normal joint and muscle integrity.
4 The child displays age-appropriate developmental behaviors.

Level of Cognitive Ability: Analysis
Client Needs: Health Promotion and Maintenance
Integrated Process: Nursing Process/Evaluation
Content Area: Child Health

Answer: 4
Rationale: By definition, *Delayed growth and development* is the state in which an individual is not performing age-appropriate tasks. Regression and inappropriate developmental behaviors may be displayed in response to immobilization and hospitalization. Options 1, 2, and 3 are appropriate evaluative statements for an immobilized child, but they do not directly address the problem of *Delayed growth and development.*

Test-Taking Strategy: The question asks for an evaluative statement that addresses the nursing diagnosis *Delayed growth and development.* All options are evaluative statements, but only option 4 addresses this particular nursing diagnosis. Review the goals of care related to *Delayed growth and development* if you had difficulty with this question.

Reference
Leifer, G. (2007). *Introduction to maternity and pediatric nursing* (5th ed., p. 468). Philadelphia: Saunders.

315. A nurse is caring for a client with deep vein thrombosis (DVT) who is on bedrest at home and has reinforced teaching about the signs of pulmonary embolism (PE), which is a complication of DVT. Which client statement indicates that the client identifies the clinical manifestations of PE?

1 "I will call you if I begin to get dizzy."
2 "I will notify you if anything unusual occurs."
3 "I will notify the doctor immediately if I become nauseous, start vomiting, and have diarrhea."
4 "I will notify the doctor immediately if I develop coughing, profuse sweating, difficulty breathing, chest pain, or a combination of any of these symptoms."

Level of Cognitive Ability: Analysis
Client Needs: Health Promotion and Maintenance
Integrated Process: Nursing Process/Evaluation
Content Area: Adult Health/Cardiovascular

Answer: 4
Rationale: The occurrence of DVT presents a risk of PE, which is when a dislodged blood clot travels to the pulmonary artery. Of the clinical manifestations of a PE, chest pain is the most common; coughing, diaphoresis, dyspnea, and apprehension are the other clinical manifestations. Pleuritic chest pain (sudden onset and aggravated by breathing) is caused by an inflammatory reaction of the lung parenchyma or when there is a pulmonary infarction or ischemia caused by an obstruction of the small pulmonary arterial branches. Options 1, 2, and 3 provide inaccurate clinical descriptions of PE.

Test-Taking Strategy: Focus on the subject and use your knowledge of the clinical manifestations of PE to answer the question. Recall that of the clinical manifestations of a PE, chest pain is the most common; this will direct you to option 4. Review the clinical manifestations of a PE if you had difficulty with this question.

Reference
Christensen, B., & Kockrow, E. (2006). *Adult health nursing* (5th ed., pp. 446-447). St. Louis: Mosby.

---

316. A client has an order to begin using nitroglycerin transdermal patches for the management of angina pectoris. The nurse provides home-care instructions for the medication and tells the client which of the following about this medication administration system?

1 Apply a new system every 7 days.
2 Wait 1 day to apply a new system if the current one becomes dislodged.
3 Place the medication system in the area of a skin fold to promote better adherence.
4 Apply the system in the morning and leave it in place for 12 to 14 hours, as directed.

Level of Cognitive Ability: Application
Client Needs: Health Promotion and Maintenance
Integrated Process: Teaching and Learning
Content Area: Pharmacology

Answer: 4
Rationale: Nitroglycerin is a coronary vasodilator used for the management of coronary artery disease and angina pectoris. The client is generally advised to apply a new system each morning and to leave it in place for 12 to 14 hours, per physician instructions; this prevents the client from developing tolerance, which happens with 24-hour use. The client should avoid placing the system in skin folds or on excoriated areas. The client can apply a new system if the current one becomes dislodged because the dose is released continuously in small amounts through the skin.

Test-Taking Strategy: Specific information about this type of medication administration system is needed to answer this question correctly. Remember that with a nitroglycerin transdermal patch, a new system is applied each morning and left in place for 12 to 14 hours, per physician instructions. Review nitroglycerin transdermal patches if you had difficulty with this question.

Reference
Kee, J., Hayes, E., & McCuistion, L. (2009). *Pharmacology: A nursing process approach* (6th ed., p. 629). St. Louis: Saunders.

---

317. A client is taking a bronchodilator by inhalation but cannot cough up secretions. The nurse teaches the client to do which of the following to best help clear the bronchial secretions?

Answer: 3
Rationale: The client should take in increased fluids (2000 to 3000 mL/day) to make secretions less viscous and for help with expectorating them. This is standard advice given to clients receiving a bronchodilator unless the client has another health problem

1 Get more exercise each day.
2 Use a dehumidifier in the home.
3 Take in increased amounts of fluids every day.
4 Administer an extra dose of medication before bedtime.

Level of Cognitive Ability: Application
Client Needs: Health Promotion and Maintenance
Integrated Process: Teaching and Learning
Content Area: Pharmacology

that could be worsened by increased fluid intake. A dehumidifier will dry secretions. The client is not advised to take additional medication. Additional exercise will not effectively clear bronchial secretions.

Test-Taking Strategy: Use the process of elimination and your knowledge of the purpose of this medication and of the adjunct measures that aid in its effectiveness. Recalling basic respiratory principles directs you to option 3. Review client teaching related to inhalation bronchodilators if you had difficulty with this question.

Reference
Hodgson, B., & Kizior, R. (2009). *Saunders nursing drug handbook 2009* (p. 28). Philadelphia: Saunders.

---

318. A client is taking an oral daily dose of amiloride hydrochloride (Midamor). The nurse gives the client which of the following home-care instructions about its use?
1 Take the dose in the morning.
2 Take the dose on an empty stomach.
3 Withhold the dose if the blood pressure is high.
4 Eat foods with extra sodium while taking this medication.

Level of Cognitive Ability: Application
Client Needs: Health Promotion and Maintenance
Integrated Process: Nursing Process/Implementation
Content Area: Pharmacology

Answer: 1
Rationale: Amiloride is a potassium-sparing diuretic used to treat edema or hypertension. A daily dose should be taken in the morning to avoid nocturia, and the dose should be taken with food to increase bioavailability. Sodium should be restricted if the medication is used as an antihypertensive. Increased blood pressure is not a reason to hold the medication, although it may be an indication for its use.

Test-Taking Strategy: Focus on the name of the medication. Recalling that this medication is a potassium-sparing diuretic will direct you to option 1. Remember that the client should take a diuretic in the morning to prevent the occurrence of nocturia. Review amiloride hydrochloride if you had difficulty with this question.

Reference
Skidmore-Roth, L. (2009). *Mosby's drug guide for nurses* (8th ed., p. 72). St. Louis: Mosby.

---

319. A nurse reinforces home-care medication instructions to a client who is taking lithium carbonate (Lithobid). The nurse determines that the client requires further instruction if the client states:
1 To take the lithium with meals
2 To decrease fluid intake while taking the lithium
3 That lithium blood levels must be monitored very closely
4 To stop taking the medication if excessive diarrhea, vomiting, or diaphoresis occurs

Level of Cognitive Ability: Analysis
Client Needs: Health Promotion and Maintenance

Answer: 2
Rationale: Lithium carbonate (Lithobid) is an antimanic and antidepressant medication. Because therapeutic and toxic dosage ranges are so close, lithium blood levels must be monitored very closely; they are reviewed more frequently at first and then once every several months. The client should be instructed to stop taking the medication if excessive diarrhea, vomiting, or diaphoresis occurs and to inform the physician. Lithium is irritating to the gastric mucosa, so it should be taken with meals. A normal diet and normal salt and fluid intake (1500 to 3000 mL/day or six 12-oz glasses) should be maintained because lithium decreases sodium reabsorption by the renal tubules, which could cause sodium depletion. A low sodium intake causes a relative increase in lithium retention and could lead to toxicity.

Integrated Process: Teaching and Learning
Content Area: Pharmacology

Test-Taking Strategy: Use the process of elimination, and note the strategic words *requires further instruction*. These words indicate a negative event query and ask you to select an option that is an incorrect statement. Remembering that it is generally important that clients be taught to maintain an adequate fluid intake directs you to option 2. Review the client teaching points related to the administration of lithium if you had difficulty with this question.

References

Hodgson, B., & Kizior, R. (2009). *Saunders nursing drug handbook 2009* (p. 693). Philadelphia: Saunders.
Lehne, R. (2007). *Pharmacology for nursing care* (6th ed., p. 361). Philadelphia: Saunders.

---

320. A nurse is reinforcing home-care instructions to a client about quinapril hydrochloride (Accupril). Which instruction should the nurse give to the client?

1 Take the medication with food only.
2 Discontinue the medication if nausea occurs.
3 Rise slowly from a lying to a sitting position.
4 A therapeutic effect will be seen immediately.

Level of Cognitive Ability: Application
Client Needs: Health Promotion and Maintenance
Integrated Process: Teaching and Learning
Content Area: Pharmacology

Answer: 3
Rationale: Quinapril hydrochloride is an angiotensin-converting enzyme inhibitor used for the treatment of hypertension. The client should be instructed to rise slowly from a lying to a sitting position and to permit the legs to dangle from the bed momentarily before standing to reduce the hypotensive effect. The medication may be given without regard to food. The client should be instructed to take a noncola carbonated beverage and salted crackers or dry toast if nausea occurs. The full therapeutic effect may take place after 1 to 2 weeks.

Test-Taking Strategy: Use the process of elimination. Eliminate option 1 because of the close-ended word *only* and option 4 because of the word *immediately.* From the remaining options, recalling that the medication is used for the treatment of hypertension directs you to option 3. Review quinapril hydrochloride if you had difficulty with this question.

Reference

Hodgson, B., & Kizior, R. (2009). *Saunders nursing drug handbook 2009* (p. 988). Philadelphia: Saunders.

---

321. Benztropine mesylate (Cogentin) is prescribed for a client with a diagnosis of Parkinson's disease. The nurse is reinforcing instructions to the client about the medication. The nurse determines that the client requires further instruction if the client states to:

1 Avoid driving if drowsiness or dizziness occurs.
2 Monitor urinary output and watch for signs of constipation.
3 Call the physician if difficulty swallowing or vomiting occurs.
4 Spend 1 hour each day sitting in the sun during rest periods to enhance the effectiveness of the medication.

Answer: 4
Rationale: Benztropine mesylate is an anticholinergic and antiparkinson medication. The client taking benztropine mesylate should be instructed to avoid driving or operating hazardous equipment if drowsy or dizzy. Tolerance to heat may be reduced as a result of a diminished ability to sweat, and the client should be instructed to plan rest periods in cool places during the day. The client should be instructed to stop taking the medication if vomiting or difficulty swallowing or speaking occurs. The client should also inform the physician if central nervous system effects occur. The client should be instructed to monitor urinary output and to watch for signs of constipation.

Level of Cognitive Ability: Analysis
Client Needs: Health Promotion and Maintenance
Integrated Process: Teaching and Learning
Content Area: Pharmacology

Test-Taking Strategy: Use the process of elimination, and note the strategic words *requires further instruction*. These words indicate a negative event query and ask you to select an option that is an incorrect statement. Recalling that this medication causes a reduced tolerance to heat directs you to option 4. Review client teaching related to benztropine mesylate if you had difficulty with this question.

Reference

Hodgson, B., & Kizior, R (2009). *Saunders nursing drug handbook 2009* (p. 125). St. Louis: Saundres.

---

322. A nurse is reinforcing home-care instructions to a client after keratoplasty. Which statement by the client indicates the need for further instruction?

1 "I should avoid bending over."
2 "Sutures are removed in 3 days."
3 "I should avoid lifting heavy objects."
4 "I should avoid crowded environments and smoke-filled areas."

Level of Cognitive Ability: Comprehension
Client Needs: Health Promotion and Maintenance
Integrated Process: Teaching and Learning
Content Area: Adult Health/Eye

Answer: 2

Rationale: Keratoplasty (corneal transplant) is the surgical removal of diseased corneal tissue followed by replacement with tissue from a human donor cornea. The client is told that the sutures are usually left in place for as long as 6 months or as prescribed by the surgeon. After the sutures are removed and complete healing has occurred, glasses or contact lenses will be prescribed. Options 1, 3, and 4 are correct discharge instructions for the client after keratoplasty.

Test-Taking Strategy: Note the strategic words *indicates the need for further instruction*. These words indicate a negative event query and ask you to select an option that is an incorrect statement. Use the process of elimination, and recall that any activities that tend to increase intraocular pressure are avoided; this will help you to eliminate options 1 and 3. Knowing that crowded environments and smoke-filled areas increase the chance of inflammation and infection will assist you with eliminating option 4. Review client teaching points after keratoplasty if you had difficulty with this question.

Reference

Linton, A. (2007). *Introduction to medical-surgical nursing* (4th ed., p. 1174). Philadelphia: Saunders.

---

323. A licensed practical nurse (LPN) is assisting with conducting a health screening clinic and is scheduled to perform hearing tests on clients. The registered nurse in charge of the clinic instructs the LPN to perform a voice test to assess the clients' hearing. Which of the following should the LPN implement to perform this screening test?

1 Face the client and whisper a statement while the client blocks both ears.
2 Quietly whisper a statement and then ask the client to repeat it to determine the hearing ability.

Answer: 2

Rationale: The nurse should stand 1 to 2 feet away from the client and ask the client to block one external ear canal. The nurse then quietly whispers a statement and asks the client to repeat it. Each ear is tested separately. Options 1, 3, and 4 are incorrect.

Test-Taking Strategy: Use the process of elimination. Eliminate options 1 and 3 because they are not measures that would effectively assess hearing. Eliminate option 4 because distance hearing is not the subject of the question. This leaves option 2 as the correct option. Review hearing screening tests if you had difficulty with this question.

Reference

Jarvis, C. (2008). *Physical examination and health assessment* (5th ed., p. 354). Philadelphia: Saunders.

3 Face the back to the client, whisper a statement, and determine whether the client can clearly repeat it.
4 Stand 4 feet away from the client when talking to him or her and determine if the client can hear at this distance.

Level of Cognitive Ability: Application
Client Needs: Health Promotion and Maintenance
Integrated Process: Nursing Process/ Implementation
Content Area: Adult Health/Ear

---

324. A nurse is reinforcing home-care instructions to a client after a hydrocelectomy. Which statement by the client would indicate the need for further instruction?
1 "I should apply ice packs to the scrotum."
2 "I should avoid sexual intercourse at this time."
3 "The sutures will be removed by the doctor in 2 weeks."
4 "I should keep the scrotum elevated until the swelling has gone away."

Level of Cognitive Ability: Comprehension
Client Needs: Health Promotion and Maintenance
Integrated Process: Teaching and Learning
Content Area: Adult Health/Renal

Answer: 3
Rationale: A hydrocele is an abnormal collection of fluid within the layers of the tunica vaginalis that surrounds the testis. It may be unilateral or bilateral, and it can occur in an infant or an adult. Hydrocelectomy is the excision of the fluid-filled sac in the tunica vaginalis. The client should be instructed that the sutures used during the hydrocelectomy are absorbable. The other options are correct.

Test-Taking Strategy: Use the process of elimination, and note the strategic words *need for further instruction.* These words indicate a negative event query and ask you to select an option that is an incorrect statement. Focus on the anatomical location of the surgical procedure to direct you to option 3. Review hydrocelectomy and the associated home-care instructions if you had difficulty with this question.

References
Ignatavicius, D., & Workman, M. (2010). *Medical-surgical nursing: Patient-centered collaborative care* (6th ed., p. 1731). St. Louis: Saunders.
Perry, A., & Potter, P. (2006). *Clinical nursing skills & techniques* (7th ed., p. 988). St. Louis: Mosby.

---

325. A nurse provides instructions to a client about administering nitroglycerin ointment (Nitro-Bid). The nurse determines that the client is using the correct technique when applying the ointment if the client:
1 Applies additional ointment if chest pain occurs
2 Applies the ointment to any nonhairy area of the body
3 Washes the ointment off when bathing and then reapplies it after the bath
4 Applies the ointment directly to the skin and then gently rubs the ointment into the skin

Answer: 2
Rationale: Nitroglycerin ointment is used on a scheduled basis and is not prescribed specifically for chest pain. The ointment is applied to a nonhairy area and is not rubbed into the skin. It is reapplied only as directed.

Test-Taking Strategy: Use the process of elimination, and focus on the subject—using the correct technique. Recalling the medication principles related to the application of ointments will direct you to option 2. Review these client teaching points if you had difficulty with this question.

Reference
Kee, J., Hayes, E., & McCuistion, L. (2009). *Phamacology: A nursing process approach* (6th ed., p. 634). St. Louis: Saunders.

Level of Cognitive Ability: Analysis
Client Needs: Health Promotion and Maintenance
Integrated Process: Nursing Process/Evaluation
Content Area: Pharmacology

---

326. A client is being discharged to home after the application of a plaster leg cast. The nurse gives the client which of the following instructions about cast care?

1 Avoid getting the cast wet.
2 Cover the casted leg with warm blankets.
3 Use the fingertips to lift and move the leg.
4 Use a soft knitting needle to scratch under the cast.

Level of Cognitive Ability: Application
Client Needs: Health Promotion and Maintenance
Integrated Process: Teaching and Learning
Content Area: Adult Health/Musculoskeletal

Answer: 1
Rationale: A plaster cast must remain dry to keep its strength. The cast should be handled with the palms of the hands (not the fingertips) until it is fully dry. Air should circulate freely around the cast to help it dry; the cast also gives off heat as it dries. The client should never scratch under the cast, although a hair dryer set at a cool setting may be used if the skin becomes itchy.

Test-Taking Strategy: Use the process of elimination, and focus on the subject—a plaster leg cast. Option 4 is dangerous to skin integrity and is immediately eliminated. Recalling that a wet cast can be dented with the fingertips causing pressure underneath will assist you with eliminating option 3. Knowing that the cast needs air circulation to dry helps you to eliminate option 2. Option 1 is correct because plaster casts should not become wet. Review home-care measures for the client with a plaster cast if you had difficulty with this question.

Reference
Linton, A. (2007). *Introduction to medical-surgical nursing* (4th ed., p. 922). Philadelphia: Saunders.

---

327. A client with an acute gastric ulcer is being discharged to home with a prescription for sucralfate (Carafate), 1 g by mouth four times daily. The nurse tells the client to take the medication at which of the following times?

1 With meals and at bedtime
2 Every 6 hours around the clock
3 1 hour after meals and at bedtime
4 1 hour before meals and at bedtime

Level of Cognitive Ability: Application
Client Needs: Health Promotion and Maintenance
Integrated Process: Teaching and Learning
Content Area: Pharmacology

Answer: 4
Rationale: Sucralfate should be scheduled for administration 1 hour before meals and at bedtime. Administration at these times allows the medication to form a protective coating over the ulcer before food intake stimulates gastric acid production and mechanical irritation. The bedtime dose protects the stomach lining during sleep. All of the other options are incorrect for these reasons.

Test-Taking Strategy: Focusing on the client's diagnosis and recalling that sucralfate protects damaged mucosa from further destruction will direct you to option 4. Review sucralfate if you had difficulty with this question.

Reference
Hodgson, B., & Kizior, R. (2009). *Saunders nursing drug handbook 2009* (p. 1082). St. Louis: Saunders.

---

328. Carbamazepine (Tegretol) is prescribed to a client for the management of generalized tonic-clonic seizures, and the nurse reinforces instructions to the client about the side effects associated with the medication. The nurse instructs the

Answer: 3
Rationale: Carbamazepine (Tegretol) is an anticonvulsant, antineuralgic, antimanic, and antipsychotic medication. Drowsiness, dizziness, nausea, and vomiting are frequent side effects associated with the medication. Adverse reactions include blood dyscrasias. The development of a fever, sore throat, mouth ulcerations,

client to inform the physician if which of the following occurs?

1 Nausea
2 Dizziness
3 Sore throat
4 Drowsiness

Level of Cognitive Ability: Application
Client Needs: Health Promotion and Maintenance
Integrated Process: Teaching and Learning
Content Area: Pharmacology

unusual bleeding or bruising, or joint pain may indicate a blood dyscrasia, and the physician should be notified.

Test-Taking Strategy: Use the process of elimination. Recalling that blood dyscrasias can occur with the use of carbamazepine directs you to option 3. Review carbamazepine and the associated adverse reactions if you had difficulty with this question.

Reference

Hodgson, B., & Kizior, R. (2009). *Saunders nursing drug handbook 2009* (p. 181). St. Louis: Saunders.

---

329. A nurse is collecting data from a client who was admitted to the hospital with complaints of anorexia, weight loss, fever, night sweats, and a persistent cough. Based on these symptoms, the nurse should specifically include which of the following in the data collection process?

1 History of smoking
2 History of recurrent bronchitis
3 Occupational exposure to asbestos
4 Past exposure to tuberculosis (TB)

Level of Cognitive Ability: Application
Client Needs: Health Promotion and Maintenance
Integrated Process: Nursing Process/Data Collection
Content Area: Adult Health/Respiratory

Answer: 4
Rationale: A diagnosis of TB should be considered for any client with a persistent cough or other symptoms that suggest TB, such as weight loss, anorexia, fatigue, night sweats, and fever. These symptoms are not compatible with bronchitis, exposure to asbestos, or smoking.

Test-Taking Strategy: Focus on the data in the question. Recalling that TB is associated with symptoms such as persistent cough, weight loss, anorexia, fatigue, night sweats, and fever will direct you to option 4. Review the signs and symptoms associated with TB if you had difficulty with this question.

Reference

Linton, A. (2007). *Introduction to medical-surgical nursing* (4th ed., p. 562). Philadelphia: Saunders.

---

330. A nurse teaches a pregnant client with human immunodeficiency virus (HIV) about measures to prevent an opportunistic infection. Which client statement indicates an understanding of these measures?

1 "I plan to have a natural childbirth experience."
2 "My husband is taking care of the cat's litter box."
3 "I know I must have a cesarean section to avoid infecting my baby."
4 "I am trying to lead a normal life. Tomorrow I will go to my niece's sixth birthday party."

Level of Cognitive Ability: Comprehension
Client Needs: Health Promotion and Maintenance
Integrated Process: Nursing Process/Evaluation
Content Area: Maternity/Antepartum

Answer: 2
Rationale: Clients should be taught proper handwashing techniques; to avoid persons who are ill; to not care for fish tanks or litter boxes; and to avoid undercooked meat, raw eggs, and unpasteurized dairy products. A pregnant client with HIV may have a normal, spontaneous vaginal delivery; however, this is not related to methods of preventing infection. It is critical to limit trauma during delivery to avoid the risk of HIV transmission to the neonate. Attending a party with a number of preschool children may increase the client's exposure to colds and opportunistic infections.

Test-Taking Strategy: Use the process of elimination, and focus on the subject—measures to prevent an opportunistic infection. Option 1 is unrelated to infection. Option 3 will increase the risk of transmission of HIV to the neonate but is not a measure to prevent an opportunistic infection. Option 4 exposes the client to the risk of infection. Review content related to the development of opportunistic infections if you had difficulty with this question.

Reference

Leifer, G. (2008). *Maternity nursing: An introductory text* (10th ed., p. 270). Philadelphia: Saunders.

---

331. A nurse has reinforced home-care instructions to a client who is about to be discharged after a prostatectomy for cancer of the prostate. Which statement by the client indicates an understanding of the instructions?

1 "I can begin to drive my car in 1 week."
2 "I cannot lift anything that weighs more than 20 pounds."
3 "If I see any clots in my urine, I should call the physician immediately."
4 "To prevent the dribbling of urine, I should limit my fluid intake to four glasses per day."

Level of Cognitive Ability: Comprehension
Client Needs: Health Promotion and Maintenance
Integrated Process: Nursing Process/Evaluation
Content Area: Adult Health/Renal

Answer: 2

Rationale: The client should be instructed to avoid lifting objects that weigh more than 20 pounds for at least 6 weeks. Small pieces of tissue or blood clots can be passed during urination for up to 2 weeks after surgery; if they are noticed, the physician does not need to be notified immediately. Driving a car and sitting for long periods of time are restricted for at least 3 weeks. A high daily fluid intake of 2 to 2.5 L/day should be maintained to limit clot formation and prevent infection.

Test-Taking Strategy: Use the process of elimination. Option 4 can be eliminated first because of the word *limit.* Eliminate option 1 next because 1 week is a rather short time period. Recalling that blood clots are expected after this type of surgery will direct you to option 2. Review the client teaching points after prostatectomy if you had difficulty with this question.

Reference

Linton, A. (2007). *Introduction to medical-surgical nursing* (4th ed., p. 1092). Philadelphia: Saunders.

---

332. A nurse is providing instructions to a client who will be discharged with an axillary drain in place after mastectomy. Which statement by the client indicates the need for further instruction?

1 "I should keep my arm elevated when I sit or lie down."
2 "I can massage the area with lotion after the incision heals."
3 "I may feel pain in the breast even though it has been removed."
4 "I should begin full range-of-motion (ROM) exercises to my upper arm as soon as I get home."

Level of Cognitive Ability: Comprehension
Client Needs: Health Promotion and Maintenance
Integrated Process: Teaching and Learning
Content Area: Adult Health/Oncology

Answer: 4

Rationale: The client should be instructed to limit upper-arm ROM to the level of the shoulder only. After the axillary drain is removed, the client can begin full ROM exercises of the upper arm if prescribed by the physician. Options 1, 2, and 3 are correct measures after a mastectomy.

Test-Taking Strategy: Use the process of elimination, and focus on the subject—that the client is being discharged with an axillary drain in place. Note the strategic words *need for further instruction.* These words indicate a negative event query and ask you to select an option that is an incorrect statement. Also note the word *full* in option 4. Review the client teaching points after mastectomy if you had difficulty with this question.

Reference

Christensen, B., & Kockrow, E. (2006). *Adult health nursing* (5th ed., p. 612). St. Louis: Mosby.

---

333. Prescriptive glasses are prescribed for a client with bilateral aphakia, and the nurse provides instructions to the client about the use of the glasses. Which statement by the client indicates the need for further instruction?

Answer: 3

Rationale: Aphakia (the absence of the lens of the eye) can be corrected with prescriptive glasses, contact lens, or intraocular lens. Only central vision is corrected with prescriptive glasses; peripheral vision is distorted. There is a magnification of the central vision of approximately 30% with prescriptive glasses;

1 "Objects that I look at may be distorted."
2 "It may be difficult to judge distances when I drive a car."
3 "The prescriptive glasses will correct my visual field of sight."
4 "The prescriptive glasses will magnify my central vision by 30%."

Level of Cognitive Ability: Comprehension
Client Needs: Health Promotion and Maintenance
Integrated Process: Teaching and Learning
Content Area: Adult Health/Eye

this requires the adjustment of daily activities and safety precautions. Because of the magnification, objects viewed centrally appear distorted, and it is difficult to judge distances when driving a car.

Test-Taking Strategy: Use the process of elimination, and note the strategic words *need for further instruction*. These words indicate a negative event query and ask you to select an option that is an incorrect statement. Think about the use of glasses and the visual field as you answer the question; this will direct you to option 3. Review the client teaching points related to the use of prescriptive glasses if you had difficulty with this question.

Reference
Ignatavicius, D., & Workman, M. (2010). *Medical-surgical nursing: Patient-centered collaborative care* (6th ed., p. 1102-1103). St. Louis: Saunders.

---

334. A client is brought to the ambulatory care department by his spouse 1 day after a cataract extraction procedure. A diagnosis of hyphema is made, which occurred as a result of the surgical procedure. The nurse provides home-care instructions to the client and his spouse regarding the treatment of the complication and tells them to:
1 Obtain assistance when ambulating.
2 Maintain rest and the patching of both eyes.
3 Resume normal activities because the hyphema will resolve on its own.
4 Return to the outpatient department for the removal of the intraocular lens implant.

Level of Cognitive Ability: Application
Client Needs: Health Promotion and Maintenance
Integrated Process: Teaching and Learning
Content Area: Adult Health/Eye

Answer: 2
Rationale: Hyphema is bleeding into the anterior chamber of the eye that can occur postoperatively as a complication of cataract surgery. Treatment includes bedrest and bilateral eye patching for 2 to 5 days during which absorption occurs. The client should be instructed to monitor for signs of increased intraocular pressure, which commonly causes sudden ocular pain. Miotics and cycloplegics may be prescribed. Occasionally the anterior chamber may be irrigated to remove the blood. Options 1, 3, and 4 are incorrect.

Test-Taking Strategy: Use the process of elimination. Eliminate options 1 and 3 first because they are comparable or alike. Eliminate option 4 because this is unnecessary and because there is no data in the question that indicates that an intraocular implant was performed. Review the treatment for a hyphema that results from surgery if you had difficulty with this question.

Reference
Ignatavicius, D., & Workman, M. (2010). *Medical-surgical nursing: Patient-centered collaborative care* (6th ed., p. 1103). St. Louis: Saunders.

---

335. A nurse reinforces home-care instructions to a client with Raynaud's phenomenon and encourages the client to engage in measures that will minimize the effects of the disorder. Which statement by the client indicates an understanding of these measures?
1 "I will take daily cool baths."
2 "I will cut down on smoking."
3 "I will eat a high-protein diet."
4 "I will keep my hands and feet warm and dry."

Answer: 4
Rationale: Raynaud's phenomenon is caused by the vasospasm of the arterioles and arteries of the upper and lower extremities. This disorder is managed by avoiding activities that promote vasoconstriction. The hands and feet are kept dry; gloves and warm fabrics should be worn in cold weather; and the client should avoid exposure to nicotine and caffeine. The avoidance of situations that trigger stress is also helpful. A high-protein diet is of no use for managing the effects of this disorder.

Level of Cognitive Ability: Comprehension
Client Needs: Health Promotion and Maintenance
Integrated Process: Nursing Process/Evaluation
Content Area: Adult Health/Cardiovascular

Test-Taking Strategy: Use the process of elimination. Recalling that the goal for managing the disorder is to avoid activities that promote vasoconstriction will direct you to option 4. Review the treatment measures for Raynaud's phenomenon if you had difficulty with this question.

Reference

Christensen, B., & Kockrow, E. (2006). *Adult health nursing* (5th ed., p. 389). St. Louis: Mosby.

---

336. Probenecid (Benemid) is prescribed to a client for the treatment of gout, and the nurse reinforces home-care instructions about the medication to the client. Which statement by the client indicates the need for further instruction?

1 "I should take the medication on an empty stomach."
2 "I should avoid any medication that contains aspirin."
3 "I should avoid alcohol because it will increase the uric acid levels."
4 "I should increase my fluid intake to maintain an adequate urine output."

Level of Cognitive Ability: Comprehension
Client Needs: Health Promotion and Maintenance
Integrated Process: Teaching and Learning
Content Area: Adult Health/Renal

Answer: 1

Rationale: Probenecid is a uricosuric medication. The client is instructed to limit high-purine foods and to administer the medication with milk or meals to prevent gastric distress. The client should be instructed to avoid alcohol because it increases the urate levels and to avoid medications that contain aspirin. Increased fluid intake is encouraged to maintain an adequate urine output and to prevent hematuria, renal colic, and stone development.

Test-Taking Strategy: Note the strategic words *need for further instruction.* These words indicate a negative event query and ask you to select an option that is an incorrect statement. Using the process of elimination and general principles related to medication therapy will direct you to option 1. Thinking about the pathophysiology associated with gout will also direct you to correct option. Review probenecid and the associated client teaching points if you had difficulty with this question.

Reference

Hodgson, B., & Kizior, R. (2009). *Saunders nursing drug handbook 2009* (p. 957). St. Louis: Saunders.

---

337. Calcium supplements have been prescribed for a client with a diagnosis of osteomalacia, and the nurse reinforces home-care instructions to the client about the supplement. Which statement by the client indicates the need for further instruction?

1 "I should drink an increased amount of water."
2 "Constipation can occur from the use of these supplements."
3 "I might experience a chalky taste in my mouth from the medication."
4 "I should take the supplements with my cereal each day in the morning."

Level of Cognitive Ability: Comprehension
Client Needs: Health Promotion and Maintenance
Integrated Process: Teaching and Learning
Content Area: Adult Health/Musculoskeletal

Answer: 4

Rationale: Calcium supplements should not be taken with whole-grain cereals, rhubarb, spinach, or bran because these foods decrease the absorption of the calcium. Most supplements should be taken on an empty stomach to promote absorption, but food may be necessary if gastric irritation develops. The client should be instructed to drink water while taking the supplements to prevent renal stones. Side effects include constipation, gastric irritation, a chalky taste in the mouth, nausea, and gastric bleeding.

Test-Taking Strategy: Note the strategic words *need for further instruction.* These words indicate a negative event query and ask you to select an option that is an incorrect statement. Use your nursing knowledge and general principles related to medication therapy to direct you to option 4. Review the client teaching points related to calcium supplement therapy if you had difficulty with this question.

References

Edmunds, M. (2010). *Introduction to clinical pharmacology* (6th ed., p. 416). St. Louis: Mosby.
Kee, J., Hayes, E., & McCuistion, L. (2009). *Pharmacology: A nursing process approach* (6th ed., p. 231). St. Louis: Saunders.

338. Fluoxetine hydrochloride (Prozac) daily is prescribed for a client, and the nurse reinforces home-care instructions about its administration. Which client statement indicates an understanding of the administration of the medication?

1 "I should take the medication right before bedtime."
2 "I should take the medication with my evening meal."
3 "I should take the medication at noontime with an antacid."
4 "I should take the medication in the morning when I first arise."

Level of Cognitive Ability: Analysis
Client Needs: Health Promotion and Maintenance
Integrated Process: Nursing Process/Evaluation
Content Area: Pharmacology

Answer: 4

Rationale: Fluoxetine hydrochloride (Prozac) is an antidepressant, antiobsessional, and antibulimic agent. A daily dose should be taken in the early morning at the same time each day, without consideration of meals. Options 1, 2, and 3 are incorrect.

Test-Taking Strategy: Knowledge of client instructions related to the use of fluoxetine hydrochloride is necessary to answer this question. Recalling that medications should generally not be administered with antacids will help you to eliminate option 3. To select from the remaining options, remember that fluoxetine hydrochloride is administered in the early morning, without consideration of meals. Review fluoxetine hydrochloride and the associated client teaching points if you had difficulty with this question.

References

deWit, S. (2009). *Medical-surgical nursing: Concepts & practice* (p. 1111). St. Louis: Saunders.

Hodgson, B., & Kizior, R. (2009). *Saunders nursing drug handbook 2009* (p. 496). St. Louis: Saunders.

---

339. A nurse is preparing to teach a client who will be self-administering insulin how to mix regular and NPH insulin in the same syringe. The nurse tells the client to:

1 Draw up the NPH insulin first into the syringe.
2 Take all of the air out of the bottle before mixing.
3 Keep both bottles stored in the refrigerator for 1 month.
4 Rotate the NPH insulin bottle in the hands before mixing.

Level of Cognitive Ability: Application
Client Needs: Health Promotion and Maintenance
Integrated Process: Teaching and Learning
Content Area: Pharmacology

Answer: 4

Rationale: Before mixing different types of insulin, the bottle should be rotated for at least 1 minute between the hands; this resuspends the insulin and helps to warm the medication. Shaking causes foaming and bubbles to form, which may trap particles of insulin and alter the dosage. Insulin may be maintained at room temperature, but additional bottles should be stored in the refrigerator for future use. Regular insulin is drawn up before NPH insulin. Air does not need to be removed from the insulin bottle.

Test-Taking Strategy: Knowledge of the procedure for mixing NPH and regular insulin in the same syringe is necessary to answer this question. Visualizing the procedure as you carefully read each option will direct you to option 4. Review the procedure for preparing NPH and regular insulin if you had difficulty with this question.

References

Ignatavicius, D., & Workman, M. (2010). *Medical-surgical nursing: Patient-centered collaborative care* (6th ed., p. 1486). St. Louis: Saunders.

Kee, J., Hayes, E., & McCuistion, L. (2009). *Pharmacology: A nursing process approach* (6th ed., p. 791). St. Louis: Saunders.

---

340. Methylphenidate hydrochloride (Ritalin) is prescribed for a child with attention-deficit/hyperactivity disorder. The nurse teaches the mother to administer the medication:

1 At bedtime
2 1 hour before bedtime
3 With the evening meal
4 With the noontime meal

Level of Cognitive Ability: Application
Client Needs: Health Promotion and Maintenance

Answer: 4

Rationale: Methylphenidate hydrochloride (Ritalin) is a central nervous system stimulant. Medications are best taken shortly before meals and not after 12 noon or 1:00 PM for children or 6:00 PM for adults because the stimulating effect may keep the client awake. Options 1, 2, and 3 are incorrect.

Test-Taking Strategy: Focus on the name of the medication. Recalling that methylphenidate hydrochloride (Ritalin) is a central nervous system stimulant will direct you to option 4. Review the client teaching points related to the administration of methylphenidate hydrochloride if you had difficulty with this question.

Integrated Process: Teaching and Learning
Content Area: Pharmacology

Reference

Hodgson, B., & Kizior, R. (2009). *Saunders nursing drug handbook 2009* (p. 746). St. Louis: Saunders.

---

341. Calcium carbonate chewable tablets are prescribed for a client with a history of duodenal ulcer. The nurse provides home-care instructions to the client and tells the client that the medication will provide relief from which disorder?

1 Flatus
2 Heartburn
3 Rectal pain
4 Muscle twitching

Level of Cognitive Ability: Application
Client Needs: Health Promotion and Maintenance
Integrated Process: Teaching and Learning
Content Area: Pharmacology

Answer: 2

Rationale: Calcium carbonate can be used as an antacid for the relief of heartburn and indigestion. It can also be used as a calcium supplement or to bind phosphorus in the gastrointestinal tract of clients with renal failure. The disorders identified in the other options are unrelated to the use of this medication.

Test-Taking Strategy: Note the strategic words *duodenal ulcer* and *relief from.* Noting the relationship between the client's diagnosis and option 2 will direct you to this option. Review the action of calcium carbonate if you had difficulty with this question.

Reference

Skidmore-Roth, L. (2009). *Mosby's drug guide for nurses* (8th ed., pp. 163-164). St. Louis: Mosby.

---

342. Aluminum hydroxide (Amphojel) tablets have been prescribed for a client with heartburn, and the nurse reinforces home-care instructions to the client. The nurse tells the client that the most common side effect with use of this medication is:

1 Dizziness
2 Excitability
3 Constipation
4 Muscle pain

Level of Cognitive Ability: Application
Client Needs: Health Promotion and Maintenance
Integrated Process: Teaching and Learning
Content Area: Pharmacology

Answer: 3

Rationale: Aluminum hydroxide is an antacid. It causes the side effect of constipation because of its aluminum base. Hypophosphatemia, which is noted by monitoring serum laboratory studies, is the other possible side effect. Options 1, 2, and 4 are incorrect.

Test-Taking Strategy: Specific knowledge of this type of antacid and its side effects is needed to answer this question. Remember that aluminum hydroxide causes the side effect of constipation because of its aluminum base. Review the side effects associated with aluminum hydroxide if you had difficulty with this question.

Reference

Hodgson, B., & Kizior, R. (2009). *Saunders nursing drug handbook 2009* (p. 46). St. Louis: Saunders.

---

343. A nurse is reinforcing home-care instructions to a client with chronic venous insufficiency secondary to deep vein thrombosis. The nurse should tell the client to avoid which of the following activities?

1 Sleeping with the foot of the bed elevated
2 Wearing elastic hose for at least 6 to 8 weeks
3 Elevating the head of the bed 6 inches during sleep

Answer: 3

Rationale: Clients with chronic venous insufficiency are advised to avoid crossing their legs, sitting in chairs in which their feet do not touch the floor, standing or sitting for prolonged periods of time, and wearing garters or sources of pressure above the legs (e.g., girdles). These clients should wear elastic hose for 6 to 8 weeks and perhaps for life, and they should sleep with the foot of the bed (not the head of the bed) elevated to promote venous return during sleep.

4 Sitting in chairs that allow the feet to touch the floor

Level of Cognitive Ability: Application
Client Needs: Health Promotion and Maintenance
Integrated Process: Teaching and Learning
Content Area: Adult Health/Cardiovascular

Test-Taking Strategy: Use the process of elimination, and note the strategic word *avoid*. This word indicates a negative event query and asks you to select an option that is an incorrect home-care measure. Use the concept of gravity when answering questions that relate to peripheral vascular problems. Venous problems are characterized by the insufficient drainage of blood from the legs returning to the heart; thus interventions should be directed toward promoting the flow of blood from the legs and to the heart. Only option 3 does not promote venous drainage, thereby making it the answer to the question as stated. Review teaching points for the client with venous insufficiency if you had difficulty with this question.

Reference

deWit, S. (2009). *Medical-surgical nursing: Concepts & practice* (pp. 449-450). St. Louis: Saunders.

---

344. A nurse has reinforced home-care instructions to a hypertensive client about nonfood items that contain sodium. The nurse determines that the client understands the information presented if the client states that which of the following may be used?

1 Toothpaste
2 Mouthwash
3 Cold remedies
4 Demineralized water

Level of Cognitive Ability: Comprehension
Client Needs: Health Promotion and Maintenance
Integrated Process: Nursing Process/Evaluation
Content Area: Adult Health/Cardiovascular

Answer: 4

Rationale: Sodium intake can be increased with use of several products, including toothpaste and mouthwashes; over-the-counter (OTC) medications such as analgesics, antacids, cough remedies, laxatives, and sedatives; and softened water, as well as some mineral waters. Clients are advised to read labels for sodium content. Water that is bottled, distilled, deionized, or demineralized may be used for drinking and cooking.

Test-Taking Strategy: Use the process of elimination. The wording of the question directs you to seek the item that is low in sodium. Remember that several OTC medications and products contain significant levels of sodium; this will assist you with eliminating options 1, 2, and 3. Finally, look at the word demineralized, which means having the minerals removed. This option would be a good choice when selecting an item that is low in sodium. Review low-sodium nonfood items if you had difficulty with this question.

Reference

Grodner, M., Long, S., & Walkingshaw, B. (2007). *Foundations and clinical applications of nutrition* (4th ed., p. 173). St. Louis: Mosby.

---

345. A nurse is reinforcing instructions with a client about how to perform the three-point gait with crutches. Which instruction should the nurse provide to the client?

1 Move both crutches forward and then swing both feet forward to the crutches.
2 Move the right crutch, the left foot, the left crutch, and then the right foot forward.
3 Advance the right crutch and the left foot forward, and then bring the right foot and left crutch forward.

Answer: 4

Rationale: A three-point gait or orthopedic gait is used for amputees and orthopedic clients. It requires that the client have normal use of one leg and both arms. The client is instructed to simultaneously move both crutches and the affected leg forward, and then the unaffected leg should be moved forward. Option 1 identifies a swing-through gait. Options 2 and 3 identify a four-point gait.

Test-Taking Strategy: Focus on the subject—a three-point gait—and read the description in each option. This will assist you with eliminating options 1, 2, and 3 because these are not three-point gaits. Review client instructions regarding a three-point gait if you had difficulty with this question.

4 Simultaneously move both crutches and the affected leg forward, and then move the unaffected leg forward.

Level of Cognitive Ability: Application
Client Needs: Health Promotion and Maintenance
Integrated Process: Teaching and Learning
Content Area: Adult Health/Musculoskeletal

Reference

deWit, S. (2009). *Medical-surgical nursing: Concepts & practice* (p. 7). St. Louis: Saunders.

---

346. A nurse is reinforcing instructions with a client about the use of crutches and teaching the client the method for ascending and descending stairs. When instructing the client about ascending the stairs, the nurse tells the client to do which of the following?

1 Move the crutches and the unaffected leg down, followed by the affected leg.
2 Move the unaffected leg up first, followed by the affected leg and the crutches.
3 Move both crutches up the stair, followed by the unaffected leg and then the affected leg.
4 Move both crutches up the stair, followed by the affected leg and then the unaffected leg.

Level of Cognitive Ability: Application
Client Needs: Health Promotion and Maintenance
Integrated Process: Teaching and Learning
Content Area: Adult Health/Musculoskeletal

Answer: 2

Rationale: To go up the stairs, the client should move the unaffected leg up first, followed by the affected leg and the crutches. When going down the stairs, the client should move the crutches and the affected leg first, followed by the unaffected leg.

Test-Taking Strategy: When answering this question, visualize the process of going up and down stairs while using crutches. If you can remember "good up and bad down," then you will be able to answer this question. When going up the stairs, the good or unaffected leg moves first. When going down the stairs, the bad or affected leg moves first. Review crutch-walking techniques if you had difficulty with this question.

Reference

deWit, S. (2009). *Medical-surgical nursing: Concepts & practice* (pp. 779-781). St. Louis: Saunders.

---

347. A client being discharged to home is prescribed enoxaparin (Lovenox) subcutaneously and will be self-administering the medication. The nurse is asked to reinforce teaching with the client about the administration of the medication and tells the client which of the following?

1 "Massage the skin after giving the injection."
2 "Aspirate the syringe before pushing down on the plunger."
3 "Push the skin flat and taut before injecting the medication."
4 "A 25- to 27-gauge, 5/8-inch needle is attached to the syringe."

Level of Cognitive Ability: Application
Client Needs: Health Promotion and Maintenance

Answer: 4

Rationale: Enoxaparin (Lovenox) is an anticoagulant administered via the subcutaneous route. With the subcutaneous injection of enoxaparin, the administration technique is the same as for subcutaneous heparin. The nurse teaches the client that a 25- to 27-gauge needle is attached to the syringe to prevent hematoma formation at the injection site. The client should use a "bunching" technique to inject the medication deep into fatty abdominal tissue. The nurse teaches the client to not aspirate the syringe before injection and to not massage the injection site.

Test-Taking Strategy: To select the correct option, recall that enoxaparin is a subcutaneously administered anticoagulant medication. With this in mind, you can select the statement that addresses standard subcutaneous injection procedure. Apply the principles related to administering heparin via subcutaneous injection to assist you with answering the question. Review the procedure for administering enoxaparin if you had difficulty with this question.

Integrated Process: Teaching and Learning
Content Area: Adult Health/Cardiovascular

References
Hodgson, B., & Kizior, R (2009). *Saunders nursing drug handbook 2009* (pp. 413-415). St. Louis: Saunders.
Perry, A., & Potter, P. (2010). *Clinical nursing skills & techniques* (7th ed., p. 621). St. Louis: Mosby .

---

348. A nurse caring for a client who experiences frequent episodes of bronchial asthma is reinforcing home-care instructions about measures to reduce the aggravation of the condition. The nurse tells the client that which of the following is least likely to help the client's condition?
1 Buying a humidifier
2 Damp dusting the furniture
3 Having the furnace serviced
4 Having the chimney cleaned

Level of Cognitive Ability: Application
Client Needs: Health Promotion and Maintenance
Integrated Process: Teaching and Learning
Content Area: Adult Health/Respiratory

Answer: 1
Rationale: Bronchial asthma is an intermittent and reversible airflow obstruction that affects only the airways and not the alveoli. Environmental allergens and organisms that can cause infection are likely to aggravate asthma. These irritants can be reduced by having the chimney cleaned and by dusting with a damp cloth. Having the furnace serviced will eliminate dirt and soot from the system and detect any carbon monoxide that is leaking or present. A humidifier will increase the moisture in the air, but it may also increase the growth of mold and mildew, which would not be helpful for this client.

Test-Taking Strategy: Use the process of elimination, and note the strategic words *least likely.* These words indicate a negative event query and ask you to select an option that will not help the client's condition. Recalling the factors that contribute to asthma will direct you to option 1. Review the home-care measures for the client with asthma if you had difficulty with this question.

Reference
deWit, S. (2009). *Medical-surgical nursing: Concepts & practice* (p. 338). St. Louis: Saunders.

---

349. A client with respiratory disease is experiencing activity intolerance at home related to fatigue and dyspnea after physical exertion. The nurse suggests which goal to the client that will best improve the client's functioning?
1 Reduce caloric intake by half to allow more energy for breathing.
2 Gradually increase ambulation and the completion of small tasks daily.
3 Stay in one room of the house to decrease episodes of fatigue and dyspnea.
4 Begin taking a light sedative medication each night to ensure a good night's sleep.

Level of Cognitive Ability: Application
Client Needs: Health Promotion and Maintenance
Integrated Process: Teaching and Learning
Content Area: Adult Health/Respiratory

Answer: 2
Rationale: The client with activity intolerance related to fatigue and dyspnea after physical exertion should try to gradually increase activity and mobility each day. The client should not reduce caloric intake by half because the client will not have sufficient energy for respiration. Rather, the client should take in adequate calories but eat small, frequent meals each day. The client needs adequate rest, but relying on a sedative each night could foster dependence. Finally, the client should not stay in one room of the house because doing so will not increase endurance and will also foster feelings of seclusion and social isolation.

Test-Taking Strategy: Use the process of elimination, and focus on the subject—the goal that will best improve the client's tolerance of activity. Option 2 is the only option that relates to activity. Review the goals for the client with activity intolerance if you had difficulty with this question.

Reference
Linton, A. (2007). *Introduction to medical-surgical nursing* (4th ed., pp. 560-561). Philadelphia: Saunders.

---

350. Captopril (Capoten) has been prescribed for a hospitalized client with hypertension, and the nurse reinforces home-care instructions to the client about the

Answer: 1
Rationale: Captopril is an antihypertensive medication (angiotensin-converting enzyme inhibitor). Orthostatic hypotension is a concern for clients taking antihypertensive medications. Clients

medication. The nurse determines that the client understands how to take this medication if the client states an intention to do which of the following?
1 Sit upright and stand slowly.
2 Drink larger amounts of water.
3 Eat foods that are high in potassium.
4 Take in large amounts of high-fiber foods.

Level of Cognitive Ability: Analysis
Client Needs: Health Promotion and Maintenance
Integrated Process: Nursing Process/Evaluation
Content Area: Adult Health/Cardiovascular

are advised to avoid standing in one position for long periods of time, to change positions slowly, and to avoid extreme warmth (e.g., shower, bath, weather). Clients are also taught to recognize the symptoms of orthostatic hypotension, including dizziness, lightheadedness, weakness, and syncope. The other options are not necessary, and option 2 could aggravate the hypertension.

Test-Taking Strategy: Use the process of elimination. Recalling that captopril is an antihypertensive will direct you to option 1 because the risk of orthostatic hypotension is present with all types of antihypertensives. Review captopril if you had difficulty with this question.

Reference

Skidmore-Roth, J. (2009). *Mosby's drug guide for nurses* (8th ed., p. 170). St. Louis: Mosby.

---

351. A client is 39 years old, has three children, and is a waitress. The nurse recognizes that this client is most at risk for developing which of the following peripheral vascular disorders?
1 Varicose veins
2 Thrombophlebitis
3 Arterial insufficiency
4 Acute arterial embolism

Level of Cognitive Ability: Analysis
Client Needs: Health Promotion and Maintenance
Integrated Process: Nursing Process/Data Collection
Content Area: Adult Health/Cardiovascular

Answer: 1
Rationale: Varicose veins are distended, protruding veins that appear darkened and tortuous. They are more common after the age of 30 years in clients who have occupations that require prolonged standing. The condition also occurs more frequently in pregnant women, obese individuals, and those with a positive family history of varicose veins or systemic problems (e.g., heart disease). The conservative treatment of these individuals focuses on promoting venous return to the heart. There is no information in the question to indicate prolonged immobility (option 2), risk of arterial insufficiency (option 3), or added risk of cardiac thrombus (option 4).

Test-Taking Strategy: Use the process of elimination and your knowledge of the risk factors for development of varicose veins. Note the strategic words *peripheral vascular* to direct you to option 1. Review the risk factors for peripheral vascular disorders if you had difficulty with this question.

Reference

Linton, A. (2007). *Introduction to medical-surgical nursing* (4th ed., pp. 708-709). Philadelphia: Saunders.

---

352. A nurse is giving a client general information about acceptable foods to include on a sodium-restricted diet. The nurse tells the client that which of the following items is lowest in sodium content?
1 Cornmeal
2 Instant rice
3 Frozen bread dough
4 Commercial stuffing

Level of Cognitive Ability: Application
Client Needs: Health Promotion and Maintenance
Integrated Process: Teaching and Learning
Content Area: Adult Health/Cardiovascular

Answer: 1
Rationale: Clients on a sodium-restricted diet should avoid the use of commercially prepared products, which often contain sodium as a preservative. Products made with natural grains (e.g., cornmeal) and that do not have added salt are the best food items to choose.

Test-Taking Strategy: Use the process of elimination. Recalling that many commercially prepared products contain sodium will direct you to option 1. Review sodium-restricted diets if you had difficulty with this question.

Reference

Christensen, B., & Kockrow, E. (2006). *Foundations of nursing* (5th ed., p. 649). St. Louis: Mosby.

---

353. A client with hyperlipidemia is advised to limit the intake of dietary cholesterol. The nurse provides dietary instructions and tells the client to choose which of the following options because it is lowest in fat?

1 Liver
2 Bacon
3 Spare ribs
4 Baked scrod

Level of Cognitive Ability: Application
Client Needs: Health Promotion and Maintenance
Integrated Process: Nursing Process/Implementation
Content Area: Adult Health/Cardiovascular

Answer: 4
Rationale: The best choices to lower the intake of cholesterol include lean cuts of beef with the fat trimmed, lamb, pork (except spare ribs), veal (except when ground), skinless poultry, and some types of fish. Meats that have larger amounts of cholesterol include prime grades of beef, pork spare ribs, goose, duck, organ meats (i.e., liver, brain, kidney), sausage, bacon, luncheon meats, frankfurters, and caviar.

Test-Taking Strategy: Use the process of elimination, and focus on the subject—the food that is lowest in fat. Remember that liver, bacon, and spare ribs are high in fat. Review low-fat foods if you had difficulty with this question.

Reference
Nix, S. (2009). *Williams' basic nutrition and diet therapy* (13th ed., p. 340). St. Louis. Mosby.

---

354. A nurse has reinforced home-care instructions about body mechanics and low back care to the client with a herniated lumbar disk. Which statement by the client indicates the need for further instruction?

1 "I should bend at the knees to pick up objects."
2 "I should swim or walk to strengthen my back muscles."
3 "I should increase the amount of fluid and fiber in my diet."
4 "I should get out of bed by sitting up straight and swinging my legs over the side."

Level of Cognitive Ability: Comprehension
Client Needs: Health Promotion and Maintenance
Integrated Process: Teaching and Learning
Content Area: Adult Health/Musculoskeletal

Answer: 4
Rationale: Clients should get out of bed by sliding toward the mattress edge. The client should then roll onto one side and push up from the bed using one or both arms. The client should keep the back straight as the legs are swung over the side. Proper body mechanics includes bending at the knees rather than at the waist to lift objects. The client should increase dietary fiber and fluids to prevent straining during stooling, which could increase intraspinal pressure. Walking and swimming are excellent exercises for strengthening the lower back muscles.

Test-Taking Strategy: Use the process of elimination, and note the strategic words *need for further instruction*. These words indicate a negative event query and ask you to select an option that is an incorrect client statement. Eliminate options 1 and 2 first because they are correct actions. Choose option 4 instead of option 3 knowing that sitting up straight causes strain on the lower back muscles or that straining during stooling increases intraspinal pressure. Review the teaching points for the client with a herniated lumbar disk if you had difficulty with this question.

Reference
Black, J., & Hawks, J. (2007). *Medical-surgical nursing: Clinical management for positive outcomes* (8th ed., pp. 1877, 1879). St. Louis: Saunders.

---

355. A nurse has reinforced home-care instructions with a client with chronic airflow limitation (CAL) about energy conservation techniques. Which statement by the client indicates the need for further instruction?

1 "I should limit activities that involve much arm movement."
2 "I should not hold my breath during activities that require exertion."

Answer: 3
Rationale: The client with CAL should alternate periods of activity with rest periods to conserve energy. The client should also sit when performing activities that do not require exertion (e.g., sewing, ironing). The client should limit activities that involve arm movements because these will increase dyspnea; the client should not hold the breath for the same reason.

3 "I should perform all activities early in the day when I am most rested."
4 "I should sit when performing activities that do not require much movement."

Level of Cognitive Ability: Comprehension
Client Needs: Health Promotion and Maintenance
Integrated Process: Teaching and Learning
Content Area: Adult Health/Respiratory

Test-Taking Strategy: Use the process of elimination, and note the strategic words *indicates the need for further instruction.* These words indicate a negative event query and ask you to select an option that is an incorrect client statement. Focus on the subject—energy conservation techniques—to direct you to option 3. Review energy conservation techniques if you had difficulty with this question.

Reference

Linton, A. (2007). *Introduction to medical-surgical nursing* (4th ed., pp. 560-561). Philadelphia: Saunders.

---

356. A nurse teaches a client with chronic airflow limitation (CAL) about positions that help breathing during dyspneic episodes. Which position, if identified by the client, indicates the need for further teaching?
1 Sitting up and leaning on a table
2 Standing and leaning against a wall
3 Sitting up with elbows resting on knees
4 Lying on the back in semi-Fowler's position

Level of Cognitive Ability: Comprehension
Client Needs: Health Promotion and Maintenance
Integrated Process: Teaching and Learning
Content Area: Adult Health/Respiratory

Answer: 4
Rationale: The client with CAL should use the positions identified in options 1, 2, and 3. These allow for maximal chest expansion and the decreased use of the accessory muscles of respiration. The client should not lie on the back because this reduces movement of a large area of the client's chest wall. Sitting is better than standing for these clients, whenever possible. If no chair is available, then leaning against a wall while standing allows accessory muscles to be used for breathing rather than posture control.

Test-Taking Strategy: Use the process of elimination, and note the strategic words *need for further teaching.* These words indicate a negative event query and ask you to select an option that is an incorrect client statement. Visualize each position described, and note that options 1, 2, and 3 are comparable or alike in that they involve a position in which the client leans forward. Review the positions that assist with breathing if you had difficulty with this question.

Reference

Linton, A. (2007). *Introduction to medical-surgical nursing* (4th ed., p. 558). Philadelphia: Saunders.

---

357. A nurse reinforces home-care instructions with a client regarding monoamine oxidase (MAO) inhibitor toxicity. The nurse determines that the client is aware of the signs of toxicity when the client tells the nurse that he will report:
1 Lethargy
2 Insomnia
3 Low-grade fever
4 Excessive fatigue

Level of Cognitive Ability: Analysis
Client Needs: Health Promotion and Maintenance
Integrated Process: Teaching and Learning
Content Area: Mental Health

Answer: 2
Rationale: Acute toxicity of MAO inhibitors is manifested by restlessness, anxiety, and insomnia. Dizziness and hypertension may also occur. Options 1, 3, and 4 are not signs of toxicity.

Test-Taking Strategy: Use the process of elimination. Options 1 and 4 can be eliminated first because they are comparable or alike. From the remaining options, it is necessary to know the signs of toxicity associated with these medications. Remember that acute toxicity of MAO inhibitors is manifested by restlessness, anxiety, and insomnia. Review these signs if you had difficulty with this question.

Reference

Varcarolis, E., & Halter, M. (2009). *Essentials of psychiatric mental health nursing: A communication approach to evidence-based care* (p. 236). St Louis: Saunders.

---

358. A nurse is reinforcing home-care instructions to the client with chronic renal failure (CRF) regarding ways to reduce pruritus caused by uremia. The nurse tells the client to avoid which of the following types of skin care products?

1 Bath oil
2 Mild soap
3 Lanolin-based lotion
4 Astringent facial cleansing pads

Level of Cognitive Ability: Application
Client Needs: Health Promotion and Maintenance
Integrated Process: Teaching and Learning
Content Area: Adult Health/Renal

Answer: 4
Rationale: The client with CRF often has dry skin that is accompanied by itching (pruritus) caused by uremia. The client should use mild soaps, lotions, and bath oils to reduce dryness without increasing skin irritation. Products that contain perfumes or alcohol increase dryness and pruritus and should be avoided.

Test-Taking Strategy: Use the process of elimination, and note the strategic word *avoid.* This word indicates a negative event query and asks you to select an option that is an incorrect item. Options 1 and 3 are comparable or alike in that they enhance skin moisture and should therefore be eliminated. From the remaining options, select option 4 instead of option 2, knowing that the client should avoid putting irritating products on the skin. Review the measures that reduce pruritus in the client with renal failure if you had difficulty with this question.

Reference
Linton, A. (2007). *Introduction to medical-surgical nursing* (4th ed., p. 1132). Philadelphia: Saunders.

---

359. A nurse has reinforced instructions to a client with chronic renal failure (CRF) about the medication therapy used for the treatment of this condition. The nurse determines that the client has a clear understanding of the medications if the client states that which of the following medications is ineffective for enhancing red blood cell (RBC) production?

1 Epoetin (Epogen)
2 Folic acid (Folvite)
3 Ferrous sulfate (Feosol)
4 Calcium carbonate (Tums)

Level of Cognitive Ability: Analysis
Client Needs: Health Promotion and Maintenance
Integrated Process: Nursing Process/Evaluation
Content Area: Adult Health/Renal

Answer: 4
Rationale: Calcium carbonate is a calcium salt that is used as a phosphate binder in the client with CRF; it has nothing to do with treatment of anemia. Folic acid is a vitamin that is needed for RBC production, and it is usually deficient in the client with CRF. Iron supplements (ferrous sulfate) are needed to produce adequate hemoglobin. Epoetin stimulates the production of RBCs because it is an external source of erythropoietin.

Test-Taking Strategy: Note the strategic word *ineffective,* and focus on the subject—enhancing RBC production. Recalling the pathophysiology and medication therapy used for the treatment of anemia in the client with CRF and the actions and uses of the medications presented in the options will direct you to option 4. Review the medications identified in the options if you had difficulty with this question.

Reference
Hodgson, B., & Kizior, R. (2009). *Saunders nursing drug handbook 2009* (pp. 170-173). Philadelphia: Saunders.

---

360. A client has been given a prescription for levothyroxine sodium (Synthroid). The nurse is asked to reinforce home-care instructions to the client regarding this medication and tells the client that an expected effect is:

1 Weight gain
2 Increased energy level
3 Decreased acid production
4 Lowered body temperature

Level of Cognitive Ability: Application
Client Needs: Health Promotion and Maintenance

Answer: 2
Rationale: Levothyroxine sodium is a synthetically prepared thyroid hormone that increases body metabolism; the client feels this effect as an increased energy level. Other effects are weight loss and increased body temperature. This medication does not affect acid production in the gastrointestinal tract.

Test-Taking Strategy: Focus on the name of the medication, and recall that this medication replaces thyroid hormone. Knowledge of the effects of thyroid hormone will direct you to option 2. Review the effects of levothyroxine sodium if you had difficulty with this question.

Integrated Process: Teaching and Learning
Content Area: Adult Health/Endocrine

Reference

Hodgson, B., & Kizior, R. (2009). *Saunders nursing drug handbook 2009* (p. 682). Philadelphia: Saunders.

---

361. A nurse has taught a client with hyperaldosteronism about the dietary changes required to manage the condition. The nurse determines that the client understands the information presented if the client states a need to decrease which of the following types of foods?

1 Oranges
2 Red meats
3 Salty snacks
4 Whole-grain breads

Level of Cognitive Ability: Comprehension
Client Needs: Health Promotion and Maintenance
Integrated Process: Nursing Process/Evaluation
Content Area: Adult Health/Endocrine

Answer: 3

Rationale: Clients with hyperaldosteronism should follow a low-sodium diet as an adjunct to medical management to decrease serum sodium levels. For this reason, salty foods are to be avoided. Potassium intake (e.g., oranges) should be maintained because the client is at risk for hypokalemia. The diet should have adequate protein, carbohydrates, and fat to maintain a normal body weight (options 2 and 4).

Test-Taking Strategy: Use the process of elimination. Recalling that aldosterone is a mineralocorticoid that helps to regulate sodium and potassium levels will assist you with eliminating options 1, 2, and 4. Review dietary measures for the client with hyperaldosteronism if you had difficulty with this question.

Reference

Christensen, B., & Kockrow, E. (2006). *Adult health nursing* (5th ed., p. 258). St. Louis: Mosby.

---

362. A client has undergone laser surgery to remove two nevi. The nurse includes which of the following statements when reinforcing home-care instructions to the client?

1 "Scrub the affected areas daily to prevent infection."
2 "Protect the areas from direct sunlight for at least 3 months."
3 "Expect frequent episodes of discomfort after the procedure."
4 "Report any swelling or redness to the physician immediately."

Level of Cognitive Ability: Application
Client Needs: Health Promotion and Maintenance
Integrated Process: Teaching and Learning
Content Area: Adult Health/Integumentary

Answer: 2

Rationale: The area should be cleansed gently with half-strength hydrogen peroxide twice a day as prescribed after the initial dressing is removed 24 hours after the procedure. There should be minimal or no discomfort after the procedure, and, if it is present, it should easily be relieved with acetaminophen (Tylenol). Redness and swelling are expected after this procedure. After the laser removal of any type of skin lesion, the skin should be protected from direct sunlight for at least 3 months.

Test-Taking Strategy: To answer this question correctly, you must be familiar with laser surgery and the elements of subsequent self-care. Read each option carefully, and use the process of elimination. The words *scrub* in option 1, *frequent* in option 3, and *immediately* in option 4 should assist you with eliminating these options. Review the client teaching points after laser therapy if you had difficulty with this question.

References

Ignatavicius, D., & Workman, M. (2010). *Medical-surgical nursing: Patient-centered collaborative care* (6th ed., p. 512). St. Louis: Saunders.
Linton, A. (2007). *Introduction to medical-surgical nursing* (4th ed., p. 1127). Philadelphia: Saunders.

---

363. A nurse is reinforcing home-care measures with the client with Addison's disease regarding ways to prevent addisonian crisis. The nurse tells the client to:

1 "Eat a diet high in protein."
2 "Eat a diet high in glucose."

Answer: 3

Rationale: Addisonian crisis (acute adrenal insufficiency) is a life-threatening event in which the need for cortisol and aldosterone is greater than the available supply. It is triggered by stressful events such as emotional crises, illness, injury, or surgery. The client should minimize the risk of infection and illness whenever

3 "Avoid stressful situations whenever possible."
4 "Stop medication therapy if infection or illness occurs."

Level of Cognitive Ability: Application
Client Needs: Health Promotion and Maintenance
Integrated Process: Teaching and Learning
Content Area: Adult Health/Endocrine

possible. If the client becomes ill, doses of adrenocortical replacement medication are increased. There are no specific dietary alterations used to manage this disorder.

Test-Taking Strategy: Use the process of elimination. Recalling that medication therapy should not be interrupted will assist you with eliminating option 4. From the remaining options, recall that stressful events will cause a crisis. Review the causes of addisonian crisis if you had difficulty with this question.

Reference

Christensen, B., & Kockrow, E. (2006). *Adult health nursing* (5th ed., p. 540). St. Louis: Mosby.

---

364. A client who has been newly diagnosed with type 1 diabetes mellitus exercises daily. When reinforcing home-care instructions about medication therapy, the nurse tells this client to inject the daily dose of insulin:
1 In any site after exercise
2 Only in the arm before exercise
3 In a site that will not be exercised
4 Only in the abdomen before exercise

Level of Cognitive Ability: Application
Client Needs: Health Promotion and Maintenance
Integrated Process: Teaching and Learning
Content Area: Adult Health/Endocrine

Answer: 3
Rationale: Exercise of a body part increases the rate of absorption of the insulin from that site. For this reason, the client should inject insulin into an area that will not be exercised. This will help the client to avoid hypoglycemia from rapid insulin absorption. Insulin should be administered at the time prescribed by the physician.

Test-Taking Strategy: Use the process of elimination. Eliminate options 2 and 4 because of the close-ended word *only.* From the remaining options, use general knowledge about principles of exercise and diabetes to choose option 3 rather than option 1. Review the client teaching points related to diabetes and exercise if you had difficulty with this question.

Reference

Christensen, B., & Kockrow, E. (2006). *Adult health nursing* (5th ed., p. 551). St. Louis: Mosby.

---

365. A nurse is reinforcing home-care instructions regarding skin care to a client receiving external radiation therapy to the chest area. The nurse tells the client to do which of the following?
1 "Use deodorants only once daily."
2 "Limit sun exposure to three times a week."
3 "Wear snug-fitting clothing to prevent irritation."
4 "Avoid the use of lotions on the area being treated."

Level of Cognitive Ability: Application
Client Needs: Health Promotion and Maintenance
Integrated Process: Teaching and Learning
Content Area: Adult Health/Oncology

Answer: 4
Rationale: The client is instructed to avoid the use of lotions on the area being treated. The client should be instructed to avoid exposure to the sun. Deodorant should not be used during treatment to the chest area. The client should wear loose-fitting clothing over the area to prevent irritation.

Test-Taking Strategy: Use the process of elimination. Focus on the subject—avoiding any substance or material that can irritate the skin in the area receiving the radiation; this will direct you to option 4. Review skin care measures for the client receiving external radiation if you had difficulty with this question.

Reference

Christensen, B., & Kockrow, E. (2006). *Adult health nursing* (5th ed., p. 828). St. Louis: Mosby.

---

366. Hyperphosphatemia has been diagnosed in a client. The nurse provides home-care instructions and teaches the client to eliminate which of the following beverages from the diet?

1 Tea
2 Coffee
3 Grape juice
4 Carbonated beverages

Level of Cognitive Ability: Application
Client Needs: Health Promotion and Maintenance
Integrated Process: Teaching and Learning
Content Area: Fundamental Skills

Answer: 4

Rationale: Foods that are naturally high in phosphates should be avoided by the client with hyperphosphatemia. These include fish, eggs, milk products, vegetables, whole grains, and carbonated beverages. Coffee, tea, and grape juice are not high in phosphates.

Test-Taking Strategy: Use the process of elimination, and focus on the client's diagnosis. Eliminate options 1 and 2 first because they are comparable or alike. From the remaining options, it is necessary to know which ones are high in phosphates. Review food items that are high in phosphates if you had difficulty with this question.

References

Black, J., & Hawks, J. (2009). *Medical-surgical nursing: Clinical management for positive outcomes* (8th ed., p. 164). St. Louis: Saunders.
Christensen, B., & Kockrow, E. (2006). *Foundations of nursing* (5th ed., p. 677). St. Louis: Mosby.

---

367. A nurse has conducted dietary teaching with a client diagnosed with iron deficiency anemia. The nurse determines that the client understands the information if the client states a need to increase the intake of which of the following foods?

1 Pineapple
2 Egg whites
3 Kidney beans
4 Refined white bread

Level of Cognitive Ability: Comprehension
Client Needs: Health Promotion and Maintenance
Integrated Process: Nursing Process/Evaluation
Content Area: Fundamental Skills

Answer: 3

Rationale: The client with iron deficiency anemia should increase the intake of foods that are naturally high in iron. The best sources of dietary iron are red meat, liver and other organ meats, blackstrap molasses, and oysters. Other good sources of iron are kidney beans, whole-wheat bread, egg yolks, spinach, kale, turnip tops, beet greens, carrots, raisins, and apricots.

Test-Taking Strategy: Use the process of elimination, and focus on the client's diagnosis. Recalling foods that are high in iron will direct you to option 3. Review the foods that are high in iron if you had difficulty with this question.

Reference

deWit, S. (2009). *Medical-surgical nursing: Concepts & practice* (p. 379). St. Louis: Saunders.

---

368. A nurse is reinforcing home-care instructions with a client who has sickle cell disease. The nurse instructs the client to avoid which of the following that could trigger a sickle cell crisis?

1 Infection
2 Mild exercise
3 Fluid overload
4 Warm weather

Level of Cognitive Ability: Application
Client Needs: Health Promotion and Maintenance
Integrated Process: Teaching and Learning
Content Area: Fundamental Skills

Answer: 1

Rationale: The client with sickle cell disease should avoid infections, which can increase metabolic demand and cause dehydration, thereby triggering a sickle cell crisis. The client should also avoid dehydration from other causes. Warm weather and mild exercise need not be avoided, but the client should take measures to avoid dehydration during these occurrences. Fluid intake is important to prevent dehydration. Finally, the client should avoid high altitudes or flying in nonpressurized aircraft because of the lesser oxygen tension.

Test-Taking Strategy: Use the process of elimination, and note the strategic word *avoid*. Recalling that infection increases metabolic demand and can cause dehydration will direct you to option 1. Review the causes of sickle cell crisis if you had difficulty with this question.

Reference
Linton, A. (2007). *Introduction to medical-surgical nursing* (4th ed., p. 584). Philadelphia: Saunders.

---

369. Which of the following clients is at lowest risk for acquiring pneumonia during hospitalization?
1 A postoperative client who had local anesthesia
2 A client with a 20-pack-year history of smoking
3 An older client with diabetes mellitus admitted to the hospital from a nursing home
4 A postoperative client who developed symptoms of a cold and upper respiratory tract irritation

Level of Cognitive Ability: Analysis
Client Needs: Health Promotion and Maintenance
Integrated Process: Nursing Process/Data Collection
Content Area: Adult Health/Respiratory

Answer: 1
Rationale: The postoperative client who had local anesthesia for a surgical procedure is at lowest risk. This client has had no direct insult to the respiratory tract. Clients who have a history of smoking, upper respiratory infection, or chronic disease (e.g., heart, lung, or kidney disease; diabetes mellitus; cancer) are more at risk for developing pneumonia. Air pollution, an insult to the respiratory tree, malnutrition, and dehydration are other miscellaneous risk factors.

Test-Taking Strategy: Use the process of elimination, and focus on the subject—risk factors for pneumonia. Apply your knowledge of these factors to the clients presented in each option. Note the strategic words *lowest risk;* these words tell you that the correct option will be the client who does not have a significant risk for developing pneumonia. This will direct you to option 1. Review the risk factors for pneumonia if you had difficulty with this question.

Reference
Linton, A. (2007). *Introduction to medical-surgical nursing* (4th ed., pp. 262-263, 537). Philadelphia: Saunders.

---

370. A nurse is collecting data from a client with a cardiovascular disorder. The nurse can best check for the presence of pallor in which of the following areas?
1 The nail beds
2 The fingertips
3 The buccal mucosa
4 Over the palms of the hands

Level of Cognitive Ability: Application
Client Needs: Health Promotion and Maintenance
Integrated Process: Nursing Process/Data Collection
Content Area: Adult Health/Cardiovascular

Answer: 3
Rationale: Pallor is best noted in the buccal mucosa or the conjunctivae, particularly in dark-skinned clients. Cyanosis is best noted in the nail beds, the conjunctivae, and the oral mucosa. Jaundice is best noted in the sclera, at the junction of the hard and soft palates, and over the palms.

Test-Taking Strategy: Focus on the subject—checking for pallor. Recalling the definition of pallor and the best techniques to use to check for pallor will direct you to option 3. Review the data collection techniques for pallor if you had difficulty with this question.

Reference
Linton, A. (2007). *Introduction to medical-surgical nursing* (4th ed., pp. 689, 1125). Philadelphia: Saunders.

---

371. A nurse is reviewing the health record of an infant who was seen in the clinic for a 6-month checkup and notes that a developmental assessment was performed. Which behavioral sign documented in the record should the nurse recognize as indicating a possible cognitive impairment that requires further developmental testing?

Answer: 4
Rationale: Developmental milestones of the 6-month-old infant include head control with no lag, an interest in environmental stimuli that includes the repetitive performance of learned skills, and motor skills. Early behavioral signs that are suggestive of cognitive impairment include diminished spontaneous activity, irritability, slow feeding, and decreased alertness to voices or movements.

1 Absence of a head lag
2 Interest in environmental stimuli
3 Repetitive performance of a new skill
4 Diminished spontaneous play activity

Level of Cognitive Ability: Comprehension
Client Needs: Health Promotion and Maintenance
Integrated Process: Nursing Process/Data Collection
Content Area: Child Health

Test-Taking Strategy: Use the process of elimination, and select the option that indicates an abnormal finding. Noting the word *diminished* in option 4 will direct you to this option. Review normal growth and development if you had difficulty with this question.

Reference

Price, D., & Gwin, J. (2008). *Pediatric nursing: An introductory text* (10th ed., p. 124). St. Louis: Saunders.

---

372. A licensed practical nurse (LPN) is employed as a camp nurse and is assisting the registered nurse with conducting a health promotion program. Which question should the LPN ask to determine if the children attending the camp are taking precautions to decrease the risk of cancer?
1 "Do you have allergies?"
2 "Do you use sunscreen?"
3 "Do you know how to swim?"
4 "Do you take baths or showers?"

Level of Cognitive Ability: Application
Client Needs: Health Promotion and Maintenance
Integrated Process: Nursing Process/Data Collection
Content Area: Child Health

Answer: 2
Rationale: The use of sunscreen will decrease the risk of skin cancer. Protective measures are warranted throughout the life span, because the harmful effects of sun exposure are cumulative, and skin damage may be severe. Although the other three options are questions that a camp nurse may ask, they do not relate specifically to cancer risk factors.

Test-Taking Strategy: Focus on the subject of the question—cancer risk. In this situation, all of the options relate to data collection; however, only option 2 is related to a cancer risk factor—exposure to the sun. Review the risks associated with skin cancer if you had difficulty with this question.

Reference

Christensen, B., & Kockrow, E. (2006). *Foundations of nursing* (5th ed., p. 1062). St. Louis: Mosby.

---

373. A woman is seen in the prenatal clinic and complains of morning sickness. Which self-care measures will the nurse suggest to the client?
1 To eat eggs for breakfast
2 To eat three well-balanced meals every day
3 To eat fatty or spicy foods only at the noontime meal
4 To eat a dry cracker before getting out of bed in the morning

Level of Cognitive Ability: Application
Client Needs: Health Promotion and Maintenance
Integrated Process: Teaching and Learning
Content Area: Maternity/Antepartum

Answer: 4
Rationale: Morning sickness is common during the first trimester of pregnancy, and it is associated with increased levels of human chorionic gonadotropin and changes in carbohydrate metabolism. It most often occurs on arising, although a few women experience it throughout the day. Self-care measures include eating a dry cracker or toast before getting out of bed; eating small, frequent meals; avoiding fatty or spicy foods; and rising slowly from a lying or sitting position to avoid orthostatic hypotension.

Test-Taking Strategy: Use the process of elimination. Focus on the subject of the question—morning sickness—to direct you to option 4. Review the measures that assist with morning sickness if you had difficulty with this question.

Reference

Leifer, G. (2008). *Maternity nursing: An introductory text* (10th ed., p. 68). Philadelphia: Saunders.

---

374. A client in her third trimester of pregnancy is seen at the clinic and complains of urinary frequency. Which self-care measure will the nurse suggest to the client?

1 Restrict fluid intake in the evening.
2 Drink at least 2000 mL of fluid per day.
3 Avoid emptying the bladder frequently.
4 Avoid large amounts of fluids during the day.

Level of Cognitive Ability: Application
Client Needs: Health Promotion and Maintenance
Integrated Process: Teaching and Learning
Content Area: Maternity/Antepartum

Answer: 2
Rationale: Urinary frequency is present during the first trimester and late in the third trimester of pregnancy because of the pressure placed on the bladder by the enlarged uterus. Self-care measures for urinary frequency include emptying the bladder frequently (every 2 hours) and drinking at least 2000 mL of fluid per day. Options 1, 3, and 4 are incorrect and could lead to urinary stasis (option 3) or a fluid volume deficit (options 1 and 4).

Test-Taking Strategy: Use the process of elimination. Eliminate options 1 and 4 first because they are comparable or alike. Eliminate option 3 next because it does not make sense to avoid emptying the bladder frequently; this action could lead to urinary stasis and cause discomfort in the woman. Review measures that will assist with the discomfort of urinary frequency if you had difficulty with this question.

Reference
Leifer, G. (2008). *Maternity nursing: An introductory text* (10th ed., p. 68). Philadelphia: Saunders.

---

375. A pregnant client is seen in the health care clinic and complains of ankle edema. The nurse reinforces self-care measures to prevent the edema. Which statement by the client indicates the need for further instruction?

1 "I should avoid frequent rest periods."
2 "I should elevate my feet during the day."
3 "I should wear supportive stockings or hose."
4 "I should avoid standing in one position or place for long periods."

Level of Cognitive Ability: Application
Client Needs: Health Promotion and Maintenance
Integrated Process: Teaching and Learning
Content Area: Maternity/Antepartum

Answer: 1
Rationale: Ankle edema is a common occurrence during pregnancy that is caused by decreased venous return from the feet as a result of gravity. It is a minor discomfort as long as hypertension and proteinuria are not present. Self-care measures for ankle edema include elevating the feet to hip level during the day, taking frequent rests, wearing supportive stockings or hose, and avoiding standing in one position or place for long periods of time.

Test-Taking Strategy: Note the strategic words *need for further instruction.* These words indicate a negative event query and ask you to select an option that is an incorrect statement. Read each option carefully and visualize its effect in relation to ankle edema; this should direct you to option 1. Review the measures to alleviate ankle edema if you had difficulty with this question.

Reference
Leifer, G. (2008). *Maternity nursing: An introductory text* (10th ed., p. 69). Philadelphia: Saunders.

---

376. A nurse working in a prenatal clinic is reviewing the records of a number of clients scheduled for prenatal visits today. The nurse recognizes that the client most at risk for abruptio placentae is the one with which characteristic?

1 Is a primipara
2 Is 26 years old
3 Exercises moderately
4 Continues to use cocaine

Answer: 4
Rationale: The highest incidence of abruptio placentae occurs in women who smoke or who use alcohol, cocaine, or caffeine during pregnancy. Other risk factors include having more than five pregnancies, advanced age, and heavy physical labor.

Test-Taking Strategy: Use the process of elimination, and focus on the subject—risk for abruptio placentae. This will direct you to option 4. Review the risk factors for abruptio placentae if you had difficulty with this question.

Level of Cognitive Ability: Analysis
Client Needs: Health Promotion and Maintenance
Integrated Process: Nursing Process/Data Collection
Content Area: Maternity/Antepartum

Reference
Leifer, G. (2008). *Maternity nursing: An introductory text* (10th ed., p. 253). Philadelphia: Saunders.

---

377. A nurse has reinforced instructions to a postpartum client regarding postpartum exercises. Which statement by the client indicates an understanding of the exercises?
1 "The postpartum exercises can result in stress urinary incontinence."
2 "Any exercises should be delayed for 4 weeks to allow for healing time."
3 "I should alternately contract and relax the muscles of the perineal area."
4 "Strenuous exercises will be started while I am in the hospital to evaluate my tolerance."

Level of Cognitive Ability: Comprehension
Client Needs: Health Promotion and Maintenance
Integrated Process: Nursing Process/Evaluation
Content Area: Maternity/Postpartum

Answer: 3
Rationale: Kegel exercises are extremely important to strengthen the muscle tone of the perineal area. Postpartum exercises can begin soon after birth. The initial exercises should be simple, with progression to increasingly strenuous exercises. Postpartum exercises will not result in stress urinary incontinence.

Test-Taking Strategy: Use the process of elimination and your knowledge of the benefit of exercise to assist you with answering the question. Eliminate options 2 and 4 because of the words *any* and *strenuous*. A careful reading of option 1 will assist you with eliminating this option. Review the purpose and benefit of postpartum exercises if you had difficulty with this question.

Reference
Leifer, G. (2008). *Maternity nursing: An introductory text* (10th ed., p. 245). Philadelphia: Saunders.

---

378. A nurse is assigned to care for a hospitalized preschooler who is in traction. The nurse determines that which of the following is the most appropriate play activity for the child?
1 Finger painting
2 Listening to music
3 Hand sewing a picture
4 Reading from a large picture book

Level of Cognitive Ability: Comprehension
Client Needs: Health Promotion and Maintenance
Integrated Process: Nursing Process/Implementation
Content Area: Child Health

Answer: 1
Rationale: A preschooler's play is simple and imaginative. Children of this age like to build and create things. For a bedridden child, the nurse should provide an activity that provides stimulation. Option 2 is most appropriate for an adolescent, option 3 is appropriate for a school-age child, and option 4 is appropriate for an infant or a young child.

Test-Taking Strategy: Use the process of elimination, and note the age group of the child. Option 4 can be eliminated because this activity is most appropriate for an infant or a young child. Eliminate option 2 next, knowing that this activity is most appropriate for an adolescent. From the remaining options, recalling that play is simple, imaginative, and creative for the preschooler will direct you to option 1. Review age-related activities and toys if you had difficulty with this question.

Reference
Price, D., & Gwin, J. (2008). *Pediatric nursing: An introductory text* (10th ed., p. 210). St. Louis: Saunders.

379. A nurse is reinforcing instructions to the parents of a 10-year-old child with hemophilia regarding appropriate activities. Which activity would be safe to suggest for the child?

1 Jogging
2 Football
3 Badminton
4 Skateboarding

Level of Cognitive Ability: Application
Client Needs: Health Promotion and Maintenance
Integrated Process: Teaching and Learning
Content Area: Child Health

Answer: 3

Rationale: Activity guidelines for children with hemophilia are categorized into those that are usually safe, those that are riskier and should be discouraged, and those in which the risks outweigh the benefits and are not recommended. Archery, badminton, fishing, golf, hiking, Ping-Pong, swimming, and walking are usually considered safe for clients with hemophilia. Options 1, 2, and 4 are riskier and are not recommended for individuals with hemophilia.

Test-Taking Strategy: Focus on the complications associated with hemophilia to assist you with answering the question. Use the process of elimination, and note that options 1, 2, and 4 are activities that present a risk of trauma and bleeding. Review the appropriate play activities for a child with hemophilia if you had difficulty with this question.

Reference

Price, D., & Gwin, J. (2008). *Pediatric nursing: An introductory text* (10th ed., p. 247). St. Louis: Saunders.

---

380. A nurse reinforces home-care instructions to a client with multiple sclerosis. Which of the following should the nurse include in the instructions?

1 Avoid pregnancy
2 Maintain a low-fiber diet.
3 Avoid taking hot baths or showers.
4 Restrict fluid intake to 1000 mL per day.

Level of Cognitive Ability: Application
Client Needs: Health Promotion and Maintenance
Integrated Process: Teaching and Learning
Content Area: Adult Health/Musculoskeletal

Answer: 3

Rationale: Because fatigue can be precipitated by warm temperatures, the client is instructed to take cool baths and to maintain a cool environmental temperature. A high-fiber diet and an adequate fluid intake of 2000 mL per day are encouraged to prevent alterations in elimination and bowel patterns. The client should not be told to avoid pregnancy, but the nurse should assist the client with making informed decisions regarding pregnancy.

Test-Taking Strategy: Use the process of elimination. Eliminate option 1 first because it is inappropriate to tell a client to avoid pregnancy. Eliminate options 2 and 4 next because these measures would be unhealthy and would promote alterations in elimination patterns for this client. Review teaching points related to the client with multiple sclerosis if you had difficulty with this question.

Reference

Christensen, B., & Kockrow, E. (2006). *Adult health nursing* (5th ed., p. 715). St. Louis: Mosby.

---

381. A client asks the nurse about the measures that will prevent Lyme disease in her children. The nurse provides which information to the client?

1 A tick should be removed by pulling it out of the skin using the fingernails.
2 If a tick falls off a pet, it will die and not be a concern for the family members.
3 Insect repellant should be applied to the entire body, except around the eyes and mouth.

Answer: 4

Rationale: Children should wear long pants, long-sleeved shirts, and hats when they are in wooded or grassy areas. Ticks should be removed with tweezers (rather than fingernails) as close to the skin as possible. Insect repellants should be used with caution and should not be applied to the hands to avoid contact with the child's eyes and mouth. Commercially prepared products should be used on pets to keep them free of ticks. If a tick falls off a pet, it can travel, contact an individual, and attach to the skin.

4 Children should wear long pants, long-sleeved shirts, and hats when they are in wooded or grassy areas.

Level of Cognitive Ability: Application
Client Needs: Health Promotion and Maintenance
Integrated Process: Teaching and Learning
Content Area: Child Health

Test-Taking Strategy: Use the process of elimination. Knowledge of the use of insect repellants will assist you with eliminating option 3. Option 1 can be eliminated next by knowing that direct contact with the tick should be avoided. From the remaining options, select option 4 because this intervention will protect children from contact with a tick. Review the preventive measures related to avoiding insect bites if you had difficulty with this question.

References

Leifer, G. (2007). *Introduction to maternity and pediatric nursing* (5th ed., p. 715). Philadelphia: Saunders.
Price, D., & Gwin, J. (2008). *Pediatric nursing: An introductory text* (10th ed., p. 266). St. Louis: Saunders.

---

382. A clinic nurse provides dietary instructions to the mother of a 3-year-old child who was seen in the health care clinic for a complaint of diarrhea. Which statement by the mother indicates the need for further instruction?

1 "It is alright to give my child active-culture yogurt."
2 "I should encourage my child to drink clear liquids."
3 "I should avoid giving my child any raw fruits or vegetables."
4 "I should give my child half a cup of chicken broth every 2 hours"

Level of Cognitive Ability: Comprehension
Client Needs: Health Promotion and Maintenance
Integrated Process: Teaching and Learning
Content Area: Child Health

Answer: 4
Rationale: When a child has diarrhea, high-sodium broths (e.g., chicken broth) are avoided to prevent electrolyte imbalance. Clear liquids are encouraged. Milk and milk products should be eliminated, except for active-culture yogurt, which restores the flora of the gastrointestinal tract. Raw fruits and vegetables, beans, spices, and any other foods that cause loose stools should be avoided.

Test-Taking Strategy: Use the process of elimination, and note the strategic words *indicates the need for further instruction.* These words indicate a negative event query and ask you to select an option that is an incorrect statement. Focusing on the child's diagnosis will direct you to option 4. Review the measures to use for a client with diarrhea if you had difficulty with this question.

References

Leifer, G. (2007). *Introduction to maternity and pediatric nursing* (5th ed., p. 643). Philadelphia: Saunders.
Price, D., & Gwin, J. (2008). *Pediatric nursing: An introductory text* (10th ed., p. 90). St. Louis: Saunders.

---

383. A school-age child with type 1 diabetes mellitus is seen in the health care clinic. The nurse reinforces instructions to the child regarding food and exercise because the child has told the nurse that she will soon begin soccer practice. Which instruction will the nurse provide to the child?

1 Avoid insulin on the day of soccer practice.
2 Eat lunch 1 hour earlier on the day of soccer practice.
3 The soccer activity should be delayed for 1 more year.
4 Eat an extra snack of carbohydrates before the soccer practice starts.

Answer: 4
Rationale: Because exercise lowers glucose levels, the child must be taught how to prevent hypoglycemia. The child should try to schedule activities to avoid exercising when an insulin dose is peaking, and she should be instructed to eat extra snacks of 15 to 30 g of carbohydrates for each 45 to 60 minutes of exercise. The extra snack before practice will avert the hypoglycemia. Options 1 and 2 are inaccurate management measures for the child with diabetes mellitus. Option 3 is unnecessary.

Test-Taking Strategy: Use the process of elimination and your knowledge of the effects of insulin to answer this question. Option 3 can be eliminated because it is inappropriate. From the remaining options, eliminate options 1 and 2 because they are inappropriate options for the management of diabetes. Review the management of diabetes mellitus in a child if you had difficulty with this question.

Level of Cognitive Ability: Application
Client Needs: Health Promotion and Maintenance
Integrated Process: Teaching and Learning
Content Area: Child Health

References
Leifer, G. (2007). *Introduction to maternity and pediatric nursing* (5th ed., p. 702). Philadelphia: Saunders.
Price, D., & Gwin, J. (2008). *Pediatric nursing: An introductory text* (10th ed., p. 300). St. Louis: Saunders.

---

384. A nurse is reinforcing home-care instructions to the mother of a child with human immunodeficiency virus (HIV) infection. Which statement by the mother indicates the need for further instruction?

1 "I should delay the polio virus vaccine."
2 "I should call the physician if my child has a fever."
3 "I should not allow my child to share toothbrushes with the other children."
4 "If any blood spills occur from a cut on my child, I should wash the spill with soap and water, rinse it with bleach and water, and allow it to air dry."

Level of Cognitive Ability: Comprehension
Client Needs: Health Promotion and Maintenance
Integrated Process: Teaching and Learning
Content Area: Child Health

Answer: 1
Rationale: The mother should be instructed to keep immunizations up to date and to not delay them. The other options are correct instructions regarding the care of the child with HIV infection.

Test-Taking Strategy: Note the strategic words *indicates the need for further instruction.* These words indicate a negative event query and ask you to select an option that is an incorrect statement. Recalling that immunizations should always be kept up to date for any child will direct you to option 1. Review the home-care measures for a child with HIV infection if you had difficulty with this question.

Reference
Price, D., & Gwin, J. (2008). *Pediatric nursing: An introductory text* (10th ed., p. 88). St. Louis: Saunders.

---

385. Which home-care instruction should be included when teaching parents how to prevent infection in their infant after the surgical repair of an inguinal hernia?

1 Restrict all of the infant's physical activity.
2 Change the diapers as soon as they become damp.
3 Soak the infant in a tub bath twice a day for the next 5 days.
4 A fever is expected to be present during the postoperative period.

Level of Cognitive Ability: Application
Client Needs: Health Promotion and Maintenance
Integrated Process: Teaching and Learning
Content Area: Child Health

Answer: 2
Rationale: Changing diapers as soon as they become damp helps to reduce the chance of irritation or infection of the incision. Parents are instructed to change diapers more frequently than usual during the day and once or twice during the night. Not all of the infant's physical activity is restricted. Parents are instructed to give the child sponge baths instead of tub baths for 2 to 5 days. A fever could indicate the presence of an infection and should be reported to the physician.

Test-Taking Strategy: Use the process of elimination. Eliminate option 1 because of the close-ended word *all.* Eliminate option 4 next because a fever indicates infection. From the remaining options, focusing on the subject and recalling the factors that cause infection will direct you to option 2. Review the measures to prevent infection if you had difficulty with this question.

Reference
Leifer, G. (2007). *Introduction to maternity and pediatric nursing* (5th ed., p. 641). Philadelphia: Saunders.

386. A client is experiencing difficulty using an incentive spirometer. The nurse teaches the client that which action may interfere with the effective use of the device?

1 Inhaling slowly
2 Breathing through the nose
3 Removing the mouthpiece to exhale
4 Forming a tight seal around the mouthpiece with the lips

Level of Cognitive Ability: Application
Client Needs: Health Promotion and Maintenance
Integrated Process: Teaching and Learning
Content Area: Adult Health/Respiratory

Answer: 2
Rationale: Incentive spirometry is not effective if the client breathes through the nose. The client should exhale, form a tight seal around the mouthpiece, inhale slowly, hold for a count of 3, and then remove the mouthpiece to exhale. The client should repeat the exercise approximately 10 times every hour for best results.

Test-Taking Strategy: Use the process of elimination, and note the strategic words *may interfere.* Visualizing the use of the incentive spirometer will direct you to option 2. Review the use of this device if you had difficulty with this question.

Reference
deWit, S. (2009). *Medical-surgical nursing: Concepts & practice* (p. 79). St. Louis: Saunders.

---

387. A client with a respiratory disorder is unsure of the position to use to breathe more easily. The nurse teaches the client to do which of the following?

1 Sit upright in bed with the arms crossed over the chest.
2 Lie on the side with the head of the bed at a 45-degree angle.
3 Sit in a reclining chair tilted back slightly and elevate the feet.
4 Sit on the edge of the bed with the arms leaning on an overbed table.

Level of Cognitive Ability: Application
Client Needs: Health Promotion and Maintenance
Integrated Process: Teaching and Learning
Content Area: Adult Health/Respiratory

Answer: 4
Rationale: Proper positioning can decrease episodes of dyspnea in a client. Such positions include sitting upright while leaning on an overbed table, sitting upright in a chair with the arms resting on the knees, and leaning against a wall while standing.

Test-Taking Strategy: Use the process of elimination. Option 2 restricts the expansion of the lateral wall of a lung and is eliminated first. From the remaining options,note that options 1 and 3 restrict movement of the anterior and posterior walls of the lung. Review the care of the client with a respiratory disorder if you had difficulty with this question.

Reference
Linton, A. (2007). *Introduction to medical-surgical nursing* (4th ed., p. 555). Philadelphia: Saunders.

---

388. A client with acquired immunodeficiency syndrome is experiencing fatigue. The nurse teaches the client which strategy to conserve energy after discharge to home?

1 Bathe before eating breakfast.
2 Sit for as many activities as possible.
3 Stand in the shower instead of taking a bath.
4 Group all tasks to be performed early in the morning.

Level of Cognitive Ability: Application
Client Needs: Health Promotion and Maintenance
Integrated Process: Teaching and Learning
Content Area: Adult Health/Respiratory

Answer: 2
Rationale: The client is taught to conserve energy by sitting for as many activities as possible, including dressing, shaving, preparing food, and ironing. The client should also sit in a shower chair instead of standing while bathing. The client should prioritize activities (e.g., eating breakfast before bathing) and should intersperse each major activity with a period of rest. Frequent short rest periods are more effective than fewer longer ones.

Test-Taking Strategy: Use the process of elimination, and answer this question by considering the amount of exertion required by the client to perform each of the activities listed in the options. Options 3 and 4 are obviously taxing for the client and are eliminated first. From the remaining options, recall that bathing may take away energy that could be used for eating. Review measures that conserve energy if you had difficulty with this question.

Reference

Christensen, B., & Kockrow, E. (2006). *Adult health nursing* (5th ed., p. 796). St. Louis: Mosby.

---

389. A nurse has reinforced instructions with a client with pleurisy about strategies to promote comfort during recuperation. The nurse determines that the client has understood the instructions if the client states that he will do which of the following?

1 Try to take only small, shallow breaths.
2 Take as much pain medication as possible.
3 Lie as much as possible on the unaffected side.
4 Splint the chest wall during coughing and deep breathing.

Level of Cognitive Ability: Comprehension
Client Needs: Health Promotion and Maintenance
Integrated Process: Nursing Process/Evaluation
Content Area: Adult Health/Respiratory

Answer: 4

Rationale: The client with pleurisy should splint the chest wall during coughing and deep breathing, which are necessary to prevent atelectasis. The client should also lie on the affected side to minimize movement of the affected chest wall. The client should not take only small, shallow breaths because this promotes atelectasis. The client should take medication prudently to allow for coughing, deep breathing, and adequate levels of comfort.

Test-Taking Strategy: Use the process of elimination. Option 2 is obviously incorrect and is eliminated first. Eliminate option 1 next because taking small, shallow breaths would promote atelectasis. Lying on the unaffected side would stretch the chest wall on the affected side, thereby increasing discomfort, so option 3 can be eliminated. Option 4 promotes lung expansion while minimizing client discomfort. Review the care of the client with pleurisy if you had difficulty with this question.

Reference

Christensen, B., & Kockrow, E. (2006). *Adult health nursing* (5th ed., p. 437). St. Louis: Mosby.

---

390. A client is to be discharged on warfarin (Coumadin) therapy, and the nurse reinforces medication instructions with the client. Which statement by the client would indicate the need for further teaching?

1 "I should have my blood levels checked in 2 weeks."
2 "I should include more foods high in vitamin K in my diet."
3 "This medicine thins my blood and allows me to clot more slowly."
4 "If I notice any increased bleeding or bruising, I should call my doctor."

Level of Cognitive Ability: Comprehension
Client Needs: Health Promotion and Maintenance
Integrated Process: Teaching and Learning
Content Area: Pharmacology

Answer: 2

Rationale: Warfarin is an oral anticoagulant that is mainly used to prevent thromboembolic events such as thrombophlebitis, pulmonary embolism, and embolism formation caused by atrial fibrillation. Oral anticoagulants prolong the clotting time and are monitored by the prothrombin time and the international normalized ratio. Client education should include signs and symptoms of toxic effects and dietary restrictions such as limiting foods high in vitamin K (e.g., leafy green vegetables, liver, cheese, egg yolks) because these food items reduce the anticoagulant effect of warfarin.

Test-Taking Strategy: Note the strategic words *the need for further teaching*. These words indicate a negative event query and ask you to select an option that is an incorrect statement. Recalling the purpose of warfarin therapy and the role that vitamin K plays in the clotting mechanism will direct you to option 2. Review client education points related to warfarin if you had difficulty with this question.

Reference

Hodgson, B., & Kizior, R. (2009). *Saunders nursing drug handbook 2009* (p. 1219). Philadelphia: Saunders.

---

391. A teenager returns to the gynecological clinic for a follow-up visit for a sexually transmitted infection (STI). Which

Answer: 4

Rationale: When a client has an STI, all sexual contacts must be notified and treated with medication. Any treatment at a

statement by the client indicates the need for further teaching?

1 "I know you won't tell my parents I'm sick."
2 "I finished all of the antibiotics, just like you said."
3 "I always make sure my boyfriend uses a condom."
4 "My boyfriend doesn't have to come in for treatment."

Level of Cognitive Ability: Comprehension
Client Needs: Health Promotion and Maintenance
Integrated Process: Teaching and Learning
Content Area: Child Health

gynecological clinic for teenagers is confidential, and parents will not be contacted, even if the client is younger than 18 years old. Clients should always finish a medication ordered by the health care provider. Clients should always use condoms with any sexual contact.

Test-Taking Strategy: Use the process of elimination, and note the strategic words *need for further teaching*. These words indicate a negative event query and ask you to select an option that is an incorrect statement. Knowledge of safe sex practices and the treatment of STIs will assist you with answering this question. Review this content if you had difficulty with this question.

Reference

Price, D., & Gwin, J. (2008). *Pediatric nursing: An introductory text* (10th ed., p. 361). St. Louis: Saunders.

---

392. A perinatal client has been instructed about the prevention of genital tract infections. Which statement by the client would indicate an understanding of the instructions?

1 "I can douche anytime I want."
2 "I can wear my tight-fitting jeans."
3 "I should avoid the use of condoms."
4 "I should choose underwear with a cotton panel liner."

Level of Cognitive Ability: Comprehension
Client Needs: Health Promotion and Maintenance
Integrated Process: Nursing Process/Evaluation
Content Area: Maternity/Antepartum

Answer: 4

Rationale: Wearing items with a cotton panel liner allows for air movement in and around the genital area and assists with the prevention of genital tract infections. Douching needs to be avoided because it places the client at risk for infection. Wearing tight clothes irritates the genital area and does not allow for air circulation. Condoms should be used to minimize the spread of sexually transmitted infectious diseases.

Test-Taking Strategy: Note the strategic words *understanding of the instructions*. Options 1, 2, and 3 are all incorrect statements regarding client self-care and the prevention of genital tract infections. Review the prevention measures associated with genital tract infections if you had difficulty with this question.

Reference

Leifer, G. (2008). *Maternity nursing: An introductory text* (10th ed., p. 345). Philadelphia: Saunders.

---

393. A client who sustained a major burn is resuming an oral diet. The nurse encourages the client to eat a variety of which types of foods to best help with continued wound healing and tissue repair?

1 High-protein and high-fat foods
2 High-fat and low-carbohydrate foods
3 High-carbohydrate and low-protein foods
4 High-protein and high-carbohydrate foods

Level of Cognitive Ability: Application
Client Needs: Health Promotion and Maintenance
Integrated Process: Nursing Process/Implementation
Content Area: Adult Health/Integumentary

Answer: 4

Rationale: To promote adequate healing and to meet continued high metabolic needs, the client with a major burn should eat a diet that is high in calories, protein, and carbohydrates. This type of diet also keeps the client in positive nitrogen balance. There is no need to increase the amount of fat in the diet.

Test-Taking Strategy: Use the process of elimination, and note the strategic words *wound healing and tissue repair*. Use the principles of nutrition as they relate to healing tissues to answer this question; this will direct you to option 4. Review the nutrition necessary for healing and tissue repair if you had difficulty with this question.

Reference

Christensen, B., & Kockrow, E. (2006). *Adult health nursing* (5th ed., p. 111). St. Louis: Mosby.

394. A nurse has taught the client with myxedema about dietary changes to help manage the disorder. The nurse determines that the client understands the information if the client states that it is permissible to continue eating which of the following foods?

1 Shrimp, green beans, and butter
2 Peanut butter, cheese, and red meat
3 Beef liver, carrots, and fried potatoes
4 Apples, whole-grain breads, and low-fat milk

Level of Cognitive Ability: Comprehension
Client Needs: Health Promotion and Maintenance
Integrated Process: Nursing Process/Evaluation
Content Area: Adult Health/Endocrine

Answer: 4
Rationale: Clients with myxedema or hypothyroidism have decreased metabolic demands from a reduced metabolic rate. For this reason, they often experience weight gain. The diet should be low in calories overall and yet be representative of all food groups. Option 4 is the only one that contains solely low-calorie foods.

Test-Taking Strategy: Remember that when there is more than one part to an option, all of the parts of the option must be correct for the option to be correct. With this in mind, analyze each option in terms of dietary content. The correct option is the one that promotes weight reduction by being low in fat and calories. Review the care of the client with myxedema if you had difficulty with this question.

Reference
Christensen, B., & Kockrow, E. (2006). *Adult health nursing* (5th ed., p. 533). St. Louis: Mosby.

---

395. A nurse demonstrates to a mother how to correctly take an axillary temperature to determine if a child has a fever. Which action by the mother would indicate the need for further teaching?

1 She holds the thermometer in place.
2 She takes the temperature only after a feeding.
3 She records the actual temperature reading and route.
4 She places the thermometer in the center of the axilla.

Level of Cognitive Ability: Comprehension
Client Needs: Health Promotion and Maintenance
Integrated Process: Teaching and Learning
Content Area: Child Health

Answer: 2
Rationale: It is not necessary to take the child's temperature only after a feeding. Options 1, 3, and 4 are correct steps for taking an axillary temperature.

Test-Taking Strategy: Note the strategic words *need for further teaching*. These words indicate a negative event query and ask you to select an option that is an incorrect action. Noting the close-ended word *only* in option 2 will direct you to this option. Review the procedure for obtaining an axillary temperature if you had difficulty with this question.

Reference
Leifer, G. (2007). *Introduction to maternity and pediatric nursing* (5th ed., p. 490). Philadelphia: Saunders.

---

396. A nurse instructs a client about a low-fat diet. The client would indicate an understanding of this diet by choosing which of the following foods?

1 Shrimp and bacon salad
2 Liver, potato salad, and sherbet
3 Turkey breast, boiled rice, and angel food cake
4 Lean hamburger steak and macaroni and cheese

Level of Cognitive Ability: Comprehension
Client Needs: Health Promotion and Maintenance
Integrated Process: Teaching and Learning
Content Area: Fundamental Skills

Answer: 3
Rationale: Major sources of fat include organ meats, red meats, salad dressings, eggs, butter, and cheese. All options except option 3 contain high-fat foods.

Test-Taking Strategy: Use the process of elimination. Eliminate options 1 and 4 first because both a hamburger steak and bacon are high in fat. From the remaining options, look at the foods closely. Option 3 does not contain any high-fat foods. Potato salad will contain mayonnaise, which is high in fat. Review the foods that contain fat if you had difficulty with this question.

Reference
Christensen, B., & Kockrow, E. (2006). *Foundations of nursing* (5th ed., p. 648). St. Louis: Mosby.

---

397. A nurse is teaching the client with acquired immunodeficiency syndrome home-care measures for preventing foodborne illnesses. The nurse teaches the client to avoid which of the following items to prevent infection?

1. Bananas
2. Raw oysters
3. Bottled water
4. Products with sorbitol

Level of Cognitive Ability: Application
Client Needs: Health Promotion and Maintenance
Integrated Process: Teaching and Learning
Content Area: Fundamental Skills

Answer: 2
Rationale: The client is taught to avoid raw or undercooked seafood, meat, poultry, and eggs. The client should also avoid unpasteurized milk and dairy products. Bottled beverages and fruits that the client peels are safe. The client may be taught to avoid sorbitol, but this is to diminish diarrhea and has nothing to do with foodborne infection.

Test-Taking Strategy: Use the process of elimination, and focus on the subject of the question—the prevention of foodborne illnesses. Sorbitol produces diarrhea but is unrelated to foodborne illness, so option 4 is eliminated first. Bottled water is safe to drink, which eliminates option 3. Eliminate option 1 because the client is taught that fruits that are peeled are safe. Review items to avoid to prevent foodborne illnesses if you had difficulty with this question.

References
Christensen, B., & Kockrow, E. (2006). *Adult health nursing* (5th ed., pp. 796, 803). St. Louis: Mosby.
deWit, S. (2009). *Medical-surgical nursing: Concepts & practice* (p. 253). St. Louis: Saunders.

---

398. A client with histoplasmosis has an order for ketoconazole (Nizoral). The nurse reinforces home-care instructions and tells the client to do which of the following while taking this medication?

1. Avoid exposure to sunlight.
2. Limit alcohol to 2 oz per day.
3. Take the medication with an antacid.
4. Take the medication on an empty stomach.

Level of Cognitive Ability: Application
Client Needs: Health Promotion and Maintenance
Integrated Process: Teaching and Learning
Content Area: Pharmacology

Answer: 1
Rationale: The client should be taught that ketoconazole is an antifungal medication. It should be taken with food or milk, and antacids should be avoided for 2 hours after it is taken. The client should avoid the concurrent use of alcohol because the medication is hepatotoxic. The client should also avoid exposure to sunlight because the medication increases photosensitivity.

Test-Taking Strategy: Use the process of elimination. Begin to answer this question by eliminating options 2 and 3. Many medications are not well absorbed if an antacid is given concurrently. There are also many medications with which alcohol use is contraindicated for the duration of the therapy. To select between options 1 and 4, you should know that this medication causes photophobia and that it should be taken with food or milk. Review ketoconazole if you had difficulty with this question.

Reference
Skidmore-Roth, L. (2009). *Mosby's drug guide for nurses* (8th ed., p. 529). St. Louis: Mosby.

---

399. A nurse is planning to teach a teenage client about sexuality. The nurse should begin the instruction by doing which of the following?

1. Determining the client's knowledge of sexuality
2. Informing the client about the dangers of pregnancy
3. Advising the client to maintain sexual abstinence until marriage
4. Providing written information about sexually transmitted diseases

Answer: 1
Rationale: The first step in the teaching and learning process is to determine the client's knowledge. The other options may be later steps, depending on the data obtained.

Test-Taking Strategy: Use the nursing process, and select the option that involves the gathering of data; this will direct you to option 1. Remember that when teaching, determining motivation, interest, and level of knowledge comes before providing information. Review the principles of teaching and learning if you had difficulty with this question.

Level of Cognitive Ability: Application
Client Needs: Health Promotion and Maintenance
Integrated Process: Teaching and Learning
Content Area: Child Health

Reference

Price, D., & Gwin, J. (2008). *Pediatric nursing: An introductory text* (10th ed., p. 333). St. Louis: Saunders.

---

400. A nurse provides suggestions to parents about the appropriate actions to take when their toddler has a temper tantrum. Which statement by the parents indicates an understanding of the actions to take?

1 "I will ignore the tantrums as long as there is no physical danger."
2 "I will give frequent reminders that only bad children have tantrums."
3 "I will send my child to a room alone for 10 minutes after every tantrum."
4 "I will reward my child with candy at the end of each day without a tantrum."

Level of Cognitive Ability: Comprehension
Client Needs: Health Promotion and Maintenance
Integrated Process: Nursing Process/Evaluation
Content Area: Child Health

Answer: 1
Rationale: Ignoring a negative attention-seeking behavior is considered to be the best way to discourage it, provided that the child is safe from injury. Option 2 is untrue and negative. Option 3 gives attention to the tantrum and also exceeds the recommended time of 1 minute per year of age for a time-out. Providing candy as a reward is unhealthy and unlikely to be effective at the end of the day.

Test-Taking Strategy: Use Maslow's Hierarchy of Needs theory. Recalling that safety is a primary concern will direct you to option 1. Review measures to discourage tantrums if you had difficulty with this question.

Reference

Price, D., & Gwin, J. (2008). *Pediatric nursing: An introductory text* (10th ed., p. 179). St. Louis: Saunders.

---

401. A nurse reinforces medication instructions to a client who has been prescribed disulfiram (Antabuse). Which statement by the client indicates the need for further instruction regarding the medication?

1 "I'll have to check my aftershave lotion."
2 "I must be careful taking cold medicines."
3 "As long as I don't drink alcohol, I'll be fine."
4 "I'll have to be more careful with the ingredients that I use for cooking."

Level of Cognitive Ability: Comprehension
Client Needs: Health Promotion and Maintenance
Integrated Process: Teaching and Learning
Content Area: Pharmacology

Answer: 3
Rationale: Clients who are taking disulfiram must be taught that substances that contain alcohol can trigger adverse reactions. Sources of hidden alcohol include foods (e.g., soups, sauces, vinegars), medicines (e.g., cold medicines, mouthwashes), and skin preparations (e.g., alcohol rubs, aftershave lotions).

Test-Taking Strategy: Use the process of elimination, and note the strategic words *need for further instruction*. These words indicate a negative event query and ask you to select an option that is an incorrect statement. Recalling that disulfiram is used with clients who have alcoholism and that any form of alcohol should be avoided with this medication will direct you to option 3. Review the client teaching points related to disulfiram if you had difficulty with this question.

Reference

Edmunds, M. (2010). *Introduction to clinical pharmacology* (6th ed., pp. 314-315). St. Louis: Mosby.

402. Which client statement indicates that the client needs further teaching about testicular self-examination (TSE)?
1 "I know to report any small lumps."
2 "I examine myself every 2 months."
3 "I examine myself after I take a warm shower."
4 "I feel a cord-like structure in back and going upward."

Level of Cognitive Ability: Comprehension
Client Needs: Health Promotion and Maintenance
Integrated Process: Teaching and Learning
Content Area: Adult Health/Oncology

Answer: 2
Rationale: A TSE should be performed every month, and small lumps or abnormalities should be reported. The spermatic cord finding is normal. After a warm bath or shower, the scrotum is relaxed, thereby making it easier to perform the TSE.

Test-Taking Strategy: Use the process of elimination, and note the strategic words *needs further teaching*. These words indicate a negative event query and ask you to select an option that is an incorrect statement. Remembering that breast self-examination should be performed monthly may assist you with recalling that the TSE is also performed monthly. Review the procedure for the TSE if you had difficulty with this question.

Reference
Christensen, B., & Kockrow, E. (2006). *Adult health nursing* (5th ed., p. 618). St. Louis: Mosby.

---

403. A nurse determines that a client with Cushing's syndrome understands the hospital discharge instructions if the client makes which of the following statements?
1 "I should eat foods low in potassium."
2 "I should check the color of my stools."
3 "I should check the temperature of my legs at least once a day."
4 "I should take aspirin rather than acetaminophen (Tylenol) for a headache."

Level of Cognitive Ability: Comprehension
Client Needs: Health Promotion and Maintenance
Integrated Process: Nursing Process/Evaluation
Content Area: Adult Health/Endocrine

Answer: 2
Rationale: Cortisol, which is secreted in clients with Cushing's syndrome, stimulates the secretion of gastric acid; this can result in peptic ulcers and gastrointestinal (GI) bleeding. The client should check the stools for signs of GI bleeding. Option 1 is incorrect because potassium-rich foods should be encouraged to correct hypokalemia. Option 3 is incorrect because Cushing's syndrome does not affect temperature changes in the lower extremities. Option 4 is incorrect because aspirin can increase the risk for gastric bleeding and skin bruising.

Test-Taking Strategy: Knowledge of the pathophysiology related to Cushing's syndrome is necessary to answer this question. Remember that cortisol stimulates the secretion of gastric acid, which can result in peptic ulcers and GI bleeding. Review Cushing's syndrome if you had difficulty with this question.

Reference
deWit, S. (2009). *Medical-surgical nursing: Concepts & practice* (p. 906). St. Louis: Saunders.

---

404. A client is on a diet that has been designed to avoid concentrated sugars. The nurse determines that the client understands the diet plan if which of the following foods are selected?
1 Strawberry yogurt, lettuce salad, and coffee
2 Chicken salad, tomato, Jell-O, tea, and honey
3 Peanut butter and jelly sandwich, sherbet, and cola
4 Tuna sandwich, lettuce salad, watermelon, and herbal tea

Answer: 4
Rationale: Concentrated sugars are found in fruit yogurt, gelatin desserts, prepared drink mixes, jelly, and sherbet.

Test-Taking Strategy: Use the process of elimination. Read all of the food items in each option, noting that options 1, 2, and 3 contain foods that are high in concentrated sugars. Review the foods that contain concentrated sugars if you had difficulty with this question.

Reference
Linton, A. (2007). *Introduction to medical-surgical nursing* (4th ed., p. 95). Philadelphia: Saunders.

Level of Cognitive Ability: Comprehension
Client Needs: Health Promotion and Maintenance
Integrated Process: Nursing Process/Evaluation
Content Area: Fundamental Skills

---

405. A nurse has reinforced instructions to a client with chronic obstructive pulmonary disease (COPD) regarding home-care measures. Which statement by the client would indicate the need for further teaching about nutrition?

1 "I will rest a few minutes before I eat."
2 "I will not eat as much cabbage as I once did."
3 "I will certainly try to drink 3 L of fluid every day."
4 "It's best to eat three large meals a day so that I will get all of my nutrients."

Level of Cognitive Ability: Comprehension
Client Needs: Health Promotion and Maintenance
Integrated Process: Teaching and Learning
Content Area: Adult Health/Respiratory

Answer: 4

Rationale: Large meals distend the abdomen and elevate the diaphragm, which may hinder breathing. Resting before eating may decrease the fatigue that is often associated with COPD. Gas-forming foods may cause bloating, which interferes with normal diaphragmatic breathing. Adequate fluid intake helps to liquefy pulmonary secretions.

Test-Taking Strategy: Use the process of elimination, and note the strategic words *need for further teaching.* These words indicate a negative event query and ask you to select an option that is an incorrect statement. Recalling that an overdistended abdomen will have harmful effects on a client's respiratory system will direct you to option 4. In addition, option 4 suggests that the only way to obtain all of the daily nutrients is by eating three large meals a day; this is a false statement. Review nutrition and the client with a chronic respiratory disorder if you had difficulty with this question.

Reference

Linton, A. (2007). *Introduction to medical-surgical nursing* (4th ed., p. 557). Philadelphia: Saunders.

---

406. A nurse is reinforcing home-care instructions to a hospitalized client with pneumonia. Which statement by the client indicates that the client requires further discharge teaching?

1 "I won't need incentive spirometry when I am discharged."
2 "I will take all of my antibiotics even if I do feel 100% better."
3 "I understand that it may be weeks before my usual sense of well-being returns."
4 "It is a good idea for me to take a nap every afternoon for the next couple of weeks."

Level of Cognitive Ability: Comprehension
Client Needs: Health Promotion and Maintenance
Integrated Process: Teaching and Learning
Content Area: Adult Health/Respiratory

Answer: 1

Rationale: Deep breathing and coughing exercises and the use of incentive spirometry should be practiced for 6 to 8 weeks after the client is discharged from the hospital to keep the alveoli expanded and to promote the removal of lung secretions. If the entire regimen of antibiotics is not taken, the client may experience a relapse. The period of convalescence with pneumonia is often lengthy, and it may be weeks before the client feels a sense of well-being. Adequate rest is needed to maintain progress toward recovery.

Test-Taking Strategy: Use the process of elimination, and note the strategic words *requires further discharge teaching.* These words indicate a negative event query and ask you to select an option that is an incorrect statement. The use of an incentive spirometer has a direct relationship to the pneumonia, which is the subject of the question. Review the teaching points for the client with pneumonia if you had difficulty with this question.

References

Christensen, B., & Kockrow, E. (2006). *Adult health nursing* (5th ed., p. 436). St. Louis: Mosby.

Ignatavicius, D., & Workman, M. (2010). *Medical-surgical nursing: Patient-centered collaborative care* (5th ed., p. 638). St. Louis: Saunders.

407. An 18-year-old client is admitted to an inpatient mental health unit with a diagnosis of anorexia nervosa. Health promotion should focus on which of the following?

1 Providing a supportive environment
2 Emphasizing social interaction with other clients
3 Examining intrapsychic conflicts and past issues
4 Helping the client identify and examine dysfunctional thoughts and beliefs

Level of Cognitive Ability: Application
Client Needs: Health Promotion and Maintenance
Integrated Process: Nursing Process/Planning
Content Area: Mental Health

Answer: 4
Rationale: Health promotion focuses on helping clients recognize and analyze dysfunctional thoughts and on identifying and examining the values and beliefs that maintain these thoughts. Providing a supportive environment is important, but it is not as critical as option 4, and it does not specifically focus on health promotion. Emphasizing social interaction is not appropriate at this time. Examining intrapsychic conflicts and past issues is not directly related to the client's problem.

Test-Taking Strategy: Use the process of elimination. Option 4 is the only option that is specifically client centered. This option also focuses on identifying client issues related to the diagnosis. Review the care of the client with anorexia nervosa if you had difficulty with this question.

Reference
Fortinash, K., & Holoday-Worret, P. (2008). *Psychiatric mental health nursing* (4th ed., p. 400). St. Louis: Mosby.

---

408. A nurse is assisting with planning home care for a client with a C5 spinal cord injury and suggests which client outcome for the plan of care?

1 Maintains intact skin
2 Regains bladder and bowel control
3 Performs activities of daily living independently
4 Independently transfers to and from a wheelchair

Level of Cognitive Ability: Application
Client Needs: Health Promotion and Maintenance
Integrated Process: Nursing Process/Planning
Content Area: Adult Health/Neurological

Answer: 1
Rationale: A C5 spinal cord injury results in quadriplegia with no sensation below the clavicle, including in most of the arms and the hands. The client may maintain partial movement of the shoulders and elbows. Maintaining intact skin is an important outcome for the client with a spinal cord injury. The remaining options are inappropriate for the client with this type of injury.

Test-Taking Strategy: Use the process of elimination. Eliminate options 3 and 4 first because they are comparable or alike. Knowledge of the effects of a C5 spinal cord injury will assist you with eliminating option 2. Review the effects of this type of injury if you had difficulty with this question.

Reference
Linton, A. (2007). *Introduction to medical-surgical nursing* (4th ed., pp. 494-495). Philadelphia: Saunders.

---

409. A client who sustained a thoracic cord injury 1 year ago returns to the physician's office with a small reddened area on the coccyx. After reinforcing home-care instructions regarding the relief of pressure on the area with the use of a turning schedule, which action by the nurse is appropriate?

1 Teach the client to feel for red and broken areas.
2 Ask a family member to check the skin daily.
3 Teach the client to use a mirror for skin assessment.
4 Have the client return to the physician's office daily for a skin check.

Answer: 3
Rationale: The client should be encouraged to be as independent as possible. The most effective method of skin self-assessment is to use a special mirror to view the skin. Options 2 and 4 involve others in performing a task that the client can perform independently. It is unrealistic to expect the client to return to the physician's office daily for a skin check. Option 1 is an inaccurate technique because redness cannot be felt. Option 3 is the only option that addresses client self-assessment of the subject of the question—redness.

Test-Taking Strategy: Use the process of elimination, and remember that independence is key in the rehabilitation of clients. Recalling this concept will direct you to option 3. Review home-care measures for the client with a spinal cord injury if you had difficulty with this question.

Level of Cognitive Ability: Application
Client Needs: Health Promotion and Maintenance
Integrated Process: Nursing Process/Implementation
Content Area: Adult Health/Neurological

Reference

Black, J., & Hawks, J. (2009). *Medical-surgical nursing: Clinical management for positive outcomes* (8th ed., p. 1966). St. Louis: Saunders.

---

410. A nurse is reinforcing home-care instructions to a client with peptic ulcer disease regarding symptom management. The nurse tells the client to do which of the following?

1 Limit the intake of water.
2 Use aspirin to relieve gastric pain.
3 Eat large meals to absorb gastric acid.
4 Eat slowly and chew food thoroughly.

Level of Cognitive Ability: Application
Client Needs: Health Promotion and Maintenance
Integrated Process: Teaching and Learning
Content Area: Adult Health/Gastrointestinal

Answer: 4

Rationale: The client with a peptic ulcer is taught to eat small, frequent meals to help keep the gastric secretions neutralized. The client should eat slowly and chew thoroughly to prevent excess gastric acid secretion. The client should drink at least 6 to 8 glasses of water per day to dilute the gastric acid. The use of aspirin is avoided because it is irritating to the gastric mucosa.

Test-Taking Strategy: Use the process of elimination. Focus on the client's diagnosis, and use your knowledge of concepts related to digestion and of substances that are known gastric irritants to direct you to option 4. Review the teaching points related to the client with peptic ulcer disease if you had difficulty with this question.

Reference

Linton, A. (2007). *Introduction to medical-surgical nursing* (4th ed., p. 767). Philadelphia: Saunders.

---

411. A client with a hiatal hernia asks the nurse about the types of juices that are acceptable to drink. The nurse instructs the client to drink which type of juice?

1 Apple juice
2 Orange juice
3 Tomato juice
4 Grapefruit juice

Level of Cognitive Ability: Application
Client Needs: Health Promotion and Maintenance
Integrated Process: Teaching and Learning
Content Area: Adult Health/Gastrointestinal

Answer: 1

Rationale: Substances that are irritating to the client with a hiatal hernia include tomato products and citrus fruits, which should be avoided. Because caffeine stimulates gastric acid secretion, beverages that contain caffeine (e.g., coffee, tea, cola, cocoa) are also eliminated from the diet.

Test-Taking Strategy: Use the process of elimination. Eliminate options 2, 3, and 4 because they are comparable or alike in that they are irritating to the gastrointestinal system. Apple juice is the least irritating substance. Review the food items that are the least irritating for the client with a hiatal hernia if you had difficulty with this question.

References

Ignatavicius, D., & Workman, M. (2010). *Medical-surgical nursing: Patient-centered collaborative care* (6th ed., pp. 1245, 1254). St. Louis: Saunders.
Nix, S. (2009). *Williams' basic nutrition and diet therapy* (13th ed., p. 342). St. Louis: Mosby.

---

412. A nurse's teaching plan for the client with seizures includes reinforcing information about the safe use of phenytoin (Dilantin). The nurse provides which information to the client?

Answer: 4

Rationale: The client should be informed about the seriousness of the condition (i.e., skipping a dose of medication places the client at risk for status epilepticus). In some well-controlled cases, the medication can eventually be discontinued. In some states, a client can drive a car if he or she has had no seizures for a year.

1 To plan on taking the anticonvulsant for life
2 To stop driving a car while taking the medication
3 That seizures can never be completely controlled
4 To avoid skipping a medication dose because it will cause seizures to occur

Level of Cognitive Ability: Application
Client Needs: Health Promotion and Maintenance
Integrated Process: Teaching and Learning
Content Area: Pharmacology

Test-Taking Strategy: Use the process of elimination. General principles related to medication administration will direct you to option 4. Review the care of the client taking phenytoin if you had difficulty with this question.

Reference

Hodgson, B., & Kizior, R. (2009). *Saunders nursing drug handbook 2009* (p. 927). Philadelphia: Saunders.

---

413. A hospitalized client with a spinal cord injury (SCI) experiences bladder spasms and reflex incontinence. When preparing for discharge, the nurse reinforces home-care instructions and tells the client to do which of the following?
1 "Avoid caffeine in the diet."
2 "Take your own temperature every day."
3 "Limit fluid intake to 1000 mL every 24 hours."
4 "Catheterize yourself every 2 hours as necessary to prevent spasm."

Level of Cognitive Ability: Application
Client Needs: Health Promotion and Maintenance
Integrated Process: Teaching and Learning
Content Area: Adult Health/Neurological

Answer: 1

Rationale: Caffeine in the diet can contribute to bladder spasms and reflex incontinence; therefore, it should be eliminated from the diet of the client with an SCI. Self-monitoring of the temperature would be useful to detect infection but does nothing to alleviate bladder spasms. Limiting fluid intake does not prevent spasm and could place the client at further risk of urinary tract infection. Self-catheterization every 2 hours is too frequent and serves no useful purpose.

Test-Taking Strategy: Use the process of elimination, and focus on the subjects—bladder spasms and reflex incontinence. Eliminate options 3 and 4 first because they increase the client's risk of urinary tract infection and are therefore not appropriate. Choose option 1 rather than option 2 because option 2 would be used to detect infection but does not deal with spasm and incontinence. Review the care of the client with an SCI if you had difficulty with this question.

Reference

Ignatavicius, D., & Workman, M. (2010). *Medical-surgical nursing: Patient-centered collaborative care* (6th ed., p. 1558). St. Louis: Saunders.

---

414. A client with atherosclerosis asks the nurse about dietary modifications to lower the risk of heart disease. The nurse encourages the client to eat which of the following foods?
1 Fresh cantaloupe
2 Broiled cheeseburger
3 Baked chicken with skin
4 Mashed potato with gravy

Level of Cognitive Ability: Application
Client Needs: Health Promotion and Maintenance
Integrated Process: Teaching and Learning
Content Area: Adult Health/Cardiovascular

Answer: 1

Rationale: To lower the risk of heart disease, the diet should be low in saturated fat and include the appropriate number of total calories. The diet should include fewer red meats and more white meat with the skin removed. The dairy products eaten should be low in fat, and foods with high amounts of empty calories should be avoided.

Test-Taking Strategy: Use the process of elimination. Eliminate options 2 and 3 first because of the fat content of the described meats. Choose option 1 rather than option 4 because fresh fruits and vegetables are naturally low in fat. Review foods that are low in fat if you had difficulty with this question.

References
Christensen, B., & Kockrow, E. (2006). *Adult health nursing* (5th ed., p. 381). St. Louis: Mosby.
Nix, S. (2009). *Williams' basic nutrition and diet therapy* (13th ed., p. 360). St. Louis: Mosby.

---

415. A client is being discharged to home after angioplasty that involved the use of the right femoral area as the catheter insertion site. The nurse reinforces home-care instructions to the client and explains that which of the following signs or symptoms may be expected after the procedure?

1 A temperature as high as 101° F
2 Mild discomfort in the right groin
3 A large area of bruising in the right groin
4 Coolness or discoloration of the right foot

Level of Cognitive Ability: Application
Client Needs: Health Promotion and Maintenance
Integrated Process: Teaching and Learning
Content Area: Adult Health/Cardiovascular

Answer: 2
Rationale: The client may feel some mild discomfort at the catheter insertion site after angioplasty. This is usually relieved by analgesics such as acetaminophen (Tylenol). The client is taught to report to the physician any neurovascular changes to the affected leg, bleeding or bruising at the insertion site, and signs of local infection (e.g., drainage at the site, increased temperature).

Test-Taking Strategy: Use the process of elimination. Knowing that bleeding and infection are complications of the procedure guides you to eliminate options 1 and 3. You would choose option 2 rather than option 4 by knowing that the neurovascular status should not be impaired by the procedure or that the area may be mildly uncomfortable. Review postprocedure expectations if you had difficulty with this question.

Reference
Christensen, B., & Kockrow, E. (2006). *Foundations of nursing* (5th ed., p. 493). St. Louis: Mosby.

---

416. A nurse is reinforcing dietary instructions to a hypertensive client. The nurse encourages which of the following snack foods as being acceptable for this client?

1 Frozen pizza
2 Cheese and crackers
3 Canned tomato soup
4 Honeydew melon slices

Level of Cognitive Ability: Application
Client Needs: Health Promotion and Maintenance
Integrated Process: Teaching and Learning
Content Area: Adult Health/Cardiovascular

Answer: 4
Rationale: Sodium should be avoided by the client with hypertension. Fresh fruits and vegetables are naturally low in sodium. Hypertensive clients are also advised to keep fat intake to less than 30% of the total daily calories. Each of the incorrect options contains high amounts of sodium.

Test-Taking Strategy: Use the process of elimination. Recall that the client with hypertension should limit sodium intake. Eliminate options 1, 2, and 3 because they are comparable or alike. The correct option is a fruit and it is also the only unprocessed food among the choices given. Review foods that are low in sodium if you had difficulty with this question.

Reference
Christensen, B., & Kockrow, E. (2006). *Foundations of nursing* (5th ed., pp. 548-549, 613). St. Louis: Mosby.

---

417. A nurse is reinforcing instructions to a client who will be discharged to home with a halo vest. Which instructions should the nurse include in the discussion?

1 Loosen the bolts once a day for bathing.

Answer: 2
Rationale: A halo vest is a device that provides stability and immobility to the cervical area in a client who sustained a cervical fracture. The client is instructed to carry the correct-size wrench in case of an emergency that requires cardiopulmonary resuscitation (CPR). In such a situation, the anterior portion of the vest,

2 Carry the correct-size wrench to loosen the bolts in an emergency.
3 Have the spouse use the metal frame to assist the client to sit upright.
4 Perform pin care three times a week using hydrogen peroxide or alcohol.

Level of Cognitive Ability: Application
Client Needs: Health Promotion and Maintenance
Integrated Process: Teaching and Learning
Content Area: Adult Health/Neurological

including the anterior bolts, must be loosened, and the posterior portion should remain in place to provide stability for the spine during the CPR. The bolts should never be loosened except in an emergency, and the physician should be notified if the bolts loosen. The metal frame is never used or pulled on for turning or lifting. Pin care should be performed at least once a day using soap and water with cotton-tipped swabs or alcohol swabs.

Test-Taking Strategy: Try to visualize the appearance of a halo vest. Eliminate option 3 because pulling on the frame will disrupt the stabilization of the fracture and possibly lead to serious complications. Eliminate option 4 because pin care should be performed at least once a day. The bolts should only be loosened in an emergency situation. Review teaching points related to the halo vest if you had difficulty with this question.

Reference

Black, J., & Hawks, J. (2009). *Medical-surgical nursing: Clinical management for positive outcomes* (8th ed., p. 1958). St. Louis: Saunders.

---

418. A client is taking iron supplements to treat iron deficiency anemia. The nurse teaches the client to do which of the following while receiving iron therapy?
1 Eat a low-fiber diet.
2 Limit the intake of fluids.
3 Limit the intake of meat, fish, and poultry.
4 Avoid taking the iron with milk or antacids.

Level of Cognitive Ability: Application
Client Needs: Health Promotion and Maintenance
Integrated Process: Teaching and Learning
Content Area: Pharmacology

Answer: 4
Rationale: The client should avoid taking iron with milk or antacids, which decrease the absorption of iron. The client should also avoid taking iron with food, if possible. The client should increase the intake of natural sources of iron (e.g., meats, fish, poultry). Finally, the client should take in sufficient fiber and fluids to prevent constipation, which is a side effect of therapy.

Test-Taking Strategy: Use the process of elimination. Begin to answer this question by eliminating options 1 and 2 by knowing that constipation is a side effect of iron therapy. From the remaining options, recalling the nutritional contents of meat products will assist you with eliminating option 3. Remember that milk products or antacids impair the absorption of certain medications. Review iron supplementation if you had difficulty with this question.

Reference

Kee, J., Hayes, E., & McCuistion, L. (2009). *Pharmacology: A nursing process approach* (6th ed., p.236). St. Louis: Saunders.

---

419. A client with a colostomy complains to the nurse of appliance odor. The nurse recommends that the client consume which of the following deodorizing foods?
1 Eggs
2 Yogurt
3 Cucumbers
4 Mushrooms

Level of Cognitive Ability: Application
Client Needs: Health Promotion and Maintenance

Answer: 2
Rationale: Foods that help to eliminate odor from a colostomy include yogurt, buttermilk, spinach, beet greens, and parsley. Foods that cause odor include alcohol, beans, turnips, radishes, asparagus, onions, cucumbers, mushrooms, cabbage, eggs, and fish.

Test-Taking Strategy: Use the process of elimination. Remember that foods that cause gas in the client with normal gastrointestinal function also cause gas in the gastrointestinal tract of the client with a colostomy. Review these gas-forming foods if you had difficulty with this question.

Integrated Process: Teaching and Learning
Content Area: Adult Health/Gastrointestinal

Reference

Ignatavicius, D., & Workman, M. (2010). *Medical-surgical nursing: Patient-centered collaborative care* (6th ed., p. 1301). St. Louis: Saunders.

---

420. A nurse is reinforcing instructions about colostomy care to a client. The nurse demonstrates the correct cutting of the appliance by making the circle how much larger than the client's stoma?

1 $1/2$ inch
2 $1/4$ inch
3 $1/8$ inch
4 $1/16$ inch

Level of Cognitive Ability: Application
Client Needs: Health Promotion and Maintenance
Integrated Process: Teaching and Learning
Content Area: Adult Health/Gastrointestinal

Answer: 3
Rationale: The size of the opening of the appliance for a client with a colostomy is generally cut $1/8$-inch larger than the size of the client's stoma. This minimizes the amount of exposed skin but does not cause pressure on the stoma itself. Options 1, 2, and 4 are incorrect.

Test-Taking Strategy: Use the process of elimination. Begin to answer this question by eliminating options 1 and 2 because they leave too much skin area exposed for possible irritation by gastrointestinal contents. From the remaining options, eliminate option 4 because $1/16$ inch is extremely small and not realistic. Review the care of the client with a colostomy if you had difficulty with this question.

Reference

Linton, A. (2007). *Introduction to medical-surgical nursing* (4th ed., p. 407). Philadelphia: Saunders.

---

421. A 10-year-old child is diagnosed with type 1 diabetes mellitus. The nurse prepares to reinforce diabetic teaching to the child and family and plans to teach:

1 The child to monitor insulin requirements and to administer his own insulin
2 The parents to always be available to monitor the child's insulin requirements
3 The child's teacher to monitor insulin requirements and to administer the child's insulin
4 All of the friends and family involved with the child's activities to monitor the child's insulin requirements

Level of Cognitive Ability: Application
Client Needs: Health Promotion and Maintenance
Integrated Process: Teaching and Learning
Content Area: Child Health

Answer: 1
Rationale: Most children 9 years old and older can understand the principles of monitoring their own insulin requirements. They are usually responsible enough to determine the appropriate intervention needed to maintain their health. Options 2, 3, and 4 do not support the growth and development level of this child.

Test-Taking Strategy: Use the process of elimination and growth and development concepts. The age of the child indicates that the child is able to control and be responsible for the health care situation. Eliminate option 4 first because of the close-ended word *all* and because this option is unrealistic. Eliminate option 3 next because the teacher will not take responsibility for health care interventions. Eliminate option 2 because the parents cannot always be available. Review the growth and development of a 10-year-old child if you had difficulty with this question.

Reference

Price, D., & Gwin, J. (2008). *Pediatric nursing: An introductory text* (10th ed., p. 299). St. Louis: Saunders.

---

422. A client has undergone surgery for glaucoma. The nurse reinforces with the client which of the following home-care safety instructions?

1 The sutures are removed after 1 week.
2 Wound healing usually takes 12 weeks.
3 A shield or eye patch should be worn to protect the eye.

Answer: 3
Rationale: After ocular surgery, the client should wear a shield or eye patch to protect the eye. Healing occurs after approximately 6 weeks. After the postoperative inflammation subsides, the client's vision should return to the preoperative level of acuity. Most sutures used for these operations are absorbable.

4 Expect that the vision will be permanently impaired to some degree.

Level of Cognitive Ability: Application
Client Needs: Health Promotion and Maintenance
Integrated Process: Teaching and Learning
Content Area: Adult Health/Eye

Test-Taking Strategy: Use Maslow's Hierarchy of Needs theory to answer this question, and note that the client has had eye surgery. Recalling the concepts related to healing after ocular surgery and focusing on the subject of safety will direct you to option 3. Review postoperative teaching points after eye surgery if you had difficulty with this question.

Reference

deWit, S. (2009). *Medical-surgical nursing: Concepts & practice* (pp. 644, 651). St. Louis: Saunders.

---

423. A client has undergone surgery for cataract removal. The nurse instructs the client to call the physician if which problem occurs?

1 A sudden decrease in vision
2 The gradual resolution of eye redness
3 Eye pain relieved by acetaminophen (Tylenol)
4 Small amounts of dried matter on the eyelashes after sleep

Level of Cognitive Ability: Application
Client Needs: Health Promotion and Maintenance
Integrated Process: Teaching and Learning
Content Area: Adult Health/Eye

Answer: 1

Rationale: After surgery for cataract removal, the client should report a noticeable or sudden decrease in vision to the physician. The client is taught to take acetaminophen, which is usually effective for the relief of discomfort. The eye may be slightly reddened postoperatively, but this should gradually resolve. Small amounts of dried material may be present on the eyelashes after sleep; this is expected, and the material should be removed with a warm, damp face cloth.

Test-Taking Strategy: Focus on the subject—the need to call the physician. Note the strategic words *sudden decrease* to direct you to option 1. Review client instructions after cataract removal if you had difficulty with this question.

Reference

deWit, S. (2009). *Medical-surgical nursing: Concepts & practice* (p. 644). St. Louis: Saunders.

---

424. A nurse reinforces dietary instructions to a client with cirrhosis and ascites and teaches the client to do which of the following?

1 Decrease fat intake.
2 Restrict sodium intake.
3 Decrease carbohydrate intake.
4 Restrict calories to 1500 daily.

Level of Cognitive Ability: Application
Client Needs: Health Promotion and Maintenance
Integrated Process: Teaching and Learning
Content Area: Adult Health/Gastrointestinal

Answer: 2

Rationale: If the client with cirrhosis has ascites, sodium and possibly fluids should be restricted in the diet. Fat restriction is not necessary. The diet should supply sufficient carbohydrates to maintain weight and ample protein to rebuild tissue but not enough protein to precipitate hepatic encephalopathy. The total daily calorie intake should range between 2000 and 3000.

Test-Taking Strategy: Focus on the client's diagnosis. Recalling the definition of ascites will direct you to option 2. Review dietary measures for the client with cirrhosis and ascites if you had difficulty with this question.

Reference

Linton, A. (2007). *Introduction to medical-surgical nursing* (4th ed., p. 814). Philadelphia: Saunders.

---

425. A nurse is preparing a client with a diagnosis of multiple myeloma for discharge. Which home-care instruction will the nurse reinforce?

1 Maintain bedrest.
2 Restrict fluid intake to 1500 mL daily.

Answer: 4

Rationale: Multiple myeloma is a malignant neoplasm of the bone marrow. Clients with multiple myeloma should be taught to watch for signs of hypercalcemia and to report them immediately to the physician. Anorexia, nausea, vomiting, polyuria, weakness, fatigue, constipation, and dehydration are signs of moderate

3 Maintain a high-calorie, low-fiber diet.
4 Notify the physician if anorexia and nausea persist.

Level of Cognitive Ability: Application
Client Needs: Health Promotion and Maintenance
Integrated Process: Teaching and Learning
Content Area: Adult Health/Oncology

hypercalcemia. A fluid intake of about 3000 mL daily is necessary to dilute the calcium overload and to prevent protein from precipitating in the renal tubules. Activity is encouraged. Although a high-calorie diet is encouraged, a diet low in fiber will lead to constipation.

Test-Taking Strategy: Use the process of elimination, and recall that hypercalcemia is a concern in clients with multiple myeloma. Eliminate option 1 first because bedrest is not indicated. Eliminate option 2 next because this amount of fluid is rather low. Finally, eliminate option 3 because a low-fiber diet is not indicated for this client. Review the care of the client with multiple myeloma and the signs of hypercalcemia if you had difficulty with this question.

Reference

Christensen, B., & Kockrow, E. (2006). *Adult health nursing* (5th ed., pp. 316-317). St. Louis: Mosby.

---

426. A nurse prepares to reinforce instructions to a postpartum client who has developed breast engorgement. Which instruction should the nurse provide to the client?

1 Avoid the use of a bra during engorgement.
2 Apply cool packs to both breasts 20 minutes before a feeding.
3 During feeding, gently massage the breast from the outer areas to the nipple.
4 Feed the infant less frequently, every 4 to 6 hours, using bottle-feeding in between.

Level of Cognitive Ability: Application
Client Needs: Health Promotion and Maintenance
Integrated Process: Teaching and Learning
Content Area: Maternity/Postpartum

Answer: 3

Rationale: The client with breast engorgement should be advised to feed frequently, at least every $2\frac{1}{2}$ hours, for 15 to 20 minutes per side. Moist heat should be applied to both breasts for about 20 minutes before a feeding. Between feedings, the mother should wear a supportive bra. During a feeding, it is helpful to gently massage the breast from the outer areas to the nipple to stimulate letdown and the flow of milk.

Test-Taking Strategy: Consider the manifestations that occur with engorgement, and eliminate those options that will not assist with increasing the flow of milk. With this concept in mind, you should be able to eliminate options 2 and 4. From the remaining options, select option 3 because massage would assist with the flow of milk. In addition, a supportive bra would reduce the discomfort that occurs with this condition. Review the measures used to treat breast engorgement if you had difficulty with this question.

Reference

Leifer, G. (2008). *Maternity nursing: An introductory text* (10th ed., p. 219). Philadelphia: Saunders.

---

427. A client in the third trimester of pregnancy arrives at the physician's office and tells the nurse that she frequently has a backache. Which instruction should the nurse provide to the client to ease the backache?

1 Maintain correct posture.
2 Eat small, frequent meals.
3 Elevate the legs when sitting.
4 Sleep in a supine position on a firm mattress.

Answer: 1

Rationale: To provide relief from backache, the nurse should advise the client to use good posture and body mechanics; to perform pelvic rock exercises; and to wear flat, supportive shoes. The client should also be instructed to avoid overexertion and to sleep in the lateral position on a firm mattress. Back massage is also helpful. Eating small meals would more specifically help relieve dyspnea. Leg elevation assists the client with varicosities.

Level of Cognitive Ability: Application
Client Needs: Health Promotion and Maintenance
Integrated Process: Teaching and Learning
Content Area: Maternity/Antepartum

Test-Taking Strategy: Use the process of elimination, and focus on the subject—backache. This should assist you with eliminating options 2 and 3. From the remaining options, recalling that the lateral position is most appropriate will direct you to option 1. Review relief measures for backache if you had difficulty with this question.

Reference

Leifer, G. (2008). *Maternity nursing: An introductory text* (10th ed., p. 69). Philadelphia: Saunders.

---

428. A nurse reinforces dietary instructions with a client receiving spironolactone (Aldactone). Which of the following foods should the nurse instruct the client to avoid while taking this medication?
1 Shrimp
2 Popcorn
3 Apricots
4 Crackers

Level of Cognitive Ability: Application
Client Needs: Health Promotion and Maintenance
Integrated Process: Teaching and Learning
Content Area: Pharmacology

Answer: 3
Rationale: Spironolactone is a potassium-sparing diuretic, and the client should avoid foods that are high in potassium, such as whole-grain cereals, legumes, meat, bananas, apricots, orange juice, potatoes, and raisins. Option 3 provides the highest source of potassium and should be avoided.

Test-Taking Strategy: Use the process of elimination, and note the strategic word *avoid*. Begin by eliminating options 2 and 4 because they are food items that are comparable or alike. Remembering that fruits, vegetables, and fresh meats are high in potassium will assist with directing you to option 3. Review foods that are high in potassium if you had difficulty with this question.

Reference

Hodgson, B., & Kizior, R. (2009). *Saunders nursing drug handbook 2009* (p. 1077). Philadelphia: Saunders.

---

429. A nurse has collected nutritional data from a client with cystitis. The nurse teaches the client that which beverage should be consumed to minimize the recurrence of cystitis?
1 Tea
2 Water
3 Coffee
4 White wine

Level of Cognitive Ability: Application
Client Needs: Health Promotion and Maintenance
Integrated Process: Teaching and Learning
Content Area: Adult Health/Renal

Answer: 2
Rationale: Cystitis is an inflammatory condition of the urinary bladder and ureters that is characterized by pain, urgency and frequency of urination, and hematuria. Caffeine and alcohol can irritate the bladder, so beverages that contain alcohol and caffeine (e.g., coffee, tea, wine) are avoided to reduce the risk of recurrence. Water helps flush bacteria out of the bladder, and an intake of 6 to 8 glasses per day is encouraged.

Test-Taking Strategy: Use the process of elimination. Option 4 should be eliminated first because alcohol intake is not encouraged for any disorder. Options 1 and 3 are comparable or alike in that both contain caffeine, and they are eliminated because it is unlikely that either is the correct answer. Review the measures that reduce the recurrence of cystitis if you had difficulty with this question.

Reference

deWit, S. (2009). *Medical-surgical nursing: Concepts & practice* (p. 838). St. Louis: Saunders.

---

430. A nurse has reinforced instructions to a female client with cystitis about measures to prevent recurrence. The nurse

Answer: 1
Rationale: Cystitis is an inflammatory condition of the urinary bladder and ureters that is characterized by pain, urgency and

determines that the client requires further instruction if the client verbalizes a need to do which of the following?

1 Take bubble baths for more effective hygiene.
2 Avoid wearing pantyhose while wearing slacks.
3 Drink a glass of water and void after intercourse.
4 Wear underwear made of cotton or with cotton panels.

Level of Cognitive Ability: Comprehension
Client Needs: Health Promotion and Maintenance
Integrated Process: Teaching and Learning
Content Area: Adult Health/Renal

frequency of urination, and hematuria. Measures to prevent cystitis include increasing fluid intake to 3 L per day; eating an acid-ash diet; wiping front to back after urination; taking showers instead of tub baths; drinking water and voiding after intercourse; avoiding bubble baths, feminine hygiene sprays, and perfumed toilet tissue and sanitary pads; and wearing clothes that "breathe" (e.g., cotton pants, no tight jeans, no pantyhose under slacks). Other measures include teaching pregnant women to void every 2 hours and instructing menopausal women to use estrogen vaginal creams to restore vaginal pH.

Test-Taking Strategy: Note the strategic words *requires further instruction*. These words indicate a negative event query and ask you to select an option that is an incorrect statement. Eliminate option 3 first because drinking water is a basic measure to prevent cystitis. Eliminate options 2 and 4 next because they are comparable or alike. Review teaching measures to prevent cystitis if you had difficulty with this question.

Reference

deWit, S. (2009). *Medical-surgical nursing: Concepts & practice* (p. 840). St. Louis: Saunders.

---

431. A client with pyelonephritis is being discharged from the hospital, and the nurse reinforces home-care instructions to prevent recurrence. The nurse determines that the client understands the information that was given if the client states an intention to do which of the following?

1 Take the prescribed antibiotics until all symptoms subside.
2 Modify fluid intake for the day based on the previous day's output.
3 Return to the physician's office for scheduled follow-up urine cultures.
4 Report signs and symptoms of urinary tract infection (UTI) if they persist for more than 1 week.

Level of Cognitive Ability: Comprehension
Client Needs: Health Promotion and Maintenance
Integrated Process: Nursing Process/Evaluation
Content Area: Adult Health/Renal

Answer: 3

Rationale: Pyelonephritis is an infection of the pelvis and of the parenchyma of the kidney. The client with pyelonephritis should take the full course of antibiotic therapy that has been prescribed and return to the physician's office for follow-up urine cultures if so instructed. The client should learn the signs and symptoms of UTI and report them immediately if they occur. The client should use all measures recommended to prevent cystitis, which includes drinking 3 L of fluids per day.

Test-Taking Strategy: Use the process of elimination. Begin to answer this question by eliminating option 4 because UTI symptoms should never go unreported for more than a week. Option 1 is eliminated next because antibiotics should be taken for the full course of treatment to adequately eliminate the infection. From the remaining options, recalling that the client needs follow-up urine cultures helps you to choose option 3 rather than option 2, which is not an appropriate option. Review the measures used to prevent UTI if you had difficulty with this question.

Reference

Christensen, B., & Kockrow, E. (2006). *Adult health nursing* (5th ed., p. 488). St. Louis: Mosby.

---

432. A client with nephrotic syndrome needs dietary teaching about how diet can help counteract the effects of altered renal function. The nurse should include which of the following statements in the instructions to the client?

Answer: 1

Rationale: Nephrotic syndrome is an abnormal condition of the kidney that is characterized by marked proteinuria, hypoalbuminemia, and edema. Sodium is limited in the nephrotic syndrome diet to help control edema, which is part of the clinical picture. Fluids are not restricted unless hyponatremia is present, but the

1 "Increase your intake of fish and other high-protein foods."
2 "Increase your intake of fatty foods to prevent protein loss."
3 "Add salt during cooking to replace sodium lost in the urine."
4 "Increase your fluid intake and drink plenty of fluids throughout the day."

Level of Cognitive Ability: Application
Client Needs: Health Promotion and Maintenance
Integrated Process: Teaching and Learning
Content Area: Adult Health/Renal

client is not encouraged to increase fluid intake and or to drink plenty of fluids throughout the day. Protein is increased unless the glomerular filtration rate is impaired; this helps to replace protein lost in the urine and ultimately helps to control edema. Hyperlipidemia, which results from the liver's synthesis of lipoproteins in response to hypoalbuminemia, is also part of the clinical picture. Increasing fatty food intake would not be helpful in this circumstance.

Test-Taking Strategy: Begin to answer this question by recalling that nephrotic syndrome is characterized by fluid retention and hypoalbuminemia; this would help you eliminate options 3 and 4. To choose between the remaining options, knowing that hyperlipidemia accompanies nephrotic syndrome would help you to choose option 1 rather than option 2. You could also choose correctly by recalling that hypoalbuminemia is part of the clinical picture and that protein intake is encouraged. Review dietary measures for the client with nephrotic syndrome if you had difficulty with this question.

Reference
Christensen, B., & Kockrow, E. (2006). *Adult health nursing* (5th ed., p. 499). St. Louis: Mosby.

---

433. A nurse has given dietary instructions to a client to minimize the risk of osteoporosis. The nurse determines that the client understands the instructions if the client verbalizes the need to increase the intake of which food item?
1 Rice
2 Bread
3 Yogurt
4 Chicken

Level of Cognitive Ability: Comprehension
Client Needs: Health Promotion and Maintenance
Integrated Process: Nursing Process/Evaluation
Content Area: Adult Health/Musculoskeletal

Answer: 3
Rationale: Osteoporosis is a disorder that is characterized by an abnormal loss of bone density and the deterioration of bone tissue. Calcium intake is important to minimize the risk of osteoporosis. The major dietary source of calcium is dairy foods, including milk, yogurt, and a variety of cheeses. Calcium may also be added to certain products (e.g., orange juice), which are then labeled as being "fortified" with calcium. Calcium supplements are available and recommended for those with typically low calcium intake. Rice, bread, and chicken are not high in calcium.

Test-Taking Strategy: Use the process of elimination. Recall that calcium is needed to minimize the risk of osteoporosis, that dairy products are rich in calcium, and that yogurt is a dairy product. Each of the incorrect options does not belong to this food group. Review the foods that are high in calcium if you had difficulty with this question.

Reference
Christensen, B., & Kockrow, E. (2006). *Adult health nursing* (5th ed., p. 142). St. Louis: Mosby.

---

434. A nurse is assisting with conducting a health screening for osteoporosis. The nurse should direct health promotion measures to which of the following clients, knowing that he or she is at the greatest risk of developing this disorder?
1 A 25-year-old female who jogs
2 A 36-year-old male who has asthma

Answer: 4
Rationale: Osteoporosis is characterized by an abnormal loss of bone density and the deterioration of bone tissue. Risk factors for osteoporosis include being female, postmenopausal, of advanced age, or sedentary; consuming a low-calcium diet; using excessive alcohol; and smoking cigarettes. The long-term use of corticosteroids, anticonvulsants, and furosemide (Lasix) also increases the risk.

3 A 70-year-old male who consumes excess alcohol
4 A sedentary 65-year-old female who smokes cigarettes

Level of Cognitive Ability: Analysis
Client Needs: Health Promotion and Maintenance
Integrated Process: Nursing Process/Data Collection
Content Area: Adult Health/Musculoskeletal

Test-Taking Strategy: Use the process of elimination. Option 1 is eliminated first, because the 25-year-old female who jogs (thereby using the long bones) has negligible risk. The 36-year-old male with asthma is eliminated next because the only risk factor may be long-term corticosteroid use. From the remaining options, the 65-year-old female has greater risk (age, gender, postmenopausal, sedentary, smoking) than the 70-year-old male (age, alcohol consumption). Review the risk factors for osteoporosis if you had difficulty with this question.

Reference

Linton, A. (2007). *Introduction to medical-surgical nursing* (4th ed., p. 904). Philadelphia: Saunders.

---

435. A nurse is providing dietary home-care instructions to a client with pancreatitis. Which of the following foods should the nurse instruct the client to avoid?
1 Chili
2 Bagel
3 Lentil soup
4 Watermelon

Level of Cognitive Ability: Application
Client Needs: Health Promotion and Maintenance
Integrated Process: Nursing Process/Implementation
Content Area: Adult Health/Gastrointestinal

Answer: 1
Rationale: Pancreatitis is an inflammatory condition of the pancreas that may be acute or chronic. The client should avoid alcohol, coffee, tea, spicy foods, and heavy meals, which stimulate pancreatic secretions and produce attacks of pancreatitis. The client is instructed regarding the benefit of eating small, frequent meals that are high in protein, low in fat, and moderate to high in carbohydrates.

Test-Taking Strategy: Note the strategic word *avoid*. Use the process of elimination, and note that options 2, 3, and 4 are foods that are moderately bland. Option 1 is a spicy food. Review the foods that should be avoided by the client with pancreatitis if you had difficulty with this question.

References

Christensen, B., & Kockrow, E. (2006). *Adult health nursing* (5th ed., p. 278). St. Louis: Mosby.
Linton, A. (2007). *Introduction to medical-surgical nursing* (4th ed., pp. 829-830). Philadelphia: Saunders.

---

436. A newborn receives the first dose of hepatitis B vaccine within 12 hours of birth. The nurse instructs the mother regarding the immunization schedule for this vaccine and tells the mother that the second vaccine is administered at which of the following times?
1 3 years of age and then during the adolescent years
2 8 months of age and then 1 year after the initial dose
3 6 months of age and then 8 months after the initial dose
4 1 to 2 months of age and then 4 months after the initial dose

Level of Cognitive Ability: Application
Client Needs: Health Promotion and Maintenance

Answer: 4
Rationale: The vaccination schedule for an infant whose mother tests negative for hepatitis B consists of a series of three immunizations given at birth, 1 to 2 months of age, and then again 4 months after the initial dose. An infant whose mother tests positive receives hepatitis B immunoglobulin along with the first dose of the hepatitis B vaccine within 12 hours of birth.

Test-Taking Strategy: Knowledge regarding the immunization schedule for hepatitis B vaccine is necessary to answer this question. Remember that the vaccination schedule for an infant whose mother tests negative consists of a series of three immunizations given at birth, 1 to 2 months of age, and then again 4 months after the initial dose. Review this schedule if you had difficulty with this question.

Reference

Leifer, G. (2008). *Maternity nursing: An introductory text* (10th ed., p. 190). Philadelphia: Saunders.

Integrated Process: Nursing Process/Implementation
Content Area: Child Health

---

437. A nurse reinforces dietary instructions with the parents of a child with a diagnosis of cystic fibrosis and tells the parents that a component of dietary management is which of the following?

1 A low-fat diet
2 A low-protein diet
3 A high-calorie diet
4 A low-sodium diet

Level of Cognitive Ability: Application
Client Needs: Health Promotion and Maintenance
Integrated Process: Teaching and Learning
Content Area: Child Health

Answer: 3

Rationale: Cystic fibrosis is an inherited autosomal-recessive disorder of the exocrine glands that causes those glands to produce abnormally thick secretions of mucus. It also causes elevation of the sweat electrolytes, increased organic and enzymatic constituents of saliva, and overactivity of the autonomic nervous system. Children with cystic fibrosis are managed with a high-calorie, high-protein diet; pancreatic enzyme replacement therapy; fat-soluble vitamin supplements; and, if nutritional problems are severe, nighttime gastrostomy feedings or total parental nutrition. Fats are not restricted unless steatorrhea cannot be controlled by increased pancreatic enzymes. Sodium intake is unrelated to this disorder.

Test-Taking Strategy: Knowledge of the digestive problems and the dietary management of children with cystic fibrosis is necessary to answer this question. If you are unfamiliar with this content, select option 3 because children require calories for growth and development. Review the digestive problems and the dietary management of children with cystic fibrosis if you had difficulty with this question.

Reference

Price, D., & Gwin, J. (2008). *Pediatric nursing: An introductory text* (10th ed., p. 157). St. Louis: Saunders.

---

438. A nurse has reinforced instructions with a client who has silicosis about the prevention of self-exposure to silica dust. The nurse determines that the client understands the instructions if the client states a need to wear a mask for which of the following hobbies?

1 Painting
2 Gardening
3 Woodworking
4 Pottery making

Level of Cognitive Ability: Comprehension
Client Needs: Health Promotion and Maintenance
Integrated Process: Nursing Process/Evaluation
Content Area: Adult Health/Respiratory

Answer: 4

Rationale: Silicosis is a lung disorder caused by the continuous long-term inhalation of the dust of the inorganic compound silicon dioxide, which is found in sands, quartzes, flints, and many other stones. Exposure to silica dust occurs with activities such as pottery making and stone masonry. Exposure to the finely ground silica, which is found in soaps, polishes, and filters, is also dangerous for these clients. Options 1, 2, and 3 are safe activities.

Test-Taking Strategy: To answer this question, it is necessary to have an understanding of the materials that could emit silica dust. Eliminate gardening first, because silica is not a pesticide, and it is not found in average soil. Recall that silica is not inhaled in fumes to help you eliminate woodworking and painting. Use the process of elimination to direct you to option 4. Review silicosis if you had difficulty with this question.

Reference

Ignatavicius, D., & Workman, M. (2010). *Medical-surgical nursing: Patient-centered collaborative care* (6th ed., p. 640). St. Louis: Saunders.

---

439. A nurse is conducting dietary teaching with a client who is hypocalcemic. The nurse encourages the client to increase the intake of which of the following foods?

1 Apples
2 Cheese
3 Cooked pasta
4 Chicken breast

Level of Cognitive Ability: Application
Client Needs: Health Promotion and Maintenance
Integrated Process: Teaching and Learning
Content Area: Fundamental Skills

Answer: 2

Rationale: Products that are naturally high in calcium are dairy products, including milk, cheese, ice cream, and yogurt. High-calcium foods generally have more than 100 mg of calcium per serving. The other options are foods that are low in calcium, which means that they have less than 25 mg of calcium per serving.

Test-Taking Strategy: Use the process of elimination and your knowledge of the calcium content of foods. As a general rule, recall that dairy products are naturally high in calcium. Review foods that are high in calcium if you had difficulty with this question.

Reference

Ignatavicius, D., & Workman, M. (2010). *Medical-surgical nursing: Patient-centered collaborative care* (6th ed., p. 191). St. Louis: Saunders.

---

440. The nurse reviews the discharge plan of care for a postoperative client who had a cystectomy and a urinary diversion (vesicostomy) created to treat bladder cancer. The nurse identifies which nursing diagnosis written in the plan as the priority?

1 *Risk for infection* related to direct opening into the bladder
2 *Risk for disturbed body image* related to the presence of a pouch
3 *Risk for toileting self-care deficit* related to poor hand–eye coordination
4 *Impaired urinary elimination* related to urinary diversion and loss of ability to void normally

Level of Cognitive Ability: Analysis
Client Needs: Health Promotion and Maintenance
Integrated Process: Nursing Process/Planning
Content Area: Delegating/Prioritizing

Answer: 4

Rationale: A urinary diversion is a surgical diversion of urinary flow from its usual path through the urinary tract. As a result, the client has impaired urinary elimination. The nursing diagnosis *Impaired urinary elimination* is the priority because it is identified as an actual problem and directly relates to the client's surgical procedure. The client is also at risk for infection because of the direct opening into the bladder. Because infection can be life-threatening if it occurs, the nursing diagnosis *Risk for infection* is the second priority. Because *Risk for toileting self-care deficit* is a physiological need, it takes priority over *Risk for disturbed body image,* which is a psychosocial need. Therefore, *Risk for toileting self-care deficit* is the third priority, followed by *Risk for disturbed body image* as the fourth priority.

Test-Taking Strategy: When presented with nursing diagnoses and asked to prioritize them, remember that, in most situations an actual nursing diagnosis is the priority. This guideline assists you with selecting *Impaired urinary elimination* as the priority. Note that options 1, 2, and 3 are not actual nursing diagnoses. Review the care of the client with a urinary diversion if you had difficulty with this question.

Reference

Linton, A. (2007). *Introduction to medical-surgical nursing* (4th ed., pp. 408-412). Philadelphia: Saunders.

---

441. A physician in a community clinic diagnoses chronic prostatitis in a client, and the nurse reinforces home-care instructions to the client. Which statement by the client would indicate the need for further instruction?

1 "There are no restrictions in my diet."
2 "The sitz baths will help my condition."
3 "I should avoid sexual activity for 1 week."

Answer: 3

Rationale: Prostatitis is an acute or chronic inflammation of the prostate gland that is usually the result of an infection. Interventions include anti-inflammatory agents or short-term antimicrobial medication, and the client should be taught about the prescribed regimen. Sitz baths are recommended. Normal sexual activity is acceptable with chronic prostatitis; with acute conditions, it should be avoided so that the prostate can rest. Dietary restrictions are not recommended unless the person finds them to be associated with manifestations.

4 "I should take the anti-inflammatory medications as prescribed."

Level of Cognitive Ability: Comprehension
Client Needs: Health Promotion and Maintenance
Integrated Process: Teaching and Learning
Content Area: Fundamental Skills

Test-Taking Strategy: Note the strategic words *need for further instruction.* These words indicate a negative event query and ask you to select an option that is an incorrect statement. Eliminate option 4 first by using the general principles associated with medication prescriptions. Option 1 can be eliminated next because there is no specific relationship between diet and this disorder. From the remaining options, eliminate option 2 because it would seem reasonable that sitz baths would provide comfort. Review the instructions for the client with prostatitis if you had difficulty with this question.

Reference

Christensen, B., & Kockrow, E. (2006). *Adult health nursing* (5th ed., p. 487). St. Louis: Mosby.

---

442. An older client is told that she has iron deficiency anemia, and she asks the nurse about the food items that are high in iron. The nurse teaches the client that which of the following food items is highest in iron?

1 Milk
2 Pork
3 Oranges
4 Broccoli

Level of Cognitive Ability: Application
Client Needs: Health Promotion and Maintenance
Integrated Process: Teaching and Learning
Content Area: Fundamental Skills

Answer: 4
Rationale: Iron is available in foods of plant and animal origin. Foods that are rich in iron include muscle meats, liver, egg yolks, brewer's yeast, green leafy vegetables, fish, fowl, beans, and cereal grains. Milk is high in calcium, pork is high in thiamine, and oranges are high in vitamin C.

Test-Taking Strategy: Focus on the subject—the food item that is highest in iron. Remembering that green leafy vegetables are high in iron will direct you to the correct option. Review the food items that are high in iron if you had difficulty with this question.

References

deWit, S. (2009). *Medical-surgical nursing: Concepts & practice* (p. 379). St. Louis: Saunders.
Wold, G. (2008). *Basic geriatric nursing* (4th ed., p. 106). St. Louis: Mosby.

---

443. A nurse reinforces discharge instructions with a client taking ticlopidine (Ticlid). Which client statement indicates the need for further instruction?

1 "I'll take my medicine as prescribed with meals."
2 "Blood work will be done every 2 weeks for the first 3 months."
3 "If I have a cold or run a fever, I will stop taking this medicine."
4 "Side effects with this medicine are different than with my aspirin."

Level of Cognitive Ability: Analysis
Client Needs: Health Promotion and Maintenance
Integrated Process: Teaching and Learning
Content Area: Pharmacology

Answer: 3
Rationale: The client is instructed to not discontinue the medication without the physician's permission. Options 1, 2, and 4 are accurate statements by the client about the medication.

Test-Taking Strategy: Note the strategic words *need for further instruction.* These words indicate a negative event query and ask you to select an option that is an incorrect client statement. Recalling basic principles related to medication administration and that the client should not stop taking the medication without the physician's approval will direct you to option 3. Review the client teaching points related to ticlopidine if you had difficulty with this question.

References

deWit, S. (2009). *Medical-surgical nursing: Concepts & practice* (p. 571). St. Louis: Saunders.
Edmunds, M. (2010). *Introduction to clinical pharmacology* (6th ed., p. 325). St. Louis: Mosby.

444. A client is taking ticlopidine (Ticlid) for the prevention of a thrombotic stroke and asks why blood work must be performed so frequently. The nurse teaches the client about the importance of blood work by making which statement?

1 "I'll have to let your physician explain that for you."
2 "Don't worry, this blood work will only be done six times."
3 "I have written information that I will give your family before you leave."
4 "These blood tests are important to check for a reversible side effect called 'neutropenia.'"

Level of Cognitive Ability: Application
Client Needs: Health Promotion and Maintenance
Integrated Process: Communication and Documentation
Content Area: Pharmacology

Answer: 4
Rationale: Option 4 provides the information that the client is requesting and teaches the client. Options 1, 2, and 3 do not address the client's concern or provide education to the client about the medication.

Test-Taking Strategy: Focus on the subject of the question, and use therapeutic communication techniques. Option 4 is the only option that addresses the client's question and that provides accurate information. The client should not be told not to worry, and options 1 and 3 place the client's question on hold. Review ticlopidine and therapeutic communication techniques if you had difficulty with this question.

Reference
Hodgson, B., & Kizior, R. (2009). *Saunders nursing drug handbook 2009* (p. 1133). St. Louis: Saunders.

---

445. Oral anticoagulant therapy is prescribed for a client. The nurse assists with preparing home-care medication instructions and includes which of the following in the plan of care?

1 The client should report any signs of bleeding.
2 The client should use a straight razor for shaving.
3 The client should take aspirin for mild discomfort.
4 The client should use a hard-bristle toothbrush for brushing the teeth.

Level of Cognitive Ability: Application
Client Needs: Health Promotion and Maintenance
Integrated Process: Teaching and Learning
Content Area: Pharmacology

Answer: 1
Rationale: An anticoagulant places the client at risk for bleeding, and the client should be instructed in the measures that will reduce the likelihood of this adverse effect. An electric razor rather than a straight razor should be used. Acetaminophen (Tylenol) should be taken for mild discomfort because aspirin has antiplatelet properties and will increase the risk of bleeding. A soft toothbrush should be used to prevent bleeding of the gums.

Test-Taking Strategy: Use the process of elimination. Recalling that an anticoagulant places the client at risk for bleeding will direct you to option 1. Review client teaching related to anticoagulants if you had difficulty with this question.

Reference
Edmunds, M. (2010). *Introduction to clinical pharmacology* (6th ed., p. 325). St. Louis: Mosby.

---

446. A client with congestive heart failure (CHF) who is taking furosemide (Lasix) is advised to eat foods that are high in potassium. The nurse teaches the client that which of these foods would meet the client's needs?

1 Potatoes and rice
2 Ham, bacon, and hot dogs
3 Fresh fruits and vegetables
4 Margarine, butter, and cheese

Answer: 3
Rationale: Fresh fruits and vegetables are a good source of potassium. Options 1, 2, and 4 identify foods that are either high in sodium or fat and thus should not be consumed by the client with CHF.

Test-Taking Strategy: Focus on the subject and the client's diagnosis. Recalling food items that are high in potassium and that foods high in sodium or fat should not be consumed by the client with CHF will assist you with eliminating options 1, 2, and 4. Review the foods that are high in potassium if you had difficulty with this question.

Level of Cognitive Ability: Application
Client Needs: Health Promotion and Maintenance
Integrated Process: Teaching and Learning
Content Area: Fundamental Skills

References

deWit, S. (2009). *Medical-surgical nursing: Concepts & practice* (p. 48). St. Louis: Saunders.

Linton, A. (2007). *Introduction to medical-surgical nursing* (4th ed., p. 107). Philadelphia: Saunders.

---

447. A 13-year-old female client is adamantly refusing to take corticosteroid therapy for the treatment of Crohn's disease. The nurse understands that this behavior may be primarily due to:

1 Fear of pain
2 A mental illness
3 Denial of the disease
4 Fear of altered body image

Level of Cognitive Ability: Comprehension
Client Needs: Health Promotion and Maintenance
Integrated Process: Nursing Process/Data Collection
Content Area: Pharmacology

Answer: 4
Rationale: Corticosteroids can greatly alter the body's appearance by causing weight gain, puffy skin, and a humped back. One of the main concerns in the teenage population is body image. Pain is not a side effect of corticosteroids. There are no data in the question to indicate denial or a mental illness.

Test-Taking Strategy: Use the concepts of growth and development and your knowledge of the side effects of corticosteroids to answer the question. Recalling that body image is a main concern of the teenager will direct you to option 4. Review the effects of corticosteroids and growth and development concepts if you had difficulty with this question.

Reference

Price, D., & Gwin, J. (2008). *Pediatric nursing: An introductory text* (10th ed., p. 305). St. Louis: Saunders.

---

448. When gathering data about a jaundiced infant, the nurse notes that the serum bilirubin levels have been increasing and that the physician has prescribed phototherapy. After explaining phototherapy to the parents, which statement would indicate the need for further instruction?

1 "We understand that home phototherapy is an option."
2 "We will be available for feedings every 2 to 3 hours."
3 "My baby will wear eye patches during this treatment."
4 "We will bring in clean clothes for my baby to wear today."

Level of Cognitive Ability: Comprehension
Client Needs: Health Promotion and Maintenance
Integrated Process: Teaching and Learning
Content Area: Maternity/Postpartum

Answer: 4
Rationale: Clean clothes are not needed because the infant will be wearing only a diaper to facilitate the benefit of the phototherapy. Eye patches will be placed on the infant's eyes. Feedings will be provided every 2 to 3 hours. Phototherapy can be performed at home.

Test-Taking Strategy: Use the process of elimination, and note the strategic words *need for further instruction*. These words indicate a negative event query and ask you to select an option that is an incorrect statement. Recalling that the infant will receive the therapy without clothing other than a diaper will direct you to option 4. Review phototherapy if you had difficulty with this question.

Reference

Leifer, G. (2008). *Maternity nursing: An introductory text* (10th ed., p. 321). Philadelphia: Saunders.

---

449. As part of the discharge planning for an infant who is to receive home phototherapy, the nurse needs to emphasize to the parents that:

1 Keeping a list of the number of wet diapers and stools is important.
2 Letting the baby sleep through feedings is acceptable.

Answer: 1
Rationale: Keeping a list of the number of wet diapers and stools is important because the infant should have 6 to 10 wet diapers a day. The infant needs to be fed every 2 to 3 hours because phototherapy can cause dehydration. The infant should receive phototherapy for 18 hours per day or for the number of hours prescribed by the physician. Patches should be placed over the infant's eyes to protect them from the light.

3 The wearing of eye patches for conventional phototherapy is optional.
4 Taking the baby away from conventional phototherapy lights for hours at a time will not interfere with the goal of the treatment.

Level of Cognitive Ability: Application
Client Needs: Health Promotion and Maintenance
Integrated Process: Teaching and Learning
Content Area: Maternity/Postpartum

Test-Taking Strategy: Use the process of elimination and your knowledge of the principles related to phototherapy to answer this question. Recalling that phototherapy can cause dehydration will direct you to the correct option. Review these important principles if you had difficulty with this question.

Reference
Price, D., & Gwin, J. (2008). *Pediatric nursing: An introductory text* (10th ed., p. 79). St. Louis: Saunders.

---

450. A nurse in a well-baby clinic is providing nutrition instructions to a mother of a 9-month-old infant. Which instruction is the most age appropriate?
1 Begin to initiate self-feeding.
2 Introduce strained fruits one at a time.
3 Introduce strained vegetables one at a time.
4 Begin to offer rice cereal mixed with breast milk or formula.

Level of Cognitive Ability: Application
Client Needs: Health Promotion and Maintenance
Integrated Process: Teaching and Learning
Content Area: Child Health

Answer: 1
Rationale: Self-feeding can be initiated at the age of approximately 9 months. Rice cereal mixed with breast milk or formula is introduced at the age of 4 months. Strained vegetables, fruits, and meats, introduced one at a time, can begin at the age of 6 months.

Test-Taking Strategy: Use the process of elimination. Focusing on the age of the infant will direct you to option 1. Options 2, 3, and 4 are initiated before the age of 9 months. Review age-appropriate nutritional measures if you had difficulty with this question.

Reference
Price, D., & Gwin, J. (2008). *Pediatric nursing: An introductory text* (10th ed., p. 126). St. Louis: Saunders.

ALTERNATE ITEM FORMAT QUESTIONS

Figure/Illustration

451. The nurse is collecting physical data from a client and is preparing to auscultate breath sounds. The nurse places the stethoscope in which area to assess bronchovesicular sounds?

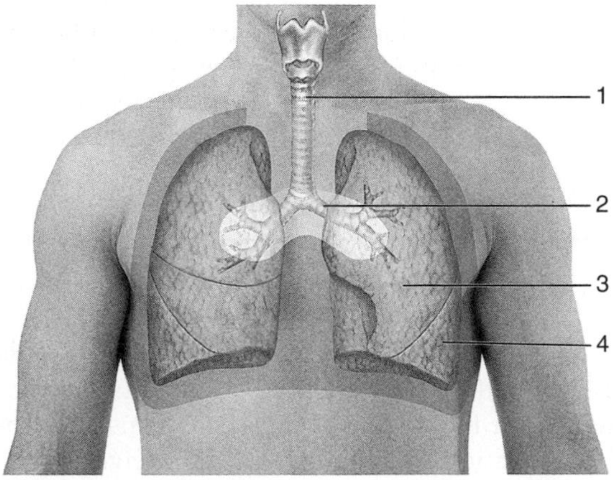

Figure 7-1 From Wilson, S., & Giddens, J. (2009). *Health assessment for nursing practice* (4th ed., p. 219). St. Louis: Mosby.

Answer: 2
Rationale: Bronchovesicular breath sounds are heard over the main bronchi. Their normal location is specifically between the first and second intercostal spaces at the sternal border anteriorly and at T4 medial to the scapula posteriorly. These sounds are moderate in pitch and medium in intensity, and the duration of inspiration and expiration is equal. Bronchial breath sounds are heard over the trachea. Vesicular breath sounds are heard over the lesser bronchi, the bronchioles, and the lobes.

Test-Taking Strategy: Focus on the locations identified. Eliminate options 3 and 4 because they identify similar locations (peripheral lung fields). From the remaining options, recall that bronchial breath sounds are heard over the trachea. Review respiratory data collection techniques if you had difficulty with this question.

Reference
Jarvis, C. (2008) *Physical examination and health assessment* (5th ed, pp. 455-456). Philadelphia: Saunders.

Answer: _____

Level of Cognitive Ability: Application
Client Needs: Health Promotion and Maintenance
Integrated Process: Nursing Process/Data Collection
Content Area: Adult Health/Respiratory

Multiple Response

452. A nurse is teaching a client about the risks of breast cancer and tells the client that which of the following are risk factors? Select all that apply.

- ❒ 1 A diet high in fat
- ❒ 2 History of late menopause
- ❒ 3 Age of more than 40 years
- ❒ 4 Menstrual history of late menarche
- ❒ 5 Previous history of cancer in one breast
- ❒ 6 Family history of any first-degree relative with breast cancer

Level of Cognitive Ability: Application
Client Needs: Health Promotion and Maintenance
Integrated Process: Teaching and Learning
Content Area: Adult Health/Oncology

Answer: 1, 2, 3, 5, 6

Rationale: Risk factors associated with breast cancer include a menstrual history of early menarche and a late menopause. Other risk factors include a previous history of breast cancer; a family history of breast cancer, including any first-degree relative (e.g., mother, sister) with breast cancer; and an age of more than 40 years (incidence increases with age and peaks during the fifth decade). A high-fat diet is associated with an increased risk of cancer.

Test-Taking Strategy: Focus on the subject—the risk factors associated with breast cancer. Remember that a diet high in fat and an early menarche are associated with breast cancer. Review the risk factors for breast cancer if you had difficulty with this question.

Reference

Ignatavicius, D., & Workman, M. (2010). *Medical-surgical nursing: Patient-centered collaborative care* (6th ed., p. 1664). St. Louis: Saunders.

Multiple Response

453. A nurse working at a health screening clinic gathers data from a client to identify the client's risk factors associated with coronary heart disease. The nurse is specifically interested in modifiable risk factors so that a health promotion and maintenance plan of care can be developed for the client. Select all risk factors that are modifiable.

- ❒ 1 Is physically inactive
- ❒ 2 Is a 45-year-old female
- ❒ 3 Is an African American
- ❒ 4 Has a family history of heart disease
- ❒ 5 Has an elevated serum cholesterol level
- ❒ 6 Has a blood pressure of 158/102 mmHg

Level of Cognitive Ability: Analysis
Client Needs: Health Promotion and Maintenance
Integrated Process: Nursing Process/Data Collection
Content Area: Adult Health/Cardiovascular

Answer: 1, 5, 6

Rationale: Modifiable risk factors for coronary artery disease are those that can be modified or reduced with treatment. These include cigarette smoking, hypertension, an elevated serum cholesterol level, physical inactivity, and obesity. Nonmodifiable risk factors are those that cannot be modified or reduced with treatment and include such factors as heredity, race, age, and gender. Clients whose parents had coronary heart disease are at higher risk. Increasing age influences both the risk and severity of the disease. Although men are at higher risk for heart attacks at a younger age, the risk for women increases significantly at menopause. The incidence of coronary heart disease is more prevalent in African-American women.

Test-Taking Strategy: Focus on the subject—modifiable risk factors. Recalling that modifiable risk factors are those that can be modified or reduced with treatment will assist you with answering this question. Look at each risk factor listed, and select those that can be changed. Review the modifiable and nonmodifiable risk factors for coronary heart disease if you had difficulty with this question.

Reference

Linton, A. (2007). *Introduction to medical-surgical nursing* (4th ed., p. 653). Philadelphia: Saunders.

Fill-in-the-Blank

454. A client at risk for urinary tract infections is told to drink 3000 mL of fluid every day to decrease the risk. The nurse explains to the client that she needs to drink how many 10-oz glasses of fluid per day to consume the prescribed 3000 mL?

Answer: _____ **10-oz glasses**

Level of Cognitive Ability: Application
Client Needs: Health Promotion and Maintenance
Integrated Process: Teaching and Learning
Content Area: Fundamental Skills

Answer: 10
Rationale: Each 10-oz glass of fluid contains 300 mL (1 oz = 30 mL; therefore, 10 oz = 300 mL). The client will need to drink ten 10-oz glasses of fluid daily (3000 mL/300 mL = 10).

Test-Taking Strategy: Focus on the subject—the number of 10-oz glasses of fluid that will equal 3000 mL. First, convert ounces to milliliters to determine the number of milliliters in each 10-oz glass of fluid. Next, divide the amount of fluid prescribed by the number of milliliters in each 10-oz glass of fluid. Review the formula for converting ounces to milliliters if you had difficulty with this question.

Reference
Kee, J., & Marshall, S. (2009). *Clinical calculations: With applications to general and specialty areas* (6th ed., p. 38). Philadelphia: Saunders.

Multiple Response

455. A nurse is providing home-care instructions to a client who has had vascular bypass surgery on a lower limb. To prevent the complications associated with the surgical procedure, the nurse teaches the client to do which of the following? Select all that apply.

- ❒ 1. Initiate a daily walking regimen.
- ❒ 2. Avoid lifting anything heavier than 20 pounds.
- ❒ 3. Take a tub bath daily to keep the incision clean.
- ❒ 4. Eat a high-fiber diet and drink plenty of liquids.
- ❒ 5. Promptly report signs of incisional infection to the physician.
- ❒ 6. Expect to feel fatigued and plan for rest periods throughout the day.

Level of Cognitive Ability: Application
Client Needs: Health Promotion and Maintenance
Integrated Process: Teaching and Learning
Content Area: Adult Health/Cardiovascular

Answer: 1, 4, 5, 6
Rationale: Vascular bypass surgery is performed to restore blood flow when a life- or limb-threatening arterial occlusion is present. To prevent complications postoperatively, the nurse teaches the client to avoid lifting anything heavier than 10 pounds until approved by the physician. Items that weigh more than 10 pounds will cause pressure and stress on the incision. To prevent complications associated with incisional healing, the client is also taught to avoid tub baths and to instead shower daily until the incision is healed. The client should advance activity gradually as tolerated and initiate a daily walk. Fatigue is expected, and the client should plan for rest periods throughout the day. A high-fiber diet and liquids will prevent constipation.

Test-Taking Strategy: Focus on the surgical procedure, and note the strategic words *lower limb.* Use general postoperative teaching guidelines to assist you with selecting the correct option. Eliminate option 2 because of the words *20 pounds.* Eliminate option 3 by focusing on the strategic words. Review the home-care instructions for the client after vascular bypass surgery on a lower limb if you had difficulty with this question.

Reference
Black, J., & Hawks, J. (2009). *Medical-surgical nursing: Clinical management for positive outcomes* (8th ed., pp. 1429-1430). St. Louis: Saunders.

REFERENCES

Black, J., & Hawks, J. (2009). *Medical surgical nursing: Clinical management for positive outcomes* (8th ed.). St. Louis: Saunders.

Christensen, B., & Kockrow, E. (2006). *Adult health nursing* (5th ed.). St. Louis: Mosby.

Christensen, B., & Kockrow, E. (2006). *Foundations of nursing* (5th ed.). St. Louis: Mosby.

deWit, S. (2009). *Medical-surgical nursing: Concepts & practice*. St. Louis: Saunders.

Edmunds, M. (2010). *Introduction to clinical pharmacology* (6th ed.). St. Louis: Mosby.

Fortinash, K., & Holoday-Worret, P. (2008). *Psychiatric mental health nursing* (4th ed.). St. Louis: Mosby.

Grodner, M., Long, S., & Walkingshaw, B. (2007). *Foundations and clinical applications of nutrition* (4th ed.). St. Louis: Mosby.

Hockenberry, M., & Wilson, D. (2007). *Nursing care of infants and children* (8th ed.). St. Louis: Mosby.

Hodgson, B., & Kizior, R. (2009). *Saunders nursing drug handbook 2009*. St. Louis: Saunders.

Ignatavicius, D., & Workman, M. (2010). *Medical-surgical nursing: Critical thinking for collaborative care* (6th ed.). St. Louis: Saunders.

Jarvis, C. (2008). *Physical examination and health assessment* (5th ed.). Philadelphia: Saunders.

Kee, J., Hayes, E., & McCuistion, L. (2009). *Pharmacology: A nursing process approach* (6th ed.). St. Louis: Saunders.

Leifer, G. (2008). *Maternity nursing: An introductory text* (10th ed.). Philadelphia: Saunders.

Leifer, G. (2007). *Introduction to maternity and pediatric nursing* (5th ed.). Philadelphia: Saunders.

Linton, A. (2007). *Introduction to medical-surgical nursing* (4th ed.). Philadelphia: Saunders.

McKinney, E., James, S., Murrary, S., & Ashwill, J. (2009). *Maternal-child nursing.* (3rd ed). St. Louis: Mosby.

Nix, S. (2009). *Williams' basic nutrition and diet therapy* (13th ed.). St. Louis: Mosby.

Perry, A., & Potter, P. (2010). *Clinical nursing skills & techniques* (7th ed.). St. Louis: Mosby.

Potter, P., & Perry, A. (2009). *Fundamentals of nursing* (7th ed.). St. Louis: Mosby.

Price, D., & Gwin, J. (2008). *Pediatric nursing: An introductory text* (10th ed.). St. Louis: Saunders.

Skidmore-Roth, L. (2008). *2008 Mosby's nursing drug reference* (21st ed.). St. Louis: Mosby.

Skidmore-Roth, L. (2009). *Mosby's drug guide for nurses* (8th ed.). St. Louis: Mosby.

Swearinger, P. (2008). *All-in-one care planning resource: Medical-surgical, pediatric, maternity, psychiatric nursing care plans* (2nd ed.). St. Louis: Mosby.

Varcarolis, E., & Halter, M. (2009). *Essentials of psychiatric mental health nursing: A communication approach to evidence-based care.* St. Louis: Saunders.

Wold, G. (2008). *Basic geriatric nursing* (4th ed). St. Louis: Mosby.

CHAPTER 8

Psychosocial Integrity

456. A nurse is collecting data from a client with a history of hypertension. The nurse determines that the client would benefit from biofeedback as an adjunctive therapy if the client makes which of the following statements?

1 "I have such a stressful job, you wouldn't believe it."
2 "It is so hard giving up all the salty foods that I enjoy."
3 "I don't have the money to pay for the pills that I take everyday."
4 "It is hard for me to get to the bus to come in to the clinic for my blood pressure checks."

Level of Cognitive Ability: Comprehension
Client Needs: Psychosocial Integrity
Integrated Process: Nursing Process/Data Collection
Content Area: Adult Health/Cardiovascular

Answer: 1

Rationale: Biofeedback is one of several stress-management techniques that may be useful for clients whose hypertension is aggravated by stress. Option 2 indicates the need for further dietary management. Options 3 and 4 relate to financial and environmental issues that are interfering with treatment.

Test-Taking Strategy: Use the process of elimination, and focus on the subject—the purpose of biofeedback training. Knowing that biofeedback is a stress-management technique enables you to eliminate each of the incorrect options. Review the basics of stress management—including methods such as relaxation, guided imagery, and biofeedback—if you had difficulty with this question.

References

Christensen, B., & Kockrow, E. (2006). *Adult health nursing* (5th ed., pp. 381-382). St. Louis: Mosby.
Christensen, B., & Kockrow, E. (2006). *Foundations of nursing* (5th ed., p. 1131). St. Louis: Mosby.

---

457. A 10-month-old infant is hospitalized for respiratory syncytial virus. The nurse knows that a 10-month-old child is in the trust versus mistrust stage of psychosocial development (Erikson) and the sensorimotor period of cognitive development (Piaget). Which of the following should the nurse do to promote the infant's development?

1 Wash hands, wear a mask, and keep the infant as quiet as possible.
2 Restrain the infant continuously to prevent tubes from being dislodged.
3 Follow the home feeding schedule and allow the infant to be held only when the parents visit.
4 Provide a consistent routine that includes touching, rocking, and cuddling throughout the hospitalization.

Level of Cognitive Ability: Application
Client Needs: Psychosocial Integrity

Answer: 4

Rationale: Hospitalization may have an adverse psychological effect on an infant. A consistent routine that is accompanied by touching, rocking, and cuddling helps the infant to develop trust and provides sensory stimulation. Option 1 identifies good infection control methods, but these measures will not help to meet the developmental task. It is important to follow the home routine, if possible, but touching and holding only when parents visit is not enough. A restrained infant may regress.

Test-Taking Strategy: Focus on the age of the child and the subject of the question—developmental needs. Eliminate options 2 and 3 because of the words *continuously* and *only,* respectively. Focusing on the subject will direct you to option 4. Review psychosocial development in an infant if you had difficulty with this question.

References

Leifer, G. (2007). *Introduction to maternity and pediatric nursing* (5th ed., pp. 577-578). Philadelphia: Saunders.
Price, D., & Gwin, J. (2008). *Pediatric nursing: An introductory text* (10th ed., p. 21). St. Louis: Saunders.

Integrated Process: Nursing Process/Implementation
Content Area: Child Health

---

458. A client with an order for a 12-lead electrocardiogram (ECG) has never had this procedure done before. The nurse most effectively reduces the client's anxiety by stating which of the following?

1 "It's important to lie still during the procedure."
2 "It should take about 30 minutes to complete the ECG tracing."
3 "The ECG tells the doctor what might be wrong with your heart."
4 "The test is painless and will record the electrical activity of your heart."

Level of Cognitive Ability: Application
Client Needs: Psychosocial Integrity
Integrated Process: Caring
Content Area: Adult Health/Cardiovascular

Answer: 4
Rationale: The ECG uses painless electrodes that are applied to the chest and limbs. It takes less than 5 minutes to complete, and the client must lie still to obtain clear tracings. The ECG measures the heart's electrical activity to determine cardiac rate and rhythm as well as a variety of abnormalities.

Test-Taking Strategy: Focus on the subject—reducing the client's anxiety. Option 2 is an incorrect statement and is eliminated first. Options 1 and 3 are factual statements but are not stated to reduce anxiety. Option 4 is the only reassuring statement, which addresses the focus of the question. Review the ECG if you had difficulty with this question.

Reference
deWit, S. (2009). *Medical-surgical nursing: Concepts & practice* (pp. 9, 412). St. Louis: Saunders.

---

459. A 16-year-old client has been diagnosed with anorexia nervosa. The nurse should further explore which of the following statements made by the client?

1 "I check my weight every day without fail."
2 "I exercise 2 to 3 hours every day to keep my figure."
3 "I've been told that I am 5% below my ideal body weight."
4 "My best friend was in the hospital with this disease a year ago."

Level of Cognitive Ability: Application
Client Needs: Psychosocial Integrity
Integrated Process: Nursing Process/Data Collection
Content Area: Mental Health

Answer: 2
Rationale: Exercising 2 to 3 hours every day is excessive physical activity and unrealistic for a 16-year-old client. The nurse should explore this statement to find out why the client feels that she should exercise this much to maintain her figure. Although it is unfortunate that the client's friend had the same disease, this is not considered a major threat to the client's physical well-being. A weight of 15% or more below the ideal body weight is characteristic of anorexia nervosa. It is not considered abnormal to check the weight every day; however, many anorexics check their weight up to 20 times a day.

Test-Taking Strategy: Note the strategic words *further explore.* Knowledge of the characteristics associated with anorexia nervosa directs you to option 2. Review these characteristics if you had difficulty with this question.

Reference
Varcarolis, E., & Halter, M. (2009). *Essentials of psychiatric mental health nursing: A communication approach to evidence-based care* (p. 250). St. Louis: Saunders.

---

460. Which of the following behaviors most strongly suggests that the client may be contemplating suicide?

1 The client reports sleep disturbances.
2 The client cries for long periods of time.
3 The client spends long periods of time alone.

Answer: 4
Rationale: Suicide precautions should be implemented if a client displays a suicidal ideation and is able to share a plan. Option 4 clearly states a plan. Options 1, 2, and 3 are indicative of depression and are not as definitive as option 4 with regard to the client contemplating suicide.

4 The client tells the nurse that he or she plans to use a belt to hang himself or herself.

Level of Cognitive Ability: Comprehension
Client Needs: Psychosocial Integrity
Integrated Process: Nursing Process/Data Collection
Content Area: Mental Health

Test-Taking Strategy: Note the strategic words *most strongly suggests* and *contemplating suicide*. Use the process of elimination, and note that option 4 identifies the formulation of a specific suicidal plan. Review the client at risk for suicide if you had difficulty with this question.

Reference
Varcarolis, E., & Halter, M. (2009). *Essentials of psychiatric mental health nursing: A communication approach to evidence-based care* (pp. 413, 416). St. Louis: Saunders.

---

461. A nurse is collecting data from a client who was admitted to the inpatient mental heath unit. The client was involved in a fire 2 months ago and is complaining of insomnia, difficulty concentrating, nervousness, and hypervigilance. In addition, the client frequently thinks about fires. The nurse recognizes these symptoms to be indicative of:

1 A phobia
2 Dissociative disorder
3 Posttraumatic stress disorder
4 Obsessive-compulsive disorder

Level of Cognitive Ability: Comprehension
Client Needs: Psychosocial Integrity
Integrated Process: Nursing Process/Data Collection
Content Area: Mental Health

Answer: 3
Rationale: Posttraumatic stress disorder is precipitated by events that are overwhelming, unpredictable, and sometimes life threatening. Typical symptoms of posttraumatic stress disorder include difficulty concentrating, sleep disturbances, intrusive recollections of the traumatic event, hypervigilance, and anxiety. Options 1, 2, and 4 are incorrect.

Test-Taking Strategy: Focus on the data in the question. Recalling that hypervigilance or hyperalertness and flashbacks of traumatic events are common symptoms of posttraumatic stress disorder directs you to option 3. Review posttraumatic stress disorder if you had difficulty with this question.

Reference
Fortinash, K., & Holoday-Worret, P. (2008). *Psychiatric mental health nursing* (4th ed., p. 451). St. Louis: Mosby.

---

462. A 16-year-old client is hospitalized with pneumonia. Which statement made by the adolescent represents a potential developmental problem and indicates the need to gather more information?

1 "I'd like my hair washed before my friends get here."
2 "Is it okay if I have a couple of friends in to visit me this evening?"
3 "Please tell my friends not to visit since I'll see them back at school next week."
4 "When my friends get here, I would like to play some computer games with them."

Level of Cognitive Ability: Comprehension
Client Needs: Psychosocial Integrity
Integrated Process: Nursing Process/Data Collection
Content Area: Child Health

Answer: 3
Rationale: Adolescents who withdraw from peers into isolation struggle with developing identity; therefore option 3 should cause the nurse to be concerned. Option 2 shows that the client is eager for companionship. Adolescents often develop special interests within their groups that may help them to maximize certain skills, such as computer skills. Personal appearance is important to many adolescents.

Test-Taking Strategy: Use the process of elimination. Options 1, 2, and 4 indicate that the adolescent is anticipating the arrival of an appropriate peer group. Option 3 indicates that the client may be withdrawing from suitable relationships. Review the concepts of growth and development if you had difficulty with this question.

Reference
Price, D., & Gwin, J. (2008). *Pediatric nursing: An introductory text* (10th ed., p. 328). St. Louis: Saunders.

463. A prenatal client is told during a physician office visit that she tested positive for human immunodeficiency virus (HIV). The client cries and is significantly distressed about this news. The nurse contributes to the formulation of a nursing diagnosis and determines that which of the following is appropriate?
1 *Acute pain*
2 *Noncompliance*
3 *Risk for infection*
4 *Anticipatory grieving*

Level of Cognitive Ability: Analysis
Client Needs: Psychosocial Integrity
Integrated Process: Nursing Process/Data Collection
Content Area: Maternity/Antepartum

Answer: 4
Rationale: A life-threatening diagnosis such as HIV stimulates the anticipatory grief response. Anticipatory grief occurs when the client, family, and loved ones know that the client will die. There are no data in the question to support options 1, 2, or 3.

Test-Taking Strategy: Focus on the data presented in the question. A client who is distressed and crying supports the nursing diagnosis of *Anticipatory grieving*. The question does not contain enough information to support options 1 or 2. Option 3 is a concern for the client with HIV, but there are no data in the question to support this nursing diagnosis. Review the defining characteristics of the nursing diagnosis of *Anticipatory grieving* if you had difficulty with this question.

Reference
Leifer, G. (2007). *Introduction to maternity and pediatric nursing* (5th ed., pp. 85, 106). Philadelphia: Saunders.

---

464. A nurse is caring for a male client recovering from a myocardial infarction. The nurse determines that the client is exhibiting signs of depression when the client:
1 Reports insomnia at night
2 Ignores activity restrictions and does not report the experience of chest pain with activity
3 Consumes only 25% of his meals and shows little interest when client education is reinforced
4 Expresses apprehension about leaving the hospital and requests someone to stay with him at night

Level of Cognitive Ability: Analysis
Client Needs: Psychosocial Integrity
Integrated Process: Nursing Process/Data Collection
Content Area: Adult Health/Cardiovascular

Answer: 3
Rationale: Signs of depression include withdrawal, crying, anorexia, and apathy. Insomnia may be a sign of anxiety or fear. Ignoring symptoms and activity restrictions is a sign of denial. Apprehension is a sign of anxiety.

Test-Taking Strategy: Use the process of elimination, and focus on the subject—signs of depression. Option 3 is the only option that identifies depression. Review the signs of depression if you had difficulty with this question.

Reference
deWit, S. (2009). *Medical-surgical nursing: Concepts & practice* (p. 499). St. Louis: Saunders.

---

465. A client who has a new feeding gastrostomy tube refuses to participate in the plan of care, will not make eye contact, and does not speak to family or visitors. The nurse recognizes that this client is using which ineffective coping mechanism?
1 Distancing
2 Self-control
3 Problem solving
4 Accepting responsibility

Level of Cognitive Ability: Comprehension
Client Needs: Psychosocial Integrity

Answer: 1
Rationale: Distancing is an unwillingness or inability to discuss events. Self-control is demonstrated by stoicism and hiding feelings. Problem solving involves making plans and verbalizing what will be done. Accepting responsibility places the responsibility for a situation on one's self.

Test-Taking Strategy: Use the process of elimination. The words *refuses, will not,* and *does not* are all indicative of ineffective coping. Option 1 is the least effective coping strategy. Review coping mechanisms if you had difficulty with this question.

Integrated Process: Nursing Process/Data Collection
Content Area: Adult Health/Gastrointestinal

Reference
Linton, A. (2007). *Introduction to medical-surgical nursing* (4th ed., p. 83). Philadelphia: Saunders.

---

466. A nurse is caring for a hospitalized client who has esophageal varices. The client says, "I deserve this. I brought it on myself by drinking too much alcohol." To gather additional data, the nurse should make which response to the client?

1 "Would you like to talk to the chaplain?"
2 "Is there some reason you feel you deserve this?"
3 "Not all esophageal varices are caused by alcohol."
4 "That is something to think about when you leave the hospital."

Level of Cognitive Ability: Application
Client Needs: Psychosocial Integrity
Integrated Process: Communication and Documentation
Content Area: Adult Health/Gastrointestinal

Answer: 2
Rationale: Esophageal varices are often a complication of cirrhosis of the liver, and the most common type of cirrhosis is caused by chronic alcohol abuse. Option 1 blocks communication. Options 3 and 4 are judgmental. Option 2 allows the client to discuss feelings.

Test-Taking Strategy: Use therapeutic communication techniques and the process of elimination to answer the question. Option 1 could block the nurse–client communication process. Options 3 and 4 are judgmental. The open-ended question in option 2 promotes the expression of feelings. Remember that the client's feelings and concerns should be addressed first. Review therapeutic communication techniques if you had difficulty with this question.

Reference
deWit, S. (2009). *Medical-surgical nursing: Concepts & practice* (pp. 9, 755-756). St. Louis: Saunders.

---

467. An older client is admitted to the hospital after falling off of a chair at home. During the night, the nurse wakes the client up to perform a neurological check. The client states, "I'm so scared. Where am I? What's happening?" Based on the findings noted in the client, the nurse should make which response?

1 "You're in the hospital after a fall. You feel scared?"
2 "Hold my hand. Try to wake up and tell me your name."
3 "You fell and hit your head. Your family brought you here."
4 "There's no reason to be scared. You're safe here in the hospital."

Level of Cognitive Ability: Application
Client Needs: Psychosocial Integrity
Integrated Process: Communication and Documentation
Content Area: Adult Health/Neurological

Answer: 1
Rationale: Reflecting is using the client's own words or feelings when responding to him or her. In option 1, the nurse gives information to the client in addition to reflecting the client's feelings. In option 2, the nurse attempts to calm the client but blocks communication by changing the subject and beginning the neurological check. In option 3, the nurse gives information but does not deal with the client's emotional needs. In option 4, the nurse does not provide the client with an opportunity to express feelings, thereby blocking communication.

Test-Taking Strategy: Use therapeutic communication techniques to answer the question. Remember to respond to the client's emotional needs. Avoid blocks to communication and focus on the client's feelings and concerns. Review therapeutic communication techniques if you had difficulty with this question.

References
deWit, S. (2009). *Medical-surgical nursing: Concepts & practice* (p. 9). St. Louis: Saunders.
Wold, G. (2008). *Basic geriatric nursing* (4th ed., pp. 191-192). St. Louis: Mosby.

---

468. The mother of a toddler who is hospitalized must leave her child to go to work. Which behavior will the nurse most likely observe in this

Answer: 2
Rationale: The stages of separation anxiety include protest, despair, and detachment. Crying loudly and kicking both legs is a protest behavior that is seen during the first stage of separation. Option

child immediately after the mother's departure?
1 Playing quietly with a favorite toy
2 Crying loudly and kicking both legs
3 Silently curled in bed with a blanket
4 Sucking the thumb and rocking back and forth

Level of Cognitive Ability: Comprehension
Client Needs: Psychosocial Integrity
Integrated Process: Nursing Process/Data Collection
Content Area: Child Health

1 is incorrect because the behavior reflects detachment, which is the third stage of separation. Options 3 and 4 are incorrect and are not likely to be noted in this situation.

Test-Taking Strategy: Note the strategic words *immediately after the mother's departure.* This directs you to look for the toddler's immediate behavioral response to separation. Review normal growth and development and the concept of separation anxiety if you had difficulty with this question.

Reference
Leifer, G. (2007). *Introduction to maternity and pediatric nursing* (5th ed., p. 401). Philadelphia: Saunders.

---

469. A preschool-age child is placed in traction for the treatment of a femur fracture. This child, who reportedly has been toilet trained for at least 1 year, begins wetting the bed. The nurse recognizes this behavior as:
1 Body-image disturbance
2 Attention-seeking behavior
3 Loss of developmental milestones
4 Regressing to earlier developmental behavior

Level of Cognitive Ability: Comprehension
Client Needs: Psychosocial Integrity
Integrated Process: Nursing Process/Data Collection
Content Area: Child Health

Answer: 4
Rationale: The monotony of immobilization can lead to sluggish intellectual and psychomotor responses. Although option 3 may seem like an appropriate response, option 4 is a more accurate description of the psychological effects of immobilization. Regressive behaviors are not uncommon in immobilized children and usually do not require professional intervention. Body image may or may not be affected by long-term immobilization, but this does not relate to the data in the question.

Test-Taking Strategy: Use the process of elimination. Eliminate option 1 because it does not relate to the question. Eliminate option 3 next because bed-wetting by an immobilized child is not unusual. To select from the remaining options, recall that regression is a normal psychological response to immobilization. Review the effects of immobilization on a preschooler if you had difficulty with this question.

Reference
Hockenberry, M., & Wilson, D. (2009). *Wong's essentials of pediatric care* (8th ed., p. 422). St. Louis: Mosby.

---

470. A nurse is reviewing the record of a client with a diagnosis of mania who has been admitted to the psychiatric unit. Which characteristic is least likely to be associated with this disorder?
1 Fatigue
2 Weight gain
3 Inflated self-esteem
4 Inability to concentrate

Level of Cognitive Ability: Comprehension
Client Needs: Psychosocial Integrity
Integrated Process: Nursing Process/Data Collection
Content Area: Mental Health

Answer: 2
Rationale: The manic client typically forgets to eat and therefore demonstrates a weight loss rather than a gain. The manic client also demonstrates fatigue, inflated self-esteem, and the inability to concentrate.

Test-Taking Strategy: Use the process of elimination, and note the strategic words *least likely.* Focusing on the name of the disorder and recalling its characteristics will direct you to option 2. Review the characteristics of mania if you had difficulty with this question.

Reference
Varcarolis, E., & Halter, M. (2009). *Essentials of psychiatric mental health nursing: A communication approach to evidence-based care* (p. 250). St. Louis: Saunders.

471. The husband of a client who has a Sengstaken-Blakemore tube states, "I thought having this tube down her nose the first time would convince my wife to quit drinking." Based on this statement, the appropriate response by the nurse is which of the following?

1 "I think you are a good person to stay with your wife."
2 "Alcoholism is a disease that affects the whole family."
3 "Have you discussed this subject at the support groups?"
4 "You sound frustrated with dealing with your wife's drinking problem."

Level of Cognitive Ability: Application
Client Needs: Psychosocial Integrity
Integrated Process: Communication and Documentation
Content Area: Adult Health/Gastrointestinal

Answer: 4
Rationale: The nurse should use therapeutic communication techniques to assist the client (in this case, the client's spouse) with expressing his feelings about his wife's chronic illness. The nurse focuses on the spouse's feelings in option 4. Expressing an opinion (option 1), stereotyping (option 2), and changing the subject (option 3) are examples of communication blocks.

Test-Taking Strategy: Use therapeutic communication techniques. With communication questions, identify the use of therapeutic tools (option 4) and blocks to communication (Options 1, 2, and 3). Remember to always focus on the client's feelings and concerns first. Review therapeutic communication techniques if you had difficulty with this question.

References
deWit, S. (2009). *Medical-surgical nursing: Concepts & practice* (p. 9). St. Louis: Saunders.
Linton, A. (2007). *Introduction to medical-surgical nursing* (4th ed., pp. 813-815). Philadelphia: Saunders.

---

472. A nurse is caring for a client on suicide precautions. The nurse gathers data about the client and recognizes that which of the following statements about suicide is true?

1 A client who talks about suicide rarely attempts it.
2 The nurse should not use the word "suicide" in front of the client.
3 The client who is unsuccessful at suicide will probably not try again.
4 The more specific the plan, the more likely that the client will be successful in the attempt.

Level of Cognitive Ability: Comprehension
Client Needs: Psychosocial Integrity
Integrated Process: Nursing Process/Data Collection
Content Area: Mental Health

Answer: 4
Rationale: The more specific the plan, the greater the likelihood of a successful suicide. Options 1, 2, and 3 are incorrect statements.

Test-Taking Strategy: Knowledge about the risks associated with suicide is necessary to answer this question. Remember that it is a priority to determine whether the client has a specific plan for suicide. Review suicide risks if you had difficulty with this question.

Reference
Stuart, G. (2009). *Principles and practices of psychiatric nursing* (9th ed., p. 316). St. Louis: Mosby.

---

473. A client is admitted to the hospital for a thyroidectomy. While preparing the client for surgery, the nurse gathers information about psychosocial problems that may cause preoperative anxiety. A primary source of anxiety related to a thyroidectomy is the fear of which of the following?

1 Sexual dysfunction and infertility
2 Imposed dietary restrictions postoperatively

Answer: 4
Rationale: Because the incision is in the neck area, clients often worry about thyroid surgery out of fear of having a large postoperative scar. Having all or part of the thyroid gland removed does not cause the client to experience gynecomastia or hirsutism. Sexual dysfunction and infertility could occur if the entire thyroid is removed and the client is not placed on thyroid replacement medications. Dietary restrictions are not prescribed.

3 Developing gynecomastia and hirsutism postoperatively
4 Changes in body image secondary to the location of the incision

Level of Cognitive Ability: Comprehension
Client Needs: Psychosocial Integrity
Integrated Process: Nursing Process/Data Collection
Content Area: Adult Health/Endocrine

Test-Taking Strategy: Use the process of elimination, and note the strategic word *primary*. Recalling the anatomical location of this surgical procedure directs you to option 4. Review thyroidectomy if you had difficulty with this question.

Reference
Linton, A. (2007). *Introduction to medical-surgical nursing* (4th ed., p. 988). Philadelphia: Saunders.

---

474. A nurse is caring for a client with type 2 diabetes mellitus who has been hospitalized for hyperglycemic hyperosmolar nonketotic syndrome. The client expresses concerns about this syndrome recurring. Based on the client's concern, which statement by the nurse is appropriate?
1 "I'm sure this won't happen again."
2 "Don't worry; your family will help you."
3 "You have concerns about this complication?"
4 "Perhaps you should consider going to a nursing home."

Level of Cognitive Ability: Application
Client Needs: Psychosocial Integrity
Integrated Process: Communication and Documentation
Content Area: Adult Health/Endocrine

Answer: 3
Rationale: The nurse should focus on the client's feelings. Options 1 and 2 are inappropriate and provide false reassurance. Option 4 is inappropriate and a premature statement. Option 3 is the only option that addresses the client's feelings.

Test-Taking Strategy: Use therapeutic communication techniques to answer the question. Remember to focus on the client's feelings; this will direct you to option 3. Review therapeutic communication techniques if you had difficulty with this question.

References
deWit, S. (2009). *Medical-surgical nursing: Concepts & practice* (p. 9). St. Louis: Saunders.
Linton, A. (2007). *Introduction to medical-surgical nursing* (4th ed., p. 1008). Philadelphia: Saunders.

---

475. While the nurse is explaining necessary lifestyle changes to a client with angina, the client continually changes the subject. The nurse determines that the client is probably exhibiting:
1 Anger
2 Denial
3 Anxiety
4 Depression

Level of Cognitive Ability: Comprehension
Client Needs: Psychosocial Integrity
Integrated Process: Nursing Process/Data Collection
Content Area: Adult Health/Cardiovascular

Answer: 2
Rationale: Denial is a defense mechanism that allows the client to minimize a threat; it may be manifested by a refusal to discuss what has happened. Denial is a common early reaction associated with chest discomfort, angina, or myocardial infarction. Anger is often manifested by "acting out" behaviors. Anxiety is usually manifested as a result of symptoms of sympathetic nervous system arousal. Depression may be manifested by passive behaviors.

Test-Taking Strategy: Focus on the strategic words *continually changes the subject.* Use the process of elimination, and select the option based on which behavior best fits the question description; this will direct you to option 2. Review the manifestations of denial if you had difficulty with this question.

Reference
deWit, S. (2009). *Medical-surgical nursing: Concepts & practice* (p. 499). St. Louis: Saunders.

---

476. A nurse is caring for a client who has verbalized suicidal ideation. Which of the following statements indicates that the client is at highest risk for suicide?

1. "I'm just useless. I want someone to take me out and shoot me!"
2. "There is nothing left for me in this life. I just wish I could die!"
3. "God has called on me to come to him. He commands me to jump off the bridge tomorrow."
4. "I tried to kill myself last year at this time by swallowing a bottle of aspirin. This time I'll swallow two bottles!"

Level of Cognitive Ability: Analysis
Client Needs: Psychosocial Integrity
Integrated Process: Nursing Process/Data Collection
Content Area: Mental Health

Answer: 3
Rationale: The formulation of a suicide plan indicates the client's serious intent. The likelihood of suicide increases when manifestations of command auditory hallucinations (voices telling the client to commit suicide) are present. In option 3, the client identifies an auditory command hallucination and a suicide plan. The nature of the psychosis is highly lethal, and the suicide plan includes an active lethal method, a time, and a place.

Test-Taking Strategy: Use the process of elimination, and note the strategic words *highest risk.* Note that option 3 identifies a suicide plan that includes an active lethal method, a time, and a place. Review risk factors for suicide if you had difficulty with this question.

Reference

Fortinash, K., & Holoday-Worret, P. (2008). *Psychiatric mental health nursing* (4th ed., p. 471). St. Louis: Mosby.

---

477. A client with cancer of the bladder has a nursing diagnosis of *Fear* related to the uncertain outcome of the upcoming cystectomy and urinary diversion. The nurse determines that this diagnosis is correct if the client makes which statement?

1. "I wish I'd never gone to the doctor at all."
2. "I'm so afraid that I won't live through all this."
3. "I'll never feel like myself once I can't go to the bathroom normally."
4. "What if I have no help at home after going through this awful surgery?"

Level of Cognitive Ability: Analysis
Client Needs: Psychosocial Integrity
Integrated Process: Nursing Process/Data Collection
Content Area: Adult Health/Renal

Answer: 2
Rationale: The client must be able to identify the object of fear for *Fear* to be an actual nursing diagnosis. This client is expressing a fear of death related to cancer. Option 1 is vague and nonspecific; further exploration is necessary to associate this statement with a nursing diagnosis. Option 3 reflects a diagnosis of *Body image disturbance.* The statement in option 4 reflects *Risk for impaired home maintenance management.*

Test-Taking Strategy: Use the process of elimination, and note that the nursing diagnosis includes wording about the uncertain outcome of surgery. Option 1 should be eliminated first because it is a general statement. Options 3 and 4 focus on the self after surgery but do not contain statements about an uncertain outcome; therefore option 2 is correct. Review the defining characteristics of the nursing diagnosis of *Fear* if you had difficulty with this question.

Reference

deWit, S. (2009). *Medical-surgical nursing: Concepts & practice* (pp. 184-185, 848-849). St. Louis: Saunders.

---

478. A nurse receives a report that a client is depressed about suffering an acute myocardial infarction (MI). The nurse verifies this information by noting:

1. That the client ignores activity restrictions
2. That the client cries off and on during the day
3. That the client talks about rehabilitation measures

Answer: 2
Rationale: The emotional and behavioral reactions of a client after MI are varied. Depression may be manifested by withdrawal, crying, or apathy. Option 1 is more indicative of denial. Option 3 indicates realistic acceptance. Option 4 is more indicative of dependence and fear.

4 The client's hesitancy to be transferred from the telemetry unit

Level of Cognitive Ability: Comprehension
Client Needs: Psychosocial Integrity
Integrated Process: Nursing Process/Data Collection
Content Area: Adult Health/Cardiovascular

Test-Taking Strategy: Focus on the subject—a client who is depressed. All options are behaviors that may be manifested in the client after an MI; however, the question is asking about depression. Note that the incorrect options indicate behavioral responses other than those associated with depression. Review manifestations of depression if you had difficulty with this question.

Reference

deWit, S. (2009). *Medical-surgical nursing: Concepts & practice* (p. 499). St. Louis: Saunders.

---

479. A nurse is caring for an older client in the home. The client is widowed and competent, but the client's son, daughter-in-law, and their three children have unexpectedly moved into the house "to care for" the client. Which of the following indicates to the nurse that the client is being exploited?

1 "Once in a while the children get to be too noisy, but overall it's been the best thing that's happened to me since my wife died."
2 "It's nice to have my family around me again. Since my wife died, I've been lonely. They're keeping me young and spoiling me rotten."
3 "My son won't let me pay for anything. They're helping me with everything. This is such a help to me, because my income has been reduced since my wife died."
4 "My son wants me to turn over the deed to the house to him. He says I'll always have a place there, but I'll feel like a tenant in my own home. What do you think?"

Level of Cognitive Ability: Analysis
Client Needs: Psychosocial Integrity
Integrated Process: Nursing Process/Data Collection
Content Area: Mental Health

Answer: 4
Rationale: The exploitation of older adults can include taking over the client's bank accounts, deeds, stock portfolios, or wills. Option 1 addresses some adjustment to the expansion of the family, but that is expected. In option 2, the client is stating positive reasons that extended families can be helpful. Option 3 states the client's complete satisfaction with the expansion of the family.

Test-Taking Strategy: Use the process of elimination. Focus on the subject of the question—exploitation. Recalling the definition of this word will assist you with eliminating options 1, 2, and 3. Review the characteristics of elder abuse if you had difficulty with this question.

Reference

Fortinash, K., & Holoday-Worret, P. (2008). *Psychiatric mental health nursing* (4th ed., p. 502). St. Louis: Mosby.

---

480. A nurse is assisting with collecting data from a family with a diagnosis of violence. Which factor should the nurse initially determine during the data collection process?

1 The coping style of each family member
2 The family's current ability to use community resources

Answer: 1
Rationale: The nurse should initially collect data about each family member. Although some family members may regard the nurse's interventions as intrusive, this is not the focus of an initial assessment of a violent family. Denial may be one of the coping styles of the family, but it is not specific to every family experiencing violence. Although the use of community resources is important, the coping style of each family member should be determined first.

3 The family's anger toward the intrusiveness of the nurse
4 The family members' denial of the violent nature of their behavior

Level of Cognitive Ability: Application
Client Needs: Psychosocial Integrity
Integrated Process: Nursing Process/Data Collection
Content Area: Mental Health

Test-Taking Strategy: Use the process of elimination, and note the strategic word *initially.* Note that options 2, 3, and 4 all relate to data collection about the family as a unit. Option 1 is the only option that addresses the individual family members. Review data collection in a family with violence if you had difficulty with this question.

References

Fortinash, K., & Holoday-Worret, P. (2008). *Psychiatric mental health nursing* (4th ed., p. 486). St. Louis: Mosby.
Varcarolis, E., & Halter, M. (2009). *Essentials of psychiatric mental health nursing: A communication approach to evidence-based care* (p. 390). St. Louis: Saunders.

---

481. A nurse is assisting with caring for a client with a diagnosis of acute pulmonary edema who is on a mechanical ventilator. The nurse should determine that the client could be anxious when the client exhibits:
1 Hypotension, confusion, and combative behaviors
2 Bradycardia, hand clenching, and startling behaviors
3 Tachycardia, clinging to family members, and pupil dilation
4 Tachypnea, a decreased level of consciousness, and palpitations

Level of Cognitive Ability: Analysis
Client Needs: Psychosocial Integrity
Integrated Process: Nursing Process/Data Collection
Content Area: Adult Health/Cardiovascular

Answer: 3
Rationale: Signs of anxiety include behaviors such as clenched hands, heightened awareness, wide eyes, pupil dilation, startle response, furrowed brow, clinging to the family or staff, or physical lashing out. Because anxiety stimulates the sympathetic nervous system, the client may also exhibit palpitations, chest pain, tachycardia, an increased respiratory rate, an elevated blood glucose level, and hand tremors. The signs noted in option 1 would be seen with hypoxia rather than anxiety. In anxious states, tachycardia is present rather than bradycardia (option 2). Anxiety produces a heightened awareness rather than a decreased level of consciousness (option 4).

Test-Taking Strategy: Use the process of elimination, and focus on the subject—anxiety. Recalling that anxiety stimulates the sympathetic nervous system and knowing the effects of sympathetic stimulation will direct you to option 3. Review the effects of this physiological process if you had difficulty with this question.

References

Christensen, B., & Kockrow, E. (2006). *Adult health nursing* (5th ed., p. 368). St. Louis: Mosby.
Linton, A. (2007). *Introduction to medical-surgical nursing* (4th ed., p. 547). Philadelphia: Saunders.

---

482. A client was just told by the physician that the client will have an exercise stress test to evaluate cardiac status after recent episodes of severe chest pain. As the nurse enters the examination room, the client states, "Maybe I shouldn't bother going. I wonder if I should just take more medication instead." Based on this information, the nurse should make which response to the client?
1 "Can you tell me more about how you're feeling?"
2 "Don't you really want to control your heart disease?"

Answer: 1
Rationale: Anxiety and fear are often present before stress testing. The nurse uses questioning as a communication method to explore a client's feelings and concerns. Only option 1 is an open-ended question that is phrased to encourage the sharing of concerns by the client. Options 2, 3, and 4 are nontherapeutic and do not focus on the client's feelings.

Test-Taking Strategy: Use therapeutic communication techniques and the process of elimination to answer the question. Only option 1 focuses on the client's feelings. Remember to focus on client feelings and concerns first. Review therapeutic communication techniques if you had difficulty with this question.

3 "Most people tolerate the procedure well without any complications."
4 "Don't worry. Emergency equipment is available if it should be needed."

Level of Cognitive Ability: Application
Client Needs: Psychosocial Integrity
Integrated Process: Communication and Documentation
Content Area: Adult Health/Cardiovascular

References
Chernecky, C., & Berger, B. (2008). *Laboratory tests and diagnostic procedures* (5th ed., pp. 1042-1043). Philadelphia: Saunders.
deWit, S. (2009). *Medical-surgical nursing: Concepts & practice* (p. 412). St. Louis: Saunders.

---

483. A newborn is diagnosed with Hirschsprung's disease based on a failure to pass meconium. The nurse observes that the parents are hesitant to hold their newborn. Based on this observation, the nurse should take which appropriate action?
1 Observe stools for color and character.
2 Help the parents adjust to the congenital disorder.
3 Stabilize the newborn's fluid and electrolyte balance.
4 Teach the parents how to administer a barium enema to their child.

Level of Cognitive Ability: Application
Client Needs: Psychosocial Integrity
Integrated Process: Nursing Process/Implementation
Content Area: Maternity/Postpartum

Answer: 2
Rationale: One of the main objectives is to help parents adjust to the congenital disorder in their child and to foster infant–parent bonding. Failure to pass meconium within 24 hours of birth is suggestive of Hirschsprung's disease. A barium enema is a diagnostic tool that would not be administered by the parents. The neonate's fluid and electrolyte status is not likely to be in an imbalanced state at this time.

Test-Taking Strategy: Focus on the subject of the question—that the parents are hesitant to hold their newborn. This may indicate a need to help the parents accept their child even though the newborn is not perfect. Only option 2 addresses this concern. Review the psychosocial issues related to disorders in a newborn if you had difficulty with this question.

Reference
Price, D., & Gwin, J. (2008). *Pediatric nursing: An introductory text* (10th ed., p. 163). St. Louis: Saunders.

---

484. A nurse is caring for a client with depression. Which of these findings, if noted in the client, should the nurse identify as most significant and thus requiring the notification of the registered nurse?
1 Verbalizing feelings of being depressed
2 Sleeping for 12 hours every night and still complaining about being tired during the day
3 Requesting to call the significant other who is supportive when the client "feels like this"
4 Getting the "old personality back" and being spontaneous and uplifted after being described as "depressed"

Level of Cognitive Ability: Analysis
Client Needs: Psychosocial Integrity
Integrated Process: Nursing Process/Data Collection
Content Area: Mental Health

Answer: 4
Rationale: The depressed individual who has a sudden mood elevation after a period of being depressed is identified as being at risk to carry out a suicide intent. Options 1, 2, and 3 would require documentation and reporting but are not the most significant findings.

Test-Taking Strategy: Use the process of elimination, and note the strategic words *most significant*. Recalling that the depressed individual who has a sudden mood elevation is at risk to carry out a suicide intent will direct you to option 4. Review the manifestations related to suicide risk if you had difficulty with this question.

References
Fortinash, K., & Holoday-Worret, P. (2008). *Psychiatric mental health nursing* (4th ed., pp. 354, 469). St. Louis: Mosby.
Varcarolis, E., & Halter, M. (2009). *Essentials of psychiatric mental health nursing: A communication approach to evidence-based care* (pp. 221, 223). St. Louis: Saunders.

485. A nurse is assisting with preparing a client for electroconvulsive therapy (ECT). The client is pacing and says to the nurse, "How do I know this will work? I really don't understand how it can help me now. It may kill me." The nurse collects additional data from the client by:

1 Exploring the meaning of the client's comment in a calm, supportive manner
2 Assisting the client with resolving ambivalence about the decision to receive ECT
3 Planning with the client how ECT will help the client's return to daily functioning
4 Asking the client to recall what the client remembers about ECT from discussions

Level of Cognitive Ability: Application
Client Needs: Psychosocial Integrity
Integrated Process: Nursing Process/Implementation
Content Area: Mental Health

Answer: 1
Rationale: In this situation, the client presents with anxiety before ECT. Only option 1 addresses the client's feelings and concerns. Although options 2, 3, and 4 may be components of caring for the client, these options do not address the subject of the question.

Test-Taking Strategy: Use therapeutic communication techniques, and note that only option 1 addresses the client's concerns. Remember to address the client's feelings and concerns first. Review therapeutic communication techniques if you had difficulty with this question.

Reference
Stuart, G. (2009). *Principles and practices of psychiatric nursing* (9th ed., pp. 27-31, 537). St. Louis: Mosby.

---

486. A mother refuses to have her child immunized because of fear that a serious injury will result. To identify the basis of the mother's concern, the nurse should make which statement to the client?

1 "Are you afraid that the child is going to die from the injection?"
2 "There will be slight discomfort at the time of the injection, and that is all."
3 "Why are you worried? Children are immunized everyday without a problem."
4 "I can see you are very concerned about your child. What do you think might happen after an immunization is given?"

Level of Cognitive Ability: Application
Client Needs: Psychosocial Integrity
Integrated Process: Communication and Documentation
Content Area: Child Health

Answer: 4
Rationale: Option 4 acknowledges the mother's concern, which provides an opportunity for the mother to respond to the nurse's open-ended question. Option 1 is an attempt to verify an assumption that is not supported by the question. Options 2 and 3 block communication.

Test-Taking Strategy: Use therapeutic communication techniques to answer the question. The correct option demonstrates empathy and helps the mother focus on specific fears so that the nurse can clarify information. These are therapeutic communication techniques. Options 1, 2, and 3 use blocking strategies by assuming what the mother fears, giving false reassurances, and devaluing the mother's feelings, respectively. Review therapeutic communication techniques if you had difficulty with this question.

References
Hockenberry, M., & Wilson, D. (2009). *Wong's essentials of pediatric care* (8th ed., p. 359). St. Louis: Mosby.
Price, D., & Gwin, J. (2008). *Pediatric nursing: An introductory text* (10th ed., p. 129). St. Louis: Saunders.

---

487. A nurse is assigned to care for a client who is dying of ovarian cancer. While receiving care, the client states, "If I can just live long enough to attend my daughter's graduation, I'll be ready to

Answer: 2
Rationale: Bargaining is the phase of coping in which the dying person tries to negotiate by making deals with their God or fate. The client's statement does not indicate isolation, depression, or acceptance.

die." The nurse identifies that the client is experiencing which phase of coping?
1 Isolation
2 Bargaining
3 Depression
4 Acceptance

Level of Cognitive Ability: Comprehension
Client Needs: Psychosocial Integrity
Integrated Process: Nursing Process/Data Collection
Content Area: Adult Health/Oncology

Test-Taking Strategy: Use the process of elimination, and focus on the client's statement. This will direct you to option 2. Review coping mechanisms if you had difficulty with this question.

References
deWit, S. (2009). *Medical-surgical nursing: Concepts & practice* (p. 185). St. Louis: Saunders.
Linton, A. (2007). *Introduction to medical-surgical nursing* (4th ed., p. 388). Philadelphia: Saunders.

---

488. A mother, who has admitted to substance abuse during the pregnancy, is holding her 1-week-old neonate. The nurse watches the mother–baby interactions because the development of this relationship is at an especially high risk. Which observed neonate behavior or need will make the mother–baby bond difficult to establish?
1 Sleeping while being cuddled
2 Need to be fed with an orogastric tube
3 Irritability in response to noise and light
4 Hyperextended posture and gaze aversion

Level of Cognitive Ability: Analysis
Client Needs: Psychosocial Integrity
Integrated Process: Nursing Process/Data Collection
Content Area: Maternity/Postpartum

Answer: 4
Rationale: A hyperextended posture and gaze aversion makes the mother–baby relationship and bond most difficult to establish. The neonate is showing its disinterest by not looking at the mother's face. Parents often feel that they do not know a child until they are able to look into the baby's eyes. In addition, the hyperextended posture makes the neonate difficult to hold and cuddle. Sleeping while being cuddled is normal. Orogastric feedings are a skill that can be taught to the parent. Irritability in response to noise and light can be assisted with environmental changes.

Test-Taking Strategy: Focus on the subject of the question—identifying the neonate behavior that will make the mother–baby bond difficult to establish. Recall that gaze aversion and hyperextension are viewed as rejection of the parent by the neonate. Review therapeutic maternal–infant bonding if you had difficulty with this question.

References
Leifer, G. (2008). *Maternity nursing: An introductory text* (10th ed., p. 242). Philadelphia: Saunders.
Price, D., & Gwin, J. (2008). *Pediatric nursing: An introductory text* (10th ed., p. 68). St. Louis: Saunders.

---

489. A client will be self-administering an anticoagulant subcutaneously at home and says to the nurse, "I'm not sure I will be able to give myself these shots." Which statement by the nurse is appropriate?
1 "Maybe your wife can give you your shot."
2 "Don't worry. Your doctor knows what's best for you."
3 "You'll be fine after you get used to giving your own shots."
4 "What are your concerns about taking this medication at home?"

Level of Cognitive Ability: Application
Client Needs: Psychosocial Integrity

Answer: 4
Rationale: Option 4 restates the client's concern and provides the opportunity to verbalize feelings. Option 1 offers advice without knowing what the client's concerns really are. Options 2 and 3 identify false reassurance, which invalidates the client's concern.

Test-Taking Strategy: Use therapeutic communication techniques to answer this question. Remember to focus on the client's feelings and concerns; this will direct you to option 4. Review therapeutic communication techniques if you had difficulty with this question.

Reference
deWit, S. (2009). *Medical-surgical nursing: Concepts & practice* (p. 9). St. Louis: Saunders.

Integrated Process: Communication and Documentation
Content Area: Fundamental Skills

---

490. A pregnant client reports that her prescribed iron supplement is causing nausea, constipation, and heartburn and that she plans to stop the medication. The nurse's best response is:
1 "In time you will get used to the side effects."
2 "Your baby needs that iron, you can't stop taking it."
3 "Do not stop taking your medication without talking to the doctor."
4 "These gastric reactions are most intense during initial therapy and become less bothersome with continued use."

Level of Cognitive Ability: Application
Client Needs: Psychosocial Integrity
Integrated Process: Communication and Documentation
Content Area: Fundamental Skills

Answer: 4
Rationale: Pregnant clients need iron supplements because the fetus places extra demands on the maternal circulation. Option 4 addresses the issues that are bothersome to the client. Option 1 places the client's issue of the side effects on hold. Options 2 and 3 show disapproval of the client's feelings.

Test-Taking Strategy: Use therapeutic communication techniques. Remember to focus on the client's feelings and concerns; this will direct you to option 4. Review therapeutic communication techniques if you had difficulty with this question.

Reference
McKinney, E., James, S., Murray, S., & Ashwill, J. (2009). *Maternal-child nursing* (3rd ed., pp. 27-29, 648). St. Louis: Mosby.

---

491. A nurse is planning a dietary regimen with an anemic client when the client states, "My iron pills will have to do; I can't afford to buy any of that fancy food." The nurse should make which response to the client?
1 "This is very important, so pay attention."
2 "Why don't you ask your family for help?"
3 "Ground beef is not very expensive right now."
4 "Would you like for me to check into some options for you?"

Level of Cognitive Ability: Application
Client Needs: Psychosocial Integrity
Integrated Process: Communication and Documentation
Content Area: Fundamental Skills

Answer: 4
Rationale: Option 4 validates the concern that the client has with income. The nurse offers help in a nonthreatening manner that will allow the client to accept or decline. Options 1 and 3 block further communication by placing the client's issues on hold. Option 2 is requesting an explanation and uses the word *why*.

Test-Taking Strategy: Use therapeutic communication techniques to answer the question. Note that option 4 is the only option that addresses the client's concern. Remember to always focus on the client's concerns. Review therapeutic communication techniques if you had difficulty with this question.

Reference
deWit, S. (2009). *Medical-surgical nursing: Concepts & practice* (pp. 9, 365). St. Louis: Saunders.

---

492. A nurse is caring for a client who is scheduled for radiation therapy. Which client statement indicates the most common concern of clients receiving this therapy?

Answer: 1
Rationale: Radiation therapy is often a source of fear and misconceptions for clients and their families. Some of the most common fears and misconceptions include fear of being burned, fear of being radioactive, radioactive treatment, treatment failure, and

1 "Will I be radioactive afterwards?"
2 "I'm certain that this will do the trick."
3 "This is just one of several options that I have for treatment."
4 "This treatment is great because it is invisible and very effective."

Level of Cognitive Ability: Comprehension
Client Needs: Psychosocial Integrity
Integrated Process: Nursing Process/Data Collection
Content Area: Adult Health/Oncology

adverse effects. Options 2, 3, and 4 identify the need to provide additional information but they do not identify the most common client concern of radiation therapy.

Test-Taking Strategy: Focus on the subject of the question—the most common concern. Note the relationship between the words *radiation* in the question and *radioactive* in the correct option. Review radiation therapy if you had difficulty with this question.

Reference

deWit, S. (2009). *Medical-surgical nursing: Concepts & practice* (p. 173). St. Louis: Saunders.

---

493. A nurse understands that becoming familiar with the cultural beliefs and practices of a childbearing woman may facilitate positive outcomes during pregnancy because:
1 Safe-sex practices are common among couples 18 years old and older in all cultures.
2 All women are comfortable discussing sexual practices with their health care providers.
3 Most males from all cultures are knowledgeable about issues related to the spread of sexually transmitted diseases.
4 Many women exist in traditional relationships with their sexual partners; thus discussing and making decisions about reproductive issues may be difficult for some.

Level of Cognitive Ability: Comprehension
Client Needs: Psychosocial Integrity
Integrated Process: Nursing Process/Implementation
Content Area: Maternity/Antepartum

Answer: 4
Rationale: The nurse providing care to women in their childbearing years must be familiar with the cultural framework within which the client lives and operates. After this is achieved, appropriate communication techniques can be used to facilitate client care and to identify health-promotion educational strategies. Options 1, 2, and 3 generalize clients.

Test-Taking Strategy: Use the process of elimination. Eliminate options 1, 2, and 3 because of the close-ended word *all* in these options. In addition, these options identify situations that generalize childbearing clients. Review concepts related to cultural practices and differences if you had difficulty with this question.

Reference

Leifer, G. (2008). *Maternity nursing: An introductory text* (10th ed., p. 59). Philadelphia: Saunders.

---

494. While counseling a prenatal client about her dietary and drinking habits, the nurse observes that the client has difficulty concentrating and appears agitated. The nurse should proceed with data collection using which guideline?
1 A nonjudgmental approach may help to gain maternal trust.
2 A discussion of possible consequences of drinking during pregnancy should be avoided.
3 Provoking maternal guilt may help the woman to recognize her problem and seek support services.

Answer: 1
Rationale: The potential effects of alcohol abuse during pregnancy for both the mother and fetus have been well documented. The nurse who expresses genuine concern with suspected abusers may motivate positive behavioral changes during the antenatal period. The maternal behaviors of lack of concentration and agitation are frequently seen in childbearing women abusing alcohol. Options 2, 3, and 4 are inappropriate and inaccurate guidelines.

Test-Taking Strategy: Use therapeutic communication techniques to answer the question. Remember to display a nonjudgmental attitude and to focus on the client's feelings. Review therapeutic communication techniques if you had difficulty with this question.

4 Women respond negatively to a hopeful message regarding the potential benefits of drinking cessation during pregnancy.

Level of Cognitive Ability: Application
Clients Needs: Psychosocial Integrity
Integrated Process: Caring
Content Area: Maternity/Antepartum

Reference

Leifer, G. (2008). *Maternity nursing: An introductory text* (10th ed., pp. 7, 79). Philadelphia: Saunders.

---

495. A nurse is told during report that an assigned male client has a nursing diagnosis of *Disturbed body image* as a result of taking the prescribed medication spironolactone (Aldactone). The nurse suspects that this nursing diagnosis is based on which side effect of the medication?

1 Edema
2 Weight gain
3 Muscle atrophy
4 Decreased libido

Level of Cognitive Ability: Analysis
Client Needs: Psychosocial Integrity
Integrated Process: Nursing Process/Data Collection
Content Area: Pharmacology

Answer: 4

Rationale: Spironolactone (Aldactone) is a potassium-sparing diuretic. The nurse should be alert to the fact that the client taking spironolactone may experience body image changes as a result of threatened sexual identity. These body image changes are related to decreased libido, gynecomastia in males, and hirsutism in females. Edema, weight gain, and muscle atrophy are unrelated to this medication and nursing diagnosis.

Test-Taking Strategy: Use the process of elimination. Focusing on the nursing diagnosis and recalling the side effects of spironolactone will direct you to option 4. Review spironolactone if you had difficulty with this question.

Reference

Hodgson, B., & Kizior, R. (2009). *Saunders nursing drug handbook 2009* (pp. 1075-1077). St. Louis: Saunders.

---

496. A nurse is caring for a client who is experiencing psychomotor agitation. Which activity is most appropriate for the nurse to plan for the client?

1 Playing chess
2 Playing Ping-Pong
3 Reading magazines
4 Playing simple card games

Level of Cognitive Ability: Application
Client Needs: Psychosocial Integrity
Integrated Process: Nursing Process/Planning
Content Area: Mental Health

Answer: 2

Rationale: With psychomotor agitation, it is best to provide activities that involve the use of the hands and gross motor movements. These activities include Ping-Pong, volleyball, finger painting, drawing, and working with clay. These activities give the client an appropriate way of discharging motor tension. Options 3 and 4 are sedentary activities. Option 1 requires concentrating and a more intensive use of the thought processes.

Test-Taking Strategy: Use the process of elimination. Note the diagnosis of the client, and recall that activities that involve the use of the hands and gross motor movements are best for this client. Eliminate option 1 because this activity will require concentration, which this client may not have. Eliminate options 3 and 4 next because they will not provide a method for discharging motor tension. Review the care of a client with psychomotor agitation if you had difficulty with this question.

Reference

Fortinash, K., & Holoday-Worret, P. (2008). *Psychiatric mental health nursing* (4th ed., pp. 219, 534). St. Louis: Mosby.

---

497. A licensed practical nurse is assigned to care for a client with depression. The nurse reviews the client's plan of care and notes that the registered nurse has documented a nursing diagnosis of *Imbalanced nutrition, less than body requirements*. Which intervention is inappropriate for this client?

1. Remaining with the client during meals
2. Completing the food menu for the client during the depressed period
3. Offering high-protein, high-calorie fluids frequently throughout the day and evening
4. Offering small, high-calorie, high-protein snacks frequently throughout the day and evening

Level of Cognitive Ability: Application
Client Needs: Psychosocial Integrity
Integrated Process: Nursing Process/Planning
Content Area: Mental Health

Answer: 2
Rationale: It is inappropriate for the nurse to complete the food menu for the client. Instead, the client should be offered dietary choices and asked which foods or drinks he or she likes. The client is more likely to eat the foods provided if he or she has selected the foods and may have foods that he or she likes. The other options are appropriate interventions for the client with depression with this nursing diagnosis.

Test-Taking Strategy: Note the strategic word *inappropriate* in the question. Use the process of elimination, and focus on the intervention that may further impair nutritional intake. Review measures to improve nutritional intake in the depressed client if you had difficulty with this question.

Reference

Varcarolis, E., & Halter, M. (2009). *Essentials of psychiatric mental health nursing: A communication approach to evidence-based care* (p. 229). St. Louis: Saunders.

---

498. A licensed practical nurse (LPN) is assigned to care for a manic client. The nurse reviews the client's plan of care and notes that the registered nurse has documented a nursing diagnosis of *Impaired social interaction* related to altered thought processes. Which activity should the LPN initially provide for the client related to this nursing diagnosis?

1. Writing
2. Playing checkers
3. Playing cards with another client
4. Playing a board game with another client

Level of Cognitive Ability: Application
Client Needs: Psychosocial Integrity
Integrated Process: Nursing Process/Implementation
Content Area: Mental Health

Answer: 1
Rationale: When the client is manic, solitary activities that require a short attention span or mild physical exertion are best initially, such as writing, painting, finger painting, woodworking, or walking with the staff. Solitary activities minimize stimuli, and mild physical activities release tension constructively. When the client is less manic, he or she may join one or two other clients in quiet, nonstimulating activities. Competitive games should be avoided because they can stimulate aggression and cause increased psychomotor activity.

Test-Taking Strategy: Use the process of elimination. Note that options 2, 3, and 4 are comparable or alike in that they are all activities that involve another individual. Option 1 is the only solitary activity that will minimize stimuli. Review appropriate activities for the manic client if you had difficulty with this question.

References

Fortinash, K., & Holoday-Worret, P. (2008). *Psychiatric mental health nursing* (4th ed., p. 534). St. Louis: Mosby.
Varcarolis, E., & Halter, M. (2009). *Essentials of psychiatric mental health nursing: A communication approach to evidence-based care* (pp. 255-256). St. Louis: Saunders.

---

499. The nurse documents that a client with schizophrenia has an inappropriate affect. Which of the following describes this type of behavioral response as observed by the nurse?

1. The client is mumbling to himself or herself.

Answer: 4
Rationale: An inappropriate affect refers to an emotional response to a situation that is not congruent with the tone of the situation. A bizarre affect such as grimacing, giggling, or mumbling to one's self is marked when the client is unable to relate logically to the environment. A blunted affect is a minimal emotional response and expresses the client's outward affect; it may not coincide with

2 The client displays minimal emotional responses.
3 The client has an immobile facial expression or a blank look.
4 The client's emotional response to a situation is not congruent with the tone of the situation.

Level of Cognitive Ability: Comprehension
Client Needs: Psychosocial Integrity
Integrated Process: Nursing Process/Data Collection
Content Area: Mental Health

the client's inner emotions. A flat affect is an immobile facial expression or a blank look.

Test-Taking Strategy: Use the process of elimination, and focus on the subject—inappropriate affect. Note the relationship between the words *inappropriate* in the question and *not congruent* in the correct option. Review the behaviors exhibited by a client with schizophrenia if you had difficulty with this question.

Reference
Fortinash, K., & Holoday-Worret, P. (2008). *Psychiatric mental health nursing* (4th ed., pp. 259, 265). St. Louis: Mosby.

---

500. A nurse is gathering data from a male client who has just been admitted to the hospital with a diagnosis of coronary artery disease. During the interviewing process, the client tells the nurse that he has been quite stressed. The nurse should take which therapeutic action first?
1 Set up a psychiatric consult for the client.
2 Tell the client that everybody is stressed these days.
3 Have the client write down the sources of stress in his life.
4 Encourage the client to verbalize the sources of stress in his life.

Level of Cognitive Ability: Application
Client Needs: Psychosocial Integrity
Integrated Process: Nursing Process/Implementation
Content Area: Adult Health/Cardiovascular

Answer: 4
Rationale: The nurse encourages the client to verbalize his stressors so that strategies for coping with unavoidable stress can be explored. Option 1 is not within the nurse's scope of practice. Option 2 does not address the client's concerns. Option 3 may be appropriate but is not the first action.

Test-Taking Strategy: Use the process of elimination. Noting the strategic words *therapeutic action first* will assist with directing you to option 4. Remember to focus on the client's feelings first. Review therapeutic communication techniques if you had difficulty with this question.

Reference
deWit, S. (2009). *Medical-surgical nursing: Concepts & practice* (pp. 9, 493-494). St. Louis: Saunders.

---

501. A nurse is caring for a female client admitted to the hospital with a diagnosis of angina pectoris. The nurse is gathering data from the client, and, during the interviewing process, the client confidentially tells the nurse that she does recreational drugs such as cocaine. Knowing the effect that this medication has on the heart, the nurse should:
1 Report the client to the police for illegal drug use.
2 Tell the client about the need to stop using the drug.
3 Explain to the client what the drug is doing to her heart.

Answer: 4
Rationale: Option 4 is the best option. In this option, the nurse teaches the client about the effects of the drug, addresses the problem, and gets the client necessary help. Option 1 is incorrect because what the client is telling the nurse is confidential; at this time, the nurse would violate the client's rights. Option 2 is incorrect because the client has an addiction and the client has to want to stop taking the drug. Option 3 does not address the fact that the client has a problem with which she needs additional help.

Test-Taking Strategy: Use the process of elimination, and select the option that provides information to the client and that assists the client with the problem; this will direct you to option 4. Review the care of the client with a drug addiction if you had difficulty with this question.

4 Teach the client about the effects that cocaine has on the heart and plan to get the client further help.

Level of Cognitive Ability: Application
Client Needs: Psychosocial Integrity
Integrated Process: Nursing Process/Implementation
Content Area: Mental Health

References

deWit, S. (2009). *Medical-surgical nursing: Concepts & practice* (p. 1122). St. Louis: Saunders.
Fortinash, K., & Holoday-Worret, P. (2008). *Psychiatric mental health nursing* (4th ed., p. 325). St. Louis: Mosby.

---

502. A male client is admitted to the hospital with a diagnosis of myocardial infarction (MI). During the interviewing process, the client tells the nurse that the pain is probably related to the greasy cheeseburger he had for lunch. The nurse knows that this response from the client is common for people experiencing an MI and will be better able to help the client because:

1 A diet high in fat causes MI.
2 The client wants to blame something else for his problem.
3 Denial is a major factor in not seeking immediate treatment.
4 The client does not understand the factors that cause the disease process.

Level of Cognitive Ability: Comprehension
Client Needs: Psychosocial Integrity
Integrated Process: Nursing Process/Planning
Content Area: Adult Health/Cardiovascular

Answer: 3

Rationale: An individual's first response to the pain that he or she is experiencing is denial because the individual cannot believe that he or she is really having an MI; this in turn keeps the individual from seeking immediate medical treatment. Knowing that this is a common response, the nurse will be better able to help the client face the reality of the situation. Option 1 is not necessarily accurate, and there is not adequate data in the question to determine that options 2 and 4 are correct.

> *Test-Taking Strategy*: Use the process of elimination and your knowledge of the psychological effects that an individual experiences during an MI. Noting the strategic word *common* will direct you to option 3. Review the psychosocial effects of an MI if you had difficulty with this question.

Reference

deWit, S. (2009). *Medical-surgical nursing: Concepts & practice* (p. 499). St. Louis: Saunders.

---

503. A nurse assigned to care for a postpartum client will promote maternal–infant bonding when the nurse instructs the parents to:

1 Avoid using a high-pitched voice to speak to the infant.
2 Hold and cuddle the infant closely each time the infant cries.
3 Allow the infant to sleep in the parental bed between the parents.
4 Allow the nursing staff to assume the infant care in the hospital so that the parents may rest.

Level of Cognitive Ability: Application
Client Needs: Psychosocial Integrity
Integrated Process: Nursing Process/Implementation
Content Area: Maternity/Postpartum

Answer: 2

Rationale: Holding and cuddling the infant closely initiates a positive experience for the mother. It is self-quieting and consoles the infant. The use of a high-pitched voice and participating in infant care are other methods of promoting maternal–infant attachment. An infant should not be allowed to sleep in the parental bed between parents because of the danger of suffocation and because the couple will require meaningful rest and time to be alone as a couple.

> *Test-Taking Strategy*: Note the strategic word *promote,* and use the process of elimination. Option 2 is the only option that addresses the issue of bonding. Review measures that promote maternal–infant bonding if you had difficulty with this question.

Reference

Leifer, G. (2008). *Maternity nursing: An introductory text* (10th ed., p. 242). Philadelphia: Saunders.

504. A nurse is assigned to care for a postpartum client. When collecting data regarding the new mother's parental anxieties, which client statement indicates a potential problem with maternal–infant attachment?

1. "I just feel weepy all the time."
2. "He has his daddy's deep blue eyes."
3. "Why did this baby have to inherit my family's ugly toes?
4. "I am too tired to feed him right now; let the nursery nurse do it this once."

Level of Cognitive Ability: Comprehension
Client Needs: Psychosocial Integrity
Integrated Process: Nursing Process/Data Collection
Content Area: Maternity/Postpartum

Answer: 3
Rationale: Negativity about the baby's features may interfere with the mother's ability to bond with and care for the infant. Positive statements and identification with family members help the mother to identify with the infant, thus promoting attachment. Fatigue and mild postpartum depression are expected responses and may cause the mother to feel weepy and to request the staff to assume care of the infant temporarily; however, after a period of rest, the mother should begin to assume the care of the infant.

Test-Taking Strategy: Focus on the subject of the question, and note the strategic words *potential problem with maternal–infant attachment.* Use the process of elimination to direct you to option 3. Review the factors that affect maternal–infant attachment if you had difficulty with this question.

References
Leifer, G. (2007). *Introduction to maternity and pediatric nursing* (5th ed., p. 220). Philadelphia: Saunders.
Leifer, G. (2008). *Maternity nursing: An introductory text* (10th ed., p. 242). Philadelphia: Saunders.

---

505. A young adult male client with spinal cord injury (SCI) tells the nurse, "It's so depressing that I'll never get to have sex again." The nurse replies in a realistic way by making which statement to the client?

1. "It must feel horrible to know you can never have sex again."
2. "It is still possible to have a sexual relationship, but it is different."
3. "You're young, so you'll adapt to this more easily than if you were older."
4. "Because of body reflexes, sexual functioning will be no different than before."

Level of Cognitive Ability: Application
Client Needs: Psychosocial Integrity
Integrated Process: Communication and Documentation
Content Area: Adult Health/Neurological

Answer: 2
Rationale: It is possible to have a sexual relationship after an SCI, but it will be different than what the client experienced before the injury. Males may experience reflex erections, although they may not ejaculate. Females can have adductor spasm. Sexual counseling may help the client to adapt to changes in sexuality after an SCI. Option 1 does not promote continued discussion of the client's concerns. Options 3 and 4 are incorrect statements.

Test-Taking Strategy: Knowledge regarding the altered physiology after SCI and therapeutic communication techniques will assist you with answering the question. Eliminate options 3 and 4 first because they are incorrect statements. Eliminate option 1 next because it is a communication block. Review the effects of an SCI and therapeutic communication techniques if you had difficulty with this question.

References
Christensen, B., & Kockrow, E. (2006). *Adult health nursing* (5th ed., p. 745). St. Louis: Mosby.
deWit, S. (2009). *Medical-surgical nursing: Concepts & practice* (p. 9). St. Louis: Saunders.

---

506. A family member of a client who was just diagnosed with a brain tumor is distraught and feeling guilty for not encouraging the client to seek medical evaluation earlier. The nurse plans to incorporate which item when formulating a response to this family member's verbal concern?

1. There are no symptoms of brain tumor.

Answer: 4
Rationale: The signs and symptoms of a brain tumor vary depending on the location of the tumor, and they may easily be attributed to another cause. Symptoms include headache, vomiting, seizures, visual disturbances, and changes in intellectual ability or personality. The family needs support to assist them during the normal grieving process. Options 1, 2, and 3 are incorrect.

2 It is true that brain tumors are easily recognizable.
3 Brain tumors are never detected until very late in their course.
4 The symptoms of brain tumor may be easily attributed to another cause.

Level of Cognitive Ability: Application
Client Needs: Psychosocial Integrity
Integrated Process: Nursing Process/Planning
Content Area: Adult Health/Neurological

Test-Taking Strategy: Use the process of elimination. Eliminate options 1 and 3 first because they contain the close-ended words *no* and *never*, respectively. From the remaining options, it is necessary to know that the symptoms of brain tumor can be vague and that they may easily be attributed to another cause. Review the signs and symptoms of a brain tumor if you had difficulty with this question.

Reference

Linton, A. (2007). *Introduction to medical-surgical nursing* (4th ed., pp. 441-442). Philadelphia: Saunders.

---

507. A client has had extensive surgery on the gastrointestinal tract and has been started on parenteral nutrition (PN).The client tells the nurse, "I think I'm going crazy. I feel like I'm starving and yet that bag is supposed to be feeding me." The best response by the nurse would be:
1 "Don't worry. Many others in your situation say the same thing."
2 "That is unusual. I wonder if the solution is being mixed correctly."
3 "Maybe you should ask your doctor about that; I've never heard of that before."
4 "That is because the empty stomach sends signals to the brain to stimulate hunger."

Level of Cognitive Ability: Application
Client Needs: Psychosocial Integrity
Integrated Process: Nursing Process/Implementation
Content Area: Fundamental Skills

Answer: 4
Rationale: When it is empty, the stomach does send signals to the brain to stimulate hunger. The client should be told that this is normal. Some clients also experience food cravings for the same reason. Options 1 and 3 will block the communication process. Option 2 will produce fear.

Test-Taking Strategy: Use the process of elimination and therapeutic communication techniques to answer the question. Begin to answer this question by eliminating option 2 first; this statement could frighten the client and lessen the client's trust in the health care team. Eliminate options 1 and 3 next because these statements block communication and do not respond to the client's concerns. Option 4 is the only response that acknowledges the client's concern and addresses it. Review therapeutic communication techniques and the physiological principles related to PN if you had difficulty with this question.

References

Black, J., & Hawks, J. (2009). *Medical-surgical nursing: Clinical management for positive outcomes* (8th ed., p. 578). St. Louis: Saunders.
Perry, A., & Potter, P. (2010). *Clinical nursing skills & techniques* (7th ed., p. 851). St. Louis: Mosby.

---

508. A licensed practical nurse (LPN) observes a nursing assistant talking in an unusually loud voice to a client with delirium. Which of these actions should the LPN take?
1 Inform the client that everything is all right.
2 Speak to the nursing assistant immediately while in the client's room to solve the problem.
3 Explain to the nursing assistant that yelling in the client's room is tolerated only if the client is talking loudly.
4 Determine the client's safety, ask the nursing assistant to step outside of the client's room, and inform the nursing assistant of the observation.

Answer: 4
Rationale: The nurse must determine that the client is safe and then discuss the matter with the nursing assistant in an area in which the conversation cannot be heard by the client. If the client hears the conversation, the client may become more confused or agitated. Option 1 is a communication block. Options 2 and 3 could add to the client's confusion. In addition, option 2 could embarrass the nursing assistant.

Test-Taking Strategy: Use Maslow's Hierarchy of Needs theory and therapeutic communication techniques. Option 1 is eliminated first because it is a communication block. Next, recall that safety needs are a priority; this will direct you to option 4. Review therapeutic communication techniques if you had difficulty with this question.

Level of Cognitive Ability: Application
Client Needs: Psychosocial Integrity
Integrated Process: Nursing Process/Implementation
Content Area: Leadership/Management

References
deWit, S. (2009). *Medical-surgical nursing: Concepts & practice* (pp. 4, 9). St. Louis: Saunders.
Fortinash, K., & Holoday-Worret, P. (2008). *Psychiatric mental health nursing* (4th ed., pp. 521-522). St. Louis: Mosby.

---

509. A teenager who has celiac disease presents with profuse watery diarrhea after a pizza party the previous night. The client states, "I don't want to be different from my friends." The nurse determines that the client is at most risk for which psychosocial problem?
1 Celiac crisis
2 Dehydration
3 Altered self-esteem
4 Lack of understanding about the disease process

Answer: 3
Rationale: The client expresses concern about being different. Data provided in the question do not support a lack of understanding about the disease process. Dehydration and celiac crisis are physiological problems.

Test-Taking Strategy: Note the strategic words *psychosocial problem.* Focus on the data in the question, and focus on the subject—the client's feelings of being different; this should direct you to option 3. Review the psychosocial issues of an adolescent with a chronic disorder if you had difficulty with this question.

Level of Cognitive Ability: Analysis
Client Needs: Psychosocial Integrity
Integrated Process: Nursing Process/Data Collection
Content Area: Child Health

Reference
Leifer, G. (2007). *Introduction to maternity and pediatric nursing* (5th ed., p. 623). Philadelphia: Saunders.

---

510. A nurse is assisting with developing a plan of care for a 1-month-old infant hospitalized for intussusception. Which measure is effective for providing psychosocial support for the parent–child relationship?
1 Provide educational materials.
2 Encourage the parents to room-in with the infant.
3 Initiate home nutritional support as early as possible.
4 Encourage the parents to go home and get some sleep.

Answer: 2
Rationale: Rooming-in is effective for reducing separation anxiety and preserving the parent–child relationship. It is stressful for the parents when a child is ill and hospitalized. Telling a parent to go home and sleep will not relieve this stress. Although they are beneficial, educational materials will not provide psychosocial support for the parent–child relationship. Home nutritional support is not usually necessary to treat intussusception.

Test-Taking Strategy: Use the process of elimination, and focus on the strategic words *providing psychosocial support.* Note that option 2 is the only option that provides an interaction between the child and the parents. Review the measures that provide psychosocial support for parents if you had difficulty with this question.

Level of Cognitive Ability: Application
Client Needs: Psychosocial Integrity
Integrated Process: Nursing Process/Planning
Content Area: Child Health

Reference
Leifer, G. (2007). *Introduction to maternity and pediatric nursing* (5th ed., pp. 474-475). Philadelphia: Saunders.

---

511. The parents of a male infant who will have an inguinal hernia repair make the following comments. Which comment requires follow-up evaluation by a nurse?

Answer: 2
Rationale: The anatomical location of hernias frequently causes more psychological concern to the parents than does the actual condition or treatment; the parents may think that the disorder affects future reproductive ability. Options 1, 3, and 4 all indicate the parents' accurate understanding.

1 "I understand that surgery will repair the hernia."
2 "I don't know if he will be able to father a child."
3 "We were told to give him sponge baths for a few days after surgery."
4 "I'll need to buy extra diapers because we need to change them more frequently now."

Level of Cognitive Ability: Analysis
Client Needs: Psychosocial Integrity
Integrated Process: Nursing Process/Data Collection
Content Area: Child Health

Test-Taking Strategy: Focus on the strategic words *requires follow-up evaluation.* Option 2 reflects parental fear and identifies a need for further assistance. Review parental concerns and the care of the infant requiring inguinal hernia repair if you had difficulty with this question.

Reference

Hockenberry, M., & Wilson, D. (2009). *Wong's essentials of pediatric care* (8th ed., p. 958). St. Louis: Mosby.

---

512. A licensed practical nurse is assisting a school nurse with conducting a crisis intervention group. The clients are high school students whose classmate recently committed suicide at the school. The students are experiencing disbelief and reviewing details about finding the student dead in a bathroom. Based on this information, the nurse should first:
1 Reinforce the students' sense of growth through this death.
2 Inquire how the students coped with death events in the past.
3 Reinforce the students' ability to work through this death event.
4 Inquire about the students' perception of their classmate's suicide.

Level of Cognitive Ability: Application
Client Needs: Psychosocial Integrity
Integrated Process: Nursing Process/Data Collection
Content Area: Mental Health

Answer: 4
Rationale: It is essential to first determine the students' perception. Inquiring about the students' perception of the death will specifically identify the appraisal of the suicide and the meaning of the perception. Options 1 and 3 are comparable or alike in that they attempt to foster clients' self-esteem; such an approach is premature at this point. Although option 2 is exploratory, it does not address the "here and now" appraisal in terms of the classmate's suicide. Although the nurse is interested in how clients have coped in the past, this inquiry should not be the most immediate.

Test-Taking Strategy: Use the process of elimination, and note the strategic word *first.* Consider the subject of the question, and select the option that deals with the here and now. The nurse must first determine the clients' perception or appraisal of the stressful event. Review the phases of crisis if you had difficulty with this question.

Reference

Varcarolis, E., & Halter, M. (2009). *Essentials of psychiatric mental health nursing: A communication approach to evidence-based care* (pp. 417, 422). St. Louis: Saunders.

---

513. A client recovering from a head injury becomes agitated at times. Which action will most likely calm this client?
1 Giving the client a soft object to hold
2 Assigning the client a new task to master
3 Turning the television on to a musical program
4 Making the client aware that the behavior is undesirable

Answer: 1
Rationale: Decreasing environmental stimuli aids in reducing agitation for the head-injured client. Option 2 does not simplify the environment; a new task may be frustrating. Option 3 increases stimuli. Option 4 identifies a nontherapeutic approach. The correct option helps to distract the client with a motor activity—holding a soft object.

Test-Taking Strategy: Use the process of elimination to identify options that may increase stimuli, agitation, and frustration; this should direct you to option 1. Review measures that will decrease agitation if you had difficulty with this question.

Level of Cognitive Ability: Application
Client Needs: Psychosocial Integrity
Integrated Process: Nursing Process/Implementation
Content Area: Adult Health/Neurological

Reference

deWit, S. (2009). *Medical-surgical nursing: Concepts & practice* (p. 549). St. Louis: Saunders.

---

514. A client recovering from a brain attack (stroke) has become irritable and angry about the associated limitations. The nurse should take which approach to help the client regain motivation to succeed?

1 Use supportive statements to correct behavior.
2 Ignore the behavior, knowing that the client is grieving.
3 Allow longer and more frequent visitation with the spouse.
4 State that nursing experience lets the nurse know how the client feels.

Answer: 1

Rationale: Clients who have had brain attacks (strokes) have many and varied needs. The client may need negative behaviors pointed out so that correction can take place, as well as support and praise for accomplishments. The client may be grieving or may have damage to cerebral inhibitory centers; however, the behavior should not be ignored. Spouses of stroke clients are often grieving, so more visits may not be helpful; short visits are often encouraged. Stating that you know how someone feels is inappropriate.

Test-Taking Strategy: Use therapeutic communication techniques. Option 1 is the only option that addresses client feelings and supportive care. Review the care of the client after a brain attack (stroke) if you had difficulty with this question.

Level of Cognitive Ability: Application
Client Needs: Psychosocial Integrity
Integrated Process: Nursing Process/Implementation
Content Area: Adult Health/Neurological

Reference

Linton, A. (2007). *Introduction to medical-surgical nursing* (4th ed., pp. 479-480). Philadelphia: Saunders.

---

515. A client is admitted to the hospital with a broken hip and is experiencing periods of confusion. The nurse assists with developing a plan of care related to disturbed thought processes. The nurse understands that the psychosocial outcome that has the highest priority is:

1 Improved sleep patterns
2 Reducing family fears and anxiety
3 Independently meeting self-care needs
4 Increased ability to concentrate and make decisions

Answer: 4

Rationale: The client should be able to concentrate and make decisions. When the client is able to do that, the nurse can work with the client to achieve the other outcomes. Options 1, 2, and 3 are goals that are secondary to option 4.

Test-Taking Strategy: Use the process of elimination, and note the strategic words *highest priority*. Look for the option that will have the greatest impact on the client's ability to function. Option 1 is unrelated to the primary issue. Option 2 can be easily eliminated because it does not address the information presented in the question. Option 3 is unrealistic at this time, considering that the word *independently* is in this option. Option 4 will make the greatest difference in the client's ability to achieve options 1, 2, and 3. Review the goals of care of the client with disturbed thought processes if you had difficulty with this question.

Level of Cognitive Ability: Analysis
Client Needs: Psychosocial Integrity
Integrated Process: Nursing Process/Planning
Content Area: Adult Health/Musculoskeletal

References

Black, J., & Hawks, J. (2009). *Medical-surgical nursing: Clinical management for positive outcomes* (8th ed., p. 529). St. Louis: Saunders.
Linton, A. (2007). *Introduction to medical-surgical nursing* (4th ed., p. 930). Philadelphia: Saunders.

---

516. The client is a young woman dying from breast cancer. A defining characteristic of anticipatory grief is present when the client:

1 Discusses thoughts and feelings related to loss
2 Has prolonged emotional reactions and outbursts
3 Verbalizes unrealistic goals and plans for the future
4 Ignores untreated medical conditions that require treatment

Level of Cognitive Ability: Analysis
Client Needs: Psychosocial Integrity
Integrated Process: Nursing Process/Data Collection
Content Area: Adult Health/Neurological

Answer: 1
Rationale: The nurse can determine the client's stage of grief by observing behavior. This is extremely important so that an appropriate plan of care can be developed. Option 1 identifies anticipatory grief. Options 2, 3, and 4 are examples of dysfunctional grieving.

Test-Taking Strategy: Use the process of elimination. Note that options 2, 3, and 4 are comparable or alike, and note the words *prolonged, unrealistic,* and *ignores* in these options, respectively. These are examples of dysfunctional grieving. Review the stages of grief and anticipatory grief if you had difficulty with this question.

Reference
deWit, S. (2009). *Medical-surgical nursing: Concepts & practice* (p. 965). St. Louis: Saunders.

---

517. A licensed practical nurse notes that a client in labor is beginning to experience signs of shock from hemorrhage secondary to a partial inversion of the uterus and immediately notifies the registered nurse. The client asks, in an apprehensive voice, "What is happening to me? I feel so funny and I know I am bleeding. Am I dying?" The nurse bases the response on the fact that the client is feeling:

1 Panic secondary to shock
2 Anticipatory grieving related to the fear of dying
3 Depression related to postpartum hormonal changes
4 Anxiety related to unexpected and ambiguous sensations

Level of Cognitive Ability: Application
Client Needs: Psychosocial Integrity
Integrated Process: Nursing Process/Implementation
Content Area: Maternity/Intrapartum

Answer: 4
Rationale: Feelings of loss of control because of the unknown are common causes of anxiety. Apprehension and feelings of impending doom are also associated with shock, but the case situation does not suggest panic at this point. Anticipatory grieving occurs when there is knowledge of an impending loss, but it is not operative in a sudden situational crisis such as this one. It is far too early for the onset of postpartum depression.

Test-Taking Strategy: Use the process of elimination, and note the strategic words *apprehensive voice* in the question. Note the relationship between the words *I feel so funny* in the question and *unexpected and ambiguous sensations* in the correct option. Review the causes of anxiety if you had difficulty with this question.

Reference
Leifer, G. (2007). *Introduction to maternity and pediatric nursing* (5th ed., pp. 184, 186). Philadelphia: Saunders.

---

518. A nurse has just assessed the fetal status of a client with a diagnosis of partial placental abruption at 20 weeks' gestation. The client is experiencing new bleeding and reports less fetal movement; the nurse informs the client that the physician has been notified. The client begins to cry quietly while holding her

Answer: 3
Rationale: Anticipatory grieving occurs when a client has knowledge of an impending loss. The first stages of anticipatory grieving may be characterized by shock, emotional numbness, disbelief, and strong emotions such as tears, screaming, or anger. Anticipatory grieving is appropriate when any signs of fetal distress accelerate. There is no indication of pain or confusion or that the death of the fetus has occurred.

abdomen with her hands, and she murmurs, "No, no, you can't go, my little man." The nurse recognizes the client's behavior as an indication of:
1 Acute confusion secondary to shock
2 Acute pain related to abdominal pain
3 Anticipatory grieving related to perceived potential loss
4 Decisional conflict related to the death of the fetus and to fear and loss

Level of Cognitive Ability: Analysis
Client Needs: Psychosocial Integrity
Integrated Process: Nursing Process/Data Collection
Content Area: Maternity/Antepartum

Test-Taking Strategy: Focus on the data in the question, and use the process of elimination. Options 1 and 2 can be eliminated because there is no indication of confusion or pain. Note that, in this situation, there is a situational crisis with feelings of grief, but no loss has occurred at this point; thus option 4 can be eliminated. Review the characteristics of anticipatory grieving if you had difficulty with this question.

Reference
Leifer, G. (2007). *Introduction to maternity and pediatric nursing* (5th ed., p. 85). Philadelphia: Saunders.

---

519. A postoperative client has been vomiting, and ileus has been diagnosed. The physician orders the insertion of a nasogastric tube. After explaining the purpose and insertion procedure to the client, the client says to the nurse, "I'm not sure I can take any more of this treatment." The appropriate response by the nurse is:
1 "Let the doctor put the tube down so you can get well."
2 "It is your right to refuse any procedure. I'll notify the physician."
3 "If you don't have this tube put down, you will just continue to vomit."
4 "You are feeling tired and frustrated with your recovery from surgery?"

Level of Cognitive Ability: Application
Client Needs: Psychosocial Integrity
Integrated Process: Communication and Documentation
Content Area: Adult Health/Gastrointestinal

Answer: 4
Rationale: Option 4 assists the client with expressing and exploring feelings, which can lead to problem solving. The other options are examples of barriers to effective communication in that the nurse does not address the client's concerns.

Test-Taking Strategy: Use therapeutic communication techniques. Option 4 is an open-ended question and a communication tool that focuses on the client's feelings. Review therapeutic communication techniques if you had difficulty with this question.

Reference
deWit, S. (2009). *Medical-surgical nursing: Concepts & practice* (pp. 9, 720). St. Louis: Saunders.

---

520. A client is admitted to the hospital with a bowel obstruction secondary to a recurrent malignancy, and the physician inserts a Miller-Abbott tube. After the procedure, the client asks the nurse, "Do you think this is worth all this trouble?" The appropriate action or response by the nurse is:
1 "Let's give this tube a chance."
2 Staying with the client and being silent
3 "Are you wondering whether you are going to get better? "
4 "I remember a case similar to yours, and the tube relieved the obstruction."

Answer: 3
Rationale: The nurse needs to use therapeutic communication tools when assisting a client with a chronic terminal illness to express feelings. The nurse should listen attentively to the client and use clarifying and focusing to assist the client with expressing his or her feelings. Changing the subject (option 1), responding with inappropriate silence (option 2), and offering false reassurance (option 4) are examples of barriers to communication.

Test-Taking Strategy: Use therapeutic communication techniques. Option 3 encourages the client to verbalize, whereas options 1, 2, and 4 are blocks to communication. Review therapeutic communication techniques if you had difficulty with this question.

Level of Cognitive Ability: Application
Client Needs: Psychosocial Integrity
Integrated Process: Communication and Documentation
Content Area: Adult Health/Oncology

References
deWit, S. (2009). *Medical-surgical nursing: Concepts & practice* (p. 9). St. Louis: Saunders.
Linton, A. (2007). *Introduction to medical-surgical nursing* (4th ed., p. 781). Philadelphia: Saunders.

---

521. A client receiving parenteral nutrition and intralipids says to the nurse, "I was always overweight until I had this illness. I'm not sure I want to get that fat. The other intravenous fluids are probably enough." The nurse should make which initial response to the client?

1 "I understand what you mean. I've dieted most of my life."
2 "I think you need to discuss this decision with the physician."
3 "Tell me how being ill has affected the way you think of yourself."
4 "Fatty acids are essential for life. You'll develop deficiencies without the fats."

Answer: 3
Rationale: Clients receiving long-term parenteral nutrition are at risk for the development of essential fatty acid deficiency. However, the client's response requires more than an informational response initially. The nurse uses tools of therapeutic communication to assist the client with expressing feelings and dealing with the aspects of illness and treatment. Blocks to communication, such as giving opinions (option 1), placing the client's feelings on hold (option 2), and giving information too soon (option 4), will not assist the client with coping effectively.

Test-Taking Strategy: Use therapeutic communication techniques. Option 3 is the only option that encourages the client to express feelings. Review therapeutic communication techniques if you had difficulty with this question.

Level of Cognitive Ability: Application
Client Needs: Psychosocial Integrity
Integrated Process: Communication and Documentation
Content Area: Fundamental Skills

References
deWit, S. (2009). *Medical-surgical nursing: Concepts & practice* (p. 9). St. Louis: Saunders.
Linton, A. (2007). *Introduction to medical-surgical nursing* (4th ed., p. 119). Philadelphia: Saunders.

---

522. A client has terminal cancer, is using opioid analgesics for pain relief, and is concerned about becoming addicted to the pain medication. The nurse allays this anxiety by:

1 Encouraging the client to hold off as long as possible between doses of pain medication
2 Telling the client to take lower doses of medications even though the pain is not well controlled
3 Explaining to the client that addiction rarely occurs in people who are taking medication to relieve pain
4 Explaining to the client that his or her fears are justified but should be of no concern during the final stages of illness

Answer: 3
Rationale: Clients who are on opioid analgesics often have well-founded fears about addiction, even in the face of pain. The nurse has a responsibility to give correct information about the likelihood of addiction while still maintaining adequate pain control. Addiction is rare for individuals who are taking medication to relieve pain. Allowing the client to be in pain, as in options 1 and 2, is not acceptable nursing practice. Option 4 is correct only in that it acknowledges the client's fear, but addressing the final stages of illness is inappropriate at this time.

Test-Taking Strategy: Use the process of elimination. Eliminate options 1 and 2 because these are not acceptable nursing practices. Eliminate option 4 because it is only partially correct. Review pain management if you had difficulty with this question.

Reference
deWit, S. (2009). *Medical-surgical nursing: Concepts & practice* (p. 145). St. Louis: Saunders.

Level of Cognitive Ability: Application
Client Needs: Psychosocial Integrity
Integrated Process: Caring
Content Area: Adult Health/Oncology

523. A client is highly anxious about receiving chest physical therapy (CPT) for the first time. When planning the client's care, the nurse reassures the client that:

1 There are no risks associated with CPT.
2 CPT will assist the client with coughing more effectively.
3 CPT will resolve all of the client's respiratory symptoms.
4 CPT will assist with mobilizing secretions to enhance more effective breathing.

Level of Cognitive Ability: Application
Client Needs: Psychosocial Integrity
Integrated Process: Nursing Process/Planning
Content Area: Adult Health/Respiratory

Answer: 4

Rationale: CPT is a respiratory treatment that will mobilize secretions to enhance more effective breathing. There are risks associated with CPT, including cardiac, gastrointestinal, neurological, and pulmonary complications. CPT will indirectly assist the client with coughing if the secretions have been mobilized and the cough stimulus is present. CPT is an intervention to assist with clearing secretions, but it will not resolve all respiratory symptoms.

Test-Taking Strategy: Use the process of elimination, and focus on the subject of the question—the purpose of CPT. Eliminate options 1 and 3 because of the close-ended words *no* and *all*, respectively. From the remaining options, focusing on the subject will direct you to option 4. Review the purpose of CPT if you had difficulty with this question.

Reference

Linton, A. (2007). *Introduction to medical-surgical nursing* (4th ed., p. 523). Philadelphia: Saunders.

---

524. A client with cardiomyopathy stops eating, takes long naps, and turns away from the nurse when the nurse is speaking. The nurse identifies that the client may be experiencing which of the following?

1 Depression
2 Intractable pain
3 Mild discomfort
4 Activity intolerance

Level of Cognitive Ability: Analysis
Client Needs: Psychosocial Integrity
Integrated Process: Nursing Process/Data Collection
Content Area: Adult Health/Cardiovascular

Answer: 1

Rationale: Depression is a common problem among clients who have long-term and debilitating illnesses. Options 2, 3, and 4 are not associated with the information in the question.

Test-Taking Strategy: Focus on the data provided in the question, and use the process of elimination. Noting the words *stops eating, takes long naps, and turns away from the nurse* will direct you to option 1. Review the signs of depression if you had difficulty with this question.

References

deWit, S. (2009). *Medical-surgical nursing: Concepts & practice* (p. 499). St. Louis: Saunders.
Linton, A. (2007). *Introduction to medical-surgical nursing* (4th ed., p. 1257). Philadelphia: Saunders.

---

525. Which short-term psychosocial intervention is important for a pregnant client who has been hospitalized for the stabilization of diabetes mellitus?

1 Be alert to the risks of early labor and birth.
2 Protect the client from risk of injury secondary to convulsions.
3 Teach the client and her family about diabetes mellitus and its implications.
4 Provide emotional support and education about interrupted family processes related to the pregnant client's hospitalization.

Level of Cognitive Ability: Analysis
Client Needs: Psychosocial Integrity

Answer: 4

Rationale: The short-term psychosocial well-being of the family is at risk because of the hospitalization of the mother. Teaching about diabetes mellitus is a long-term intervention and is more physiological in nature. Options 1 and 2 are unrelated to diabetes mellitus, are physiological, and are more related to gestational hypertension (pregnancy-induced hypertension).

Test-Taking Strategy: Use the process of elimination, and note the strategic word *psychosocial.* Eliminate options 1 and 2 because they are unrelated to diabetes mellitus and are physiological. From the remaining options, note the words *short-term psychosocial intervention;* this should direct you to option 4. Review the psychosocial aspects of the care of a pregnant client with diabetes mellitus if you had difficulty with this question.

Integrated Process: Nursing Process/Planning
Content Area: Maternity/Antepartum

Reference

Leifer, G. (2007). *Introduction to maternity and pediatric nursing* (5th ed., p. 101). Philadelphia: Saunders.

---

526. A new parent is trying to decide whether or not to have her baby boy circumcised. The nurse should make which statement to the mother to assist her with making this decision?

1 "I had my son circumcised, and I am so glad."
2 "Circumcision is a difficult decision. Let's discuss the questions that you have."
3 "You know, they say it prevents cancer and sexually transmitted infections, so I would definitely have my son circumcised."
4 "Circumcision is a difficult decision, but your physician is the best, and you know it's better to get it done now rather than later."

Level of Cognitive Ability: Application
Client Needs: Psychosocial Integrity
Integrated Process: Communication and Documentation
Content Area: Maternity/Postpartum

Answer: 2

Rationale: Circumcision can be a difficult decision for parents, and the nurse should provide the client with the opportunity to discuss feelings and concerns and to ask questions. Options 1, 3, and 4 identify nontherapeutic communication techniques in that they offer personal opinion and advice to the client. The nurse's personal thoughts and feelings should not be part of the educational process.

Test-Taking Strategy: Use the process of elimination. Eliminate options 1 and 3 because they are comparable or alike. In addition, options 1, 3, and 4 are communication blocks because the nurse is providing a personal opinion to the client. Informed decision making is the key point to consider when selecting the correct option in this question. Review therapeutic communication techniques and teaching and learning principles if you had difficulty with this question.

Reference

Leifer, G. (2008). *Maternity nursing: An introductory text* (10th ed., p. 195). Philadelphia: Saunders.

---

527. A nurse is assisting with planning care for a client who is experiencing anxiety after a myocardial infarction. Which nursing intervention should be included in the plan of care?

1 Answer questions with factual information.
2 Provide detailed explanations of all procedures.
3 Limit family involvement during the acute phase.
4 Administer antianxiety medication at least every 4 hours around the clock.

Level of Cognitive Ability: Application
Client Needs: Psychosocial Integrity
Integrated Process: Nursing Process/Planning
Content Area: Adult Health/Cardiovascular

Answer: 1

Rationale: Accurate information reduces fear, strengthens the nurse–client relationship, and assists the client with dealing realistically with the situation. Providing detailed information may increase the client's anxiety; the information provided should be simple and clear. Limiting family involvement may or may not be helpful, because the client's family may be a source of support for the client. Although antianxiety medication may be helpful, administering it at least every 4 hours around the clock is excessive.

Test-Taking Strategy: Use the process of elimination. Eliminate option 4 because medication should not be the first intervention used to alleviate anxiety. In addition, administering antianxiety medication at least every 4 hours around the clock is excessive. Eliminate option 2 next because of the word *detailed.* From the remaining options, eliminate option 3 because limiting family involvement does not reduce anxiety in all situations. Review measures to use to relieve anxiety if you had difficulty with this question.

References

deWit, S. (2009). *Medical-surgical nursing: Concepts & practice* (pp. 499, 1105). St. Louis: Saunders.
Ignatavicius, D., & Workman, M. (2010). *Medical-surgical nursing: Patient-centered collaborative care* (6th ed., p. 713). St. Louis: Saunders.

---

528. A client recovering from an acute myocardial infarction will be discharged from the hospital the next day. Which client action on the evening before discharge suggests that the client is in the denial phase of grieving?

1 Expresses hesitancy to leave the hospital
2 Requests a sedative for sleep at 10:00 PM
3 Consumes 25% of the foods and fluids given for supper
4 Walks up and down three flights of stairs without supervision

Level of Cognitive Ability: Analysis
Client Needs: Psychosocial Integrity
Integrated Process: Nursing Process/Data Collection
Content Area: Adult Health/Cardiovascular

Answer: 4
Rationale: Ignoring activity limitations and avoiding lifestyle changes are signs of denial during the process of grieving. Walking up and down three flights of stairs should be a supervised activity during the rehabilitation process. Option 1 may be a manifestation of anxiety or fear rather than denial. Option 2 is an appropriate client action on the evening before discharge. Option 3 is a manifestation of depression rather than denial.

Test-Taking Strategy: Use the process of elimination, and focus on the subject—the denial phase. Option 1 identifies anxiety or fear. Option 2 is an appropriate client action. Option 3 identifies depression. Option 4 is the only option that suggests denial in the client. Review the signs of denial if you had difficulty with this question.

Reference
deWit, S. (2009). *Medical-surgical nursing: Concepts & practice* (p. 499). St. Louis: Saunders.

---

529. Which statement by a client indicates a positive coping mechanism to be used during treatment for Hodgkin's disease?

1 "I will not leave the house bald."
2 "I know losing my hair won't bother me."
3 "I will be one of the few who don't lose their hair."
4 "I have selected a wig even though I will miss my own hair."

Level of Cognitive Ability: Analysis
Client Needs: Psychosocial Integrity
Integrated Process: Nursing Process/Evaluation
Content Area: Adult Health/Oncology

Answer: 4
Rationale: A combination of radiation and chemotherapy often causes alopecia in clients with Hodgkin's disease. To use positive coping mechanisms, the client must identify personal feelings and use problem-solving positive interventions to deal with the side effects of treatment. Option 4 is the only option that indicates a positive coping mechanism.

Test-Taking Strategy: Use the process of elimination, and note the strategic words *positive coping mechanism.* Options 1 and 3 involve avoidance, and option 2 indicates denial. Option 4 is the only option that addresses a positive coping mechanism. Review positive coping mechanisms if you had difficulty with this question.

Reference
Christensen, B., & Kockrow, E. (2006). *Adult health nursing* (5th ed., pp. 318-319, 834-835). St. Louis: Mosby.

---

530. A client is admitted to the hospital with diabetic ketoacidosis (DKA). The client's daughter says to the nurse, "My mother died last month, and now this. I've been trying to follow all of the instructions from the doctor. What have I done wrong?" The nurse should make which therapeutic response to the client?

1 "Tell me what you think you did wrong."
2 "Maybe we can keep your father in the hospital for a while longer to give you a rest."
3 "You should talk to the social worker about getting you someone at home who is more capable of managing a diabetic's care."

Answer: 4
Rationale: Environment, infection, or an emotional stressor can initiate the pathophysiological mechanism of DKA. Option 2 is inappropriate and not cost effective. Options 1 and 3 substantiate the daughters' feelings of guilt.

Test-Taking Strategy: Use the process of elimination. Note that the client's daughter (rather than the client himself) is the subject of the question; this will assist you with eliminating option 2, in addition to the fact that this option is inappropriate and not cost effective. Options 1 and 3 devalue the client (the daughter) and block therapeutic communication. Review therapeutic communication techniques if you had difficulty with this question.

4 "An emotional stress such as your mother's death can trigger DKA even though you are following your father's prescribed regimen to the letter."

Level of Cognitive Ability: Application
Client Needs: Psychosocial Integrity
Integrated Process: Communication and Documentation
Content Area: Adult Health/Endocrine

References

deWit, S. (2009). *Medical-surgical nursing: Concepts & practice* (pp. 9, 1101). St. Louis: Saunders.
Linton, A. (2007). *Introduction to medical-surgical nursing* (4th ed., p. 1007). Philadelphia: Saunders.

---

531. A nurse is assisting with planning goals for a victim of rape. Which short-term initial goal is inappropriate?

1 The client will verbalize feelings about the rape event.
2 The client will resolve feelings of fear and anxiety related to the rape trauma.
3 The client will experience physical healing of the wounds that were incurred at the time of the rape.
4 The client will participate in the treatment plan by keeping appointments and following through with treatment options.

Level of Cognitive Ability: Analysis
Client Needs: Psychosocial Integrity
Integrated Process: Nursing Process/Planning
Content Area: Mental Health

Answer: 2

Rationale: Short-term goals will include the beginning stages of dealing with the rape trauma. Clients will initially be expected to keep appointments, participate in care, begin to explore feelings, and begin to heal the physical wounds that were inflicted at the time of the rape. The resolution of feelings is a long-term goal.

Test-Taking Strategy: Note the strategic words *short-term initial goal* and *inappropriate.* The word *resolve* in option 2 indicates that this is a long-term goal. Review the care of the client who is a victim of rape if you had difficulty with this question.

Reference

Varcarolis, E., & Halter, M. (2009). *Essentials of psychiatric mental health nursing: A communication approach to evidence-based care* (p. 403). St. Louis: Saunders.

---

532. A client with a diagnosis of cancer is scheduled for surgery in the morning. When the nurse enters the room and begins the surgical preparation, the client states, "I'm not having surgery, you must have the wrong person! My test results were negative. I'll be going home tomorrow." The nurse recognizes that the defense mechanism that the client is exhibiting is:

1 Denial
2 Delusions
3 Psychosis
4 Displacement

Level of Cognitive Ability: Comprehension
Client Needs: Psychosocial Integrity
Integrated Process: Nursing Process/Data Collection
Content Area: Adult Health/Oncology

Answer: 1

Rationale: Defense mechanisms protect against anxiety. Denial is the defense mechanism that blocks out painful or anxiety-inducing events or feelings. In this case, the client cannot deal with the upcoming surgery for cancer and therefore denies that he or she is ill. Displacement is acting out in anger or frustration with people who did not arouse those feelings. Options 2 and 3 are not defense mechanisms.

Test-Taking Strategy: Use the process of elimination, and focus on the subject—defense mechanisms. Options 2 and 3 are eliminated first because these are not defense mechanisms. From the remaining options, focusing on the data in the question will direct you to option 1. Review defense mechanisms if you had difficulty with this question.

Reference

Linton, A. (2007). *Introduction to medical-surgical nursing* (4th ed., p. 386). Philadelphia: Saunders.

---

533. A nurse who works in an industrial setting is given a memo that indicates that a large number of employees will be laid off during the next 2 weeks. A review of previous layoffs suggested that workers experienced role crises, indecision, and depression. Using this data, the nurse assists with planning for the layoff by suggesting the need for which of the following?

1 Helping the workers acquire unemployment benefits to avoid a gap in income
2 Reducing the staff in the occupational health department of the industrial setting
3 Notifying insurance carriers of the upcoming event to assist with potential health alterations
4 Identifying referral, counseling, and vocational rehabilitative services for the employees being laid off

Level of Cognitive Ability: Analysis
Client Needs: Psychosocial Integrity
Integrated Process: Nursing Process/Planning
Content Area: Mental Health

Answer: 4
Rationale: A review of data should lead to a comprehensive conclusion based directly on the data. In this case, option 4 is the only conclusion; the other options may or may not need to occur. The nurse would need to know more about the industry to determine whether option 1, 2, or 3 would be necessary or possible.

Test-Taking Strategy: Use the process of elimination, and focus on the data in the question. Options 1, 2, and 3 are more industry specific, and one would need to know more about the industrial setting than is presented in the question. In addition, option 4 is the umbrella option. Review the purpose of referral, counseling, and rehabilitative services if you had difficulty with this question.

Reference

Fortinash, K., & Holoday-Worret, P. (2008). *Psychiatric mental health nursing* (4th ed., p. 215). St. Louis: Mosby.

---

534. During the discharge planning of a small-for-gestational-age (SGA) infant, the nurse makes an appointment for the infant to be evaluated by a developmental specialist. The mother says to the nurse, "I am not sure that going to a specialist is necessary just because the baby is small." Which of the following is the appropriate response by the nurse?

1 "Your baby is very small and needs to be evaluated by the developmental specialist."
2 "A lot of parents have to have their baby's evaluated by the developmental specialist."
3 "I feel that it is the best thing for you to have the baby evaluated by the developmental specialist."
4 "You have questions about the appointment for your baby to be evaluated by the developmental specialist?"

Level of Cognitive Ability: Application
Client Needs: Psychosocial Integrity
Integrated Process: Communication and Documentation
Content Area: Maternity/Postpartum

Answer: 4
Rationale: SGA infants are at risk for poor postnatal growth and for neurological and developmental handicaps. By paraphrasing the mother's message, the nurse uses a therapeutic communication technique and addresses the mother's need for understanding. Options 1, 2, and 3 are nontherapeutic responses.

Test-Taking Strategy: Use therapeutic communication techniques to answer the question. Only option 4 addresses the mother's concern. Options 1 and 3 provide advice from the nurse's viewpoint and opinion. Option 2 is a generalized statement that does not address the mother's individual concern. Review therapeutic communication techniques if you had difficulty with this question.

Reference

Leifer, G. (2008). *Maternity nursing: An introductory text* (10th ed., pp. 7, 311-312). Philadelphia: Saunders.

---

535. A toddler is admitted to the hospital with a fever of unknown origin. The mother has three other children for whom she must care, and the father is out of town on business. The mother's time at the hospital is limited to the hours that the other children are in school. The nurse demonstrates an understanding of the toddler's psychosocial development by making which statement to the mother?

1 "Your child is egocentric, which allows a child to self-comfort."
2 "It is better to leave without saying good-bye so that your child will not be upset."
3 "Games such as peekaboo and hide-and-seek will help your child understand that you will return."
4 "Your child is too old to be having separation anxiety. Crying is just a way children have of controlling their parents."

Level of Cognitive Ability: Application
Client Needs: Psychosocial Integrity
Integrated Process: Communication and Documentation
Content Area: Child Health

Answer: 3

Rationale: In option 3, the nurse suggests ways in which the child can be helped to develop object permanence. Options 1, 2, and 4 do not meet the psychosocial needs of a toddler.

Test-Taking Strategy: Focus on the age of the child and the psychosocial development that occurs during this time, and use the process of elimination. Review the psychosocial development of a toddler if you had difficulty with this question.

Reference

Price, D., & Gwin, J. (2008). *Pediatric nursing: An introductory text* (10th ed., pp. 21, 24-25). St. Louis: Saunders.

---

536. A nurse is caring for a client diagnosed with angina. When entering the client's room, the nurse should be most concerned about which finding?

1 The client's lunch tray has not been touched.
2 The client is laughing loudly at a television program.
3 The client is transacting business with his laptop computer while in bed.
4 The client is resting with both eyes closed, and the television is on at moderate volume.

Level of Cognitive Ability: Comprehension
Client Needs: Psychosocial Integrity
Integrated Process: Nursing Process/Data Collection
Content Area: Adult Health/Cardiovascular

Answer: 3

Rationale: Rest and relaxation are crucial for clients with angina because stress and emotional tension can trigger episodes of pain. The volume of the television and client laughter are not related to triggering episodes of pain. Although nutrition is important, the nurse is most concerned with the finding related to stress.

Test-Taking Strategy: Use the process of elimination. Focusing on the client's diagnosis and the factors that can trigger anginal pain will direct you to option 3. Review these factors if you had difficulty with this question.

Reference

deWit, S. (2009). *Medical-surgical nursing: Concepts & practice* (p. 500). St. Louis: Saunders.

---

537. A stillborn infant was delivered a few hours ago. After the birth, the family has remained together, holding and touching the baby. Which statement by the

Answer: 1

Rationale: Nurses should explore measures that assist the family with creating memories of a stillborn infant so that the existence of the child is confirmed and the parents can complete the grieving

nurse will further assist the family during their initial period of grief?
1 "What did you name your baby?"
2 "You seem upset. Do you need a tranquilizer?"
3 "I feel so bad. I don't understand why this happened either."
4 "You can hold the baby for another 15 minutes, then I should take the baby away."

Level of Cognitive Ability: Application
Client Needs: Psychosocial Integrity
Integrated Process: Caring
Content Area: Maternity/Postpartum

process. Option 1 identifies this measure and also demonstrates a caring and empathetic response. Option 2 devalues the parents' feelings and is inappropriate. Option 3 is inappropriate and reflects a lack of knowledge on the nurse's part. Option 4 is uncaring.

Test-Taking Strategy: Use therapeutic communication techniques, and note the strategic words *further assist the family during their initial period of grief.* Choose the option that demonstrates a caring and empathetic nursing response and that meets the psychosocial needs of the client and family. Review therapeutic communication techniques and the grief process if you had difficulty with this question.

References

Leifer, G. (2007). *Introduction to maternity and pediatric nursing* (5th ed., pp. 212-213). Philadelphia: Saunders.
Leifer, G. (2008). *Maternity nursing: An introductory text* (10th ed., pp. 273-274). Philadelphia: Saunders.

---

538. A primigravida client is seen by the physician, and a urinary tract infection is diagnosed. The client has repeatedly verbalized concern regarding the safety of the fetus. The nurse determines that which of the following is the priority client concern at this time?
1 Fear
2 Pain
3 Embarrassment
4 Nutritional requirements

Level of Cognitive Ability: Analysis
Client Needs: Psychosocial Integrity
Integrated Process: Nursing Process/Data Collection
Content Area: Maternity/Antepartum

Answer: 1
Rationale: The primary concern for this client is fear for the safety of her fetus (rather than for her own safety). There is no information in the question to support options 2, 3, and 4.

Test-Taking Strategy: Focus on the subject of the question and the data provided in the question. There is no information in the question to support options 2, 3, and 4. Review the defining characteristics of fear if you had difficulty with this question.

References

Leifer, G. (2007). *Introduction to maternity and pediatric nursing* (5th ed., pp. 107, 239). Philadelphia: Saunders.
Leifer, G. (2008). *Maternity nursing: An introductory text* (10th ed., p. 271). Philadelphia: Saunders.

---

539. A pregnant client is newly diagnosed with sickle cell anemia. Which of the following is the most important psychosocial intervention at this time?
1 Providing emotional support
2 Avoiding discussing the topic of the disease
3 Allowing the client to be alone if she is crying
4 Providing all available information about the disease

Level of Cognitive Ability: Application
Client Needs: Psychosocial Integrity
Integrated Process: Nursing Process/Implementation
Content Area: Maternity/Antepartum

Answer: 1
Rationale: The most important psychosocial intervention is providing emotional support to the client and family. Option 3 is only appropriate if the client asks to be alone. Option 2 is similar to option 3 and is nontherapeutic. Option 4 overwhelms the client with information while the client is trying to cope with the news of the disease. Supportive therapy allows the client to express feelings, explore alternatives, and make decisions in a safe, caring environment.

Test-Taking Strategy: Use the process of elimination. Eliminate options 2 and 4 because of the words *avoiding* and *all*, respectively. In addition, these actions are nontherapeutic. From the remaining options, remember that the client's feelings are the priority and that an important role of the nurse is to provide emotional support. Review psychosocial issues related to sickle cell anemia if you had difficulty with this question.

Reference

Leifer, G. (2007). *Introduction to maternity and pediatric nursing* (5th ed., p. 104). Philadelphia: Saunders.

---

540. A nurse is assisting with caring for a newborn with a suspected diagnosis of erythroblastosis fetalis immediately after delivery. The nurse makes which therapeutic statement to the parents at this time?

1 "You must have many concerns. Please ask me any questions."
2 "Your newborn is very sick. The next 24 hours are most crucial."
3 "This is a common neonatal problem; you shouldn't be concerned."
4 "There is no need to worry. We have the most updated equipment in this hospital."

Level of Cognitive Ability: Application
Clients Needs: Psychosocial Integrity
Integrated Process: Communication and Documentation
Content Area: Maternity/Postpartum

Answer: 1

Rationale: Erythroblastosis fetalis is a type of hemolytic anemia that results from maternal–fetal blood group incompatibility involving the Rh factor and the ABO blood groups. Parental concern and anxiety are expected and are related to the care of the newborn with erythroblastosis fetalis. This anxiety results from a lack of knowledge about the disease process, treatment, and expected outcomes. Parents need to be encouraged to verbalize their concerns and to participate in care as appropriate.

Test-Taking Strategy: Use the process of elimination. Eliminate options 3 and 4 because they are comparable or alike in that they say basically the same thing. In addition, they are blocks to communication. The wording in option 2 would frighten the parents. Remember to address clients' feelings and concerns. Review therapeutic communication techniques if you had difficulty with this question.

Reference

Leifer, G. (2008). *Maternity nursing: An introductory text* (10th ed., pp. 7, 256, 320). Philadelphia: Saunders.

---

541. A licensed practical nurse (LPN) is assisting a school nurse with weighing all the high school students. One of the teenagers who has type 1 diabetes mellitus has gained 15 pounds since last year with no gain in height. This client tells the nurse that he eats alone in the cafeteria at lunch time. Based on this data, the LPN is most concerned that the student may have:

1 Depression
2 Bulimia nervosa
3 An insulin deficiency
4 An alcohol abuse problem

Level of Cognitive Ability: Analysis
Client Needs: Psychosocial Integrity
Integrated Process: Nursing Process/Data Collection
Content Area: Child Health

Answer: 1

Rationale: Diabetic teenagers are at risk for depression and suicide, which is frequently manifested by changing insulin and eating patterns. Social isolation is another clue. Remember that weight loss is a symptom of type 1 diabetes and that an insulin deficiency would have the same effect. Bulimic clients may be of normal weight, but they control weight gain by purging. Alcohol abuse is more likely to be related to weight loss.

Test-Taking Strategy: Use the process of elimination, and focus on the data presented in the question. Eliminate options 2, 3, and 4 because weight gain would not occur in these conditions. Review the signs associated with depression if you had difficulty with this question.

Reference

Price, D., & Gwin, J. (2008). *Pediatric nursing: An introductory text* (10th ed., p. 302). St. Louis: Saunders.

---

542. A nurse is conducting a session with a class of high school students about the risk of sexually transmitted infections (STIs). What opening statement will best encourage participation within the group?

Answer: 4

Rationale: The correct option states the rules for confidentiality, which will help the high school students to develop trust when sharing sensitive issues with the group. Option 1 offers the opportunity to share personal experiences but no promise of

1 "Please feel free to share your personal experiences with the group."
2 "At the end of the class, condoms will be distributed to everyone in the class."
3 "Our goal today is to describe ways to prevent acquiring a sexually transmitted infection."
4 "The topic today is very personal. For this reason, anything shared with the group will remain confidential."

Level of Cognitive Ability: Application
Client Needs: Psychosocial Integrity
Integrated Process: Nursing Process/ Implementation
Content Area: Child Health

confidentiality. Option 2 may be an incentive for those attending to stay but infers that participation during the class is not required to get the reward. Option 3 is a good introduction to the topic but does not foster trust, especially among those who may already have an STI.

Test-Taking Strategy: Use the process of elimination, and focus on the subject—confidentiality, trust building, and sharing. Eliminate option 3, which focuses on content, and option 1, which addresses format. From the remaining options, note that option 4 is the umbrella option and that it addresses the subject of confidentiality. Review teaching and learning principles if you had difficulty with this question.

Reference

Price, D., & Gwin, J. (2008). *Pediatric nursing: An introductory text* (10th ed., pp. 332-333). St. Louis: Saunders.

---

543. A client tells the nurse, "My doctor says I can have the surgery and go home the same day, but I'm afraid. My husband's dead, and my son lives 500 miles away. I'm alone. What happens if something goes wrong? I'm not supposed to be up walking unless absolutely necessary." Which nursing response is therapeutic?
1 "Don't worry. This procedure is done all the time without any problems. You'll be fine."
2 "You seem very concerned about going home without help. Have you discussed your concerns with your doctor?"
3 "Your concern is well voiced. I advise you to call your son and insist that he come home immediately. You can't be too careful."
4 "Do you have an alarm system so that, if you fall, it will alert someone to come? If worst comes to worst, call me and I'll come immediately."

Level of Cognitive Ability: Application
Client Needs: Psychosocial Integrity
Integrated Process: Communication and Documentation
Content Area: Fundamental Skills

Answer: 2
Rationale: In option 2, the nurse uses reflection to direct the client's feelings and concerns. In option 1, the nurse provides false reassurance and then minimizes the client's concerns. In option 3, the nurse is projecting the client's own fears, and the problem solving suggested by the nurse is histrionic and provokes fear and anxiety. In option 4, the nurse is trying to solve problems for the client but is overly controlling and takes the decision making out of the client's hands.

Test-Taking Strategy: Use therapeutic communication techniques. Eliminate options 1, 3, and 4 because they are nontherapeutic and do not address the client's feelings. Remember that the priority is to address the client's feelings. Review therapeutic communication techniques if you had difficulty with this question.

Reference

deWit, S. (2009). *Medical-surgical nursing: Concepts & practice* (p. 9). St. Louis: Saunders.

---

544. A client with severe preeclampsia is admitted to the hospital. She is a student at a local college and insists on continuing her studies while in the hospital despite being instructed to rest.

Answer: 2
Rationale: Option 2 involves the client in the decision making. In options 1 and 4, the nurse is judging the client's decisions and asking probing questions; this will cause a breakdown in communication. Option 3 persuades the client's significant others

The nurse notes that the client studies several hours a day between numerous visits from fellow students, family, and friends. Which nursing approach should initially be included in the plan of care?

1 Asking the client why she is not complying with the order of rest
2 Developing a routine with the client to balance studies and rest needs
3 Including a significant other in helping the client understand the need for rest
4 Instructing the client that the health of the baby is more important than her studies at this time

Level of Cognitive Ability: Application
Client Needs: Psychosocial Integrity
Integrated Process: Nursing Process/Implementation
Content Area: Maternity/Antepartum

to disagree with the client's actions; this could cause problems with the client's self-esteem and also affect the nurse–client relationship.

Test-Taking Strategy: Use therapeutic communication techniques and the process of elimination. Eliminate options 1, 3, and 4 because these are blocks to communication. Option 2 is therapeutic and the most thorough nursing action because it addresses rest and studies and involves the client in the decision-making process. Review therapeutic communication techniques if you had difficulty with this question.

Reference

Leifer, G. (2008). *Maternity nursing: An introductory text* (10th ed., pp. 5, 260). Philadelphia: Saunders.

---

545. A pregnant client is newly diagnosed with gestational diabetes. She is crying, and she keeps repeating, "What have I done to cause this? If I could only live my life over." The nurse identifies the client as experiencing which problem?

1 A risk for injury to the fetus related to maternal distress
2 A disturbance in body image related to complications of pregnancy
3 A disturbance in self-concept related to complications of pregnancy
4 A lack of understanding regarding diabetic self-care during pregnancy

Level of Cognitive Ability: Comprehension
Client Needs: Psychosocial Integrity
Integrated Process: Nursing Process/Data Collection
Content Area: Maternity/Antepartum

Answer: 3

Rationale: The client is putting the blame for the diabetes on herself, thus lowering her self-concept or image. She is expressing fear and grief. There is no information in the question to support options 1, 2, and 4.

Test-Taking Strategy: Use the data presented in the question to assist you with selecting the correct option. The words *what have I done* should help you to eliminate options 2 and 4. From the remaining options, focusing on the data in the question should direct you to option 3. Review the defining characteristics of a disturbance in self-concept if you had difficulty with this question.

Reference

Leifer, G. (2008). *Maternity nursing: An introductory text* (10th ed., pp. 101, 239). Philadelphia: Saunders.

---

546. A client says to the nurse, "I'm going to die, and I wish my family would stop hoping for a cure! I get so angry when they carry on like this! After all, I'm the one who's dying." The nurse should make which therapeutic response to the client?

1 "Have you shared your feelings with your family?"
2 "Well, it sounds like you're being pretty pessimistic."

Answer: 4

Rationale: Reflection is the therapeutic communication technique that redirects the client's feelings back to validate what the client is saying. In option 3, the nurse attempts to use focusing but the attempt addresses a premature statement. In option 2, the nurse makes a judgment and is nontherapeutic. In option 1, the nurse is attempting to assess the client's ability to openly discuss feelings with family members.

3 "I think we should talk more about your anger with your family."
4 "You're feeling angry that your family continues to hope for you to be cured?"

Level of Cognitive Ability: Application
Client Needs: Psychosocial Integrity
Integrated Process: Communication and Documentation
Content Area: Mental Health

Test-Taking Strategy: Use therapeutic communication techniques to eliminate options 1, 2, and 3. Option 4 is the only option that address a therapeutic communication technique and that redirects the client's feelings back to validate what the client is saying. Review therapeutic communication techniques if you had difficulty with this question.

References
Fortinash, K., & Holoday-Worret, P. (2008). *Psychiatric mental health nursing* (4th ed., p. 72). St. Louis: Mosby.
Stuart, G. (2009). *Principles and practices of psychiatric nursing* (9th ed., pp. 27-31). St. Louis: Mosby.

---

547. A nurse is caring for an older adult client who says, "I don't want to talk with you. You're only a nurse, I'll wait for my doctor." Which nursing response is therapeutic?
1 "I'll leave you now and call your physician."
2 "Are you saying that you want to talk to your physician?"
3 "I'm assigned to work with you. Your doctor placed you in my hands."
4 "I'm angry with the way you've dismissed me. I am your nurse not your servant."

Level of Cognitive Ability: Application
Client Needs: Psychosocial Integrity
Integrated Process: Communication and Documentation
Content Area: Fundamental Skills

Answer: 2
Rationale: In option 2, the nurse uses the therapeutic communication of reflection to redirect the client's feelings back for validation. Note that the nurse does not reflect a negative in option 2 but instead focuses on the client's desire to talk with the physician. Options 1, 3, and 4 are nontherapeutic. Remember that the nurse places the client's well-being first and foremost while engaged in nursing care.

Test-Taking Strategy: Focus on the subject—therapeutic communication for clients who are using defensive statements to drive others away. You can easily eliminate options 3 and 4 because these are nontherapeutic responses. Option 1 is a social response and intervention that reinforces the continuation of this behavior. Review therapeutic communication techniques if you had difficulty with this question.

References
deWit, S. (2009). *Medical-surgical nursing: Concepts & practice* (p. 9). St. Louis: Saunders.
Wold, G. (2008). *Basic geriatric nursing* (4th ed., p. 95). St. Louis: Mosby.

---

548. A female client and her newborn infant have undergone human immunodeficiency virus (HIV) testing, and the test results for both clients are positive. The news is devastating, and the mother is crying. The appropriate nursing action at this time is to:
1 Examine with the mother how she got HIV.
2 Listen quietly while the mother talks and cries.
3 Describe the progressive stages and treatments of HIV.
4 Call an HIV counselor to make an appointment for the mother and baby.

Level of Cognitive Ability: Application
Client Needs: Psychosocial Integrity
Integrated Process: Nursing Process/Implementation
Content Area: Maternity/Postpartum

Answer: 2
Rationale: This client has just received devastating news and needs to have someone present with her as she begins to cope with this issue. The nurse needs to sit and actively listen while the mother talks and cries. Calling an HIV counselor may be helpful but is not what the client needs at this time. The other options are not appropriate for this stage of coping with the news that both she and the infant are HIV positive.

Test-Taking Strategy: Use the process of elimination. Noting the strategic words *at this time* will assist you with eliminating options 3 and 4. From the remaining options, remember to address the client's feelings and to support the client. Review therapeutic communication techniques if you had difficulty with this question.

Reference
Leifer, G. (2008). *Maternity nursing: An introductory text* (10th ed., pp. 5, 105-106). Philadelphia: Saunders.

---

549. A nurse employed in a home-care agency is assigned to provide care to a recently widowed and retired military man who is estranged from his only son because the son was discharged from the service for being homosexual. When the nurse arrives at the client's home, the ordinarily immaculate house is in chaos, and the client is disheveled, with alcohol on his breath. Which statement by the nurse is therapeutic?

1 "This probably isn't a good time to visit."
2 "You seem to be having a very troubling time."
3 "Do you think your wife would want you to behave like this?"
4 "What are you doing? How much have you been drinking and for how long?"

Level of Cognitive Ability: Application
Client Needs: Psychosocial Integrity
Integrated Process: Communication and Documentation
Content Area: Mental Health

Answer: 2

Rationale: The therapeutic statement is the one that helps the client to explore his situation and to express his feelings. Option 2 identifies the use of reflection and will assist the client with beginning to express his feelings. As this happens, the nurse can assist the client with discussing the reasons behind his alienation from his only child. In option 1, the nurse uses humor to avoid therapeutic intimacy and effective problem solving. In option 3, the nurse uses social communication. In option 4, the nurse uses admonishment and tries to shame the client, which is not therapeutic; this belittles the client, causes anger, and may evoke acting out by the client.

> ***Test-Taking Strategy***: Use therapeutic communication techniques. Option 2 is the only option that addresses the client's feelings. Review therapeutic communication techniques if you had difficulty with this question.

Reference

Wold, G. (2008). *Basic geriatric nursing* (4th ed., pp. 95-96). St. Louis: Mosby.

---

550. A client says to the nurse, "I don't do anything right. I'm such a loser." The therapeutic response is:

1 "Everything will get better."
2 "You don't do anything right?"
3 "You do things right all the time."
4 "You are not a loser, you are sick."

Level of Cognitive Ability: Application
Client Needs: Psychosocial Integrity
Integrated Process: Communication and Documentation
Content Area: Mental Health

Answer: 2

Rationale: Option 2 allows the client to verbalize feelings. With this question, the nurse can learn more about what the client really means. This option repeats the client's statement and allows the communication to stay open. Options 1, 3, and 4 are closed statements and do not encourage the client to further explore feelings.

> ***Test-Taking Strategy***: Use therapeutic communication techniques. Remember to address the client's feelings. Option 2 is the only option that identifies a therapeutic response and that allows the client to verbalize feelings. Review therapeutic communication techniques if you had difficulty with this question.

Reference

Stuart, G. (2009). *Principles and practices of psychiatric nursing* (9th ed., pp. 27-31). St. Louis: Mosby.

---

551. A client who is experiencing suicidal thoughts says to the nurse, "It just doesn't seem worth it anymore. Why not just end it all?" The nurse would gather data from the client by using which response?

1 "Did you sleep at all last night?"
2 "Tell me what you mean by that."

Answer: 2

Rationale: Option 2 allows the client to tell the nurse more about his or her current thoughts. Options 1 and 3 change the subject and block communication. Option 4 is false reassurance and may also block communication.

3 "I know you have had a stressful night."
4 "I'm sure your family is worried about you."

Level of Cognitive Ability: Application
Client Needs: Psychosocial Integrity
Integrated Process: Communication and Documentation
Content Area: Mental Health

Test-Taking Strategy: Use therapeutic communication techniques. Note the strategic words *gather data*. Options 3 and 4 can be eliminated because they do not reflect data collection. Both options 1 and 2 relate to further data collection, but option 2 is directly related to the subject of the question and provides the opportunity for the client to express his or her thoughts. Review therapeutic communication techniques if you had difficulty with this question.

Reference

Stuart, G. (2009). *Principles and practices of psychiatric nursing* (9th ed., pp. 27-31, 322). St. Louis: Mosby.

---

552. A mother says to the nurse, "I am afraid that my child may have another febrile seizure." Which response by the nurse is therapeutic?
1 "Tell me what frightens you the most about seizures."
2 "Why worry about something that you cannot control?"
3 "Most children will never experience a second seizure."
4 "Acetaminophen (Tylenol) can prevent another seizure from occurring."

Level of Cognitive Ability: Application
Client Needs: Psychosocial Integrity
Integrated Process: Communication and Documentation
Content Area: Child Health

Answer: 1
Rationale: Option 1 is the only response that is an open-ended statement and that provides the mother with an opportunity to express her feelings. Option 2 is incorrect because it blocks communication by giving a flippant response to an expressed fear. Options 3 and 4 are incorrect because the nurse is giving false assurance that a seizure will not reoccur or that it can be prevented in this woman's child.

Test-Taking Strategy: Note the strategic word *therapeutic*. Use the process of elimination, and determine which option encourages the client to express her feelings. Options 2, 3, and 4 are nontherapeutic and block communication. Review therapeutic communication techniques if you had difficulty with this question.

References

Leifer, G. (2007). *Introduction to maternity and pediatric nursing* (5th ed., p. 536). Philadelphia: Saunders.
Price, D., & Gwin, J. (2008). *Pediatric nursing: An introductory text* (10th ed., p. 256). St. Louis: Saunders.

---

553. A mother has just given birth to a baby who has a cleft lip and palate. When planning to talk to this mother, the nurse should recognize that this client needs to be allowed to work through which of the following emotions before mother–infant bonding can occur?
1 Guilt
2 Grief
3 Anger
4 Depression

Level of Cognitive Ability: Comprehension
Client Needs: Psychosocial Integrity
Integrated Process: Nursing Process/Planning
Content Area: Maternity/Postpartum

Answer: 2
Rationale: The mother must first be assisted with grieving for the anticipated perfect child that she did not have. After this happens, the mother can begin to focus on bonding with the infant to which she gave birth. Options 1, 3, and 4 are incorrect because they are each only one component of the grief process.

Test-Taking Strategy: Use the process of elimination. The strategic words are *to work through. . . before mother–infant bonding can occur.* Options 1, 3, and 4 are incorrect because each is only one component of the grief process; option 2 is the umbrella option. Review the grief process if you had difficulty with this question.

Reference

Price, D., & Gwin, J. (2008). *Pediatric nursing: An introductory text* (10th ed., pp. 103, 404). St. Louis: Saunders.

---

554. A client scheduled for cardiac stress testing expresses a fear of his heart "giving out" during the procedure. The nurse attempts to discuss these fears with the client. Which client behavior indicates a barrier to communication?

1 The client does not talk about the procedure.
2 The client asks numerous questions about the stress test.
3 The client verbally expresses fears about his own mortality.
4 The client is frustrated because the test needs to be performed.

Level of Cognitive Ability: Comprehension
Client Needs: Psychosocial Integrity
Integrated Process: Nursing Process/Data Collection
Content Area: Adult Health/Cardiovascular

Answer: 1

Rationale: Expressions of fear, anxiety, and frustration are examples of effective client communication. These expressions are identified in options 2, 3, and 4. Not wanting to talk about the procedure is a barrier to effective communication.

Test-Taking Strategy: Use the process of elimination, and note the strategic words *barrier to communication.* Options 2, 3, and 4 contain evidence of communication on the client's part. Not talking indicates a barrier. Review the barriers to communication if you had difficulty with this question.

References

deWit, S. (2009). *Medical-surgical nursing: Concepts & practice* (p. 412). St. Louis: Saunders.
Linton, A. (2007). *Introduction to medical-surgical nursing* (4th ed., pp. 53-54). Philadelphia: Saunders.

---

555. After the vaginal delivery of a large-for-gestational-age (LGA) male infant, the nurse wraps the infant in a warm blanket and hands him to his mother. The mother demonstrates reluctance to touch the baby and verbalizes concern about the infant's facial bruising. To enhance maternal–infant attachment, the nurse responds:

1 "It is a normal finding in large babies and nothing to be concerned about."
2 "The bruising is temporary, and it is important to interact with your infant."
3 "The bruising is caused by polycythemia, which usually leads to jaundice."
4 "Because the bruising is painful, it is advisable that you not touch the baby's face."

Level of Cognitive Ability: Application
Client Needs: Psychosocial Integrity
Integrated Process: Nursing Process/Implementation
Content Area: Maternity/Postpartum

Answer: 2

Rationale: The mother of an LGA infant with facial bruising may be reluctant to interact with the infant because of concern about causing additional pain to the infant. The bruising is temporary. Option 1 appears to be an appropriate response but does not address the subject of the question. The LGA infant may have polycythemia, which can contribute to bruising, but the bruising is not caused by the polycythemia. Option 4 involves advising the mother to not touch the baby's face because the bruising is painful; however, touch is an important component of the attachment process. Touching the infant gently with the fingertips should be encouraged.

Test-Taking Strategy: Use the process of elimination. Note the relationship of the word *attachment* in the question and the word *interact* in the correct option. Review the concepts related to maternal–infant attachment if you had difficulty with this question.

Reference

Leifer, G. (2008). *Maternity nursing: An introductory text* (10th ed., p. 138). Philadelphia: Saunders.

---

556. A client with myasthenia gravis is ready to return home and confides that she is concerned that her husband will no longer find her physically attractive. The nurse should plan to:

1 Tell the client to not dwell on the negative.

Answer: 4

Rationale: Encouraging the client to share her feelings with her husband directly addresses the subject of the question. Encouraging the client to start a support group will not address the client's immediate and individual concern. Options 1 and 3 are blocks to communication and avoid the client's concern.

2 Encourage the client to start a support group.
3 Insist that the client reach out and face this fear.
4 Encourage the client to share her feelings with her husband.

Level of Cognitive Ability: Application
Client Needs: Psychosocial Integrity
Integrated Process: Nursing Process/Planning
Content Area: Adult Health/Neurological

Test-Taking Strategy: Focus on the subject, and use the process of elimination. Option 4 is the only option that addresses the client's immediate concern. Remember to address the client's feelings first. Review therapeutic communication techniques if you had difficulty with this question.

Reference

deWit, S. (2009). *Medical-surgical nursing: Concepts & practice* (pp. 9, 608). St. Louis: Saunders.

---

557. A 9-year-old child is hospitalized for 2 months after a car accident. The best way to promote the psychosocial development of this child is to plan for:
1 A phone to call family and friends
2 A portable radio and tape player with headphones
3 Tutoring to keep the child up-to-date with schoolwork
4 Computer games, television, and videos at the bedside

Level of Cognitive Ability: Application
Client Needs: Psychosocial Integrity
Integrated Process: Nursing Process/Planning
Content Area: Child Health

Answer: 3
Rationale: The developmental task of the school-age child is industry versus inferiority. The child achieves success by mastering skills and knowledge. Maintaining schoolwork provides for accomplishment and prevents feelings of inferiority that may result from lagging behind the class. The other options provide diversion and are of lesser importance for a child of this age.

Test-Taking Strategy: Note the age of the child, and determine the developmental task for this child. Options 1, 2, and 4 address social and diversional issues, whereas option 3 specifically addresses psychosocial development. Review the growth and development of the school-age child if you had difficulty with this question.

Reference

Price, D., & Gwin, J. (2008). *Pediatric nursing: An introductory text* (10th ed., p. 27). St. Louis: Saunders.

---

558. A client who is in halo traction says to the nurse, "I can't get used to this contraption. I can't see properly on the side, and I keep misjudging where everything is." The nurse should make which therapeutic response to the client?
1 "If I were you, I would have had the surgery rather than suffer like this."
2 "No one ever gets used to that thing! It's horrible. Many of our sports people who are in it complain vigorously."
3 "Halo traction involves many difficult adjustments. Practice scanning with your eyes after standing up and before you move."
4 "Why do you feel like this when you could have died from a broken neck? This is the way it is for several months. You need to accept it more, don't you think?"

Level of Cognitive Ability: Application
Client Needs: Psychosocial Integrity

Answer: 3
Rationale: The therapeutic communication technique that the nurse uses in option 3 is reflection. The nurse then offers a problem-solving strategy that helps to increase the client's peripheral vision. In option 1, the nurse provides a social response that contains emotionally charged language and that could increase the client's anxiety. In option 2, the nurse undermines the client's faith in the medical treatment being used by giving advice that is insensitive and unprofessional. In option 4, the nurse uses excessive questioning and gives advice, which is nontherapeutic.

Test-Taking Strategy: Use the process of elimination, and look for the option that represents a therapeutic communication technique. The therapeutic communication technique that the nurse uses in option 3 is reflection. Review therapeutic communication techniques if you had difficulty with this question.

Reference

deWit, S. (2009). *Medical-surgical nursing: Concepts & practice* (pp. 9, 553). St. Louis: Saunders.

Integrated Process: Communication and Documentation
Content Area: Adult Health/Neurological

---

559. An older client has been admitted to the hospital with a hip fracture. The nurse assists with preparing a plan for the client and identifies desired outcomes. Which client statement supports a positive adjustment to the experienced alterations in mobility?

1 "Hurry up and go away. I want to be alone."
2 "What took you so long? I called for you 30 minutes ago."
3 "I wish you nurses would leave me alone! You're always telling me what to do!"
4 "I find it difficult to concentrate since the doctor talked with me about the surgery tomorrow."

Level of Cognitive Ability: Comprehension
Client Needs: Psychosocial Integrity
Integrated Process: Nursing Process/Evaluation
Content Area: Adult Health/Musculoskeletal

Answer: 4
Rationale: Option 4 is reflective of a person with moderate anxiety. This client statement appropriately supports a positive adjustment. Option 1 demonstrates withdrawal behavior. Option 2 is a demanding response. Option 3 demonstrates acting out by the client. Demanding, acting-out, and withdrawn clients have not coped with or adjusted to injury or disease.

Test-Taking Strategy: Focus on the subject—positive adjustment. Remember that age, limited mobility, and medications often contribute to anxiety and confusion; this should direct you to option 4. Review the characteristics of positive adjustment if you had difficulty with this question.

Reference
Linton, A. (2007). *Introduction to medical-surgical nursing* (4th ed., pp. 54, 929). Philadelphia: Saunders.

---

560. The best way to help the parents of a premature infant develop attachment behaviors is to:

1 Place family pictures in the infant's view.
2 Encourage the parents to touch and speak to their infant.
3 Report only positive qualities and progress to the parents.
4 Provide information about infant development and stimulation.

Level of Cognitive Ability: Application
Client Needs: Psychosocial Integrity
Integrated Process: Nursing Process/Implementation
Content Area: Maternity/Postpartum

Answer: 2
Rationale: The parents' involvement through touch and voice establishes and initiates the attachment process in the relationship. Their active participation builds confidence and supports the parenting role. Family pictures are ineffective for an infant. Providing information and emphasizing only positives do not relate to the attachment process.

Test-Taking Strategy: Use the process of elimination. The clients of the question are the parents, and the subject is attachment. The only option that addresses attachment behaviors is option 2. Review parent–infant bonding concepts if you had difficulty with this question.

Reference
Leifer, G. (2007). *Introduction to maternity and pediatric nursing* (5th ed., p. 316). Philadelphia: Saunders.

---

561. A client angrily tells the nurse that the doctor purposefully provided wrong information. Which nursing response hinders therapeutic communication?

1 "I'm certain the doctor would not lie to you."

Answer: 1
Rationale: Option 1 hinders communication by disagreeing with the client; this technique could make the client defensive and block further communication. Options 2 and 4 attempt to clarify what the client is referring. Option 3 attempts to explore whether the client is comfortable talking to the doctor about this issue and encourages direct confrontation.

2 "I'm not sure what information you are referring to."
3 "Are you comfortable talking to your doctor about this?"
4 "Can you describe the information that you are talking about?"

Level of Cognitive Ability: Application
Client Needs: Psychosocial Integrity
Integrated Process: Communication and Documentation
Content Area: Fundamental Skills

Test-Taking Strategy: Use the process of elimination, and note the strategic word *hinders.* Disagreeing with or challenging a client's response will hinder or block therapeutic communication. Therapeutic communication addresses client concerns, seeks clarification, acknowledges feelings, or encourages open and direct communication. Review therapeutic communication techniques if you had difficulty with this question.

Reference

Linton, A. (2007). *Introduction to medical-surgical nursing* (4th ed., p. 54). Philadelphia: Saunders.

---

562. A client with major depression says to the nurse, "I should have died. I've always been a failure." The nurse should make which therapeutic response to the client?

1 "I see a lot of positive things in you."
2 "You still have a great deal to live for."
3 "Feeling like a failure is part of your illness."
4 "You've been feeling like a failure for some time now?"

Level of Cognitive Ability: Application
Client Needs: Psychosocial Integrity
Integrated Process: Communication and Documentation
Content Area: Mental Health

Answer: 4

Rationale: Responding to the feelings expressed by a client is an effective therapeutic communication technique. The correct option is an example of the use of restating. Options 1, 2, and 3 block communication because they minimize the client's experience and do not facilitate the exploration of the client's expressed feelings.

Test-Taking Strategy: Use therapeutic communication techniques. Select the option that directly addresses client feelings and concerns. Option 4 is the only option that is stated in the form of an open-ended question that will encourage the verbalization of feelings. Review therapeutic communication techniques if you had difficulty with this question.

Reference

Stuart, G. (2009). *Principles and practices of psychiatric nursing* (9th ed., pp. 27-31, 285-286). St. Louis: Mosby.

---

563. Two months after a right mastectomy for breast cancer, a client comes to the physician's office for a follow-up appointment. The client was told that the risk for cancer in the left breast existed. When asked about her breast self-examination (BSE) practices since the surgery, the client replies, "I don't need to do that any more." This response may indicate:

1 Denial
2 Grief and mourning
3 Change in family role
4 Change in body image

Level of Cognitive Ability: Comprehension
Client Needs: Psychosocial Integrity
Integrated Process: Nursing Process/Evaluation
Content Area: Adult Health/Oncology

Answer: 1

Rationale: The coping strategy of denying or minimizing a health problem is manifested in anxiety-producing health situations, especially those that may be life threatening. Denial can lead to the avoidance of self-care measures such as the BSE. Options 2, 3, and 4 are not associated with the information in the client's statement.

Test-Taking Strategy: Use the data presented in the question to select the correct option. Note the strategic words *I don't need to do that any more.* Eliminate options 2, 3, and 4 because they are not directly related to the client's statement. Option 1 is based on the client's statement, which reflects denial. Review the indicators of denial if you had difficulty with this question.

Reference

Linton, A. (2007). *Introduction to medical-surgical nursing* (4th ed., pp. 386, 1062). Philadelphia: Saunders.

---

564. When planning the care of a client dying of cancer, one of the nurse's goals is to have the client verbalize his or her acceptance of impending death. Which client statement indicates to the nurse that this goal has been met?

1 "I just want to live until my one-hundredth birthday."
2 "I'd like to have my family here when I die."
3 "I'll be ready to die when my children finish school."
4 "I want to go to my daughter's wedding. Then I'll be ready to die."

Level of Cognitive Ability: Comprehension
Client Needs: Psychosocial Integrity
Integrated Process: Nursing Process/Evaluation
Content Area: Adult Health/Oncology

Answer: 2
Rationale: Acceptance is often characterized by plans for death; often the client wants loved ones near. Options 1, 3, and 4 all reflect the bargaining stage of coping in which the client tries to negotiate with his or her God or with fate.

Test-Taking Strategy: Use the process of elimination. Note that options 1, 3, and 4 are comparable or alike in that they all demonstrate negotiating for something else to happen before death occurs. Option 2 is the option that reflects acceptance. Review the stages of death and dying if you had difficulty with this question.

Reference
Christensen, B., & Kockrow, E. (2006). *Foundations of nursing* (5th ed., p. 193). St. Louis: Mosby.

---

565. Which intervention should the nurse implement for the oncology client who has a body image disturbance related to alopecia?

1 Teach the client the importance of rinsing the mouth after eating.
2 Tell the client to use cosmetics to hide medication-induced rashes.
3 Teach the client proper dental hygiene with the use of a foam toothbrush.
4 Tell the client about the use of wigs, which are often paid for by health insurance.

Level of Cognitive Ability: Application
Client Needs: Psychosocial Integrity
Integrated Process: Nursing Process/Implementation
Content Area: Adult Health/Oncology

Answer: 4
Rationale: The temporary or permanent thinning or loss of hair known as alopecia is common among oncology clients receiving chemotherapy. This often causes a body image disturbance that can be addressed with the use of wigs, hats, or scarves. Options 1, 2, and 3 are unrelated to alopecia.

Test-Taking Strategy: Use the process of elimination. Eliminate options 1 and 3 because they are comparable or alike in that they are addressing a subject other than alopecia. Select option 4 over option 2 because cosmetics are not always prescribed when a client has a rash. Knowledge of the definition of alopecia will direct you to option 4. Review the effects of alopecia if you had difficulty with this question.

Reference
deWit, S. (2009). *Medical-surgical nursing: Concepts & practice* (pp. 182-183). St. Louis: Saunders.

---

566. A client with hyperparathyroidism says to the nurse, "I can't stay on this diet. It is too difficult for me." When intervening in this situation, how should the nurse respond?

1 "Why do you think you find this diet plan difficult to adhere to?"
2 "You are having a difficult time staying on this plan. Let's discuss this."
3 "It really isn't difficult to stick to this diet. Just avoid milk products."
4 "It is very important that you stay on this diet to avoid forming renal calculi."

Answer: 2
Rationale: By paraphrasing the client's statement, the nurse can encourage the client to express feelings. The nurse also sends feedback to the client that the message was understood. An open-ended statement or question such as this prompts an informative response. Option 1 is requesting information that the client may not be able to express. Option 3 is giving advice, which blocks communication. Option 4 devalues the client's feelings.

Test-Taking Strategy: Use therapeutic communication techniques. Option 2 is the only option that paraphrases the client's statement and addresses the client's feelings. Review therapeutic communication techniques if you had difficulty with this question.

Level of Cognitive Ability: Application
Client Needs: Psychosocial Integrity
Integrated Process: Communication and Documentation
Content Area: Adult Health/Endocrine

References
Christensen, B., & Kockrow, E. (2006). *Adult health nursing* (5th ed., pp. 535-536). St. Louis: Mosby.
deWit, S. (2009). *Medical-surgical nursing: Concepts & practice* (p. 9). St. Louis: Saunders.

---

567. A nurse is caring for a client who recently had a bilateral adrenalectomy. Which intervention is essential for the nurse to include in the client's plan of care?
1 Prevent social isolation.
2 Avoid stressful situations.
3 Consider occupational therapy.
4 Discuss changes in body image.

Level of Cognitive Ability: Application
Client Needs: Psychosocial Integrity
Integrated Process: Nursing Process/Planning
Content Area: Adult Health/Endocrine

Answer: 2
Rationale: Adrenalectomy can lead to adrenal insufficiency. Adrenal hormones are essential for maintaining homeostasis in response to stressors. Options 1, 3, and 4 are not directly related to the client's diagnosis.

Test-Taking Strategy: Focus on the client's diagnosis. Recalling that an adrenalectomy can lead to adrenal insufficiency and recalling the relationship of an adrenalectomy to the stress response will direct you to option 2. Review the effects of an adrenalectomy if you had difficulty with this question.

Reference
Christensen, B., & Kockrow, E. (2006). *Adult health nursing* (5th ed., p. 541). St. Louis: Mosby.

---

568. Which statement made by a client with anorexia nervosa indicates that treatment has been effective?
1 "I'll eat until I don't feel hungry."
2 "I no longer have a weight problem."
3 "I don't want to starve myself anymore."
4 "My friends and I went out and ate lunch today."

Level of Cognitive Ability: Analysis
Client Needs: Psychosocial Integrity
Integrated Process: Nursing Process/Evaluation
Content Area: Mental Health

Answer: 4
Rationale: Anorexia nervosa is usually seen in adolescent girls who try to establish identity and control by self-imposed starvation. Options 1, 2, and 3 are verbalizations of the client's intentions. Option 4 is a measurable action that can be verified.

Test-Taking Strategy: Use the process of elimination, and note the strategic words *treatment has been effective.* Select the option that is measurable and that can be verified. Option 4 is the only measurable action. Review the goals of care for the client with anorexia nervosa if you had difficulty with this question.

Reference
Varcarolis, E., & Halter, M. (2009). *Essentials of psychiatric mental health nursing: A communication approach to evidence-based care* (p. 202). St. Louis: Saunders.

---

569. A nurse is reinforcing home-care instructions to a client with left-sided heart failure. The client interrupts by saying, "What's the use? I'll never remember all of this, and I'll probably die anyway!" The nurse responds, understanding that the client's response is most likely a result of:
1 Anger about the new medical regimen
2 The teaching strategies used by the nurse
3 Insufficient financial resources to pay for the medications
4 Anxiety about the ability to manage the disease process at home

Answer: 4
Rationale: Anxiety often develops after heart failure. The fear of death can persist, and there is often a long and difficult period of adjustment. Anxiety and fear further tax the failing heart. The nurse should take time to explore the concerns and fears of the client. The client's statement is not associated with options 1, 2, and 3.

Test-Taking Strategy: Use the process of elimination, and note that the client's statement comes suddenly in the middle of receiving home-care instructions. There is no evidence in the question to support options 1, 2, or 3. Note the strategic words *I'll never remember all of this* to direct you to option 4. Review the causes of anxiety if you had difficulty with this question.

Level of Cognitive Ability: Comprehension
Client Needs: Psychosocial Integrity
Integrated Process: Nursing Process/Implementation
Content Area: Adult Health/Cardiovascular

Reference

Christensen, B., & Kockrow, E. (2006). *Adult health nursing* (5th ed., p. 361). St. Louis: Mosby.

---

570. A client who is to be discharged with a temporary colostomy says to the nurse, "I know I've changed this thing once, but I just don't know how I'll do it by myself when I'm home alone. Can't I stay here until the doctor puts it back?" The nurse should make which therapeutic response to the client?

1 "This is only temporary, but you need to hire a nurse companion until your surgery."
2 "So you're saying that you don't feel comfortable on your own yet even though you've practiced changing your colostomy bag once?"
3 "Well, your insurance will not pay for a longer stay just to practice changing your colostomy, so you'll have to fight it out with them."
4 "Going home to care for yourself still feels pretty overwhelming? I will ask the registered nurse to schedule you for home visits until you're feeling more comfortable."

Level of Cognitive Ability: Application
Client Needs: Psychosocial Integrity
Integrated Process: Communication and Documentation
Content Area: Adult Health/Gastrointestinal

Answer: 4

Rationale: The client is expressing feelings of helplessness and abandonment. Option 4 assists with meeting these needs. Option 1 provides information that the client already knows and then helps with problem solving by using a client-centered action that would probably overwhelm the client. Option 2 restates but focuses on the subject of helplessness. Option 3 provides what is probably accurate information but the words *just to practice* can be interpreted by the client as belittling.

Test-Taking Strategy: Use the process of elimination, and focus on the subject of the question—fear and dependency. Eliminate options 1 and 3 first. From the remaining options, look for the one that addresses the client's feelings and concerns. Option 2 involves restating but focuses on the subject of helplessness. Option 4 addresses both fear and dependency needs. Review the psychosocial issues related to a colostomy if you had difficulty with this question.

Reference

Linton, A. (2007). *Introduction to medical-surgical nursing* (4th ed., pp. 407, 409, 1241). Philadelphia: Saunders.

---

571. A client is diagnosed with schizophrenia and is unable to speak, although nothing is wrong with the organs of communication. The nurse understands that this condition is referred to as:

1 Mutism
2 Verbigeration
3 Pressured speech
4 Poverty of speech

Level of Cognitive Ability: Comprehension
Client Needs: Psychosocial Integrity
Integrated Process: Nursing Process/Data Collection
Content Area: Mental Health

Answer: 1

Rationale: Mutism is the absence of verbal speech. The client does not communicate verbally despite an intact physical structural ability to speak. Verbigeration is the purposeless repetition of words or phrases. Pressured speech refers to a rapidity of speech that reflects the client's racing thoughts. Poverty of speech means diminished amounts of speech or monotonic replies.

Test-Taking Strategy: Use the process of elimination, and focus on the subject—the inability to speak. This should assist you with eliminating options 2 and 3. Knowledge that poverty of speech indicates a diminished amount of speech will help you to eliminate option 4. Review these altered thought and speech patterns if you had difficulty with this question.

Reference

Stuart, G. (2009). *Principles and practices of psychiatric nursing* (9th ed., pp. 350, 354). St. Louis: Mosby.

---

572. A client tells the nurse, "I am a spy for the FBI. I am an eye, an eye in the sky." The nurse recognizes that this is an example of:

1 Echolalia
2 Tangential speech
3 Clang associations
4 Loosened associations

Level of Cognitive Ability: Comprehension
Client Needs: Psychosocial Integrity
Integrated Process: Nursing Process/Data Collection
Content Area: Mental Health

Answer: 3

Rationale: Repetition of words or phrases that are similar in sound and in no other way (rhyming) is one of the patterns of altered thought and language noted in clients with schizophrenia. Clang associations often take the form of rhyming. Echolalia is an involuntary parrot-like repetition of words spoken by others. Tangential speech is characterized by a tendency to digress from an original topic of discussion using a common word that connects two unrelated thoughts. Loosened associations are a sign of disordered thought processes in which the person speaks with frequent changes of subject; the content is related only obliquely (if at all) to the subject matter.

Test-Taking Strategy: Use the process of elimination. Recalling that rhyming occurs in clang associations will direct you to option 3. Review altered thought and language patterns in schizophrenia if you had difficulty with this question.

Reference

Stuart, G. (2009). *Principles and practices of psychiatric nursing* (9th ed., p. 338). St. Louis: Mosby.

---

573. A nurse is assisting with planning the hospital discharge of a young male client who has been newly diagnosed with type 1 diabetes mellitus. The client tells the nurse that he is concerned about self-administering insulin while in school with other students around. Which statement by the nurse supports the client's need at this time?

1 "Oh, don't worry about that! You'll do fine!"
2 "You could leave school early and take your insulin at home."
3 "You shouldn't be embarrassed by your diabetes. Lots of people have this disease."
4 "You could contact the school nurse, who could provide a private area for you to take your insulin."

Level of Cognitive Ability: Application
Client Needs: Psychosocial Integrity
Integrated Process: Communication and Documentation
Content Area: Child Health

Answer: 4

Rationale: In the therapeutic caring relationship, the nurse offers information that will promote or assist the client to reach a decision that optimizes a sense of well-being. Option 2 requires a change in lifestyle. Options 1 and 3 are inappropriate statements and blocks to communication.

Test-Taking Strategy: Use the process of elimination, and note the subject—concern about self-administering insulin while in school. Eliminate options 1 and 3 because they are nontherapeutic responses and not supportive to the client. Select option 4 because it promotes the client's ability to continue his present lifestyle, whereas option 2 requires a change in his lifestyle. Review the psychosocial issues associated with diabetes mellitus if you had difficulty with this question.

Reference

Price, D., & Gwin, J. (2008). *Pediatric nursing: An introductory text* (10th ed., pp. 299, 301-302). St. Louis: Saunders.

---

574. A client who was admitted to the hospital for recurrent thyroid storm is preparing for discharge. The client is anxious about the illness and at times emotionally labile. Which approach is appropriate for the nurse to suggest including in the care plan for this client?

1 Assist the client with identifying coping skills, support systems, and potential stressors.
2 Avoid teaching the client anything about the disease until he or she is emotionally stable.
3 Reassure the client that everything will be fine when he or she is in the home environment.
4 Confront the client and explain that he or she must control the anxiety if he or she wants to go home.

Level of Cognitive Ability: Application
Client Needs: Psychosocial Integrity
Integrated Process: Nursing Process/Planning
Content Area: Adult Health/Endocrine

Answer: 1
Rationale: It is normal for clients who experience thyroid storm to continue to be anxious and emotionally labile at the time of discharge. Confrontation in option 4 will only heighten the client's anxiety. Option 2 avoids the subject, and option 3 provides false reassurance. The best intervention is to help the client cope with these changes in behavior and to perhaps anticipate potential stressors so that symptoms will not be as severe.

Test-Taking Strategy: Use therapeutic communication techniques, and focus on the subject—anxiety; this will direct you to option 1. Review the care of the client with anxiety if you had difficulty with this question.

Reference
deWit, S. (2009). *Medical-surgical nursing: Concepts & practice* (pp. 897-898). St. Louis: Saunders.

---

575. A client newly diagnosed with tuberculosis (TB) will be on respiratory isolation in the hospital for at least 2 weeks. Which of the following is vital to prevent social isolation?

1 Note whether the client has visitors.
2 Instruct all staff to not touch the client.
3 Give the client a roommate with TB who persistently tries to talk to the client.
4 Remove the calendar and clock from the room so that the client will not obsess about time.

Level of Cognitive Ability: Application
Client Needs: Psychosocial Integrity
Integrated Process: Nursing Process/Implementation
Content Area: Adult Health/Respiratory

Answer: 1
Rationale: The nurse should note whether the client has adequate visitation and social contact because the presence of others can offer positive stimulation. Touch may be important to help the client feel socially acceptable. A roommate who insists on talking could create sensory overload, and the client with TB should be in a private room. The calendar and clock are needed to facilitate the client's orientation to time.

Test-Taking Strategy: Use the process of elimination, and note the strategic words *prevent social isolation*. Remembering the basic principles related to sensory deprivation will direct you to option 1. Review the psychosocial issues related to the hospitalized client with TB if you had difficulty with this question.

References
deWit, S. (2009). *Medical-surgical nursing: Concepts & practice* (p. 328). St. Louis: Saunders.
Linton, A. (2007). *Introduction to medical-surgical nursing* (4th ed., pp. 563-564). Philadelphia: Saunders.

---

576. A client was injured after drinking alcohol and falling into the coals of a fire, which resulted in a circumferential burn wound to the left leg. During report, the nurse is told that the client has just signed a consent form for the

Answer: 1
Rationale: Reflection statements tend to elicit a deeper awareness of feelings. In addition, option 1 validates the perception that the client is upset. Option 3 is inappropriate and a block to communication. Options 2 and 4 initiate interventions prematurely.

amputation of the limb, and the procedure is scheduled for the next day. While caring for the client, the nurse notes that the client is upset and withdrawn. The nurse should take which appropriate action at this time?

1 Reflect back to the client that he or she appears upset.
2 Let the client have some time alone to grieve over the future loss of the limb.
3 Remind the client that the injury was a result of alcohol abuse and refer him or her for counseling.
4 Inform the physician of the client's depression and request medication to assist the client with coping with the diagnosis.

Level of Cognitive Ability: Application
Client Needs: Psychosocial Integrity
Integrated Process: Nursing Process/ Implementation
Content Area: Mental Health

Test-Taking Strategy: Use therapeutic communication techniques. Select the option that encourages the client to express feelings; this will direct you to option 1. Review therapeutic communication techniques if you had difficulty with this question.

References

Keltner, N., Schwecke, L., & Bostrom, C. (2007). *Psychiatric nursing* (5th ed., pp. 90-91). St. Louis: Mosby.

Varcarolis, E., Halter, M. (2009). *Essentials of psychiatric mental helath nursing: A communication approach to evidence-based care* (pp. 93-94). St. Louis: Saunders.

---

577. Which statement made by a client with left-sided Bell's palsy requires further exploration by the nurse?

1 "My left eye is tearing a lot."
2 "I have trouble closing my left eyelid."
3 "I can't taste anything on the left side."
4 "I don't know how I'll live with the effects of this stroke for the rest of my life."

Level of Cognitive Ability: Comprehension
Client Needs: Psychosocial Integrity
Integrated Process: Nursing Process/Evaluation
Content Area: Adult Health/Neurological

Answer: 4

Rationale: Bell's palsy is an inflammatory condition that involves the facial nerve (cranial nerve VII). The condition is usually temporary, with symptoms resolving after several weeks to months. Many clients fear that they have had a stroke when the symptoms of Bell's palsy appear, and they commonly believe that the paralysis is permanent. It is important for the nurse to identify these fears and to formulate a plan for helping clients deal with them. Options 1, 2, and 3 are expected findings in a client with Bell's palsy.

Test-Taking Strategy: Use the process of elimination, and note the strategic words *requires further exploration*. Options 1, 2, and 3 identify expected findings in clients with Bell's palsy. Option 4 identifies an inaccurate understanding of the disorder and requires further exploration. Review Bell's palsy if you had difficulty with this question.

Reference

Black, J., & Hawks, J. (2009). *Medical-surgical nursing: Clinical management for positive outcomes* (8th ed., p. 1886). St. Louis: Saunders.

---

578. A nurse is assisting with caring for a client newly diagnosed with diabetes mellitus who is anxious about the self-administration of insulin. Initially, the nurse should:

1 Teach a family member to give the client the insulin.

Answer: 3

Rationale: Some clients find it difficult to insert a needle into their own skin. For these clients, the nurse might assist by selecting the injection site and inserting the needle. Then, as a first step in self-injection, the client can push in the plunger and remove the needle. Options 1 and 4 place the client into a dependent role. Option 2 is not realistic in view of the subject of the question.

2 Have the client practice giving injections to an orange until he or she is less anxious.
3 Insert the needle into the client and then have the client push in the plunger and remove the needle.
4 Give the client the injection until the client feels confident enough to do so by himself or herself.

Level of Cognitive Ability: Application
Client Needs: Psychosocial Integrity
Integrated Process: Nursing Process/Implementation
Content Area: Adult Health/Endocrine

Test-Taking Strategy: Use the process of elimination, and note the strategic word *initially*. Focus on the subject—the self-administration of insulin; this will direct you to option 3. Review the psychosocial issues related to the self-administration of insulin if you had difficulty with this question.

Reference
deWit, S. (2009). *Medical-surgical nursing: Concepts & practice* (pp. 917-918). St. Louis: Saunders.

---

579. A 16-year-old client is admitted to the hospital with hyperglycemia from a failure to follow the prescribed diet, insulin, and glucose-monitoring regimen. The client states, "I'm fed up with having my life ruled by doctors' orders and machines!" The nurse identifies that the client is experiencing which problem?
1 Confusion related to the chronic illness
2 Anxiety related to the personal crisis
3 Failure to allow the prescribed regimen related to feelings of loss of control
4 Nutritional intake greater than needed related to the high blood glucose level

Level of Cognitive Ability: Analysis
Client Needs: Psychosocial Integrity
Integrated Process: Nursing Process/Data Collection
Content Area: Child Health

Answer: 3
Rationale: Adolescents strive for identity and independence, and this question describes a common fear of loss of control. The correct option relates to the subjects of the question—failure to follow the prescribed regimen and feelings of powerlessness. There is no indication of confusion or anxiety, and there are no data to support the problem related to nutrition.

Test-Taking Strategy: Use the process of elimination, and focus on the data in the question. Eliminate option 1 because there are no data to support confusion. Eliminate option 2 because, although the client may be experiencing a personal crisis, there is no evidence of anxiety. Eliminate option 4 because there are no data to support that the client is consuming more calories than the body requires. Review the needs of the adolescent with a chronic illness if you had difficulty with this question.

Reference
Price, D., & Gwin, J. (2008). *Pediatric nursing: An introductory text* (10th ed., pp. 330-331). St. Louis: Saunders.

---

580. The parents of a newborn with congenital hypothyroidism and Down syndrome tell the nurse how sad they are that their child was born with these problems. They had many plans for a normal child, and now these plans will need to be adjusted. Based on these statements, the nurse should address which problem?
1 Impaired adjustment
2 Anticipatory grieving
3 Dysfunctional grieving
4 Disabled family coping

Answer: 2
Rationale: Anticipatory grieving involves the intellectual and emotional responses and behaviors that individuals and families use to work through the process of modifying their self-concept with the perception of potential loss. Defining characteristics include expressions of sorrow and distress. Dysfunctional grieving and impaired adjustment are abnormal responses to changes in health status. Disabled family coping is identified when a usually supportive person is providing insufficient, ineffective, or compromised support, comfort, assistance, or encouragement.

Level of Cognitive Ability: Analysis
Client Needs: Psychosocial Integrity
Integrated Process: Nursing Process/Planning
Content Area: Maternity/Postpartum

Test-Taking Strategy: Use the process of elimination. Noting the word *sad* in the question should immediately lead you to one of the options related to grieving. From this point, eliminate option 3 because there is no data in the question to indicate that the grieving is dysfunctional. Review the characteristics of anticipatory grieving if you had difficulty with this question.

References

Leifer, G. (2007). *Introduction to maternity and pediatric nursing* (5th ed., p. 334). Philadelphia: Saunders.
Leifer, G. (2008). *Maternity nursing: An introductory text* (10th ed., p. 317). Philadelphia: Saunders.

---

581. A nurse is preparing a client for a parathyroidectomy. The client states, "I guess I'll have to learn to love wearing a scarf after this surgery!" The nurse determines that the client is experiencing which psychosocial problem?

1 Avoidance related to poor coping mechanisms
2 Acute pain related to surgical interruption of body tissue
3 Altered physical appearance related to the perceived negative effect of the surgical incision
4 Decreased physical mobility related to limited movement secondary to neck surgery

Level of Cognitive Ability: Analysis
Client Needs: Psychosocial Integrity
Integrated Process: Nursing Process/Data Collection
Content Area: Fundamental Skills

Answer: 3
Rationale: The client's statement reflects a psychosocial concern about appearance after surgery; thus altered physical appearance would be a potential problem. Option 1 is inappropriate because the client is addressing the concern rather than avoiding or denying it. Options 2 and 4 identify physiological problems.

Test-Taking Strategy: Use the process of elimination. The client is expressing a concern, so option 1 can be eliminated. Options 2 and 4 are physiological rather than psychosocial problems and are eliminated next. Review the psychosocial problems related to parathyroidectomy if you had difficulty with this question.

Reference

Ignatavicius, D., & Workman, M. (2010). *Medical-surgical nursing: Patient-centered collaborative care* (6th ed., pp. 682-683). St. Louis: Saunders.

---

582. The husband of a client with Graves' disease expresses concern about his wife's health. During the past 3 months, she has been experiencing nervousness, an inability to concentrate on even trivial tasks, and outbursts of temper. Based on this information, the nurse determines that the client is experiencing:

1 Grieving
2 Social isolation
3 Ineffective coping
4 Disturbed sensory perception

Level of Cognitive Ability: Analysis
Client Needs: Psychosocial Integrity
Integrated Process: Nursing Process/Data Collection
Content Area: Adult Health/Endocrine

Answer: 3
Rationale: Family and friends may report that the client with Graves' disease has become more irritable or depressed, especially after discharge from the hospital. The signs and symptoms in the question support data for the problem of ineffective coping and are not related to options 1, 2, and 4.

Test-Taking Strategy: Use the process of elimination, and focus on the data in the question. There is no information in the question that supports options 1, 2, or 4. Review the characteristics of ineffective coping if you had difficulty with this question.

Reference

Christensen, B., & Kockrow, E. (2006). *Adult health nursing* (5th ed., pp. 527-530, 535). St. Louis: Mosby.

---

583. A nurse is caring for a client with hypoparathyroidism. When assisting with planning for the client's discharge from the hospital, the nurse identifies which of the following as a potential psychosocial problem?

1 Skin breakdown related to edema
2 Acute pain related to cold intolerance secondary to decreased metabolic rate
3 Anxiety related to the need for lifelong dietary interventions to control the disease
4 Constipation related to decreased peristaltic action secondary to decreased metabolic rate

Level of Cognitive Ability: Analysis
Client Needs: Psychosocial Integrity
Integrated Process: Nursing Process/Data Collection
Content Area: Adult Health/Endocrine

Answer: 3

Rationale: The medical management of hypoparathyroidism is aimed at correcting the hypocalcemia. This is accomplished with prescribed medications and lifelong compliance with dietary guidelines, which include the consumption of foods high in calcium but low in phosphorus. Knowing that the interventions are lifelong can create some anxiety for the client, and this problem needs to be addressed before discharge. Options 1, 2, and 4 are unrelated to this disorder and are physiological problems rather than psychosocial concerns.

Test-Taking Strategy: Use the process of elimination. Noting the subject of the question and the words *psychosocial problem* will direct you to option 3. Options 1, 2, and 4 address physiological needs. Review hypoparathyroidism if you had difficulty with this question.

References

Christensen, B., & Kockrow, E. (2006). *Adult health nursing* (5th ed., p. 537). St. Louis: Mosby.
Linton, A. (2007). *Introduction to medical-surgical nursing* (4th ed., p. 999). Philadelphia: Saunders.

---

584. A client in labor has human immunodeficiency virus (HIV) and says to the nurse, "I know I will have a sick-looking baby." The nurse should make which therapeutic response to the client?

1 "You are very sick, but your baby may not be."
2 "All babies are beautiful. I am sure your baby will be, too."
3 "You have concerns about how HIV will affect your baby?"
4 "There is no reason to worry. Our neonatal unit offers the latest treatments available."

Level of Cognitive Ability: Application
Client Needs: Psychosocial Integrity
Integrated Process: Communication and Documentation
Content Area: Maternity/Postpartum

Answer: 3

Rationale: Option 3 is a therapeutic response and the response that will elicit the best information from the client. It addresses the therapeutic communication technique of paraphrasing. The mother should know that her baby will not look sick at birth and that there will be a period of uncertainty before it is known whether the baby has acquired HIV. Options 1 and 2 provide false reassurances. The nurse should not tell the client that there is no reason to worry.

Test-Taking Strategy: Use therapeutic communication techniques. Options 1 and 2 provide false reassurance. Eliminate option 4 because the nurse would not tell the client that there is no reason to worry. Option 3 is an open-ended question that will provide an opportunity for the client to verbalize her concerns. Review therapeutic communication techniques if you had difficulty with this question.

Reference

Leifer, G. (2007). *Introduction to maternity and pediatric nursing* (5th ed., p. 106). Philadelphia: Saunders.

---

585. A client who is scheduled for an abdominal peritoneoscopy says to the nurse, "The doctor told me to restrict food and liquids for at least 8 hours before this procedure and to use a Fleet enema 4 hours before coming to the hospital. Do people ever get into trouble with this procedure?" The nurse should

Answer: 2

Rationale: Abdominal peritoneoscopy is performed to directly visualize the liver, gallbladder, spleen, and stomach after the insufflation of carbon dioxide. During the procedure, a rigid laparoscope is inserted through a small incision in the abdomen. A microscope allows for the visualization of the organs and provides a way to collect a specimen for biopsy or to remove small tumors. A therapeutic response is one that facilitates the client's expression

make which therapeutic response to the client?
1 "Any invasive procedure brings risk with it. You need to report any shoulder pain immediately."
2 "You seem to understand the preparation very well. Are you having concerns about the procedure?"
3 "Trouble? There is never any trouble with this procedure. That's why the surgeon will use local anesthesia."
4 "There are relatively few problems, especially if you are having local anesthesia, but vaginal bleeding should be reported immediately."

Level of Cognitive Ability: Application
Client Needs: Psychosocial Integrity
Integrated Process: Communication and Documentation
Content Area: Adult Health/Gastrointestinal

of feelings and directly addresses the client's concerns. Options 1 and 4 will cause anxiety about the procedure. Option 3 is an inaccurate statement.

Test-Taking Strategy: Use therapeutic communication techniques. Option 2 is the therapeutic response because it supports the data provided in the question and provides an opportunity for the client to verbalize concerns. Review therapeutic communication techniques if you had difficulty with this question.

References

Chernecky, C., & Berger, B. (2008). *Laboratory tests and diagnostic procedures* (5th ed., pp. 700-701). Philadelphia: Saunders.
deWit, S. (2009). *Medical-surgical nursing: Concepts & practice* (p. 9). St. Louis: Saunders.

---

586. When planning care to meet the client's emotional needs during a precipitate labor, the nurse can anticipate the client having:
1 Fewer fears regarding the effect on the infant
2 Less pain and anxiety than with a normal labor
3 A sense of satisfaction regarding the quick labor
4 A need for support in maintaining a sense of control

Level of Cognitive Ability: Comprehension
Client Needs: Psychosocial Integrity
Integrated Process: Nursing Process/Planning
Content Area: Maternity/Intrapartum

Answer: 4
Rationale: The client experiencing a precipitate labor may have more difficulty maintaining control because of the abrupt onset of labor and its quick progression. This may be very different from previous labor experiences; therefore the client needs support from the nurse to understand and adapt to the rapid progression. The contractions often increase in intensity quickly, thus adding to the client's pain, anxiety, and lack of control. The client may also have an increased amount of concern about the effect of labor on the baby. Lack of control over the situation in combination with increased pain and anxiety can result in a decreased level of satisfaction with the labor and delivery experience. Options 1, 2, and 3 imply positive effects of the experience of precipitate labor.

Test-Taking Strategy: Use the process of elimination, and recall that precipitate labor has an abrupt onset and a quick progression. Note the strategic words *need for support* in option 4. Psychosocial questions often address the client's needs for support. Review the psychosocial issues related to precipitate labor if you had difficulty with this question.

References

Leifer, G. (2007). *Introduction to maternity and pediatric nursing* (5th ed., p. 192). Philadelphia: Saunders.
Leifer, G. (2008). *Maternity nursing: An introductory text* (10th ed., pp. 7, 291). Philadelphia: Saunders.

---

587. A nurse is assisting with planning care for a client who presents in active labor with a history of a previous cesarean delivery. The client complains of a

Answer: 4
Rationale: Pregnant clients have concern for the safety of their babies during labor and delivery, especially when a problem arises. A calm attitude with realistic reassurances is an important

tearing sensation in the lower abdomen. She is upset and expresses concern for the safety of her baby. The appropriate response from the nurse is:

1 "Don't worry, you are in good hands."
2 "I don't have time to answer questions now. We'll talk later."
3 "You'll have to talk to your doctor about the tearing sensation."
4 "I can understand that you are fearful. We are doing everything possible for your baby."

Level of Cognitive Ability: Application
Client Needs: Psychosocial Integrity
Integrated Process: Communication and Documentation
Content Area: Maternity/Intrapartum

aspect of client care. Dismissing or ignoring the client's concerns (options 1, 2, and 3) can lead to increased fear and lack of cooperation.

Test-Taking Strategy: Use therapeutic communication techniques, and avoid options that block therapeutic communication. Option 1 involves the use of a cliché and false reassurance. Options 2 and 3 place the client's feelings on hold. Look for the option that reflects acceptance of the client's feelings and provides realistic reassurances; this will direct you to option 4. Review therapeutic communication techniques if you had difficulty with this question.

References

Leifer, G. (2007). *Introduction to maternity and pediatric nursing* (5th ed., p. 142). Philadelphia: Saunders.

Leifer, G. (2008). *Maternity nursing: An introductory text* (10th ed., p. 7). Philadelphia: Saunders.

---

588. During an initial physical examination of a newborn male, undescended testes (cryptorchidism) are discovered, and these findings are shared with the parents. The nurse understands that if this condition is not corrected, which of the following could have a psychosocial impact?

1 Atrophy
2 Infertility
3 Malignancy
4 Feminization

Level of Cognitive Ability: Comprehension
Client Needs: Psychosocial Integrity
Integrated Process: Nursing Process/Planning
Content Area: Child Health

Answer: 2

Rationale: Infertility could occur with this disorder because sperm production is decreased in the undescended testes. The psychological effects of an "empty scrotum" could affect the client's self-perception as well as his ability to reproduce. Options 1 and 3 are physiological concerns. Option 4 is not associated with this condition.

Test-Taking Strategy: Note the strategic words *psychosocial impact.* Options 1 and 3 are possible physical consequences of a failure to treat cryptorchidism, so they can be eliminated. Because all hormones responsible for secondary sex characteristics continue to be secreted directly into the bloodstream, option 4 is not correct. Review the psychosocial effects of cryptorchidism if you had difficulty with this question.

References

Leifer, G. (2007). *Introduction to maternity and pediatric nursing* (5th ed., p. 672). Philadelphia: Saunders.

Price, D., & Gwin, J. (2008). *Pediatric nursing: An introductory text* (10th ed., p. 167). St. Louis: Saunders.

---

589. Cranial surgery is performed on an adolescent who sustained a head injury. Which psychosocial issue is of the most concern in the adolescent?

1 Residual headaches
2 Short-term memory loss
3 Head area being shaved for the surgical procedure
4 Administration of phenobarbital (Luminal) medication

Answer: 3

Rationale: Body image is a main focus for an adolescent; appearance is very important and is linked with peer acceptance in this age group. A loss of hair in the head area alters the adolescent's appearance. Residual headaches can be controlled with medication and stress-reduction techniques. Option 2 could be a problem if memory loss interferes with remembering friends' names or directions or with school performance, but these are not as obvious as hair loss. Phenobarbital administration does not have psychosocial implications unless the adolescent refuses to take the medication.

Level of Cognitive Ability: Comprehension
Client Needs: Psychosocial Integrity
Integrated Process: Nursing Process/Planning
Content Area: Child Health

Test-Taking Strategy: Use the process of elimination. Remember that adolescents' focus at this stage of growth and development is body image and how peers perceive them. Based on this focus, you can easily eliminate options 1 and 4. From the remaining options, select option 3 because this is the most obvious alteration in body image. Review psychosocial issues related to the adolescent if you had difficulty with this question.

Reference

Leifer, G. (2007). *Introduction to maternity and pediatric nursing* (5th ed., p. 533). Philadelphia: Saunders.

---

590. A mother with an infant with hydrocephalus is concerned about the complication of mental retardation. The mother states, "I'm not sure if I can care for my baby at home." Which of the following is the appropriate response by the nurse?

1 "All babies have individual needs."
2 "Mothers instinctively know what is best for their babies."
3 "You have concerns about your baby's condition and care?"
4 "There is no reason to worry. You have a good pediatrician."

Level of Cognitive Ability: Application
Client Needs: Psychosocial Integrity
Integrated Process: Communication and Documentation
Content Area: Maternity/Postpartum

Answer: 3

Rationale: Paraphrasing is restating the mother's message in the nurse's own words. Option 3 involves the therapeutic technique of paraphrasing. In option 1, the nurse is minimizing the social needs involved with the baby's diagnosis, which is harmful for the nurse–parent relationship. In options 2 and 4, the nurse is offering false reassurance; these types of responses will block communication.

Test-Taking Strategy: Use therapeutic communication techniques and the process of elimination. Option 3 is the only therapeutic technique, and it includes paraphrasing; this is the only option that will provide the client with an opportunity to verbalize her concerns. Review therapeutic communication techniques if you had difficulty with this question.

References

Leifer, G. (2007). *Introduction to maternity and pediatric nursing* (5th ed., p. 323). Philadelphia: Saunders.
Leifer, G. (2008). *Maternity nursing: An introductory text* (10th ed., p. 7). Philadelphia: Saunders.

---

591. A preschooler has just been diagnosed with impetigo. The child's mother tells the nurse, "But my children take baths every day." Which of the following is the appropriate response by the nurse?

1 "You are concerned about how your child got impetigo?"
2 "There is no need to worry, we will not tell day care why your child is absent."
3 "Not only do you have to do a better job of keeping your children clean, you also need to wash your hands more frequently."
4 "You should have seen the doctor before the wound became infected, then you would not have had to worry about your child having impetigo."

Answer: 1

Rationale: By paraphrasing what the parent tells the nurse, the nurse is addressing the parent's thoughts. Option 1 involves the therapeutic technique of paraphrasing. All of the other options are blocks to communication because they make the parent feel guilty for the child's illness.

Test-Taking Strategy: Use therapeutic communication techniques and the process of elimination. Option 1 is the only therapeutic option, and it includes the technique of paraphrasing; this is the only option that will provide the client with an opportunity to verbalize her concerns. Options 2, 3, and 4 are blocks to communication. Review therapeutic communication techniques if you had difficulty with this question.

References

deWit, S. (2009). *Medical-surgical nursing: Concepts & practice* (p. 9). St. Louis: Saunders.
Price, D., & Gwin, J. (2008). *Pediatric nursing: An introductory text* (10th ed., pp. 138, 140). St. Louis: Saunders.

Level of Cognitive Ability: Application
Client Needs: Psychosocial Integrity
Integrated Process: Communication and Documentation
Content Area: Child Health

---

592. Which is the best way to address the cultural needs of a child and family when the child is admitted to a health care facility?

1 Address only those issues that directly affect the nurse's care of the child.
2 Ignore cultural needs because they are not important to health care professionals.
3 Ask questions about cultural needs, and explain to the family why the questions are being asked.
4 Explain to the family that while the child is being treated, they need to discontinue cultural practices because they may be harmful to the child.

Level of Cognitive Ability: Comprehension
Client Needs: Psychosocial Integrity
Integrated Process: Nursing Process/Implementation
Content Area: Child Health

Answer: 3
Rationale: When caring for individuals from different cultures, it is important to ask questions about specific cultural needs and means of treatment. An understanding of the family's beliefs and health practices is essential to successful interventions for that particular family. Options 1, 2, and 4 ignore the cultural beliefs and values of the client.

Test-Taking Strategy: Use the process of elimination, and focus on the subject—cultural needs. Options 1, 2, and 4 are comparable or alike in that they ignore the cultural practices and values of the client. Option 3 addresses the cultural needs of the family and the child. Review the concepts related to cultural needs if you had difficulty with this question.

Reference
Leifer, G. (2007). *Introduction to maternity and pediatric nursing* (5th ed., pp. 468, 470-471). Philadelphia: Saunders.

---

593. A client with a T1 spinal cord injury has just learned that the cord was completely severed. The client says, "I'm no good to anyone. I might as well be dead." The appropriate response by the nurse is:

1 "You're not a useless person at all."
2 "I'll ask the psychologist to see you about this."
3 "You are feeling pretty bad about things right now."
4 "It makes me uncomfortable when you talk this way."

Level of Cognitive Ability: Application
Client Needs: Psychosocial Integrity
Integrated Process: Communication and Documentation
Content Area: Adult Health/Neurological

Answer: 3
Rationale: Restating and reflecting keeps the communication open and shows interest that will encourage the client to expand on the current feelings of unworthiness and loss that require exploration. The nurse blocks communication by showing disapproval (option 1) or discomfort (option 4) or by postponing a discussion of issues (option 2). Options 1, 2, and 4 block communication.

Test-Taking Strategy: Use therapeutic communication techniques and the process of elimination. Review the options and consider the effect that they may have on the client. Options 1, 2, and 4 clearly block communication. Option 3 identifies the therapeutic communication technique of restating and reflecting. Review therapeutic communication techniques if you had difficulty with this question.

Reference
Linton, A. (2007). *Introduction to medical-surgical nursing* (4th ed., pp. 54, 503-504). Philadelphia: Saunders.

---

594. A nurse enters the room of a client with coronary artery disease and finds the client quietly crying. After determining that

Answer: 2
Rationale: Clients with heart disease often experience anxiety or fear. The nurse encourages the client to express concerns by

there is no physiological reason for the client's distress, the nurse replies:
1 "Do you want me to call your daughter?"
2 "Can you tell me a little about what has you so upset?"
3 "Try not to be so upset. Psychological stress is bad for your heart."
4 "I understand how you feel. I'd cry too if I had a major heart attack."

Level of Cognitive Ability: Application
Client Needs: Psychosocial Integrity
Integrated Process: Communication and Documentation
Content Area: Adult Health/Cardiovascular

showing genuine interest and by facilitating communication using therapeutic communication techniques. Options 1, 3, and 4 do not address the client's feelings or promote client verbalization.

Test-Taking Strategy: Use therapeutic communication techniques. Select the option that has an exploratory approach because the question does not identify why the client is upset. Review therapeutic communication techniques if you had difficulty with this question.

Reference
deWit, S. (2009). *Medical-surgical nursing: Concepts & practice* (p. 499). St. Louis: Saunders.

---

595. A male client with a recent complete T4 spinal cord transection tells the nurse that he will walk as soon as spinal shock abates. Which of the following will provide the most accurate basis for planning the nurse's response?
1 The client is projecting by insisting that walking is the goal of rehabilitation.
2 To speed acceptance, the client needs reinforcement that he will not walk again.
3 The client should move through the grieving process rapidly to benefit from rehabilitation.
4 Denial can be protective while the client deals with the anxiety created by the new disability.

Level of Cognitive Ability: Analysis
Client Needs: Psychosocial Integrity
Integrated Process: Nursing Process/Planning
Content Area: Adult Health/Neurological

Answer: 4
Rationale: During the adjustment period that occurs for the first few weeks after a spinal cord injury, clients may use denial as a defense mechanism. Denial may temporarily decrease anxiety, and it is a normal part of grieving. After spinal shock abates, denial may impair rehabilitation if its use is prolonged or excessive. However, rehabilitation programs include psychological counseling to deal with grief. Options 1, 2, and 3 are inaccurate.

Test-Taking Strategy: Use the process of elimination. The words *walking is the goal of rehabilitation, speed acceptance,* and *move through the grieving process rapidly* should be indicators that options 1, 2, and 3, respectively, are incorrect. Focus on the client's statement, which is an indication of denial. Review the characteristics of denial if you had difficulty with this question.

References
Christensen, B., & Kockrow, E. (2006). *Foundations of nursing* (5th ed., pp. 1133-1134). St. Louis: Mosby.
deWit, S. (2009). *Medical-surgical nursing: Concepts & practice* (p. 554). St. Louis: Saunders.

---

596. Maladaptive coping behavior can occur in response to a loss or change in the body associated with surgery. In this situation, the nurse should include which action in the nursing care plan?
1 Explain to the client that open grieving is abnormal.
2 Encourage the client to express feelings about body changes.
3 Advise the client to seek psychological treatment immediately.
4 Discourage sharing feelings with others who have had similar experiences.

Answer: 2
Rationale: Surgery can alter a client's body image. The onset of problems with coping with these changes may occur during the immediate or extended postoperative stage. Nursing interventions primarily involve providing psychological support, and the nurse should encourage the client to express feelings. Options 1, 3, and 4 are inaccurate interventions.

Test-Taking Strategy: Use therapeutic communication techniques. Remember that options that block communication (e.g., giving advice, as shown in option 3) and that show disapproval (options 1 and 4) are incorrect. Always focus on the client's feelings first. Review therapeutic communication techniques if you had difficulty with this question.

Level of Cognitive Ability: Application
Client Needs: Psychosocial Integrity
Integrated Process: Nursing Process/Planning
Content Area: Fundamental Skills

Reference

Linton, A. (2007). *Introduction to medical-surgical nursing* (4th ed., p. 275). Philadelphia: Saunders.

---

597. A client with pulmonary edema exhibits severe anxiety. The nurse is preparing to carry out the medically prescribed orders. Which approach should the nurse plan to meet the needs of the client in a holistic manner?

1 Ask a family member to stay with the client.
2 Give the client the call bell and encourage its use if the client feels worse.
3 Leave the client alone while gathering required equipment and medications.
4 Stay with the client and ask another nurse to gather the equipment and supplies that are not already in the room.

Level of Cognitive Ability: Application
Client Needs: Psychosocial Integrity
Integrated Process: Nursing Process/Planning
Content Area: Adult Health/Respiratory

Answer: 4

Rationale: Pulmonary edema is accompanied by extreme fear and anxiety. Because the client typically experiences a sense of impending doom, the nurse should remain with the client as much as possible. Options 2 and 3 do not provide for the psychological needs of the client in distress. Family members (option 1) can emotionally support the client but are not able to respond to physiological needs and symptoms. In fact, they are typically in psychological distress themselves.

Test-Taking Strategy: Use the process of elimination. The word *holistic* in the question guides you to consider both the physical and emotional needs of the client; this will direct you to option 4. Review the care of the client with pulmonary edema if you had difficulty with this question.

References

deWit, S. (2009). *Medical-surgical nursing: Concepts & practice* (p. 470). St. Louis: Saunders.

Ignatavicius, D., & Workman, M. (2010). *Medical-surgical nursing: Patient-centered collaborative care* (6th ed., pp. 682-683). St. Louis: Saunders.

---

598. The family of a client with myocardial infarction is visibly anxious and upset about the client's condition. The nurse should plan to do which of the following to provide support for the family?

1 Offer them coffee and other beverages on a regular basis.
2 Insist that they go home to sleep at night to keep up their strength.
3 Ask the hospital chaplain to sit with them until the client's condition stabilizes.
4 Provide flexibility with visiting times according to the client's condition and family needs.

Level of Cognitive Ability: Application
Client Needs: Psychosocial Integrity
Integrated Process: Nursing Process/Planning
Content Area: Adult Health/Cardiovascular

Answer: 4

Rationale: The use of flexible visiting hours meets the needs of the client and family by reducing the anxiety levels of both. Offering the family beverages does not provide support. Although the chaplain may provide support, it is unrealistic for the chaplain to stay until the client stabilizes; in addition, the religious preference of the family may not be compatible with this option. Insisting that the family go home is non-therapeutic.

Test-Taking Strategy: Use the process of elimination. The question asks for the method of support. Options 2 and 3 may or may not be helpful, depending on the client and family situation. Coffee and beverages, while probably helpful for many visitors, do not provide support and can also be obtained in the hospital cafeteria. This leaves option 4 as the intervention with the most value. Review the measures that provide support to the client and family if you had difficulty with this question.

Reference

deWit, S. (2009). *Medical-surgical nursing: Concepts & practice* (p. 498). St. Louis: Saunders.

---

599. A client with unstable angina says to the nurse, "I'm so afraid something bad will happen." Which action by the nurse provides the most immediate help to the client?

1 Staying with the client
2 Telephoning the client's family
3 Using television to distract the client
4 Giving reassurance that nothing will happen to the client

Level of Cognitive Ability: Application
Client Needs: Psychosocial Integrity
Integrated Process: Nursing Process/Implementation
Content Area: Adult Health/Cardiovascular

Answer: 1

Rationale: When a client experiences fear, the nurse can provide a calm, safe environment by offering appropriate reassurance with the therapeutic use of touch and by remaining with the client as much as possible. The actions in options 2 and 3 avoid the client and do not provide direct support. Option 4 provides false reassurance.

Test-Taking Strategy: Use the process of elimination. Options 2 and 3 can be eliminated first because they do not provide direct support to the client. From the remaining options, focus on the strategic words *most immediate help;* this will direct you to option 1. Remember to provide support to the client. Review the measures that provide support to the client if you had difficulty with this question.

Reference

Christensen, B., & Kockrow, E. (2006). *Adult health nursing* (5th ed., p. 358). St. Louis: Mosby.

---

600. A male client with Raynaud's disease tells the nurse that he has a stressful job and that he does not handle stressful situations well. The nurse should encourage the client to:

1 Change jobs.
2 Seek help from a psychologist.
3 Consider a stress-management program.
4 Use earplugs to minimize environmental noise.

Level of Cognitive Ability: Application
Client Needs: Psychosocial Integrity
Integrated Process: Nursing Process/Implementation
Content Area: Adult Health/Cardiovascular

Answer: 3

Rationale: Stress can trigger the vasospasm that occurs with Raynaud's disease, so referral to a stress-management program or the use of biofeedback training may be helpful. These measures teach clients a variety of techniques to reduce or minimize stress. Option 1 is unrealistic. Option 2 is not necessarily required at this time. Option 4 does not specifically address the subject.

Test-Taking Strategy: Use the process of elimination, and focus on the subject—managing stress. Note the word *consider* in option 3. This option provides the client with both assistance and the opportunity to make an independent decision. Review the care of the client with Raynaud's disease if you had difficulty with this question.

Reference

Christensen, B., & Kockrow, E. (2006). *Adult health nursing* (5th ed., p. 389). St. Louis: Mosby.

---

601. A client has an oral endotracheal tube attached to a mechanical ventilator and is about to begin the weaning process. The nurse who is assisting with caring for the client determines that which item, which was previously useful to minimize the client's anxiety, should be limited?

1 Radio
2 Television
3 Family visitors
4 Antianxiety medications

Level of Cognitive Ability: Comprehension
Client Needs: Psychosocial Integrity
Integrated Process: Nursing Process/Implementation
Content Area: Adult Health/Respiratory

Answer: 4

Rationale: Antianxiety medications and opioid analgesics are used cautiously in the client being weaned from a mechanical ventilator. These medications may interfere with the weaning process by suppressing the respiratory drive. The client may exhibit anxiety during the weaning process for a variety of reasons; therefore distractions such as radio, television, and visitors are still very useful.

Test-Taking Strategy: To answer this question accurately, you should identify the item that could interfere with the client's strength, endurance, and respiratory drive when maintaining independent ventilation. Using this as the guideline will direct you to option 4. Side effects of antianxiety medications can include sedation, which could interfere with optimal respiratory function. Review the psychosocial effects of weaning from a mechanical ventilator if you had difficulty with this question.

Reference

Black, J., & Hawks, J. (2009). *Medical-surgical nursing: Clinical management for positive outcomes* (8th ed., pp. 1651-1652). St. Louis: Saunders.

---

602. A client scheduled for pulmonary angiography is fearful about the procedure and asks the nurse if the procedure involves significant pain and radiation exposure. The nurse gives a response to the client that provides reassurance, understanding that:

1 The procedure is somewhat painful, but there is minimal exposure to radiation.
2 Discomfort may occur with needle insertion, and there is minimal exposure to radiation.
3 There is very mild pain throughout the procedure, and the exposure to radiation is negligible.
4 There is absolutely no pain, although a moderate amount of radiation must be used to obtain accurate results.

Level of Cognitive Ability: Comprehension
Client Needs: Psychosocial Integrity
Integrated Process: Nursing Process/Implementation
Content Area: Adult Health/Respiratory

Answer: 2

Rationale: Pulmonary angiography involves minimal exposure to radiation. The procedure is painless, although the client may feel discomfort with the insertion of the needle for the catheter that is used for dye injection. Options 1, 3, and 4 are incorrect.

Test-Taking Strategy: Use the process of elimination. Knowing that radiation exposure is minimal with this procedure helps you to eliminate option 4 first. It is also helpful to know that the only discomfort occurs with needle insertion; this will direct you to option 2. Review pulmonary angiography if you had difficulty with this question.

Reference

Chernecky, C., & Berger, B. (2008). *Laboratory tests and diagnostic procedures* (5th ed., pp. 936-937). Philadelphia: Saunders.

---

603. A client has an initial positive result of an enzyme-linked immunosorbent assay (ELISA) test for human immunodeficiency virus (HIV). The client begins to cry and asks the nurse what this means. The nurse is able to provide support to the client, using knowledge that:

1 The client is HIV positive but the client's CD4 cell count is high.
2 The client is HIV positive but the disease has been detected early.
3 There are occasional false-positive readings with this test, which can be cleared up by repeating it one more time.
4 There is a high rate of false-positive results with this test, so more testing is needed before diagnosing the client as being HIV positive.

Level of Cognitive Ability: Comprehension
Client Needs: Psychosocial Integrity
Integrated Process: Nursing Process/Implementation
Content Area: Adult Health/Respiratory

Answer: 4

Rationale: If the ELISA test results are positive, the test is repeated. If the test is positive a second time, then a Western blot test, which is more specific, is performed to confirm the finding. The client is not considered HIV positive unless the Western blot test is positive. The ELISA is a fast and relatively inexpensive test, but it carries a high false-positive rate.

Test-Taking Strategy: Use the process of elimination, and recall that HIV infection is not diagnosed with a single laboratory test. With this in mind, eliminate options 1 and 2 first. To choose correctly between options 3 and 4, it is necessary to understand that the ELISA would be repeated and that a Western blot test would be done to confirm these results. Review HIV testing if you had difficulty with this question.

Reference

deWit, S. (2009). *Medical-surgical nursing: Concepts & practice* (pp. 237, 240). St. Louis: Saunders.

604. A client is hospitalized during an acute period of mania. The client is restless and pacing in the hallway and slaps another client who is walking down the hall to a group meeting. Which statement by the nurse regarding the client's behavior is the least therapeutic?

1 "You're lucky that you didn't get hit right back!"
2 "You cannot hit other people. Come with me to your room now."
3 "I understand that you are not feeling well, but you cannot hurt others."
4 "If you are having difficulty controlling yourself right now, I will help you."

Level of Cognitive Ability: Application
Client Needs: Psychosocial Integrity
Integrated Process: Communication and Documentation
Content Area: Mental Health

Answer: 1
Rationale: The client with mania may exhibit aggression. The nurse should respond using therapeutic communication techniques and should set limits on the client's behavior. Option 1 is the least therapeutic because it could aggravate the client and escalate the client's aggressive behavior. The statements in options 3 and 4 convey understanding and set limits on the client's behavior. The statement in option 2 sets limits on the client's behavior.

Test-Taking Strategy: Use the process of elimination, and note the strategic words *least therapeutic*. Option 1 could aggravate the client and escalate the client's behavior. Review therapeutic communication techniques if you had difficulty with this question.

Reference
Varcarolis, E., & Halter, M. (2009). *Essentials of psychiatric mental health nursing: A communication approach to evidence-based care* (pp. 251-252). St. Louis: Saunders.

---

605. A client with renal cell carcinoma of the left kidney is scheduled for nephrectomy. The client is told that the right kidney appears normal at this time, but the client is anxious about whether dialysis will ultimately be a necessity. The nurse should plan to use which of the following information during discussions with the client?

1 There is a strong likelihood that the client will need dialysis within 5 to 10 years.
2 There is absolutely no chance of needing dialysis because of the nature of the surgery.
3 One kidney is adequate to meet the needs of the body as long as it has normal function.
4 Dialysis could become likely, but it depends on how well the client complies with fluid restriction after surgery.

Level of Cognitive Ability: Application
Client Needs: Psychosocial Integrity
Integrated Process: Nursing Process/Planning
Content Area: Adult Health/Oncology

Answer: 3
Rationale: Fears about having only one functioning kidney are common among clients who must undergo nephrectomy for renal cancer. These clients need emotional support and reassurance that the remaining kidney should be able to fully meet the body's metabolic needs as long as it has normal function. Options 1, 2, and 4 are incorrect statements.

Test-Taking Strategy: Use the process of elimination. Eliminate option 2 first because it contains the close-ended words *absolutely no chance.* Knowing that there is no need for fluid restriction with a functioning kidney guides you to eliminate option 4 next. From the remaining options, remember that an individual can donate a kidney without adverse consequences or the need for dialysis. Review the psychosocial effects of a nephrectomy if you had difficulty with this question.

Reference
Linton, A. (2007). *Introduction to medical-surgical nursing* (4th ed., pp. 863-864). Philadelphia: Saunders.

---

606. A psychosocial plan of care for a client with a diagnosis of acute pulmonary edema should include strategies for:

1 Reducing anxiety
2 Increasing fluid volume

Answer: 1
Rationale: When cardiac output falls as a result of acute pulmonary edema, the sympathetic nervous system is stimulated. Stimulation of the sympathetic nervous system results in the fight-or-flight reaction, which further impairs cardiac function. The goal

3 Decreasing cardiac output
4 Promoting a positive body image

Level of Cognitive Ability: Application
Client Needs: Psychosocial Integrity
Integrated Process: Nursing Process/Planning
Content Area: Adult Health/Cardiovascular

of treatment is to increase cardiac output. Fluid volume should be decreased. Disturbed body image is not a common problem among clients with acute pulmonary edema.

Test-Taking Strategy: Use the process of elimination. Considering the physiological manifestations of this condition will assist you with eliminating options 2 and 3. From the remaining options, recalling that severe dyspnea occurs will direct you to option 1. Review the psychosocial manifestations associated with acute pulmonary edema if you had difficulty with this question.

Reference

Christensen, B., & Kockrow, E. (2006). *Adult health nursing* (5th ed., p. 445). St. Louis: Mosby.

---

607. A client with acute renal failure (ARF) is having trouble remembering information and instructions because of an elevated blood urea nitrogen (BUN) level. The nurse should avoid doing which of the following when communicating with this client?

1 Giving simple, clear directions
2 Including the family in discussions related to care
3 Explaining treatments using understandable language
4 Giving thorough, complete explanations of treatment options

Level of Cognitive Ability: Application
Client Needs: Psychosocial Integrity
Integrated Process: Communication and Documentation
Content Area: Adult Health/Renal

Answer: 4

Rationale: The client with ARF may have difficulty remembering information and instructions because of an increased BUN level and anxiety. Communication should be clear, simple, and understandable. The family is included whenever possible. It is the physician's responsibility to explain treatment options.

Test-Taking Strategy: Use the process of elimination, and note the strategic word *avoid*. Recalling the basic principles of effective communication will help you to recognize that options 1, 2, and 3 are helpful for maintaining effective communication. Review effective communication techniques if you had difficulty with this question.

Reference

deWit, S. (2009). *Medical-surgical nursing: Concepts & practice* (pp. 853-854). St. Louis: Saunders.

---

608. A nurse is assisting with planning care for a client who has been newly diagnosed with active tuberculosis (TB). When addressing the psychosocial needs of the client, which of the following is the primary goal?

1 The client will list all instructions for care and explain when to use each.
2 The client will verbalize ways to lessen the risk of transmitting the infection.
3 The client will ask questions and actively seek information about the disease and its care.
4 The client will share with the nurse or another support person his or her fears about the disease.

Answer: 4

Rationale: Addressing psychosocial needs relates to helping the client deal with his or her own feelings. Goals for the client focus on the open expression of feelings and fears and the development of coping skills for dealing with the illness and the care required. Options 1, 2, and 3 do not address psychosocial needs.

Test-Taking Strategy: Focus on the strategic words *psychosocial needs*. Use the process of elimination, and note the word *fears* in option 4. Review psychosocial care needs for the client with TB if you had difficulty with this question.

Reference

Linton, A. (2007). *Introduction to medical-surgical nursing* (4th ed., p. 564). Philadelphia: Saunders.

Level of Cognitive Ability: Application
Client Needs: Psychosocial Integrity
Integrated Process: Nursing Process/Planning
Content Area: Adult Health/Respiratory

---

609. When collecting data during the psychosocial assessment of a client with human immunodeficiency virus (HIV), the nurse should focus primarily on:
1 The presence of any concerns or fears
2 Why the client waited so long to seek treatment
3 What type of career the client would like to pursue
4 Which family member will assume the client's care on discharge

Level of Cognitive Ability: Application
Client Needs: Psychosocial Integrity
Integrated Process: Nursing Process/Data Collection
Content Area: Fundamental Skills

Answer: 1
Rationale: When collecting data about the psychosocial needs of a client with HIV, the nurse should address the issue of client concerns or fears. Asking why someone did or did not do something tends to produce defensiveness rather than trust. Career choices are not the priority issue at this time. Asking about care at home is an important discharge planning issue, but it is not the primary concern among the options provided.

Test-Taking Strategy: Use the process of elimination, and note the strategic word *psychosocial*. Recalling that the primary intervention when addressing psychosocial needs is addressing the client's feelings will direct you to option 1. Review the psychosocial needs of the client with HIV if you had difficulty with this question.

Reference
Christensen, B., & Kockrow, E. (2006). *Adult health nursing* (5th ed., pp. 797-799). St. Louis: Mosby.

---

610. A client with hyperparathyroidism talks to the nurse about the dietary changes prescribed by the physician. The client states, "I guess I'll never be able to eat ice cream and yogurt again." The nurse appropriately responds by stating:
1 "Why do you say that?"
2 "There are lots of other foods you can eat."
3 "Ice cream has too much fat content, anyway."
4 "You don't think you will be able to eat them at all?"

Level of Cognitive Ability: Application
Client Needs: Psychosocial Integrity
Integrated Process: Communication and Documentation
Content Area: Fundamental Skills

Answer: 4
Rationale: Treatment for clients with hyperparathyroidism includes a low-calcium diet. Ice cream and yogurt are high in calcium and should be restricted. The nurse should respond by rephrasing the client's statement. Options 1, 2, and 3 are examples of communication blocks (e.g., giving advice, requesting an explanation).

Test-Taking Strategy: Use therapeutic communication techniques to answer the question. Options 1, 2, and 3 are communication blocks. Option 4 seeks to validate what the nurse heard to determine whether additional instruction is needed. Review therapeutic communication techniques if you had difficulty with this question.

References
Christensen, B., & Kockrow, E. (2006). *Adult health nursing* (5th ed., p. 536). St. Louis: Mosby.
deWit, S. (2009). *Medical-surgical nursing: Concepts & practice* (p. 9). St. Louis: Saunders.

---

611. A client scheduled for chorionic villus sampling tells the nurse, "I'm not sure I should have this test." Which response by the nurse is appropriate?
1 "It's your decision."
2 "Tell me what concerns you have."

Answer: 2
Rationale: The nurse needs to gather more data and assist the client with exploring her feelings about the test. The nurse should not disregard the client's feelings. Options 1, 3, and 4 are nontherapeutic.

3 "Don't worry. Everything will be fine."
4 "Why don't you want to have this test?"

Level of Cognitive Ability: Application
Client Needs: Psychosocial Integrity
Integrated Process: Communication and Documentation
Content Area: Fundamental Skills

Test-Taking Strategy: Use therapeutic communication techniques to answer the question. Options 1, 3, and 4 are blocks to communication. Option 2 addresses the client's concern. Review therapeutic communication techniques if you had difficulty with this question.

References

Chernecky, C., & Berger, B. (2008). *Laboratory tests and diagnostic procedures* (5th ed., pp. 339-340). Philadelphia: Saunders.
deWit, S. (2009). *Medical-surgical nursing: Concepts & practice* (p. 9). St. Louis: Saunders.

---

612. A client states, "It will be so hard to wait for the results of this amniocentesis. I don't know what I will do if something goes wrong." The nurse should make which therapeutic response to the client?
1 "You are in good hands; your doctor is the best."
2 "You sound concerned about having this test done."
3 "It's not good for your baby when you become upset or worry."
4 "This test has been done for many years with few reported complications."

Level of Cognitive Ability: Application
Client Needs: Psychosocial Integrity
Integrated Process: Communication and Documentation
Content Area: Fundamental Skills

Answer: 2
Rationale: The nurse needs to gather more data and assist the client with exploring her feelings about the test. The nurse should not disregard the client's feelings. Options 1, 3, and 4 are incorrect; they do not focus on the client's feelings and concerns.

Test-Taking Strategy: Use therapeutic communication techniques to answer the question. Options 1, 3, and 4 are blocks to communication. Option 2 addresses the client's concern. Review therapeutic communication techniques if you had difficulty with this question.

Reference

Leifer, G. (2008). *Maternity nursing: An introductory text* (10th ed., pp. 7, 64, 66). Philadelphia: Saunders.

---

613. A hospitalized client is being prepared for discharge to home in 2 days. The client has been eating a regular diet for a week but is still receiving intermittent enteral tube feedings; he expresses concern that he will not be able to do the tube feedings at home. The nurse should make which appropriate response at this time?
1 "Do you want to stay in the hospital?"
2 "Have you discussed your feelings with your doctor?"
3 "Tell me more about your concerns with your diet after going home."
4 "Your tube feedings will no longer be necessary after your discharge."

Level of Cognitive Ability: Application
Client Needs: Psychosocial Integrity
Integrated Process: Communication and Documentation
Content Area: Fundamental Skills

Answer: 3
Rationale: A client often has fears about leaving the secure, cared-for environment of the hospital. This client is concerned about not being able to care for himself at home and not being able to perform his tube feedings. Option 1 is not related to the client's concern. Option 2 places the client's concern on hold. There are no data to indicate that the tube feedings will be discontinued.

Test-Taking Strategy: Use therapeutic communication techniques to answer the question. Remember to always focus on the client's concerns. Option 3 is the only option that addresses the client's concerns. Review therapeutic communication techniques if you had difficulty with this question.

References

Christensen, B., & Kockrow, E. (2006). *Foundations of nursing* (5th ed., pp. 228, 230-231). St. Louis: Mosby.
dewit, S. (2009). *Medical surgical nursing: Concepts & practice* (p. 9). St. Louis: Saunders.

614. A client will be receiving continuous parenteral nutrition at home for long-term nutritional therapy. Which potential problem is a priority concern?

1 Hopelessness
2 Social isolation
3 Low self-esteem
4 Fluid volume deficit

Answer: 2

Rationale: This client will be receiving continuous parenteral nutrition for the long term and thus isolated from psychological and physical stimuli outside of the home. Social isolation leads to depression, poor healing, and decreased compliance with medical regimens. Fluid volume excess (rather than deficit) is most likely to occur. There are no data in the question to support options 1 or 3.

Test-Taking Strategy: Focus on the data provided in the question, and note the strategic words *long-term*. The careful reading of option 4 will assist you with eliminating this option. Next, eliminate options 1 and 3 because there are no data in the question to support these options. Review the psychosocial impact of long-term continuous parenteral nutrition if you had difficulty with this question.

Level of Cognitive Ability: Analysis
Client Needs: Psychosocial Integrity
Integrated Process: Nursing Process/Data Collection
Content Area: Fundamental Skills

Reference

Perry, A., & Potter, P. (2010). *Clinical nursing skills & techniques* (7th ed., p. 856). St. Louis: Mosby.

---

615. A nurse is collecting data about a client's psychosocial adjustment to a newly applied body cast. The nurse should first collect data about which of the following?

1 Home environment
2 Usual coping techniques
3 Ability to perform activities of daily living
4 Type of transportation available for discharge

Answer: 2

Rationale: When collecting data about the client's psychosocial adjustment, the nurse should first address the client's usual coping techniques. Options 1, 3, and 4 do not address psychosocial issues.

Test-Taking Strategy: Use the process of elimination, and focus on the strategic word *psychosocial*. Option 2 is the only option that addresses the client's psychosocial needs. Review data collection techniques related to psychosocial assessment if you had difficulty with this question.

Level of Cognitive Ability: Application
Client Needs: Psychosocial Integrity
Integrated Process: Nursing Process/Data Collection
Content Area: Fundamental Skills

Reference

Ignatavicius, D., & Workman, M. (2010). *Medical-surgical nursing: Patient-centered collaborative care* (6th ed., p. 1194). St. Louis: Saunders.

---

616. A client who has been on bedrest in a private room for 1 week is exhibiting periods of confusion. The physician has ordered progressive walking as tolerated. Which of the following interventions would best decrease the confusion?

1 Progressive ambulation in the hall three times a day
2 Range-of-motion exercises three times a day to increase strength
3 Ambulating the client to the bathroom in his or her room three times a day
4 Ambulating the client in his or her room and increasing the distance by 5 feet each time

Answer: 1

Rationale: Confusion in this situation is probably due to decreased sensory stimulation as a result of being in a private room. Ambulating the client in the hall will increase sensory stimulation and may decrease confusion. Options 3 and 4 do not provide the best methods for increasing sensory stimulation. The question addresses ambulation rather than range-of-motion exercises.

Test-Taking Strategy: Use the process of elimination, and focus on the subject—decreased sensory stimulation. Eliminate options 3 and 4 first because they are comparable or alike in that they both address ambulating the client in his or her room. Eliminate option 2 next because it is unrelated to the data in the question. Review measures to increase sensory stimulation if you had difficulty with this question.

Level of Cognitive Ability: Application
Client Needs: Psychosocial Integrity
Integrated Process: Nursing Process/Implementation
Content Area: Fundamental Skills

Reference

deWit, S. (2009). *Medical-surgical nursing: Concepts & practice* (p. 195). St. Louis: Saunders.

---

617. A client with a history of pulmonary emboli is scheduled for the insertion of an inferior vena cava filter. The nurse checks on the client 1 hour after the physician has explained the procedure and obtained informed consent. The client is lying in bed, wringing her hands, and she says to the nurse, "I'm not sure about this. What if it doesn't work and I'm just as bad off as before?" The nurse addresses which primary concern of the client?

1 Anxiety related to the possibility of death
2 Ineffective coping related to the treatment regimen
3 Lack of knowledge related to the surgical procedure
4 Fear related to the potential risks and outcome of surgery

Level of Cognitive Ability: Analysis
Client Needs: Psychosocial Integrity
Integrated Process: Nursing Process/Implementation
Content Area: Fundamental Skills

Answer: 4

Rationale: This client has indicated fear regarding the surgical procedure and its outcome. Anxiety is present when the client cannot identify the source of the uneasy feelings. Deficient knowledge is characterized by a lack of appropriate information. Ineffective coping is appropriate when the client is not making necessary adaptations to deal with daily life.

Test-Taking Strategy: Use the process of elimination. Focus on the client's statement and the data provided in the question to assist with directing you to option 4. The client's statement supports fear related to the potential risks and outcome of surgery. Review the defining characteristics of fear if you had difficulty with this question.

Reference

deWit, S. (2009). *Medical-surgical nursing: Concepts & practice* (pp. 104-105). St. Louis: Saunders.

---

618. According to the standard orders after a myocardial infarction (MI), the client with an uncomplicated MI may begin progressive activity after 3 days. A male client who experienced an MI 4 days previously refuses to let his legs dangle at the bedside and says, "If my doctor tells me to do it, I will." The nurse determines that the client is likely displaying:

1 Anger
2 Denial
3 Depression
4 Dependency

Level of Cognitive Ability: Analysis
Client Needs: Psychosocial Integrity
Integrated Process: Nursing Process/Data Collection
Content Area: Adult Health/Cardiovascular

Answer: 4

Rationale: Clients may experience numerous emotional and behavioral responses after an MI. Dependency is one response that may be manifested by the client's refusal to perform any tasks or activities unless they have been approved by the physician. Anger is displayed by verbal and nonverbal acting-out behaviors. Performing activities that may seem harmful is indicative of denial, which is commonly noted after MI. Depression is identified by withdrawal behaviors.

Test-Taking Strategy: Use the process of elimination, and focus on the data identified in the question. Begin by eliminating options 2 and 3 first. Although the client's statement may express anger to some degree, it most specifically addresses dependency. Review the characteristics of the behaviors identified in the options if you had difficulty with this question.

Reference

deWit, S. (2009). *Medical-surgical nursing: Concepts & practice* (p. 500). St. Louis: Saunders.

619. A nurse is collecting data from a client admitted to the hospital with a diagnosis of renal calculi. The client states to the nurse, "I'm scared to death that it'll come back. That was the worst pain I ever had, like a knife going from my right side to my groin." The nurse identifies which of the following as the most appropriate client problem?

1 Fear related to anticipation of recurrent severe pain
2 Pain related to presence of calculus in the right ureter
3 Urinary retention related to obstruction of the urinary tract by calculi
4 Lack of knowledge related to lack of information about the disease process

Level of Cognitive Ability: Analysis
Client Needs: Psychosocial Integrity
Integrated Process: Nursing Process/Data Collection
Content Area: Mental Health

Answer: 1
Rationale: The anticipation of the recurring pain is the client's concern. There is no evidence that the client has a calculus in the right ureter or that urinary retention or a knowledge deficit exists.

Test-Taking Strategy: Use the process of elimination and the data presented in the question. Note the strategic words *I'm scared to death that it'll come back*. Note the relationship of these words to the word *fear* in option 1. Review the definition of fear if you had difficulty with this question.

Reference
Linton, A. (2007). *Introduction to medical-surgical nursing* (4th ed., pp. 861, 1239). Philadelphia: Saunders.

---

620. A nurse observes parents at the bedside of their female infant, who was born at 27 weeks' gestation and is small for gestational age (SGA). The infant's mother states, "She is so tiny and fragile. I'll never be able to hold her with all those tubes." The nurse interprets the mother's statement as being relevant to which problem?

1 Nonacceptance
2 Risk for altered parenting abilities
3 Compromised family coping
4 Lack of coping mechanisms

Level of Cognitive Ability: Analysis
Client Needs: Psychosocial Integrity
Integrated Process: Nursing Process/Data Collection
Content Area: Maternity/Postpartum

Answer: 2
Rationale: One of the problems for the parents of a high-risk neonate is the risk for altered parenting abilities. The initial focus of intervention for parents of a preterm SGA infant is assisting parent–infant bonding. Option 1 addresses nonacceptance of a health status change or an inability to solve problems or set goals. Option 3 involves the identification of lacking coping mechanisms. Option 4 addresses the strain of a caregiver, which, during the initial hospitalization, is too early to apply. At this time, there is inadequate data to accurately identify these problems, although they may become relevant at a later time.

Test-Taking Strategy: Use the process of elimination, and focus on the data presented in the question. Eliminate options 1 and 3 first because these options identify actual problems that do not exist. When selecting from the remaining options, note the strategic words *I'll never be able to hold her*. Note the relationship between these words and the words *altered parenting* abilities in the correct option. Review parental reactions related to high-risk neonates if you had difficulty with this question.

Reference
Leifer, G. (2008). *Maternity nursing: An introductory text* (10th ed., p. 242). Philadelphia: Saunders.

---

621. A nurse is caring for a client who will be wearing a cast for several weeks. The client expresses concern about the ability

Answer: 3
Rationale: Illness can present a unique and often frustrating challenge for clients. Activities may need to be planned around the

to care for herself. The nurse determines that the appropriate client problem is:
1 Anxiety
2 Powerlessness
3 Self-care deficit
4 Compromised family coping

Level of Cognitive Ability: Analysis
Client Needs: Psychosocial Integrity
Integrated Process: Nursing Process/Data Collection
Content Area: Adult Health/Musculoskeletal

availability of assistance. There is no evidence in the question that anxiety exists or that there is compromised family coping. Although a client facing several weeks of limited mobility may experience powerlessness, no data support this problem.

Test-Taking Strategy: Use the process of elimination. Note the relationship between the words *ability to care for herself* in the question and option 3. Review the defining characteristics of a self-care deficit if you had difficulty with this question.

References
deWit, S. (2009). *Medical-surgical nursing: Concepts & practice* (p. 776). St. Louis: Saunders.
Linton, A. (2007). *Introduction to medical-surgical nursing* (4th ed., p. 927). Philadelphia: Saunders.

---

622. A nurse working in a rehabilitation center witnesses a postoperative coronary artery bypass graft client and his spouse arguing after a rehabilitation session. The appropriate statement by the nurse to identify the feelings of the client is:
1 "You seem upset."
2 "Oh, don't let this get you down."
3 "It will seem better tomorrow. Smile."
4 "You shouldn't get upset. It will affect your heart."

Level of Cognitive Ability: Application
Client Needs: Psychosocial Integrity
Integrated Process: Communication and Documentation
Content Area: Adult Health/Cardiovascular

Answer: 1
Rationale: Therapeutic communication techniques assist with the flow of communication and always focus on the client. Open-ended statements allow the client to verbalize, thus giving the nurse some direction for clarifying the client's true feelings. In addition, acknowledging the client's feelings without inserting personal values or judgments is a method of therapeutic communication. Options 2, 3, and 4 do not encourage verbalization by the client.

Test-Taking Strategy: Use therapeutic communication techniques. Remember to always focus on the client's feelings; this will direct you to option 1. Review therapeutic communication techniques if you had difficulty with this question.

Reference
Linton, A. (2007). *Introduction to medical-surgical nursing* (4th ed., pp. 54, 657-658). Philadelphia: Saunders.

---

623. As the nurse approaches a client who was recently admitted to the inpatient unit of a psychiatric hospital, the client says, "Quit following me. You're with the FBI or with some other crazy police department, I can tell by the way you're walking." This is an example of which alteration in thinking?
1 Delusion
2 Hallucination
3 Circumstantiality
4 Loose association

Level of Cognitive Ability: Comprehension
Client Needs: Psychosocial Integrity
Integrated Process: Nursing Process/Data Collection
Content Area: Mental Health

Answer: 1
Rationale: Delusions are false fixed beliefs that cannot be corrected with reasoning. Most commonly, delusional thinking involves themes of reference, persecution, grandiosity, jealousy, and control. Hallucinations are defined as sensory perceptions for which there is no external stimulus. The most common types of hallucinations are auditory, visual, olfactory, and tactile. Circumstantiality is a pattern of speech characterized by indirectness and delay before a person gets to the point or answers a question; the client gets caught up in countless details and explanations. Associative looseness is an alteration in speech that consists of threads (associations) that tie one thought or concept to another.

Test-Taking Strategy: Focus on the subject of the question—a client who is exhibiting disturbed thought processes. Next, determine what type of altered thought process the client is expressing. Recalling the definitions of each item in the options will direct you to option 1. Review the definition of delusions if you had difficulty with this question.

Reference

Varcarolis, E., & Halter, M. (2009). *Essentials of psychiatric mental health nursing: A communication approach to evidence-based care* (pp. 279-280). St. Louis: Saunders.

---

624. A client on the psychiatric unit is displaying manipulative behavior. The nurse should avoid which of the following when working with this client?

1 Communicating to the client the behaviors that are expected
2 Identifying the manipulative behaviors that the client exhibits
3 Arguing with the client to ensure that views of a situation are shared
4 Describing clearly the consequences of not staying within identified limits

Level of Cognitive Ability: Application
Client Needs: Psychosocial Integrity
Integrated Process: Nursing Process/Implementation
Content Area: Mental Health

Answer: 3

Rationale: The nurse should avoid getting into arguments with the manipulative client. The other options listed are helpful interventions that will eventually assist the client with setting limits on his or her own behavior.

Test-Taking Strategy: Use the process of elimination, and note the strategic word *avoid.* This word indicates a negative event query and asks you to select an option that is an incorrect action on the part of the nurse. Use your knowledge of the characteristics of this personality type to direct you to option 3. Review the interventions described in the options if you had difficulty with this question.

References

Keltner, N., Schwecke, L., & Bostrom, C. (2007). *Psychiatric nursing* (5th ed., p. 106). St. Louis: Mosby.

Varcarolis, E., & Halter, M. (2009). *Essentials of psychiatric mental health nursing: A communication approach to evidence-based care* (p. 189). St. Louis: Saunders.

---

625. A client who has never been hospitalized before is having trouble initiating the stream of urine. Knowing that there is no pathological reason for this difficulty, the nurse avoids which of the following because it is the least helpful method of assisting the client?

1 Encouraging fluid intake
2 Providing privacy during voiding
3 Closing the bathroom door during voiding
4 Assisting the client to a commode behind a closed curtain

Level of Cognitive Ability: Application
Client Needs: Psychosocial Integrity
Integrated Process: Nursing Process/Implementation
Content Area: Adult Health/Renal

Answer: 4

Rationale: A lack of privacy may inhibit the ability of the client to void. Using a commode behind a curtain may inhibit voiding in some people. Providing privacy and the use of a bathroom and encouraging fluid intake will aid in urinary elimination.

Test-Taking Strategy: Use the process of elimination. Note the strategic words *avoids* and *least helpful.* Option 1 is most helpful and therefore is eliminated first. Knowing that options 2 and 3 are general nursing measures will direct you to option 4 as the least helpful method of assisting the client with elimination. Review urinary elimination measures if you had difficulty with this question.

Reference

Potter, P., & Perry, A. (2009) *Fundamentals of nursing* (7th ed., pp. 1135-1136). St. Louis: Mosby.

---

626. While the nurse is providing care, the client says, "My doctor just told me that my cancer has spread and that I have less than 6 months to live." The nurse should make which therapeutic response to the client?

1 "I am sorry. Would you like to discuss this with me some more?"
2 "I am sorry. There are no easy answers in times like this, are there?"

Answer: 1

Rationale: The client has just received very distressing news. In the correct option, the nurse encourages the client to ventilate feelings. Option 2 expresses the nurse's feelings rather than facilitating the client's feelings. Option 3 is patronizing and stereotypical. Option 4 provides a social communication and false hope.

3 "I hope you'll focus on the fact that your doctor says you have 6 months to live and that you'll think of how you'd like to live it."
4 "I know it seems desperate but there have been a lot of breakthroughs. Something might come along in a month or so to change your status drastically."

Level of Cognitive Ability: Application
Client Needs: Psychosocial Integrity
Integrated Process: Communication and Documentation
Content Area: Adult Health/Oncology

Test-Taking Strategy: Use therapeutic communication techniques. Note that option 1 is the only option that provides the opportunity for the client to express feelings. Review therapeutic communication techniques if you had difficulty with this question.

Reference
deWit, S. (2009). *Medical-surgical nursing: Concepts & practice* (pp. 9, 169). St. Louis: Saunders.

---

627. A client with an endotracheal tube gets frustrated easily when trying to communicate personal needs to the nurse. The best method for communication for this client is:
1 The use of a pad and paper
2 The use of a picture or word board
3 The use of a system of hand signals
4 Having the family interpret the client's needs

Level of Cognitive Ability: Comprehension
Client Needs: Psychosocial Integrity
Integrated Process: Communication and Documentation
Content Area: Adult Health/Respiratory

Answer: 2
Rationale: The client with an endotracheal tube in place cannot speak, and the nurse needs to devise an alternative communication system with the client. The use of a picture or word board is the simplest method of communication because it only requires the client to point at a word or object. A pad and pencil is an acceptable alternative, but it requires more client effort and time. The family does not need to bear the burden of communicating the client's needs, and they may not understand them either. The use of hand signals may not be a reliable method; it may not meet all of the client's needs, and it is subject to misinterpretation.

Test-Taking Strategy: Use the process of elimination, and focus on the strategic words *frustrated easily* and *best*. Options 1 and 3 are obviously not the easiest and therefore are eliminated first. Because the family may not necessarily know what the client is trying to communicate, option 4 could add to the client's frustration. Thus, the picture or word board is the easiest and least frustrating method of communication for the client. Review these alternative methods of communication if you had difficulty with this question.

Reference
deWit, S. (2009). *Medical-surgical nursing: Concepts & practice* (p. 309). St. Louis: Saunders.

---

628. A client has been receiving protriptyline (Vivactil). The nurse notifies the health care provider if which of the following client responses to the medication is noted?
1 Increased appetite
2 Increased drowsiness
3 Reported decrease in anxiety
4 Increased sense of well-being

Level of Cognitive Ability: Application
Client Needs: Psychosocial Integrity

Answer: 2
Rationale: Protriptyline is an antidepressant used to treat various forms of depression and anxiety. The client is also often in psychotherapy while taking this medication. Expected effects of the medication include improved sense of well-being, appetite, and sleep, as well as a reduced level of anxiety. If the client experiences increased drowsiness, the health care provider should be notified.

Test-Taking Strategy: Note the strategic words *notifies the health care provider.* Recall that the medication is an antidepressant. With this in mind, note that options 1, 3, and 4 are positive client responses. Review protriptyline if you had difficulty with this question.

Integrated Process: Nursing Process/Implementation
Content Area: Pharmacology

Reference
Kee, J., Hayes, E., & McCuistion, L. (2009). *Pharmacology: A nursing process approach* (6th ed., p. 416). St. Louis: Saunders.

---

629. A client who is to undergo thoracentesis is afraid of not being able to tolerate the procedure. The nurse provides support and reassurance with which of the following statements?

1 "I'll be right by your side, but the procedure will be totally painless as long as you don't move."
2 "The procedure takes only 1 to 2 minutes, so you might try to get through it by mentally counting up to 120."
3 "The needle may be painful when it goes in, but you must remain still. I'll stay with you throughout the entire procedure and help you hold your position."
4 "The needle is a little uncomfortable going in, but the pain can be controlled by rhythmically breathing in and out. I'll be with you to coach your breathing."

Level of Cognitive Ability: Application
Client Needs: Psychosocial Integrity
Integrated Process: Communication and Documentation
Content Area: Adult Health/Respiratory

Answer: 3
Rationale: The needle insertion for thoracentesis is painful for the client. The nurse tells the client how important it is to remain still during the procedure so that the needle does not injure visceral pleura or lung tissue. The procedure takes longer than 1 to 2 minutes and may take up to 1 hour, depending on the client's condition. The client may also need to hold his or her breath at certain points during the procedure. The nurse reassures the client during the procedure and helps the client to hold the proper position.

Test-Taking Strategy: Use the process of elimination. Knowing that the client must remain still during the procedure helps you to eliminate option 4 first. Knowing that the procedure may be painful for the client and that it takes longer than 1 to 2 minutes helps you to eliminate options 1 and 2. Review thoracentesis if you had difficulty with this question.

References
Chernecky, C., & Berger, B. (2008). *Laboratory tests and diagnostic procedures* (5th ed., pp. 1063-1064). Philadelphia: Saunders.
Christensen, B., & Kockrow, E. (2006). *Foundations of nursing* (5th ed., p. 500). St. Louis: Mosby.
deWit, S. (2009). *Medical-surgical nursing: Concepts & practice* (p. 288). St. Louis: Saunders.

---

630. A client with chronic respiratory failure is dyspneic and responds to the dyspnea with anxiety, which worsens the condition. The nurse should teach the client which methods to best interrupt the dyspnea–anxiety–dyspnea cycle?

1 Guided imagery and limiting fluids
2 Relaxation and breathing techniques
3 Biofeedback and coughing techniques
4 Distraction and increased dietary carbohydrates

Level of Cognitive Ability: Application
Client Needs: Psychosocial Integrity
Integrated Process: Nursing Process/Implementation
Content Area: Adult Health/Respiratory

Answer: 2
Rationale: The anxious client with dyspnea should be taught interventions to decrease anxiety. These methods include relaxation, biofeedback, guided imagery, and distraction, and they will stop the escalation of feelings of dyspnea. The dyspnea can be further controlled by teaching the client respiratory techniques, including pursed-lip and diaphragmatic breathing. Coughing techniques are useful, but breathing techniques are more effective. Limiting fluids will thicken secretions and is contraindicated. Increased dietary carbohydrates will increase the production of carbon dioxide by the body and are also contraindicated.

Test-Taking Strategy: Use the process of elimination, and note the strategic words *best interrupt*. Because the first part of every option is helpful for anxiety reduction, focus on the second part to select the correct option. Limiting fluids and increasing carbohydrates are contraindicated; therefore options 1 and 4 can be eliminated. Breathing techniques are more effective than coughing techniques, which helps you to choose option 2. Review the care of the client with chronic respiratory failure if you had difficulty with this question.

Reference

Linton, A. (2007). *Introduction to medical-surgical nursing* (4th ed., p. 557). Philadelphia: Saunders.

---

631. A client who has undergone the drainage of a pleural effusion is in pain. The nurse avoids which intervention when providing support to this client?

1 Providing pain medication for the client
2 Offering verbal support and reassurance
3 Leaving the client alone for an extended rest period
4 Assisting the client with finding positions of comfort

Level of Cognitive Ability: Application
Client Needs: Psychosocial Integrity
Integrated Process: Caring
Content Area: Fundamental Skills

Answer: 3

Rationale: The pain associated with the drainage of a pleural effusion is minimized by positioning the client for comfort and administering analgesics for pain relief. The nurse also offers verbal support and understanding. All of these measures help the client to cope with the pain and discomfort associated with this problem. It is least helpful to leave the client alone for extended periods because the pain may be augmented by isolation.

Test-Taking Strategy: Use the process of elimination, and note the strategic word *avoids*. Basic knowledge of pain management techniques and of the principles of nursing care will direct you to option 3. Review effective pain management techniques if you had difficulty with this question.

References

Christensen, B., & Kockrow, E. (2006). *Adult health nursing* (5th ed., p. 439). St. Louis: Mosby.
deWit, S. (2009). *Medical-surgical nursing: Concepts & practice* (p. 144). St. Louis: Saunders.

---

632. A nurse is caring for a client who has just experienced a pulmonary embolism and who is restless and very anxious. The nurse plans to use which approach when communicating with this client?

1 Explaining each treatment in great detail
2 Giving simple, clear directions and explanations
3 Having the family reinforce the nurse's directions
4 Speaking very little to the client until the crisis is over

Level of Cognitive Ability: Application
Client Needs: Psychosocial Integrity
Integrated Process: Nursing Process/Planning
Content Area: Adult Health/Respiratory

Answer: 2

Rationale: The client who has suffered pulmonary embolism is fearful and apprehensive. The nurse effectively communicates with this client by staying with the client; providing simple, clear, and accurate information; and acting in a calm, efficient manner. Options 1, 3, and 4 will produce more anxiety for the client and the client's family.

Test-Taking Strategy: Use the process of elimination. Options 1 and 4 represent the least effective communication strategies and may be eliminated first. Having the family reinforce the directions may place stress on the family. The nurse gives simple, clear information to the client who is in distress. Review the care of the anxious client if you had difficulty with this question.

Reference

deWit, S. (2009). *Medical-surgical nursing: Concepts & practice* (p. 342). St. Louis: Saunders.

---

633. A nurse is collecting data from a confused older client admitted to the hospital with a hip fracture. Which of the following data obtained by the nurse least likely places the client at more risk for disturbed thought processes?

Answer: 4

Rationale: Confusion in the older client with a hip fracture could result from the unfamiliar hospital setting, stress caused by the fracture, concurrent systemic diseases, cerebral ischemia, or side effects of medications. The use of eyeglasses and hearing aids enhances the client's interaction with the environment and can reduce disorientation and confusion.

1 Eyeglasses left at home
2 Unfamiliar hospital setting
3 Stress induced by the fracture
4 Hearing aid available and in working order

Level of Cognitive Ability: Comprehension
Client Needs: Psychosocial Integrity
Integrated Process: Nursing Process/Data Collection
Content Area: Fundamental Skills

Test-Taking Strategy: Use the process of elimination, and note the strategic words *least likely*. The wording of the question asks you to look for an option that will keep the client at the highest possible level of functioning from a cognitive perspective. An unfamiliar setting (option 2) and stress from the fracture (option 3) are not likely to help the client's functional level and are eliminated first. Both eyeglasses and hearing aids are useful adjuncts for communicating with this client. Because the client's eyeglasses were left at home, they are of no use at the current time. Review the causes of confusion and disorientation in the hospitalized client if you had difficulty with this question.

Reference

Linton, A. (2007). *Introduction to medical-surgical nursing* (4th ed., p. 930). Philadelphia: Saunders.

---

634. A client is admitted to the nursing unit after a below-the-knee amputation after sustaining a crush injury to the left foot and lower leg. The client tells the nurse, "I think I'm going crazy. I can feel my left foot itching." The nurse responds, understanding that the client's statement is:

1 A normal response that indicates the presence of phantom limb pain
2 A normal response that indicates the presence of phantom limb sensation
3 An abnormal response that indicates that the client is in denial about the limb loss
4 An abnormal response that indicates that the client needs more psychological support

Level of Cognitive Ability: Comprehension
Client Needs: Psychosocial Integrity
Integrated Process: Nursing Process/Implementation
Content Area: Adult Health/Neurological

Answer: 2

Rationale: Phantom limb sensations are felt in the area of the amputated limb and can include itching, warmth, and cold. The sensations are caused by intact peripheral nerves in the area that has been amputated. Whenever possible, clients should be prepared for these normal sensations. The client may also feel painful sensations in the amputated limb, which is called phantom limb pain. The origin of the pain is less understood, but, whenever possible, the client should also be prepared for this occurrence.

Test-Taking Strategy: Use the process of elimination. Knowing that sensation and pain may be felt in the amputated limb helps you to eliminate options 3 and 4 first because the sensations are not abnormal responses. Select option 2 instead of option 1 because the client has described an itching sensation but has not complained of pain. Review the care of the client after amputation if you had difficulty with this question.

Reference

Christensen, B., & Kockrow, E. (2006). *Adult health nursing* (5th ed., pp. 186-187). St. Louis: Mosby.

---

635. A client who has had a spinal fusion and the insertion of hardware is extremely concerned about the perceived lengthy rehabilitation period. The client expresses concerns about finances and the ability to return to prior employment. The nurse understands that the client's needs could best be addressed by referral to the:

1 Surgeon
2 Social worker
3 Physical therapist
4 Clinical nurse specialist

Answer: 2

Rationale: After spinal surgery, concerns about finances and employment are best handled by referral to a social worker; this health care member is aware of the best information about resources available to the client. The physical therapist has knowledge of techniques for increasing mobility and endurance. An occupational therapist would have knowledge of techniques for activities of daily living and items related to occupation, but this is not one of the options. The clinical nurse specialist and surgeon are not the best resources for providing specific information related to financial resources.

Level of Cognitive Ability: Comprehension
Client Needs: Psychosocial Integrity
Integrated Process: Nursing Process/Planning
Content Area: Fundamental Skills

Test-Taking Strategy: An understanding of the roles of the various members of the health care team helps you to answer this question. Focus on the subject—concern about finances; this will direct you to the social worker as the optimal resource in this situation. Review the role of the social worker if you had difficulty with this question.

Reference

deWit, S. (2009). *Medical-surgical nursing: Concepts & practice* (pp. 210, 559). St. Louis: Saunders.

---

636. A client is fearful about having an arm cast removed. Which action by the nurse is helpful?

1. Telling the client that the saw makes a frightening noise
2. Reassuring the client that no one has had an arm lacerated yet
3. Stating that the hot cutting blades only cause burns very rarely
4. Showing the client the cast cutter and explaining how it works

Level of Cognitive Ability: Application
Client Needs: Psychosocial Integrity
Integrated Process: Nursing Process/Implementation
Content Area: Adult Health/Musculoskeletal

Answer: 4

Rationale: Because of misconceptions about the cast-cutting blade, clients may be fearful about having a cast removed. The nurse should show the cast cutter to the client before it is used and explain that the client may feel heat, vibration, and pressure. The cast cutter resembles a small electric saw with a circular blade. The nurse should reassure the client that the blade does not cut like a saw but instead cuts the cast by vibrating side to side.

Test-Taking Strategy: Use the process of elimination, and note the strategic word *helpful*. Option 2 provides no information and may increase fear. Options 1 and 3 give accurate information but are not reassuring. Option 4 gives the client the most reassurance because it best prepares the client for what will occur when the cast is removed. Review the care of the client preparing for cast removal if you had difficulty with this question.

Reference

Christensen, B., & Kockrow, E. (2006). *Adult health nursing* (5th ed., p. 173). St. Louis: Mosby.

---

637. A client is admitted to the mental health unit with a diagnosis of panic disorder. The nurse anticipates that the physician's order for a benzodiazepine would indicate:

1. Doxepin (Sinequan)
2. Alprazolam (Xanax)
3. Imipramine (Tofranil)
4. Bupropion (Wellbutrin)

Level of Cognitive Ability: Analysis
Client Needs: Psychosocial Integrity
Integrated Process: Nursing Process/Planning
Content Area: Pharmacology

Answer: 2

Rationale: Options 1, 3, and 4 are classified as antidepressants and act by stimulating the central nervous system (CNS) to elevate mood. Alprazolam, which is a benzodiazepine antianxiety agent, depresses the CNS and induces relaxation in clients with panic disorders.

Test-Taking Strategy: Use the process of elimination. Eliminate options 1, 3, and 4 because they are comparable or alike in that they are antidepressants. Review the medications listed in the options if you had difficulty with this question.

Reference

Hodgson, B., & Kizior, R. (2009). *Saunders nursing drug handbook 2009* (pp. 39-41). St. Louis: Saunders.

---

638. A client scheduled for an implanted port for intermittent chemotherapy treatments says, "I'm not sure if I can

Answer: 3

Rationale: What the client says in this situation indicates that the client should be educated about the implanted port. An implanted

handle having a tube coming out of me all the time. What will my friends think?" The appropriate nursing action is to:

1 Notify the physician of the client's concerns.
2 Show the client various central line tubes and catheters.
3 Explain that an implanted port is not visible under the skin.
4 Explain that the client's friends probably will not see the tube under the client's clothing.

Level of Cognitive Ability: Application
Client Needs: Psychosocial Integrity
Integrated Process: Nursing Process/Implementation
Content Area: Fundamental Skills

port is placed under the skin and is not visible, and there is no visible tubing. Tubing is used only when the port is accessed intermittently and the intravenous line is connected. Showing the client various other tubes will not be beneficial because the client will not be using them. It is premature to notify the physician. Option 4 does not correct the client's confusion regarding the implanted port.

Test-Taking Strategy: Use the process of elimination, and focus on the subject—an implanted port. Recalling that a port is placed under the skin will direct you to option 3. Review the concepts related to implanted ports and the teaching and learning process if you had difficulty with this question.

Reference

Ignatavicious, D., & Workman, M. (2010). *Medical-surgical nursing: Patient-centered collaborative care* (6th ed., p. 872). St. Louis: Saunders.

---

639. A client displays signs of anxiety because of pain at an intravenous (IV) site. When explaining to the client that the IV line will need to be discontinued because of an infiltration, the nurse should say which of the following?

1 "This will be a totally painless experience. It is nothing to worry about."
2 "I'm sure it will be a real relief for you just as soon as I discontinue this IV for good."
3 "Just relax and take a deep breath. This procedure will not take long and will be over soon."
4 "I can see that you're anxious. The removal of the IV shouldn't be painful; however, the IV will need to be restarted in another location by the registered nurse."

Level of Cognitive Ability: Application
Client Needs: Psychosocial Integrity
Integrated Process: Communication and Documentation
Content Area: Fundamental Skills

Answer: 4

Rationale: Although discontinuing an IV line is a painless experience, it is not therapeutic to tell a client not to worry. Option 2 does not acknowledge the client's feelings and does not let the client know that an infiltrated IV line will need to be restarted. Option 3 does not address the client's feelings. The correct option addresses the client's anxiety and honestly informs the client that the IV line will need to be restarted. This option uses the therapeutic technique of giving information, and it also acknowledges the client's feelings.

Test-Taking Strategy: When answering communication questions, remember to use therapeutic techniques. Option 4 is the only option that addresses the client's feelings. Remember to always focus on the client's feelings. Review therapeutic communication techniques if you had difficulty with this question.

Reference

deWit, S. (2009). *Medical-surgical nursing: Concepts & practice* (pp. 9, 59). St. Louis: Saunders.

---

640. A toddler with suspected conjunctivitis is crying and refuses to sit still during the eye examination. The nurse should make which therapeutic statement to the child?

Answer: 1

Rationale: Fears in this age group can be decreased by getting the child actively involved in the examination. Option 2 tells the child how to feel. Option 3 gives advice and ignores the child's feelings. Although option 4 acknowledges feelings, it puts off the inevitable.

1 "Would you like to see the flashlight?"
2 "Don't be scared, the light won't hurt you."
3 "If you will sit still, the exam will be over soon."
4 "I know you are upset. We can do this exam later."

Level of Cognitive Ability: Application
Client Needs: Psychosocial Integrity
Integrated Process: Communication and Documentation
Content Area: Child Health

Test-Taking Strategy: Note that the child is a toddler. Using the child's developmental level and the techniques of therapeutic communication will direct you to option 1. Review the growth and development of the toddler if you had difficulty with this question.

References

deWit, S. (2009). *Medical-surgical nursing: Concepts & practice* (p. 9). St. Louis: Saunders.
Leifer, G. (2007). *Introduction to maternity and pediatric nursing* (5th ed., pp. 526-527). Philadelphia: Saunders.

---

641. A client with acute pyelonephritis is scheduled for a voiding cystourethrogram. The client has had other diagnostic tests, and the nurse observed that the client is timid and shy. The nurse interprets that this client could most likely benefit from increased support and teaching about the procedure because:
1 Radioactive contrast is injected into the bladder.
2 Radiopaque contrast is injected into the bloodstream.
3 The client must lie on an x-ray table in a cold, barren room.
4 The client must void while the micturition process is filmed.

Level of Cognitive Ability: Comprehension
Client Needs: Psychosocial Integrity
Integrated Process: Nursing Process/Planning
Content Area: Adult Health/Renal

Answer: 4
Rationale: Having to void in the presence of others can be very embarrassing for clients and may actually interfere with the client's ability to void. The nurse teaches the client about the procedure to try to minimize stress from a lack of preparation and gives the client encouragement and emotional support. Screens may be used in the radiology department to provide privacy during this procedure. The contrast material is inserted into the bladder by means of a catheter.

Test-Taking Strategy: Use the process of elimination. Begin to answer this question by eliminating options 1 and 2 because the contrast material is inserted into the bladder with a catheter. From the remaining options, it is necessary to know that the client has to void to allow for the filming of the movement of urine through the lower urinary tract. Review the voiding cystourethrogram if you had difficulty with this question.

Reference

Chernecky, C., & Berger, B. (2008). *Laboratory tests and diagnostic procedures* (5th ed., pp. 420-421). Philadelphia: Saunders.

---

642. A female client in a manic state emerges from her room. She is topless and making sexual remarks and gestures toward the staff and her peers. The best initial nursing action is to:
1 Approach the client in the hallway and insist that she go to her room.
2 Quietly approach the client, escort her to her room, and assist her with getting dressed.
3 Confront the client about the inappropriateness of her behavior and offer her a time-out.
4 Ask the other clients to ignore her behavior because eventually she will return to her room.

Answer: 2
Rationale: A person who is experiencing mania lacks insight and judgment, has poor impulse control, and is highly excitable. The nurse must take control without creating increased stress or anxiety in the client. A quiet, firm approach while distracting the client (i.e., walking her to her room and assisting her with dressing) achieves the goals of having the client dressed appropriately and preserving her psychosocial integrity. Options 1, 3, and 4 are inappropriate actions.

Test-Taking Strategy: Use the process of elimination. The goal of the interaction is to have the client dressed appropriately, so option 4 is eliminated. Insisting that the client go to her room may be met with a great deal of resistance. Confronting the client and offering her a consequence of a time-out may be meaningless to her. Review the care of the client with mania if you had difficulty with this question.

Level of Cognitive Ability: Application
Client Needs: Psychosocial Integrity
Integrated Process: Nursing Process/Implementation
Content Area: Mental Health

Reference

Keltner, N., Schwecke, L., & Bostrom, C. (2007). *Psychiatric nursing* (5th ed., p. 405). St. Louis: Mosby.

---

643. A client who had cardiac surgery and the client's family express anxiety regarding how to cope with the recuperative process after the client is discharged and they are home alone. The nurse should plan to tell the client and family about which available resource?

1 The United Way
2 The local library
3 The American Cancer Society Reach for Recovery
4 The American Heart Association Mended Heart's Club

Level of Cognitive Ability: Application
Client Needs: Psychosocial Integrity
Integrated Process: Nursing Process/Planning
Content Area: Adult Health/Cardiovascular

Answer: 4
Rationale: Most clients and families benefit from knowing that there are available resources to help them cope with the stress of self-care management at home. These can include telephone contact with the surgeon, the cardiologist, and the nurse; cardiac rehabilitation programs; and community support groups such as the American Heart Association Mended Heart's Club, which is a nationwide program with local chapters. The United Way provides resources for clients with various disorders and is not specific to the client with a cardiac problem. The American Cancer Society Reach for Recovery assists clients with breast cancer who have undergone breast surgery. The local library provides resources but does not provide support via an interactive process.

Test-Taking Strategy: Use the process of elimination. Of the four options, three list organizations, and one lists a library. Eliminate the library first because the client and family need resources for coping, which implies the need for an interactive process. From the remaining options, focusing on the type of surgery addressed in the question will direct you to option 4. Review the purpose of the American Heart Association Mended Heart's Club if you had difficulty with this question.

Reference

Ignatavicius, D., & Workman, M. (2010). *Medical-surgical nursing: Patient-centered collaborative care* (6th ed., p. 872). Philadelphia: Saunders.

---

644. A client diagnosed with obsessive-compulsive disorder is upset and agitated. She is walking repeatedly around the unit and following the same route each time. The client asks the nurse working the 3 PM to 11 PM shift to walk with him. Which response by the nurse is appropriate?

1 "Go to sleep now, we can talk tomorrow afternoon."
2 "No, it is bedtime. Let me walk you back to your room."
3 "I can see that you're upset. I will walk with you and we can talk for awhile."
4 "I'm sorry, but I'm too busy right now. Let me find someone else to do that with you."

Level of Cognitive Ability: Application
Client Needs: Psychosocial Integrity

Answer: 3
Rationale: This response in option 3 acknowledges the client's feelings and provides an avenue for a release of the client's anxieties. Each of the incorrect options represents a block to communication. The wording of these responses does not indicate that the client is valued or acknowledge the client's feelings.

Test-Taking Strategy: Use therapeutic communication techniques. Eliminate each of the incorrect options because they do not deal with the client's concerns or promote further communication. Remember that the client's feelings need to be addressed first. Review therapeutic communication techniques if you had difficulty with this question.

References

Fortinash, K., & Holoday-Worret, P. (2008). *Psychiatric mental health nursing* (4th ed., pp. 185-186). St. Louis: Mosby.
Varcarolis, E., & Halter, M. (2009). *Essentials of psychiatric mental health nursing: A communication approach to evidence-based care* (pp. 95-98). St. Louis: Saunders.

Integrated Process: Communication and Documentation
Content Area: Mental Health

---

645. A client with superficial varicose veins says to the nurse, "I hate these things. They're so ugly. I wish I could get them to go away." The nurse should make which therapeutic response to the client?
1 "You should try sclerotherapy, it's great."
2 "There's not much you can do after you get them."
3 "What have you been told about varicose veins and their management?"
4 "I understand how you feel, but you know, they really don't look too bad."

Level of Cognitive Ability: Application
Client Needs: Psychosocial Integrity
Integrated Process: Communication and Documentation
Content Area: Adult Health/Cardiovascular

Answer: 3
Rationale: The client is expressing distress about the physical appearance and has a risk for body image disturbance. The nurse collects data regarding what the client has been told. Options 1, 2, and 4 are nontherapeutic responses.

Test-Taking Strategy: Use the nursing process and therapeutic communication techniques to answer the question; this will direct you to option 3. Remember that data collection is the first step of the nursing process. Review therapeutic communication techniques if you had difficulty with this question.

References
Christensen, B., & Kockrow, E. (2006). *Adult health nursing* (5th ed., 392-393). St. Louis: Mosby.
deWit, S. (2009). *Medical-surgical nursing: Concepts & practice* (p. 9). St. Louis: Saunders.

---

646. A client who has been diagnosed with chronic renal failure has been told that hemodialysis will be required. The client becomes angry and states, "I'll never be the same now." The nurse determines that the client is experiencing which problem?
1 Fear
2 Anxiety
3 Depression
4 Disturbed body image

Level of Cognitive Ability: Comprehension
Client Needs: Psychosocial Integrity
Integrated Process: Nursing Process/Data Collection
Content Area: Adult Health/Renal

Answer: 4
Rationale: The client with renal failure may become angry because of the need for dialysis and the permanence of the alteration. Because of the physical change and the change in lifestyle that may be required to manage a severe renal condition, the client may experience body image disturbance. Although options 1, 2, and 3 may occur, these problems are not associated with the data in the question.

Test-Taking Strategy: Use the process of elimination, and focus on the strategic words *I'll never be the same now.* Note that the client's statement focuses on the self, which is consistent with a disturbance in body image; this will direct you to option 4. Review the characteristics associated with a body image disturbance if you had difficulty with this question.

Reference
deWit, S. (2009). *Medical-surgical nursing: Concepts & practice* (pp. 851-854). St. Louis: Saunders.

---

647. A nurse observes that a client who is recovering from a myocardial infarction is crying silently. What action by the nurse explores the client's feelings?
1 Sitting quietly by the client
2 Assuring the client that the condition will improve

Answer: 1
Rationale: Sitting quietly by the client conveys caring and acceptance. Option 3 may not encourage the client to express feelings because the nurse does not take an active part in identifying the client's feelings. Options 2 and 4 do not address the client's feelings and instead ignore the client's behavior.

3 Entering the room and standing quietly at the bedside
4 Sitting by the client and discussing the news of the day

Level of Cognitive Ability: Application
Client Needs: Psychosocial Integrity
Integrated Process: Caring
Content Area: Adult Health/Cardiovascular

Test-Taking Strategy: Use therapeutic communication techniques to answer this question. Options 2 and 4 can be easily eliminated because they ignore the client's feelings. From the remaining options, option 1 is the option that conveys caring and acceptance. Review therapeutic communication techniques if you had difficulty with this question.

References
Christensen, B., & Kockrow, E. (2006). *Adult health nursing* (5th ed., p. 358). St. Louis: Mosby.
deWit, S. (2009). *Medical-surgical nursing: Concepts & practice* (p. 9). St. Louis: Saunders.

---

648. A nurse caring for a client with newly diagnosed diabetes mellitus is assisting with developing a teaching plan. The nurse assesses the client for which of the following first?
1 Fear of administering insulin
2 Knowledge of the diabetic diet
3 Denial regarding having diabetes
4 Depression regarding lifestyle changes

Level of Cognitive Ability: Comprehension
Client Needs: Psychosocial Integrity
Integrated Process: Nursing Process/Data Collection
Content Area: Adult Health/Endocrine

Answer: 3
Rationale: When diabetes mellitus is diagnosed, the client will usually go through the phases of grief, including denial, fear, anger, bargaining, depression, and acceptance. Denial is the phase that is the most detrimental to the teaching and learning process. If the client is denying the fact that he or she has diabetes mellitus, then he or she probably will not listen to discussions about the disease or how to manage it. Denial must be identified before the nurse can develop a teaching plan.

Test-Taking Strategy: Use the process of elimination, and note the strategic word *first*. All of the options may be appropriate; however, note that options 1, 2, and 4 are related to very specific components of teaching. Option 3 is the umbrella option, and, considering the principles of teaching and learning, this aspect needs to be determined before teaching begins. Review the teaching and learning principles if you had difficulty with this question.

References
deWit, S. (2009). *Medical-surgical nursing: Concepts & practice* (p. 924). St. Louis: Saunders.
Linton, A. (2007). *Introduction to medical-surgical nursing* (4th ed., pp. 1242-1243). Philadelphia: Saunders.

---

649. A nurse is reinforcing teaching with a client taking conjugated estrogen (Premarin). The nurse plans to address which psychosocial issue related to the medication?
1 The client should notify the physician if migraine headaches occur.
2 Estrogen should be used with caution by individuals with a family history of breast or reproductive cancer.
3 Estrogen may cause mood and affect changes, and the medication may need to be discontinued if depression occurs.
4 Estrogen may cause hyperglycemia, and the client should be informed about signs and symptoms to report to the physician.

Answer: 3
Rationale: Conjugated estrogen can cause changes in client affect, mood, and behavior. Aggression, depression, or both can also occur. Options 1, 2, and 4 are correct but address physiological needs. Option 3 is the only psychosocial need noted.

Test-Taking Strategy: Use the process of elimination, and note the strategic word *psychosocial*. Eliminate options 1, 2, and 4 because they address physiological issues. Review the psychosocial effects of conjugated estrogen if you had difficulty with this question.

Reference
Hodgson, B., & Kizior, R. (2009). *Saunders nursing drug handbook 2009* (p. 285). St. Louis: Saunders.

Level of Cognitive Ability: Application
Client Needs: Psychosocial Integrity
Integrated Process: Nursing Process/Planning
Content Area: Pharmacology

---

650. A client with newly diagnosed diabetes mellitus has been seen in the clinic for 3 consecutive days because of hyperglycemia. The client says to the nurse, "I'm sorry to keep bothering you every day, but I just can't give myself those awful shots." The nurse should make which therapeutic response to the client?

1 "I couldn't give myself a shot either."
2 "You must learn to give yourself the shots."
3 "Let me see if the doctor can change your medication."
4 "I'm sorry you are having trouble with your injections. Has someone given you instructions on them?"

Level of Cognitive Ability: Application
Client Needs: Psychosocial Integrity
Integrated Process: Communication and Documentation
Content Area: Adult Health/Endocrine

Answer: 4

Rationale: It is important to determine and deal with a client's underlying fear of self-injection. The nurse should determine whether a client needs additional instructions. Positive reinforcement is necessary instead of focusing on negative behaviors (option 1). Scare tactics (option 2) should not be used. The nurse should not offer a change in regimen that cannot be accomplished (option 3).

Test-Taking Strategy: Use therapeutic communication techniques, and focus on the subject of the question. Options 1 and 2 are not therapeutic, and option 3 may give false reassurance about a change in medication. Option 4 focuses on the subject and is the therapeutic response. Review therapeutic communication techniques if you had difficulty with this question.

References

Christensen, B., & Kockrow, E. (2006). *Adult health nursing* (5th ed., p. 554). St. Louis: Mosby.
deWit, S. (2009). *Medical-surgical nursing: Concepts & practice* (p. 9). St. Louis: Saunders.

---

651. A nurse asks a client with diabetes mellitus to ask her significant others to attend an educational conference about the self-administration of insulin. The client asks why the significant others need to be included. The nurse should make which response to the client?

1 "Family members can take you to the doctor."
2 "Family members are at risk of developing diabetes."
3 "Nurses need someone to call to check on a client's progress."
4 "Clients and families often work together to develop strategies for the management of diabetes."

Level of Cognitive Ability: Application
Client Needs: Psychosocial Integrity
Integrated Process: Nursing Process/Implementation
Content Area: Adult Health/Endocrine

Answer: 4

Rationale: Families or significant others may be included in diabetes education to assist with adjustment to the diabetic regimen. Although options 1 and 2 may be accurate, they are not the most appropriate response in relation to the subject of the question. Option 3 devalues the client, disregards the subject of independence, and promotes powerlessness.

Test-Taking Strategy: Use the process of elimination, your knowledge of diabetes mellitus, and therapeutic communication techniques. Option 4 involves a collaborative response and addresses the client. Review psychosocial issues related to teaching if you had difficulty with this question.

References

Linton, A. (2007). *Introduction to medical-surgical nursing* (4th ed., pp. 1020-1021). Philadelphia: Saunders.
Perry, A., & Potter, P. (2010). *Clinical nursing skills & techniques* (7th ed., p. 594). St. Louis: Mosby.

---

652. A 22-year-old female client has recently been diagnosed with polycystic kidney disease. The nurse plans a series of discussions with the client that are intended to help her adjust to the disorder. The nurse should include which item as part of one of these discussions?
1 Ongoing fluid restriction
2 Need for genetic counseling
3 Risk for hypotensive episodes
4 Depression regarding massive edema

Level of Cognitive Ability: Application
Client Needs: Psychosocial Integrity
Integrated Process: Nursing Process/Planning
Content Area: Adult Health/Renal

Answer: 2
Rationale: Adult polycystic kidney disease is a hereditary disorder that is inherited as an autosomal-dominant trait. Because of this, the client and her extended family should have genetic counseling. Ongoing fluid restriction is unnecessary. The client is likely to have hypertension rater than hypotension. Massive edema is not a symptom of this disorder.

Test-Taking Strategy: Use the process of elimination. Because massive edema and the need for fluid restriction are not part of the clinical picture of the client with polycystic kidney disease, options 1 and 4 are eliminated first. From the remaining options, you would need to know either that this disorder is hereditary in nature or that the client would exhibit hypertension rather than hypotension. Review polycystic kidney disease if you had difficulty with this question.

Reference
Christensen, B., & Kockrow, E. (2006). *Adult health nursing* (5th ed., pp. 492-493). St. Louis: Mosby.

---

653. A nurse is caring for an older adult client with mild depression who says, "What do you think I should do about my home? My son thinks I should sell it and move into something smaller now that I'm alone." The nurse should make which therapeutic response to the client?
1 "I agree with your son. As you age, you will find that smaller, one-floor living is best."
2 "Oh no, I'm not getting into the middle of this. This is something only you can decide."
3 "Why not wait until you're feeling less depressed to make such an important decision? You've only been taking your medication for 4 months."
4 "What would you like to do? Do you feel you'd be happier in a smaller place? As your depression lifts, you'll be more able to decide what's best for you."

Level of Cognitive Ability: Application
Client Needs: Psychosocial Integrity
Integrated Process: Communication and Documentation
Content Area: Mental Health

Answer: 4
Rationale: The therapeutic response is the one that encourages the client to make his or her own decisions. This approach provides the client with a sense of personal empowerment that will relieve his or her powerlessness. If the client is moderately or severely depressed, decision making is difficult. Option 1 is incorrect because the nurse agrees with the client's son and makes a judgment, which is unprofessional and not therapeutic. Option 2 is incorrect because the nurse provides a social response rather than a therapeutic one, which may undermine the client's confidence, sense of support, and mutuality. Option 3 is incorrect because the nurse provides procrastination and avoidance as models for problem solving.

Test-Taking Strategy: Use the process of elimination and therapeutic communication techniques that focus on the client's feelings and concerns. Option 4 addresses the client's concerns directly. Review therapeutic communication techniques if you had difficulty with this question.

References
Fortinash, K., & Holoday-Worret, P. (2008). *Psychiatric mental health nursing* (4th ed., p. 219). St. Louis: Mosby.
Varcarolis, E., & Halter, M. (2009). *Essentials of psychiatric mental health nursing: A communication approach to evidence-based care* (pp. 95-98). St. Louis: Saunders.

---

654. A dying client's spouse says to the nurse, "I don't think I can come anymore and watch her die. It's chewing me up too much!" The nurse should make which therapeutic response to the client?

Answer: 3
Rationale: The husband is the subject of this question. The therapeutic response is the one that reflects the nurse's understanding of the husband's stress and emotional pain. Option 1 makes a statement that the nurse cannot know is true (the wife may in fact not

1 "I know it's hard for you, but she would know if you're not there, and you'd feel guilty all the rest of your days."
2 "I think you're making the right decision. Your wife knows you love her. You don't have to come. I'll take care of her."
3 "It's hard to watch someone you love die. You've been here with your wife every day. Are you taking any time for yourself?"
4 "I wish you'd focus on your wife's pain rather than yours. I know it's hard, but this isn't about what's happening to you, you know."

Level of Cognitive Ability: Application
Client Needs: Psychosocial Integrity
Integrated Process: Caring
Content Area: Fundamental Skills

know whether the husband visits), and predicting feelings of guilt is not appropriate. Option 2 is inappropriate because it fosters dependency and gives advice, which is nontherapeutic. Option 4 is an example of a nontherapeutic and judgmental attitude.

Test-Taking Strategy: Use the process of elimination and therapeutic communication techniques. Option 3 is the only option that addresses the client's feelings. Review therapeutic communication techniques if you had difficulty with this question.

Reference

Linton, A. (2007). *Introduction to medical-surgical nursing* (4th ed., pp. 48, 53). Philadelphia: Saunders.

---

655. An older client at a retirement center spits her food out and throws it on the floor during a Thanksgiving dinner in the community dining room. The client yells, "This turkey is dry and cold! I can't stand the food here!" The nurse should make which therapeutic response to the client?

1 "I think you had better return to your apartment, where a new meal will be served to you."
2 "Now look what you've done! You're ruining this meal for the whole community. Aren't you ashamed of yourself?"
3 "Let me get you another serving that is more to your liking. Would you like to come visit the chef and select your own serving?"
4 "One of the things that the residents of this group agreed on was that anyone who did not use appropriate behavior would be asked to leave the dining room. Please leave now."

Level of Cognitive Ability: Application
Client Needs: Psychosocial Integrity
Integrated Process: Communication and Documentation
Content Area: Fundamental Skills

Answer: 3

Rationale: The therapeutic response identifies that the client's behavior stems from some troubled feelings with which the client is struggling. Option 1 could provoke a regressive struggle between the nurse and client and cause more explosive behavior on the client's part. Option 2 is an angry, aggressive, nontherapeutic response, and it is humiliating to the client. In option 4, the nurse is authoritative, but trying to expel the client would not be appropriate, and it might set up an aggressive struggle between the nurse and the client. Asking the client to accompany the nurse to the kitchen respects the client's need for control, removes the angry client from the dining room, and may offer the nurse an opportunity to identify what is happening to the client.

Test-Taking Strategy: Use therapeutic communication techniques. Option 3 is the only option that focuses on the client's feelings. Review therapeutic communication techniques if you had difficulty with this question.

Reference

deWit, S. (2009). *Medical-surgical nursing: Concepts & practice* (p. 9). St. Louis: Saunders.

---

656. An older adult client with emphysema is at a physician's office for a follow-up visit. When it is time for the client to see the physician, the nurse finds the client smoking at the front door of the office complex. Which statement by the nurse is therapeutic?

1 "Well, I can see you never got to the stop-smoking clinic!"
2 "I'm glad I caught you smoking! Now that your secret is out, let's decide what you are going to do."
3 "I notice that you are smoking. Did you explore the stop-smoking program at the senior citizens' center?"
4 "I wonder if you realize that you are slowly killing yourself. Why prolong the agony? You can just jump off the bridge!"

Level of Cognitive Ability: Application
Client Needs: Psychosocial Integrity
Integrated Process: Communication and Documentation
Content Area: Adult Health/Respiratory

Answer: 3
Rationale: Option 3 places the decision making in the client's hands and provides an avenue for the client to share what may be expressions of frustration at an inability to stop what is essentially a physiological addiction. Option 1 is a disciplinary remark that places a barrier between the nurse and client within the therapeutic relationship. Option 2 is preachy and judgmental, and it is an example of a countertransference issue for the nurse. Option 4 is an intrusive use of sarcastic humor that demeans the client.

Test-Taking Strategy: This question tests your knowledge of the therapeutic communication techniques for the nurse to use with a client who is failing to make adaptive decisions about health. Use the process of elimination and therapeutic communication techniques to direct you to option 3. Review therapeutic communication techniques if you had difficulty with this question.

References
deWit, S. (2009). *Medical-surgical nursing: Concepts & practice* (p. 9). St. Louis: Saunders.
Linton, A. (2007). *Introduction to medical-surgical nursing* (4th ed., p. 557). Philadelphia: Saunders.

---

657. A client is to have blood drawn by the respiratory therapist to test arterial blood gas levels. While the respiratory therapist is performing Allen's test, the client says to the nurse, "What is he doing? No one else has done that!" On the basis of the understanding of this test, the nurse should make which appropriate response to the client?

1 "I assure you that this is the correct procedure. I cannot account for what others do."
2 "This step is crucial to safe blood withdrawal. I would not let anyone take my blood until they did this."
3 "This is a routine precautionary step that makes sure that your circulation is intact before a blood sample is obtained."
4 "Oh, you have questions about this? You should insist that everyone does this procedure before drawing your blood."

Level of Cognitive Ability: Application
Client Needs: Psychosocial Integrity
Integrated Process: Communication and Documentation
Content Area: Adult Health/Cardiovascular

Answer: 3
Rationale: Allen's test is performed to assess collateral circulation in the hand before blood is drawn from an artery. The nurse's most therapeutic response gives information. Option 1 is defensive and nontherapeutic in that it offers false reassurance. Option 2 demonstrates client advocacy that is overly controlling, quite aggressive, and undermining of treatment. Option 4 is aggressive, controlling, and nontherapeutic with its disapproving stance.

Test-Taking Strategy: Use the process of elimination and therapeutic communication techniques. Option 3 is the only therapeutic response, and it provides information to the client. Review therapeutic communication techniques if you had difficulty with this question.

References
Chernecky, C., & Berger, B. (2008). *Laboratory tests and diagnostic procedures* (5th ed., pp. 210-214). Philadelphia: Saunders.
deWit, S. (2009). *Medical-surgical nursing: Concepts & practice* (p. 9). St. Louis: Saunders.

658. A client reports difficulty concentrating, outbursts of anger, and constantly feeling "keyed up." The nurse obtaining data from the client discovers that the symptoms started approximately 6 months ago after the client witnessed his best friend being killed during a drive-by shooting while the two were sitting on the porch talking. The nurse suspects that the client is experiencing:

1 Panic disorder
2 Social phobia
3 Posttraumatic stress disorder
4 Obsessive-compulsive disorder

Level of Cognitive Ability: Comprehension
Client Needs: Psychosocial Integrity
Integrated Process: Nursing Process/Data Collection
Content Area: Mental Health

Answer: 3

Rationale: Posttraumatic stress disorder is a response to an event that would be markedly distressing to almost anyone. Characteristic symptoms include a sustained level of anxiety, difficulty sleeping, irritability, difficulty concentrating, or outbursts of anger. Panic disorder and social phobia are characterized by the specific fear of an object or situation. Obsessive-compulsive disorder refers to repetitive thoughts and behaviors.

Test-Taking Strategy: Use the process of elimination and your knowledge of the disorders identified in the options. Options 1 and 2 are disorders that have similar symptoms and thus are eliminated first. The information described in the question is not characteristic of an obsessive-compulsive disorder, so option 4 can be eliminated. Review the disorders listed in the options if you had difficulty with this question.

Reference

Fortinash, K., & Holoday-Worret, P. (2008). *Psychiatric mental health nursing* (4th ed., pp. 184, 451). St. Louis: Mosby.

---

659. A client who is reported by the staff to be very demanding says to the nurse, "I can't get any help with my care! I call and call but the nurses never answer my light. Last night one of them told me she had other patients besides me! I'm very sick, but the nurses don't care!" The nurse should make which therapeutic response to the client?

1 "You poor thing! I'm so sorry this happened to you. That nurse should be reported!"
2 "It's hard to be in bed and have to ask for help. You call for a nurse who never seems to come."
3 "I think you are being very impatient. The nurses work very hard and come as quickly as they can."
4 "I can hear your anger. That nurse had no right to speak to you that way. I will report her to the director. It won't happen again."

Level of Cognitive Ability: Application
Client Needs: Psychosocial Integrity
Integrated Process: Communication and Documentation
Content Area: Fundamental Skills

Answer: 2

Rationale: In option 2, the nurse displays empathy as she shares her perceptions. Sharing perceptions asks the client to validate the nurse's understanding of what the client is feeling and thinking. It opens the door for the client to share concerns, fears, and anxieties. Option 1 is sympathetic but inappropriate because of the negative comment about another nurse. In option 3, the nurse is assertive and certainly defends the nursing staff. In option 4, the nurse expresses the client's frustration by labeling the client's feelings as angry and disapproving of the nursing staff.

Test-Taking Strategy: Use therapeutic communication techniques and the process of elimination. Option 2 is the only option that encourages the client to express feelings. Review therapeutic communication techniques if you had difficulty with this question.

References

deWit, S. (2009). *Medical-surgical nursing: Concepts & practice* (p. 9). St. Louis: Saunders.
Christensen, B., & Kockrow, E. (2006). *Foundations of nursing* (5th ed., p. 1134). St. Louis: Mosby.

---

660. A nurse is caring for a hospitalized client with an alcohol abuse disorder. When reviewing the client's discharge

Answer: 4

Rationale: All of the outcomes deserve support by the nurse, but option 4 will help the client to abstain from alcohol and provide

outcomes, the most positive outcome is that the client states that he or she will:

1 Learn to play golf.
2 Take a biofeedback class.
3 Start an exercise program.
4 Continue to attend Alcoholics Anonymous (AA) meetings.

Level of Cognitive Ability: Analysis
Client Needs: Psychosocial Integrity
Integrated Process: Nursing Process/Evaluation
Content Area: Mental Health

the client with a support group. Option 4 is the most positive outcome.

Test-Taking Strategy: Use the process of elimination, and focus on the subject of the question—the most positive outcome. From the options presented, option 4 addresses the client's disorder. AA has the greatest potential to provide impulse control. Review the care of the client with an alcohol abuse disorder if you had difficulty with this question.

Reference

Varcarolis, E., & Halter, M. (2009). *Essentials of psychiatric mental health nursing: A communication approach to evidence-based care* (pp. 353-354). St. Louis: Saunders.

---

661. An English-speaking Hispanic male has a long leg cast applied because of a right proximal fractured tibia. During rounds that night, the nurse finds the client restless, withdrawn, and quiet. Which initial statement by the nurse is appropriate?

1 "Are you uncomfortable?"
2 "Tell me what you are feeling."
3 "You'll feel better in the morning."
4 "I'll get your pain medication right away."

Level of Cognitive Ability: Application
Client Needs: Psychosocial Integrity
Integrated Process: Communication and Documentation
Content Area: Adult Health/Musculoskeletal

Answer: 2
Rationale: Option 2 is an open-ended statement and makes no assumptions about the client's physiological or emotional state. Option 1 is incorrect because the Hispanic male may deny feeling any pain when asked. False reassurance is never therapeutic, which makes option 3 incorrect. Data collection is necessary before intervention, so option 4 would be incorrect.

Test-Taking Strategy: Use the process of elimination. The word *initial* in the question tells you that data collection and prioritization with a therapeutic communication technique is needed. Remember to focus on the client's feelings. Review therapeutic communication techniques if you had difficulty with this question.

Reference

deWit, S. (2009). *Medical-surgical nursing: Concepts & practice* (pp. 9, 140). St. Louis: Saunders.

---

662. A client was started on oral anticoagulant therapy while hospitalized. The client is now being discharged to home and is intermittently confused. The nurse determines that the client has the best support system for successful anticoagulant therapy monitoring if the client:

1 Lives with a daughter and son-in-law
2 Has a home health aide coming to the house for 9 weeks
3 Will have blood work drawn in the home by a local laboratory
4 Has a good friend living next door who will take the client to the doctor

Level of Cognitive Ability: Analysis
Client Needs: Psychosocial Integrity
Integrated Process: Nursing Process/Evaluation
Content Area: Adult Health/Cardiovascular

Answer: 1
Rationale: Successful anticoagulant therapy has three components: taking the medication properly, having proper follow-up medical care, and doing serial follow-up blood work. Option 2 facilitates only reminding the client to take the medication, option 3 facilitates only blood work, and option 4 facilitates only medical care. The client who is intermittently confused may need support systems in place to enhance compliance with therapy. Option 1 addresses the best support system.

Test-Taking Strategy: Use the process of elimination, and note that the client is intermittently confused. Focus on the subject—the best support system for the client; this will direct you to option 1. Review appropriate support systems if you had difficulty with this question.

References

Christensen, B., & Kockrow, E. (2006). *Adult health nursing* (5th ed., p. 391). St. Louis: Mosby.
Potter, P., & Perry, A. (2009). *Fundamentals of nursing* (7th ed., p. 456). St. Louis: Mosby.

663. A client who has undergone successful femoral-popliteal bypass grafting to the leg says to the nurse, "I hope everything goes well after this and that I don't lose my leg. I'm so afraid that I'll have gone through this for nothing." The nurse should make which therapeutic response to the client?

1 "I can understand what you mean. I'd be nervous, too, if I were in your shoes."
2 "This surgery is so successful that I wouldn't be concerned at all if I were you."
3 "Stress isn't helpful for you. You should probably just relax and try not to worry unless something actually happens."
4 "Complications are possible, but you have a good deal of control if you make the lifestyle adjustments we talked about."

Level of Cognitive Ability: Application
Client Needs: Psychosocial Integrity
Integrated Process: Communication and Documentation
Content Area: Adult Health/Cardiovascular

Answer: 4

Rationale: Clients frequently fear that they will ultimately lose a limb or become debilitated in some other way. The nurse reassures the client that participation in exercise, diet, and medication therapy, along with smoking cessation, can limit further plaque development. Option 1 feeds into the client's anxiety and is not therapeutic. Option 2 gives false reassurance, which is incorrect. Option 3 is meant to be reassuring but offers no suggestions to empower the client.

Test-Taking Strategy: Use the process of elimination and therapeutic communication techniques. Option 4 acknowledges the client's concerns and empowers the client to improve health, which will ultimately reduce concern about the risk of complications. Review therapeutic communication techniques if you had difficulty with this question.

References

Christensen, B., & Kockrow, E. (2006). *Adult health nursing* (5th ed., p. 384). St. Louis: Mosby.
deWit, S. (2009). *Medical-surgical nursing: Concepts & practice* (pp. 9, 444-445). St. Louis: Saunders.

---

664. A client is scheduled to undergo pericardiocentesis for pericardial effusion. The nurse plans to alleviate the client's apprehension by:

1 Telling the client to watch television during the procedure as a distraction
2 Talking to the client from the foot of the bed so as to be available to get added supplies
3 Staying beside the client and giving information and encouragement during the procedure
4 Telling the client that the nurse will take care of another assigned client during the procedure so as to be available when the procedure is complete

Level of Cognitive Ability: Application
Client Needs: Psychosocial Integrity
Integrated Process: Nursing Process/Implementation
Content Area: Adult Health/Cardiovascular

Answer: 3

Rationale: Staying with the client and giving information and encouragement is most supportive to the client. Options 1 and 4 distance the nurse from a client in the psychosocial as well as the physical sense. The nurse should ask another caregiver to be available to get extra supplies, if needed.

Test-Taking Strategy: Use the process of elimination and therapeutic communication techniques. Remember to provide support to the client and to always address the client's feelings and concerns. This will direct you to option 3. Review measures to provide client support if you had difficulty with this question.

References

Chernecky, C., & Berger, B. (2008). *Laboratory tests and diagnostic procedures* (5th ed., pp. 861-863). Philadelphia: Saunders.
Christensen, B., & Kockrow, E. (2006). *Adult health nursing* (5th ed., p. 371). St. Louis: Mosby.

---

665. An adolescent is hospitalized for the evaluation and treatment of Tourette's syndrome. The nurse reviews the client's record and notes that the client is exhibiting motor tics. The nurse most likely expects to note which of the following in the client?

1 Grunting sounds
2 Tongue protrusion
3 Uttering of obscenities
4 Consistent yelping sounds

Level of Cognitive Ability: Comprehension
Client Needs: Psychosocial Integrity
Integrated Process: Nursing Process/Data Collection
Content Area: Mental Health

Answer: 2
Rationale: Tourette's syndrome involves motor and verbal tics that cause marked distress and significant impairment in a client's social and occupational functioning. Motor tics usually involve the head but can also involve the torso and limbs. The most frequent first symptom is a single tic such as eye blinking. Other motor tics include tongue protrusion, touching, squatting, hopping, skipping, retracing steps, and twirling when walking. Vocal tics include words and sounds such as barks, grunts, yelps, clicks, snorts, sniffs, and coughs. Coprolalia, which is the uttering of obscenities, is present in a small number of cases.

Test-Taking Strategy: Note the strategic words *motor tics* in the question. Use the process of elimination, and note that options 1, 3, and 4 all address verbal behaviors. Review the manifestations of Tourette's syndrome if you had difficulty with this question.

Reference
Fortinash, K., & Holoday-Worret, P. (2008). *Psychiatric mental health nursing* (4th ed., p. 373). St. Louis: Mosby.

---

666. Which statement is appropriate for the nurse to make when talking with a hospitalized client who is recovering from the signs and symptoms of autonomic dysreflexia?

1 "How could your home-care nurse let this happen?"
2 "Now that this problem is taken care of, I'm sure you'll be fine."
3 "I have some time if you would like to talk about what happened to you."
4 "I'm sure you now understand the importance of preventing this from occurring."

Level of Cognitive Ability: Application
Client Needs: Psychosocial Integrity
Integrated Process: Communication and Documentation
Content Area: Adult Health/Neurological

Answer: 3
Rationale: Offering time to the client encourages the client to discuss feelings. Options 1, 2, and 4 are blocks to communication. Options 1 and 4 show disapproval, and option 2 gives false reassurance.

Test-Taking Strategy: Use the process of elimination, and select the option that is therapeutic. Always address the client's concerns and feelings first. Review therapeutic communication techniques if you had difficulty with this question.

References
Christensen, B., & Kockrow, E. (2006). *Adult health nursing* (5th ed., p. 746). St. Louis: Mosby.
deWit, S. (2009). *Medical-surgical nursing: Concepts & practice* (p. 9). St. Louis: Saunders.

---

667. A nurse is assisting a client with a spinal cord injury with activities of daily living. The client states, "I can't do this; I wish I were dead." The nurse should make which therapeutic response to the client?

1 "Why do you say that?"
2 "You wish you were dead?"
3 "Let's wash your back now."
4 "I'm sure you are frustrated, but things will work out just fine for you."

Answer: 2
Rationale: Clarifying is a therapeutic technique that involves restating what was said to obtain additional information. By using the word *why* in option 1, the nurse puts the client on the defensive. Option 3 changes the subject. Option 4 provides false reassurance. Options 1, 3, and 4 are nontherapeutic and block communication.

Test-Taking Strategy: Use therapeutic communication techniques. Option 2 involves clarifying and restating and is the only option that will encourage the client to verbalize feelings and concerns. Review therapeutic communication techniques if you had difficulty with this question.

Level of Cognitive Ability: Application
Client Needs: Psychosocial Integrity
Integrated Process: Communication and Documentation
Content Area: Adult Health/Neurological

Reference
Linton, A. (2007). *Introduction to medical-surgical nursing* (4th ed., pp. 503-504). Philadelphia: Saunders.

---

668. A client says to the nurse, "I want to die. I think about it sometimes, but I don't know how in the world to do it. My mother gave me this ring, and I love it so. I think I'll give it to my grandchildren." Based on the client's statement, the nurse determines that:
1 There is minimal suicide risk.
2 There is no suicide risk noted.
3 Suicide has been attempted unsuccessfully.
4 The risk for suicide exists; continued data collection is needed.

Level of Cognitive Ability: Analysis
Client Needs: Psychosocial Integrity
Integrated Process: Nursing Process/Data Collection
Content Area: Mental Health

Answer: 4
Rationale: The words *I want to die* indicate a suicide risk. Any self-harm language must be viewed as serious. This situation gives no data related to a history of self-harm. Options 1, 2, and 3 are inaccurate interpretations.

Test-Taking Strategy: Use the process of elimination. Focus on the statement made by the client to direct you to option 4. Review suicide assessment if you had difficulty with this question.

Reference
Varcarolis, E., & Halter, M. (2009). *Essentials of psychiatric mental health nursing: A communication approach to evidence-based care* (p. 415). St. Louis: Saunders.

---

669. Family members awaiting the outcome of a suicide attempt are tearful. Which response by the nurse is therapeutic to the family at this time?
1 "I can see you are worried."
2 "Everything possible is being done."
3 "Don't worry, you have nothing to feel guilty about."
4 "Let me check to see how long it will be before you can see your loved one."

Level of Cognitive Ability: Application
Client Needs: Psychosocial Integrity
Integrated Process: Communication and Documentation
Content Area: Mental Health

Answer: 1
Rationale: The nursing statement in option 1 uses the therapeutic technique of clarifying. Options 2, 3, and 4 are communication blocks. Option 2 uses clichés and false reassurance. Option 3 labels the family's behavior without their validation. Option 4 focuses on an important subject at an inappropriate time (i.e., when family members are tearful).

Test-Taking Strategy: Use therapeutic communication techniques. Option 1 identifies clarifying and is the only option that will encourage the family to verbalize feelings and concerns. Review therapeutic communication techniques if you had difficulty with this question.

References
Fortinash, K., & Holoday-Worret, P. (2008). *Psychiatric mental health nursing* (4th ed., p. 469). St. Louis: Mosby.
Varcarolis, E., & Halter, M. (2009). *Essentials of psychiatric mental health nursing: A communication approach to evidence-based care* (pp. 95-98). St. Louis: Saunders.

---

670. Which of the following is appropriate to include when caring for an 11-year-old child who has been abused?
1 Encourage the child to fear the abuser.
2 Provide a care environment that allows for the development of trust.

Answer: 2
Rationale: The abused child usually requires long-term therapeutic support. The environment during the child's healing must include one in which trust and caring are provided for the child. Options 3 and 4 ask the child to behave with a maturity beyond that which would be expected for an 11-year-old child. Option 1 reinforces fear.

3 Teach the child to make wise choices when confronted with an abusive situation.
4 Have the child point out the abuser if that person should visit while the child is hospitalized.

Level of Cognitive Ability: Application
Client Needs: Psychosocial Integrity
Integrated Process: Caring
Content Area: Child Health

Test-Taking Strategy: Use the process of elimination and the components of a therapeutic nurse–client relationship. Option 2 is the option that is appropriate because it provides the child with a nurturing and supportive environment in which to begin the healing process. Review the psychosocial issues related to an abused child if you had difficulty with this question.

Reference
Leifer, G. (2007). *Introduction to maternity and pediatric nursing* (5th ed., p. 568). Philadelphia: Saunders.

---

671. A nurse collects data from an older client and monitors for signs of potential abuse. The nurse understands that which of the following psychosocial factors place the client at risk for abuse?
1 The client has a chronic illness.
2 The client resides in a low-income neighborhood.
3 The client shows signs and symptoms of depression.
4 The client is completely dependent on family members for receiving food and medicine.

Level of Cognitive Ability: Comprehension
Client Needs: Psychosocial Integrity
Integrated Process: Nursing Process/Data Collection
Content Area: Mental Health

Answer: 4
Rationale: Elder abuse is sometimes the result of frustration of adult children who find themselves caring for dependent parents. Increasing demands by parents for care and financial support can cause resentment and may be burdensome. Option 1 is a physiological condition. Issues of abuse are not bound to socioeconomic status. Signs and symptoms of depression do not specifically indicate abuse.

Test-Taking Strategy: Use the process of elimination, and focus on the words *psychosocial factors*. Note the strategic word *dependent* in option 4 to direct you to this option. Review the risk factors associated with elder abuse if you had difficulty with this question.

Reference
Fortinash, K., & Holoday-Worret, P. (2008). *Psychiatric mental health nursing* (4th ed., p. 501). St. Louis: Mosby.

---

672. The nurse is caring for a dying client who says, "What would you say if I asked you to be the executor of my will?" Which nursing response is appropriate?
1 "Why, I'd be honored to be the executor of your will."
2 "Is there any money in it? I adore money, but I am honest."
3 "I'd say, 'Great!' Don't worry. I'll carry out your will just as you want me to."
4 "Your confidence in me is an honor, but I would like to understand more about your thinking."

Level of Cognitive Ability: Application
Client Needs: Psychosocial Integrity
Integrated Process: Communication and Documentation
Content Area: Fundamental Skills

Answer: 4
Rationale: In option 4, the nurse uses the therapeutic communication of seeking clarification. In option 1, the nurse responds with a social communication with no assessment of the consequences, which demonstrates a lack of critical thinking and of the exploration of the client's motivation or needs. In option 2, the nurse uses histrionic language and crass ideation. In option 3, the nurse provides false reassurance, which is nontherapeutic.

Test-Taking Strategy: Use therapeutic communication techniques. Option 4 is the only option that is therapeutic and that seeks to clarify the client's request. Review therapeutic communication techniques if you had difficulty with this question.

Reference
deWit, S. (2009). *Medical-surgical nursing: Concepts & practice* (p. 9). St. Louis: Saunders.

---

673. A client who is suffering from urticaria (hives) and pruritus says to the nurse, "What am I going to do? I'm getting married next week and I'll probably be covered in this rash and itching like crazy." Which of the following is a therapeutic response by the nurse?

1 "It's probably just due to prewedding jitters."
2 "I hope your husband-to-be has a sense of humor."
3 "You're very troubled that this will extend into your wedding?"
4 "The antihistamine will help a great deal, just you wait and see."

Level of Cognitive Ability: Application
Client Needs: Psychosocial Integrity
Integrated Process: Communication and Documentation
Content Area: Adult Health/Integumentary

Answer: 3

Rationale: The therapeutic communication technique that the nurse uses is reflection. In option 1, the nurse minimizes the client's anxiety and fears. In option 4, the nurse talks about antihistamines and asks the client to wait; this is nontherapeutic because the nurse is making promises that may not be kept and because the response is close-ended and shuts off the client's expression of feelings. In option 2, the nurse uses humor inappropriately and with insensitivity.

Test-Taking Strategy: Use therapeutic communication techniques. Option 3 is the only option that encourages the client to express feelings. Review therapeutic communication techniques if you had difficulty with this question.

Reference

deWit, S. (2009). *Medical-surgical nursing: Concepts & practice* (pp. 9, 263, 1043). St. Louis: Saunders.

---

674. A client with a spinal cord injury (SCI) makes the following comments. Which comment warrants additional intervention by the nurse?

1 "I'm so angry that this happened to me."
2 "I'm really looking forward to going home."
3 "I know I will have to make major adjustments in my life."
4 "I would like my family members to be here for my teaching sessions."

Level of Cognitive Ability: Analysis
Client Needs: Psychosocial Integrity
Integrated Process: Nursing Process/Evaluation
Content Area: Adult Health/Neurological

Answer: 1

Rationale: It is important to allow a client with an SCI to verbalize feelings. If the client indicates a desire to discuss feelings, the nurse should respond therapeutically. The words *I'm so angry that this happened to me* indicate the client's need to discuss feelings. Options 2 and 3 indicate that the client understands that changes will be occurring and that family involvement is best. Option 4 does not require further intervention.

Test-Taking Strategy: Use the process of elimination, and note the strategic words *warrants additional intervention.* Options 2, 3, and 4 are comparable or alike in that the client expresses positive acceptance of the injury. In option 1, the client expresses a feeling that warrants a need for more information. Review psychosocial concerns related to an SCI if you had difficulty with this question.

References

deWit, S. (2009). *Medical-surgical nursing: Concepts & practice* (p. 9). St. Louis: Saunders.
Linton, A. (2007). *Introduction to medical-surgical nursing* (4th ed., p. 499). Philadelphia: Saunders.

---

675. A nurse is preparing to collect data from a client who is suspected of having Alzheimer's disease. The nurse enters the client's room and asks the client, "How was your weekend?" The client responds by saying "It was great. I discussed politics with the President, and he took me out to dinner." The nurse interprets that the client is exhibiting which defensive maneuver?

Answer: 4

Rationale: Confabulation is a defensive maneuver and an unconscious attempt to maintain self-esteem. Hiding is a form of denial and an unconscious protective defense against the terrifying reality of losing one's place in the world. Apraxia is not a defensive maneuver; it is characterized by the loss of purposeful movement in the absence of motor or sensory impairment. Perseveration is the repetition of phrases or behaviors that is often intensified under stress.

1 Hiding
2 Apraxia
3 Perseveration
4 Confabulation

Level of Cognitive Ability: Comprehension
Client Needs: Psychosocial Integrity
Integrated Process: Nursing Process/Data Collection
Content Area: Mental Health

Test-Taking Strategy: Use the process of elimination, and focus on the strategic words *defensive maneuvers*. Eliminate option 2 first because this is not a defensive maneuver. From the remaining options, focus on the client's statement to direct you to option 4. Review defensive maneuvers if you had difficulty with this question.

References

deWit, S. (2009). *Medical-surgical nursing: Concepts & practice* (p. 1138). St. Louis: Saunders.
Wold, G. (2008). *Basic geriatric nursing* (4th ed., p. 60). St. Louis: Mosby.

---

676. An agoraphobic client has been hospitalized for a relatively prolonged time. The client has become cooperative and communicative with peers and has also begun to make appropriate suggestions during group discussions. The nurse concludes that the client's behavior is representative of:
1 Acting out
2 Manipulation
3 Improvement
4 Attention seeking

Level of Cognitive Ability: Comprehension
Client Needs: Psychosocial Integrity
Integrated Process: Nursing Process/Evaluation
Content Area: Mental Health

Answer: 3
Rationale: The behavior demonstrated by the client during hospitalization is appropriate. There is no evidence in the question to indicate that the client is acting out (which is an attention-seeking behavior), seeking attention, or being manipulative.

Test-Taking Strategy: Use the process of elimination, and focus on the data in the question. This should direct you to option 3. Review the indications of improvement in a client with a phobia if you had difficulty with this question.

Reference

Keltner, N., Schwecke, L., & Bostrom, C. (2007). *Psychiatric nursing* (5th ed., p. 423). St. Louis: Mosby.

---

677. An examination of a 14-year-old child reveals bruises and bleeding in the genital area, cigarette burns on the chest, rope burns on the buttocks, and multiple old fractures. The child says, "I'm afraid to go home! My stepfather will be angry with me for telling on him!" The nurse should make which therapeutic response to the child?
1 "You can't go back there with that man. How do you think your mother will react?"
2 "You must know that your presence in the house will only tease your stepfather more."
3 "Let's keep this between you, me, and the physician until we can formulate further plans to assist you."
4 "I am sorry that this has happened to you, but you will be safe here. Your physician has admitted you until further plans can be made."

Answer: 4
Rationale: A child who is found to be physically and sexually assaulted should be admitted to the hospital. This will provide time for a more comprehensive evaluation while simultaneously protecting the child from further abuse. Option 2 accuses the victim of "teasing" the stepfather and is incorrect; it is also judgmental, controlling, and demeaning. In option 1, the nurse does not respond with a calm and reassuring communication style or maintain a professional attitude. The nurse's suggestion in option 3 is inappropriate, and the statement is collusive and passive in its stance.

Test-Taking Strategy: Use the process of elimination. Recalling that the priority issue is to protect the victim from the abuser will direct you to option 4. Review the care of the abused child if you had difficulty with this question.

References

deWit, S. (2009). *Medical-surgical nursing: Concepts & practice* (p. 9). St. Louis: Saunders.
Price, D., & Gwin, J. (2008). *Pediatric nursing: An introductory text* (10th ed., p. 174). St. Louis: Saunders.

Level of Cognitive Ability: Application
Client Needs: Psychosocial Integrity
Integrated Process: Communication and Documentation
Content Area: Child Health

---

678. A nurse is caring for a 15-year-old female client admitted to the hospital with a diagnosis of physical and sexual abuse by her father. That evening, the father angrily approaches the nurse and says, "I'm taking my daughter home. She's told me what you people are up to, and we're out of here!" The nurse should make which appropriate response to the father?

1 "Listen to me. If you attempt to take your daughter from this unit, the police will only bring her back."
2 "Over my dead body you will! She's here and here she stays until the doctor says differently, so get off my floor or I'll call hospital security and the police!"
3 "You seem very upset. Let's talk at the nurse's station. I want to help you. I know you're very concerned and want to help your daughter. It will be best if you agree to let your daughter stay here for now."
4 "Your daughter is ill and needs to be here. I know you want to help her to recover and that you will work to help everyone straighten out the circumstances that caused this. Go to the chapel and pray for your daughter and for your soul."

Level of Cognitive Ability: Application
Client Needs: Psychosocial Integrity
Integrated Process: Communication and Documentation
Content Area: Child Health

Answer: 3
Rationale: When a child suspected of being abused is admitted to the hospital for further evaluation and protection, the physician usually attempts to get the parents to agree to the admission. If the parents refuse, the hospital can request an immediate court order to retain the child for a specific length of time. In option 1, the command to listen is somewhat demanding. In option 2, the nurse is angry and verbally abusive, and it is clear that the nurse has decided that the father is guilty of child abuse. In addition, the nurse is so aggressive and challenging that she may antagonize the father and become a victim of violence as well. Option 4 is pompous and lecturing.

Test-Taking Strategy: Use therapeutic communication techniques, and focus on the subject—the father. Option 3 is the only option that addresses the father's behavior. Review therapeutic communication techniques if you had difficulty with this question.

References
deWit, S. (2009). *Medical-surgical nursing: Concepts & practice* (p. 9). St. Louis: Saunders.
Price, D., & Gwin, J. (2008). *Pediatric nursing: An introductory text* (10th ed., p. 174). St. Louis: Saunders.

---

679. A 12-year-old client is seen in the health care clinic, and the nurse collects data from the client. Which data suggests to the nurse that the client is experiencing disruption in the development of self-concept?

1 The client interacts well with the peer group.
2 The client enjoys a part-time babysitting job.

Answer: 3
Rationale: A sense of industry is appropriate for this age group and may be exhibited by having a part-time job. The increase in self-esteem associated with skill mastery is an important part of development for the school-age child. Positive peer interaction is also appropriate. The formation of an intimate relationship would not be expected until early adulthood.

3 The client has an intimate relationship with a significant other.
4 The client enjoys playing chess and mastering new skills with this game.

Level of Cognitive Ability: Analysis
Client Needs: Psychosocial Integrity
Integrated Process: Nursing Process/Data Collection
Content Area: Child Health

Test-Taking Strategy: Use the process of elimination, and focus on normal growth and development. Note the age of the client in the question; this will assist you with eliminating options 1, 2, and 4. Review normal growth and development and developmental tasks associated with this age group if you had difficulty with this question.

Reference

Price, D., & Gwin, J. (2008). *Pediatric nursing: An introductory text* (10th ed., p. 276). St. Louis: Saunders.

---

680. The nurse is caring for an infant with hyaline membrane disease. The infant will require surfactant replacement therapy via an endotracheal tube, and the parents will be present during the procedure. The father states that he is not sure about having this done to his baby. Before the procedure, the nurse helps to prepare the parents by stating:

1 "Don't worry. We do this all the time."
2 "You have concerns about this procedure for your baby?"
3 "You have a wonderful physician who has made the right decision for your baby."
4 "We are going to be busy with the baby, so why don't you wait outside during the procedure?"

Level of Cognitive Ability: Application
Client Needs: Psychosocial Integrity
Integrated Process: Communication and Documentation
Content Area: Maternity/Postpartum

Answer: 2
Rationale: When planning for this infant's care and for the well-being of the parents, it is important to apply the techniques of therapeutic communication. By paraphrasing the father's concern, the message is restated in the nurse's own words. Option 1 involves false reassurance, which will block communication. Option 3 is a communication block that denies the parents the right to their opinion. Option 4 is incorrect because the parents have every right to be present during the procedure.

Test-Taking Strategy: Use therapeutic communication techniques to answer the question. Select the option that enhances communication. Only option 2 addresses the use of a therapeutic communication technique because it addresses the needs of the parents. Review therapeutic communication techniques if you had difficulty with this question.

References

Leifer, G. (2007). *Introduction to maternity and pediatric nursing* (5th ed., pp. 306-307). Philadelphia: Saunders.
Leifer, G. (2008). *Maternity nursing: An introductory text* (10th ed., p. 7). Philadelphia: Saunders.

---

681. The parents of a postmature infant ask the nurse, "Why does our baby have such a worried facial expression?" Which of the following is the appropriate response by the nurse?

1 "I think you are right to be concerned."
2 "Don't worry, all babies look like that."
3 "Have you decided on a name for your baby?"
4 "You have concerns about the baby's worried facial expression?"

Level of Cognitive Ability: Application
Client Needs: Psychosocial Integrity
Integrated Process: Communication and Documentation
Content Area: Maternity/Postpartum

Answer: 4
Rationale: Paraphrasing is restating the parents' message in the nurse's own words. In option 1, the nurse is expressing approval, which can be harmful to the nurse–parent relationship. In option 2, the nurse is offering false reassurance, which blocks communication. Option 3 involves a communication block as well because it does not address the subject of the clients' concern.

Test-Taking Strategy: Use therapeutic communication techniques to answer the question. Only option 4 reflects the use of a therapeutic communication technique and addresses the clients' concern. Review therapeutic communication techniques if you had difficulty with this question.

Reference

Leifer, G. (2008). *Maternity nursing: An introductory text* (10th ed., pp. 7, 303-304). Philadelphia: Saunders.

ALTERNATE ITEM FORMAT QUESTIONS

Multiple Response

682. A nurse is caring for a client who is at risk for violent behavior. Select all interventions that will assist with preventing violent behavior if the client becomes agitated.

❒ 1 Speak in a calm, low voice.
❒ 2 Use short, simple sentences.
❒ 3 Maintain intense direct eye contact.
❒ 4 Avoid laughing and smiling inappropriately.
❒ 5 Assume a supportive stance that is at least 3 feet from the client.
❒ 6 Face the client with the arms across the chest so that the client will be assured that the nurse is in control of the situation.

Level of Cognitive Ability: Application
Client Needs: Psychosocial Integrity
Integrated Process: Nursing Process/ Implementation
Content Area: Mental Health

Answer: 1, 2, 4, 5

Rationale: Speaking to the client in a calm, low voice can help to decrease the client's agitation. Agitated clients often speak loudly and use profanity. It is important that nurses not respond by raising their voices because doing so will probably be perceived as competition and will further escalate a volatile situation. The nurse should use short, simple sentences and avoid laughing and smiling inappropriately. The nurse can help reduce agitation by acknowledging the client's feelings and reassuring the client that the staff is there to help. A posture that avoids intimidation should be assumed by the nurse. Placing the hands on the hips and crossing the arms across the chest are intimidating and communicate emotional distance and an unwillingness to help. The nurse should avoid intense direct eye contact. However, altering position so that the nurse's eyes are at the same level as those of the client allows the client to communicate from an equal rather than an inferior position. In addition, the nurse should assume a supportive stance that is at least 3 feet from the client because intrusion into a client's personal space can be perceived as a threat and provoke aggression and violence.

Test-Taking Strategy: Focus on the subject—preventing violent behavior. Recalling that interventions are aimed at strengthening the therapeutic alliance with the client will assist you with identifying the correct interventions. Review interventions for violent situations if you had difficulty with this question.

Reference

Fortinash, K., & Holoday-Worret, P. (2008). *Psychiatric mental health nursing* (4th ed., p. 279). St. Louis: Mosby.

Fill-in-the-Blank

683. The nurse notes an order for clorazepate (Tranxene T-Tab) 15 mg twice daily. The nurse prepares to administer how many tablets to administer one dose?

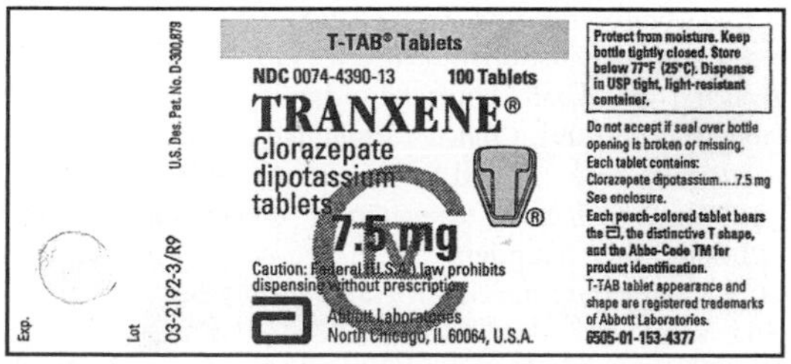

Figure 8-1 From Kee, J., & Marshall, S. (2009). *Clinical calculations: With applications to general and specialty areas* (6th ed., p. 366). Philadelphia: Saunders.

Answer: _____ tablet(s)

Answer: 2 tablets

Rationale: Use the formula for calculating medication dosages.

Formula

$$\frac{\text{Desired}}{\text{Available}} \times \text{tablet} = \text{Tablet(s) per dose}$$

$$\frac{15\text{ mg}}{7.5\text{ mg}} \times 1\text{ tablet} = 2\text{ tablets}$$

Test-Taking Strategy: Identify the components of the question and what the question is asking. In this case, the question asks for the number of tablets per dose. Set up the formula, knowing that the desired dose is 15 mg and that the available amount is 7.5 mg per 1 tablet; then perform the calculation. Verify the answer using a calculator. Review medication calculations if you had difficulty with this question.

Level of Cognitive Ability: Application
Client Needs: Psychosocial Integrity
Integrated Process: Nursing Process/ Implementation
Content Area: Mental Health

References
Kee, J., & Marshall, S. (2009). *Clinical calculations: With applications to general and specialty areas* (6th ed., p. 366). Philadelphia: Saunders.
Potter, P., & Perry, A. (2009). *Fundamentals of nursing* (7th ed., p. 697). St. Louis: Mosby.

Prioritizing (Ordered Response)

684. A nurse who is caring for a client who is dying reviews the client's plan of care and notes a nursing diagnosis of *Fear* and appropriate nursing interventions. List the nursing interventions in order of priority. (Number 1 is the first priority.)

____ Help the client express his fears.
____ Identify the nature of the client's fears.
____ Assist the client with implementing coping methods to deal with fear.
____ Evaluate the effectiveness of the coping method used to deal with fear.
____ Help the client identify methods that were used to cope with fear in the past.
____ Document verbal and nonverbal expressions of fear and other significant data.

Level of Cognitive Ability: Application
Client Needs: Psychosocial Integrity
Integrated Process: Nursing Process/ Implementation
Content Area: Delegating/Prioritizing

Answer: 2, 1, 4, 5, 3, 6
Rationale: Fear can range from a paralyzing, overwhelming feeling to a mild concern, so the nurse would first identify the nature of the client's fears to know how to best help the client. Next, the nurse would help the client to express fears. The client's fear may not be limited to the fear of dying, and the nurse needs this information to help the client appropriately. When the nurse is aware of the client's fears, the methods that the client used to cope with fear in the past are identified. At this point, the nurse assists the client with implementing coping methods and then evaluates their effectiveness. The nurse would lastly document the client's verbal and nonverbal expressions of fear and any other significant data.

Test-Taking Strategy: Use the steps of the nursing process to assist you with determining the order of priority of the nursing interventions. This will help you to determine that identifying the nature of the client's fears is the first priority. Identify the last priority as documenting the verbal and nonverbal expressions of fear and other significant data; the nurse would not be aware of this information until he or she performed an assessment and provided care to the client. It would be necessary to help the client express fears before methods used to cope with fear could be determined, implemented, and evaluated. Review the care of the dying client who is experiencing fear if you had difficulty with this question.

Reference
Linton, A. (2007). *Introduction to medical-surgical nursing* (4th ed., pp. 356-357). Philadelphia: Saunders.

REFERENCES

Black., J, & Hawks, J. (2009). *Medical-surgical nursing: Clinical management for positive outcomes* (8th ed.). St. Louis: Saunders.
Chernecky, C., & Berger, B. (2008). *Laboratory tests and diagnostic procedures* (5th ed.). Philadelphia: Saunders.
Christensen, B., & Kockrow, E. (2006). *Adult health nursing* (5th ed.). St. Louis: Mosby.
Christensen, B., & Kockrow, E. (2006). *Foundations of nursing* (5th ed.). St. Louis: Mosby.
deWit, S. (2009). *Medical-surgical nursing: Concepts & practice*. St. Louis: Saunders.
Fortinash, K., & Holoday-Worret, P. (2008). *Psychiatric mental health nursing* (4th ed.). St. Louis: Mosby.
Hodgson, B., & Kizior, R. (2009). *Saunders nursing drug handbook 2009*. St. Louis: Saunders.
Hockenberry, M., & Wilson, D. (2009). *Wong's essentials of pediatric care* (8th ed.). St. Louis: Mosby.
Ignatavicius, D., & Workman, M. (2010). *Medical-surgical nursing: Patient-centered collaborative care.* (6th ed.). St. Louis: Saunders.
Kee, J., Hayes, E., & McCuistion L. (2009). *Pharmacology: A nursing process approach* (6th ed.). St. Louis: Saunders.
Kee, J., & Marshall, S. (2009). *Clinical calculations: With applications to general and specialty areas* (6th ed.). St. Louis: Saunders.
Leifer, G. (2007). *Introduction to maternity and pediatric nursing* (5th ed.). Philadelphia: Saunders.
Leifer, G. (2008). *Maternity nursing: An introductory text* (10th ed.). Philadelphia: Saunders.
Linton, A. (2007). *Introduction to medical-surgical nursing* (4th ed.). Philadelphia: Saunders.
McKinney, E., James, S., Murray, S., & Ashwill, J. (2009). *Maternal-child nursing* (3rd ed.). St. Louis: Mosby.
Perry, A., & Potter, P. (2010). *Clinical nursing skills & techniques* (7th ed.). St. Louis: Mosby.

Potter, P., & Perry, A. (2009). *Fundamentals of nursing* (7th ed.). St. Louis: Mosby.
Price, D., & Gwin, J. (2008). *Pediatric nursing: An introductory text* (10th ed.). St. Louis: Saunders.
Stuart, G. (2009). *Principles & practice of psychiatric nursing* (9th ed.). St. Louis: Mosby.
Varcarolis, E., & Halter., M. (2009). *Essentials of psychiatric mental health nursing: A communication approach to evidence-based care.* St. Louis: Saunders.
Wold, G. (2008). *Basic geriatric nursing* (4th ed.). St. Louis: Mosby.

CHAPTER
9

Physiological Integrity

685. A nurse is caring for a client receiving hemodialysis who has an internal arteriovenous fistula. Which finding indicates to the nurse that the fistula is patent?

1 The lack of a bruit at the radial pulse
2 White fibrin specks noted in the fistula
3 A feeling of warmth at the site of the fistula
4 The palpation of a thrill over the site of the fistula

Level of Cognitive Ability: Analysis
Client Needs: Physiological Integrity
Integrated Process: Nursing Process/Data Collection
Content Area: Adult Health/Renal

Answer: 4
Rationale: An internal arteriovenous fistula is created through a surgical procedure in which an artery in the arm is anastomosed to a vein. The fistula is internal. To determine patency, the nurse palpates over the fistula for a thrill and auscultates for a bruit. The presence of a bruit or a thrill indicates a patent fistula. The nurse would not note white fibrin specks in the fistula because the fistula is internal. A feeling of warmth may indicate a potential inflammatory process.

Test-Taking Strategy: Use the process of elimination. Recalling that the presence of a bruit or a thrill indicates a patent fistula helps you to eliminate option 1. Option 2 can be eliminated because the nurse would not note white fibrin specks in the fistula because the fistula is internal. Option 3 can be eliminated because a feeling of warmth may indicate a potential inflammatory process. Review the normal findings in clients with hemodialysis access devices if you had difficulty with this question.

Reference
Linton, A. (2007). *Introduction to medical-surgical nursing* (4th ed., p. 874). Philadelphia: Saunders.

---

686. A nurse is reviewing the record of a client with cancer and notes that the client's calcium level is 14 mg/dL. The nurse determines that this calcium level is consistent with which oncological emergency?

1 Hyperkalemia
2 Hypercalcemia
3 Spinal cord compression
4 Superior vena cava syndrome

Level of Cognitive Ability: Analysis
Client Needs: Physiological Integrity
Integrated Process: Nursing Process/Evaluation
Content Area: Adult Health/Oncology

Answer: 2
Rationale: Hypercalcemia is characterized by greater than normal amounts of calcium in the blood. One potentially life-threatening complication of cancer is hypercalcemia, which is characterized by calcium levels of more than 11 mg/dL. Although spinal cord compression and superior vena cava syndrome are also oncological emergencies, they are not characterized by high calcium levels.

Test-Taking Strategy: Use the process of elimination. Note the relationship between the calcium level in the question and *hypercalcemia* in the correct option. Review normal calcium levels and oncological emergencies if you had difficulty with this question.

References
Chernecky, C., & Berger, B. (2008). *Laboratory tests and diagnostic procedures* (5th ed., p. 279). Philadelphia: Saunders.
Linton, A. (2007). *Introduction to medical-surgical nursing* (4th ed., p. 393). Philadelphia: Saunders.

---

687. A licensed practical nurse (LPN) is gathering data about a postpartum client. Which finding indicates hemorrhage and the need to notify the registered nurse?

1 Multiparity
2 Prolonged labor
3 Soft or "boggy" uterus
4 Precipitous labor and delivery

Level of Cognitive Ability: Comprehension
Client Needs: Physiological Integrity
Integrated Process: Nursing Process/Data Collection
Content Area: Maternity/Postpartum

Answer: 3

Rationale: Uterine atony accounts for most of the cases of immediate postpartum hemorrhage. A soft uterus indicates that the uterus is flaccid or "boggy" and that bleeding is not controlled. Options 1, 2, and 4 identify potential causes of hemorrhage rather than findings that indicate hemorrhage.

Test-Taking Strategy: Use the process of elimination, and focus on the subject—the finding that indicates hemorrhage. Note that options 1, 2, and 4 are risk factors for uterine atony and hemorrhage but not findings that indicate hemorrhage. Review the signs of hemorrhage in a postpartum client if you had difficulty with this question.

Reference

Leifer, G. (2008). *Maternity nursing: An introductory text* (10th ed., pp. 340-341). Philadelphia: Saunders.

---

688. A licensed practical nurse (LPN) is caring for a client after a cystoscopy. Which finding, if noted in the client, indicates the need to notify the registered nurse?

1 Back pain
2 Bladder spasms
3 Bright red clots in the urine
4 Complaints of fullness and burning in the bladder

Level of Cognitive Ability: Analysis
Client Needs: Physiological Integrity
Integrated Process: Nursing Process/Data Collection
Content Area: Adult Health/Renal

Answer: 3

Rationale: Cystoscopy is the direct visualization of the urinary tract by means of a cystoscope inserted into the urethra. Back pain, bladder spasms, and feelings of fullness and burning in the bladder may be experienced by the client after a cystoscopy; warm tub baths, mild analgesics, and antispasmodics will provide relief. Pink-tinged urine is common, but any bright red bleeding or clots in the urine should be reported to the registered nurse.

Test-Taking Strategy: Use the process of elimination. Note that option 3 indicates clots, which suggest hemorrhage; this should alert you to a potential complication. Review postprocedure care after a cystoscopy if you had difficulty with this question.

Reference

Chernecky, C., & Berger, B. (2008). *Laboratory tests and diagnostic procedures* (5th ed., p. 420). Philadelphia: Saunders.

---

689. A nurse assigned to care for a newborn reviews the newborn's record and determines that the newborn is at risk for hypoglycemia if which of the following are documented?

1 Polydactyly and moist skin
2 Cephalohematoma, 40 weeks' gestation, and mongolian spots
3 Hypothermia; weak, high-pitched cry; and meconium-stained skin
4 One-minute Apgar score of 7, acrocyanosis, and moist breath sounds

Level of Cognitive Ability: Analysis
Client Needs: Physiological Integrity
Integrated Process: Nursing Process/Data Collection
Content Area: Maternity/Postpartum

Answer: 3

Rationale: Hypothermia may result in hypoglycemia because of the increased demands on the newborn's metabolism to generate heat. A weak, high-pitched cry is both a neurological symptom and a symptom of hypoglycemia that results from a lack of glucose to the brain. Meconium-stained skin indicates fetal distress in utero, which places the infant at risk for hypoglycemia. A full-term gestation (40 weeks), an Apgar score of 7 or more, acrocyanosis, mongolian spots, and moist breath sounds are normal findings in a newborn who is an hour old. Moist skin is a normal finding, cephalohematoma is a sign of birth trauma to the skull, and polydactyly is a congenital anomaly characterized by the presence of more than the normal number of fingers or toes; none of these conditions place the newborn at risk for hypoglycemia.

Test-Taking Strategy: Focus on the subject—the risk factors associated with hypoglycemia. Note that option 3 is the only option that contains all abnormal findings. Review the risk factors for hypoglycemia if you had difficulty with this question.

Reference
Leifer, G. (2008). *Maternity nursing: An introductory text* (10th ed., p. 323). Philadelphia: Saunders.

---

690. A nurse is caring for a client diagnosed with Parkinson's disease who is receiving bromocriptine (Parlodel) daily. Which finding indicates to the nurse that the client is experiencing an adverse reaction to the medication?

1 Nausea
2 Confusion
3 Hypotension
4 Auditory hallucinations

Level of Cognitive Ability: Analysis
Client Needs: Physiological Integrity
Integrated Process: Nursing Process/Evaluation
Content Area: Pharmacology

Answer: 4

Rationale: Bromocriptine (Parlodel) is an antiparkinson prolactin inhibitor. Frequent side effects include hypotension, dizziness, lightheadedness, nausea, and confusion. Adverse reactions include visual and auditory hallucinations.

Test-Taking Strategy: Use the process of elimination. Focus on the subject—an adverse reaction; this will direct you to option 4. Review bromocriptine if you had difficulty with this question.

Reference
Hodgson, B., & Kizior, R. (2009). *Saunders nursing drug handbook 2009* (pp. 151-153). St. Louis: Saunders.

---

691. A nurse is caring for a client after a modified radical mastectomy. Which finding indicates that the client is experiencing a complication related to the surgery?

1 Pain at the incision site
2 Arm edema on the operative side
3 Bloody drainage in the Jackson Pratt tube
4 Complaints of numbness near the operative site

Level of Cognitive Ability: Analysis
Client Needs: Physiological Integrity
Integrated Process: Nursing Process/Data Collection
Content Area: Adult Health/Oncology

Answer: 2

Rationale: A mastectomy is the surgical removal of the breast, which is most commonly performed to remove a malignant tumor. After a modified radical mastectomy, a drain is placed in the wound and connected to gentle suction to prevent blood or serum from collecting in the operative site. After surgery, it is expected that bloody fluid will collect in the drain. Pain at the incision site is an expected occurrence. In addition, numbness may occur, but it will resolve with time. Arm edema is a common complication that can occur immediately postoperatively or months or even years after surgery.

Test-Taking Strategy: Use the process of elimination, and focus on the subject—a complication. Knowing that pain, bloody drainage, and numbness are expected during the postoperative period will direct you to option 2. Review the postoperative care of the client after a mastectomy if you had difficulty with this question.

References
Christensen, B., & Kockrow, E. (2006). *Adult health nursing* (5th ed., pp. 611-612). St. Louis: Mosby.
Linton, A. (2007). *Introduction to medical-surgical nursing* (4th ed., p. 1066). Philadelphia: Saunders.

---

692. A nurse is caring for a client with a seizure disorder who is receiving phenytoin sodium (Dilantin) three times daily. Which of the following indicates to the nurse that the client is experiencing a side effect related to the medication?

1 Constipation
2 Bleeding gums

Answer: 2

Rationale: Phenytoin sodium is an anticonvulsant. Frequent side effects include drowsiness, lethargy, irritability, headache, restlessness, joint aches, vertigo, anorexia, nausea, gastric distress, and gingival hyperplasia. Gingival hyperplasia is indicated by the bleeding, tenderness, or swelling of the gums. The urine may appear pink, red, or red-brown while taking this medication, but this is not a concern. Options 1 and 4 are not side effects.

3 Brown-colored urine
4 Difficulty swallowing

Level of Cognitive Ability:: Analysis
Client Needs: Physiological Integrity
Integrated Process: Nursing Process/Data Collection
Content Area: Pharmacology

Test-Taking Strategy: Use the process of elimination, and focus on the subject—a side effect of the medication. Remember that gingival hyperplasia is a common side effect of this medication. Review phenytoin sodium if you had difficulty with this question.

Reference

Hodgson, B., & Kizior, R. (2009). *Saunders nursing drug handbook 2009* (p. 927). St. Louis: Saunders.

---

693. A nurse is assisting with data collection at a health screening clinic for skin cancer. The nurse recognizes that moles with a variegated color, irregular borders, an irregular surface, or any combination of these characteristics should be considered:
1 Normal
2 Common
3 Malignant
4 Suspicious

Level of Cognitive Ability: Comprehension
Client Needs: Physiological Integrity
Integrated Process: Nursing Process/Data Collection
Content Area: Adult Health/Integumentary

Answer: 4
Rationale: The description indicated in the question suggests the possibility of malignant melanoma; moles with these characteristics should be considered suspicious. This description is not normal or common, and the diagnosis of malignancy can only be made by histopathology.

Test-Taking Strategy: Use the process of elimination. Eliminate options 1 and 2 first because they are comparable or alike. From the remaining options, recalling that malignancy can only be determined by histopathology will direct you to option 4. Review the normal appearance of moles if you had difficulty with this question.

Reference

Linton, A. (2007). *Introduction to medical-surgical nursing* (4th ed., p. 1125). Philadelphia: Saunders.

---

694. A nurse is gathering data from a client who is admitted to the hospital for diagnostic studies to rule out the presence of Hodgkin's disease. Which question should the nurse ask the client to elicit information specifically related to this disease?
1 "Are you tiring easily?"
2 "Do you have any weakness?"
3 "Have you gained any weight?"
4 "Have you noticed any swollen lymph nodes?"

Level of Cognitive Ability: Application
Client Needs: Physiological Integrity
Integrated Process: Nursing Process/Data Collection
Content Area: Adult Health/Oncology

Answer: 4
Rationale: Hodgkin's disease is a chronic, progressive, neoplastic disorder of the lymphoid tissue that is characterized by the painless enlargement of the lymph nodes and progression to extralymphatic sites (e.g., spleen, liver). Fatigue and weakness may occur but are not significantly related to the disease. Weight loss (rather than weight gain) is most likely to be noted.

Test-Taking Strategy: Use the process of elimination. Option 3 can be eliminated first because, with such a disorder, weight loss is most likely to occur. Options 1 and 2 are comparable or alike in that they are rather vague symptoms that can occur with many disorders. Recalling that Hodgkin's disease affects the lymph nodes will direct you to option 4. Review the manifestations associated with Hodgkin's disease if you had difficulty with this question.

Reference

Christensen, B., & Kockrow, E. (2006). *Adult health nursing* (5th ed., p. 319). St. Louis: Mosby.

---

695. A nurse is collecting admission data from a client who is suspected of having ovarian cancer. Which question should the nurse ask the client to elicit information specifically related to this disorder?

Answer: 4
Rationale: Ovarian cancer is a malignant neoplasm of the ovaries that is rarely detected in its early stages and that is usually far advanced when diagnosed. Clinical manifestations of ovarian cancer include abdominal distension, urinary frequency and urgency,

1 "Have you been having diarrhea?"
2 "Have you had any abnormal vaginal bleeding?"
3 "Are you having any excessive vaginal bleeding?"
4 "Does your abdomen feel as though it is swollen?"

Level of Cognitive Ability: Application
Client Needs: Physiological Integrity
Integrated Process: Nursing Process/Data Collection
Content Area: Adult Health/Oncology

pleural effusion, malnutrition, pain from pressure caused by the growing tumor or from the effects of urinary or bowel obstruction, and constipation. Ascites with dyspnea and ultimately general severe pain will occur as the disease progresses. Abnormal bleeding that often results in hypermenorrhea is associated with uterine cancer.

Test-Taking Strategy: Use the process of elimination. Eliminate options 2 and 3 first because they are comparable or alike. From the remaining options, consider the anatomical location of the diagnosis; this will assist with directing you to option 4. Review the manifestations associated with ovarian cancer if you had difficulty with this question.

Reference
Christensen, B., & Kockrow, E. (2006). *Adult health nursing* (5th ed., pp. 600-601). St. Louis: Mosby.

---

696. A nurse is collecting admission data from a client with Ménière's disease. Which question would elicit information specific to the attacks that occur with this disorder?
1 "Do you feel unusually tired?"
2 "Are you having any headaches?"
3 "Do you have difficulty sleeping at night?"
4 "Do you have a feeling of fullness in your ear?"

Level of Cognitive Ability: Application
Client Needs: Physiological Integrity
Integrated Process: Nursing Process/Data Collection
Content Area: Adult Health/Ear

Answer: 4
Rationale: Ménière's disease is a chronic disease of the inner ear that results from a disturbance in the fluid of the endolymphatic system. The cause of the disturbance is unknown, and it is characterized by recurrent attacks of vertigo, progressive sensorineural hearing loss, and tinnitus. Attacks may be preceded by a feeling of fullness in the ear or by tinnitus. Headaches are not associated with this disorder. Options 1 and 3 are also unrelated to Ménière's disease.

Test-Taking Strategy: Focus on the subject, and recall the pathophysiology associated with Ménière's disease. It is necessary to know that attacks are preceded by either a feeling of fullness in the ear or by tinnitus. In addition, knowing that this disorder is associated with the ear will direct you to option 4. Review Ménière's disease if you had difficulty with this question.

References
Ignatavicius, D., & Workman, M. (2010). *Medical-surgical nursing: Patient-centered collaborative care* (6th ed., p. 1127). St. Louis: Saunders.
Linton, A. (2007). *Introduction to medical-surgical nursing* (4th ed., p. 1203). Philadelphia: Saunders.

---

697. A nurse is reviewing data collected from a client with mastoiditis. Which finding should the nurse expect to be documented in the client's record?
1 Swelling behind the ear
2 Nontender lymph nodes
3 A pink-colored tympanic membrane on otoscopic examination
4 A transparent and clear tympanic membrane on otoscopic examination

Level of Cognitive Ability: Comprehension
Client Needs: Physiological Integrity

Answer: 1
Rationale: Mastoiditis is an infection of one of the mastoid bones, and it is usually an extension of a middle-ear infection. Otoscopic examination in a client with mastoiditis reveals a red, dull, thick, and immobile tympanic membrane with or without perforation. The postauricular lymph nodes are tender and enlarged. In addition, clients have a low-grade fever, malaise, anorexia, swelling behind the ear, and pain with minimal movement of the head.

Test-Taking Strategy: Focus on the subject—the clinical manifestations associated with mastoiditis. Eliminate options 2, 3, and 4 because they are comparable or alike in that they are normal findings. Review the findings associated with mastoiditis if you had difficulty with this question.

Integrated Process: Nursing Process/Data Collection
Content Area: Adult Health/Ear

Reference

Linton, A. (2007). *Introduction to medical-surgical nursing* (4th ed., pp. 1200-1201). Philadelphia: Saunders.

---

698. A client returns to the clinic for follow-up treatment after a skin biopsy of a suspicious lesion that was performed 1 week ago. The biopsy report indicates that the lesion is a squamous cell carcinoma. The nurse recognizes that this type of lesion:

1 Is encapsulated
2 Is highly metastatic
3 Does not metastasize
4 Is characterized by local invasion

Level of Cognitive Ability: Comprehension
Client Needs: Physiological Integrity
Integrated Process: Nursing Process/Data Collection
Content Area: Adult Health/Integumentary

Answer: 4

Rationale: Squamous cell carcinomas are malignant neoplasms of the epidermis; they are characterized by local invasion and the potential for metastasis. Melanomas are pigmented malignant lesions that originate in the melanin-producing cells of the epidermis; this type of skin cancer is highly metastatic, and a person's survival depends on early diagnosis and treatment. Basal cell carcinomas arise in the basal cell layer of the epidermis. Early malignant basal cell lesions often go unnoticed, and, although metastasis is rare, underlying tissue destruction can progress to include vital structures.

Test-Taking Strategy: Use the process of elimination and your knowledge of the various types of skin cancers. Eliminate options 1 and 3, knowing that the potential for metastasis exists with this type of carcinoma. Noting the word *highly* in option 2 will assist in eliminating this option. Review the characteristics of skin cancers if you had difficulty with this question.

Reference

Christensen, B., & Kockrow, E. (2006). *Adult health nursing* (5th ed., p. 100). St. Louis: Mosby.

---

699. A nurse is reviewing the record of a client with pemphigus and notes that the physician has documented the presence of Nikolsky's sign. Based on this documentation, which of the following should the nurse expect to note in the client?

1 A carpal spasm can be elicited by compressing the client's upper arm.
2 The epidermis of the client's skin can be rubbed off with slight friction or injury.
3 The client complains of discomfort behind the knee on forced dorsiflexion of the foot.
4 A spasm of the client's facial muscles is elicited by tapping the facial nerve in the region of the parotid gland.

Level of Cognitive Ability: Comprehension
Client Needs: Physiological Integrity
Integrated Process: Nursing Process/Data Collection
Content Area: Adult Health/Integumentary

Answer: 2

Rationale: Pemphigus is a severe disease of the skin and mucous membranes that is characterized by thin-walled bullae that arise from apparently normal skin or mucous membranes. A hallmark sign of pemphigus is Nikolsky's sign, which is when the epidermis can be rubbed off with slight friction or injury. Other characteristics of pemphigus include flaccid bullae that rupture easily, that emit a foul-smelling drainage, and that leave crusted, denuded skin. The lesions are common on the face, back, chest, groin, and umbilicus. Even slight pressure on an intact blister may cause it to spread to adjacent skin. Trousseau's sign is a sign of tetany in which a carpal spasm can be elicited by compressing the upper arm and causing ischemia to the nerves distally. Homans' sign, which is a sign of thrombosis in the leg, involves discomfort behind the knee on forced dorsiflexion of the foot. Chvostek's sign is seen in clients with tetany; it is a spasm of the facial muscles that is elicited by tapping the facial nerve in the region of the parotid gland.

Test-Taking Strategy: Use the process of elimination. Eliminate options 1 and 4 first because they are comparable or alike in that they test for tetany. Next, eliminate option 3, recalling that Homans' sign involves discomfort behind the knee on forced dorsiflexion of the foot and indicates the presence of thrombophlebitis. Review the characteristic findings of pemphigus if you had difficulty with this question.

References
Copstead, L., & Banasik, J. (2010). *Pathophysiology* (4th ed., p. 1235). St. Louis: Mosby.
Ignatavicius, D., & Workman, M. (2010). *Medical-surgical nursing: Patient-centered collaborative care* (6th ed., p. 516). St. Louis: Saunders.

---

700. Which finding is a characteristic of scabies?
1 The appearance of vesicles or pustules
2 Patchy hair loss and round, red macules with scales
3 The presence of white patches scattered about the trunk
4 Multiple straight or wavy, thread-like lines beneath the skin

Level of Cognitive Ability: Comprehension
Client Needs: Physiological Integrity
Integrated Process: Nursing Process/Data Collection
Content Area: Adult Health/Integumentary

Answer: 4
Rationale: Scabies is a contagious disease caused by *Sarcoptes scabiei*, which is the human itch mite. The condition is characterized by intense itching of the skin and excoriation from scratching. It can be identified by the multiple straight or wavy, thread-like lines noted beneath the skin. The skin lesions are caused by the female, which burrows beneath the skin and lays its eggs. The eggs hatch in a few days, and the baby mites find their way to the skin surface, where they mate and complete the life cycle. Options 1, 2, and 3 are not characteristics of this contagious disease.

Test-Taking Strategy: Focus on the subject—a characteristic of scabies. Recalling that scabies involves mites burrowing beneath the skin surface will direct you to option 4. Review the characteristics associated with scabies if you had difficulty with this question.

Reference
Linton, A. (2007). *Introduction to medical-surgical nursing* (4th ed., p. 1142). Philadelphia: Saunders.

---

701. A nurse is assigned to care for a client suspected of having herpes zoster. Which finding should the nurse expect to note if herpes zoster is present?
1 Clustered and grouped skin vesicles
2 A generalized red body rash that causes pruritus
3 A fiery red edematous rash on the cheeks and neck
4 Small bluish-white spots with red bases on the extremities

Level of Cognitive Ability: Comprehension
Client Needs: Physiological Integrity
Integrated Process: Nursing Process/Data Collection
Content Area: Adult Health/Integumentary

Answer: 1
Rationale: Herpes zoster is an acute infection caused by the reactivation of the latent varicella zoster virus. The primary lesion of herpes zoster is a vesicle. The classic presentation is grouped vesicles on an erythematous base along a dermatome. Because they follow nerve pathways, the lesions do not cross the body's midline. Options 2, 3, and 4 are not characteristics of herpes zoster.

Test-Taking Strategy: Use the process of elimination. Remembering that these lesions occur as grouped vesicles along a nerve pathway will assist you with answering the question. Review the characteristics of herpes zoster lesions if you had difficulty with this question.

Reference
Christensen, B., & Kockrow, E. (2006). *Adult health nursing* (5th ed., p. 79). St. Louis: Mosby.

---

702. A nurse is collecting data from a client admitted to the hospital with a fever of unknown origin. After data collection, the appropriate nursing action is to:
1 Write the information on a worksheet.
2 Record the information in the client's record.

Answer: 2
Rationale: After data collection, the nurse should record the data in the client's record. Verbal information and notes on worksheets are not part of the client's permanent record. In addition, it may or may not be appropriate to share client information with another nurse.

3 Inform the supervisor of the client's vital signs.
4 Tell another nurse that the client has a high fever.

Level of Cognitive Ability: Application
Client Needs: Physiological Integrity
Integrated Process: Communication and Documentation
Content Area: Fundamental Skills

Test-Taking Strategy: Use the process of elimination. Eliminate options 3 and 4 first because they are comparable or alike. From the remaining options, select option 2 because the client's record is a permanent document. Review the importance of documentation if you had difficulty with this question.

Reference

Christensen, B., & Kockrow, E. (2006). *Foundations of nursing* (5th ed., pp. 111-112). St. Louis: Mosby.

---

703. A nurse is reviewing the health record of a prenatal client at risk of contracting a perinatal infection. The nurse uses knowledge of which of the following when planning care for the client?
1 The mother's immune system is depressed during pregnancy.
2 The placenta functions as a filtering system, thus prohibiting the transplacental spread of all organisms.
3 The vaginal pH is decreased during pregnancy, thus reducing the risk of the client acquiring a bacterial infection.
4 The vaginal walls become hypertrophied during pregnancy, which reduces the exposure of the epithelium cell layer to microorganisms.

Level of Cognitive Ability: Comprehension
Client Needs: Physiological Integrity
Integrated Process: Nursing Process/Planning
Content Area: Maternity/Antepartum

Answer: 1
Rationale: The acquisition of neonatal infections can occur during the antenatal, intrapartal, or neonatal period. Infections can occur via two routes: by transfer of the infecting agent across the placenta or by the ascending of bacteria from the vagina. Three common alterations during pregnancy may further make the mother or fetus more susceptible to infection: the vaginal wall becomes hypertrophied, thus exposing more cells to microorganisms; the vaginal epithelium produces more glycogen, which increases the pH of the vagina and results in an increased risk for bacterial infection; and the maternal immune system is depressed as evidenced by suppressed lymphocyte function and decreased counts of CD4+ T lymphocytes.

Test-Taking Strategy: Use the process of elimination. Recalling the normal maternal physiological changes that occur during pregnancy will direct you option 1. Remember that the mother's immune system is depressed during pregnancy. Review the normal maternal physiological changes that occur during pregnancy if you had difficulty with this question.

Reference

McKinney, E., James, S., Murray, S., & Ashwill, J. (2009). *Maternal-child nursing* (3rd ed., p. 258). St. Louis: Mosby.

---

704. A client has just had an insertion of skeletal pins and an application of leg traction. Initially, the nurse should monitor the neurovascular status of the client's affected leg:
1 Daily
2 Hourly
3 Every shift
4 Every 4 hours

Level of Cognitive Ability: Application
Client Needs: Physiological Integrity
Integrated Process: Nursing Process/Implementation
Content Area: Adult Health/Musculoskeletal

Answer: 2
Rationale: Immediately after the application of skeletal traction, neurovascular assessment of the affected limb should be performed every hour. The client is told to report any changes in movement or sensation so that any complications can be detected and treated quickly.

Test-Taking Strategy: Use the process of elimination, and note the strategic word *initially.* This is a clue that the frequency should be greater than usual, and it will assist with directing you to option 2. Review the care of the client in traction if you had difficulty with this question.

Reference

Ignatavicius, D., & Workman, M. (2010). *Medical-surgical nursing: Patient-centered collaborative care* (6th ed., p. 1190). St. Louis: Saunders.

---

705. A nurse is looking at an electrocardiogram (ECG) rhythm strip of a client. The P waves and the QRS complexes are regular, and the overall heart rate is 64 beats/min. The nurse identifies this cardiac rhythm as:

1 Sinus bradycardia
2 Sinus tachycardia
3 A normal sinus rhythm
4 A slow and abnormal rate

Level of Cognitive Ability: Analysis
Client Needs: Physiological Integrity
Integrated Process: Nursing Process/Data Collection
Content Area: Adult Health/Cardiovascular

Answer: 3

Rationale: A normal sinus rhythm is defined as a regular rhythm with an overall rate of 60 to 100 beats/min and with normal P-R and QRS measurements. Sinus bradycardia is defined as a heart rate of less than 60 beats/min. Sinus tachycardia is defined as a heart rate of more than 100 beats/min.

Test-Taking Strategy: Use the process of elimination. Eliminate options 1 and 4 first because they are comparable or alike. Note the strategic word *regular* in the question to direct you to the correct option. Review the basics of ECG monitoring if you had difficulty with this question.

Reference

Linton, A. (2007). *Introduction to medical-surgical nursing* (4th ed., pp. 634, 675). Philadelphia: Saunders.

---

706. A client with a peripheral intravenous (IV) site tells the nurse that the IV site is swollen. The nurse inspects the IV site and notes that it is also cool and pale and that the IV has stopped running. Which of the following has probably occurred?

1 Phlebitis
2 Infection
3 Infiltration
4 Thrombosis

Level of Cognitive Ability: Analysis
Client Needs: Physiological Integrity
Integrated Process: Nursing Process/Data Collection
Content Area: Fundamental Skills

Answer: 3

Rationale: An infiltrated IV line is one that has dislodged from the vein and that is lying in subcutaneous tissue. The pallor, coolness, and swelling result from IV fluid being deposited in the subcutaneous tissue. The flow of the IV solution stops when the pressure in the tissue exceeds the pressure in the tubing. The corrective actions are to remove the catheter and to have a new IV line started. The other three options are likely to be accompanied by warmth (rather than coolness) at the site.

Test-Taking Strategy: To answer this question accurately, it is necessary to be familiar with the signs and symptoms of IV therapy complications. Focus on the data in the question to direct you to option 3. Note that options 1, 2, and 4 are comparable or alike in that they are likely to be accompanied by warmth (rather than coolness) at the site. Review the signs of infiltration if you had difficulty with this question.

Reference

deWit, S. (2009). *Medical-surgical nursing: Concepts & practice* (p. 59). St. Louis: Saunders.

---

707. A nursing student is assigned to care for a client with presbycusis. The student reviews the client's record, expecting to note which of the following documentation?

1 The client has a conductive hearing loss.
2 The client has a sensorineural hearing loss.
3 The client experiences continuous nystagmus.
4 The client has been experiencing dizziness and ringing in the ears.

Level of Cognitive Ability: Comprehension
Client Needs: Physiological Integrity

Answer: 2

Rationale: Presbycusis is a type of hearing loss that occurs with aging. It is a gradual sensorineural loss caused by the nerve degeneration of the inner ear or the auditory nerve. It is not a conductive hearing loss, and it is not specifically associated with nystagmus, dizziness, or ringing in the ears.

Test-Taking Strategy: Use the process of elimination. Recalling that presbycusis occurs with aging will direct you to option 2. Review this age-related disorder if you had difficulty with this question.

Reference

Linton, A. (2007). *Introduction to medical-surgical nursing* (4th ed., p. 135). Philadelphia: Saunders.

Integrated Process: Nursing Process/Data Collection
Content Area: Adult Health/Ear

---

708. A nurse should expect a client with an acute myocardial infarction (MI) to first manifest:
1 Nausea
2 Vomiting
3 Chest pain
4 Elevated serum creatine kinase (CK)-MB isoenzyme level

Level of Cognitive Ability: Analysis
Client Needs: Physiological Integrity
Integrated Process: Nursing Process/Data Collection
Content Area: Adult Health/Cardiovascular

Answer: 3
Rationale: The client with an MI will initially experience chest pain. Although nausea and vomiting may be part of the clinical picture, these symptoms usually do not occur first. The CK-MB isoenzyme level begins to rise 3 to 6 hours after an MI.

Test-Taking Strategy: Use the process of elimination, and note the strategic word *first.* Although all of the options generally occur with acute MI, the first manifestation that is likely to occur is chest pain. Review the characteristics of MI if you had difficulty with this question.

Reference
Christensen, B., & Kockrow, E. (2006). *Adult health nursing* (5th ed., p. 353). St. Louis: Mosby.

---

709. A nurse is caring for a large-for-gestational-age (LGA) infant who has polycythemia and hyperviscosity. The nurse anticipates that the physician will prescribe which of the following if the infant becomes symptomatic?
1 Exchange transfusion
2 Radiographic kidney evaluation
3 Ultrasound evaluation of the brain
4 Enteral feedings instead of oral feedings

Level of Cognitive Ability: Analysis
Client Needs: Physiological Integrity
Integrated Process: Nursing Process/Planning
Content Area: Maternity/Postpartum

Answer: 1
Rationale: An LGA infant is an infant whose fetal growth was accelerated and whose size and weight at birth fall above the ninetieth percentile of appropriate-for-gestational-age infants, whether delivered prematurely, at term, or postterm. The most likely intervention for an infant with symptomatic polycythemia and hyperviscosity is an exchange transfusion. This treatment improves cerebral blood flow, systemic blood flow, and oxygen transport. Options 2, 3, and 4 are not indicated in this situation.

Test-Taking Strategy: Use the process of elimination. Note the relationship between the words *polycythemia and hyperviscosity* in the question and *transfusion* in the correct option. Review the treatment for these disorders if you had difficulty with this question.

Reference
Leifer, G. (2008). *Maternity nursing: An introductory text* (10th ed., p. 304). Philadelphia: Saunders.

---

710. A nurse determines that which of the following clients is the least likely candidate for the implantation of an internal automatic cardioverter defibrillator (AICD)?
1 A client with syncopal episodes related to ventricular tachycardia
2 A client with ventricular dysrhythmias despite medication therapy
3 A client with one episode of cardiac arrest related to myocardial infarction

Answer: 3
Rationale: An AICD consists of a pulse generator and a sensor that continuously monitors the heart rhythm; it detects and delivers an electric shock to terminate life-threatening episodes of ventricular tachycardia and ventricular fibrillation. These devices are implanted in clients who are considered high risk, including those who have survived sudden cardiac arrest that is unrelated to myocardial infarction, those who are refractive to medication therapy, and those who have syncopal episodes related to ventricular tachycardia.

4 A client with three episodes of cardiac arrest unrelated to myocardial infarction

Level of Cognitive Ability: Analysis
Client Needs: Physiological Integrity
Integrated Process: Nursing Process/Data Collection
Content Area: Adult Health/Cardiovascular

Test-Taking Strategy: Note the strategic words *least likely*. Eliminate options 1 and 2 first because they are comparable or alike. From the remaining options, select option 3. The client who is most likely to be responsive to AICD would be the client without myocardial infarction because those dysrhythmias are spontaneous. Review the purpose and use of AICD if you had difficulty with this question.

Reference
Ignatavicius, D., & Workman, M. (2010). *Medical-surgical nursing: Patient-centered collaborative care* (6th ed., p. 758). St. Louis: Saunders.

---

711. A client was hospitalized 5 days previously and has developed thrombophlebitis in the right lower extremity. The nurse reviews the client's record and expects to note the documentation of which characteristic of this disorder?
1 Unilateral edema
2 Bilateral calf tenderness
3 Diminished distal peripheral pulses
4 Coolness and pallor of the affected limb

Level of Cognitive Ability: Comprehension
Client Needs: Physiological Integrity
Integrated Process: Nursing Process/Data Collection
Content Area: Adult Health/Cardiovascular

Answer: 1
Rationale: Thrombophlebitis is the inflammation of a vein accompanied by the formation of a clot. The client with thrombophlebitis exhibits redness, warmth, or both of the affected leg; tenderness at the affected site; possible dilated veins (if superficial); low-grade fever; edema distal to the obstruction; and possible positive Homans' sign in the affected extremity. Pedal pulses are unchanged from baseline because this is a venous (rather than arterial) problem.

Test-Taking Strategy: Use the process of elimination. Begin by eliminating options 3 and 4, which are symptoms of arterial (rather than venous) problems. Remember that thrombophlebitis is usually a unilateral problem. In addition, the question states that the client has thrombophlebitis in the right lower extremity; this should direct you to option 1. Review the signs of thrombophlebitis if you had difficulty with this question.

Reference
deWit, S. (2009). *Medical-surgical nursing: Concepts & practice* (pp. 456-457). St. Louis: Saunders.

---

712. A nurse is collecting data about a lethargic client who was brought to the emergency department by the emergency medical service. The nurse notes a fruity odor to the client's breath and immediately suspects:
1 Hypoglycemia
2 Ethanol oxide intoxication
3 Diabetic ketoacidosis (DKA)
4 Hyperglycemic hyperosmolar nonketotic syndrome

Level of Cognitive Ability: Analysis
Client Needs: Physiological Integrity
Integrated Process: Nursing Process/Data Collection
Content Area: Adult Health/Endocrine

Answer: 3
Rationale: DKA is an acute, life-threatening complication of diabetes mellitus. With this condition, urinary loss of water, potassium, ammonium, and sodium results in hypovolemia, electrolyte imbalance, extremely high blood glucose levels, and the breakdown of free fatty acids; this results in acidosis, often with coma. Clients with DKA accumulate large amounts of ketone bodies in the extracellular fluids. A fruity odor to the breath develops as a result of the volatile nature of acetone; this odor is not a characteristic of the disorders listed in the other options.

Test-Taking Strategy: Use the process of elimination. Remember to associate a fruity breath odor with DKA. Review the characteristics of DKA if you had difficulty with this question.

Reference
deWit, S. (2009). *Medical-surgical nursing: Concepts & practice* (p. 926). St. Louis: Saunders.

---

713. A client arrives at the health care clinic and complains of severe pain in the right large toe. The joint of the toe is red, warm, shiny, and swollen, and it is extremely sensitive to the slightest touch. A diagnosis of gout is suspected, and laboratory blood studies are performed. Which of the following should the nurse expect to note with a diagnosis of gout?

1 An increased serum uric acid level
2 A decreased white blood cell count
3 A decreased erythrocyte sedimentation rate
4 An increased blood urea nitrogen (BUN) level

Level of Cognitive Ability: Comprehension
Client Needs: Physiological Integrity
Integrated Process: Nursing Process/Data Collection
Content Area: Adult Health/Musculoskeletal

Answer: 1

Rationale: Gout is associated with an inborn error of uric acid metabolism that increases production or interferes with the excretion of uric acid. A diagnosis of gout is made on the basis of clinical manifestations, hyperuricemia, and the presence of uric acid crystals in the synovial fluid of the inflamed joint. Blood studies show an increased serum uric acid level of more than 7 mg/dL (normal: 4.5 to 6.2 mg/dL). The erythrocyte sedimentation rate and the white blood cell count may be elevated during an acute episode. The BUN level is unrelated to the diagnosis of gout.

Test-Taking Strategy: Use the process of elimination. Recalling that gout is caused by a buildup of uric acid in the blood will direct you to option 1. Review the etiology and pathophysiology of gout if you had difficulty with this question.

Reference

Christensen, B., & Kockrow, E. (2006). *Adult health nursing* (5th ed., pp. 139-140). St. Louis: Mosby.

---

714. A nurse is reviewing the record of a client with cervical cancer. Which of the following should the nurse expect to note in the client's record related to a risk factor associated with this type of cancer?

1 Single female, no children
2 Intercourse with circumcised males
3 Intercourse with a single sex partner
4 History of genital herpesvirus infection

Level of Cognitive Ability: Comprehension
Client Needs: Physiological Integrity
Integrated Process: Nursing Process/Data Collection
Content Area: Adult Health/Oncology

Answer: 4

Rationale: Cervical cancer is a neoplasm of the uterine cervix that can be detected in the early, curable stage with a Papanicolaou test. Risk factors associated with cervical cancer include intercourse with uncircumcised males; early, frequent intercourse with multiple sexual partners; multiparity; chronic cervicitis; and a history of genital herpes or human papillomavirus infection.

Test-Taking Strategy: Focus on the subject—the risk factors associated with cervical cancer. Remember that cervical cancer is associated with a history of genital herpes or human papillomavirus infection. Review the risk factors for cervical cancer if you had difficulty with this question.

Reference

Linton, A. (2007). *Introduction to medical-surgical nursing* (4th ed., pp. 1066-1067). Philadelphia: Saunders.

---

715. A nurse is monitoring the intravenous (IV) site of a client receiving an IV solution and suspects thrombophlebitis. Which sign indicates that thrombophlebitis has occurred?

1 Inflammation at the IV site
2 Coolness around the IV site
3 Edema and coolness at the IV site
4 A hard or cord-like feeling along the vein

Level of Cognitive Ability: Comprehension
Client Needs: Physiological Integrity

Answer: 4

Rationale: Thrombophlebitis is the inflammation of a vein accompanied by a clot. If thrombophlebitis is present, the nurse notes heat, redness, tenderness, and swelling along the course of the vein. The vein may feel hard or cord-like with thrombophlebitis. Edema and coolness occur with infiltration. Inflammation at the site occurs with a local infection.

Test-Taking Strategy: Use the process of elimination, and focus on the subject—thrombophlebitis. Eliminate options 2 and 3 first because they are comparable or alike. Recalling that inflammation is a sign of infection assists you with eliminating option 1 and directs you to option 4. Review the signs of thrombophlebitis if you had difficulty with this question.

Integrated Process: Nursing Process/Data Collection
Content Area: Fundamental Skills

References
deWit, S. (2009). *Medical-surgical nursing: Concepts & practice* (p. 59). St. Louis: Saunders.
Linton, A. (2007). *Introduction to medical-surgical nursing* (4th ed., p. 287). Philadelphia: Saunders.

---

716. A nurse is preparing to provide instructions to a client with glaucoma about prescribed treatment measures for the disorder. The nurse understands that the goal of treatment is:
1 Producing mydriasis in the eyes
2 Promoting the dilation of the pupil
3 Increasing the formation of aqueous humor
4 Maintaining intraocular pressure at a reduced level

Level of Cognitive Ability: Comprehension
Client Needs: Physiological Integrity
Integrated Process: Nursing Process/Planning
Content Area: Adult Health/Eye

Answer: 4
Rationale: Glaucoma is an abnormal condition of elevated pressure within the eye caused by the obstruction of the outflow of aqueous humor. The goal of treatment of the client with glaucoma is maintaining intraocular pressure at a reduced level to prevent further damage to the intraocular structures. Medications are used to create miosis (constriction of the pupil) and to reduce the formation of aqueous humor by the ciliary body.

Test-Taking Strategy: Use the process of elimination. Eliminate options 1 and 2 first because they are comparable or alike. Recalling that glaucoma is characterized by increased intraocular pressure will assist you with eliminating option 3. Review the goals of treatment for the client with glaucoma if you had difficulty with this question.

Reference
Christensen, B., & Kockrow, E. (2006). *Adult health nursing* (5th ed., pp. 658-659). St. Louis: Mosby.

---

717. A nurse is reviewing the record of a client recently diagnosed with a cataract. Which clinical manifestation associated with this disorder should the nurse expect to be documented in the client's record?
1 Color blindness
2 Loss of central vision only
3 Constant dull, achy pain in the eyes
4 Painless, progressive loss of peripheral vision

Level of Cognitive Ability: Comprehension
Client Needs: Physiological Integrity
Integrated Process: Nursing Process/Data Collection
Content Area: Adult Health/Eye

Answer: 4
Rationale: A cataract is an opacity of the crystalline lens of the eye. The classic symptom of cataract is a painless, progressive loss of peripheral vision in one or both eyes. Some individuals also complain of glare from bright lights. Occasionally pain can result when the lens becomes swollen and blocks the normal flow of aqueous fluid, thereby causing increased intraocular pressure. Color blindness is not an associated symptom.

Test-Taking Strategy: Use the process of elimination. Eliminate option 2 first because of the close-ended word *only*. Next, eliminate option 1, knowing that color blindness is not an associated manifestation. From the remaining options, recalling that a cataract is an opacity of the lens of the eye will direct you to option 4. Review the manifestations associated with cataract if you had difficulty with this question.

Reference
Christensen, B., & Kockrow, E. (2006). *Adult health nursing* (5th ed., p. 651). St. Louis: Mosby.

---

718. A nurse is caring for a client after enucleation of the eye. When collecting data, the nurse notes staining and bleeding on the dressing. Which nursing action is appropriate?
1 Reinforce the dressing.
2 Document the findings.

Answer: 3
Rationale: The enucleation of the eye involves the removal of the eyeball. Postoperative nursing care includes observing the dressing and reporting any staining or bleeding. The nurse would notify the RN, who would then contact the surgeon. Options 1, 2, and 4 are inaccurate nursing actions if staining or bleeding is present on the dressing after enucleation.

3 Notify the registered nurse (RN).
4 Mark the amount of staining with a black pen and continue to monitor the client.

Level of Cognitive Ability: Application
Client Needs: Physiological Integrity
Integrated Process: Nursing Process/Implementation
Content Area: Adult Health/Eye

Test-Taking Strategy: Use the process of elimination. Noting the strategic words *bleeding on the dressing* will direct you to option 3. Review postoperative care after the enucleation of the eye if you had difficulty with this question.

Reference

Christensen, B., & Kockrow, E. (2006). *Adult health nursing* (5th ed., p. 664). St. Louis: Mosby.

---

719. A nurse reviews the chart of an assigned client and notes that the physician has documented that the client is legally blind. The nurse plans care knowing that this condition is characterized by which of the following?

1 The client has no light perception at all.
2 The client retains some perception of light and movement.
3 The client can perform some work that requires visual ability.
4 The client has a severe visual impairment with some visual ability.

Level of Cognitive Ability: Comprehension
Client Needs: Physiological Integrity
Integrated Process: Nursing Process/Planning
Content Area: Adult Health/Eye

Answer: 2

Rationale: The person who is legally blind usually retains some perception of light and movement. Legal blindness also implies that the person cannot perform work that requires visual ability. Total blindness means the absence of all light perception. Low vision refers to a legally blind person or a person with severe vision impairment who still has some visual ability.

Test-Taking Strategy: Knowledge of the definition of legal blindness is necessary to answer this question. Remember that the person who is legally blind usually retains some perception of light and movement. Review the definition of legal blindness if you had difficulty with this question.

Reference

Christensen, B., & Kockrow, E. (2006). *Adult health nursing* (5th ed., pp. 642-643). St. Louis: Mosby.

---

720. A client wishes to donate blood for a family member for an upcoming surgery and asks the nurse, "How will I know if our blood types match?" When formulating a response, the nurse states that which test is used to test compatibility?

1 Monocyte count
2 Eosinophil count
3 Direct Coombs' test
4 Indirect Coombs' test

Level of Cognitive Ability: Application
Client Needs: Physiological Integrity
Integrated Process: Nursing Process/Implementation
Content Area: Fundamental Skills

Answer: 4

Rationale: The indirect Coombs' test detects circulating antibodies against red blood cells (RBCs). It is the screening component of a physician's order to type and screen a client's blood. This test is used in addition to the ABO typing, which is normally done to determine blood type. The direct Coombs' test is used to detect idiopathic hemolytic anemia by detecting the presence of autoantibodies against the client's RBCs. Eosinophil and monocyte counts are part of a complete blood cell (CBC) count, which is a routine hematological screening test.

Test-Taking Strategy: Use the process of elimination. Begin to answer this question by eliminating options 1 and 2, which are part of a routine CBC test. From the remaining options, remember that the indirect Coombs' test detects circulating antibodies against RBCs. Review these different blood tests if you had difficulty with this question.

Reference

Chernecky, C., & Berger, B. (2008). *Laboratory tests and diagnostic procedures* (5th ed., p. 381). Philadelphia: Saunders.

721. A client has a history of hypothyroidism. The nurse asks the client about which complaint that is associated with this disorder?
1 Diarrhea
2 Weight loss
3 Increased sleep
4 Heat intolerance

Level of Cognitive Ability: Application
Client Needs: Physiological Integrity
Integrated Process: Nursing Process/Data Collection
Content Area: Adult Health/Endocrine

Answer: 3
Rationale: Hypothyroidism is characterized by the decreased activity of the thyroid gland. The client with hypothyroidism has decreased function of the thyroid gland, which often results in weight gain, constipation, cold intolerance, and an increased need for sleep. The nurse questions the client regarding any of these manifestations.

Test-Taking Strategy: Use the process of elimination. Noting the prefix *hypo-* and recalling the function of the thyroid gland assists with directing you to the correct option. Review the symptoms of hypothyroidism if you had difficulty with this question.

References
Christensen, B., & Kockrow, E. (2006). *Adult health nursing* (5th ed., pp. 530-531). St. Louis: Mosby.
deWit, S. (2009). *Medical-surgical nursing: Concepts & practice* (p. 898). St. Louis: Saunders.

---

722. A nursing instructor asks a nursing student to demonstrate the procedure for performing an otoscopic examination on an adult client. Which observation, if made by the instructor, indicates the correct procedure?
1 The nursing student obtains a small speculum to decrease the discomfort of the exam.
2 The nursing student tilts the client's head forward and down before inserting the speculum.
3 The nursing student pulls the pinna up and back to assist with the insertion of the speculum.
4 The nursing student pulls the earlobe down and back to assist with the insertion of the speculum.

Level of Cognitive Ability: Comprehension
Client Needs: Physiological Integrity
Integrated Process: Teaching and Learning
Content Area: Adult Health/Ear

Answer: 3
Rationale: The correct procedure for performing the otoscopic examination on an adult client is to pull the pinna up and back and to visualize the external canal while slowly inserting the speculum. The nurse tilts the client's head slightly away and holds the otoscope upside down as if it were a large pen. A small speculum may not provide adequate visualization of the ear canal and would be more appropriately used in a pediatric setting.

Test-Taking Strategy: Use the process of elimination, and note that the question involves an adult client. Recalling that, for an adult client, the pinna is pulled up and back will direct you to option 1. Review the procedure for an otoscopic examination if you had difficulty with this question.

Reference
Jarvis, C. (2008) *Physical examination and health assessment* (5th ed., pp. 351-352). Philadelphia: Saunders.

---

723. A client is seen in the health care clinic, and the physician suspects the presence of herpes zoster. The nurse who is preparing the items needed to perform the diagnostic test that will confirm this diagnosis obtains which item?
1 A biopsy kit
2 A patch test kit
3 A Wood's light
4 A culture swab and tube

Answer: 4
Rationale: Herpes zoster is caused by a reactivation of the varicella zoster virus, which is the cause of chickenpox. With a classic presentation of herpes zoster, the clinical examination is diagnostic. A viral culture of the lesion provides the definitive diagnosis. A biopsy determines tissue type. In a Wood's light examination, the skin is viewed under ultraviolet light to identify superficial infections of the skin. A patch test is a skin test that involves the administration of an allergen to the skin's surface to identify specific allergies.

Level of Cognitive Ability: Application
Client Needs: Physiological Integrity
Integrated Process: Nursing Process/Planning
Content Area: Adult Health/Integumentary

Test-Taking Strategy: Eliminate options 2 and 3 first, recalling that herpes zoster is caused by a virus. From the remaining options, remember that a biopsy will determine tissue type whereas a culture will identify an organism. Review herpes zoster if you had difficulty with this question.

References

Chernecky, C., & Berger, B. (2008). *Laboratory tests and diagnostic procedures* (5th ed., pp. 410-411). Philadelphia: Saunders.
Christensen, B., & Kockrow, E. (2006). *Adult health nursing* (5th ed., p. 79). St. Louis: Mosby.

---

724. A client with multiple sclerosis is being treated with diazepam (Valium) for painful muscle spasms. The nurse monitors the client, knowing that a common side effect of diazepam is:

1 Headache
2 Incoordination
3 Urinary frequency
4 Increased salivation

Level of Cognitive Ability: Analysis
Client Needs: Physiological Integrity
Integrated Process: Nursing Process/Data Collection
Content Area: Pharmacology

Answer: 2
Rationale: Diazepam is a centrally acting skeletal muscle relaxant. Incoordination and drowsiness are common side effects that result from the large doses of the medication that must be used to achieve the desired effects. Options 1, 3, and 4 are not side effects of this medication.

Test-Taking Strategy: Use the process of elimination. Recalling that diazepam is used for muscle spasms helps you to remember that this medication relaxes muscles. The only option that directly relates to this medication action is option 2. Review the action and side effects of diazepam if you had difficulty with this question.

Reference

Hodgson, B., & Kizior, R. (2009). *Saunders nursing drug handbook 2009* (p. 347). St. Louis: Saunders.

---

725. A client is taking the prescribed dose of phenytoin (Dilantin) to control seizures. A Dilantin blood level is drawn, and the nurse is told that the results reveal a level of 35 mg/mL. The nurse expects to note which of the following as a result of this laboratory result?

1 Lethargy
2 Nystagmus
3 Tachycardia
4 No effect; this is a normal therapeutic level

Level of Cognitive Ability: Analysis
Client Needs: Physiological Integrity
Integrated Process: Nursing Process/Data Collection
Content Area: Pharmacology

Answer: 1
Rationale: The therapeutic phenytoin level is 10 to 20 mg/mL. Blood levels of phenytoin of more than 30 mg/mL produce lethargy.

Test-Taking Strategy: Knowledge of the normal phenytoin level and of the signs that occur in the client when the level rises is necessary to answer this question. Remember that blood levels of phenytoin of more than 30 mg/mL produce lethargy. Review phenytoin if you had difficulty with this question.

Reference

Hodgson, B., & Kizior, R. (2009). *Saunders nursing drug handbook 2009* (p. 927). St. Louis: Saunders.

---

726. To reduce the risk of aspiration, which of the following is the best position in which to place a child with cleft palate repair after feeding?

Answer: 4
Rationale: A cleft palate repair is the surgical correction of a congenital fissure in the midline of the partition that separates the oral and nasal cavities. The child with cleft palate repair is placed

1 Prone
2 On the stomach
3 On the left side
4 Upright in an infant seat

Level of Cognitive Ability: Application
Client Needs: Physiological Integrity
Integrated Process: Nursing Process/ Implementation
Content Area: Child Health

on his or her right side after feeding or in an upright position in an infant seat to reduce the chance of aspirating regurgitated formula. Options 1, 2, and 3 are incorrect positions.

Test-Taking Strategy: Use the process of elimination. Visualize the anatomical location of the stomach when answering this question; this will help you to eliminate options 1 and 2. From the remaining options, remember that positioning on the right side aids in absorption and reduces the risk of aspiration. Review the care of the child after cleft palate repair if you had difficulty with this question.

References

Leifer, G. (2007). *Introduction to maternity and pediatric nursing* (5th ed., p. 326). Philadelphia: Saunders.

McKinney, E., James, S., Murray, S., & Ashwill, J. (2009). *Maternal-child nursing* (3rd ed., p. 1095). St. Louis: Mosby.

---

727. A nurse is providing dietary instructions to a client with hyperparathyroidism. Which statement by the client indicates the need for further instruction?

1 "I should consume foods high in fiber."
2 "I should consume foods high in vitamin D."
3 "I should consume 3000 mL of fluid per day."
4 "I should drink cranberry juice on a daily basis."

Level of Cognitive Ability: Comprehension
Client Needs: Physiological Integrity
Integrated Process: Teaching and Learning
Content Area: Adult Health/Endocrine

Answer: 2

Rationale: Hyperparathyroidism is an abnormal endocrine condition characterized by the hyperactivity of any of the four parathyroid glands with excessive secretion of parathyroid hormone. The client with hyperparathyroidism should consume at least 3000 mL of fluid per day. Dehydration is dangerous because it increases the serum calcium levels and promotes the formation of renal stones. Cranberry juice and prune juice help make the urine more acidic. A high urinary acidity helps prevent renal stone formation because calcium is more soluble in an acidic urine than in an alkaline urine. Clients should maintain a diet that is low in calcium and vitamin D. High-fiber foods are important to prevent constipation and fecal impaction, which can result from the hypercalcemia that occurs with this disorder.

Test-Taking Strategy: Use the process of elimination. Note the strategic words *need for further instruction.* These words indicate a negative event query and ask you to select an option that is an incorrect statement. Recalling the pathophysiology of hyperparathyroidism and the dietary measures used to treat the disorder assists you with answering this question. Review the dietary measures associated with hyperparathyroidism if you had difficulty with this question.

Reference

Christensen, B., & Kockrow, E. (2006). *Adult health nursing* (5th ed., p. 536). St. Louis: Mosby.

---

728. A nurse is assigned to care for a child with hemophilia. The nurse reviews the child's health record and expects that which laboratory result will be abnormal?

1 Bleeding time
2 Sedimentation rate
3 Clot retraction time
4 Partial thromboplastin time (PTT)

Answer: 4

Rationale: The PTT measures the activity of thromboplastin, which is dependent on intrinsic factors. The intrinsic clotting factor VIII (antihemophilic factor) is deficient in clients with hemophilia, which results in a prolonged PTT. Options 1, 2, and 3 will not necessarily be abnormal in clients with this disorder.

Level of Cognitive Ability: Comprehension
Client Needs: Physiological Integrity
Integrated Process: Nursing Process/Data Collection
Content Area: Child Health

Test-Taking Strategy: Focus on the diagnosis of hemophilia, and recall the pathophysiology associated with this disorder. Remember that the intrinsic clotting factor VIII (antihemophilic factor) is deficient in clients with hemophilia, which results in a prolonged PTT. Review these laboratory tests if you had difficulty with this question.

Reference

Price, D., & Gwin, J. (2008). *Pediatric nursing: An introductory text* (10th ed., p. 246). St. Louis: Saunders.

---

729. A nurse assigned to assist with caring for a client after a gastric resection is monitoring the drainage from a nasogastric (NG) tube. No drainage has been noted for the past 4 hours, and the client complains of severe nausea. Which of the following is the appropriate nursing action?

1 Irrigate the tube.
2 Reposition the tube.
3 Medicate for nausea.
4 Notify the registered nurse (RN).

Level of Cognitive Ability: Application
Client Needs: Physiological Integrity
Integrated Process: Nursing Process/Implementation
Content Area: Adult Health/Gastrointestinal

Answer: 4

Rationale: Nausea and vomiting should not occur if the NG tube is patent. The NG tube should not be repositioned after gastric surgery because it is placed directly over the suture line. Only with a physician's order may the RN gently irrigate the NG tube with saline. In this situation, the RN should be notified.

Test-Taking Strategy: Use the process of elimination. Note that this client had a surgical procedure that involved the gastric area. In addition, remember that a nasogastric tube is placed near the surgical site. Note the strategic words *severe nausea;* this should direct you to option 4. Review postoperative nursing care after gastric surgery if you had difficulty with this question.

Reference

Linton, A. (2007). *Introduction to medical-surgical nursing* (4th ed., p. 743). Philadelphia: Saunders.

---

730. A client with diabetes mellitus is receiving prenatal care, and the nurse teaches the client about the early signs of hyperglycemia. The nurse determines that the teaching is effective when the client states that an early sign of hyperglycemia is which of the following?

1 Hunger
2 Polyuria
3 Shakiness
4 Nervousness

Level of Cognitive Ability: Comprehension
Client Needs: Physiological Integrity
Integrated Process: Nursing Process/Evaluation
Content Area: Maternity/Antepartum

Answer: 2

Rationale: Polyuria is an early sign of hyperglycemia. Other signs can include polydipsia; polyphagia; dry mouth; increased appetite; fatigue; nausea; hot, flushed skin; rapid, deep breathing; abdominal cramps; acetone breath; headache; drowsiness; depressed reflexes; oliguria; anuria; stupor; and coma. Options 1, 3, and 4 are signs of hypoglycemia.

Test-Taking Strategy: Use the process of elimination. Options 3 and 4 should be eliminated first because they are comparable or alike in that they are signs of hypoglycemia. Recalling that hunger is also a sign of hypoglycemia assists you with eliminating option 1. Review the signs of both hypoglycemia and hyperglycemia if you had difficulty with this question.

References

Hockenberry, M., & Wilson, D. (2009). *Wong's essentials of pediatric care* (8th ed., p. 1044). St. Louis: Mosby.
Leifer, G. (2008). *Maternity nursing: An introductory text* (10th ed., p. 266). Philadelphia: Saunders.

---

731. An older client is brought to the emergency department by a family member with whom she lives. The nurse notes that the client has poor hygiene, contractures, and pressure ulcers on the sacrum, scapula, and heels. The nurse suspects that the client is a victim of which type of abuse?

1. Sexual
2. Physical
3. Emotional
4. Psychological

Level of Cognitive Ability: Comprehension
Client Needs: Physiological Integrity
Integrated Process: Nursing Process/Data Collection
Content Area: Mental Health

Answer: 2

Rationale: Victimization in the family takes many forms. When collecting data about a specific client situation, it is important to understand which form of abuse is being considered. Physical abuse can take the form of battering (hitting, slapping, striking), or it can be more subtle, such as neglect (the failure to meet basic needs). The data in the question do not indicate sexual, emotional, or psychological abuse.

Test-Taking Strategy: Use the process of elimination, and focus on the data provided in the question. Option 2 is the only option that addresses the data in the question. Review the signs of physical abuse if you had difficulty with this question.

References

Fortinash, K., & Holoday-Worret, P. (2008). *Psychiatric mental health nursing* (4th ed., p. 500). St. Louis: Mosby.
Varcarolis, E., & Halter, M. (2009). *Essentials of psychiatric mental health nursing: A communication approach to evidence-based care* (p. 390). St. Louis: Saunders.

---

732. A client recovering from a craniotomy complains of a runny nose. The nurse should take which important action in this situation?

1. Provide the client with tissues.
2. Notify the registered nurse (RN).
3. Monitor the client for signs of a cold.
4. Tell the client to pat the drainage with the tissue.

Level of Cognitive Ability: Application
Client Needs: Physiological Integrity
Integrated Process: Nursing Process/Implementation
Content Area: Adult Health/Neurological

Answer: 2

Rationale: A craniotomy is any surgical opening into the skull that is made to relieve intracranial pressure, to control bleeding, or to remove a tumor. If the client has sustained a craniocerebral injury or is recovering from a craniotomy, careful observation of any drainage from the eyes, ears, nose, or traumatic area is critical. Cerebrospinal fluid is colorless and generally nonpurulent, and its presence indicates a serious breach of cranial integrity. Any suspicious drainage should be reported to the RN immediately. Options 1, 3, and 4 are inappropriate nursing actions.

Test-Taking Strategy: Use the process of elimination. Eliminate options 1 and 4 because they are comparable or alike. From the remaining options, recalling the signs of complications associated with craniotomy should direct you to option 2. Review postoperative nursing care after craniotomy if you had difficulty with this question.

Reference

Linton, A. (2007). *Introduction to medical-surgical nursing* (4th ed., p. 430). Philadelphia: Saunders.

---

733. A nurse is assigned to assist with caring for a client who has returned from the postanesthesia care unit after prostatectomy. The client has a three-way urinary catheter with an infusion of continuous bladder irrigation. The nurse determines that the flow rate is adequate if the color of the urinary drainage is which of the following?

1. Dark cherry
2. Clear as water
3. Pale yellow or slightly pink
4. Concentrated yellow with small clots

Answer: 3

Rationale: A prostatectomy is the surgical removal of a part of the prostate gland. The infusion of a bladder irrigant is not done at a preset rate; rather, the rate is increased or decreased to maintain urine that is a clear, pale, yellow color or that has just a slight pink tinge. The infusion rate should be increased if the drainage is cherry colored or if clots are seen. Alternatively, the rate can be slowed down slightly if the returns are as clear as water.

Level of Cognitive Ability: Comprehension
Client Needs: Physiological Integrity
Integrated Process: Nursing Process/Evaluation
Content Area: Adult Health/Renal

Test-Taking Strategy: Use the process of elimination. Eliminate option 4 as the least realistic of the described urine characteristics. Eliminate options 1 and 2 because they reflect inadequate and excessive flow, respectively. The urine should be pale yellow or pale pink with the proper flow rate of bladder irrigant. Review postoperative expectations after prostatectomy if you had difficulty with this question.

Reference

Linton, A. (2007). *Introduction to medical-surgical nursing* (4th ed., p. 1091). Philadelphia: Saunders.

---

734. A nurse is teaching a client with asthma how to use a peak-flow meter. The nurse should tell the client which of the following?

1 Inhale an average-size breath.
2 Blow out as slowly as possible.
3 Record the final position of the indicator.
4 Form a loose seal with the mouth around the mouthpiece.

Level of Cognitive Ability: Application
Client Needs: Physiological Integrity
Integrated Process: Teaching and Learning
Content Area: Adult Health/Respiratory

Answer: 3

Rationale: A peak-flow meter is used to give an objective measure of the client's peak expiratory flow. The client is instructed to take the deepest possible breath, to form a tight seal around the mouthpiece with the lips, and to exhale forcefully and rapidly. The final position of the indicator on the meter is recorded.

Test-Taking Strategy: To answer this question correctly, it is necessary to be familiar with this piece of equipment and its use. Visualize the use of the peak-flow meter to direct you to option 3. Review the peak-flow meter, which may be used to determine when medication adjustments are needed, if you had difficulty with this question.

References

Christensen, B., & Kockrow, E. (2006). *Adult health nursing* (5th ed., p. 459). St. Louis: Mosby.
deWit, S. (2009). *Medical-surgical nursing: Concepts & practice* (pp. 289-290). St. Louis: Saunders.

---

735. A mother of a child with celiac disease asks how long a special diet is necessary for the child. The nurse should tell the mother which of the following?

1 A gluten-free diet must be followed for life.
2 A lactose-free diet must be followed temporarily.
3 Adequate nutritional status helps to prevent celiac crisis.
4 Supplemental vitamins, iron, and folate prevent complications.

Level of Cognitive Ability: Application
Client Needs: Physiological Integrity
Integrated Process: Nursing Process/Implementation
Content Area: Child Health

Answer: 1

Rationale: Celiac disease is an inborn error of metabolism that is characterized by the inability to hydrolyze the peptides that are contained in gluten. The main nursing consideration with celiac disease is helping the child to adhere to dietary management. The treatment of celiac disease consists primarily of dietary management with a gluten-free diet. Options 2, 3, and 4 are all true statements, but they do not answer the mother's question. Children with untreated celiac disease may have lactose intolerance that usually improves with gluten withdrawal. Nutritional deficiencies that result from malabsorption are treated with appropriate supplements.

Test-Taking Strategy: Use the process of elimination. Focus on the subject—the length of time that a special diet is necessary; this will direct you to option 1. Review dietary requirements for celiac disease if you had difficulty with this question.

Reference

Price, D., & Gwin, J. (2008). *Pediatric nursing: An introductory text* (10th ed., p. 250). St. Louis: Saunders.

---

736. When providing the health history, the parents report that their 6-month-old baby has been screaming and drawing his knees up to his chest. The parents state that the infant is passing jelly-like stools mixed with blood and mucus. The nurse recognizes these signs and symptoms as indicative of which of the following?

1 Peritonitis
2 Appendicitis
3 Intussusception
4 Hirschsprung's disease

Level of Cognitive Ability: Analysis
Client Needs: Physiological Integrity
Integrated Process: Nursing Process/Data Collection
Content Area: Child Health

Answer: 3

Rationale: Intussusception is the prolapse of one segment of the bowel into the lumen of another segment. The classic signs and symptoms of intussusception are acute, colicky abdominal pain and currant-jelly–like stools. Peritonitis is a serious complication that may follow intestinal obstruction and perforation. The most common symptom of appendicitis is colicky periumbilical or lower abdominal pain in the right quadrant. Clinical manifestations of Hirschsprung's disease include constipation, abdominal distention, and ribbon-like, foul-smelling stools.

Test-Taking Strategy: Use the process of elimination and your knowledge of this disorder to answer the question. Focusing on the data and recalling that the classic signs and symptoms of intussusception are acute, colicky abdominal pain and currant-jelly–like stools will direct you to option 3. Review the clinical manifestations of intussusception if you had difficulty with this question.

Reference

Price, D., & Gwin, J. (2008). *Pediatric nursing: An introductory text* (10th ed., p. 161). St. Louis: Saunders.

---

737. A nurse is caring for a client who has sustained thoracic burns and smoke inhalation and who is at risk for impaired gas exchange. The nurse avoids which action as the least helpful when caring for this client?

1 Suctioning the airway on an as-needed basis
2 Repositioning the client from side to side every 2 hours
3 Providing humidified oxygen and incentive spirometry, as prescribed
4 Positioning the client on the back only with the head of the bed at a 45-degree angle

Level of Cognitive Ability: Application
Client Needs: Physiological Integrity
Integrated Process: Nursing Process/Implementation
Content Area: Adult Health/Integumentary

Answer: 4

Rationale: Aggressive pulmonary measures are used to prevent respiratory complications in the client who has impaired gas exchange as a result of a burn injury. These include turning and repositioning, positioning for comfort, using humidified oxygen, providing incentive spirometry, and suctioning the client on an as-needed basis. The least helpful measure is to keep the client in a single position; this ultimately leads to atelectasis and possible pneumonia.

Test-Taking Strategy: Note the strategic word *avoids*. This word indicates a negative event query and asks you to select an option that is an incorrect nursing action. Use basic nursing knowledge of respiratory support measures to eliminate each of the incorrect options. In addition, note the close-ended word *only* in the correct option. Review aggressive pulmonary measures if you had difficulty with this question.

References

Ignatavicius, D., & Workman, M. (2010). *Medical-surgical nursing: Patient-centered collaborative care* (6th ed., p. 530). St. Louis: Saunders.
Linton, A. (2007). *Introduction to medical-surgical nursing* (4th ed., p. 1151). Philadelphia: Saunders.

---

738. After the delivery of a newborn infant, a nurse assists with performing an initial assessment. The nurse obtains and documents an Apgar score of 8. This score indicates which of the following?

1 The infant is adjusting well to extrauterine life.

Answer: 1

Rationale: One of the earliest indicators of the successful adaptation of the newborn is the Apgar score. Scores range from 0 to 10. A score of 8 to 10 indicates that the infant is adjusting well to extrauterine life. A score of 4 to 7 often indicates that the infant requires some resuscitative intervention, such as oxygen. A score of less than 4 indicates that the infant is having

2 The infant requires some resuscitative intervention.
3 The infant is having difficulty adjusting to extrauterine life.
4 This is an inaccurate score that should be immediately repeated.

Level of Cognitive Ability: Comprehension
Client Needs: Physiological Integrity
Integrated Process: Nursing Process/Evaluation
Content Area: Maternity/Postpartum

difficulty adjusting to extrauterine life and requires vigorous resuscitation.

Test-Taking Strategy: Use the process of elimination, and remember that Apgar scores range from 0 to 10. Option 4 can be eliminated first. From the remaining options, note that the score is 8 and that options 2 and 3 are comparable or alike. Review the Apgar score if you had difficulty with this question.

Reference

Leifer, G. (2008). *Maternity nursing: An introductory text* (10th ed., p. 137). Philadelphia: Saunders.

---

739. A client with a history of rheumatic heart disease asks the nurse why he must tell the dentist about this condition before dental cleaning or other work. The nurse's response is based on the knowledge that:
1 The client is at risk for episodes of heart failure triggered by stressful events.
2 The dentist should use a lidocaine solution that does not contain epinephrine.
3 The dentist should be aware that the vibration of the drill could cause dysrhythmias.
4 The client is susceptible to reinfection unless prophylactic antibiotic therapy is given before treatment.

Level of Cognitive Ability: Comprehension
Client Needs: Physiological Integrity
Integrated Process: Nursing Process/Implementation
Content Area: Adult Health/Cardiovascular

Answer: 4
Rationale: Rheumatic heart disease is a disorder in which damage to the heart muscle and heart valves has occurred as a result of episodes of rheumatic fever. The client with a history of rheumatic heart disease is at risk for developing infective endocarditis. The client notifies all physicians and dentists about the history so that prophylactic antibiotic therapy can be given before any invasive procedure or if there is risk of bleeding. Options 1, 2, and 3 are incorrect.

Test-Taking Strategy: Use the process of elimination. Remember that prophylactic antibiotic treatment before any type of invasive procedure is indicated to prevent an episode of endocarditis. Knowledge of this concept should help you to eliminate the incorrect options. Review prophylactic antibiotic treatment for rheumatic heart disease if you had difficulty with this question.

Reference

Christensen, B., & Kockrow, E. (2006). *Adult health nursing* (5th ed., p. 370). St. Louis: Mosby.

---

740. A nurse interprets a Mantoux tuberculin skin test as demonstrating a significant finding. To most accurately diagnose tuberculosis (TB), the nurse should plan to consult with the physician to follow up the skin test with which procedure?
1 Sputum culture
2 Chest radiograph
3 Complete blood cell count
4 Computerized tomography (CT) scan of the chest

Level of Cognitive Ability: Analysis
Client Needs: Physiological Integrity
Integrated Process: Nursing Process/Planning
Content Area: Adult Health/Respiratory

Answer: 1
Rationale: TB is a chronic granulomatous infection that usually infects the lungs and that is caused by an acid-fast bacillus, *Mycobacterium tuberculosis*. The demonstration of tubercle bacilli bacteriologically is essential for establishing a diagnosis. The microscopic examination of stained sputum smears for acid-fast bacilli is usually the first bacteriologic evidence of the presence of tubercle bacilli. Although the findings of a chest x-ray are important, it is not possible to make a diagnosis of tuberculosis solely on the basis of this examination because other diseases can mimic the appearance of tuberculosis. A complete blood cell count or CT scan of the chest will not confirm the diagnosis.

Test-Taking Strategy: Use the process of elimination, and note the strategic words *to most accurately diagnose tuberculosis*. Analyze the probability of each option being the most accurate method of diagnosing TB as a follow-up to the Mantoux skin test. Review the tests used to diagnose TB if you had difficulty with this question.

Reference

Christensen, B., & Kockrow, E. (2006). *Adult health nursing* (5th ed., p. 428). St. Louis: Mosby.

---

741. A nurse has an order to suction the airway of an adult client and is using a wall suction unit. The nurse begins the procedure by setting the suction control dial at which of the following levels?

1 80 mm Hg
2 150 mm Hg
3 180 mm Hg
4 220 mm Hg

Level of Cognitive Ability: Application
Client Needs: Physiological Integrity
Integrated Process: Nursing Process/Implementation
Content Area: Adult Health/Respiratory

Answer: 1

Rationale: The correct pressure during the suctioning of an adult using a wall suction unit is 80 to 120 mm Hg. The correct suction pressure for infants and children is 60 to 110 mm Hg.

Test-Taking Strategy: Use the process of elimination, and focus on the subject—an adult client. Recall the fundamental principles associated with suctioning a client's airway, and select option 1 because it is the lowest level identified in the options. Review the essentials of suctioning a client's airway if you had difficulty with this question.

Reference

deWit, S. (2009). *Medical-surgical nursing: Concepts & practice* (p. 293). St. Louis: Saunders.

---

742. A nurse is assisting with obtaining an Apgar score for an infant immediately after birth. The nurse notes that the infant's heart rate is less than 100 beats/min, the respiratory effort is good, and the muscle tone indicates some extremity flexion. The newborn sneezes when suctioned by the bulb syringe, and the extremities are cyanotic. The nurse should document which of the following Apgar scores for this newborn?

1 3
2 5
3 7
4 10

Level of Cognitive Ability: Comprehension
Client Needs: Physiological Integrity
Integrated Process: Communication and Documentation
Content Area: Maternity/Postpartum

Answer: 3

Rationale: One of the earliest indicators of the successful adaptation of the newborn is the Apgar score. Scores range from 0 to 10. The test assesses five areas to measure the infant's adaptation: heart rate (absent = 0; less than 100 beats/min = 1; more than 100 beats/min = 2); respiratory effort (absent = 0; slow or irregular weak cry = 1; good, crying lustily = 2); muscle tone (limp or hypotonic = 0; some extremity flexion = 1; active, moving, and well flexed = 2); irritability or reflexes as measured by bulb suctioning (no response = 0; grimace = 1; cough, sneeze, or vigorous cry = 2); and color (cyanotic or pale = 0; acrocyanotic, cyanosis of extremities = 1; pink = 2).

Test-Taking Strategy: Knowledge that Apgar scores range from 0 to 10 and of the measurements used to determine the score assists you with answering this question. Focus on the data in the question to direct you to option 3. Review Apgar scoring if you had difficulty with this question.

Reference

Leifer, G. (2008). *Maternity nursing: An introductory text* (10th ed., p. 137). Philadelphia: Saunders.

743. A nurse in the newborn nursery is obtaining admission vital signs from a newborn. Which finding indicates a normal axillary temperature?

1 35.5° C (95.9° F)
2 37.5° C (99.5° F)
3 38.5° C (101.3° F)
4 39.5° C (103.1° F)

Level of Cognitive Ability: Comprehension
Client Needs: Physiological Integrity
Integrated Process: Nursing Process/Data Collection
Content Area: Maternity/Postpartum

Answer: 2

Rationale: The normal axillary temperature for a newborn ranges from 36.5° C to 37.5° C (97.7° F to 99.5° F). The normal rectal temperature ranges from 36.5° C to 37.6° C (97.7° F to 99.6° F).

Test-Taking Strategy: Knowledge of the normal axillary temperature of a newborn is necessary to answer this question. Remember that the normal axillary temperature for a newborn ranges from 36.5° C to 37.5° C (97.7° F to 99.5° F). Review the normal ranges for newborn vital signs if you had difficulty with this question.

Reference

Leifer, G. (2008). *Maternity nursing: An introductory text* (10th ed., p. 166). Philadelphia: Saunders.

---

744. An instructor asks a nursing student who is collecting data from a newborn admitted to the nursery after birth about the anterior fontanel. Which response by the student indicates inaccurate information regarding the fontanel?

1 "It is diamond shaped."
2 "It should be flat and soft."
3 "It normally closes by 2 to 3 months of age."
4 "It normally closes by 12 to 18 months of age."

Level of Cognitive Ability: Comprehension
Client Needs: Physiological Integrity
Integrated Process: Teaching and Learning
Content Area: Maternity/Postpartum

Answer: 3

Rationale: The anterior fontanel is diamond shaped and located on the top of the head. It should be flat and soft, and it may range in size from almost nonexistent to 4 to 5 cm across. It normally closes by 12 to 18 months of age. The posterior fontanel closes by 2 to 3 months of age.

Test-Taking Strategy: Note the strategic word *inaccurate.* This word indicates a negative event query and asks you to select an option that is an incorrect student response. Use the process of elimination, and note that options 3 and 4 both address a time frame regarding the closure of the fontanel; therefore it is likely that one of these options is correct. Knowledge that the anterior fontanel normally closes by 12 to 18 months of age is necessary to answer the question correctly. Review normal newborn findings if you had difficulty with this question.

Reference

Leifer, G. (2008). *Maternity nursing: An introductory text* (10th ed., p. 170). Philadelphia: Saunders.

---

745. A client is admitted to the hospital with a diagnosis of Cushing's syndrome. The nurse interprets that which laboratory result is consistent with this health problem?

1 Potassium: 3.4 mEq/L
2 Blood glucose: 205 mg/dL
3 Blood urea nitrogen (BUN): 16 mg/dL
4 White blood cell (WBC) count: 3200/mm^3

Level of Cognitive Ability: Comprehension
Client Needs: Physiological Integrity
Integrated Process: Nursing Process/Data Collection
Content Area: Adult Health/Endocrine

Answer: 2

Rationale: Cushing's syndrome is characterized by an excess of adrenocorticosteroid hormones. Abnormal laboratory findings that occur with this disorder are hyperkalemia, hyperglycemia, an elevated WBC count, and elevated plasma cortisol and adrenocorticotropic hormone levels. These effects are the result of excess glucocorticoids and mineralocorticoids in the body. The potassium and WBC levels identified in the options are low, whereas the BUN is normal and is an unrelated finding. Only the blood glucose level is elevated.

Test-Taking Strategy: To answer this question accurately, you must understand Cushing's syndrome and its effects on the body. Recalling that Cushing's syndrome is characterized by an excess of adrenocorticosteroid hormones will assist you with answering this question. Review the clinical manifestations associated with Cushing's syndrome if you had difficulty with this question.

Reference

Ignatavicius, D., & Workman, M. (2010). *Medical-surgical nursing: Patient-centered collaborative care* (6th ed., pp. 1472, 1474-1475). St. Louis: Saunders.

---

746. A client has just undergone the trans-sphenoidal resection of a pituitary adenoma. The nurse includes which of the following in the plan of care?

1 Remove the nasal packing in 12 hours.
2 Observe the client for frequent swallowing.
3 Remind the client to cough and breathe deeply.
4 Administer acetylsalicylic acid (aspirin) for a severe headache.

Level of Cognitive Ability: Application
Client Needs: Physiological Integrity
Integrated Process: Nursing Process/Planning
Content Area: Adult Health/Endocrine

Answer: 2

Rationale: After trans-sphenoidal surgery, the client should be observed for frequent swallowing, which could indicate postnasal drip; this drainage could be cerebrospinal fluid. The nurse should report severe headache to the physician because it could indicate increased intracranial pressure. In most cases, the surgeon removes the nasal packing after 24 hours. The client should be allowed to breathe deeply but not cough because coughing could increase the intracranial pressure.

Test-Taking Strategy: Use the process of elimination. Recalling the anatomical location of trans-sphenoidal surgery assists you with eliminating options 3 and 4. From the remaining options, recall that packing is removed by the physician; noting the time frame in option 1 helps you to eliminate this option. Review the care of the client after the trans-sphenoidal resection of a pituitary adenoma if you had difficulty with this question.

Reference

Ignatavicius, D., & Workman, M. (2010). *Medical-surgical nursing: Patient-centered collaborative care* (6th ed., p. 1431). St. Louis: Saunders.

---

747. A client with Cushing's disease is admitted to the hospital after a motor vehicle crash that resulted in multiple lacerations. The nurse identifies which problem as the highest priority concern based on the history of Cushing's disease?

1 Risk for infection
2 Fluid volume deficit
3 Altered health maintenance
4 Sensory-perceptual alterations

Level of Cognitive Ability: Analysis
Client Needs: Physiological Integrity
Integrated Process: Nursing Process/Data Collection
Content Area: Adult Health/Endocrine

Answer: 1

Rationale: Cushing's syndrome is characterized by an excess of adrenocorticosteroid hormones. The client with lacerations has a break in the body's first line of defense against infection. The client with Cushing's disease has a heightened risk for infection because of excess cortisol secretion, impaired antibody function, and decreased proliferation of lymphocytes. This client is at risk for fluid volume excess rather than fluid volume deficit. The client may have altered health maintenance but there is insufficient information in the question to determine this. Sensory-perceptual alterations are an unrelated concern.

Test-Taking Strategy: Use the process of elimination. The strategic words in the question are *highest priority*. Recall the pathophysiology of this disorder and note the words *multiple lacerations* to direct you to option 1. Review Cushing's syndrome if you had difficulty with this question.

References

deWit, S. (2009). *Medical-surgical nursing: Concepts & practice* (p. 906). St. Louis: Saunders.

Linton, A. (2007). *Introduction to medical-surgical nursing* (4th ed., p. 976). Philadelphia: Saunders.

---

748. A client arrives at the nursing unit after abdominal surgery. A nasogastric (NG) tube is in place, and the physician has instructed that the NG tube be attached to intermittent suction. The nurse monitors the client, knowing that the client with an NG tube attached to suction is at risk for which acid-base disorder?

1 Metabolic acidosis
2 Metabolic alkalosis
3 Respiratory acidosis
4 Respiratory alkalosis

Level of Cognitive Ability: Analysis
Client Needs: Physiological Integrity
Integrated Process: Nursing Process/Data Collection
Content Area: Adult Health/Gastrointestinal

Answer: 2
Rationale: Metabolic alkalosis can occur from vomiting or gastric suction because of the loss of acid through the suctioning. Options 1, 3, and 4 are incorrect because they are not likely to occur as a result of gastrointestinal (GI) suction.

Test-Taking Strategy: Use the process of elimination. Recalling that the loss of acid occurs through GI suctioning assists you with determining that an alkalosis can occur. Note that the situation described in the question is not a respiratory disorder; this will direct you to option 2. Review the complications associated with GI suctioning if you had difficulty with this question.

Reference
Ignatavicius, D., & Workman, M. (2010). *Medical-surgical nursing: Patient-centered collaborative care* (6th ed., p. 1278). St. Louis: Saunders.

---

749. A client has returned to the nursing unit after undergoing computerized tomography (CT) scanning with a contrast medium. The nurse instructs the client to do which of the following after the procedure?

1 Drink extra fluids during the day.
2 Eat lightly for the remainder of the day.
3 Rest quietly for the remainder of the day.
4 Do not take any medications for at least 8 hours.

Level of Cognitive Ability: Application
Client Needs: Physiological Integrity
Integrated Process: Nursing Process/Implementation
Content Area: Fundamental Skills

Answer: 1
Rationale: After CT scanning, the client may resume all usual activities and diet. The contrast dye will cause diuresis, so the client should consume extra fluids to replace those that will be lost. Options 2, 3, and 4 are unnecessary.

Test-Taking Strategy: Use the process of elimination. Note the words *contrast medium* in the question to direct you to option 1. Review the postprocedural care after CT scanning if you had difficulty with this question.

Reference
Christensen, B., & Kockrow, E. (2006). *Foundations of nursing* (5th ed., p. 490). St. Louis: Mosby.

---

750. A nurse is assigned to assist with caring for a client receiving peritoneal dialysis and notes a brownish color to the dialysate output. The nurse interprets that this finding could result from which of the following conditions?

1 Early infection
2 Bowel perforation
3 Bladder perforation
4 Insufficient fluid instillation

Level of Cognitive Ability: Analysis
Client Needs: Physiological Integrity

Answer: 2
Rationale: Brown-colored or bloody drainage could indicate the perforation of the bowel by the peritoneal dialysis catheter. If this is noted, it must be reported to the physician immediately. Early signs of infection include cloudy dialysate output, fever, and most likely abdominal discomfort. Bladder perforation could yield yellow or bloody drainage. Insufficient fluid instillation is an incorrect option. The client would have no signs of insufficient fluid instillation except for the outflow of smaller amounts of dialysate.

Test-Taking Strategy: Use the process of elimination. Focus on the data in the question to direct you to option 2. Review the complications of peritoneal dialysis if you had difficulty with this question.

Integrated Process: Nursing Process/Data Collection
Content Area: Adult Health/Renal

References

Ignatavicius, D., & Workman, M. (2010). *Medical-surgical nursing: Patient-centered collaborative care* (6th ed., p. 1630). St. Louis: Saunders.
Linton, A. (2007). *Introduction to medical-surgical nursing* (4th ed., p. 875). Philadelphia: Saunders.

---

751. A client is scheduled to have a serum glycosylated hemoglobin level drawn. The nurse determines that the client understands the nature of the test if the client makes which statement about preparation?

1 "I shouldn't eat anything after midnight."
2 "I can eat and drink as usual before the test."
3 "I shouldn't eat red meat for 3 days before the test."
4 "I shouldn't eat very fatty foods the day before the test."

Level of Cognitive Ability: Comprehension
Client Needs: Physiological Integrity
Integrated Process: Nursing Process/Evaluation
Content Area: Adult Health/Endocrine

Answer: 2
Rationale: No special dietary preparation is necessary for this diagnostic test, which measures the amount of diabetic control during the previous 3 months. When circulating glucose levels are elevated, glucose molecules permanently attach themselves to red blood cells (RBCs). They remain on the RBCs for the rest of their life span (up to 120 days), thus giving some estimate of a client's long-term diabetic control.

Test-Taking Strategy: Use the process of elimination. Recalling that the purpose of the test is to measure long-term glucose control helps you to eliminate options 1, 3, and 4. Review serum glycosylated hemoglobin level testing if you had difficulty with this question.

Reference

Chernecky, C., & Berger, B. (2008). *Laboratory tests and diagnostic procedures* (5th ed., p. 594). Philadelphia: Saunders.

---

752. A nurse is collecting data from a client with hypoparathyroidism. The nurse should do which of the following to check for Chvostek's sign?

1 Dorsiflex the foot briskly.
2 Tap the cheek over the facial nerve.
3 Stroke upward on the soles of the feet.
4 Inflate a blood pressure cuff on the arm for 3 minutes.

Level of Cognitive Ability: Application
Client Needs: Physiological Integrity
Integrated Process: Nursing Process/Data Collection
Content Area: Adult Health/Endocrine

Answer: 2
Rationale: Hypoparathyroidism is a condition that involves the insufficient secretion of parathyroid hormone by the parathyroid gland, which results in low serum calcium levels, which can cause tetany. This can be assessed by testing for Chvostek's sign (option 2), which is an abnormal spasm of the facial muscles elicited by light taps on the facial nerve. Option 1 describes a method of checking for Homans' sign. Option 3 describes the assessment of the Babinski reflex. Option 4 describes Trousseau's sign, which is another indication of tetany.

Test-Taking Strategy: To answer this question accurately, you must be familiar with data collection techniques and the manifestations of hypoparathyroidism. Remember that Chvostek's sign is an abnormal spasm of the facial muscles that is elicited by light taps on the facial nerve. Review the various techniques of assessing for tetany if you had difficulty with this question.

Reference

Christensen, B., & Kockrow, E. (2006). *Foundations of nursing* (5th ed., p. 676). St. Louis: Mosby.

---

753. A client with right-sided weakness has been taught how to use a cane. The nurse determines that the client is using the cane correctly if the client positions the cane by holding it:

Answer: 3
Rationale: The client is taught to hold the cane on the opposite side of the weakness because the opposite arm and leg move together (reciprocal motion) with normal walking. The cane is placed 6 inches lateral to the fifth toe.

1 In the left hand and in front of the left foot
2 In the right hand and in front of the right foot
3 In the left hand and 6 inches lateral to the left foot
4 In the right hand and 6 inches lateral to the right foot

Level of Cognitive Ability: Comprehension
Client Needs: Physiological Integrity
Integrated Process: Nursing Process/Evaluation
Content Area: Adult Health/Musculoskeletal

Test-Taking Strategy: Use the process of elimination. Knowing that the cane is held at the client's side (not in front) helps you to eliminate options 1 and 2 first. Recalling that the cane is positioned on the stronger side helps you to eliminate option 4. Review client instructions for the use of a cane if you had difficulty with this question.

Reference

deWit, S. (2009). *Medical-surgical nursing: Concepts & practice* (p. 779). St. Louis: Saunders.

---

754. A client has a long arm cast applied after a severe fracture of the left radius. The nurse monitors for which sign or symptom of compartment syndrome?
1 Pain that is relieved by opioid analgesics
2 Aggravation of pain with elevation of the left arm
3 Paralysis of the left hand not preceded by paresthesias
4 Absence of pain with passive movement of the left arm

Level of Cognitive Ability: Application
Client Needs: Physiological Integrity
Integrated Process: Nursing Process/Data Collection
Content Area: Adult Health/Musculoskeletal

Answer: 2

Rationale: Compartment syndrome is caused by the progressive development of arterial compression and the consequent reduction of blood supply. The pain of compartment syndrome is aggravated by limb elevation, which further impairs blood supply. This pain is not relieved by opioid analgesics, and the compartment is painful when moved. Paresthesias occur early in the syndrome and progress to paralysis unless pressure in the compartment is relieved.

Test-Taking Strategy: Use the process of elimination. Recall that compartment syndrome impairs arterial circulation. Knowing that this pain would be aggravated by antigravity measures (e.g., elevating the limb) directs you to option 2. Review the signs of compartment syndrome if you had difficulty with this question.

Reference

Christensen, B., & Kockrow, E. (2006). *Adult health nursing* (5th ed., pp. 164-165). St. Louis: Mosby.

---

755. A client is learning to use a walker to aid in mobility after the internal fixation of a hip fracture. The nurse corrects the client if the nurse notes that the client does which of the following?
1 Holds the walker using the hand grips
2 Advances the walker with reciprocal motion
3 Leans forward slightly when moving the walker
4 Supports body weight on the hands while moving the weaker leg

Level of Cognitive Ability: Application
Client Needs: Physiological Integrity
Integrated Process: Nursing Process/Implementation
Content Area: Adult Health/Musculoskeletal

Answer: 2

Rationale: The client should place the hands on the hand grips for stability. The client should lift the walker to advance it and lean forward slightly while moving it. The client walks into the walker, supporting the body weight on the hands while moving the weaker leg. A disadvantage of the walker is that it does not allow for reciprocal walking motion. If the client were to try to use this type of motion with a walker, the walker would advance forward one side at a time as the client was walking. This is incorrect because the client would not be supporting the weaker leg with the walker during ambulation.

Test-Taking Strategy: Use the process of elimination, and note the strategic words *corrects the client*. These words indicate a negative event query and ask you to select an option that is an incorrect movement. Holding the hand grips of the walker is obviously correct, so option 1 is eliminated first. Because the client must lean forward slightly to move the walker forward, option 3 is eliminated next. From the remaining options, recalling that the purpose of a walker is to provide support directs you to option 2. Review client instructions regarding the use of a walker if you had difficulty with this question.

References

deWit, S. (2009). *Medical-surgical nursing: Concepts & practice* (p. 779). St. Louis: Saunders.

Linton, A. (2007). *Introduction to medical-surgical nursing* (4th ed., p. 924). Philadelphia: Saunders.

---

756. A nurse is caring for a client with a left leg cast. The nurse suspects that the client has an infection under the cast if which sign is noted?

1 Weakened left pedal pulse
2 Dependent left foot edema
3 Coolness and pallor of the left foot
4 Presence of a "hot spot" on the cast

Level of Cognitive Ability: Comprehension
Client Needs: Physiological Integrity
Integrated Process: Nursing Process/Data Collection
Content Area: Adult Health/Musculoskeletal

Answer: 4

Rationale: Signs and symptoms of infection under a casted area include odor or purulent drainage from the cast and the presence of "hot spots," which are areas of the cast that are warmer than others. The physician should be notified if any of these occur. Signs of impaired circulation in the distal limb include coolness and pallor of the skin, diminished pulse, and edema.

Test-Taking Strategy: Use the process of elimination. Recall that the typical signs of infection include redness, swelling, heat, and purulent drainage. With these signs in mind, you can eliminate options 1 and 3. From the remaining options, recall that dependent edema does not necessarily indicate infection. Swelling would be continuous. The "hot spot" on the cast could signify infection underneath that area and is the correct answer to the question. Review the signs of infection if you had difficulty with this question.

References

deWit, S. (2009). *Medical-surgical nursing: Concepts & practice* (p. 791). St. Louis: Saunders.

Ignatavicius, D., & Workman, M. (2010). *Medical-surgical nursing: Patient-centered collaborative care* (6th ed., p. 1189). St. Louis: Saunders.

---

757. Treatment for a client with asthma has been changed from oral to inhalation therapy with beclomethasone dipropionate. The client complains of weakness and anorexia. The client's blood glucose level is 58 mg/dL, and his blood pressure (BP) drops to 102/70 mm Hg from 118/78 mm Hg. The nurse interprets that the client may be experiencing which of the following adverse medication effects?

1 Diabetes mellitus
2 Circulatory collapse
3 Adrenal insufficiency
4 Exacerbation of gastritis

Answer: 3

Rationale: Beclomethasone dipropionate is a corticosteroid inhalant that is used to treat asthma. The nurse should monitor for signs of adrenal insufficiency whenever a client is switched from oral to inhalation glucocorticoid therapy (e.g., beclomethasone). Signs of adrenal insufficiency include anorexia, nausea, weakness, fatigue, hypotension, and hypoglycemia. Options 1, 2, and 4 are not associated with the use of this medication.

Test-Taking Strategy: Focus on the name of the medication, and recall that medication names that end with *-sone* are corticosteroids. Recalling the signs and symptoms of adrenal insufficiency and the adverse effects of beclomethasone will direct you to option 3. Review beclomethasone if you had difficulty with this question.

Level of Cognitive Ability: Analysis
Client Needs: Physiological Integrity
Integrated Process: Nursing Process/Data Collection
Content Area: Pharmacology

References

Kee, J., Hayes, E., & McCuistion, L. (2009). *Pharmacology: A nursing process approach* (6th ed., p. 787). St. Louis: Saunders.
Linton, A. (2007). *Introduction to medical-surgical nursing* (4th ed., p. 533). Philadelphia: Saunders.

---

758. A client has been given a prescription for erythromycin stearate to treat a respiratory infection, and the nurse reinforces medication instructions to the client. The nurse determines that the client requires further instruction if the client states that it is necessary to report which of the following while taking the medication?

1 Loss of appetite
2 Foul-smelling diarrhea
3 Vaginal itching or discharge
4 Furry overgrowth on the tongue

Level of Cognitive Ability: Analysis
Client Needs: Physiological Integrity
Integrated Process: Teaching and Learning
Content Area: Pharmacology

Answer: 1

Rationale: Erythromycin stearate is a macrolide antibiotic. The client is taught to report signs of superinfection while taking an antibiotic such as Erythrocin stearate. These signs include furry overgrowth on the tongue, vaginal itching or discharge, and loose or foul-smelling stools. Loss of appetite is not a sign of superinfection and does not warrant reporting if it occurs.

Test-Taking Strategy: Note the strategic words *requires further instruction*. These words indicate a negative event query and ask you to select an option that is an incorrect statement. Recalling that superinfection occurs with antibiotic therapy and recalling the common signs of superinfection will direct you to option 1. Review the adverse effects of erythromycin stearate if you had difficulty with this question.

Reference

Hodgson, B., & Kizior, R. (2009). *Saunders nursing drug handbook 2009* (p. 437). St. Louis: Saunders.

---

759. A client has just returned to the nursing unit after having a bone scan. The nurse tells the client to do which of the following after this procedure?

1 Increase fluid intake.
2 Eat small, frequent meals.
3 Walk in the hallway as much as possible.
4 Call the nurse if nausea or flushing is felt.

Level of Cognitive Ability: Application
Client Needs: Physiological Integrity
Integrated Process: Nursing Process/ Implementation
Content Area: Adult Health/Musculoskeletal

Answer: 1

Rationale: There are no special restrictions for diet or activity after a bone scan. The client is encouraged to drink large amounts of water for 24 to 48 hours to flush the radioisotope from the system. Options 2 and 3 are unnecessary. Option 4 is unrelated to this procedure.

Test-Taking Strategy: Use the process of elimination. There is no purpose for options 2 and 3, so these are eliminated first. Eliminate option 4 next for two reasons. First, the question relates to postprocedural concerns, and nausea and flushing accompany dye injection during a procedure. Second, this procedure involves the use of radioisotopes rather than dye. The only option left is increasing fluids, which speeds up the elimination of the isotope from the client's system. Review postprocedural instructions after a bone scan if you had difficulty with this question.

Reference

Chernecky, C., & Berger, B. (2008). *Laboratory tests and diagnostic procedures* (5th ed., p. 246). Philadelphia: Saunders.

---

760. A nurse is collecting data from a client with a left arm fracture and checking for impaired venous return distal to the fracture. Which sign indicates that this is occurring?

Answer: 1

Rationale: Impaired venous return is often marked by edema and can occur distal to the site of a fracture. Signs of arterial damage can result if an artery becomes contused, thrombosed, lacerated, or spastic. The other options are signs of arterial damage, which

1 Edema of the left hand
2 Weakened left radial pulse
3 Pallor with blotchy cyanosis
4 Continued pain despite medication

Level of Cognitive Ability: Analysis
Client Needs: Physiological Integrity
Integrated Process: Nursing Process/Data Collection
Content Area: Adult Health/Musculoskeletal

include pallor or blotchy cyanosis; variable, weakened, or absent distal pulse; pain; poor capillary refill; and distal paralysis or loss of sensation.

Test-Taking Strategy: Use the process of elimination, and focus on the strategic words *impaired venous return.* Recalling the signs that accompany impairments of arterial and venous circulation directs you to option 1. Review data collection techniques for circulatory status after fracture if you had difficulty with this question.

Reference
Linton, A. (2007). *Introduction to medical-surgical nursing* (4th ed., p. 918). Philadelphia: Saunders.

---

761. A nurse is checking an intravenous (IV) site of a client, and an infiltration is suspected. The nurse notes which of the following if an infiltration has occurred?
1 Warmth at the site
2 Redness at the site
3 Coolness at the site
4 Inflammation at the site

Level of Cognitive Ability: Comprehension
Client Needs: Physiological Integrity
Integrated Process: Nursing Process/Data Collection
Content Area: Fundamental Skills

Answer: 3
Rationale: Infiltration occurs when fluid extravasates into tissue. Signs of infiltration include edema and coolness at the site of insertion. The nurse should compare the site with the opposite extremity to note any swelling. Warmth and redness are noted in phlebitis, inflammation at the site, and infection.

Test-Taking Strategy: Use the process of elimination. Note that options 1, 2, and 4 are comparable or alike in that they all indicate phlebitis or inflammation. Recalling that coolness at the IV insertion site indicates infiltration directs you to option 3. Review the signs of infiltration if you had difficulty with this question.

Reference
Linton, A. (2007). *Introduction to medical-surgical nursing* (4th ed., pp. 285, 287). Philadelphia: Saunders.

---

762. A nurse is assisting with caring for a client with a central intravenous (IV) line who is receiving IV solutions. The client suddenly develops tachycardia, and dyspnea and cyanosis are noted. The nurse suspects an air embolism. Which initial nursing action should the nurse take?
1 Slow the IV rate.
2 Provide emotional support for the client.
3 Elevate the head of the bed and monitor the vital signs.
4 Turn the client on the left side and lower the head of the bed.

Level of Cognitive Ability: Application
Client Needs: Physiological Integrity
Integrated Process: Nursing Process/Implementation
Content Area: Delegating/Prioritizing

Answer: 4
Rationale: If an air embolism is suspected, the initial nursing actions are to turn the client on the left side and to lower the head of the bed to trap the air in the right atrium. The tubing should be clamped, the vital signs should be monitored, and the physician should be notified. Oxygen should be administered as prescribed, and emotional support should be given to the client. However, the initial nursing action is to position the client.

Test-Taking Strategy: Use the process of elimination, and note the strategic word *initial.* Eliminate option 2 first, recalling that physiological needs are the priority. Eliminate option 1 next because the IV flow is stopped rather than slowed. Use the concepts of gravity to assist you with selecting option 4 from the remaining options. Review the initial nursing actions that must be taken if an air embolism is suspected if you had difficulty with this question.

Reference
Linton, A. (2007). *Introduction to medical-surgical nursing* (4th ed., p. 288). Philadelphia: Saunders.

763. A client's serum digoxin level is 1.2 ng/mL. The nurse interprets that this level is:
1 Incorrectly reported
2 Above the therapeutic range
3 Below the therapeutic range
4 Within the therapeutic range

Level of Cognitive Ability: Comprehension
Client Needs: Physiological Integrity
Integrated Process: Nursing Process/Data Collection
Content Area: Pharmacology

Answer: 4
Rationale: The normal therapeutic range for digoxin is 0.8 to 2.0 ng/mL (although some laboratory resources indicate 0.5 to 2.0 ng/mL). A level of 1.2 ng/mL is within the therapeutic range.

Test-Taking Strategy: To answer this question correctly, you must know the therapeutic range of digoxin, which is 0.8 to 2.0 ng/mL. Review the therapeutic range of digoxin if you had difficulty with this question.

Reference
Hodgson, B., & Kizior, R. (2009). *Saunders nursing drug handbook 2009* (p. 356). St. Louis: Saunders.

---

764. A client has been diagnosed with hyperthyroidism. The nurse asks the client about which complaint that is associated with this disorder?
1 Lethargy
2 Weight gain
3 Constipation
4 Heat intolerance

Level of Cognitive Ability: Application
Client Needs: Physiological Integrity
Integrated Process: Nursing Process/Data Collection
Content Area: Adult Health/Endocrine

Answer: 4
Rationale: Hyperthyroidism is characterized by the hyperactivity of the thyroid gland. The client with hyperthyroidism has the metabolic manifestations of heat intolerance as well as an increased metabolic rate and a low-grade fever. Some of the other symptoms include weight loss, restlessness, and diarrhea, which are the opposite of the symptoms presented in options 1, 2, and 3.

Test-Taking Strategy: Use the process of elimination. Note the prefix *hyper-* and recall the function of the thyroid gland to direct you to option 4. Review the symptoms of hyperthyroidism if you had difficulty with this question.

Reference
Christensen, B., & Kockrow, E. (2006). *Adult health nursing* (5th ed., p. 527). St. Louis: Mosby.

---

765. A client is being treated for diabetic ketoacidosis (DKA). The nurse monitors for which of the following as the most serious electrolyte disturbance that can accompany the treatment of this disorder?
1 Hypokalemia
2 Hyponatremia
3 Hypocalcemia
4 Hypomagnesemia

Level of Cognitive Ability: Analysis
Client Needs: Physiological Integrity
Integrated Process: Nursing Process/Data Collection
Content Area: Adult Health/Endocrine

Answer: 1
Rationale: DKA is an acute, life-threatening complication of uncontrolled diabetes mellitus. The client who is being treated for DKA may experience hypokalemia. Potassium attaches to the insulin–glucose complex and is carried into the cell with it. As the client's serum glucose falls during treatment, hypokalemia can also occur. The nurse monitors the serum potassium results during this treatment. Hypokalemia can lead to cardiac dysrhythmias.

Test-Taking Strategy: Use the process of elimination, and recall the pathophysiology of DKA and its treatment. Recalling the process of glucose transport into the cells assists with directing you to option 1. Review the treatment of DKA if you had difficulty with this question.

Reference
Linton, A. (2007). *Introduction to medical-surgical nursing* (4th ed., p. 1008). Philadelphia: Saunders.

---

766. A client has an order to receive glyburide (Micronase) once per day. The nurse schedules this medication so that it is

Answer: 4
Rationale: Glyburide is an oral hypoglycemic agent that is administered once per day. It should be given 15 to 30 minutes before

administered at which of the following times?
1 At bedtime
2 With the noon meal
3 2 hours after breakfast
4 30 minutes before breakfast

Level of Cognitive Ability: Application
Client Needs: Physiological Integrity
Integrated Process: Nursing Process/Implementation
Content Area: Adult Health/Endocrine

breakfast to most effectively prevent postprandial hyperglycemia. The other options are incorrect.

Test-Taking Strategy: Use the process of elimination. Recalling that this medication is an oral hypoglycemic agent and that it should be given before the first meal of the day directs you to option 4. Review oral hypoglycemic therapy and glyburide if you had difficulty with this question.

Reference
Skidmore-Roth, L. (2009). *Mosby's drug guide for nurses* (8th ed., p. 458). St. Louis: Mosby.

---

767. A client with abdominal pain has a history of duodenal ulcer. To assist with determining whether the etiology of the pain is a recurrence of the ulcer, the nurse asks the client which of the following about the pain?
1 If it is relieved with eating
2 If it radiates down the right arm
3 If it is experienced just after a meal
4 If it is accompanied by nausea and vomiting

Level of Cognitive Ability: Application
Client Needs: Physiological Integrity
Integrated Process: Nursing Process/Data Collection
Content Area: Adult Health/Gastrointestinal

Answer: 1
Rationale: A duodenal ulcer is an ulcer in the duodenum. The most frequent manifestation of a duodenal ulcer is pain that is relieved by food intake. Clients with this condition generally describe the pain as a burning, heavy, sharp, or "hungry" pain that often localizes in the midepigastric area. Pain that occurs after a meal characterizes a gastric ulcer. Nausea and vomiting are also more typical in the client with a gastric ulcer. Option 2 is unrelated to a duodenal ulcer.

Test-Taking Strategy: Use the process of elimination. Eliminate option 2 first because it is unrelated to a duodenal ulcer. From the remaining options, recalling the differences between the symptoms of duodenal and gastric ulcer directs you to option 1. Review these differences if you had difficulty with this question.

Reference
Linton, A. (2007). *Introduction to medical-surgical nursing* (4th ed., p. 766). Philadelphia: Saunders.

---

768. A client has undergone esophagogastroduodenoscopy (EGD). The nurse checks which of the following items immediately upon the client's return to the clinical nursing unit?
1 Temperature
2 Return of the gag reflex
3 Complaints of heartburn
4 Complaints of a sore throat

Level of Cognitive Ability: Application
Client Needs: Physiological Integrity
Integrated Process: Nursing Process/Data Collection
Content Area: Delegating/Prioritizing

Answer: 2
Rationale: An EGD is an endoscopic test that permits the direct visualization of the upper gastrointestinal tract. The nurse immediately checks the return of the client's gag reflex, which protects the client's airway. The client's vital signs are also monitored. A sudden sharp increase in temperature could indicate the perforation of the gastrointestinal tract, which would be accompanied by other signs (e.g., pain). Monitoring for sore throat and heartburn is also important; however, the client's airway is still the priority.

Test-Taking Strategy: Use the process of elimination and the ABCs—airway, breathing, and circulation. Note that the question contains the strategic word *immediately.* This tells you that more than one or all of the options may be partially or totally correct. Review the care of the client after EGD if you had difficulty with this question.

Reference
Chernecky, C., & Berger, B. (2008). *Laboratory tests and diagnostic procedures* (5th ed., p. 484). Philadelphia: Saunders.

---

769. A nurse is checking for stoma retraction in a client who has recently undergone colostomy. The nurse should inspect to see if the stoma is:

1 Sunken and hidden
2 Protruding and swollen
3 Narrowed and flattened
4 Dark and bluish in color

Level of Cognitive Ability: Application
Client Needs: Physiological Integrity
Integrated Process: Nursing Process/Data Collection
Content Area: Adult Health/Gastrointestinal

Answer: 1

Rationale: Stoma retraction is characterized by the sinking of the stoma, which makes it harder to see. A prolapsed stoma is one in which bowel protrudes through the stoma, which causes an elongated and swollen appearance. A stoma with a narrowed opening at the level of either the skin or the fascia is said to be stenosed. Ischemia of the stoma would be associated with a dusky or bluish color.

Test-Taking Strategy: Use the process of elimination. Noting the strategic words *stoma retraction* assists with directing you to the correct option. Review the complications associated with a stoma if you had difficulty with this question.

Reference

Linton, A. (2007). *Introduction to medical-surgical nursing* (4th ed., p. 398). Philadelphia: Saunders.

---

770. A nurse reviews the record of a client who is scheduled for the removal of a skin lesion. The record indicates that the lesion is an irregularly shaped pigmented papule with a blue-toned color. The nurse interprets that the description of the lesion is characteristic of:

1 Actinic keratosis
2 Basal cell carcinoma
3 Malignant melanoma
4 Squamous cell carcinoma

Level of Cognitive Ability: Comprehension
Client Needs: Physiological Integrity
Integrated Process: Nursing Process/Data Collection
Content Area: Adult Health/Integumentary

Answer: 3

Rationale: A melanoma is an irregularly shaped pigmented papule or plaque with a red-, white-, or blue-toned color. Actinic keratosis, which is a premalignant lesion, appears as a small macule or papule with dry, rough, adherent yellow or brown scale. Basal cell carcinoma appears as a pearly papule with a central crater and rolled waxy border. Squamous cell carcinoma is a firm nodular lesion that is topped with a crust or a central area of ulceration.

Test-Taking Strategy: Knowledge of the characteristics of melanoma is necessary to answer this question. Recalling that these types of lesions are irregularly shaped will assist with directing you to the correct option. Review the characteristics of malignant skin lesions if you had difficulty with this question.

Reference

Christensen, B., & Kockrow, E. (2006). *Adult health nursing* (5th ed., pp. 100-101). St. Louis: Mosby.

---

771. A nurse is caring for a client with viral hepatitis. The client reports to the nurse that his appetite is poor and that the presence of food causes nausea. Which nursing intervention is appropriate?

1 Encourage the client to consume foods that are high in protein.
2 Encourage the client to consume a low-calorie diet with numerous snacks.
3 Encourage the client to consume the majority of calories during the morning hours.
4 Encourage the client to consume high-fat foods because they are usually better tolerated.

Answer: 3

Rationale: Hepatitis is an inflammatory condition of the liver. It is important to explain to the client that the majority of calories should be eaten during the morning hours because nausea most often occurs during the afternoon and evening. The nurse would also plan a referral to a nutritionist to assist the client with meal planning. Protein should be limited. Clients should select a diet that is high in calories and carbohydrates because energy is necessary for healing. Changes in bilirubin interfere with fat absorption, so low-fat diets are better tolerated in these clients.

Test-Taking Strategy: Use the process of elimination. Focus on the client's diagnosis and the data in the question to direct you to option 3. Review the care of the client with viral hepatitis if you had difficulty with this question.

Level of Cognitive Ability: Application
Client Needs: Physiological Integrity
Integrated Process: Nursing Process/Implementation
Content Area: Adult Health/Gastrointestinal

Reference

Black, J., & Hawks, J. (2009). *Medical-surgical nursing: Clinical management for positive outcomes* (8th ed., p. 1143). St. Louis: Saunders.

---

772. A nurse is collecting data from a client with Bell's palsy. Which finding should the nurse expect to note in the client?

1 Complaints of hearing loss
2 Complaints of dizziness and vertigo
3 Inability to close the eye on the affected side
4 The presence of muscle spasms in the jaw and cheek areas

Level of Cognitive Ability: Comprehension
Client Needs: Physiological Integrity
Integrated Process: Nursing Process/Data Collection
Content Area: Adult Health/Neurological

Answer: 3

Rationale: Bell's palsy is a unilateral paralysis of the facial nerve. With Bell's palsy, the client experiences weakness in one entire half of the face. The client is unable to close the eye on the affected side and experiences paralysis of the ipsilateral facial muscles. The client also experiences pain, drooling, decreased taste, and increased tearing. Tinnitus, vertigo, and deafness are not associated with Bell's palsy, but they may be seen with Ménière's disease. Muscle spasms in the jaw and cheek area are most likely associated with trigeminal neuralgia.

Test-Taking Strategy: Use the process of elimination. Note the strategic word *palsy* in the name of the diagnosis. This word should assist with directing you to option 3. Review the manifestations associated with Bell's palsy if you had difficulty with this question.

Reference

Christensen, B., & Kockrow, E. (2006). *Adult health nursing* (5th ed., p. 735). St. Louis: Mosby.

---

773. A nurse is assigned to care for a client who underwent an above-the-knee amputation of the right leg 2 days ago. The nurse assists with developing a plan of care and includes measures to prevent hip contractures. Which of the following should the nurse suggest be included in the plan of care?

1 Maintain a supine position.
2 Elevate the residual limb on a pillow.
3 Maintain a high-Fowler's position when the client is in bed.
4 Position the client on the abdomen for 30 minutes every 4 to 6 hours.

Level of Cognitive Ability: Application
Client Needs: Physiological Integrity
Integrated Process: Nursing Process/Planning
Content Area: Adult Health/Musculoskeletal

Answer: 4

Rationale: To prevent hip contractures after amputation, the client should be positioned on the abdomen for 30-minute periods every 4 to 6 hours. For the first 24 hours after amputation, the nurse should elevate the residual limb as prescribed to decrease swelling and promote comfort. Elevation is then performed at intervals because elevation for longer periods may cause flexion contractures of the hip.

Test-Taking Strategy: Use the process of elimination, and note the strategic words *2 days ago*. Focus on the subject—preventing hip contractures. Visualize each of the options to direct you to option 4. Review the care of the client after amputation if you had difficulty with this question.

References

Christensen, B., & Kockrow, E. (2006). *Adult health nursing* (5th ed., p. 187). St. Louis: Mosby.
Ignatavicius, D., & Workman, M. (2010). *Medical-surgical nursing: Patient-centered colaborative care* (6th ed., p. 1202). St. Louis: Saunders.

---

774. A client is receiving external radiation to the neck for cancer of the larynx. The nurse instructs the client that the most likely side effect to expect is:

Answer: 4

Rationale: In general, only the area in the treatment field is affected by radiation. Skin reactions, fatigue, nausea, and anorexia may occur with radiation to any site, whereas other

1 Dyspnea
2 Diarrhea
3 Headache
4 Sore throat

Level of Cognitive Ability: Application
Client Needs: Physiological Integrity
Integrated Process: Teaching and Learning
Content Area: Adult Health/Oncology

side effects occur only when specific areas are involved in treatment. A client who is receiving radiation to the larynx is most likely to experience a sore throat. Dyspnea may occur with lung involvement. Diarrhea may occur with radiation to the gastrointestinal tract. Headache may occur with radiation to the head.

Test-Taking Strategy: Use the process of elimination. Consider the anatomical location of the radiation therapy to direct you to option 4. Review the effects of radiation therapy if you had difficulty with this question.

References

deWit, S. (2009). *Medical-surgical nursing: Concepts & practice* (p. 175). St. Louis: Saunders.

Ignatavicius, D., & Workman, M. (2010). *Medical-surgical nursing: Patient-centered colaborative care* (6th ed., p. 420). St. Louis: Saunders.

---

775. A client with acute pancreatitis is experiencing severe pain from the disorder. The nurse should avoid placing the client in which of the following positions?

1 Recumbent
2 Semi-Fowler's
3 Side lying with legs flexed
4 Upright and leaning forward

Level of Cognitive Ability: Application
Client Needs: Physiological Integrity
Integrated Process: Nursing Process/Implementation
Content Area: Adult Health/Gastrointestinal

Answer: 1

Rationale: The pain of pancreatitis is aggravated by both lying supine and walking because the pancreas is located retroperitoneally, and the edema and inflammation intensify the irritation of the posterior peritoneal wall with these positions. Positions such as the semi-Fowler's position, being upright, leaning forward, and having the legs flexed (especially the left leg) may reduce some of the pain associated with pancreatitis.

Test-Taking Strategy: Use the process of elimination, and note the strategic word *avoid*. This word indicates a negative event query and asks you to select an option that is an incorrect position. Eliminate options 2 and 4 because they are comparable or alike. From the remaining options, visualize the pancreas and the potential effects of stretching associated with the various positions listed; this will direct you to option 1. Review pancreatitis if you had difficulty with this question.

Reference

Christensen, B., & Kockrow, E. (2006). *Adult health nursing* (5th ed., p. 278). St. Louis: Mosby.

---

776. A nurse is completing the preprocedural checklist before a client is sent for bronchoscopy. The nurse determines that the client is not adequately prepared for the procedure if which of the following is noted?

1 Dentures have been removed.
2 Sedation has been administered.
3 There is no signed informed consent.
4 The client has had nothing by mouth since midnight.

Level of Cognitive Ability: Comprehension
Client Needs: Physiological Integrity

Answer: 3

Rationale: Bronchoscopy is the visualization of the tracheobronchial tree with the use of a bronchoscope. The client must sign an informed consent because the procedure is invasive. The client is not allowed to eat or drink for 6 hours before the procedure. If the client wears contact lenses, dentures, or other prostheses, they are removed before the client receives preprocedural sedation.

Test-Taking Strategy: Use the process of elimination, and note the strategic words *not adequately prepared*. Recalling that this procedure is invasive and that invasive procedures require an informed consent directs you to option 3. Review preprocedural care before bronchoscopy if you had difficulty with this question.

Integrated Process: Nursing Process/Evaluation
Content Area: Adult Health/Respiratory

Reference

Chernecky, C., & Berger, B. (2008). *Laboratory tests and diagnostic procedures* (5th ed., p. 262). Philadelphia: Saunders.

---

777. A client is told that a tuberculin skin test yielded positive results and asks the nurse what this means. The nurse tells the client that the test results indicate which of the following?

1 No tuberculosis
2 Active tuberculosis
3 Exposure to tuberculosis
4 A history of tuberculosis

Level of Cognitive Ability: Application
Client Needs: Physiological Integrity
Integrated Process: Nursing Process/Implementation
Content Area: Adult Health/Respiratory

Answer: 3

Rationale: A test in a client who is not immunosuppressed and who is considered low risk is considered positive for tuberculosis if there is an area of induration that measures 10 mm or more. The reading is generally done 48 to 72 hours after the testing solution is planted in the forearm. A positive result indicates that the client has been exposed to tuberculosis and requires further diagnostic workup; it does not indicate the presence of active disease.

Test-Taking Strategy: To answer this question accurately, you must know the significance of positive results of tuberculosis skin testing. Remember that a positive result indicates that the client has been exposed to tuberculosis and requires further diagnostic workup. Review the procedure for interpreting tuberculin skin test results if you had difficulty with this question.

Reference

Christensen, B., & Kockrow, E. (2006). *Adult health nursing* (5th ed., p. 428). St. Louis: Mosby.

---

778. A client is wearing an oxygen cannula that delivers a flow rate of 2 L/min. The nurse is told that the physician has requested that a set of arterial blood gas (ABG) levels be drawn with the client breathing room air. The nurse interprets this to mean that there is a need to do which of the following with the oxygen?

1 Remove the oxygen just before the ABG levels are drawn.
2 Leave the oxygen unchanged when the ABG levels are drawn.
3 Remove the oxygen at least 1 hour before the ABG levels are drawn.
4 Change the oxygen cannula to a Venturi face mask before the ABG levels are drawn.

Level of Cognitive Ability: Comprehension
Client Needs: Physiological Integrity
Integrated Process: Nursing Process/Implementation
Content Area: Adult Health/Respiratory

Answer: 1

Rationale: A request for ABG levels drawn on room air indicates that the client should have the oxygen removed before the blood is drawn for these tests. When the physician is deciding whether to discontinue oxygen therapy, ABG levels will be obtained with the client breathing room air, and the levels will be evaluated to see how the client tolerates oxygen removal. Options 2, 3, and 4 are incorrect.

Test-Taking Strategy: Use the process of elimination. Noting the strategic words *room air* directs you to option 1. Review the procedures for obtaining ABG levels if you had difficulty with this question.

References

Black, J., & Hawks, J. (2009). *Medical-surgical nursing: Clinical management for positive outcomes* (8th ed., p. 181). St. Louis: Saunders.
Chernecky, C., & Berger, B. (2008). *Laboratory tests and diagnostic procedures* (5th ed., p. 213). Philadelphia: Saunders.

---

779. A client with emphysema has arterial blood gas (ABG) levels drawn. The results indicate a pH of 7.31. Based on this pH result, the nurse interprets that which condition is present?

Answer: 1

Rationale: Acidosis is defined as a pH of less than 7.35, whereas alkalosis is defined as a pH of more than 7.45. There are not adequate data in the question to determine compensation or decompensation.

1 Acidosis
2 Alkalosis
3 Compensation
4 Decompensation

Level of Cognitive Ability: Comprehension
Client Needs: Physiological Integrity
Integrated Process: Nursing Process/Data Collection
Content Area: Adult Health/Respiratory

Test-Taking Strategy: Use the process of elimination. Recalling the physiology related to the body pH directs you to option 1. Review the interpretation of ABG levels if you had difficulty with this question.

Reference

Christensen, B., & Kockrow, E. (2006). *Adult health nursing* (5th ed., p. 411). St. Louis: Mosby.

---

780. A nurse is caring for a child with erythema infectiosum (fifth disease). Which clinical manifestations does the nurse expect to note in this child?

1 Reddish, pinpoint petechiae on the soft palate
2 An intense, fiery red edematous rash on the cheeks
3 Small bluish-white spots with red bases on the buccal mucosa
4 A pinkish-red maculopapular rash on the face, neck, and scalp

Level of Cognitive Ability: Comprehension
Client Needs: Physiological Integrity
Integrated Process: Nursing Process/Data Collection
Content Area: Child Health

Answer: 2

Rationale: Erythema infectiosum is an acute benign infectious disease that occurs mainly during childhood and that is characterized by the presence of an intense, fiery red edematous rash on the cheeks that gives an appearance that the client with the condition has been slapped. Options 1 and 4 are clinical manifestations of rubella (German measles). Option 3 describes Koplik spots, which are found in clients with rubeola (red measles).

Test-Taking Strategy: Use the process of elimination. Recalling the slapped cheek appearance associated with erythema infectiosum directs you to the correct option. Review the clinical manifestations of erythema infectiosum if you had difficulty with this question.

Reference

Leifer, G. (2007). *Introduction to maternity and pediatric nursing* (5th ed., p. 713). Philadelphia: Saunders.

---

781. A nurse is caring for a child admitted to the hospital with nonspecific symptoms of headache, fever, anorexia, and restlessness. A rash is noted on the palms and soles of the child's feet and on the remainder of the child's body. The child is diagnosed with Rocky Mountain spotted fever (RMSF). Which medication does the nurse anticipate will be prescribed for the child?

1 Thioguanine
2 Thiotepa (Thioplex)
3 Ticlopidine hydrochloride (Ticlid)
4 Tetracycline hydrochloride (Sumycin)

Level of Cognitive Ability: Analysis
Client Needs: Physiological Integrity
Integrated Process: Nursing Process/Planning
Content Area: Pharmacology

Answer: 4

Rationale: RMSF is a tick-borne infectious disease. With early detection, tetracycline hydrochloride and chloramphenicol (Chloromycetin) have been found to be effective treatment. These medications inhibit the growth of the associated organism. However, if vascular damage has already occurred, the medications may not alter the course of the disease. Antibiotic therapy is continued until the child has had no fever for at least 2 to 3 days. The usual duration of therapy is 6 to 10 days. Thioguanine and thiotepa are antineoplastic medications. Ticlopidine hydrochloride is a platelet aggregation inhibitor.

Test-Taking Strategy: Knowledge regarding the treatment of RMSF is necessary to answer this question. If you are familiar with the classifications of the medications identified in the options, you will be directed to option 4. Tetracycline hydrochloride is the only antibiotic listed. Review the treatment of RMSF if you had difficulty with this question.

Reference

Hodgson, B., & Kizior, R. (2009). *Saunders nursing drug handbook 2009* (pp. 1118-1119). St. Louis: Saunders.

---

782. A nurse is caring for a child with human immunodeficiency virus (HIV). The nurse plans care based on which accurate description of this disorder?

1 It is a febrile generalized vasculitis of unknown etiology.
2 It is an acquired cell-mediated immunodeficiency disorder.
3 It is a chronic multisystem autoimmune disease that is characterized by the inflammation of the connective tissue.
4 It is an inflammatory autoimmune disease that affects the connective tissue of the heart, the joints, and the subcutaneous tissues.

Level of Cognitive Ability: Comprehension
Client Needs: Physiological Integrity
Integrated Process: Nursing Process/Planning
Content Area: Child Health

Answer: 2

Rationale: HIV infection is an acquired cell-mediated immunodeficiency disorder that causes a wide spectrum of illnesses in children, ranging from no symptoms to mild and moderate symptoms to severe symptoms. Acquired immunodeficiency syndrome represents the most severe illness that results from HIV infection. Option 1 identifies Kawasaki disease. Option 3 identifies systemic lupus erythematosus. Option 4 identifies rheumatic fever.

Test-Taking Strategy: Use the process of elimination, and focus on the subject—HIV infection. Note the relationship between immunodeficiency in the question and the correct option. Review information about HIV if you had difficulty with this question.

Reference

Price, D., & Gwin, J. (2008). *Pediatric nursing: An introductory text* (10th ed., p. 86). St. Louis: Saunders.

---

783. A nurse is collecting data about a child who is suspected of having rheumatic fever (RF). The nurse plans to obtain specific data about the child's recent illnesses and asks the parent which question?

1 "Has the child had a recent ear infection?"
2 "Has the child had a recent case of pneumonia?"
3 "Has the child had a recent case of otitis media?"
4 "Has the child had a recent streptococcal infection of the throat?"

Level of Cognitive Ability: Comprehension
Client Needs: Physiological Integrity
Integrated Process: Nursing Process/Data Collection
Content Area: Child Health

Answer: 4

Rationale: RF is a systemic inflammatory disease that characteristically presents 1 to 3 weeks after an untreated or partially treated group A beta-hemolytic streptococcal infection of the upper respiratory tract. The questions asked in options 1, 2, and 3 are not specifically related to RF, although they may be part of the data collection process.

Test-Taking Strategy: Use the process of elimination. Options 1 and 3 can be eliminated first because they are comparable or alike. From the remaining options, remember that RF can follow a streptococcal infection of the upper respiratory tract. Review the etiology of RF if you had difficulty with this question.

Reference

Price, D., & Gwin, J. (2008). *Pediatric nursing: An introductory text* (10th ed., pp. 308, 311). St. Louis: Saunders.

---

784. A nurse is preparing to care for a hospitalized child with rheumatic fever (RF) and is told that the child has erythema marginatum. Which of the following does the nurse expect to see documented in the child's record?

1 Involuntary movements of the legs, arms, and face
2 Inflammation of all parts of the heart, primarily the mitral valve

Answer: 4

Rationale: RF is a systemic inflammatory disease that may develop as a delayed reaction to an untreated or partially treated group A beta-hemolytic streptococcal infection of the upper respiratory tract. Erythema marginatum is a clinical manifestation of RF that is characterized by red skin lesions that start as flat or slightly raised macules (usually over the trunk) and that spread peripherally. Option 1 identifies chorea. Option 2 identifies carditis. Option 3 identifies polyarthritis.

3 Tender and painful joints, especially the elbows, knees, ankles, and wrists
4 Red skin lesions that started as flat or slightly raised macules over the trunk and that spread peripherally

Level of Cognitive Ability: Comprehension
Client Needs: Physiological Integrity
Integrated Process: Nursing Process/Data Collection
Content Area: Child Health

Test-Taking Strategy: Use the process of elimination. Noting the relationship between the words *erythema* in the question and *red* in option 4 assists you with answering this question. Review the manifestations of RF if you had difficulty with this question.

Reference

Leifer, G. (2007). *Introduction to maternity and pediatric nursing* (5th ed., p. 603). Philadelphia: Saunders.

---

785. The nurse reviews a child's health care record and notes that the laboratory values indicate a potassium level of 3.2 mEq/L. Which clinical manifestation does the nurse expect to note in this child?

1 Nausea
2 Muscle weakness
3 Increased bowel sounds
4 Elevated blood pressure

Level of Cognitive Ability: Analysis
Client Needs: Physiological Integrity
Integrated Process: Nursing Process/Data Collection
Content Area: Child Health

Answer: 2

Rationale: Hypokalemia is indicated by a potassium level of less than 3.5 mEq/L. Clinical manifestations include muscle weakness, paralysis, leg cramps, decreased bowel sounds, a weak and irregular pulse, and cardiac dysrhythmias (tachycardia or bradycardia). Clinical manifestations may also include hypotension, ileus, irritability, and fatigue. Nausea may or may not occur.

Test-Taking Strategy: Knowledge of the normal potassium level assists you with determining that the child is experiencing hypokalemia. Recall the clinical manifestations associated with hypokalemia to direct you to option 2. Remember that muscle weakness occurs in clients with hypokalemia. Review the manifestations of hypokalemia if you had difficulty with this question.

Reference

McKinney, E., James, S., Murray, S., & Ashwill, J. (2009). *Maternal-child nursing* (3rd ed., pp. 1069). St. Louis: Mosby.

---

786. A nurse is preparing to administer an intramuscular injection to an 11-year-old child. Which site should the nurse select as the best area for administering the injection?

1 Deltoid muscle
2 Ventral gluteal muscle
3 Anterolateral aspect of the thigh
4 Posterolateral aspect of the thigh

Level of Cognitive Ability: Application
Client Needs: Physiological Integrity
Integrated Process: Nursing Process/Implementation
Content Area: Child Health

Answer: 2

Rationale: The ventral gluteal site may be used for intramuscular injections in older children. In children who have not yet developed the gluteal muscle (those younger than 2 years of age), the preferred site for intramuscular injections is the anterolateral aspect of the thigh. The deltoid muscle can be used in children 18 months old or older; however, in an 11-year-old child, the ventral gluteal muscle is the preferred site. Option 4 is an inappropriate site for an injection.

Test-Taking Strategy: Use the process of elimination. Option 4 can be easily eliminated first. Note the age of the child in the question and the strategic word *best*. Visualize each of these body areas to help you to choose the correct option. Review the sites for intramuscular injections if you had difficulty with this question.

Reference

Price, D., & Gwin, J. (2008). *Pediatric nursing: An introductory text* (10th ed., p. 384). St. Louis: Saunders.

787. A nurse employed in a physician's office is administering immunizations to a child. The nurse ensures that which of the following is available as the priority item during the administration of a vaccine?

1 A 7/8-inch needle
2 Pediatric syringes
3 Epinephrine (Adrenalin)
4 Diphenhydramine hydrochloride (Benadryl)

Level of Cognitive Ability: Application
Client Needs: Physiological Integrity
Integrated Process: Nursing Process/Planning
Content Area: Delegating/Prioritizing

Answer: 3
Rationale: Any immunization may cause an anaphylactic reaction. All physicians' offices and clinics that administer immunizations must have epinephrine 1:1000 available. Pediatric syringes are needed to administer the immunization. Generally, a needle that is 7/8 of an inch or longer is adequate to administer immunizations for a normal 4-month-old infant. Diphenhydramine hydrochloride is not normally needed unless it is specifically prescribed by the physician. However, the priority item is the epinephrine.

Test-Taking Strategy: Use the process of elimination. Note the strategic word *priority,* and recall the risk associated with the potential for an anaphylactic reaction; this should direct you to option 3. Review the risks associated with the administration of immunizations if you had difficulty with this question.

Reference
Leifer, G. (2007). *Introduction to maternity and pediatric nursing* (5th ed., p. 720). Philadelphia: Saunders.

---

788. A nurse is monitoring a client with hypoparathyroidism for signs of hypocalcemia. The nurse wraps a blood pressure (BP) cuff around the client's upper arm, fills the cuff, and monitors for spasms of the wrist and the hand. The nurse documents the findings, knowing that this test signifies the presence of which of the following?

1 Homans' sign
2 Chvostek's sign
3 Trousseau's sign
4 Positive Allen's test

Level of Cognitive Ability: Comprehension
Client Needs: Physiological Integrity
Integrated Process: Nursing Process/Data Collection
Content Area: Adult Health/Endocrine

Answer: 3
Rationale: Hypocalcemia is a deficiency of calcium in the serum. Trousseau's sign occurs when spasms of the wrist and hand occur after the compression of the upper arm with a BP cuff. Homans' sign is the presence of pain in the calf area when the foot is dorsiflexed. Chvostek's sign is present when spasms of the facial muscles occur after a tap over a facial nerve, which signifies facial hyperirritability. Allen's test indicates adequate circulation to the hand before arterial blood gas levels are obtained.

Test-Taking Strategy: Use the process of elimination. Eliminate option 1 because this sign is noted in the client with thrombophlebitis. Eliminate option 4 because this test is performed to determine the adequacy of the circulation before drawing arterial blood gas levels. Knowledge of the techniques used for each of the remaining options directs you to option 3. Review the techniques used to elicit the listed diagnostic signs if you had difficulty with this question.

Reference
Christensen, B., & Kockrow, E. (2006). *Adult health nursing* (5th ed., p. 537). St. Louis: Mosby.

---

789. A client who experienced a single rib fracture 3 days earlier is breathing shallowly and splinting the injured area by leaning against a chair and other supports. The nurse plans care, knowing that the client is at risk for developing which complications of the injury?

1 Hemoptysis and fever
2 Atelectasis and pneumonia
3 Pneumothorax and infection
4 Deep vein thrombosis and atelectasis

Answer: 2
Rationale: The client with fractured ribs is predisposed to atelectasis and pneumonia because of the effects of shallow breathing, which leads to decreased coughing, the accumulation of secretions, and subsequent pneumonia. The client could have hemoptysis or pneumothorax at the time of injury if the rib pierced lung tissue or the pleural cavity, but these complications are not likely to occur beyond the first 24 to 48 hours after injury. Fever is a symptom rather than a complication. Deep vein thrombosis is often a result of immobility, which is not indicated in the question.

Level of Cognitive Ability: Comprehension
Client Needs: Physiological Integrity
Integrated Process: Nursing Process/Planning
Content Area: Adult Health/Respiratory

Test-Taking Strategy: Focus on the data in the question, and note the strategic words *shallowly and splinting*. These words tell you that the client is not fully expanding the lungs, which should lead you to conclude that the client is at risk for atelectasis and pneumonia. Review the fundamental principles of lung expansion if you had difficulty with this question.

Reference

Ignatavicius, D., & Workman, M. (2010). *Medical-surgical nursing: Patient-centered collaborative care* (6th ed., p. 698). St. Louis: Saunders.

---

790. A client is recovering from flail chest. The nurse determines that the client status is most favorable if which of the following respiratory data are noted?

1 Respiratory rate, 16 breaths per minute; oxygen saturation, 90%
2 Respiratory rate, 18 breaths per minute; oxygen saturation, 98%
3 Respiratory rate, 22 breaths per minute; oxygen saturation, 93%
4 Respiratory rate, 24 breaths per minute; oxygen saturation, 99%

Level of Cognitive Ability: Analysis
Client Needs: Physiological Integrity
Integrated Process: Nursing Process/Evaluation
Content Area: Adult Health/Respiratory

Answer: 2

Rationale: The normal respiratory rate ranges from 12 to 20 breaths per minute, whereas the normal oxygen saturation range is 95% to 100%. Options 1, 3, and 4 do not represent normal values. Option 2 is the only option that identifies values that fall within normal parameters.

Test-Taking Strategy: Use the process of elimination, and note the strategic words *most favorable*. Recall the normal respiratory rate and the normal oxygen saturation level to direct you to option 2. Review these normal values if you had difficulty with this question.

References

Christensen, B., & Kockrow, E. (2006). *Foundations of nursing* (5th ed., p. 252). St. Louis: Mosby.
Linton, A. (2007). *Introduction to medical-surgical nursing* (4th ed., p. 545). Philadelphia: Saunders.

---

791. A nurse is assisting with planning care for a client with a respiratory disorder. The highest priority of the nurse is to plan care that focuses on which of the following?

1 Conserving energy
2 Optimizing nutrition
3 Maintaining fluid balance
4 Preventing Valsalva's maneuver

Level of Cognitive Ability: Application
Client Needs: Physiological Integrity
Integrated Process: Nursing Process/Planning
Content Area: Adult Health/Respiratory

Answer: 1

Rationale: The care of the client with a respiratory disorder is focused on maintaining effective respirations and conserving energy. Nutrition and fluid balance are important, but energy conservation takes priority. Energy conservation conserves oxygen. Option 4 is unrelated to the subject of the question.

Test-Taking Strategy: Use the process of elimination, and note the strategic words *respiratory disorder* and *highest priority*. Recall that energy conservation conserves oxygen to direct you to option 1. Review the care to the client with a respiratory disorder if you had difficulty with this question.

Reference

Christensen, B., & Kockrow, E. (2006). *Adult health nursing* (5th ed., p. 450). St. Louis: Mosby.

---

792. A nurse is collecting urine for a culture and sensitivity screening for a 1-year-old child. The nurse attaches a urine specimen bag to the child's perineum after cleansing the perineum meticulously.

Answer: 2

Rationale: For infants and children who are not toilet trained, a urine specimen may be collected by attaching a bag to the perineum. The perineal area must be meticulously cleansed, and the specimen must be collected within 30 minutes. If

After 30 minutes, the nurse checks the child to see whether the specimen has been obtained and notes that the child has not voided. Which action is most appropriate?

1 Catheterize the child.
2 Change the urine collection bag.
3 Check in 1 hour to see whether the child has voided.
4 Notify the physician that the specimen cannot be obtained.

Level of Cognitive Ability: Application
Client Needs: Physiological Integrity
Integrated Process: Nursing Process/ Implementation
Content Area: Child Health

the child or infant does not void within 30 minutes, the bag should be changed. Urine can be collected by urethral catheterization, but this is not the best method because it may introduce bacteria into the bladder. It is not necessary to notify the physician.

Test-Taking Strategy: Use the process of elimination, and note the strategic words *culture and sensitivity.* Eliminate option 4 first because there is no indication that the physician should be notified. Eliminate option 1 next because of the invasive nature of this procedure. Focus on the strategic words to direct you to option 2. Review the procedure for obtaining a urine specimen for culture from an infant or a child if you had difficulty with this question.

Reference

Price, D., & Gwin, J. (2008). *Pediatric nursing: An introductory text* (10th ed., p. 377). St. Louis: Saunders.

---

793. A child is diagnosed with glomerulonephritis, and the child's mother asks the nurse what the diagnosis means. The nurse bases the response on which of the following?

1 It is a condition in which the child is unable to control bladder functions.
2 It is characterized by the inflammation of the capillaries in the glomerulus.
3 It occurs when one or both testes fail to descend through the inguinal canal and into the scrotal sac.
4 It is the backflow or reflux of urine from the bladder into the ureters and possibly into the kidneys.

Level of Cognitive Ability: Comprehension
Client Needs: Physiological Integrity
Integrated Process: Nursing Process/ Implementation
Content Area: Child Health

Answer: 2

Rationale: Glomerulonephritis is characterized by the inflammation of the capillaries in the glomerulus. It can result from different causes, such as an infection, a systemic disease process, or a primary defect in the glomerulus itself. Option 1 describes enuresis. Option 3 describes cryptorchidism. Option 4 describes vesicoureteral reflux.

Test-Taking Strategy: Use the process of elimination. Note the relationship between the words *glomerulonephritis* in the question and *glomerulus* in option 2. Review the physiology associated with glomerulonephritis if you had difficulty with this question.

Reference

Price, D., & Gwin, J. (2008). *Pediatric nursing: An introductory text* (10th ed., pp. 257-258). St. Louis: Saunders.

---

794. A client with rheumatoid arthritis has been prescribed 1000 mg of aspirin (acetylsalicylic acid) daily in divided doses, and the nurse has reinforced instructions with the client regarding the medication. Which statement by the client indicates the need for further instruction?

1 "I will watch for signs of bleeding."
2 "I will take the aspirin 1 hour before meals."

Answer: 2

Rationale: Aspirin (acetylsalicylic acid) is an anti-inflammatory medication. The client with rheumatoid arthritis may be prescribed a dose of aspirin of 1000 to 1600 mg per day. At these high doses, aspirin is frequently toxic. In addition, aspirin must be taken four times per day to sustain therapeutic blood levels, and such frequent doses often lead to problems with compliance with the medication regimen. Clients should be instructed to take aspirin with food and to watch for the clinical manifestations of gastrointestinal bleeding, easy bruising, and tinnitus (ringing in the ears).

3 "I will avoid activities that may cause bruising."
4 "I will call my doctor if ringing in my ears occurs."

Level of Cognitive Ability: Analysis
Client Needs: Physiological Integrity
Integrated Process: Teaching and Learning
Content Area: Pharmacology

Test-Taking Strategy: Use the process of elimination, and note the strategic words *need for further instruction*. These words indicate a negative event query and ask you to select an option that is an incorrect statement. Eliminate options 1 and 3 first because they are comparable or alike in that they both relate to the potential for bleeding. Select option 2 instead of option 4 as the answer because aspirin taken on an empty stomach can produce gastrointestinal irritation and possible bleeding. Review the teaching points related to the administration of aspirin if you had difficulty with this question.

Reference
Hodgson, B., & Kizior, R. (2009). *Saunders nursing drug handbook 2009* (p. 95). St. Louis: Saunders.

---

795. A nurse is caring for a large-for-gestational-age (LGA) infant and gathering data about the infant. A major complication associated with LGA infants can be observed when the nurse does which of the following?
1 Weighs the infant
2 Takes the infant's blood pressure
3 Tests the infant's blood glucose level
4 Measures the infant's head circumference

Level of Cognitive Ability: Comprehension
Client Needs: Physiological Integrity
Integrated Process: Nursing Process/Data Collection
Content Area: Maternity/Postpartum

Answer: 3
Rationale: An LGA infant is an infant whose fetal growth was accelerated and whose size and weight at birth fall above the ninetieth percentile of appropriate-for-gestational-age infants, whether delivered prematurely, at term, or later than term. LGA infants are at risk for hypoglycemia; this is a major metabolic complication associated with LGA infants, and it can cause brain damage. Although options 1, 2, and 4 are components of data collection, they are not associated with a major complication.

Test-Taking Strategy: Use the process of elimination. Recalling that the LGA infant is at risk for hypoglycemia directs you to option 3. In addition, noting the strategic words *major complication* assists you with answering the question correctly. Options 1, 2, and 4 are data collection techniques for any infant. Review the complications associated with the LGA infant if you had difficulty with this question.

Reference
Leifer, G. (2007). *Introduction to maternity and pediatric nursing* (5th ed., p. 343). Philadelphia: Saunders.

---

796. Hypospadias is diagnosed in a newborn infant, and the mother asks the nurse about the disorder. The nurse bases the response on which of the following?
1 It occurs when one or both testes fail to descend through the inguinal canal into the scrotal sac.
2 It is a congenital anomaly characterized by the extrusion of the urinary bladder to the outside of the body.
3 It is a congenital anomaly in which the actual opening of the urethral meatus is located on the dorsal surface of the penis.
4 It is a congenital anomaly in which the actual opening of the urethral meatus is below the normal placement on the glans penis.

Answer: 4
Rationale: Hypospadias is a congenital anomaly in which the actual opening of the urethral meatus is below the normal placement on the glans penis. Option 1 describes cryptorchidism. Option 2 describes bladder exstrophy. Option 3 describes epispadias.

Test-Taking Strategy: Use the process of elimination. Note the relationship between the prefix *hypo-* in the name of the disorder and the word *below* in the correct option; this will direct you to option 4. Review hypospadias if you had difficulty with the question.

Reference
Price, D., & Gwin, J. (2008). *Pediatric nursing: An introductory text* (10th ed., pp. 167-168). St. Louis: Saunders.

Level of Cognitive Ability: Comprehension
Client Needs: Physiological Integrity
Integrated Process: Nursing Process/Implementation
Content Area: Child Health

---

797. A nurse is reviewing the record of an infant admitted to the newborn nursery and notes that the physician has documented bladder exstrophy. Which of the following does the nurse expect to note in the infant?

1 Undescended or hidden testes
2 The urinary bladder on the outside of the body
3 The opening of the urethral meatus on the ventral side of the glans penis
4 The opening of the urethral meatus below the normal placement on the glans penis

Level of Cognitive Ability: Comprehension
Client Needs: Physiological Integrity
Integrated Process: Nursing Process/Data Collection
Content Area: Child Health

Answer: 2
Rationale: Bladder exstrophy is a congenital anomaly characterized by the extrusion of the urinary bladder to the outside of the body through a defect in the lower abdominal wall. Option 1 describes cryptorchidism. Option 3 describes epispadias. Option 4 describes hypospadias.

Test-Taking Strategy: Use the process of elimination. Note the relationship between the prefix *ex-* in the name of the disorder and the word *outside* in the correct option; this will direct you to option 2. Review bladder exstrophy if you had difficulty with this question.

Reference
Leifer, G. (2007). *Introduction to maternity and pediatric nursing* (5th ed., p. 663). Philadelphia: Saunders.

---

798. A nurse is reinforcing discharge instructions to the parents of a child who underwent a myringotomy with the insertion of tympanostomy tubes. Which of the following should the nurse include in the instructions?

1 Encourage the child to blow the nose gently.
2 If any reddish drainage occurs, call the physician immediately.
3 Notify the physician if the child complains of any pain or has a fever.
4 Allow the child to swim as long as it is in a chlorinated swimming pool.

Level of Cognitive Ability: Application
Client Needs: Physiological Integrity
Integrated Process: Teaching and Learning
Content Area: Child Health

Answer: 3
Rationale: A myringotomy is the surgical incision of the eardrum, which is performed to relieve pressure and to release pus or fluid from the middle ear. A small amount of reddish drainage is normal for the first few days after surgery; however, the parents should report any heavier bleeding or bleeding that occurs more than 3 days postoperatively. The parents should also be instructed to report any fever or increased pain. The child should not blow the nose for 7 to 10 days. Baths and lake water are potential sources of bacterial contamination, and chlorinated swimming pools can be irritative to the tympanic membranes. The child should place earplugs or cotton balls covered with petroleum jelly in the ears during baths and shampoos. Swimming is allowed only with earplugs and with a physician's approval. Diving and swimming deeply underwater are prohibited.

Test-Taking Strategy: Use the process of elimination. Note both the anatomical location of this surgical procedure and the strategic words *insertion of tympanostomy tubes* to direct you to option 3. Remember that a general teaching guideline is to notify the physician if a fever occurs. Review the teaching points related to myringotomy with the insertion of tympanostomy tubes if you had difficulty with this question.

Reference
McKinney, E., James, S., & Ashwill, J. (2009). *Maternal-child nursing* (3rd ed., pp. 1181). St. Louis: Mosby.

799. A nurse is assisting with preparing a plan of care for a client with hyperthyroidism and is instructing the client regarding dietary measures. Which of the following foods are included in the plan of care?

1 Those low in calories
2 Those high in calories
3 Those high in bulk and fiber
4 Those low in carbohydrates and fats

Level of Cognitive Ability: Application
Client Needs: Physiological Integrity
Integrated Process: Teaching and Learning
Content Area: Adult Health/Endocrine

Answer: 2
Rationale: Hyperthyroidism is a condition that is characterized by the hyperactivity of the thyroid gland. The client with hyperthyroidism is usually extremely hungry as a result of an increased metabolism. The client should be instructed to consume a high-calorie diet with six full meals a day. The client should be instructed to eat foods that are nutritious and that contain ample amounts of protein, carbohydrates, fats, and minerals. Clients should be discouraged from eating foods that increase peristalsis and thus result in diarrhea, such as highly seasoned, bulky, and fibrous foods.

Test-Taking Strategy: Use the process of elimination. Recalling that metabolic processes are increased in clients with this condition assists you with eliminating options 1, 3, and 4. Review the dietary measures for the client with hyperthyroidism if you had difficulty with this question.

Reference
deWit, S. (2009). *Medical-surgical nursing: Concepts & practice* (p. 894). St. Louis: Saunders.

---

800. A nurse has reinforced instructions to a mother regarding the care of her 10-year-old child with pharyngitis. Which statement by the mother indicates the need for further instruction?

1 "I should encourage my child to gargle with saline."
2 "I should apply warm compresses to my child's throat."
3 "Antibiotics should be taken for the entire prescribed course."
4 "I should bring my child to the clinic in 2 days for a repeat throat culture."

Level of Cognitive Ability: Comprehension
Client Needs: Physiological Integrity
Integrated Process: Teaching and Learning
Content Area: Child Health

Answer: 4
Rationale: Pharyngitis is an inflammation or infection of the pharynx that usually causes a sore throat. The older child may gargle with saline, and warm or cool compresses may be applied to the throat. Antibiotics should be taken for the entire prescribed course, even if the child is feeling better and is free of symptoms. A follow-up with a repeat throat culture may be ordered for 3 to 5 days after the course of antibiotics is completed.

Test-Taking Strategy: Note the strategic words *need for further instruction.* These words indicate a negative event query and ask you to select an option that is an incorrect statement. Use the process of elimination and general principles related to the effects of antibiotic therapy to answer the question. Careful reading of option 4 indicates that a throat culture after 2 days will provide useful information regarding the resolution of the infection; this is an incorrect statement. Review the teaching guidelines related to pharyngitis if you had difficulty with this question.

Reference
Leifer, G. (2007). *Introduction to maternity and pediatric nursing* (5th ed., pp. 574-575). Philadelphia: Saunders.

---

801. Fluids are prescribed for a child after a tonsillectomy. The nurse should offer which appropriate item to the child?

1 Ice cream
2 Apple juice
3 Orange juice
4 A carbonated beverage

Level of Cognitive Ability: Application
Client Needs: Physiological Integrity

Answer: 2
Rationale: A tonsillectomy is the surgical excision of the palatine tonsils, which is performed to prevent recurrent tonsillitis. Clear, cool liquids are offered to the child when the child is fully awake. Citrus, carbonated, and extremely hot or cold liquids are avoided because they irritate the throat. Milk and milk products, including puddings and ice cream, are avoided initially until the child has tolerated clear liquids well. This is done because milk products can coat the throat and cause the child to clear it, thus increasing the risk of bleeding.

Integrated Process: Nursing Process/Implementation
Content Area: Child Health

Test-Taking Strategy: Focus on the surgical procedure, and use the process of elimination. Eliminate option 4 first because of the word *carbonated.* Eliminate option 3 next because an orange is a citrus product. Eliminate option 1 because milk products can coat the throat and cause the child to attempt to clear it. Review nursing care after tonsillectomy if you had difficulty with this question.

Reference
Price, D., & Gwin, J. (2008). *Pediatric nursing: An introductory text* (10th ed., p. 249). St. Louis: Saunders.

---

802. Ribavirin (Virazole) is prescribed for a child with respiratory syncytial virus. The nurse prepares to administer this medication by which route?

1 Oral
2 Inhalation
3 Intravenous
4 Subcutaneous

Level of Cognitive Ability: Application
Client Needs: Physiological Integrity
Integrated Process: Nursing Process/Planning
Content Area: Child Health

Answer: 2
Rationale: Ribavirin is an antiviral respiratory medication that is used to inhibit viral replication. Administration is by the inhalation route via hood, face mask, or oxygen tent. It is not administered via the oral, intravenous, or subcutaneous routes.

Test-Taking Strategy: Knowledge of the route of administration of ribavirin is necessary to answer this question. Remember that this medication is administered via inhalation. Review ribavirin if you had difficulty with this question.

Reference
Leifer, G. (2007). *Introduction to maternity and pediatric nursing* (5th ed., p. 578). Philadelphia: Saunders.

---

803. A client seen in the health care clinic is scheduled for several diagnostic procedures. An abdominal aorta sonogram, a barium enema, an upper gastrointestinal (GI) series, and a small bowel series have been ordered. Which procedure should the nurse schedule first?

1 The barium enema
2 The upper GI series
3 The small bowel series
4 The abdominal aorta sonogram

Level of Cognitive Ability: Application
Client Needs: Physiological Integrity
Integrated Process: Nursing Process/Implementation
Content Area: Delegating/Prioritizing

Answer: 4
Rationale: The abdominal aorta sonogram should be performed before intestinal barium tests because the barium obstructs the view when the abdominal aorta sonogram is obtained. The tests identified in options 1, 2, and 3 involve the use of barium for the visualization of these organs.

Test-Taking Strategy: Use the process of elimination, and note the strategic word *first.* Note that options 1, 2, and 3 are comparable or alike in that they all involve the use of barium for the visualization of the associated organs. With this in mind, consider the effect of barium on the visualization of structures when a sonogram is performed. Review the diagnostic tests presented in the options if you had difficulty with this question.

Reference
Chernecky, C., & Berger, B. (2008). *Laboratory tests and diagnostic procedures* (5th ed., p. 84). Philadelphia: Saunders.

---

804. A nurse is assigned to care for a child with a diagnosis of atrial septal defect. The nurse plans care knowing that which of the following is characteristic of this type of defect?

1 It occurs because of the inappropriate fetal development of the endocardial cushions.

Answer: 3
Rationale: Atrial septal defect is an opening between the two atria that allows oxygenated blood and unoxygenated blood to mix. The left-to-right shunting of blood occurs because of higher pressure on the left side of the heart. Atrioventricular canal defect occurs as a result of the inappropriate fetal development of the endocardial cushions. Patent ductus arteriosus involves an artery that connects the aorta and the pulmonary artery during fetal life.

2 It involves an artery that connects the aorta and the pulmonary artery during fetal life.
3 It is an opening between the two atria, and it allows oxygenated and unoxygenated blood to mix.
4 It is an opening between the two ventricles, and it allows oxygenated and unoxygenated blood to mix.

Level of Cognitive Ability: Comprehension
Client Needs: Physiological Integrity
Integrated Process: Nursing Process/Planning
Content Area: Child Health

Ventricular septal defect is an opening between the two ventricles that allows oxygenated and unoxygenated blood to mix.

Test-Taking Strategy: Use the process of elimination. Noting the words *atrial* in the question and *atria* in the correct option will direct you to option 3. Review the characteristics of atrial septal defect if you had difficulty with this question.

Reference
Price, D., & Gwin, J. (2008). *Pediatric nursing: An introductory text* (10th ed., p. 94). St. Louis: Saunders.

---

805. A client has been prescribed isoniazid (INH) for the treatment of tuberculosis. While the client is receiving this medication, the nurse plans to monitor the results of the periodic measurement of which of the following?
1 Vision
2 Hepatic enzymes
3 Hemoglobin and hematocrit
4 Blood urea nitrogen (BUN) and creatinine

Level of Cognitive Ability: Analysis
Client Needs: Physiological Integrity
Integrated Process: Nursing Process/Data Collection
Content Area: Pharmacology

Answer: 2
Rationale: INH is an antitubercular medication. The client taking INH is at risk for hepatotoxicity. For this reason, the client's hepatic enzymes are measured before and periodically during medication therapy. The BUN and creatinine levels are measured during therapy with streptomycin, which is a nephrotoxic medication. Vision testing is performed during treatment with ethambutol (Myambutol). Streptomycin and ethambutol (Myambutol) are also antitubercular medications. The hemoglobin and hematocrit values are unrelated to the medication addressed in the question.

Test-Taking Strategy: Use the process of elimination. Knowledge of the various medications that are used to treat tuberculosis and their associated adverse or toxic effects is required to answer this question correctly. Remember that antitubercular the client who is taking INH is at risk for hepatotoxicity. Review medications if you had difficulty with this question.

Reference
Hodgson, B., & Kizior, R. (2009). *Saunders nursing drug handbook 2009* (pp. 631-633). St. Louis: Saunders.

---

806. A client is at risk for pulmonary embolism because of a postoperative state and immobility. The nurse monitors the client for which most common symptom of pulmonary embolism?
1 Dry cough
2 Diaphoresis
3 Apprehension
4 Sudden onset of chest pain

Level of Cognitive Ability: Analysis
Client Needs: Physiological Integrity
Integrated Process: Nursing Process/Data Collection
Content Area: Adult Health/Respiratory

Answer: 4
Rationale: A pulmonary embolism is the blockage of a pulmonary artery by fat, air, tumor tissue, or a thrombus that usually arises from a peripheral vein (most frequently one of the deep veins of the legs). The most common symptom of pulmonary embolism is a sudden onset of chest pain. The next most frequent symptoms are dyspnea and tachypnea. Other manifestations include tachycardia, diaphoresis, cough, fever, hemoptysis, and syncope.

Test-Taking Strategy: Use the process of elimination, and note the strategic words *most common*. Recall the manifestations associated with pulmonary embolism to direct you to option 4. Review these manifestations if you had difficulty with this question.

Reference
Christensen, B., & Kockrow, E. (2006). *Adult health nursing* (5th ed, p. 446). St. Louis: Mosby.

807. A nurse is preparing to administer quinapril hydrochloride (Accupril) to a client with hypertension. The nurse understands that this medication belongs to which medication classification?

1 Loop diuretic
2 Thiazide diuretic
3 Calcium-channel blocker
4 Angiotensin-converting enzyme (ACE) inhibitor

Level of Cognitive Ability: Comprehension
Client Needs: Physiological Integrity
Integrated Process: Nursing Process/Planning
Content Area: Pharmacology

Answer: 4
Rationale: Quinapril hydrochloride is an ACE inhibitor. It suppresses the renal angiotensin–aldosterone system and reduces peripheral arterial resistance and blood pressure. It is used for the treatment of hypertension, either alone or in combination with other antihypertensive agents. Quinapril hydrochloride is not a diuretic or a calcium-channel blocker.

Test-Taking Strategy: Use the process of elimination. Eliminate options 1 and 2 first because they are comparable or alike. From the remaining options, recall that most ACE inhibitor medication names end with *-pril;* this will direct you to option 4. Review the characteristics of ACE inhibitors if you had difficulty with this question.

Reference

Hodgson, B., & Kizior, R. (2009). *Saunders nursing drug handbook 2009* (p. 987). St. Louis: Saunders.

---

808. Quinidine (Quinaglute Dura-Tabs) is prescribed for a client. Which of the following should the nurse specifically plan to monitor before administering this medication?

1 Temperature
2 Respirations
3 Blood pressure
4 Pulse oximetry

Level of Cognitive Ability: Analysis
Client Needs: Physiological Integrity
Integrated Process: Nursing Process/Data Collection
Content Area: Pharmacology

Answer: 3
Rationale: Quinidine is an antidysrhythmic medication, so the blood pressure should be monitored before the medication is administered. Although temperature, respirations, and pulse oximetry may be components of the data collection process, monitoring the blood pressure is specific to the administration of this medication. The nurse would also check the rate and rhythm of the apical heart rate by listening and counting for 1 full minute.

Test-Taking Strategy: Knowledge of the actions and nursing interventions associated with the administration of this medication is necessary to answer this question. Recalling that quinidine is an antidysrhythmic medication will direct you to option 3. Review quinidine if you had difficulty with this question.

Reference

Hodgson, B., & Kizior, R. (2009). *Saunders nursing drug handbook 2009* (pp. 989-990). St. Louis: Saunders.

---

809. Quinine sulfate is prescribed for a client, and the client asks the nurse about the purpose of this medication. The nurse bases the response on the fact that this medication is classified as which of the following?

1 Antimalarial
2 Antimicrobial
3 Antispasmodic
4 Antidysrhythmic

Level of Cognitive Ability: Analysis
Client Needs: Physiological Integrity
Integrated Process: Nursing Process/Implementation
Content Area: Pharmacology

Answer: 1
Rationale: Quinine sulfate is an antimalarial, antimyotonic medication. Its antimalarial effect elevates the pH in the intracellular organelles of parasites, thus producing parasitic death. It relaxes the skeletal muscle by increasing the refractory period, decreasing the excitability of motor end plates, and affecting the distribution of calcium within the muscle fibers. Options 2, 3, and 4 are incorrect.

Test-Taking Strategy: Knowledge of the action of quinine sulfate is necessary to answer this question. Focus carefully on the name of the medication, and recall that it is an antimalarial, antimyotonic medication. Review the characteristics of quinine sulfate if you had difficulty with this question.

Reference

Hodgson, B., & Kizior, R. (2009). *Saunders nursing drug handbook 2009* (pp. 991-992). St. Louis: Saunders.

810. A client has been given instructions for taking nitrofurantoin (Macrodantin) in the oral suspension form. The nurse determines that the client does not fully understand the medication information given if the client states which of the following?

1 "This medication turns the urine a brownish color."
2 "I should rinse my mouth with water to avoid staining my teeth."
3 "If a dose is missed, I should double the dose at the next scheduled time."
4 "I should avoid driving while taking this medication because it can cause dizziness."

Level of Cognitive Ability: Analysis
Client Needs: Physiological Integrity
Integrated Process: Teaching and Learning
Content Area: Adult Health/Renal

Answer: 3

Rationale: Nitrofurantoin (Macrodantin) is an antibacterial medication that is used to treat urinary tract infections. Doses should not be skipped or doubled. The client should avoid driving until tolerance to the medication is known because the medication can cause dizziness and drowsiness. It is recommended that the client rinse the mouth with water after a dose because the oral suspension may stain the teeth. The medication does discolor the urine, but this is not significant.

Test-Taking Strategy: Use the process of elimination, and note the strategic words *does not fully understand.* These words indicate a negative event query and ask you to select an option that is an incorrect statement. Knowledge of general principles regarding client instructions related to medication therapy will direct you to option 3. Review nitrofurantoin if you had difficulty with this question.

Reference

Hodgson, B., & Kizior, R. (2009). *Saunders nursing drug handbook 2009* (pp. 837-839). St. Louis: Saunders.

---

811. A licensed practical nurse (LPN) is assisting with developing a plan of care for a pregnant woman with an amniotic fluid embolism (AFE). The registered nurse has formulated a nursing diagnosis of *Impaired gas exchange* related to blockage of the lungs from AFE. Which outcome should the LPN consider appropriate for this client?

1 The woman will verbalize an understanding of the complications of AFE.
2 The woman will demonstrate a normal cardiac rate, blood pressure, and skin color.
3 The woman will demonstrate an effective respiratory rate and have a normal gas exchange.
4 The woman will show no complications of hemorrhage, hypovolemia, or disseminated intravascular coagulation.

Level of Cognitive Ability: Analysis
Client Needs: Physiological Integrity
Integrated Process: Nursing Process/Planning
Content Area: Maternity/Antepartum

Answer: 3

Rationale: Impaired gas exchange is defined as an excess or deficit of oxygenation, carbon dioxide elimination, or both at the alveolar–capillary membrane. Option 3 identifies the appropriate outcome for the nursing diagnosis of *Impaired gas exchange.* Option 1 relates to *Deficient knowledge,* option 2 relates to *Impaired tissue perfusion,* and option 4 relates to *Risk for deficient fluid volume.*

Test-Taking Strategy: Use the process of elimination. Focus on the strategic words *impaired gas exchange* and use the ABCs—airway, breathing, and circulation—to direct you to option 3. Also note the relationship between the words *Impaired gas exchange* in the question and *normal gas exchange* in option 3. Review the care of the client with AFE if you had difficulty with this question.

Reference

Leifer, G. (2007). *Introduction to maternity and pediatric nursing* (5th ed., p. 197). Philadelphia: Saunders.

---

812. A mother is admitted to the postpartum unit after the delivery of a healthy newborn. During the immediate postpartum period, how often does the nurse plan to take the mother's vital signs?

Answer: 1

Rationale: During the immediate postpartum period, vital signs are normally taken every 15 minutes during the first hour after birth, every 30 minutes for the next 2 hours, and every hour for the next 2 to 6 hours or as designated by agency policy. The

1 Every 15 minutes during the first hour after birth
2 Every 30 minutes during the first hour after birth
3 When the client arrives at the unit and 60 minutes later
4 When the client arrives at the unit and every 4 hours thereafter

Level of Cognitive Ability: Application
Client Needs: Physiological Integrity
Integrated Process: Nursing Process/Planning
Content Area: Maternity/Postpartum

vital signs are monitored thereafter every 4 hours for the first 24 hours and every 8 to 12 hours for the remainder of the hospital stay.

Test-Taking Strategy: Use the process of elimination, and note the strategic words *immediate postpartum* in the question. This should direct you to option 1 because this option addresses the most frequent time frame for monitoring the vital signs. Review postpartum assessments if you had difficulty with this question.

Reference
McKinney, E., James, S., Murray, S., & Ashwill, J. (2009). *Maternal-child nursing* (3rd ed., pp 462, 465). St. Louis: Mosby.

---

813. A nurse is monitoring the vital signs of a client after the delivery of a healthy newborn and notes that the mother's apical pulse rate is 50 beats/min. Based on this finding, the nurse should take which appropriate action?
1 Increase oral fluids.
2 Notify the physician.
3 Document the finding.
4 Encourage the mother to ambulate and then reassess the apical pulse.

Level of Cognitive Ability: Application
Client Needs: Physiological Integrity
Integrated Process: Nursing Process/Implementation
Content Area: Maternity/Postpartum

Answer: 3
Rationale: During the first week after birth, transient episodes of bradycardia are common. The woman's pulse may be as low as 40 to 50 beats/min for the first 1 to 2 days after delivery. It is not necessary to notify the physician. Options 1, 2, and 4 are not related to the data in the question.

Test-Taking Strategy: Use the process of elimination, and focus on the data in the question. Recall the normal findings during the postpartum period to direct you to option 3. Review normal postpartum assessment findings if you had difficulty with this question.

Reference
McKinney, E., James, S., Murray, S., & Ashwill, J. (2009). *Maternal-child nursing* (3rd ed., p. 465). St. Louis: Mosby.

---

814. A nurse is caring for a woman in the postpartum unit. When the nurse checks the position of the client's fundus, the nurse notes that it is displaced to one side. Based on this finding, the nurse should take which appropriate action?
1 Encourage fluids.
2 Massage the fundus.
3 Notify the physician.
4 Assist the client with emptying her bladder.

Level of Cognitive Ability: Application
Client Needs: Physiological Integrity
Integrated Process: Nursing Process/Implementation
Content Area: Maternity/Postpartum

Answer: 4
Rationale: The position of the fundus should be midline; displacement to the side indicates that the bladder may be full. The administration of fluids is important during the postpartum period, but this action is unrelated to the subject of the question. Fundal massage is performed when the uterus is soft and boggy. It is not necessary to notify the physician.

Test-Taking Strategy: Use the process of elimination. Focus on the information provided in the question to direct you to option 4. Remember that the position of the fundus should be midline and that displacement to the side indicates that the bladder may be full. Review normal postpartum assessment findings if you had difficulty with this question.

Reference
Leifer, G. (2008). *Maternity nursing: An introductory text* (10th ed., p. 227). Philadelphia: Saunders.

815. A nurse is assigned to care for a client with acquired immunodeficiency syndrome (AIDS) and notes that a nursing diagnosis of *Risk for infection* is documented in the client's care plan. The nurse determines that the client has not yet met expected outcomes if the client demonstrates which of the following?

1. Has negative urine and sputum cultures
2. Maintains a body temperature of less than 99° F
3. Has a shift to the left in white blood cells (WBCs)
4. Has a blood pressure (BP) of 128/86 mm Hg and a pulse rate of 82 breaths/min

Level of Cognitive Ability: Analysis
Client Needs: Physiological Integrity
Integrated Process: Nursing Process/Evaluation
Content Area: Adult Health/Respiratory

Answer: 3

Rationale: Signs of infection include a fever of more than 100° F; increased pulse and BP rates; a high WBC count with a shift to the left, which indicates the rapid proliferation of WBCs; and positive cultures for things such as wounds, urine, sputum, or blood. If the client meets the expected outcomes, then he or she is free of the signs and symptoms of infection.

Test-Taking Strategy: Note the strategic words *has not yet met.* These words indicate a negative event query and ask you to select an option that indicates infection. Use the process of elimination, and remember the basic concepts related to infection. Note that options 1, 2, and 4 are relatively normal findings. Review the indications of infection if you had difficulty with this question.

References

deWit, S. (2009). *Medical-surgical nursing: Concepts & practice* (p. 251). St. Louis: Saunders.

Ignatavicius, D., & Workman, M. (2010). *Medical-surgical nursing: Patient-centered collaborative care* (6th ed., pp. 373, 375). St. Louis: Saunders.

Linton, A. (2007). *Introduction to medical-surgical nursing* (4th ed., p. 624). Philadelphia: Saunders.

---

816. A client with emphysema is at risk for infection related to chronic respiratory disease. The nurse collects data regarding which factor that predisposes this client to infection?

1. Limited fluid intake
2. Pursed-lip breathing
3. Avoidance of crowds
4. Controlled cough technique

Level of Cognitive Ability: Comprehension
Client Needs: Physiological Integrity
Integrated Process: Nursing Process/Data Collection
Content Area: Adult Health/Respiratory

Answer: 1

Rationale: Emphysema is an abnormal condition of the pulmonary system that is characterized by overinflation and destructive changes in the alveolar walls. It results in a loss of lung elasticity and decreased gas exchange. A limited fluid intake can predispose the client to dehydration and respiratory infection because dehydration impairs the action of the cilia in the respiratory tree. Pursed-lip breathing and controlled cough technique are taught to clients to help make breathing easier and to assist with the expectoration of secretions. The avoidance of crowds is an important measure to prevent infection in the client with emphysema.

Test-Taking Strategy: Use the process of elimination and knowledge of the risk factors that predispose the client with emphysema to infection. Eliminate options 2 and 4 because these are comparable or alike in that they are breathing techniques. Recalling the effect of limiting fluid intake directs you to option 1 from the remaining options. Review the predisposing risk factors for infection if you had difficulty with this question.

Reference

Christensen, B., & Kockrow, E. (2006). *Adult health nursing* (5th ed., p. 452). St. Louis: Mosby.

---

817. A client is diagnosed with polycythemia vera and asks the nurse about the disorder. The nurse plans to base the response on which characteristic of this condition?

Answer: 2

Rationale: Polycythemia vera is defined as an increase in both the number of circulating erythrocytes and the concentration of hemoglobin within the blood. It is classified as a myeloproliferative disorder, which means that there is an overgrowth of bone

1 It occurs as a result of a hereditary factor.
2 It is classified as a myeloproliferative disorder.
3 It occurs as a result of a lack of the intrinsic factor.
4 It is an anemia that occurs as the result of poor iron intake.

Level of Cognitive Ability: Comprehension
Client Needs: Physiological Integrity
Integrated Process: Teaching and Learning
Content Area: Fundamental Skills

marrow. It usually develops in middle-aged people, particularly Jewish men. The cause remains unknown, although it is possibly a form of malignancy similar to leukemia. It is often considered a premalignant condition, and it is sometimes referred to as myeloproliferative dyscrasia. A lack of the intrinsic factor produces pernicious anemia. Iron deficiency anemia occurs as a result of a poor intake of iron.

Test-Taking Strategy: Use the process of elimination, and focus on the name of the disorder to answer the question. Note the relationship between the word *polycythemia* in the question and *myeloproliferative* in option 2. Review polycythemia if you had difficulty with this question.

Reference
Christensen, B., & Kockrow, E. (2006). *Adult health nursing* (5th ed., p. 304). St. Louis: Mosby.

---

818. A nurse is caring for a client with a diagnosis of suspected leukemia. The nurse prepares the client for which test that will confirm this diagnosis?
1 Lumbar puncture
2 Lymphangiogram
3 Radiographic tests
4 Bone marrow aspiration biopsy

Level of Cognitive Ability: Application
Client Needs: Physiological Integrity
Integrated Process: Nursing Process/Planning
Content Area: Adult Health/Oncology

Answer: 4
Rationale: Leukemia is a malignant disease that is characterized by the diffuse replacement of bone marrow with proliferating leukocyte precursors; abnormal numbers and forms of immature white blood cells in the circulation; and the infiltration of the lymph nodes, spleen, and liver. Bone marrow aspiration biopsy is a strategic diagnostic tool for confirming the diagnosis of leukemia and for identifying malignant cell types. Lumbar puncture may determine the presence of blast cells in the central nervous system. A lymphangiogram may be performed to locate malignant lesions and to accurately classify the disease. Radiographic tests may detect lesions and sites of infection.

Test-Taking Strategy: Use the process of elimination. Focus on the strategic word *confirm* to direct you to option 4. Review the diagnostic tests for leukemia if you had difficulty with this question.

Reference
Christensen, B., & Kockrow, E. (2006). *Adult health nursing* (5th ed., p. 307). St. Louis: Mosby.

---

819. A nurse is caring for a client who is receiving chemotherapy for leukemia. The nurse reviews the laboratory results and notes that the client's neutrophil count is less than $500/mm^3$. Based on this laboratory result, the nurse should implement which intervention for the client?
1 Using an electric shaver for shaving
2 Providing a soft toothbrush for oral care
3 Providing meticulous skin decontamination before venipuncture
4 Avoiding overinflation of the blood pressure (BP) cuff and rotating the cuff to different sites when checking the BP

Answer: 3
Rationale: Leukemia is a malignant disease that is characterized by the diffuse replacement of bone marrow with proliferating leukocyte precursors; abnormal numbers and forms of immature white blood cells in the circulation; and the infiltration of the lymph nodes, spleen, and liver. Chemotherapy causes neutropenia and other blood dyscrasias. When the neutrophil count is less than $1000/mm^3$, the client is at risk for infection. Options 1, 2, and 4 address nursing interventions if the client is at risk for bleeding. Providing meticulous skin decontamination before venipuncture, maintaining sterile occlusion of intravenous and central venous catheters, and monitoring the oral temperature are critical nursing interventions for the client who is at risk for infection.

Level of Cognitive Ability: Application
Client Needs: Physiological Integrity
Integrated Process: Nursing Process/Implementation
Content Area: Adult Health/Oncology

Test-Taking Strategy: Use the process of elimination. Recalling the relationship between a low neutrophil count and the risk for infection assists with directing you to option 3. Review the nursing plan of care for a client with leukemia if you had difficulty with this question.

Reference

Christensen, B., & Kockrow, E. (2006). *Adult health nursing* (5th ed., p. 310). St. Louis: Mosby.

---

820. A pregnant client arrives at the prenatal clinic and is complaining that her breasts are very tender. She is concerned about what is causing this discomfort. The nurse plans to base the response to the client on the fact that tender breasts during pregnancy occur as a result of which of the following?

1 Increased levels of prolactin
2 Decreased levels of prolactin
3 Increased levels of estrogen and progesterone
4 Decreased levels of estrogen and progesterone

Level of Cognitive Ability: Comprehension
Client Needs: Physiological Integrity
Integrated Process: Nursing Process/Planning
Content Area: Maternity/Antepartum

Answer: 3

Rationale: The breasts become tender early in pregnancy because of increased levels of estrogen and progesterone. Self-care measures for breast tenderness include sleeping with a pillow and wearing a well-fitting brassiere that provides support for the breasts and that decreases discomfort. Breast tenderness is not due to increased or decreased levels of prolactin or to decreased levels of estrogen and progesterone.

Test-Taking Strategy: Knowledge of the physiological alterations that occur during pregnancy assists you with answering this question. Remember that the breasts become tender early in pregnancy because of increased levels of estrogen and progesterone. Review the hormonal changes that occur as a result of pregnancy if you had difficulty with this question.

Reference

Leifer, G. (2008). *Maternity nursing: An introductory text* (10th ed., p. 47). Philadelphia: Saunders.

---

821. A client has just been told by the physician that a cerebral angiogram will be obtained. The nurse will then need to collect data from the client regarding which condition?

1 Allergy to eggs
2 Claustrophobia
3 Excessive weight
4 Allergy to iodine or shellfish

Level of Cognitive Ability: Application
Client Needs: Physiological Integrity
Integrated Process: Nursing Process/Data Collection
Content Area: Fundamental Skills

Answer: 4

Rationale: An angiography is the visualization of the internal anatomy of the blood vessels after the introduction of a radiopaque contrast material. The client undergoing angiography is assessed for possible allergy to the contrast dye, which can be determined by questioning the client about allergies to iodine or shellfish. Allergy to eggs is irrelevant to this test. Claustrophobia and excessive weight are areas of concern with magnetic resonance imaging.

Test-Taking Strategy: Use the process of elimination. Remember that a primary concern is allergy to iodine or shellfish; this concept is fundamental for angiography of any group of blood vessels. Review angiography if you had difficulty with this question.

Reference

Chernecky, C., & Berger, B. (2008). *Laboratory tests and diagnostic procedures* (5th ed., p. 310). Philadelphia: Saunders.

---

822. A client is being prepared for a lumbar puncture. The nurse assists the client into which position for the procedure?

Answer: 4

Rationale: The client undergoing a lumbar puncture is positioned lying on his or her side with the legs pulled up against

1 Side lying, with a pillow under the hip
2 Prone, with a pillow under the abdomen
3 Prone, in slight Trendelenburg's position
4 Side lying, with the legs pulled up and the head bent down onto the chest

Level of Cognitive Ability: Application
Client Needs: Physiological Integrity
Integrated Process: Nursing Process/Implementation
Content Area: Adult Health/Neurological

the abdomen and with the head bent down toward the chest. This position helps to widen the spaces between the vertebrae. The positions identified in options 1, 2, and 3 will not widen the spaces between the vertebrae.

Test-Taking Strategy: Use the process of elimination. Because a lumbar puncture is the introduction of a needle into the subarachnoid space, it is reasonable to assume that the position of the client must facilitate this. The correct option is the only position that flexes the vertebrae for easier needle insertion. Review lumbar puncture if you had difficulty with this question.

Reference

Chernecky, C., & Berger, B. (2008). *Laboratory tests and diagnostic procedures* (5th ed., p. 730). Philadelphia: Saunders.

---

823. A nurse notes fine involuntary movements of a client's eyes. The nurse documents in the medical record that the client has which of the following?
1 Ataxia
2 Nystagmus
3 Pronator drift
4 Hyperreflexia

Level of Cognitive Ability: Application
Client Needs: Physiological Integrity
Integrated Process: Communication and Documentation
Content Area: Adult Health/Neurological

Answer: 2
Rationale: Nystagmus is characterized by fine involuntary eye movements. Ataxia is a disturbance in gait. Pronator drift occurs when a client cannot maintain the hands in a supinated position with the arms extended and the eyes closed; this data collection technique may be done to detect small changes in muscle strength that might not otherwise be noted. Hyperreflexia is an excessive reflex action.

Test-Taking Strategy: To answer this question accurately, you must be familiar with abnormal findings of the neurological system. Remember that nystagmus is characterized by fine involuntary eye movements. Review the description of nystagmus if you had difficulty with this question.

Reference

Christensen, B., & Kockrow, E. (2006). *Adult health nursing* (5th ed., pp. 714-715). St. Louis: Mosby.

---

824. A nurse is caring for a client with a cerebellar lesion. The nurse plans to obtain which device to assist the client with adapting to this problem?
1 Walker
2 Slider board
3 Raised toilet seat
4 Adaptive eating utensils

Level of Cognitive Ability: Application
Client Needs: Physiological Integrity
Integrated Process: Nursing Process/Planning
Content Area: Adult Health/Neurological

Answer: 1
Rationale: The cerebellum is responsible for balance and coordination. A walker provides stability for the client during ambulation. A slider board is useful for transferring a client who cannot move from a bed to a stretcher or wheelchair. A raised toilet seat is useful if the client does not have the mobility or ability to flex the hips. Adaptive eating utensils may be useful if the client has partial paralysis of the hand.

Test-Taking Strategy: Use the process of elimination. Recalling that the cerebellum controls balance and coordination will assist you with answering this question. Look for the option that will assist the client in one of these areas; this helps you to eliminate options 2 and 3. From the remaining options, recall that adaptive eating utensils are used when there is a loss of fine motor coordination (e.g., after a stroke). The walker will help the client to maintain balance. Review the care of the client with a cerebellar lesion if you had difficulty with this question.

References
Christensen, B., & Kockrow, E. (2006). *Adult health nursing* (5th ed., p. 688). St. Louis: Mosby.
deWit, S. (2009). *Medical-surgical nursing: Concepts & practice* (p. 779). St. Louis: Saunders.

---

825. A client with Bell's palsy has a dysfunction of cranial nerve VII. The nurse monitors the client for which sign and symptom of this disorder?
1 Facial droop and excessive drooling
2 Double vision and excessive tearing
3 Eye pain and heightened sense of taste
4 Sharp facial pain and muscle twitching

Level of Cognitive Ability: Analysis
Client Needs: Physiological Integrity
Integrated Process: Nursing Process/Data Collection
Content Area: Adult Health/Neurological

Answer: 1
Rationale: The facial nerve (cranial nerve VII) has both motor and sensory divisions. Common symptoms of dysfunction of this nerve include an inability to close the eye or to blink automatically; facial asymmetry; drooling and the inability to swallow secretions; the loss of the ability to form tears; and a possible loss of taste on the anterior two thirds of the tongue. Bell's palsy, fracture of the temporal bone, and parotid lacerations or contusions are often responsible for these symptoms. Options 2, 3, and 4 do not occur as a result of a dysfunction of the facial nerve.

Test-Taking Strategy: Questions related to cranial nerves are difficult unless you know the differences among these nerves. If you remember that cranial nerve VII is the facial nerve, you can eliminate each of the incorrect options. Review Bell's palsy if you had difficulty with this question.

Reference
Christensen, B., & Kockrow, E. (2006). *Adult health nursing* (5th ed., p. 735). St. Louis: Mosby.

---

826. A pregnant client arrives at a prenatal clinic for a regularly scheduled prenatal visit. The client tells the nurse that she has been having a clear and slightly whitish vaginal discharge. Which action by the nurse is appropriate?
1 Obtain a culture of the vaginal discharge.
2 Inform the client that she should see the physician immediately.
3 Inform the client that this is a common occurrence during pregnancy.
4 Inform the client that sexual intercourse should be avoided until the discharge has been further evaluated.

Level of Cognitive Ability: Application
Client Needs: Physiological Integrity
Integrated Process: Nursing Process/Implementation
Content Area: Maternity/Antepartum

Answer: 3
Rationale: Vaginal discharge called leukorrhea is common in pregnant women because of the increased mucus production by the endocervical gland. The mucus should be clear or slightly whitish and mucoid in appearance. Option 1 is unnecessary. Option 2 is unnecessary and may alarm the client. Option 4 is inaccurate based on the subject stated in the question.

Test-Taking Strategy: Use the process of elimination. Recall that a clear or slightly whitish vaginal discharge is normal during pregnancy to direct you to option 3. Review the physiological changes that occur during pregnancy if you had difficulty with this question.

Reference
Leifer, G. (2008). *Maternity nursing: An introductory text* (10th ed., p. 68). Philadelphia: Saunders.

---

827. A pregnant woman is suspected of alcohol abuse, and the nurse checks the client for clinical manifestations associated with this practice. Which of the

Answer: 4
Rationale: Clinical manifestations that are indicative of alcohol abuse during the prenatal period include poor weight gain, hypoglycemia, tremors at rest, nausea, weakness, anxiety, slurred

following would least likely be noted in the client?

1 Sweating
2 Slurred speech
3 Hypoglycemia
4 Increased weight gain

Level of Cognitive Ability: Comprehension
Client Needs: Physiological Integrity
Integrated Process: Nursing Process/Data Collection
Content Area: Maternity/Antepartum

speech, unsteady gait, obvious sweating of the palms and forehead, and generalized sweating.

Test-Taking Strategy: Use the process of elimination. Focus on the strategic words *least likely* and the subject of the question to direct you to option 4. Review alcohol abuse during pregnancy if you had difficulty with this question.

Reference

McKinney, E., James, S., Murray, S., & Ashwill, J. (2009). *Maternal-child nursing* (3rd ed., p. 277). St. Louis: Mosby.

---

828. A nurse is checking for the presence of pitting edema in a prenatal client. The nurse presses the tips of the index and middle fingers against the skin of the client and holds pressure for 2 to 3 seconds. Upon releasing the pressure, the nurse notes a slight indentation. Which determination should the nurse make based on this finding?

1 1+ edema
2 2+ edema
3 3+ edema
4 4+ edema

Level of Cognitive Ability: Comprehension
Client Needs: Physiological Integrity
Integrated Process: Nursing Process/Data Collection
Content Area: Maternity/Antepartum

Answer: 1

Rationale: After assessment for pitting edema, if the nurse notes a slight indentation, then the condition is documented as 1+ edema. A determination of 2+ edema is made if the indentation is approximately 1/4-inch deep. The presence of 3+ edema is noted if the indentation is approximately 1/2-inch deep, and 4+ edema is present if the indentation is approximately 1-inch deep.

Test-Taking Strategy: Use the process of elimination. Focus on the strategic words *slight indentation;* this should direct you to option 1. Review data collection for and the evaluation of pitting edema if you had difficulty with this question.

References

Leifer, G. (2007). *Introduction to maternity and pediatric nursing* (5th ed., p. 91). Philadelphia: Saunders.
McKinney, E., James, S., Murray, S., & Ashwill, J. (2009). *Maternal-child nursing* (3rd ed., p. 623). St. Louis: Mosby.

---

829. A nurse is caring for a client with a diagnosis of chronic pancreatitis. The nurse collects data about the client, knowing that which symptom indicates the poor absorption of dietary fats?

1 Steatorrhea
2 Bloody diarrhea
3 Electrolyte disturbances
4 Gastrointestinal reflux disease

Level of Cognitive Ability: Comprehension
Client Needs: Physiological Integrity
Integrated Process: Nursing Process/Data Collection
Content Area: Adult Health/Gastrointestinal

Answer: 1

Rationale: Pancreatitis is an inflammatory condition of the pancreas that may be acute or chronic. The pancreas makes digestive enzymes that aid in the absorption of food and nutrients. Chronic pancreatitis interferes with the absorption of nutrients. Fat absorption is limited because of the lack of pancreatic lipase. Steatorrhea involves fatty stools that often result from malabsorption problems. Options 2, 3, and 4 are incorrect.

Test-Taking Strategy: Use the process of elimination, and focus on the client's diagnosis. Recall the definition of steatorrhea to direct you to option 1. In addition, options 2, 3, and 4 are rarely associated with chronic pancreatitis. Review the manifestations of pancreatitis if you had difficulty with this question.

Reference

deWit, S. (2009). *Medical-surgical nursing: Concepts & practice* (p. 760). St. Louis: Saunders.

830. A nurse is assigned to care for a client who is recovering from a burn injury that affects 60% of the total body surface area. On the fourth hospital day, the nurse notes that the client's temperature is 102.8° F, the pulse is 98 beats/min, the respirations are 24 breaths/min, and the blood pressure is 105/64 mm Hg. Parenteral nutrition is infusing at 82 mL per hour. Which initial nursing action is appropriate?

1 Continue to monitor the client.
2 Check the client for signs of infection.
3 Prepare to change the parenteral nutrition solution and intravenous tubing.
4 Prepare to discontinue the parenteral nutrition solution and to culture the tip of the catheter and the insertion site.

Level of Cognitive Ability: Application
Client Needs: Physiological Integrity
Integrated Process: Nursing Process/Implementation
Content Area: Delegating/Prioritizing

Answer: 2

Rationale: The client is recovering from serious burns. The client with burns is prone to several complications, such as infection, dehydration, and sepsis. A temperature of 102.8° F is significant. If this occurs on the fourth hospital day, infection may be the problem. The cause of the infection may be the burns, the parenteral nutrition infusion, the parenteral nutrition site, or another problem. As an initial action, the nurse should check the client for signs of infection and then notify the registered nurse. Options 3 and 4 may follow after notification of the registered nurse. Continuing to monitor the client delays necessary intervention.

Test-Taking Strategy: Use the process of elimination. Note the strategic words *on the fourth hospital day* and *initial nursing action*. Recall that data collection is the first step of the nursing process. Only option 2 addresses data collection. Review the signs of infection in a client with a burn injury if you had difficulty with this question.

References

deWit, S. (2009). *Medical-surgical nursing: Concepts & practice* (pp. 1045-1046). St. Louis: Saunders.
Linton, A. (2007). *Introduction to medical-surgical nursing* (4th ed., p. 1149). Philadelphia: Saunders.

---

831. A client has parenteral nutrition that is infusing, per the physician's order, at 75 mL per hour. The nurse prepares to care for the client and plans to do which of the following?

1 Monitor the urine output hourly.
2 Monitor the vital signs every hour.
3 Monitor for dependent edema every hour.
4 Monitor the blood glucose level every 4 to 6 hours.

Level of Cognitive Ability: Application
Client Needs: Physiological Integrity
Integrated Process: Nursing Process/Planning
Content Area: Fundamental Skills

Answer: 4

Rationale: Parenteral nutrition delivers high concentrations of glucose, so standard protocol for a client on parenteral nutrition is the monitoring of the blood glucose levels. The client may become hypoglycemic because of the addition of insulin to the parenteral nutrition solution, or he or she may become hyperglycemic and require supplemental insulin. Options 1, 2, and 3 may be parts of the plan, but the frequency noted in these options is not necessary unless a specific complication has occurred.

Test-Taking Strategy: Use the process of elimination. Recall the complications associated with parenteral nutrition and note the frequency in each of the options to direct you to option 4. Review the care of the client receiving parenteral nutrition if you had difficulty with this question.

References

deWit, S. (2009). *Medical-surgical nursing: Concepts & practice* (p. 62). St. Louis: Saunders.
Linton, A. (2007). *Introduction to medical-surgical nursing* (4th ed., p. 744). Philadelphia: Saunders.

---

832. A pregnant client is prescribed magnesium sulfate by intramuscular injection. The nurse understands that this medication is most likely prescribed to do which of the following?

Answer: 3

Rationale: Magnesium sulfate is administered to pregnant women to control seizures that result from hypomagnesemia (e.g., due to eclampsia). A secondary effect of magnesium sulfate is that it acts as a laxative by increasing the water content of feces. Magnesium

1 Increase the amount of water in the feces.
2 Increase the conduction time in the myocardium.
3 Control the seizures caused by low magnesium levels.
4 Increase the sinoatrial (SA) node impulse formulation.

Level of Cognitive Ability: Analysis
Client Needs: Physiological Integrity
Integrated Process: Nursing Process/Implementation
Content Area: Pharmacology

sulfate decreases SA node impulse formation and myocardial conduction time.

Test-Taking Strategy: Use the process of elimination. Note the relationship between the name of the medication and option 3. Administering magnesium sulfate will most likely be necessary if the magnesium level is low. Review the action of magnesium sulfate if you had difficulty with this question.

Reference

Leifer, G. (2008). *Maternity nursing: An introductory text* (10th ed., p. 259). Philadelphia: Saunders.

---

833. Sitz baths are prescribed for a postpartum client. The nurse understands that the purpose of the sitz baths is to assist with which of the following?
1 Promoting healing and providing comfort
2 Reducing the edema and numbing the tissue
3 Reducing infection and stimulating peristalsis
4 Cleansing the perineum and preventing hemorrhoids

Level of Cognitive Ability: Comprehension
Client Needs: Physiological Integrity
Integrated Process: Nursing Process/Implementation
Content Area: Maternity/Postpartum

Answer: 1
Rationale: Warm, moist heat is used during the first 24 hours postpartum after vaginal birth to provide comfort, promote healing, and reduce the incidence of infection. Ice is used to reduce the edema and numb the tissue. The stimulation of peristalsis is better achieved by ambulation. A sitz bath may provide comfort for hemorrhoids but does not prevent them.

Test-Taking Strategy: Use the process of elimination. Eliminate option 2 because heat from the sitz bath will not numb the tissue. Eliminate option 4 because of the word *preventing*. From the remaining options eliminate option 3 because a sitz bath will not necessarily stimulate peristalsis. Review the purpose of a sitz bath if you had difficulty with this question.

Reference

Leifer, G. (2008). *Maternity nursing: An introductory text* (10th ed., pp. 229, 240). Philadelphia: Saunders.

---

834. A nurse is preparing to administer a first dose of an antiretroviral agent to a client. The nurse provides medication instructions to the client and tells the client about the need to have serial monitoring of which test to determine the effectiveness of therapy?
1 Western blot
2 CD4+ cell count
3 Enzyme-linked immunosorbent assay (ELISA)
4 Complete blood cell (CBC) count with differential

Level of Cognitive Ability: Analysis
Client Needs: Physiological Integrity
Integrated Process: Nursing Process/Implementation
Content Area: Pharmacology

Answer: 2
Rationale: An antiretroviral agent slows the progression of human immunodeficiency virus (HIV) disease by improving the CD4+ cell count. The Western blot test and the ELISA are performed to diagnose HIV initially. A CBC with differential may be performed as part of an ongoing monitoring of the status of the client with HIV and to detect adverse effects of other medications.

Test-Taking Strategy: Focus on the classification of the medication. Recall that this type of medication slows the progression of HIV disease by improving the CD4+ cell count to direct you to the correct option. Review antiretroviral agents if you had difficulty with this question.

Reference

Ignatavicius, D., & Workman, M. (2010). *Medical-surgical nursing: Patient-centered collaborative care* (6th ed., p. 376). St. Louis: Saunders.

---

835. During the initial mother–infant bonding period after the delivery of the placenta, the nurse's primary responsibility is which of the following?

1 Make sure the siblings are involved with the process.
2 Help the mother to begin breast-feeding the infant immediately.
3 Protect the infant from infection by maintaining isolation of the infant.
4 Make sure that the infant stays warm and is in no danger of slipping from the parents' grasp.

Level of Cognitive Ability: Application
Client Needs: Physiological Integrity
Integrated Process: Nursing Process/Implementation
Content Area: Maternity/Postpartum

Answer: 4
Rationale: During the early interactions between parents and their infants, the safety of the infant is the initial concern. Not all mothers breast-feed, and not all families have siblings. The protection of the infant is important, but it is not done by isolating the infant.

Test-Taking Strategy: Use the process of elimination, and focus on the subject. Use Maslow's Hierarchy of Needs theory to assist with answering the question. Option 4 addresses both a physiological and a safety need. Review the concepts of mother–infant bonding if you had difficulty with this question.

References

Leifer, G. (2007). *Introduction to maternity and pediatric nursing* (5th ed., p. 220). Philadelphia: Saunders.
Leifer, G. (2008). *Maternity nursing: An introductory text* (10th ed., p. 138). Philadelphia: Saunders.

---

836. A nurse assigned to care for a lactating postpartum client plans to instruct the client to do which of the following?

1 Resume the prepregnancy diet.
2 Increase caloric intake by 500 calories a day.
3 Limit fluid intake to 32 ounces of water a day to prevent engorgement.
4 Continue folate and iron supplements at the same dosage as during the pregnancy.

Level of Cognitive Ability: Application
Client Needs: Physiological Integrity
Integrated Process: Teaching and Learning
Content Area: Maternity/Postpartum

Answer: 2
Rationale: Lactating women require at least 500 additional calories above that consumed during pregnancy to ensure an adequate milk supply. Women are encouraged to increase their normal fluid intake (six to eight 8-ounce glasses per day) to provide an additional 24 to 32 ounces of milk. Folate and iron requirements are lower than during pregnancy.

Test-Taking Strategy: Use the process of elimination. Focus on the strategic word *lactating;* this word implies that additional calories are needed and directs you to option 2. Review the nutritional needs of a lactating postpartum client if you had difficulty with this question.

Reference

McKinney, E., James, S., Murray, S., & Ashwill, J. (2009). *Maternal-child nursing* (3rd ed., pp. 315-316). St. Louis: Mosby.

---

837. A nurse determines that a breast-feeding mother is at risk of developing mastitis if the nurse observes the mother doing which of the following?

1 Offering only one breast per feeding
2 Manually expressing the remaining breast milk after each feeding
3 Placing her finger in the infant's mouth to break suction on her nipple
4 Gently pressing breast tissue away from the infant's nose while nursing

Level of Cognitive Ability: Comprehension
Client Needs: Physiological Integrity

Answer: 1
Rationale: Offering only one breast per feeding causes milk stasis, which is a risk factor for mastitis. The mother is encouraged to allow the infant to empty one breast completely and to then continue feeding the infant on the opposite breast. Newborns frequently tire and do not completely empty the second breast. The mother is instructed to express the remaining milk manually until an adequate milk supply is established and to offer the second breast first at the next feeding. A safety pin attached to the brassiere cup reminds the mother which breast should be offered first at the subsequent feeding. Breaking the infant's suction before removing the infant from the breast reduces nipple trauma, which is another risk factor for mastitis. Gentle pressure placed on the tissue does not influence the development of mastitis. It is recommended to allow the infant to breathe through the nose unobstructed while he or she is nursing.

Integrated Process: Nursing Process/Data Collection
Content Area: Maternity/Postpartum

Test-Taking Strategy: Use the process of elimination. Focus on the strategic words *at risk of developing mastitis.* Visualize each of the mother's actions and use your knowledge regarding the risk factors for mastitis to direct you to option 1. In addition, note the close-ended word *only* in option 1. Review the risk factors for mastitis if you had difficulty with this question.

Reference

McKinney, E., James, S., Murray, S., & Ashwill, J. (2009). *Maternal-child nursing* (3rd ed., p. 708). St. Louis: Mosby.

---

838. Erythromycin base (Ilotycin) ophthalmic ointment is prescribed for a newborn. The nurse understands which of the following about this medication?

1 It is more irritating to the newborn's eyes than silver nitrate.
2 It may stain the infant's skin and must be wiped off immediately.
3 It must be administered at room temperature to prevent side effects.
4 It is useful to protect the newborn from both *Neisseria gonorrhoeae* and *Chlamydia*.

Level of Cognitive Ability: Analysis
Client Needs: Physiological Integrity
Integrated Process: Nursing Process/Implementation
Content Area: Maternity/Postpartum

Answer: 4

Rationale: Erythromycin base is effective against both *Neisseria gonorrhea* and *Chlamydia.* It is less irritating to the newborn's eyes than silver nitrate, it does not stain, and it may be administered at any safe temperature.

Test-Taking Strategy: Knowledge of erythromycin base is necessary to answer this question. Remember that this medication is useful to protect the newborn from both *Neisseria gonorrhoeae* and *Chlamydia.* In addition, note that option 4 is the umbrella option. Review erythromycin base if you had difficulty with this question.

Reference

Leifer, G. (2008). *Maternity nursing: An introductory text* (10th ed., p. 139). Philadelphia: Saunders.

---

839. A client who was tested for human immunodeficiency virus (HIV) after a recent exposure had a negative test result. Which item should the nurse plan to include during posttest counseling?

1 The test should be repeated in 6 months.
2 The client probably has immunity to HIV.
3 The client no longer needs to protect sexual partners.
4 The test ensures that the client is not infected with the HIV virus.

Level of Cognitive Ability: Application
Client Needs: Physiological Integrity
Integrated Process: Nursing Process/Implementation
Content Area: Fundamental Skills

Answer: 1

Rationale: HIV is a retrovirus that causes acquired immunodeficiency syndrome. A negative test result indicates that no HIV antibodies were detected in the blood sample. A repeat test in 6 months is recommended because false-negative results can occur early during the course of the infection. Options 2, 3, and 4 are incorrect.

Test-Taking Strategy: Use the process of elimination. Begin to answer this question by eliminating options 2 and 3 because they are incorrect statements. Even without specific knowledge of the implications of certain test results, you should choose option 1 instead of option 4 because of the closed-ended words *ensures* and *not.* Review HIV testing procedures if you had difficulty with this question.

References

Chernecky, C., & Berger, B. (2008). *Laboratory tests and diagnostic procedures* (5th ed., p. 99). Philadelphia: Saunders.
Linton, A. (2007). *Introduction to medical-surgical nursing* (4th ed., p. 620). Philadelphia: Saunders.

840. A nurse notes signs of restlessness, dyspnea, anxiety, and a rapid pulse in a client who is at risk for acute respiratory distress syndrome. Which of the following is the priority nursing action?

1 Checking the client's medical record for a history of anxiety attacks
2 Staying with the client and positioning him or her to relieve dyspnea
3 Preparing to medicate the client with the PRN medication for anxiety
4 Reassuring the client by checking his or her vital signs every 10 minutes

Level of Cognitive Ability: Analysis
Client Needs: Physiological Integrity
Integrated Process: Nursing Process/Implementation
Content Area: Adult Health/Respiratory

Answer: 2

Rationale: Acute respiratory distress syndrome is a severe pulmonary congestion characterized by diffuse injury to the alveolar–capillary membranes. Signs of respiratory distress are often accompanied by a fear of suffocation. In addition to immediate interventions to improve the client's respiratory status, the nurse's presence can provide reassurance and ease the client's anxiety. The vital signs should be monitored, but reassuring the client that this will be done will not relieve the anxiety. The client may receive medication if prescribed, but this is not the priority. Option 3 will not relieve the client's distress.

Test-Taking Strategy: Use the process of elimination, and note the strategic word *priority.* Focus on the signs provided in the question and on the need to reassure the client. Option 2 is the priority because it addresses both the client's dyspnea and the anxiety. Review the care of the client with acute respiratory distress syndrome if you had difficulty with this question.

References

Christensen, B., & Kockrow, E. (2006). *Adult health nursing* (5th ed., p. 54). St. Louis: Mosby.
deWit, S. (2009). *Medical-surgical nursing: Concepts & practice* (p. 289). St. Louis: Saunders.

---

841. A nurse is teaching a client about the care of a right leg cast that was just applied to treat a fracture. The nurse tells the client which of the following?

1 There is no danger of complications related to the cast after the cast has dried completely.
2 Elevation of the right leg above heart level should relieve foot swelling, which occurs while the leg is dependent.
3 Foul odors coming from the cast should be reported only if there also is visible drainage on the outside of the cast.
4 Swelling, blue-tinged toes, and pain in the right leg and foot with any movement are expected during the healing process.

Level of Cognitive Ability: Application
Client Needs: Physiological Integrity
Integrated Process: Teaching and Learning
Content Area: Adult Health/Musculoskeletal

Answer: 2

Rationale: Dependent edema may occur when the casted extremity is in the dependent position or when there is prolonged hip flexion while the client is sitting. Dependent edema caused by sluggish venous return should decrease when the leg is elevated above the level of the heart. If the edema is related to the potentially serious complication of compartment syndrome, pressure in the compartment is not decreased by elevating the leg above the heart; in fact, the pressure and swelling may increase with elevation. Therefore, swelling that does not resolve after elevation of the extremity should be reported to the physician. Blue skin color and persistent pain are not typical and could be signs of compartment syndrome. Foul odors with or without drainage may indicate infection and should be reported to the physician.

Test-Taking Strategy: Use the process of elimination. Eliminate option 3 because of the words *only if there also is visible drainage.* Eliminate option 4 because these signs are not normal. Note the strategic words *no danger* in option 1 to assist you with eliminating this option. Review the care of the client with a cast if you had difficulty with this question.

Reference

Christensen, B., & Kockrow, E. (2006). *Adult health nursing* (5th ed., p. 172). St. Louis: Mosby.

---

842. A nurse receives a telephone call from the parent of a toddler with acute lymphocytic leukemia (ALL). The parent tells the nurse that the child has developed

Answer: 3

Rationale: Epistaxis is a nosebleed. Keeping a child calm and quiet decreases blood flow. Laying the child down and applying a warm washcloth to the bridge of the nose increases blood flow.

epistaxis. The nurse advises the parent to do which of the following immediately?

1 Call 911.
2 Have the child lie down.
3 Keep the child calm and quiet.
4 Apply a warm washcloth to the bridge of the child's nose.

Level of Cognitive Ability: Application
Client Needs: Physiological Integrity
Integrated Process: Nursing Process/Implementation
Content Area: Child Health

In addition, the child should sit up and lean forward (not lie down). Although bleeding in a child with ALL can be an emergency, steps should be taken immediately to resolve the nosebleed before calling 911.

Test-Taking Strategy: Use the process of elimination, and note the strategic word *immediately.* Use principles related to gravity to assist you with eliminating option 2. Use principles related to the effects of warmth to eliminate option 4. Focus on the strategic word *immediately* and recall the steps that should be taken to resolve a nosebleed to eliminate option 1. Review the care of the child with epistaxis if you had difficulty with this question.

Reference

Hockenberry, M., & Wilson, D. (2009). *Wong's essentials of pediaric care* (8th ed., pp. 929-930). St. Louis: Mosby.

---

843. A client recently diagnosed with tuberculosis (TB) is being admitted to the hospital. When collecting data from the client, a primary consideration is to identify which of the following?

1 The religious affiliation or church of preference
2 The names of close friends and family members
3 What medications are ordered and what the client knows about their side effects
4 Who the client contracted TB from so that the person can be reported for follow-up care

Level of Cognitive Ability: Comprehension
Client Needs: Physiological Integrity
Integrated Process: Nursing Process/Data Collection
Content Area: Adult Health/Respiratory

Answer: 2

Rationale: TB is a contagious disease that is spread through respiratory droplets. A primary consideration of the nurse is to identify the names of close friends and family members of the client so that these individuals can be tested for exposure to TB. The client may not know from whom the disease was contracted. It is premature to determine the client's knowledge of medications because treatment measures may not have been prescribed. The religious affiliation or church of preference is part of the data collection process but is not the primary consideration of the options provided.

Test-Taking Strategy: Use the process of elimination, and note the strategic word *primary.* Recall the route of transmission of TB to direct you to option 2. Review data collection techniques for the client who has been recently diagnosed with TB if you had difficulty with this question.

References

Christensen, B., & Kockrow, E. (2006). *Adult health nursing* (5th ed., p. 429). St. Louis: Mosby.
deWit, S. (2009). *Medical-surgical nursing: Concepts & practice* (p. 328). St. Louis: Saunders.

---

844. A nurse in the prenatal clinic is taking a nutritional history from a 16-year-old adolescent. Which statement made by the client would suggest a possible problem?

1 "I should eat more foods that I am used to."
2 "I don't like milk but I do like other dairy products."
3 "I will continue eating my afternoon snack of popcorn."
4 "I only want to gain 7 to 10 pounds because I want a small, petite baby girl."

Answer: 4

Rationale: Pregnant adolescents are at higher risk for complications than are mature women. Adolescents are often concerned about their body image. If weight is a major focus, the client is more likely to restrict calories to avoid weight gain. Option 4 is the only option that suggests a possible problem because it indicates the potential for a nursing diagnosis of *Imbalance nutrition, less than body requirements.*

Test-Taking Strategy: Use the process of elimination, and note the strategic word *adolescent.* Recall that body image is a concern of an adolescent to direct you to option 4. Review pregnancy in the adolescent if you had difficulty with this question.

Level of Cognitive Ability: Analysis
Client Needs: Physiological Integrity
Integrated Process: Nursing Process/Data Collection
Content Area: Maternity/Antepartum

Reference

Leifer, G. (2008). *Maternity nursing: An introductory text* (10th ed., p. 79). Philadelphia: Saunders.

---

845. A nurse is providing information to a client with hepatitis about the convalescence stage. Recognizing the need for psychosocial support for this client, the nurse suggests which of the following?

1 That the client join an aerobic exercise class
2 That the client stay in his or her room to facilitate resting
3 That the client participate in diversionary activities that are not physically taxing
4 That the client speak with his or her doctor about a prescription for antidepressant medications

Level of Cognitive Ability: Application
Client Needs: Physiological Integrity
Integrated Process: Nursing Process/Planning
Content Area: Adult Health/Gastrointestinal

Answer: 3

Rationale: Hepatitis is an inflammatory condition of the liver. The process of convalescence with hepatitis is long and slow; the client becomes easily fatigued and needs additional rest. However, as the client recovers, there is an equally important need for some diversion from the long days of bedrest. Option 1 is a much too strenuous activity for the client. Option 2 socially isolates the client. The use of antidepressant medications is contraindicated in a client with decreased liver function.

Test-Taking Strategy: Use the process of elimination, and recall that rest is needed to heal the liver of the client with hepatitis. Eliminate option 1 because this activity is strenuous. Eliminate option 2 because this intervention socially isolates the client. Eliminate option 4 because the use of antidepressant medications is contraindicated for a client with decreased liver function. Review the care of the client with hepatitis if you had difficulty with this question.

Reference

Linton, A. (2007). *Introduction to medical-surgical nursing* (4th ed., pp. 806-807). Philadelphia: Saunders.

---

846. A nurse is monitoring the intravenous (IV) site of a client receiving an IV solution that contains potassium chloride. The nurse notes heat, redness, and tenderness at the site and suspects phlebitis. The nurse understands that which of the following is the most likely cause of the phlebitis?

1 The inflammation of the vein
2 The collection of blood in the tissues
3 The infusion of solution into the subcutaneous tissue
4 A local growth of microorganisms that gain entry through the venipuncture site

Level of Cognitive Ability: Comprehension
Client Needs: Physiological Integrity
Integrated Process: Nursing Process/Data Collection
Content Area: Fundamental Skills

Answer: 1

Rationale: Phlebitis is caused by the inflammation of a vein from chemical irritants in the IV solution or medication, by mechanical irritation from the needle or cannula, or by accompanying local infection. A hematoma is the collection of blood in the tissues that occurs during unsuccessful venipuncture or after the venipuncture site is discontinued. Infiltration is the infusion of solution into the subcutaneous tissue. Infection is the local or systemic growth of microorganisms that gain entry into the body through the venipuncture site.

Test-Taking Strategy: Use the process of elimination, and note the strategic words *most likely.* Focus on the subject—phlebitis; the definition of this term should direct you to option 1. Review the causes of phlebitis if you had difficulty with this question.

Reference

Linton, A. (2007). *Introduction to medical-surgical nursing* (4th ed., p. 287). Philadelphia: Saunders.

847. A client with diabetes mellitus who takes NPH insulin tells the nurse, "I usually begin to feel sick late in the afternoon. Is there something wrong with me?" The appropriate response by the nurse is which of the following?

1 "Let me know if that happens today."
2 "Most people feel tired late in the afternoon."
3 "Can you describe what you mean by 'feeling sick?'"
4 "Don't worry about that. Most diabetics feel that way."

Level of Cognitive Ability: Application
Client Needs: Physiological Integrity
Integrated Process: Communication and Documentation
Content Area: Adult Health/Endocrine

Answer: 3
Rationale: An excess of insulin relative to the amount of blood glucose induces hypoglycemia. Depending on when the NPH insulin is administered, the risk of hypoglycemia may be greatest during the late afternoon. The nurse should collect more data to determine if the client is actually experiencing hypoglycemia. Asking the client to describe the feeling provides the nurse with more data. Options 1, 2, and 4 are nontherapeutic communication techniques.

Test-Taking Strategy: Use the process of elimination and therapeutic communication techniques to answer the question. Option 3 identifies data collection, which is the first step of the nursing process. Review the effects of insulin and hypoglycemic reactions if you had difficulty with this question.

References
deWit, S. (2009). *Medical-surgical nursing: Concepts & practice* (p. 9). St. Louis: Saunders.
Linton, A. (2007). *Introduction to medical-surgical nursing* (4th ed., pp. 1017, 1019). Philadelphia: Saunders.

---

848. A nurse is caring for a client with diabetes mellitus and gathering data from the client about the events that led to the client's request for medical attention. The nurse identifies which of the following as the major symptoms of diabetes mellitus?

1 Polydipsia, polyuria, and polyphagia
2 Dyspepsia, polyuria, and polyphagia
3 Hypoglycemia, polyuria, and dysphagia
4 Hypoglycemia, polyuria, and dysphasia

Level of Cognitive Ability: Comprehension
Client Needs: Physiological Integrity
Integrated Process: Nursing Process/Data Collection
Content Area: Adult Health/Endocrine

Answer: 1
Rationale: Polydipsia, polyuria, and polyphagia are the classic signs and symptoms of diabetes mellitus. Dyspepsia, dysphagia, and dysphasia are associated with the gastrointestinal and neurological body systems.

Test-Taking Strategy: Focus on the subject—the major symptoms of diabetes mellitus. Remember the "three Ps" of diabetes mellitus: polydipsia, polyuria, and polyphagia. Review the signs of diabetes mellitus if you had difficulty with this question.

Reference
Linton, A. (2007). *Introduction to medical-surgical nursing* (4th ed., p. 1002). Philadelphia: Saunders.

---

849. A client is being discharged from the hospital in 2 days, and the physician tells the client to maintain a low-fat diet at home. The client demonstrates an understanding of a low-fat diet by choosing which of the following foods from the hospital breakfast menu?

1 Bran muffin
2 Peanut butter sandwich
3 Bagel with cream cheese
4 Dry toast and strawberry jelly

Answer: 4
Rationale: Among the foods mentioned in the options, bread (toast without butter or margarine) contains the least amount of fat. Strawberry jelly contains calories but nominal fats. Bran muffins may be high in residue but are made with shortenings, which are high in fat. Peanut butter and cheese contain significant amounts of fat.

Test-Taking Strategy: Use the process of elimination and your knowledge of those food items that are low in fat; this will direct you to option 4. Review food items that are high in fat if you had difficulty with this question.

Level of Cognitive Ability: Comprehension
Client Needs: Physiological Integrity
Integrated Process: Nursing Process/Evaluation
Content Area: Fundamental Skills

References

Christensen, B., & Kockrow, E. (2006). *Foundations of nursing* (5th ed., p. 648). St. Louis: Mosby.
deWit, S. (2009). *Medical-surgical nursing: Concepts & practice* (p. 491). St. Louis: Saunders.

---

850. A licensed practical nurse (LPN) is assisting a registered nurse (RN) with caring for a client who is receiving lidocaine (Xylocaine) for the treatment of ventricular tachycardia. The LPN assists with planning care knowing that this medication is classified as which of the following?
1 A diuretic
2 An antihypertensive
3 An antidysrhythmic
4 A calcium-channel blocker

Level of Cognitive Ability: Analysis
Client Needs: Physiological Integrity
Integrated Process: Nursing Process/Planning
Content Area: Pharmacology

Answer: 3
Rationale: Lidocaine is classified as an antidysrhythmic, and it is used to treat cardiac dysrhythmias. It is not classified as a diuretic, an antihypertensive, or a calcium-channel blocker.

Test-Taking Strategy: Use the process of elimination. Note the diagnosis of the client to direct you to option 3. Review the action of lidocaine if you had difficulty with this question.

References

Lehne, R. (2007). *Pharmacology for nursing care* (6th ed., p. 536). Philadelphia: Saunders.
Hodgson, B., & Kizior, R. (2009). *Saunders nursing drug handbook 2009* (p. 684). St. Louis: Saunders.

---

851. A nurse is monitoring a child with a head injury for signs of complications. Which of the following indicates to the nurse that notification of the registered nurse is necessary?
1 A urine specific gravity of 1.015
2 A urine specific gravity of 1.020
3 A urine specific gravity of 1.030
4 A urine specific gravity of 1.035

Level of Cognitive Ability: Analysis
Client Needs: Physiological Integrity
Integrated Process: Nursing Process/Data Collection
Content Area: Child Health

Answer: 4
Rationale: Urine specific gravity is normally 1.005 to 1.030. The nurse should monitor the specific gravity of a child with a head injury or brain tumor or a child who is at risk for increased intracranial pressure (ICP) every 4 to 6 hours. The registered nurse should be notified (who in turn will notify the physician) if the urine specific gravity is above 1.030 or less than 1.005. With increasing ICP, diabetes insipidus or the syndrome of inappropriate antidiuretic hormone may occur.

Test-Taking Strategy: Recall that the urine specific gravity is normally 1.005 to 1.030 to direct you to option 4. This is the only option that represents an abnormal value. Review urine specific gravity values and the care of a child with a head injury if you had difficulty with this question.

Reference

Hockenberry, M., & Wilson, D. (2009). *Wong's essentials of pediaric care* (8th ed., pp. 1030-1031). St. Louis: Mosby.

---

852. The nurse expects to note which clinical manifestations in the client with trigeminal neuralgia?
1 Paralysis on one side of the face
2 Decreased pain after gentle massage
3 Sharp, knife-like pain after brushing the teeth
4 Decreased pain after drinking a cold beverage

Answer: 3
Rationale: Trigeminal neuralgia is a neurological condition of the trigeminal facial nerve. Clients with trigeminal neuralgia report excruciating, sharp, knife-like facial pain (usually unilateral) after brushing their teeth and with exposure to extremes of hot or cold, touch, and chewing. Paralysis of one side of the face is seen with Bell's palsy. Massage and drinking cold beverages would not decrease the pain of trigeminal neuralgia.

Level of Cognitive Ability: Comprehension
Client Needs: Physiological Integrity
Integrated Process: Nursing Process/Data Collection
Content Area: Adult Health/Neurological

Test-Taking Strategy: Use the process of elimination, and focus on the data in the question. The word *neuralgia* in the name of this disorder assists with directing you to the correct option. Review trigeminal neuralgia if you had difficulty with this question.

References

Christensen, B., & Kockrow, E. (2006). *Adult health nursing* (5th ed., p. 734). St. Louis: Mosby.
Linton, A. (2007). *Introduction to medical-surgical nursing* (4th ed., p. 456). Philadelphia: Saunders.

---

853. A nurse is caring for a client with a small venous stasis ulcer who has a new order to be out of bed. The nurse plans to obtain which of the following for use in the client's room to best enhance the circulatory status of the affected area?

1 Reclining chair
2 Overbed trapeze
3 Bedside commode
4 Warm, heavy blankets

Level of Cognitive Ability: Application
Client Needs: Physiological Integrity
Integrated Process: Nursing Process/Planning
Content Area: Adult Health/Cardiovascular

Answer: 1

Rationale: A venous stasis ulcer occurs as a result of slowing or halted blood flow through a vein. The client should have a reclining chair to allow the legs to be elevated when the client is not resting in bed. Positioning the client with the legs elevated allows gravity to drain the extremities while the client is at rest, thereby increasing venous drainage from the affected leg. An overbed trapeze is used for a client who needs assistance with repositioning himself or herself in bed. A bedside commode may be helpful for a client with limited mobility, but it does not increase circulation to the leg. Warm, heavy blankets could put extra weight on the ulcer and actually reduce venous drainage by causing additional vasodilatation.

Test-Taking Strategy: Use the process of elimination, and note the strategic words *best enhance the circulatory status.* Recall that the client with a venous problem has impaired venous drainage from the extremity to help you to eliminate each of the options that does not assist with venous drainage through leg elevation. Review the care of the client with a venous problem if you had difficulty with this question.

References

Christensen, B., & Kockrow, E. (2006). *Adult health nursing* (5th ed., p. 394). St. Louis: Mosby.
Linton, A. (2007). *Introduction to medical-surgical nursing* (4th ed., p. 711). Philadelphia: Saunders.

---

854. A client with acquired immunodeficiency syndrome is diagnosed with *Pneumocystis jiroveci* pneumonia. Which of the following will the nurse most likely note when gathering data about the client?

1 Temperature, 98.6° F; pulse, 80 beats/min; respirations, 18 breaths/min
2 Temperature, 98.6° F; pulse, 80 beats/min; respirations, 32 breaths/min
3 Temperature, 101.5° F; pulse, 80 beats/min; respirations, 18 breaths/min
4 Temperature, 101.5° F; pulse, 120 beats/min; respirations, 32 breaths/min

Answer: 4

Rationale: Pneumocystis jiroveci pneumonia is a fungal infection of the lung that is usually seen in clients with human immunodeficiency virus infection. Signs and symptoms of *Pneumocystis jiroveci* pneumonia include fever, dyspnea on exertion, tachypnea, tachycardia, and persistent dry cough. Therefore, options 1, 2, and 3 are incorrect.

Test-Taking Strategy: Note the strategic words *most likely,* and select the option that contains abnormal vital signs. Options 1, 2, and 3 all contain two or more vital signs that are within the normal range. Option 4 contains only abnormal vital signs. Review the signs of *Pneumocystis jiroveci* pneumonia if you had difficulty with this question.

Level of Cognitive Ability: Comprehension
Client Needs: Physiological Integrity
Integrated Process: Nursing Process/Data Collection
Content Area: Adult Health/Respiratory

Reference
Ignatavicius, D., & Workman, M. (2010). *Medical-surgical nursing: Patient-centered collaborative care* (6th ed., p. 371). St. Louis: Saunders.

---

855. A nurse is reviewing the record of a mother who is 2 days postpartum and who has been diagnosed with thrombophlebitis. The nurse expects to note which finding in the client's record?
1 Homans' sign is positive.
2 Intake is slightly greater than output.
3 The leg circumference of both legs is equal.
4 The fundal height is 2 cm below the umbilicus.

Level of Cognitive Ability: Analysis
Client Needs: Physiological Integrity
Integrated Process: Nursing Process/Data Collection
Content Area: Maternity/Postpartum

Answer: 1
Rationale: Thrombophlebitis is the inflammation of a vein accompanied by the formation of a clot. Homans' sign is positive when the client feels pain in the calf when dorsiflexing the foot; this indicates irritation of the blood vessels caused by clot formation and is indicative of thrombophlebitis. The findings in options 2, 3, and 4 are normal findings.

Test-Taking Strategy: Focus on the subject—findings in a client with thrombophlebitis. Noting the word *positive* in option 1 will direct you to this option. Review the assessment of thrombophlebitis if you had difficulty with this question.

Reference
Leifer, G. (2008). *Maternity nursing: An introductory text* (10th ed., p. 343). Philadelphia: Saunders.

---

856. The nurse reviewing the record of an infant expects to note the documentation of which earliest symptom if the infant has the human immunodeficiency (HIV)?
1 Lethargy
2 Respiratory distress
3 Hepatosplenomegaly
4 Purulent eye drainage

Level of Cognitive Ability: Analysis
Client Needs: Physiological Integrity
Integrated Process: Nursing Process/Data Collection
Content Area: Maternity/Postpartum

Answer: 3
Rationale: Most infants at risk for HIV infection have no evidence of the condition at birth. The earliest symptom in an HIV-positive infant is hepatosplenomegaly. This occurs because the liver and spleen are the target areas of the virus, and the increased activity in these organs increases their size. Lethargy, respiratory distress, and purulent eye drainage are not specific symptoms related to HIV.

Test-Taking Strategy: Focus on the subject—the earliest symptom in an HIV-positive infant. Remember that the earliest symptom present in an HIV-positive infant is hepatosplenomegaly and that this occurs because the liver and spleen are the target areas of the virus; the increased activity in these organs increases their size. Review the clinical manifestations of HIV in an infant if you had difficulty with this question.

Reference
Hockenberry, M., & Wilson, D. (2009). *Wong's essentials of pediatric care* (8th ed., p. 940). St. Louis: Mosby.

---

857. A nurse is interviewing a client with chronic obstructive pulmonary disease (COPD) who has a respiratory rate of 35 breaths/min and who is experiencing extreme dyspnea. Which nursing diagnosis should the nurse identify as a barrier to collecting data?

Answer: 3
Rationale: COPD is a progressive and irreversible condition that is characterized by the diminished inspiratory and expiratory capacity of the lungs. A client may suffer physical or psychological alterations that impair communication. To speak spontaneously and clearly, a person must have an intact respiratory system. Extreme dyspnea is a physical condition that affects speech.

1 *Ineffective coping* related to COPD
2 *Impaired verbal communication* related to a neurological deficit
3 *Impaired verbal communication* related to the physical condition
4 *Ineffective coping* related to client's inability to handle a crisis situation

Level of Cognitive Ability: Analysis
Client Needs: Physiological Integrity
Integrated Process: Nursing Process/Data Collection
Content Area: Adult Health/Respiratory

Option 1 is a medical diagnosis. There is nothing to indicate that the client has a neurological deficit. Option 4 is judgmental and inappropriate.

Test-Taking Strategy: Use the process of elimination, and focus on the data provided in the question. Option 3 clearly addresses the problem that the client is experiencing. Review the care of the client with COPD and the barriers to communication if you had difficulty with this question.

References

Christensen, B., & Kockrow, E. (2006). *Adult health nursing* (5th ed., p. 454). St. Louis: Mosby.
Ignatavicius, D., & Workman, M. (2010). *Medical-surgical nursing: Patient-centered collaborative care* (6th ed., p. 626). St. Louis: Saunders.

---

858. A client with late-stage emphysema complains of an occipital headache, drowsiness, and difficulty concentrating. The nurse interprets that these symptoms are compatible with which complication of emphysema?
1 Encephalopathy
2 Cerebral embolism
3 Carbon dioxide narcosis
4 Carbon monoxide poisoning

Level of Cognitive Ability: Analysis
Client Needs: Physiological Integrity
Integrated Process: Nursing Process/Data Collection
Content Area: Adult Health/Respiratory

Answer: 3
Rationale: Emphysema is an abnormal condition of the pulmonary system that is characterized by overinflation and destructive changes in the alveolar walls. With late-stage emphysema, the retention of carbon dioxide can lead to carbon dioxide narcosis; this is manifested by occipital headache, drowsiness, and an inability to concentrate. Other signs that may occur are a bounding pulse, an arterial carbon dioxide level of more than 75 mm Hg, confusion, coma, and asterixis (flap tremor). Options 1, 2, and 4 are incorrect interpretations.

Test-Taking Strategy: To answer this question accurately, you must be familiar with the complications of emphysema. Recall that emphysema is characterized by high carbon dioxide levels to direct you to option 3. Review the manifestations of emphysema if you had difficulty with this question.

References

deWit, S. (2009). *Medical-surgical nursing: Concepts & practice* (p. 280). St. Louis: Saunders.
Ignatavicius, D., & Workman, M. (2010). *Medical-surgical nursing: Patient-centered collaborative care* (6th ed., p. 573, 623). St. Louis: Saunders.

---

859. A nurse witnesses an accident in which a pedestrian is hit by an automobile. The nurse stops at the scene and checks the victim, noting that the client is responsive and has possibly suffered a flail chest involving at least three ribs. The nurse should do which of the following to assist the victim's respiratory status until help arrives?
1 Assist the victim to sit up.
2 Remove the victim's shirt.
3 Turn the victim onto the side with the flail chest.
4 Apply firm but gentle pressure with the hands to the flail segment.

Answer: 4
Rationale: Flail chest occurs when multiple rib fractures cause instability in part of the chest wall. Paradoxical breathing, with the lung underlying the injured area contracting on inspiration and bulging on expiration, occurs. With flail chest, the nurse applies firm yet gentle pressure to the flail segments of the ribs to stabilize the chest wall, which will ultimately help the victim's respiratory status. The nurse does not move an injured person for fear of worsening an undetected spinal injury. Removing the victim's shirt is of no value in this situation and could chill the victim, which is counterproductive. Injured persons should be kept warm until help arrives.

Level of Cognitive Ability: Application
Client Needs: Physiological Integrity
Integrated Process: Nursing Process/ Implementation
Content Area: Adult Health/Respiratory

Test-Taking Strategy: Use your knowledge of the principles of respiration and emergency nursing to answer this question. Eliminate option 2 first because this action is of no value to the victim. Eliminate options 1 and 3 next because a victim of injury should not be moved until the extent of the injury is determined. Review the emergency care of a client with flail chest if you had difficulty with this question.

References

deWit, S. (2009). *Medical-surgical nursing: Concepts & practice* (pp. 342-343). St. Louis: Saunders.
Ignatavicius, D., & Workman, M. (2010). *Medical-surgical nursing: Patient-centered collaborative care* (6th ed., p. 698). St. Louis: Saunders.

---

860. A nurse notes bilateral 2+ edema in the lower extremities of a client with known cardiac disease who was admitted to the hospital 2 days ago. The nurse plans to do which of the following first?

1 Order daily weights starting on the following morning.
2 Review the intake and output records for the last 2 days.
3 Request a sodium restriction of 1 g per day from the physician.
4 Change the time of diuretic administration from morning to evening.

Level of Cognitive Ability: Application
Client Needs: Physiological Integrity
Integrated Process: Nursing Process/ Implementation
Content Area: Adult Health/Cardiovascular

Answer: 2

Rationale: Edema is the accumulation of excess fluid in the interstitial spaces, which can be determined by intake that is greater than output and by a sudden increase in weight. Diuretics should be given in the morning, whenever possible, to avoid nocturia. Strict sodium restrictions are reserved for clients with severe symptoms.

Test-Taking Strategy: Use the process of elimination, and note the strategic word *first.* Note that option 2 can give the nurse immediate information about fluid balance and that it reflects the process of data collection. Review the care of the client with cardiac disease and edema if you had difficulty with this question.

Reference

deWit, S. (2009). *Medical-surgical nursing: Concepts & practice* (p. 428). St. Louis: Saunders.

---

861. A nurse is caring for a client with chest pain in the emergency department. Which observation by the nurse helps determine that this pain is caused by myocardial infarction?

1 The client experienced no nausea or vomiting.
2 The pain was described as substernal and radiating to the left arm.
3 The client reports that the pain began while pushing a lawnmower.
4 The pain is unrelieved with nitroglycerin but relieved with morphine sulfate.

Level of Cognitive Ability: Analysis
Client Needs: Physiological Integrity

Answer: 4

Rationale: The pain of angina may radiate to the left arm; it is often precipitated by exertion or stress, it has few associated symptoms, and it is relieved by rest and nitroglycerin. The pain of myocardial infarction may radiate to the left arm, the left shoulder, the jaw, and the neck. It typically begins spontaneously, it lasts longer than 30 minutes, it is frequently accompanied by associated symptoms (e.g., nausea, vomiting, dyspnea, diaphoresis, anxiety), and it requires opioid analgesics for relief.

Test-Taking Strategy: Use the process of elimination. The question seeks to differentiate the pain of angina from that of myocardial infarction, which may be similar at the onset. Remember that a classic hallmark of myocardial infarction pain is that rest and nitroglycerin provide no relief. Review the manifestations associated with myocardial infarction if you had difficulty with this question.

Integrated Process: Nursing Process/Data Collection
Content Area: Adult Health/Cardiovascular

Reference
deWit, S. (2009). *Medical-surgical nursing: Concepts & practice* (p. 497). St. Louis: Saunders.

---

862. A nurse is assisting with positioning a client for pericardiocentesis to treat cardiac tamponade. The nurse places the client in which position?
1 Supine and in slight Trendelenburg's position
2 Lying on the right side with a pillow under the head
3 Lying on the left side with a pillow under the chest wall
4 Supine with the head of the bed elevated 45 to 60 degrees

Level of Cognitive Ability: Application
Client Needs: Physiological Integrity
Integrated Process: Nursing Process/Implementation
Content Area: Adult Health/Cardiovascular

Answer: 4
Rationale: Pericardiocentesis is a procedure for aspirating fluid from the pericardial sac. The client undergoing pericardiocentesis is positioned supine with the head of the bed elevated 45 to 60 degrees. This places the heart in close proximity to the chest wall for easier insertion of the needle into the pericardial sac.

Test-Taking Strategy: Visualize each of the positions described to answer this question. Evaluate how the heart is sitting in the chest with each position and how easily the pericardial sac could be accessed with a needle. This should help you to eliminate all of the incorrect options. Review positioning for pericardiocentesis if you had difficulty with this question.

Reference
Chernecky, C., & Berger, B. (2008). *Laboratory tests and diagnostic procedures* (5th ed., pp. 862-863). Philadelphia: Saunders.

---

863. A nurse explains to a mother that her newborn is being admitted to the neonatal intensive care unit with a probable diagnosis of fetal alcohol syndrome (FAS). The nurse explains FAS to the mother and determines an understanding of the condition when the mother states which of the following?
1 "Mental retardation is unlikely to happen."
2 "Withdrawal symptoms will occur after 3 days."
3 "The reason the child is so large is because of the FAS."
4 "Withdrawal symptoms are tremors, crying, and seizures."

Level of Cognitive Ability: Comprehension
Client Needs: Physiological Integrity
Integrated Process: Nursing Process/Evaluation
Content Area: Maternity/Postpartum

Answer: 4
Rationale: FAS is a set of congenital psychological, behavioral, and physical abnormalities that tend to appear in infants whose mothers consumed alcohol during pregnancy. The long-term prognosis for newborns with FAS is poor. Symptoms of withdrawal include tremors, sleeplessness, seizures, abdominal distention, hyperactivity, and uncontrollable crying. Central nervous system (CNS) disorders are the most common problems associated with FAS. Because of the associated CNS disorders, children born with FAS are often hyperactive and have a high incidence of speech and language disorders. Symptoms of withdrawal often occur within 6 to 12 hours after birth or, at the latest, within 3 days of birth. Most newborns with FAS are mildly to severely mentally retarded. The newborn is usually growth deficient at birth.

Test-Taking Strategy: Use the process of elimination. Think about the effects of FAS to help you to eliminate options 1 and 3. From the remaining options, you must know that withdrawal symptoms can appear within 6 to 12 hours after birth or, at the latest, within 3 days of birth. Review the manifestations associated with FAS if you had difficulty with this question.

Reference
Leifer, G. (2007). *Introduction to maternity and pediatric nursing* (5th ed., pp. 108-109, 343). Philadelphia: Saunders.

---

864. Ferrous sulfate (iron) is prescribed for a pregnant client. Before beginning this medication, the nurse reviews which

Answer: 3
Rationale: Ferrous sulfate (iron) is an iron supplement. Generally, a healthy diet provides adequate sources of iron. Because of

laboratory result that will provide the necessary baseline data for monitoring the therapeutic effect of the medication?
1 Clotting time
2 Prothrombin time
3 Hemoglobin level
4 Iron binding levels

Level of Cognitive Ability: Application
Client Needs: Physiological Integrity
Integrated Process: Nursing Process/Data Collection
Content Area: Maternity/Antepartum

the expansion of maternal blood volume and the production of fetal red blood cells, iron requirements increase during pregnancy. Hemoglobin measures oxygen carrying capacity of the blood. Options 1 and 2 identify tests performed for clients with bleeding disorders. Option 4 identifies a measurement test used to diagnose various anemias and blood diseases.

Test-Taking Strategy: Use the process of elimination, and focus on the subject of the question. Recall that the hemoglobin level identifies the presence of iron deficiency anemia to direct you to option 3. Review hemoglobin level testing if you had difficulty with this question.

Reference
McKinney, E., James, S., Murray, S., & Ashwill, J. (2009). *Maternal-child nursing* (3rd ed., p. 253). St. Louis: Mosby.

---

865. A client is receiving warfarin sodium (Coumadin) therapy, and the nurse is monitoring the client for bleeding. The nurse understands that which of the following is the antidote to this medication if an overdose occurs?
1 Heparin sodium
2 Protamine sulfate
3 Phytonadione (vitamin K)
4 Oral potassium supplements

Level of Cognitive Ability: Comprehension
Client Needs: Physiological Integrity
Integrated Process: Nursing Process/Planning
Content Area: Pharmacology

Answer: 3
Rationale: Warfarin sodium (Coumadin) is an anticoagulant, and the effects of warfarin sodium overdose can be overcome with phytonadione (vitamin K). Vitamin K is an antagonist of warfarin sodium that can reverse the warfarin-induced inhibition of clotting factor synthesis. Heparin sodium is an anticoagulant. Protamine sulfate is the antidote for heparin sodium. Oral potassium is used to treat potassium deficiency.

Test-Taking Strategy: Knowledge of the antidote for warfarin sodium is necessary to answer this question. Remember that the antidote for warfarin sodium is phytonadione (vitamin K). Review the effects of warfarin sodium and the antidote if you had difficulty with this question.

Reference
Hodgson, B., & Kizior, R. (2009). *Saunders nursing drug handbook 2009* (p. 1219). St. Louis: Saunders.

---

866. A client who takes aspirin every day reports to the nurse that dental surgery is recommended. The nurse appropriately tells the client which of the following?
1 "Dental surgery is contraindicated."
2 "Ask your pharmacist about the surgery."
3 "Dental surgery can safely be done 48 hours after you stop taking your aspirin."
4 "There is no risk to having such a minor surgery while continuing your aspirin therapy."

Level of Cognitive Ability: Application
Client Needs: Physiological Integrity
Integrated Process: Nursing Process/Implementation
Content Area: Pharmacology

Answer: 3
Rationale: Aspirin is an antiplatelet medication. For an elective procedure such as dental surgery, aspirin therapy should be stopped approximately 48 hours before the surgery to prevent bleeding complications. Options 1 and 4 are incorrect. Option 2 is an inappropriate response and places the client's concern on hold.

Test-Taking Strategy: Use the process of elimination and therapeutic communication techniques to answer the question. Eliminate options 1 and 4 first because of the words *contraindicated* and *no risk*, respectively. Eliminate option 2 next because it is nontherapeutic and places the client's concerns on hold. Review the effects of aspirin if you had difficulty with this question.

Reference
Kee, J., Hayes, E., & McCuistion, L. (2009). *Pharmacology: A nursing process approach* (6th ed., p. 360). St. Louis: Saunders.

---

867. A nurse is monitoring a client who is at risk for developing acute renal failure (ARF). The nurse should become most concerned if which of the following is noted during data collection?

1 Urine output, 20 mL/hour for the last 3 hours; blood urea nitrogen, 35 mg/dL; creatinine, 2.1 mg/dL
2 Urine output, 30 mL/hour for the last 3 hours; blood urea nitrogen, 10 mg/dL; creatinine, 1.2 mg/dL
3 Urine output, 40 mL/hour for the last 3 hours; blood urea nitrogen, 15 mg/dL; creatinine, 0.8 mg/dL
4 Urine output, 60 mL/hour for the last 3 hours; blood urea nitrogen, 20 mg/dL; creatinine, 1.1 mg/dL

Level of Cognitive Ability: Analysis
Client Needs: Physiological Integrity
Integrated Process: Nursing Process/Data Collection
Content Area: Adult Health/Renal

Answer: 1

Rationale: ARF is the inability of the kidneys to excrete waste, concentrate urine, and conserve electrolytes. The client is often oliguric or anuric with ARF, although he or she may have nonoliguric renal failure. The blood urea nitrogen and serum creatinine levels also rise, which is indicative of defective kidney function. Normal serum blood urea nitrogen levels are usually 5 to 20 mg/dL; normal creatinine levels range from 0.6 to 1.3 mg/dL. The greatest abnormality in urine output and laboratory values is described in option 1 and indicates the client who is most at risk for developing ARF.

Test-Taking Strategy: To answer this question accurately, you must know that the client with ARF becomes oliguric or anuric and that serum blood urea nitrogen and creatinine levels rise. With this in mind, options 3 and 4 are eliminated first, because the urine output is above the minimum required level. From the remaining options, option 2 meets the minimum required hourly output, whereas option 1 falls below it. In addition, recall the normal serum blood urea nitrogen and creatinine levels to help you to definitively choose option 1 instead of option 2. Review the findings associated with ARF if you had difficulty with this question.

References

deWit, S. (2009). *Medical-surgical nursing: Concepts & practice* (pp. 851, 853). St. Louis: Saunders.
Linton, A. (2007). *Introduction to medical-surgical nursing* (4th ed., pp. 867-868). Philadelphia: Saunders.

---

868. A client with acute renal failure (ARF) has been treated with sodium polystyrene sulfonate (Kayexalate) by mouth. The nurse determines that this therapy is effective if which of the following values is noted on follow-up laboratory testing?

1 Calcium, 9.8 mg/dL
2 Sodium, 142 mEq/L
3 Potassium, 4.9 mEq/L
4 Phosphorus, 3.9 mg/dL

Level of Cognitive Ability: Analysis
Client Needs: Physiological Integrity
Integrated Process: Nursing Process/Evaluation
Content Area: Adult Health/Renal

Answer: 3

Rationale: ARF is the inability of the kidneys to excrete waste, concentrate urine, and conserve electrolytes. Of all of the electrolyte imbalances that accompany renal failure, hyperkalemia is the most dangerous, because it can lead to cardiac dysrhythmias and death. If the potassium level rises too high, sodium polystyrene sulfonate (a cation exchange resin and antihyperkalemic) may be given to cause the excretion of potassium through the gastrointestinal tract. Each of the electrolyte levels noted in the options falls within the normal reference range for that electrolyte. The potassium level is measured after the administration of this medication to determine the extent of the medication's effectiveness.

Test-Taking Strategy: To answer this question, you must know that the potassium level rises in ARF and that this condition is treated with the medication identified in the question. This will direct you to option 3. Review the therapeutic effects of sodium polystyrene sulfonate and the care of the client with ARF if you had difficulty with this question.

Reference

Linton, A. (2007). *Introduction to medical-surgical nursing* (4th ed., p. 196). Philadelphia: Saunders.

869. A nurse is caring for a client with chronic renal failure (CRF) and monitors for which most frequent cardiovascular finding associated with this condition?

1 Bradycardia
2 Tachycardia
3 Hypotension
4 Hypertension

Level of Cognitive Ability: Comprehension
Client Needs: Physiological Integrity
Integrated Process: Nursing Process/Data Collection
Content Area: Adult Health/Renal

Answer: 4

Rationale: CRF is the inability of the kidneys to excrete waste, concentrate urine, and conserve electrolytes. Hypertension is the most common cardiovascular finding in the client with CRF. It is caused by a number of mechanisms, including volume overload, renin–angiotensin system stimulation, vasoconstriction from sympathetic stimulation, and the absence of prostaglandins. Hypertension also may be the cause of the renal failure. It is important to monitor hypertension because it can lead to heart failure in the CRF client as a result of an increased cardiac workload in conjunction with fluid overload. Bradycardia and tachycardia are not specifically associated with renal failure.

Test-Taking Strategy: Use the process of elimination, and recall the pathophysiology of renal failure as well as its causes. Note that the options are broken into two sets: pulse and blood pressure. Knowing that blood pressure is the strategic item to monitor in a client with this condition helps you to eliminate options 1 and 2. Recall that hypertension (not hypotension) is associated with CRF to direct you to option 4. Review the cardiovascular signs of CRF if you had difficulty with this question.

Reference

Linton, A. (2007). *Introduction to medical-surgical nursing* (4th ed., p. 868). Philadelphia: Saunders.

---

870. A client with a closed fracture has just had a cast applied to the affected arm and is complaining of intense pain. The nurse has elevated the limb, applied an ice bag, and administered an analgesic that has provided very little relief. The nurse interprets that this pain may be caused by which of the following?

1 Infection under the cast
2 The anxiety of the client
3 Impaired tissue perfusion
4 The newness of the fracture

Level of Cognitive Ability: Analysis
Client Needs: Physiological Integrity
Integrated Process: Nursing Process/Data Collection
Content Area: Adult Health/Musculoskeletal

Answer: 3

Rationale: Most pain associated with fractures can be minimized with rest, elevation, the application of cold, and the administration of analgesics. Pain that is not relieved with these measures should be reported to the physician because it may result from impaired tissue perfusion, tissue breakdown, or necrosis. Because this is a new closed fracture, cast infection would not have had time to set in. Based on the signs and symptoms in the question, anxiety is not the cause.

Test-Taking Strategy: Use the process of elimination. Focus on the data in the question to assist you with eliminating options 2 and 4. Because the fracture and cast are new, it is extremely unlikely that infection could have set in. The most likely option is impaired tissue perfusion because pain from ischemia is not relieved by comfort measures and analgesics. Review the signs of impaired tissue perfusion in a client with a cast if you had difficulty with this question.

Reference

Linton, A. (2007). *Introduction to medical-surgical nursing* (4th ed., p. 927). Philadelphia: Saunders.

---

871. A nurse is caring for a client with a history of renal insufficiency who is having captopril (Capoten) added to the medication regimen. Before administering the first dose, the nurse reviews the medical

Answer: 2

Rationale: Captopril is an angiotensin-converting enzyme (ACE) inhibitor that is used for clients who do not respond to first-line antihypertensive agents. ACE inhibitors are used cautiously in clients with renal impairment. Before treatment is begun, baseline

record for the results of urinalysis, especially noting the presence of which of the following?
1 Casts
2 Protein
3 Red blood cells (RBCs)
4 White blood cells (WBCs)

Level of Cognitive Ability: Analysis
Client Needs: Physiological Integrity
Integrated Process: Nursing Process/Data Collection
Content Area: Pharmacology

assessments of blood pressure, and urine protein are done. The client with renal insufficiency may develop nephrotic syndrome and should be monitored for proteinuria on a monthly basis for 9 months and then periodically afterward.

Test-Taking Strategy: Use the process of elimination. The question tells you that the client has renal impairment and directs you to look at the client's urinalysis results. RBCs and WBCs could be indications of trauma, infection, or both, so these options should be eliminated first. Casts are mineral deposits that form along the renal tubules and that occasionally appear in the urine. Normally the kidneys conserve large protein molecules, which can make proteinuria abnormal; therefore this is the best indicator and the correct option. Review captopril if you had difficulty with this question.

Reference
Kee, J., Hayes, E., & McCuistion, L. (2009). *Pharmacology: A nursing process approach* (6th ed., p. 668). St. Louis: Saunders.

---

872. A nurse is caring for a client with chronic arterial insufficiency. The client complains of leg pain and cramping after walking 3 blocks, which is relieved when the client stops and rests. The nurse documents that the client is experiencing which of the following?
1 Venous insufficiency
2 Deep vein thrombosis
3 Arteriovenous shunting
4 Intermittent claudication

Level of Cognitive Ability: Application
Client Needs: Physiological Integrity
Integrated Process: Communication and Documentation
Content Area: Adult Health/Cardiovascular

Answer: 4
Rationale: Intermittent claudication is a classic symptom of peripheral vascular disease; it is described as a cramp-like pain that occurs with exercise and that is relieved by rest. Intermittent claudication is caused by ischemia and is very reproducible; in other words, a predictable amount of exercise causes the pain each time. The characteristics described in the question are not associated with venous insufficiency, deep vein thrombosis, or arteriovenous shunting.

Test-Taking Strategy: Use the process of elimination. The question tells you that this is an arterial disorder, so options 1 and 2 can be eliminated first. The word *intermittent* in option 4 is a clue that it is the correct option because it matches the timing cited in the question. Arteriovenous shunting is not an intermittent type of problem. Review the manifestations of arterial disease and the definition of intermittent claudication if you had difficulty with this question.

Reference
Linton, A. (2007). *Introduction to medical-surgical nursing* (4th ed., p. 688). Philadelphia: Saunders.

---

873. A nurse has been assigned to admit a 14-year-old female client to the family planning clinic. The client explains that she has missed several periods and has been gaining weight. To improve the client's nutritional status, the nurse gathers which of the following pieces of information?
1 The identity of the father and whether or not the client is planning to keep the baby
2 Whether this is the client's first pregnancy and what plans she has made for the baby

Answer: 4
Rationale: Because the client is several months pregnant and this is her first prenatal visit, the nurse's primary concern is the client's health status and her estimated date of delivery. Options 1 and 2 do not provide information that is helpful for planning prenatal care. The type of insurance coverage is information that a clinic or social worker may need, but it should not have any effect on the care provided to the client.

3 The client's type of insurance, whether she has had morning sickness, and what her normal diet consists of
4 The date of the client's last menstrual period; her weight, blood pressure, and urine test results; and resources available regarding a proper pregnancy diet

Level of Cognitive Ability: Analysis
Client Needs: Physiological Integrity
Integrated Process: Nursing Process/Data Collection
Content Area: Maternity/Antepartum

Test-Taking Strategy: Use the process of elimination. Note the strategic words *missed several periods.* Focus on the subject—improving the client's nutritional status. Eliminate options 1 and 2 first because they are comparable or alike. From the remaining options, select option 4 because it elicits objective data as a baseline for planning and focuses on the subject of the question. Review the care of the pregnant adolescent if you had difficulty with this question.

Reference

Leifer, G. (2008). *Maternity nursing: An introductory text* (10th ed., pp. 370-371). Philadelphia: Saunders.

---

874. A client is admitted for elective surgery and lists the home medications that were taken that day. The nurse collects data about the medications taken and is most concerned if the client took which of the following?
1 A β-blocker
2 An antibiotic
3 An anticoagulant
4 A calcium-channel blocker

Level of Cognitive Ability: Analysis
Client Needs: Physiological Integrity
Integrated Process: Nursing Process/Data Collection
Content Area: Fundamental Skills

Answer: 3

Rationale: An anticoagulant suppresses coagulation by inhibiting clotting factors. A client who is admitted for elective surgery should have been instructed to discontinue the anticoagulant preoperatively. The nurse should notify the physician even if this is unscheduled surgery. An antidote may be given to reverse the effects of the medication, but the client may still remain at risk for bleeding. The medications listed in options 1, 2, and 4 do not place the client at risk.

Test-Taking Strategy: Use the process of elimination. Eliminate options 1 and 4 first because they are comparable or alike in that both are cardiac medications. Eliminate option 2 next because antibiotics are often prescribed during the preoperative period. Review anticoagulant therapy and its associated risks if you had difficulty with this question.

Reference

Christensen, B., & Kockrow, E. (2006). *Adult health nursing* (5th ed., p. 43). St. Louis: Mosby.

---

875. Streptokinase (Streptase) is administered to a client in the emergency department after the diagnosis of a myocardial infarction. The nurse understands which of the following about this medication?
1 Thrombolytics suppress the production of fibrin.
2 Thrombolytics act to prevent thrombus formation.
3 Thrombolytics act to dissolve thrombi that have already formed.
4 Streptokinase has been proved to reverse all detrimental effects of heart attacks.

Level of Cognitive Ability: Analysis
Client Needs: Physiological Integrity
Integrated Process: Nursing Process/Planning
Content Area: Pharmacology

Answer: 3

Rationale: Thrombolytics (e.g., streptokinase) are most effective when started within 4 to 6 hours of the symptom onset of a myocardial infarction. Streptokinase acts to dissolve existing thrombi that are causing a blockage. Options 1, 2, and 4 are incorrect.

Test-Taking Strategy: Use the process of elimination and your knowledge of the action of this medication. Eliminate option 4 because of the words *proved* and *all.* From the remaining options, recalling the action of this medication directs you to option 3. Review streptokinase if you had difficulty with this question.

Reference

Hodgson, B., & Kizior, R. (2009). *Saunders nursing drug handbook 2009* (p. 1080). St. Louis: Saunders.

---

876. A nurse is assigned to care for a client who is receiving heparin intravenously. When planning care for the client, which of the following is the important consideration?

1 Using an electric razor for shaving
2 Providing complete care to the client
3 Not allowing the client to brush the teeth
4 Allowing the client to sit only at the bedside

Level of Cognitive Ability: Application
Client Needs: Physiological Integrity
Integrated Process: Nursing Process/Planning
Content Area: Pharmacology

Answer: 1

Rationale: Heparin is an anticoagulant. Clients receiving heparin should have extra considerations taken when planning care because these clients are at risk for bleeding. An electric shaver rather than a straight razor should be used for shaving. Options 2, 3, and 4 are not necessary.

Test-Taking Strategy: Use the process of elimination and your knowledge of the side effects of an anticoagulant to assist you with answering the question. Options 3 and 4 include the close-ended words *not* and *only*, respectively, and thus should be eliminated. From the remaining options, select option 1 because this action will reduce the risk of bleeding. In addition, it is best to allow the client to participate in care, if possible. Review the characteristics of heparin if you had difficulty with this question.

Reference

Edmunds, M. (2010). *Introduction to clinical pharmacology* (6th ed., p. 325). St. Louis: Mosby.

---

877. A client who is taking an anticoagulant reports to the laboratory for scheduled follow-up laboratory work. The results indicate an international normalized ratio (INR) of 2.5. The nurse evaluates these results as:

1 Normal
2 Insignificant findings
3 Lower than normal, so the anticoagulant dose should be increased
4 Higher than normal, so the anticoagulant dose should be decreased

Level of Cognitive Ability: Comprehension
Client Needs: Physiological Integrity
Integrated Process: Nursing Process/Evaluation
Content Area: Pharmacology

Answer: 1

Rationale: The normal INR is 2.0 to 3.0. A value of 2.5 indicates a normal value. Therefore, options 2, 3, and 4 are incorrect.

Test-Taking Strategy: Knowledge of the normal therapeutic value of the INR for a client who is taking an anticoagulant will direct you to option 1. Review this laboratory test if you had difficulty with this question.

Reference

Chernecky, C., & Berger, B. (2008). *Laboratory tests and diagnostic procedures* (5th ed., p. 927). Philadelphia: Saunders.

---

878. A nurse is collecting data from a client who is receiving weekly cyanocobalamin (vitamin B_{12}) injections. Which client statement indicates that the client is receiving the desired effects from the medication?

1 "I'm pain free now."
2 "My nausea is better."
3 "I get dizzy when I stand up."
4 "I feel stronger and have an increased appetite."

Level of Cognitive Ability: Analysis
Client Needs: Physiological Integrity
Integrated Process: Nursing Process/Evaluation
Content Area: Pharmacology

Answer: 4

Rationale: Cyanocobalamin is a vitamin that is essential for DNA synthesis. It can take up to 3 years for vitamin B_{12} stores to be depleted and symptoms of pernicious anemia to be noticed. These symptoms include weakness, fatigue, anorexia, loss of taste, and diarrhea. To correct deficiencies, a crystalline form of vitamin B_{12} (cyanocobalamin) can be given intramuscularly. Options 1, 2, and 3 are unrelated to the use or effects of this medication.

Test-Taking Strategy: Use the process of elimination. Focus on the medication identified in the question, and note that it is a vitamin. With this in mind, eliminate options 1, 2, and 3. Review the desired effects of cyanocobalamin injection if you had difficulty with this question.

Reference

Hodgson, B., & Kizior, R. (2009). *Saunders nursing drug handbook 2009* (p. 292). St. Louis: Saunders.

879. Ticlopidine (Ticlid), which is an antiplatelet medication, is prescribed for a client. The nurse reviews the client's record for the documentation of which baseline data before administering the medication?

1 History of stroke
2 Sedimentation rate
3 Most recent vital signs
4 White blood cell (WBC) differential results

Level of Cognitive Ability: Analysis
Client Needs: Physiological Integrity
Integrated Process: Nursing Process/Data Collection
Content Area: Pharmacology

Answer: 4

Rationale: Ticlopidine is an antiplatelet medication that is used to assist with the prevention of thrombotic stroke. Ticlopidine can cause neutropenia, which is an abnormally small number of mature white blood cells. Baseline data are necessary before initiating therapy. A complete blood count with WBC differential is necessary to determine neutropenia, and therapy may be stopped if this adverse effect occurs. The effects of neutropenia are reversible within 1 to 3 weeks after the discontinuation of the medication. The sedimentation rate and the vital signs are not associated with this medication.

Test-Taking Strategy: Knowledge of the adverse effects of this medication is necessary to answer this question. Remember that ticlopidine is an antiplatelet medication that can cause neutropenia. Review ticlopidine if you had difficulty with this question.

Reference

Hodgson, B., & Kizior, R. (2009). *Saunders nursing drug handbook 2009* (pp. 1135). St. Louis: Saunders.

---

880. A nurse is caring for a client who has had a transient ischemic attack. In the event that an ischemic stroke occurs, the nurse anticipates that which medication will most likely be prescribed initially?

1 A β-blocker
2 An oral anticoagulant
3 An antiplatelet medication
4 A thrombolytic medication

Level of Cognitive Ability: Analysis
Client Needs: Physiological Integrity
Integrated Process: Nursing Process/Planning
Content Area: Pharmacology

Answer: 4

Rationale: An ischemic stroke is a cerebrovascular disorder that is caused by the deprivation of blood flow to an area of the brain, generally as a result of thrombosis, embolism, or reduced blood pressure. Alteplase (Activase), which is a thrombolytic medication, may be prescribed for clients who experience ischemic strokes. For clients who are treated within 6 hours of the onset of symptoms, progression of the stroke frequently can be halted. Many of the symptoms that are present can also be reversed. A β-blocker is used for cardiac and hypertensive conditions. An oral anticoagulant and an antiplatelet medication may be used to assist with the prevention of an ischemic stroke.

Test-Taking Strategy: Use the process of elimination, and focus on the subject—a client who has had an ischemic stroke. Knowledge of the action of a β-blocker assists you with eliminating option 1. Focus on the subject of the question to direct you to option 4 from the remaining options. Review pharmacological treatments for a client with a stroke if you had difficulty with this question.

References

Christensen, B., & Kockrow, E. (2006). *Adult health nursing* (5th ed., p. 731). St. Louis: Mosby.
Hodgson, B., & Kizior, R. (2009). *Saunders nursing drug handbook 2009* (p. 43). St. Louis: Saunders.

---

881. After receiving replacement surfactant therapy, the infant with respiratory distress syndrome (RDS) requires frequent arterial blood gas monitoring. Which statement by the infant's mother indicates that she understands the reason that frequent blood sampling is needed?

Answer: 2

Rationale: RDS is an acute lung disease of the newborn that is characterized by airless alveoli, inelastic lungs, a respiration rate of more than 60 breaths/min, nasal flaring, intercostal and subcostal retractions, grunting on expiration, and peripheral edema. Frequent monitoring may be necessary during the acute stages of RDS in the newborn and especially after replacement surfactant therapy has occurred. This

1 "You just keep taking blood from my baby for all these tests."
2 "Frequent blood gas tests help to monitor my baby's respiratory patterns."
3 "Taking blood samples is the hospital's policy after giving this medication."
4 "My baby will require frequent blood gas tests throughout the hospital stay."

Level of Cognitive Ability: Comprehension
Client Needs: Physiological Integrity
Integrated Process: Nursing Process/Evaluation
Content Area: Maternity/Postpartum

allows for the trending of the respiratory status and assists with decision making during further management. Options 1, 3, and 4 do not reflect an understanding of the purpose of the blood gas tests.

Test-Taking Strategy: Use the process of elimination and your knowledge of surfactant replacement therapy to answer this question. Note the relationship between the subject of the question and option 2. Review the care of the infant with RDS if you had difficulty with this question.

Reference

Leifer, G. (2007). *Introduction to maternity and pediatric nursing* (5th ed., pp. 305, 317). Philadelphia: Saunders.

---

882. A nurse reads the radiology report of the initial chest radiograph taken of an infant who is experiencing respiratory distress syndrome (RDS) and who has received replacement surfactant therapy. The report states that both lung fields have a "ground-glass" appearance. How does the nurse evaluate this report?
1 Indicative of a pneumothorax
2 Insignificant and unrelated to respiratory distress syndrome
3 Consistent with a diagnosis of bronchopulmonary dysplasia
4 Characteristic of RDS secondary to hyaline membrane disease

Level of Cognitive Ability: Analysis
Client Needs: Physiological Integrity
Integrated Process: Nursing Process/Evaluation
Content Area: Maternity/Postpartum

Answer: 4
Rationale: RDS is an acute lung disease of the newborn that is characterized by airless alveoli, inelastic lungs, a respiration rate of more than 60 breaths/min, nasal flaring, intercostal and subcostal retractions, grunting on expiration, and peripheral edema. Chest radiographs in infants with respiratory distress syndrome related to hyaline membrane disease show a "ground-glass" appearance that is characteristic of the disease process. This finding is significant; it is not consistent with a diagnosis of bronchopulmonary dysplasia or indicative of a pneumothorax.

Test-Taking Strategy: Use the process of elimination. Focus on the subject of the question, and note the relationship between the words *experiencing respiratory distress syndrome* in the question and *characteristic of RDS* in the correct option. Review the findings associated with RDS if you had difficulty with this question.

Reference

Leifer, G. (2007). *Introduction to maternity and pediatric nursing* (5th ed., pp. 305-306). Philadelphia: Saunders.

---

883. A nurse is caring for an infant with respiratory distress syndrome (RDS) secondary to hyaline membrane disease. The nurse is gathering data about the client and looking for a major finding associated with RDS when he or she does which of the following?
1 Weighs the infant
2 Takes the infant's blood pressure
3 Tests the infant's urine for glucose
4 Reviews the results of the arterial blood gas testing

Level of Cognitive Ability: Application
Client Needs: Physiological Integrity
Integrated Process: Nursing Process/Data Collection
Content Area: Maternity/Postpartum

Answer: 4
Rationale: RDS is an acute lung disease of the newborn that is characterized by airless alveoli, inelastic lungs, a respiration rate of more than 60 breaths/min, nasal flaring, intercostal and subcostal retractions, grunting on expiration, and peripheral edema. Acidosis is a major manifestation of RDS that develops because of the hypoxemia associated with RDS. The results of the arterial blood gas test would indicate an acid–base imbalance. Options 1 and 2 may be components of the data collection, but they are not specifically associated with RDS. Option 3 is unrelated to RDS.

Test-Taking Strategy: Use the process of elimination. Focus on the diagnosis of RDS to direct you to the only option that addresses a respiratory assessment technique. Review the clinical manifestations associated with RDS and the appropriate data collection techniques if you had difficulty with this question.

Reference

Leifer, G. (2007). *Introduction to maternity and pediatric nursing* (5th ed., p. 305). Philadelphia: Saunders.

884. A nurse is reviewing laboratory results for a preterm infant with respiratory distress syndrome (RDS) and suspected hyaline membrane disease. The results of the lecithin–sphingomyelin (L/S) ratio drawn at 30 weeks' gestation are reported as less than 2:1. The nurse evaluates these results as:
1 Normal
2 Insignificant
3 Lower than normal
4 Higher than normal

Level of Cognitive Ability: Analysis
Client Needs: Physiological Integrity
Integrated Process: Nursing Process/Evaluation
Content Area: Maternity/Postpartum

Answer: 3
Rationale: RDS is an acute lung disease of the newborn that is characterized by airless alveoli, inelastic lungs, a respiration rate of more than 60 breaths/min, nasal flaring, intercostal and subcostal retractions, grunting on expiration, and peripheral edema. The presence of surfactant in the amniotic fluid is an indicator of fetal lung maturity. Sampling may be done by amniocentesis or by the removal of a fluid sample from the vagina after the rupture of the membranes. Pulmonary status is generally considered to be mature with an L/S ratio of at least 2:1.

Test-Taking Strategy: Use the process of elimination. Knowing that the L/S ratio can be an indicator of lung maturity, expect that the level would be less than normal in an infant with RDS. In addition, select the option that is similar to the information in the question. In this case, *less than 2:1* and *lower than normal* are comparable or alike. Review the L/S ratio if you had difficulty with this question.

Reference
Leifer, G. (2007). *Introduction to maternity and pediatric nursing* (5th ed., pp. 81, 305). Philadelphia: Saunders.

---

885. A nurse caring for a small-for-gestational-age (SGA) infant reviews the results of a total serum calcium level and notes that the result is reported as 5.9 mg/dL. How does the nurse evaluate these results?
1 Insignificant
2 Lower than normal
3 Higher than normal
4 Within normal limits

Level of Cognitive Ability: Comprehension
Client Needs: Physiological Integrity
Integrated Process: Nursing Process/Evaluation
Content Area: Maternity/Postpartum

Answer: 2
Rationale: An SGA infant is an infant whose weight and size at birth fall below the tenth percentile of appropriate-for-gestational-age infants, whether delivered at term or earlier or later than term. SGA infants are at risk for developing hypocalcemia. The normal range for a total serum calcium level is 7.0 mg/dL to 8.5 mg/dL; therefore, options 1, 3, and 4 are incorrect.

Test-Taking Strategy: Focus on the data in the question. Recalling that the normal range for a total serum calcium level is 7.0 mg/dL to 8.5 mg/dL will direct you to option 2. Review total serum calcium level testing if you had difficulty with this question.

References
Chernecky, C., & Berger, B. (2008). *Laboratory tests and diagnostic procedures* (5th ed., p. 280). Philadelphia: Saunders.
Leifer, G. (2007). *Introduction to maternity and pediatric nursing* (5th ed., p. 309). Philadelphia: Saunders.

---

886. A nurse is caring for a small-for-gestational-age (SGA) infant. When evaluating the infant's growth and determining whether the infant is asymmetrically or symmetrically SGA, the nurse collects data regarding which of the following?
1 Temperature, pulse, and blood pressure
2 Head circumference, length, and weight
3 Weight, respiratory rate, and urine output

Answer: 2
Rationale: An SGA infant is an infant whose weight and size at birth fall below the tenth percentile of appropriate-for-gestational-age infants, whether delivered at term or earlier or later than term. Symmetrical versus asymmetrical growth determines whether the growth restriction began early or late in the pregnancy; it is determined by collecting information about head circumference, length, and weight. Options 1, 3 and 4 do not provide information about growth.

4 Chest circumference, hematocrit level, and blood glucose

Level of Cognitive Ability: Comprehension
Client Needs: Physiological Integrity
Integrated Process: Nursing Process/Data Collection
Content Area: Maternity/Postpartum

Test-Taking Strategy: Use the process of elimination, and focus on the subject of the question. Note that the subject addresses growth to assist with directing you to option 2. Review the techniques for determining growth factors in the SGA infant if you had difficulty with this question.

Reference

Leifer, G. (2007). *Introduction to maternity and pediatric nursing* (5th ed., p. 305). Philadelphia: Saunders.

---

887. A nurse is monitoring a small-for-gestational-age (SGA) infant. Which data indicates a potential complication in this infant?

1 Intolerance of oral feedings
2 An axillary temperature of 99° F
3 A blood glucose level of 45 to 60 mg/dL
4 A urinary output of less than 3 to 4 mL/kg per hour

Level of Cognitive Ability: Comprehension
Client Needs: Physiological Integrity
Integrated Process: Nursing Process/Data Collection
Content Area: Maternity/Postpartum

Answer: 1
Rationale: An SGA infant is an infant whose weight and size at birth fall below the tenth percentile of appropriate-for-gestational-age infants, whether delivered at term or earlier or later than term. One of the complications associated with SGA infants is an intolerance of oral feedings. All of the other options are values that are within normal limits and therefore are not complications. It is important to recognize that nutrition in the SGA infant is a primary consideration. If the infant is intolerant of oral feedings, an alternate form of nutritional support should be implemented.

Test-Taking Strategy: Use the process of elimination and your knowledge of the normal vital signs and laboratory values for an infant to direct you to option 1. Review the normal values and complications in an SGA infant if you had difficulty with this question.

Reference

Leifer, G. (2008). *Maternity nursing: An introductory text* (10th ed., pp. 303, 309). Philadelphia: Saunders.

---

888. A nurse can best prevent a fluid volume deficit after the administration of a diuretic to a disoriented client by doing which of the following?

1 Frequently offering fluids
2 Leaving water at the bedside
3 Keeping the client on bedrest
4 Advising the client to drink lots of fluids

Level of Cognitive Ability: Application
Client Needs: Physiological Integrity
Integrated Process: Nursing Process/Implementation
Content Area: Fundamental Skills

Answer: 1
Rationale: A disoriented client should be offered fluid by the caregiver to increase fluid intake and prevent dehydration. Options 2 and 4 do not ensure that the client will drink the needed fluids. Option 3 is unrelated to the subject of the question.

Test-Taking Strategy: Use the process of elimination, and focus on the subject of the question. Note the strategic words *disoriented client*. Eliminate option 3 because it is unrelated to the subject of the question. Eliminate options 2 and 4 because these actions cannot ensure that the client will drink the needed fluids. Review the care of the client with a fluid volume deficit if you had difficulty with this question.

Reference

Wold, G. (2008). *Basic geriatric nursing* (4th ed., pp. 256-257, 259). St. Louis: Mosby.

---

889. A nurse is preparing to administer captopril (Capoten), which is an angiotensin-converting enzyme (ACE) inhibitor. Which data would be important to collect before administering the medication?

Answer: 4
Rationale: Captopril (Capoten) is an ACE inhibitor. ACE inhibitors are potent antihypertensive medications. A baseline blood pressure is needed to evaluate the outcome of this therapy. Options 1, 2, and 3 are generally not affected by the action of ACE inhibitors.

1 Temperature
2 Lung sounds
3 Mental status
4 Blood pressure

Level of Cognitive Ability: Analysis
Client Needs: Physiological Integrity
Integrated Process: Nursing Process/Data Collection
Content Area: Pharmacology

Test-Taking Strategy: Use the process of elimination. Recall that ACE inhibitors are most often used to treat hypertension to direct you to option 4. Review the actions and uses of ACE inhibitors if you had difficulty with this question.

Reference

Hodgson, B., & Kizior, R. (2009). *Saunders nursing drug handbook 2009* (p. 179). St. Louis: Saunders.

---

890. The nurse is preparing to administer an intramuscular injection to a toddler. Which of the following is the safest body site to use to administer this injection?
1 Deltoid muscle
2 Dorsogluteal muscle
3 Ventrogluteal muscle
4 Vastus lateralis muscle

Level of Cognitive Ability: Application
Client Needs: Physiological Integrity
Integrated Process: Nursing Process/Implementation
Content Area: Child Health

Answer: 4
Rationale: The vastus lateralis muscle is large enough to handle an intramuscular injection in a toddler. Options 1, 2, and 3 are not appropriate sites because they are not large muscle groups.

Test-Taking Strategy: Use the process of elimination and your knowledge of the administration of intramuscular injections to a toddler to answer the question. Recall the anatomy of muscle groups to direct you to option 4. Review intramuscular injection techniques for the toddler if you had difficulty with this question.

Reference

Hockenberry, M., & Wilson, D. (2009). *Wong's essentials of pediaric care* (8th ed., p. 720). St. Louis: Mosby.

---

891. A nurse is caring for a postmature infant who had a venous hematocrit level of more than 65% when he was 2 hours old. The nurse reviews the results of the laboratory tests, knowing that, during the next 24 hours, the priority laboratory value to monitor is which of the following?
1 Bilirubin
2 Creatinine
3 Urine for protein
4 Blood urea nitrogen

Level of Cognitive Ability: Analysis
Client Needs: Physiological Integrity
Integrated Process: Nursing Process/Data Collection
Content Area: Maternity/Postpartum

Answer: 1
Rationale: A postmature infant is an infant who is born after the end of the forty-second week of gestation and who bears the physical signs of placental insufficiency. Postmature infants are at risk for inadequate oxygen in utero, which predisposes them to polycythemia. Polycythemia then makes the infant prone to hyperbilirubinemia. In this infant, the priority is to monitor the bilirubin level.

Test-Taking Strategy: Use the process of elimination and your knowledge of the care of the postmature infant. Note that options 2, 3, and 4 are comparable or alike in that they all relate to the renal system. Review the care of the postmature infant if you had difficulty with this question.

References

Leifer, G. (2007). *Introduction to maternity and pediatric nursing* (5th ed., p. 287). Philadelphia: Saunders.
Hockenberry, M. & Wilson, D. (2009). *Wong's essentials of pediatric care* (8th ed., pp. 274-275). St. Louis: Mosby.

---

892. An anticholinergic medication is prescribed for preoperative client. The nurse prepares to administer the medication, knowing that it has which action?
1 It increases the heart rate and helps to prevent shock.

Answer: 2
Rationale: Anticholinergic medications dry up secretions, which helps to prevent aspiration. Options 1 and 3 are inaccurate actions of the medication. Although the medication may relax the urinary bladder, this is not the purpose for administering the medication during the preoperative period. In addition, this medication does not prevent urinary tract infections.

2 It reduces respiratory tract secretions and helps to prevent aspiration.
3 It prolongs blood clotting time and helps to prevent thrombophlebitis.
4 It relaxes the urinary bladder and helps to prevent urinary tract infections.

Level of Cognitive Ability: Analysis
Client Needs: Physiological Integrity
Integrated Process: Nursing Process/Implementation
Content Area: Fundamental Skills

Test-Taking Strategy: Use the process of elimination, and recall that one of the risks associated with surgery is aspiration; this will direct you to option 2. Review the actions of anticholinergics if you had difficulty with this question.

Reference

Kee, J., Hayes, E., & McCuistion, L. (2009). *Pharmacology: A nursing process approach* (6th ed., pp. 602-603). St. Louis: Saunders.

---

893. A nurse is gathering data about a postmature infant born after 42 weeks' gestation. The most significant information is obtained when the nurse does which of the following?
1 Obtains the Apgar scores
2 Obtains the infant's footprints
3 Determines the maternal blood type
4 Estimates the actual gestational age by recording the infant's weight, length, and head circumference on standard growth charts

Level of Cognitive Ability: Analysis
Client Needs: Physiological Integrity
Integrated Process: Nursing Process/Data Collection
Content Area: Maternity/Postpartum

Answer: 4
Rationale: A postmature infant is an infant who is born after the end of the forty-second week of gestation and who bears the physical signs of placental insufficiency. The medical management of a postmature infant is different than that of a preterm or term infant. The documentation of the actual estimated gestational age is an important factor for determining the management of the infant. Although options 1, 2, and 3 identify data that would be obtained, option 4 specifically identifies information that is necessary for the care of the postmature infant.

Test-Taking Strategy: Focus on the subject—the postmature infant. Although all of the options identify information that would be collected, only option 4 identifies information related to the postmature infant. Review the initial care of the postmature infant if you had difficulty with this question.

Reference

Hockenberry, M., & Wilson, D. (2009). *Wong's essentials of pediatric nursing* (8th ed., pp. 273-274). St. Louis: Mosby.

---

894. A client is admitted to the hospital with complications of celiac disease. Which question would be most helpful when obtaining information for the initial plan of care?
1 "What types of pasta can you eat?"
2 "What is your understanding of celiac disease?"
3 "Tell me about the types of foods that you like to eat."
4 "Have you eliminated whole-wheat bread from your diet?"

Level of Cognitive Ability: Application
Client Needs: Physiological Integrity
Integrated Process: Nursing Process/Data Collection
Content Area: Fundamental Skills

Answer: 2
Rationale: Celiac disease also is known as gluten-induced enteropathy. It causes diseased intestinal villi, which results in fewer absorptive surfaces and malabsorption syndrome. Clients with celiac disease must maintain a gluten-free diet, which eliminates all products made from wheat, rye, barley, and oats. Beer, pasta, crackers, cereals, and many more substances contain gluten. To plan care, it is most important to determine the client's understanding of the disease.

Test-Taking Strategy: Use the process of elimination and the principles related to teaching and learning concepts. Option 2 focuses on the client's disorder and is the umbrella option. Review teaching and learning principles and celiac disease if you had difficulty with this question.

Reference

Linton, A. (2007). *Introduction to medical-surgical nursing* (4th ed., p. 777). Philadelphia: Saunders.

895. A client with a duodenal ulcer asks the nurse why an antibiotic has been prescribed. The nurse responds by telling the client that this medication will do which of the following?

1 Reduce the inflammation
2 Prevent secondary infections
3 Soothe the irritated mucosal surface
4 Eliminate a germ that impairs mucosal function

Level of Cognitive Ability: Analysis
Client Needs: Physiological Integrity
Integrated Process: Nursing Process/Implementation
Content Area: Adult Health/Gastrointestinal

Answer: 4

Rationale: A duodenal ulcer is an ulcer in the duodenum. Duodenal ulcers are strongly associated with *Helicobacter pylori* infection. It is believed that these bacteria colonize in the mucous cells and impair their function. Antibiotics are given to control this infection. Options 1 and 3 are not effects of antibiotics. Option 2 is a rare occurrence with duodenal ulcers.

Test-Taking Strategy: Use the process of elimination and your knowledge of the actions of antibiotics to assist you with eliminating options 1 and 3. Recall the pathophysiology related to duodenal ulcers and their probable causes to direct you to option 4. Review duodenal ulcers if you had difficulty with this question.

Reference

Linton, A. (2007). *Introduction to medical-surgical nursing* (4th ed., p. 766). Philadelphia: Saunders.

---

896. A nurse is caring for a client who is receiving prednisone (Deltasone). The nurse plans to most closely monitor the client for the development of which of the following?

1 Weight loss
2 Hypoglycemia
3 Hyperglycemia
4 Adrenal insufficiency

Level of Cognitive Ability: Analysis
Client Needs: Physiological Integrity
Integrated Process: Nursing Process/Planning
Content Area: Pharmacology

Answer: 3

Rationale: Prednisone (Deltasone) is a corticosteroid. Exogenously administered corticosteroids have profound systemic effects because they mimic naturally occurring adrenal hormones. Hyperglycemia occurs because of the stimulation of gluconeogenesis and the decreased use of glucose by the cells. Option 1 is an incorrect effect because weight gain is often experienced by clients receiving prednisone. Option 4 identifies a condition in which corticosteroids may be administered.

Test-Taking Strategy: Note the strategic words *most closely monitor.* Remember that corticosteroids can cause hyperglycemia. Review the side effects of corticosteroids if you had difficulty with this question.

Reference

Kee, J., Hayes, E., & McCuistion, L. (2009). *Pharmacology: A nursing process approach* (6th ed., p. 787). St. Louis: Saunders.

---

897. A nurse is admitting a client with a diagnosis of a nasal polyp to the surgical nursing unit. Which of the following should the nurse expect the client to describe when collecting data from the client?

1 Coryza
2 Headaches
3 Runny nose
4 Nasal obstruction

Level of Cognitive Ability: Comprehension
Client Needs: Physiological Integrity
Integrated Process: Nursing Process/Data Collection
Content Area: Adult Health/Respiratory

Answer: 4

Rationale: A nasal polyp is a rounded, elongated piece of pulpy, dependent mucosa that projects into the nasal cavity. The primary symptom of a nasal polyp is nasal obstruction. Coryza and headache are not symptoms of a nasal tumor. A runny nose is suggestive of a cold or sinus drainage.

Test-Taking Strategy: Use the process of elimination, and focus on the diagnosis of nasal polyp. Visualize this disorder and the effect that it may have on the client to direct you to option 4. Review the manifestations associated with nasal polyps if you had difficulty with this question.

Reference

Linton, A. (2007). *Introduction to medical-surgical nursing* (4th ed., p. 1219). Philadelphia: Saunders.

898. A licensed practical nurse (LPN) is assisting a registered nurse (RN) with preparing to insert a nasogastric (NG) tube into a client. The RN asks the LPN to assist with determining the appropriate length of the tube needed for insertion. The LPN does which of the following to provide the requested measurement?

1 Places the tube at the tip of the nose and measures by extending the tube to the sternum and then to the earlobe
2 Places the tube at the tip of the earlobe and measures by extending the tube to the nose and down to the umbilicus
3 Places the tube at the tip of the earlobe and measures by extending the tube to the nose and then to the xiphoid process
4 Places the tube at the tip of the nose and measures by extending the tube to the earlobe and then down to the xiphoid process

Level of Cognitive Ability: Application
Client Needs: Physiological Integrity
Integrated Process: Nursing Process/Implementation
Content Area: Adult Health/Gastrointestinal

Answer: 4
Rationale: The appropriate method of measuring the length of the tube needed for NG tube insertion is to place the tube at the tip of the nose and measure by extending the tube to the earlobe and then down to the xiphoid process; the tube should be marked at that length. Options 1, 2, and 3 are inaccurate measurement procedures.

Test-Taking Strategy: Use the process of elimination and your knowledge of the appropriate procedure for measuring the length of an NG tube required for insertion to answer this question. Visualize the description in each of the options to help you to answer the question correctly. Review this procedure if you had difficulty with this question.

Reference
Christensen, B., & Kockrow, E. (2006). *Foundations of nursing* (5th ed., p. 590). St. Louis: Mosby.

---

899. A nurse is monitoring a client after endoscopic retrograde cholangiopancreatography for complications of the procedure. Which of the following indicates a potential complication?

1 Lethargy
2 Abdominal pain
3 Lack of a gag reflex
4 Lack of a cough reflex

Level of Cognitive Ability: Analysis
Client Needs: Physiological Integrity
Integrated Process: Nursing Process/Data Collection
Content Area: Adult Health/Gastrointestinal

Answer: 2
Rationale: An endoscopic retrograde cholangiopancreatography is an endoscopic test that provides radiographic visualization of the bile and pancreatic ducts. Postprocedural care after endoscopic retrograde cholangiopancreatography include monitoring the vital signs and maintaining an NPO status until the gag reflex returns. The client probably received sedating medication before the procedure; consequently, lethargy is expected. A local anesthetic is sprayed into the client's throat, so it is possible that the gag and cough reflexes will not be present. The client should be monitored for signs of cholangitis and perforation, which include fever, abdominal pain (especially in the right upper quadrant), hypotension, and tachycardia.

Test-Taking Strategy: Use the process of elimination, and note the strategic words *potential complication.* Eliminate options 3 and 4 first because the test is endoscopic in nature and because a local anesthetic is sprayed into the client's throat. Recall that medication is administered before the procedure to help you to eliminate option 1. Review the complications of an endoscopic retrograde cholangiopancreatography if you had difficulty with this question.

Reference
Chernecky, C., & Berger, B. (2008). *Laboratory tests and diagnostic procedures* (5th ed., p. 474). Philadelphia: Saunders.

900. A nurse is assisting a physician who is performing abdominal paracentesis on a client. The nurse should assist with placing the client into which of the following positions for this procedure?
1 Supine
2 Left lateral position
3 Right lateral position
4 Upright or high-Fowler's position

Level of Cognitive Ability: Application
Client Needs: Physiological Integrity
Integrated Process: Nursing Process/Implementation
Content Area: Adult Health/Gastrointestinal

Answer: 4
Rationale: A paracentesis is a procedure in which fluid is withdrawn from a body cavity. During abdominal paracentesis, the nurse should support the client in an upright or high-Fowler's position. This position allows the intestine to float posteriorly, and it helps to prevent laceration during catheter insertion. Options 1, 2, and 3 are incorrect.

Test-Taking Strategy: Use the process of elimination. Eliminate options 1, 2, and 3 because they are comparable or alike positions. In addition, visualizing this procedure and each of the positions identified in the options directs you to option 4. Review the procedure for abdominal paracentesis if you had difficulty with this question.

References
Chernecky, C., & Berger, B. (2008). *Laboratory tests and diagnostic procedures* (5th ed., p. 845). Philadelphia: Saunders.
Linton, A. (2007). *Introduction to medical-surgical nursing* (4th ed., p. 810). Philadelphia: Saunders.

---

901. A client is seen in the health care clinic, and a diagnosis of hypothyroidism is suspected. Which finding does the nurse expect to note in this client?
1 Bradycardia
2 Hyperactivity
3 Exophthalmos
4 Profuse diaphoresis

Level of Cognitive Ability: Comprehension
Client Needs: Physiological Integrity
Integrated Process: Nursing Process/Data Collection
Content Area: Adult Health/Endocrine

Answer: 1
Rationale: Hypothyroidism is a condition that is characterized by decreased activity of the thyroid gland. Clinical manifestations associated with hypothyroidism include bradycardia; obesity; dry, sparse hair; flaky, dry, inelastic skin; and a lowered basal body temperature. The client's ability to sweat also diminishes. Constipation and fecal impaction occur, and the client has an increased susceptibility to infection. The blood pressure may be normal or slightly elevated, and the temperature is normal to subnormal. Options 2, 3, and 4 are findings noted in clients with hyperthyroidism.

Test-Taking Strategy: Use the process of elimination. Recall that metabolic processes are decreased in clients with hypothyroidism to direct you to option 1. Options 2, 3, and 4 are findings that are noted in clients with hyperthyroidism. Review the findings associated with hypothyroidism if you had difficulty with this question.

Reference
Christensen, B., & Kockrow, E. (2006). *Adult health nursing* (5th ed., p. 531). St. Louis: Mosby.

---

902. A nurse is monitoring a client with hypothyroidism for neurological manifestations. Which of the following does the nurse expect to note in the client?
1 Fine tremors
2 Restlessness
3 Slow, deliberate speech
4 Increased deep tendon reflexes

Level of Cognitive Ability: Comprehension
Client Needs: Physiological Integrity

Answer: 3
Rationale: Hypothyroidism is a condition that is characterized by decreased activity of the thyroid gland. The neurological manifestations of hypothyroidism include decreased deep tendon reflexes, muscle sluggishness, fatigue, slow and deliberate speech, apathy, depression, impaired short-term memory, and lethargy. Options 1, 2, and 4 are signs of hyperthyroidism.

Integrated Process: Nursing Process/Data Collection
Content Area: Adult Health/Endocrine

Test-Taking Strategy: Use the process of elimination. Recall that metabolic processes are decreased in clients with hypothyroidism to direct you to option 3. Options 1, 2, and 4 are findings that are noted in clients with hyperthyroidism. Review the findings associated with hypothyroidism if you had difficulty with this question.

Reference
Christensen, B., & Kockrow, E. (2006). *Adult health nursing* (5th ed., p. 531). St. Louis: Mosby.

---

903. A nurse is caring for a client with a diagnosis of thyroid crisis (thyroid storm). Which of the following should the nurse include in the plan of care for this client?

1 A high-fiber diet
2 Use of a hypothermic blanket
3 Administration of levothyroxine (Synthroid)
4 Administration of enemas and stool softeners

Level of Cognitive Ability: Application
Client Needs: Physiological Integrity
Integrated Process: Nursing Process/Planning
Content Area: Adult Health/Endocrine

Answer: 2
Rationale: Thyroid crisis is a potentially fatal acute episode of thyroid overactivity that is characterized by high fever, severe tachycardia, delirium, dehydration, and extreme irritability. Because thyroid storm is an emergency, it requires immediate interventions for control. The high fever is treated with hypothermic blankets, and dehydration is reversed with intravenous fluids. The other options are treatment measures for hypothyroidism.

Test-Taking Strategy: Use the process of elimination. Recall that thyroid crisis is an acute episode of thyroid overactivity to help you to eliminate options 1, 3, and 4. Review thyroid crisis if you had difficulty with this question.

Reference
Ignatavicius, D., & Workman, M. (2010). *Medical-surgical nursing: Patient-centered collaborative care* (6th ed., p. 1455). St. Louis: Saunders.

---

904. The nurse is caring for a client after thyroidectomy and monitoring for complications. Which of the following, if noted in the client, indicates the need for physician notification?

1 Voice hoarseness
2 Weakness of the voice
3 Surgical pain in the neck area
4 Numbness and tingling around the mouth

Level of Cognitive Ability: Analysis
Client Needs: Physiological Integrity
Integrated Process: Nursing Process/Data Collection
Content Area: Adult Health/Endocrine

Answer: 4
Rationale: Thyroidectomy is the surgical removal of the thyroid gland. Hypocalcemia can develop after thyroidectomy if the parathyroid glands are accidentally removed or traumatized during surgery. The physician should be called immediately if the client develops twitching, muscle spasms, or numbness and tingling around the mouth or in the fingertips or toes. A hoarse or weak voice may occur temporarily if there has been unilateral injury to the laryngeal nerve during surgery. Pain is expected during the postoperative period. Calcium gluconate ampules should be available at the bedside, and the client should have a patent intravenous line in the event that hypocalcemic tetany occurs.

Test-Taking Strategy: Use the process of elimination. Eliminate options 1 and 2 first because they are comparable or alike. Note that surgical pain is expected after thyroidectomy to direct you to option 4 from the remaining options. Review the complications associated with thyroidectomy if you had difficulty with this question.

Reference
Linton, A. (2007). *Introduction to medical-surgical nursing* (4th ed., pp. 987-988). Philadelphia: Saunders.

---

905. A nurse is assisting with monitoring a client for signs of hypocalcemia. Which of the following should the nurse note on data collection if hypocalcemia is present?

1 Positive Homans' sign
2 Positive Trousseau's sign
3 Negative Chvostek's sign
4 Hypoactive deep tendon reflexes

Level of Cognitive Ability: Comprehension
Client Needs: Physiological Integrity
Integrated Process: Nursing Process/Data Collection
Content Area: Adult Health/Endocrine

Answer: 2

Rationale: Hypocalcemia is a deficiency of calcium in the serum. Data collection findings from the client who is hypocalcemic include a positive Chvostek's sign and Trousseau's sign, hyperactive deep tendon reflexes, circumoral paresthesia, and numbness and tingling of the fingers. A positive Homans' sign is noted in a client with thrombophlebitis.

Test-Taking Strategy: Use the process of elimination, and focus on the subject—hypocalcemia. Recall the findings from a hypocalcemic client and that a positive Chvostek's sign is noted in this condition to direct you to option 2. Review the findings associated with hypocalcemia if you had difficulty with this question.

Reference

Ignatavicius, D., & Workman, M. (2010). *Medical-surgical nursing: Patient-centered collaborative care* (6th ed., pp. 192-193). St. Louis: Saunders.

---

906. A client reports to the health care clinic and tells the nurse that she felt a lump in her breast. The nurse prepares for further data collection, knowing that which of the following is a clinical manifestation of breast cancer?

1 A tender mass
2 A painful mass
3 Nipple discharge
4 A soft, mobile mass

Level of Cognitive Ability: Comprehension
Client Needs: Physiological Integrity
Integrated Process: Nursing Process/Data Collection
Content Area: Adult Health/Oncology

Answer: 3

Rationale: Clinical manifestations associated with breast cancer include a mass that is usually painless, nontender, hard, irregular in shape, and nonmobile. Nipple discharge and retraction, edema with peau d'orange skin, and dimpling may be present.

Test-Taking Strategy: Use the process of elimination. Eliminate options 1 and 2 first because they are comparable or alike. Recall that breast cancer is most often associated with a mass that is hard to direct you to option 3 from the remaining options. Review the clinical manifestations associated with breast cancer if you had difficulty with this question.

Reference

Christensen, B., & Kockrow, E. (2006). *Adult health nursing* (5th ed., p. 605). St. Louis: Mosby.

---

907. A client with breast cancer is scheduled for a simple mastectomy. The client asks the nurse what this type of surgery involves. The nurse plans to include which of the following in the response?

1 It involves the removal of the breast, the axillary lymph nodes, and the overlying skin.
2 It involves the removal of the cancerous mass and some normal tissue to produce clean margins.
3 It involves the removal of the breast, the overlying skin, the pectoral muscles, and the axillary nodes.
4 It involves the resection of breast tissue and some skin from the clavicle to the costal margin and from the midline to the latissimus dorsi.

Answer: 4

Rationale: A simple mastectomy involves the resection of breast tissue and some skin from the clavicle to the costal margin and from the midline to the latissimus dorsi. The axillary tail and pectoral fascia are also removed, but the axillary nodes are not removed. Option 1 describes a modified radical mastectomy. Option 2 describes a lumpectomy, and option 3 describes a standard radical mastectomy.

Test-Taking Strategy: Use the process of elimination. Eliminate options 1 and 3 first because they are comparable or alike. Focus on the words *simple mastectomy* in the question to direct you to option 4 from the remaining options. Review the various types of mastectomies if you had difficulty with this question.

Reference

Christensen, B., & Kockrow, E. (2006). *Adult health nursing* (5th ed., p. 608). St. Louis: Mosby.

Level of Cognitive Ability: Comprehension
Client Needs: Physiological Integrity
Integrated Process: Nursing Process/Planning
Content Area: Adult Health/Oncology

---

908. A nurse is reviewing the nursing care plan of a client who has a stage 4 pressure ulcer. Which of the following does the nurse expect to note during data collection for this client?

1 Intact skin
2 A deep ulcer that extends into muscle and bone
3 An area in which the top layer of skin is missing
4 A reddened area that returns to normal skin color after 15 to 20 minutes of pressure relief

Level of Cognitive Ability: Comprehension
Client Needs: Physiological Integrity
Integrated Process: Nursing Process/Data Collection
Content Area: Adult Health/Integumentary

Answer: 2
Rationale: A stage 4 pressure ulcer is a deep ulcer that extends into muscle and bone. It has a foul smell, and the eschar is brown or black. Purulent drainage is common. With a stage 1 ulcer, the skin is intact, but the area may appear pale when pressure is first removed; this type of ulcer is also identified by a reddened area that returns to normal skin color after 15 to 20 minutes of pressure relief. A stage 2 ulcer is an area in which the top layer of skin is missing.

Test-Taking Strategy: Use the process of elimination. Note the strategic words *stage 4 pressure ulcer.* Recall that a stage 4 pressure ulcer is the most extensive type of ulcer to direct you to option 2. Review the stages of decubitus ulcers if you had difficulty with this question.

Reference
Linton, A. (2007). *Introduction to medical-surgical nursing* (4th ed., p. 317). Philadelphia: Saunders.

---

909. A client is seen in the health care clinic, and a biopsy is performed on a skin lesion that the physician suspects is malignant melanoma. The nurse assists with preparing a plan of care based on which characteristic of this type of skin cancer?

1 It is the most common form of skin cancer.
2 It is a slow-growing cancer that seldom metastasizes.
3 It is an aggressive cancer that requires aggressive therapy to control its rapid spread.
4 It can grow so large that an entire area (e.g., nose, lip, ear) must be removed and reconstructed if it occurs on the face.

Level of Cognitive Ability: Comprehension
Client Needs: Physiological Integrity
Integrated Process: Nursing Process/Planning
Content Area: Adult Health/Integumentary

Answer: 3
Rationale: Malignant melanoma, which is commonly just called melanoma, is a cancer of the melanocyte cells of the skin. It is an aggressive cancer that requires aggressive therapy to control its spread. Basal cell carcinoma, which is also known as basal cell epithelioma, is the most common form of skin cancer. It is a slow-growing cancer that seldom metastasizes, but it can grow so large that an entire affected area must be removed and reconstructed.

Test-Taking Strategy: Knowledge of the various types of skin cancer is necessary to answer this question. Remember that malignant melanoma is an aggressive cancer that requires aggressive therapy to control its spread. Review malignant melanoma if you had difficulty with this question.

Reference
Christensen, B., & Kockrow, E. (2006). *Adult health nursing* (5th ed., pp. 101-102). St. Louis: Mosby.

---

910. A nurse is assisting with caring for a client brought to the emergency department after a burn injury that occurred

Answer: 3
Rationale: Inhalation injuries are most common when a fire occurs in a closed space. Initial findings include facial burns,

in the basement of the home. The nurse should suspect an inhalation injury based on which initial finding?

1 Bradycardia
2 Expectoration of mucus
3 The presence of singed nasal hairs
4 Clear breath sounds in the lower lobes bilaterally

Level of Cognitive Ability: Analysis
Client Needs: Physiological Integrity
Integrated Process: Nursing Process/Data Collection
Content Area: Adult Health/Integumentary

singed nasal hairs, and sputum tinged with carbon. In addition, the auscultation of wheezing suggests an inhalation injury. Options 1, 2, and 4 are not specific findings associated with an inhalation injury.

Test-Taking Strategy: Use the process of elimination, and note the strategic word *initial* in the question. Think about each of the options and note the relationship between the client's injury and option 3. The initial observation that the nurse would make is singed nasal hairs. Review the findings associated with an inhalation injury if you had difficulty with this question.

Reference

deWit, S. (2009). *Medical-surgical nursing: Concepts & practice* (p. 1040). St. Louis: Saunders.

---

911. A nurse is assisting with caring for a client who arrived at the emergency department with the emergency medical services team after a severe burn injury from an explosion. After the initial assessment has been performed by the physician and life-threatening dysfunctions have been addressed, the nurse reviews the physician's orders, anticipating that which pain medication will be prescribed?

1 Intravenous (IV) morphine sulfate
2 IV meperidine hydrochloride (Demerol)
3 Morphine sulfate via the subcutaneous route
4 Aspirin with oxycodone (Percodan) via nasogastric tube

Level of Cognitive Ability: Analysis
Client Needs: Physiological Integrity
Integrated Process: Nursing Process/Planning
Content Area: Adult Health/Integumentary

Answer: 1

Rationale: After an initial assessment has been made and life-threatening dysfunctions have been addressed, pain medication can be administered. IV opioids are the initial medications of choice because absorption from the musculature is erratic and because an ileus can be present in the burn client. The initial medication of choice is morphine sulfate, although other medications may also be used. IV opioids are given until fluid resuscitation is complete and gastric motility is restored.

Test-Taking Strategy: Use the process of elimination, and note the strategic words *severe burn injury;* this assists you with eliminating option 3. Recall the potential complication of ileus associated with a burn injury; this will help you to eliminate option 4. From the remaining options, you must know that morphine sulfate is the medication of choice. Review the therapeutic management of a burn injury if you had difficulty with this question.

Reference

Christensen, B., & Kockrow, E. (2006). *Adult health nursing* (5th ed., p. 107). St. Louis: Mosby.

---

912. A nurse is collecting data regarding the operative site of a client who underwent breast reconstruction. The nurse is inspecting the flap and the areola of the nipple and notes that the areola is a dusky color around the edge. Which nursing action is appropriate?

1 Elevate the breast.
2 Document the findings.
3 Encourage nipple massage.
4 Notify the registered nurse.

Level of Cognitive Ability: Analysis
Client Needs: Physiological Integrity

Answer: 4

Rationale: After breast reconstruction, the flap is inspected for color, temperature, and capillary refill. An assessment of the nipple areola is made, and dressings are designed so that this area can be observed. An areola that is deep red, purple, dusky, or black around the edge is reported to the registered nurse, who will then contact the physician. This finding can indicate ischemia of the tissue.

Test-Taking Strategy: Use the process of elimination. Note the strategic words *dusky color* to direct you to option 4. Review the complications associated with breast reconstruction if you had difficulty with this question.

Integrated Process: Nursing Process/ Implementation
Content Area: Adult Health/Integumentary

References

Ignatavicius, D., & Workman, M. (2010). *Medical-surgical nursing: Patient-centered collaborative care* (6th ed., p. 1677). St. Louis: Saunders.
Linton, A. (2007). *Introduction to medical-surgical nursing* (4th ed., p. 1065). Philadelphia: Saunders.

---

913. A nurse is caring for a client who has had intermaxillary fixation for mandibular fractures that occurred during a motor vehicle accident. The client is complaining of a runny nose and asks the nurse for something to relieve this discomfort. Which nursing action is appropriate?

1 Administering an antihistamine
2 Checking the discharge for the presence of glucose
3 Assuring the client that this is a normal occurrence after surgery
4 Providing the client with additional tissues for the discharge from the nose

Level of Cognitive Ability: Application
Client Needs: Physiological Integrity
Integrated Process: Nursing Process/ Implementation
Content Area: Adult Health/Musculoskeletal

Answer: 2

Rationale: When rhinorrhea (a thin, watery discharge from the nose) or otorrhea (ear inflammation with serum discharge) is noted, cerebrospinal fluid (CSF) may be leaking through the fractures. The nurse checks the fluid for glucose using a test tape or Ketostix. CSF contains glucose, whereas rhinorrhea does not. CSF dries on gauze as a concentric halo-like ring and does not crust. Options 1, 3, and 4 are inappropriate actions.

Test-Taking Strategy: Focus on the anatomical location of this type of surgery to direct you to option 2. Remember that drainage from a client's ears or nose after head surgery may indicate the presence of CSF. In addition, option 2 is the only option that addresses data collection, which is the first step of the nursing process. Review the complications associated with this type of surgery if you had difficulty with this question.

References

Ignatavicius, D., & Workman, M. (2010). *Medical-surgical nursing: Patient-centered collaborative care* (6th ed., pp. 591, 593). St. Louis: Saunders.
Linton, A. (2007). *Introduction to medical-surgical nursing* (4th ed., p. 430). Philadelphia: Saunders.

---

914. A nurse is reinforcing teaching about the signs of peritonitis with a client who has begun peritoneal dialysis. The nurse instructs the client to report which finding to the physician?

1 Heartburn
2 Cloudy dialysate output
3 Increased abdominal girth
4 A temperature of 99° F orally

Level of Cognitive Ability: Application
Client Needs: Physiological Integrity
Integrated Process: Teaching and Learning
Content Are: Adult Health/Renal

Answer: 2

Rationale: Peritonitis is an inflammation of the peritoneum. Typical symptoms of peritonitis include fever, nausea, malaise, rebound abdominal tenderness, and cloudy dialysate output. The client does not need to measure abdominal girth. A low-grade temperature may or may not indicate that the client is developing peritonitis. The complaint of heartburn is too vague to be correct.

Test-Taking Strategy: Use the process of elimination. Note the strategic words *peritonitis* and *report;* these words imply that the correct answer is a sign or symptom of peritonitis, which will assist you with eliminating options 1 and 3. From the remaining options, recall that infection would cause white blood cells to be present in the dialysate (thus yielding cloudy dialysate output) and that the fever would be high grade rather than low grade. Review the signs of peritonitis if you had difficulty with this question.

Reference

Christensen, B., & Kockrow, E. (2006). *Adult health nursing* (5th ed., p. 508). St. Louis: Mosby.

915. Ofloxacin (Floxin) is prescribed for a client. The nurse provides which information to the client about this medication?

1. Take the medication with food.
2. Take the medication with an antacid.
3. Drink at least three glasses of milk per day.
4. Drink at least 1500 to 2000 mL of fluid per day.

Level of Cognitive Ability: Application
Client Needs: Physiological Integrity
Integrated Process: Teaching and Learning
Content Area: Adult Health/Renal

Answer: 4

Rationale: Ofloxacin (Floxin) is an anti-infective medication. The client should drink at least 1500 to 2000 mL of fluid per day. Food, antacids, and milk interfere with the absorption of this medication.

Test-Taking Strategy: Use the process of elimination. Note that options 1, 2, and 3 are comparable or alike in that they indicate administering the medication with a substance. Review ofloxacin if you had difficulty with this question.

Reference

Hodgson, B., & Kizior, R. (2009). *Saunders nursing drug handbook 2009* (p. 855). St. Louis: Saunders.

---

916. A client receiving streptogramin (Synercid) by intravenous intermittent infusion for the treatment of a bone infection develops diarrhea. Which nursing action should the licensed practical nurse (LPN) caring for the client implement first?

1. Stop the infusion.
2. Notify the registered nurse (RN).
3. Monitor the client's temperature.
4. Administer an antidiarrheal agent.

Level of Cognitive Ability: Application
Client Needs: Physiological Integrity
Integrated Process: Nursing Process/Implementation
Content Area: Pharmacology

Answer: 2

Rationale: Streptogramin is an antimicrobial agent. One adverse effect of the medication is superinfection, including antibiotic-associated colitis, which may result from a bacterial imbalance. The medication should be withheld if the client develops diarrhea. The LPN should notify the RN, who should then take the necessary actions and contact the physician. The LPN should not make a decision to stop the infusion and should not administer an antidiarrheal agent. Although the LPN may monitor the client's temperature, the first action is to notify the RN.

Test-Taking Strategy: Note the strategic word *first,* and use your knowledge of the adverse effects and nursing interventions related to this medication. From the options presented, the first action would be to notify the RN. Remember that the RN is notified if adverse effects from a medication occur. Review the adverse effects of streptogramin if you had difficulty with this question.

Reference

Gahart, B., & Nazareno, A. (2009). *Intravenous medications* (25th ed., p. 1138). St. Louis: Mosby.

---

917. A nurse is reviewing the record of a newborn in the nursery and notes that the physician has documented the presence of a suture split of more than 1 cm. On the basis of this documentation, the nurse expects to monitor the newborn for which of the following?

1. Craniosynostosis
2. Increased intracranial pressure
3. Swelling of the soft tissues of the head and scalp
4. Edema as a result of bleeding below the periosteum of the cranium

Level of Cognitive Ability: Comprehension
Client Needs: Physiological Integrity

Answer: 2

Rationale: Normal suture lines may be approximated or overriding, and they are also mobile. A split in the sutures of as much as 1 cm is considered normal. Overriding suture lines are most often caused by the birthing process and resolve spontaneously. A suture split of more than 1 cm may indicate increased intracranial pressure. Option 3 describes a caput succedaneum. Option 4 describes a cephalhematoma. A hard, rigid, immobile suture line can be associated with premature closure or craniosynostosis and should be investigated further.

Test-Taking Strategy: Use the process of elimination. Focus on the data in the question and recall normal and abnormal newborn findings to answer this question. Note the strategic words *more than* to direct you to the correct option. Review normal and abnormal newborn findings if you had difficulty with this question.

Integrated Process: Nursing Process/Data Collection
Content Area: Maternity/Postpartum

References

Hockenberry, M., & Wilson, D. (2009). *Wong's essentials of pediaric nursing* (8th ed., p. 976). St. Louis: Mosby.
Leifer, G. (2008). *Maternity nursing: An introductory text* (10th ed., p. 177). Philadelphia: Saunders.

---

918. A nurse is reviewing the laboratory results of an infant who is suspected of having pyloric stenosis. Which of the following does the nurse expect to note in this infant?

1 An elevated blood pH
2 A decreased blood pH
3 An elevated serum chloride level
4 An elevated serum potassium level

Level of Cognitive Ability: Analysis
Client Needs: Physiological Integrity
Integrated Process: Nursing Process/Data Collection
Content Area: Child Health

Answer: 1
Rationale: Pyloric stenosis is a narrowing of the pyloric sphincter at the outlet of the stomach, which causes an obstruction that blocks the flow of food into the small intestine. Laboratory findings for an infant with pyloric stenosis include metabolic alkalosis caused by vomiting and decreased serum potassium, sodium, and chloride levels. Increased pH and bicarbonate levels indicate metabolic alkalosis. Options 2, 3, and 4 are not typically noted in an infant with this disorder.

Test-Taking Strategy: Remember that metabolic alkalosis occurs as a result of vomiting. Recall that progressive projectile nonbilious vomiting occurs in clients with pyloric stenosis. Remember the concepts related to acid–base balance and the clinical manifestations of this disorder to direct you to option 1. In clients with metabolic alkalosis, the pH and the bicarbonate levels are elevated. Review metabolic alkalosis if you had difficulty with this question.

Reference

McKinney, E., James, S., Murray, S., & Ashwill, J. (2009). *Maternal-child nursing* (3rd ed., pp. 1120-1121). St. Louis: Mosby.

---

919. A nurse is caring for a client with colorectal cancer who had a colostomy performed. The nurse inspects the stoma postoperatively and expects to note which of the following?

1 A pink, dry stoma
2 A red, moist stoma
3 A pale-colored stoma
4 A dark-colored stoma

Level of Cognitive Ability: Comprehension
Client Needs: Physiological Integrity
Integrated Process: Nursing Process/Data Collection
Content Area: Adult Health/Oncology

Answer: 2
Rationale: After a colostomy procedure, the stoma should be red and moist. The registered nurse should be notified if the stoma is dry (a fluid volume deficit), pale (a lack of blood supply), or dark (necrosis).

Test-Taking Strategy: Focus on the subject—the expected findings regarding the appearance of a stoma after a colostomy. Remember that the stoma should be red and moist. Review postoperative care after the creation of a stoma if you had difficulty with this question.

Reference

deWit, S. (2009). *Medical-surgical nursing: Concepts & practice* (p. 731). St. Louis: Saunders.

---

920. A client reports to the health care clinic for an eye examination, and a diagnosis of primary open-angle glaucoma is suspected. Which nursing question will elicit information about the initial clinical manifestation associated with this disorder?

1 "Is your central vision blurred?"
2 "Do bright lights cause a glare?"

Answer: 4
Rationale: Glaucoma is an abnormal condition of elevated pressure within the eye that is caused by the obstruction of the outflow of aqueous humor. Because glaucoma is usually symptom free, the client may first note changes in peripheral visual acuity. If pain occurs with glaucoma, it is usually late in the course of structural changes, with an intraocular pressure of 40 to 50 mm Hg or higher. Most severe pain is characteristic of absolute glaucoma

3 "Do you have any pain in your eyes?"
4 "Have you had difficulty with peripheral vision?"

Level of Cognitive Ability: Application
Client Needs: Physiological Integrity
Integrated Process: Nursing Process/Data Collection
Content Area: Adult Health/Eye

(total vision loss). Blurred central vision occurs with macular degeneration. Glare from bright lights is a complaint of a client with a cataract.

Test-Taking Strategy: Focus on the subject—the clinical manifestations of glaucoma. Remember that because glaucoma is usually symptom free, the client may first note changes in peripheral visual acuity. Review the clinical manifestations of glaucoma if you had difficulty with this question.

Reference

deWit, S. (2009). *Medical-surgical nursing: Concepts & practice* (p. 646). St. Louis: Saunders.

---

921. A client reports to the nurse that, when performing a testicular self-examination (TSE), he found a lump the size and shape of a pea. Based on this finding, the nurse's best response is:

1 "Lumps like that are normal, don't worry."
2 "Let me know if it gets bigger next month."
3 "That could be cancer. I'll ask the doctor to examine you."
4 "That's important to report even though it might not be serious."

Level of Cognitive Ability: Application
Client Needs: Physiological Integrity
Integrated Process: Nursing Process/Implementation
Content Area: Adult Health/Oncology

Answer: 4
Rationale: A pea-like lump found during a TSE could be an infection or a tumor. The correct option reinforces the appropriate behavior of reporting the finding without heightening client anxiety. The finding should be investigated, because it could be an infection or a tumor, so delays are not appropriate. Telling the client that he could have cancer could increase his anxiety.

Test-Taking Strategy: Use therapeutic communication techniques and your knowledge of testicular cancer to answer this question. By the process of elimination, only option 4 is the appropriate choice. Review therapeutic communication techniques and the signs of testicular cancer if you had difficulty with this question.

Reference

Christensen, B., & Kockrow, E. (2006). *Adult health nursing* (5th ed., pp. 618-619). St. Louis: Mosby.

---

922. A client is seen in the health care clinic and shows the nurse an area on the skin that has a flat brown circular nevus that is less than 1 cm in diameter. The client asks the nurse, "Is this cancer?" Based on the observation, the appropriate response is:

1 "This indicates malignancy."
2 "This is are probably verruca."
3 "This is likely to be a benign mole."
4 "This requires immediate attention because it is probably cancer."

Level of Cognitive Ability: Application
Client Needs: Physiological Integrity
Integrated Process: Communication and Documentation
Content Area: Adult Health/Integumentary

Answer: 3
Rationale: The description is of a classic benign mole. If the client stated that the color of the lesion changed, if the size of the lesion was more than 1 cm, or if the mole was raised or itchy, it should be considered suspicious. The description of the lesion indicates that the lesion is a nevus (mole) and not a verruca (wart).

Test-Taking Strategy: Use the process of elimination. Eliminate options 1 and 4 because they are comparable or alike in that they indicate that the description is consistent with cancer. From the remaining options, remember to use therapeutic communication techniques; a client would not understand the terminology used in option 2. Review the description of nevi if you had difficulty with this question.

References

Christensen, B., & Kockrow, E. (2006). *Adult health nursing* (5th ed., p. 99). St. Louis: Mosby.
Linton, A. (2007). *Introduction to medical-surgical nursing* (4th ed., p. 1125). Philadelphia: Saunders.

---

923. A breast-feeding mother has developed a temperature of 104° F and shaking chills. The nurse collects additional data from the client about symptoms of mastitis, which include:

1 Bilateral breast engorgement
2 Reddened and tender breast tissue
3 Scant lactation with bloody discharge
4 A hard, warm, nodular area in the outer breast quadrant

Level of Cognitive Ability: Comprehension
Client Needs: Physiological Integrity
Integrated Process: Nursing Process/Data Collection
Content Area: Maternity/Postpartum

Answer: 2

Rationale: Mastitis is an inflammatory condition of the breast tissue. Reddened and tender breast tissue along with shaking chills and fever are the major symptoms of mastitis. Bilateral breast engorgement (option 1), scant milk production with bloody discharge (option 3), and a hard, warm, nodular area in the outer breast quadrant (option 4) are symptoms of other lactation problems.

Test-Taking Strategy: Use the process of elimination, and focus on the subject—mastitis. This will direct you to option 2. Review the signs of mastitis if you had difficulty with this question.

Reference

Leifer, G. (2008). *Maternity nursing: An introductory text* (10th ed., p. 345). Philadelphia: Saunders.

---

924. A nurse is assigned to care for a client who was admitted to the hospital with a musculoskeletal injury. The nurse gathers data about a major symptom associated with progressive neurovascular compromise when the nurse:

1 Counts the client's apical pulse for 1 full minute
2 Takes the client's blood pressure on the unaffected side
3 Observes for drainage on the dressing of the affected extremity
4 Determines if pain is experienced with passive motion of the affected extremity

Level of Cognitive Ability: Analysis
Client Needs: Physiological Integrity
Integrated Process: Nursing Process/Data Collection
Content Area: Adult Health/Musculoskeletal

Answer: 4

Rationale: Neurovascular compromise in a client with a musculoskeletal injury is created by increased pressure within a compartment. It is characterized by pain and diminished sensation or pulses in the affected extremity. The pressure occurs because the fascia is unable to expand when muscle swelling occurs. The only option that addresses neurovascular compromise is option 4.

Test-Taking Strategy: Use the process of elimination, and focus on the subject—neurovascular compromise. This will direct you to option 4. Review the complications related to neurovascular injuries if you had difficulty with this question.

Reference

Christensen, B., & Kockrow, E. (2006). *Adult health nursing* (5th ed., p. 189). St. Louis: Mosby.

---

925. A nurse is gathering data from a client admitted to the hospital with a diagnosis of hemarthrosis. The nurse determines that which medication, if taken by the client, would contribute to this diagnosis?

1 Phenothiazine
2 Anticoagulant
3 Corticosteroid
4 Anticonvulsant

Level of Cognitive Ability: Analysis
Client Needs: Physiological Integrity

Answer: 2

Rationale: Hemarthrosis is the extravasation of blood into a joint. High doses of an anticoagulant can produce bleeding in the joints. Phenothiazines may produce gait disturbances. Corticosteroids can precipitate necrosis of the head of the femur. Anticonvulsants may cause osteomalacia.

Test-Taking Strategy: Use your knowledge of medical terminology to identify the definition of hemarthrosis. Recalling the side effects of each medication in the options will direct you to option 2. Review these medications if you had difficulty with this question.

Integrated Process: Nursing Process/Data Collection
Content Area: Adult Health/Musculoskeletal

Reference
deWit, S. (2009). *Medical-surgical nursing: Concepts & practice* (pp. 392-393). St. Louis: Saunders.

---

926. A nurse is reviewing the record of a client with human immunodeficiency virus (HIV) infection. The nurse notes that the client complains of dyspnea on exertion and tachypnea. The client has a dry cough, and, during auscultation of the lungs, crackles were heard. The nurse determines that the most likely cause of these symptoms is:
1 Toxoplasmosis
2 Cryptosporidiosis
3 Malignant lymphoma
4 *Pneumocystis jiroveci* pneumonia

Level of Cognitive Ability: Analysis
Client Needs: Physiological Integrity
Integrated Process: Nursing Process/Data Collection
Content Area: Adult Health/Respiratory

Answer: 4
Rationale: *Pneumocystis jiroveci* pneumonia is a fungal infection of the lung that is usually seen in clients with HIV infection. Signs and symptoms of *Pneumocystis jiroveci* pneumonia include fever, dyspnea on exertion, tachypnea, and persistent dry cough. Crackles are heard on auscultation. Signs and symptoms of toxoplasmosis include changes in mental status, neurological deficits, headaches, and fever. Signs and symptoms of cryptosporidiosis range from mild diarrhea to a cholera-like syndrome with body wasting and electrolyte imbalances. There can be a voluminous diarrhea with a volume loss of up to 15 to 20 L/day. Signs and symptoms of malignant lymphoma include weight loss, fever, and night sweats.

Test-Taking Strategy: Focus on the signs and symptoms presented in the question. Note that *Pneumocystis jiroveci* is a type of pneumonia and hence affects the respiratory system. The incorrect options do not contain data related to the respiratory system. Review the assessment signs and symptoms related to the disorders presented in the options if you had difficulty with this question.

Reference
Linton, A. (2007). *Introduction to medical-surgical nursing* (4th ed., p. 616). Philadelphia: Saunders.

---

927. A woman who gave birth 2 days ago complains of severe pain and an intense feeling of swelling and pressure in the vaginal area. After hearing these complaints, the nurse's first priority is to collect additional data by checking the:
1 Vagina for lacerations
2 Vulva for a hematoma
3 Episiotomy for drainage
4 Rectum for hemorrhoids

Level of Cognitive Ability: Application
Client Needs: Physiological Integrity
Integrated Process: Nursing Process/Data Collection
Content Area: Maternity/Postpartum

Answer: 2
Rationale: A hematoma is a collection of extravasated blood that is trapped in the tissues. Hematoma is suspected when pain or pressure in the vaginal area is reported by the client. Massive hemorrhaging can occur into the tissues and result in hypovolemia and shock. Options 1, 3, and 4 are not associated with the client's complaint.

Test-Taking Strategy: Note the strategic words *first priority* and focus on the client's complaints to assist with directing you to the correct option. In addition, option 2 indicates a bleeding disorder, which is a priority. Review the signs and symptoms of hematoma if you had difficulty with this question.

Reference
Leifer, G. (2008). *Maternity nursing: An introductory text* (10th ed., p. 336). Philadelphia: Saunders.

---

928. A newborn of a mother with diabetes mellitus displays irregular respirations, grunting, substernal retractions, and lethargy. Respiratory distress syndrome (RDS) is suspected based on the results

Answer: 4
Rationale: RDS is an acute lung disease of the newborn that is most often noted in premature infants and that is characterized by respiratory distress. Hyperglycemia during pregnancy delays fetal lung maturity. An L/S ratio is needed to determine the presence

of which of the following tests performed during the week before delivery?
1 Ultrasound series
2 Biophysical profile
3 A reassuring nonstress test
4 Lecithin-to-sphingomyelin (L/S) ratio

Level of Cognitive Ability: Analysis
Client Needs: Physiological Integrity
Integrated Process: Nursing Process/Data Collection
Content Area: Maternity/Postpartum

of sufficient surfactant to prevent RDS. An ultrasound would not indicate RDS, but it would reflect the size of the infant and other anatomical findings. Both the reassuring nonstress test and the biophysical profile indicate the well-being of the fetus and would not be predictors of RDS.

Test-Taking Strategy: Use the process of elimination. This question relates to respiratory distress, so select the option that identifies the test that would identify a potential respiratory problem. Review prenatal testing if you had difficulty with this question.

Reference
Leifer, G. (2007). *Introduction to maternity and pediatric nursing* (5th ed., p. 81). Philadelphia: Saunders.

---

929. When caring for a pregnant client who is at risk for disseminated intravascular coagulation (DIC), the nurse recognizes that one of the first signs may be:
1 Continuous abdominal pain
2 An increase in peripheral edema
3 A decrease in the level of consciousness
4 The presence of purpura on the lower extremities and abdomen

Level of Cognitive Ability: Analysis
Client Needs: Physiological Integrity
Integrated Process: Nursing Process/Data Collection
Content Area: Maternity/Antepartum

Answer: 4
Rationale: DIC is a coagulopathy that results from the overstimulation of clotting and anticlotting processes in response to disease or injury. The presence of purpura on the lower extremities and abdomen, which reflects fibrin deposits in the capillaries, is a common first sign. An increase in peripheral edema is a symptom of a gestational hypertensive disorder such as preeclampsia. A decrease in the level of consciousness can occur as preeclampsia progresses. Continuous abdominal pain is a symptom of abruptio placentae, which may be a precipitating cause of DIC.

Test-Taking Strategy: Note the strategic words *first signs*, and focus on the subject—disseminated intravascular coagulation. Note the relationship between the subject and option 4. Review the signs of disseminated intravascular coagulation if you had difficulty with this question.

Reference
Leifer, G. (2008). *Maternity nursing: An introductory text* (10th ed., p. 255). Philadelphia: Saunders.

---

930. A nurse is preparing to administer an intramuscular injection to a 10-year-old child in the vastus lateralis muscle. The nurse understands that which of the following is the maximum volume of medication that can be safely administered into this muscle?
1 0.5 mL
2 1.5 mL
3 2.5 mL
4 3.0 mL

Level of Cognitive Ability: Comprehension
Client Needs: Physiological Integrity
Integrated Process: Nursing Process/Implementation
Content Area: Child Health

Answer: 2
Rationale: In a child between the ages of 6 and 15 years, the maximum volume of intramuscular medication that can be safely administered into the vastus lateralis muscle is 1.5 mL to 2.0 mL.

Test-Taking Strategy: Note the age of the child, and visualize each of the amounts in the options. Option 1 represents a small amount and options 3 and 4 represent large amounts of medication for intramuscular injection into this muscle. Review intramuscular administration techniques if you had difficulty with this question.

Reference
Price, D., & Gwin, J. (2008). *Pediatric nursing: An introductory text* (10th ed., p. 385). St. Louis: Saunders.

---

931. A client who is taking albuterol sulfate (Proventil HFA) experiences a severe episode of wheezing, which the nurse interprets as bronchospasm. A telephone call is made to the physician's office. The nurse tells the client to do which of the following while waiting for the physician to call?

1 Take half the dose.
2 Take a double dose.
3 Withhold the next dose.
4 Take the next dose as scheduled.

Level of Cognitive Ability: Application
Client Needs: Physiological Integrity
Integrated Process: Nursing Process/Implementation
Content Area: Pharmacology

Answer: 3

Rationale: Albuterol sulfate is an inhalation powder device and a sympathomimetic bronchodilator. If bronchospasm occurs, the nurse instructs the client to withhold the medication, and the physician is called immediately. This adverse effect is often caused by the excessive use of adrenergic bronchodilators.

Test-Taking Strategy: Use the process of elimination. To answer this question correctly, it is necessary to know the expected and untoward effects of bronchodilators. Note the word *bronchospasm* in the question to direct you to option 3. Review the adverse effects of albuterol sulfate if you had difficulty with this question.

Reference

Kee, J., Hayes, E., & McCuistion, L. (2009). *Pharmacology: A nursing process approach* (6th ed., pp. 609-610). St. Louis: Saunders.

---

932. A client has begun medication therapy with hydrochlorothiazide (HydroDIURIL). The nurse interprets that which item, if reported by the client, indicates that the client is experiencing a side effect of the medication?

1 Hypoglycemia
2 Photosensitivity
3 Weight loss of 4 pounds
4 Decreased blood pressure

Level of Cognitive Ability: Analysis
Client Needs: Physiological Integrity
Integrated Process: Nursing Process/Data Collection
Content Area: Pharmacology

Answer: 2

Rationale: Hydrochlorothiazide is a thiazide diuretic. The intended effects of the medication are the promotion of fluid loss and the reduction of blood pressure; photosensitivity and hyperglycemia are side effects. Hypoglycemia is not a side effect of this medication. Although some weight loss may occur as a result of the diuretic effect, this is not a side effect.

Test-Taking Strategy: Focus on the name of the medication. Recall that this medication is a potassium-wasting diuretic and remember its associated side effects to direct you to option 2. Remember that photosensitivity and hyperglycemia are side effects. Review the side effects of hydrochlorothiazide if you had difficulty with this question.

Reference

Hodgson, B., & Kizior, R. (2009). *Saunders nursing drug handbook 2009* (p. 571). St. Louis: Saunders.

---

933. A licensed practical nurse (LPN) says to the registered nurse, "I think my client's closed chest drainage system has some kind of leak in it." The LPN bases this interpretation on which observation of the closed chest drainage system?

1 Continuous bubbling in the water seal chamber
2 Intermittent bubbling in the water seal chamber
3 Continuous bubbling in the suction control chamber
4 Intermittent bubbling in the suction control chamber

Level of Cognitive Ability: Analysis
Client Needs: Physiological Integrity

Answer: 1

Rationale: Continuous bubbling in the water seal chamber through both inspiration and expiration indicates that there is an air leak in the system. A resolving pneumothorax is indicated by intermittent bubbling with respiration in the water seal chamber. Continuous bubbling in the suction control chamber indicates that suction is attached to the system and is working as expected. There cannot be intermittent bubbling in the suction control chamber; either the suction is turned on (bubbling) or off (no bubbling).

Test-Taking Strategy: To answer this question accurately, you must be familiar with closed chest drainage systems and indications of proper and improper function. Remember that continuous bubbling through both inspiration and expiration in the water seal chamber indicates that there is air leaking into the system. Review chest tube drainage systems if you had difficulty with this question.

Integrated Process: Nursing Process/Data Collection
Content Area: Adult Health/Respiratory

Reference
Christensen, B., & Kockrow, E. (2006). *Adult health nursing* (5th ed., p. 439). St. Louis: Mosby.

---

934. A licensed practical nurse (LPN) is asked by the registered nurse to obtain the supplies necessary to initiate an intravenous (IV) line for a client who will receive peripheral fat (lipid) infusions. Which device should the LPN select for the initiation of the IV?
1 A 14-gauge needle
2 A 19-gauge needle
3 A 23-gauge needle
4 A 25-gauge needle

Level of Cognitive Ability: Application
Client Needs: Physiological Integrity
Integrated Process: Nursing Process/Implementation
Content Area: Fundamental Skills

Answer: 2
Rationale: For peripheral fat infusions, a 19- to 20-gauge needle is used. A 14-, 16-, 18-, or 19-gauge needle is used for the administration of blood products. A 22- or 23-gauge needle is used for standard IV solutions. A 25-gauge needle is most often used to administer subcutaneous injections.

Test-Taking Strategy: Remember that the smaller the gauge number, the larger the needle. When answering questions like to this one, specifically note the type of solution to be infused. It seems reasonable that an adequate-sized needle is necessary for the administration of a fat solution. Options 3 and 4 can be eliminated first because the needles described in these options are too small. Eliminate option 1 next, recalling that a 14-gauge needle is extremely large and that it is used primarily for blood products or for rapid emergency fluid administration. Review infusion concepts if you had difficulty with this question.

Reference
Perry, A. & Potter, P. (2010). *Clinical nursing skills & techniques* (7th ed., p. 576). St. Louis: Mosby.

---

935. A nurse is caring for an older client who is receiving an intravenous (IV) infusion and who is at risk for IV infiltration. The nurse inspects the IV site and plans the client's care knowing that which of the following will place the client at greatest risk for infiltration?
1 The use of an armboard
2 Looping of the IV tubing
3 Anchoring the venipuncture cannula
4 An IV line placed in the antecubital area

Level of Cognitive Ability: Comprehension
Client Needs: Physiological Integrity
Integrated Process: Nursing Process/Planning
Content Area: Fundamental Skills

Answer: 4
Rationale: Infiltration occurs when fluid seeps into tissues. Older clients are at an increased risk for infiltration because they have fragile veins. Preventive measures include avoiding venipuncture over an area of flexion, anchoring the venipuncture cannula, and looping the IV tubing securely. The use of an armboard or splint is especially helpful for an active or restless person.

Test-Taking Strategy: Use the process of elimination, and note the strategic words *greatest risk* in the question. Visualize each of the options to identify the one that would not assist with the prevention of an infiltration. Note the word *antecubital* in option 4 to direct you to this option. Review preventive measures related to infiltration if you had difficulty with this question.

Reference
Christensen, B., & Kockrow, E. (2006). *Foundations of nursing* (5th ed., pp. 548-549). St. Louis: Mosby.

---

936. A nurse is collecting data about a client with Brown-Séquard syndrome. Which finding does the nurse expect to note?
1 Loss of touch and vibration sensation
2 Bilateral loss of pain and temperature sensation
3 Contralateral paralysis and loss of touch and vibration sensation

Answer: 1
Rationale: Brown-Séquard syndrome results from the hemisection of the spinal cord, which results in ipsilateral paralysis and a loss of touch, pressure sensation, vibration sensation, and proprioception. Contralaterally, sensations of pain and temperature are lost because the fibers associated with them decussate after entering the spinal cord. Options 2, 3, and 4 are not characteristics of this syndrome.

4 Complete paraplegia or quadriplegia, depending on the level of injury

Level of Cognitive Ability: Analysis
Client Needs: Physiological Integrity
Integrated Process: Nursing Process/Data Collection
Content Area: Adult Health/Neurological

Test-Taking Strategy: Knowledge of Brown-Séquard syndrome is necessary to answer this question correctly. Remember that Brown-Séquard syndrome results from the hemisection of the spinal cord and results in ipsilateral paralysis and a loss of touch, pressure sensation, vibration sensation, and proprioception. Review the findings and nursing care associated with Brown-Séquard syndrome if you had difficulty with this question.

Reference
Linton, A. (2007). *Introduction to medical-surgical nursing* (4th ed., p. 491). Philadelphia: Saunders.

---

937. A nurse is collecting data about a client who has a suspected spinal cord injury. Which of the following is the priority?
1 Pain
2 Mobility
3 Respiratory status
4 Pupillary response

Level of Cognitive Ability: Application
Client Needs: Physiological Integrity
Integrated Process: Nursing Process/Data Collection
Content Area: Delegating/Prioritizing

Answer: 3
Rationale: A spinal cord injury is a traumatic disruption of the spinal cord that is often associated with extensive musculoskeletal involvement. All of the items in the options would be assessed for a client with a suspected spinal cord injury; however, the respiratory status is the priority.

Test-Taking Strategy: Use the ABCs—airway, breathing, and circulation—to answer this question. Option 3 addresses the airway. Review the care of the client with a spinal cord injury if you had difficulty with this question.

Reference
Linton, A. (2007). *Introduction to medical-surgical nursing* (4th ed., pp. 491-492). Philadelphia: Saunders.

---

938. A nurse is caring for a client with acquired immunodeficiency syndrome (AIDS). The nurse plans care, knowing that it is important to monitor for which of the following findings?
1 Bradypnea
2 Jaundiced skin
3 Urine specific gravity of 1.010
4 White patches in the oral cavity

Level of Cognitive Ability: Application
Client Needs: Physiological Integrity
Integrated Process: Nursing Process/Planning
Content Area: Fundamental Skills

Answer: 4
Rationale: AIDS involves a defect in cell-mediated immunity. Clients with AIDS frequently have opportunistic infections. *Candida albicans,* which is the causative organism of thrush, is a common opportunistic infection. Thrush and hairy leukoplakia both present as white patches in the oral cavity. Jaundice is a symptom of hepatic disease. Clients with AIDS frequently develop pneumonia and thus may present with tachypnea (not bradypnea). Clients with AIDS frequently have inadequate nutrition and hydration and thus may present with dehydration; this results in a high rather than a low specific gravity.

Test-Taking Strategy: Recall the pathophysiology of AIDS to answer this question correctly. Eliminate options 2 and 3 because they are not associated with the disease. Clients with AIDS do have respiratory problems; however, the problem is an increased rather than decreased respiratory rate. Review the manifestations associated with AIDS if you had difficulty with this question.

Reference
Linton, A. (2007). *Introduction to medical-surgical nursing* (4th ed., p. 752). Philadelphia: Saunders.

---

939. A nurse is caring for a client who has been involved in a motor vehicle crash. The nurse monitors the client closely, knowing that the need to prepare for chest tube insertion will be necessary if the client exhibits which symptoms?

1 Chest pain and shortness of breath
2 Peripheral cyanosis and hypotension
3 Shortness of breath and tracheal deviation
4 Decreasing oxygen saturation on pulse oximetry and bradypnea

Level of Cognitive Ability: Analysis
Client Needs: Physiological Integrity
Integrated Process: Nursing Process/Data Collection
Content Area: Adult Health/Respiratory

Answer: 3
Rationale: Shortness of breath and tracheal deviation result when lung tissue and alveoli have collapsed. The trachea deviates to the unaffected side in the presence of a tension pneumothorax. Air entering the pleural cavity causes the lung to lose its normal negative pressure. The increasing pressure in the affected side displaces contents to the unaffected side. Shortness of breath results from a decreased area being available for the diffusion of gases. Chest pain and shortness of breath are more commonly associated with myocardial ischemia or infarction. Clients who require chest tubes exhibit decreasing oxygen saturation but will more likely experience tachypnea related to the hypoxia. Peripheral cyanosis is caused by circulatory disorders. Hypotension may be a result of a tracheal shift and the impedance of venous return to the heart or of other problems (e.g., a failing heart).

Test-Taking Strategy: Focus on the subject—the need for chest tub insertion. Tracheal deviation is a manifestation that indicates a tension pneumothorax, which is treated with closed chest drainage. Review the signs associated with tension pneumothorax and the conditions that require closed chest drainage if you had difficulty with this question.

Reference
Linton, A. (2007). *Introduction to medical-surgical nursing* (4th ed., pp. 233, 235, 543). Philadelphia: Saunders.

---

940. A client has a serum sodium level of 129 mEq/L as a result of hypervolemia. The nurse reviews the physician's orders to determine whether which measure is prescribed?

1 Restricting fluids
2 Restricting sodium intake to 2 g/day
3 Restricting sodium intake to 4 g/day
4 Administering intravenous hypertonic saline

Level of Cognitive Ability: Analysis
Client Needs: Physiological Integrity
Integrated Process: Nursing Process/Planning
Content Area: Fundamental Skills

Answer: 1
Rationale: Hyponatremia is defined as a serum sodium level of less than 135 mEq/L. When this condition is caused by hypervolemia, it may be treated with fluid restriction. The low serum sodium level is caused by hemodilution. Intravenous hypertonic saline is reserved for hyponatremia when the serum sodium level is less than 125 mEq/L. A 4-g sodium diet is a no-added-salt diet; a 2-g sodium restriction would not raise the serum sodium level.

Test-Taking Strategy: Use the process of elimination, and focus on the serum sodium level, knowing that it is low. With this in mind, you can eliminate option 2. Knowing that hypervolemia causes the hemodilution of serum sodium guides you to choose option 1 instead of options 3 and 4. Review treatment measures for hyponatremia if you had difficulty with this question.

Reference
deWit, S. (2009). *Medical-surgical nursing: Concepts & practice* (p. 892). St. Louis: Saunders.

---

941. A nurse is preparing to apply a pulse oximeter to a client. To ensure the accurate monitoring of the client's oxygenation status, the nurse implements which of the following?

Answer: 2
Rationale: The pulse oximeter passes a beam of light through the tissue, and a sensor attached to the fingertip, toe, or earlobe measures the amount of light absorbed by the oxygen-saturated hemoglobin. The oximeter then gives a reading of the percentage of hemoglobin that is saturated with oxygen. Motion at the

1 Tapes the sensor to the client's finger
2 Instructs the client to not move the sensor
3 Places the sensor on a finger below the blood pressure cuff
4 Notifies the physician immediately of an oxygen saturation of less than 92%

Level of Cognitive Ability: Application
Client Needs: Physiological Integrity
Integrated Process: Nursing Process/Implementation
Content Area: Adult Health/Respiratory

sensor site changes light absorption. The motion mimics the pulsatile motion of blood, and results can be inaccurate because the detector cannot distinguish between the movement of blood and the movement of the finger. The sensor should not be placed distal to blood pressure cuffs, pressure dressings, arterial lines, or any invasive catheters. The sensor should not be taped to the client's finger because vasoconstriction may reduce arterial blood flow to the sensor. If values fall below preset norms (usually 90%), the client should be instructed to breathe deeply, if this is appropriate.

Test-Taking Strategy: Use the process of elimination, and focus on the subject—ensuring accurate monitoring. Eliminate option 4 because, although reporting low oxygen saturations to the physician is important, it is unrelated to the subject of the question. Option 3 is unreasonable, so eliminate it also. When considering the remaining options, recall that motion at the sensor site changes light absorption to help you to select the correct option. Review the principles associated with pulse oximetry if you had difficulty with this question.

Reference

Christensen, B., & Kockrow, E. (2006). *Adult health nursing* (5th ed., pp. 411-412). St. Louis: Mosby.

---

942. A nurse is working in a renal unit in a local hospital. The nurse interprets that which of the following clients in the unit is best suited for peritoneal dialysis as a treatment option?

1 A client with severe congestive heart failure
2 A client with a history of ruptured diverticuli
3 A client with a history of herniated lumbar disk
4 A client with a history of three previous abdominal surgeries

Level of Cognitive Ability: Analysis
Client Needs: Physiological Integrity
Integrated Process: Nursing Process/Data Collection
Content Area: Adult Health/Renal

Answer: 1

Rationale: Peritoneal dialysis is a dialysis procedure in which the peritoneum is used as a diffusible membrane. Peritoneal dialysis may be the treatment option of choice for clients with severe cardiovascular disease, which is worsened by the rapid shifts in fluid, electrolytes, urea, and glucose that occur with hemodialysis. For the same reason, peritoneal dialysis may be indicated for clients with diabetes mellitus. Relative contraindications to peritoneal dialysis include diseases of the abdomen (e.g., ruptured diverticuli, malignancy), extensive abdominal surgeries, history of peritonitis, obesity, and a history of back problems, which could be aggravated by the fluid weight of the dialysate. Severe disease of the vascular system may also be a relative contraindication.

Test-Taking Strategy: Use the process of elimination. Note that the question asks you which of the clients presented is the best candidate for peritoneal dialysis. This implies that you must understand the advantages and disadvantages of peritoneal dialysis and use priority setting to eliminate each of the incorrect options. Options 2 and 4 can be eliminated first. Knowledge of the concepts related to fluid weight and fluid shifts in the body is needed to select between options 1 and 3. Review the indications for peritoneal dialysis if you had difficulty with this question.

Reference

Ignatavicius, D., & Workman, M. (2010). *Medical-surgical nursing: Patient-centered collaborative care* (6th ed., pp. 771, 1611). St. Louis: Saunders.

943. A client undergoing long-term peritoneal dialysis is currently experiencing a problem with reduced outflow from the dialysis catheter. The nurse collecting data from the client inquires whether the client has had a recent problem with which of the following?

1 Diarrhea
2 Vomiting
3 Flatulence
4 Constipation

Level of Cognitive Ability: Analysis
Client Needs: Physiological Integrity
Integrated Process: Nursing Process/Data Collection
Content Area: Adult Health/Renal

Answer: 4
Rationale: Peritoneal dialysis is a dialysis procedure in which the peritoneum is used as a diffusible membrane. Reduced outflow may be caused by catheter positioning, adherence to the omentum, infection, or constipation. Constipation may contribute to reduced outflow in part because peristalsis, which is slowed in constipation, seems to aid in drainage. For this reason, bisacodyl suppositories are sometimes used prophylactically, even without a history of constipation. The other options are unrelated to impaired catheter drainage.

Test-Taking Strategy: Use the process of elimination. Evaluate each option in terms of its effect on gut motility, which affects catheter outflow. Each of the incorrect options involves the hypermotility of the gastrointestinal tract, which should facilitate outflow. Only constipation is related to decreased gut motility, which could impair fluid drainage. Review the factors that can cause reduced outflow if you had difficulty with this question.

Reference
Linton, A. (2007). *Introduction to medical-surgical nursing* (4th ed., p. 878). Philadelphia: Saunders.

---

944. A nurse is teaching a client who is taking medications by inhalation about the advantages of a newly prescribed spacer. Which statement by the client identifies the need for further teaching?

1 "Medication is dispersed more deeply and uniformly."
2 "It reduces the frequency of medication to only once per day."
3 "The need to coordinate timing between pressing the inhaler and inspiration is reduced."
4 "It reduces the chance of yeast infection because large drops aren't deposited on mouth tissues."

Level of Cognitive Ability: Comprehension
Client Needs: Physiological Integrity
Integrated Process: Teaching and Learning
Content Area: Adult Health/Respiratory

Answer: 2
Rationale: There are key advantages to the use of a spacer for medications that are administered by inhalation. One is that it reduces the incidence of yeast infections, because large medication droplets are not deposited on oral tissues. The medication is also dispensed more deeply and uniformly than without a spacer. There is less need to coordinate the effort of inhalation with pressing on the canister of the inhaler. Finally, the use of a spacer may decrease either the number or volume of the puffs taken. Option 2 is too absolute and limiting.

Test-Taking Strategy: Use the process of elimination, and note the strategic words *need for further teaching.* These words indicate a negative event query and ask you to select an option that is an incorrect statement. In addition, note the use of the close-ended word *only* in option 2. Review the principles related to the use of a spacer if you had difficulty with this question.

Reference
Christensen, B., & Kockrow, E. (2006). *Adult health nursing* (5th ed., p. 459). St. Louis: Mosby.

---

945. A nurse is caring for a client with a tentative diagnosis of emphysema. The nurse monitors the client for which sign that distinguishes emphysema from chronic bronchitis?

1 Marked dyspnea
2 Minimal weight loss
3 Copious sputum production
4 Cough that began before the onset of dyspnea

Answer: 1
Rationale: Emphysema is an abnormal condition of the pulmonary system that is characterized by overinflation and destructive changes in the alveolar walls. Key features of emphysema include dyspnea that is often marked, late cough (after the onset of dyspnea), scant mucus production, and marked weight loss. By contrast, chronic bronchitis is characterized by an early onset of cough (before dyspnea); copious, purulent mucus production; minimal weight loss; and milder severity of dyspnea.

Level of Cognitive Ability: Analysis
Client Needs: Physiological Integrity
Integrated Process: Nursing Process/Data Collection
Content Area: Adult Health/Respiratory

Test-Taking Strategy: To answer this question accurately, you must understand the differences between and the associated manifestations of emphysema and chronic bronchitis. Remember that the key features of emphysema include dyspnea that is often marked, late cough (after the onset of dyspnea), scant mucus production, and marked weight loss. Review the manifestations of emphysema if you had difficulty with this question.

Reference

Christensen, B., & Kockrow, E. (2006). *Adult health nursing* (5th ed., p. 451). St. Louis: Mosby.

---

946. A client is diagnosed with vitamin K deficiency. The nurse should collect data from the client about which of the following that results from this deficiency?
1 Scaly skin
2 Skeletal pain
3 Night blindness
4 Clotting problems

Level of Cognitive Ability: Comprehension
Client Needs: Physiological Integrity
Integrated Process: Nursing Process/Data Collection
Content Area: Fundamental Skills

Answer: 4
Rationale: Vitamin K is associated with the production of prothrombin, which helps the blood to properly clot. Vitamin B_2 (riboflavin) deficiency is associated with scaly skin. Vitamin D deficiency is associated with skeletal pain. Vitamin A deficiency is associated with night blindness.

Test-Taking Strategy: Use the process of elimination. Recall that vitamin K is associated with the production of prothrombin to direct you to option 4. Review vitamin deficiencies if you had difficulty with this question.

References

deWit, S. (2009). *Medical-surgical nursing: Concepts & practice* (p. 747). St. Louis: Saunders.
Linton, A. (2007). *Introduction to medical-surgical nursing* (4th ed., p. 106). Philadelphia: Saunders.

---

947. A client has been diagnosed with goiter. The nurse should expect to note which of the following documented in the client's record?
1 Heart damage
2 Chronic fatigue
3 Enlarged thyroid gland
4 Decreased wound healing

Level of Cognitive Ability: Comprehension
Client Needs: Physiological Integrity
Integrated Process: Nursing Process/Data Collection
Content Area: Adult Health/Endocrine

Answer: 3
Rationale: Goiter is an enlargement of the thyroid gland. Enlargement occurs in an attempt to compensate for hormone deficiency. Heart damage, chronic fatigue, and decreased wound healing are not specifically associated with goiter.

Test-Taking Strategy: Focus on the client's diagnosis, and consider the anatomical location of goiter; this will direct you to option 3. Review goiter if you had difficulty with this question.

Reference

Christensen, B., & Kockrow, E. (2006). *Adult health nursing* (5th ed., p. 534). St. Louis: Mosby.

---

948. An 85-year-old client is hospitalized with a fractured right hip, and surgery is performed. The client refuses to get out of bed during the postoperative period. The nurse should make which appropriate statement to the client?

Answer: 3
Rationale: If the client does not increase activity, the bones will suffer from a loss of calcium. Iron (not iodine) is recommended for hemoglobin synthesis because oxygen is necessary for wound healing. An 85-year-old postoperative client should be turned every 2 hours by the nursing staff. Increasing calcium intake only

1 "It is necessary to give you iodine to help with hemoglobin synthesis."
2 "You should remember to turn yourself in bed to keep from getting so stiff."
3 "It is important for you to get out of bed so that calcium will go back into the bone."
4 "It is necessary to increase your calcium intake because you are spending too much time in bed."

Level of Cognitive Ability: Application
Client Needs: Physiological Integrity
Integrated Process: Nursing Process/Implementation
Content Area: Fundamental Skills

leads to elevated amounts in the blood, which could cause kidney stones.

Test-Taking Strategy: Focus on the subject, and use therapeutic communication techniques. Recall the effects of immobility to direct you to option 3. Review the effects of immobility if you had difficulty with this question.

References

Christensen, B., & Kockrow, E. (2006). *Foundations of nursing* (5th ed., pp. 1106-1107). St. Louis: Mosby.
Linton, A. (2007). *Introduction to medical*-surgical *nursing* (4th ed., p. 929). Philadelphia: Saunders.

---

949. A client has an abdominal aortic aneurysm. The nurse best detects bleeding from the aneurysm by:
1 Palpating the pedal pulses every 4 hours
2 Measuring abdominal girth every 4 hours
3 Checking the pulses with a Doppler every 4 hours
4 Asking the client about mild pain in the area PRN

Level of Cognitive Ability: Application
Client Needs: Physiological Integrity
Integrated Process: Nursing Process/Data Collection
Content Area: Adult Health/Cardiovascular

Answer: 2
Rationale: An aneurysm is a localized dilation of the wall of a blood vessel. Bleeding from an aneurysm causes blood to accumulate in the retroperitoneal area, which can most directly be detected by measuring abdominal girth. Palpation and auscultation of the pulses determines patency and may be of some use for detecting bleeding if the pulses are diminished because of reduced circulating volume. However, other signs of hypovolemic shock may also be apparent by that time. The assessment of pain is done routinely, and mild regional discomfort is expected.

Test-Taking Strategy: Note the strategic words *bleeding, aneurysm,* and *best detects.* Select option 2 by looking for an abdominal assessment because the aneurysm is located in the peritoneal cavity. Review postprocedural care if you had difficulty with this question.

Reference

Ignatavicius, D., & Workman, M. (2010). *Medical-surgical nursing: Patient-centered collaborative care* (6th ed., pp. 812, 1223). St. Louis: Saunders.

---

950. A nurse is assigned to care for a client who underwent peripheral arterial bypass surgery 16 hours previously. When collecting data from the client, the client complains of increasing pain in the leg at rest that worsens with movement and that is accompanied by paresthesias. The nurse should take which action?
1 Notify the registered nurse (RN).
2 Apply warm, moist heat for comfort.
3 Administer a prescribed opioid analgesic.
4 Apply ice to minimize any developing swelling.

Answer: 1
Rationale: Compartment syndrome can occur after peripheral arterial bypass surgery. The condition is characterized by increased pressure within a muscle compartment that is caused by bleeding or excessive edema. It compresses the nerves in the area and can cause vascular compromise. The classic signs are pain at rest that intensifies with movement and the development of paresthesias. The RN is notified immediately. The RN then contacts the physician because the client could require an emergency fasciotomy. Options 2, 3, and 4 are incorrect.

Level of Cognitive Ability: Application
Client Needs: Physiological Integrity
Integrated Process: Nursing Process/Implementation
Content Area: Adult Health/Cardiovascular

Test-Taking Strategy: Use the process of elimination, and note the strategic words *increasing pain*. The signs and symptoms described in the case situation indicate a new problem about which the RN needs to be notified. Review the complications of peripheral arterial bypass surgery if you had difficulty with this question.

Reference

Ignatavicius, D., & Workman, M. (2010). *Medical-surgical nursing: Patient-centered collaborative care* (6th ed., p. 809). St. Louis: Saunders.

---

951. A client returned from the postanesthesia care unit 8 hours ago after having a femoral–popliteal bypass graft of the left leg. The client exhibits increasing pallor and coolness in the left foot. The capillary refill time is 5 seconds, with a weakly palpable pedal pulse. The client complains of left leg pain that resembles the pain experienced before surgery. The nurse concludes which of the following about the client?

1 The client is experiencing graft occlusion.
2 The client has developed deep vein thrombosis.
3 The client is in need of immediate pain medication.
4 The client has dislodged an embolus from the left atrium.

Level of Cognitive Ability: Analysis
Client Needs: Physiological Integrity
Integrated Process: Nursing Process/Data Collection
Content Area: Adult Health/Cardiovascular

Answer: 1
Rationale: The most frequent indication that a graft is occluding is the return of pain that is similar to that experienced preoperatively. Signs of impaired neurovascular status accompany the occlusion and include pallor, cool temperature, diminished capillary refill, and diminished or absent pedal pulses. If graft occlusion is suspected, the surgeon is notified. The symptoms described do not resemble those of deep vein thrombosis. There is no indication that the client has a history of atrial fibrillation, which can result in an arterial embolus caused by left atrial thrombus.

Test-Taking Strategy: Use the process of elimination. Eliminate option 3 first because the clinical manifestations indicate that a complication is occurring. Eliminate options 2 and 4 next because the problem is not venous in nature (option 2) and because there is no history of atrial fibrillation (predisposing to an embolus) mentioned in the question. Review the signs of graft occlusion if you had difficulty with this question.

Reference

Christensen, B., & Kockrow, E. (2006). *Adult health nursing* (5th ed., pp. 384-385). St. Louis: Mosby.

---

952. A nurse is evaluating the status of a client who is taking spironolactone (Aldactone). The nurse determines that this medication is ineffective if the client demonstrates which of the following?

1 Increased edema
2 Increased urine output
3 Stable potassium level
4 Decreased blood pressure

Level of Cognitive Ability: Analysis
Client Needs: Physiological Integrity
Integrated Process: Nursing Process/Evaluation
Content Area: Pharmacology

Answer: 1
Rationale: Spironolactone (Aldactone) is a potassium-sparing diuretic that is used to treat edema, hypertension, and hyperaldosteronism. Thus, it should decrease the blood pressure, increase the urine output, maintain stable potassium levels, and decrease edema.

Test-Taking Strategy: Use the process of elimination, and note the strategic word *ineffective*. Recall that this medication is a potassium-sparing diuretic to direct you to option 1. Review the characteristics of spironolactone if you had difficulty with this question.

Reference

Kee, J., Hayes, E., & McCuistion, L. (2009). *Pharmacology: A nursing process approach* (6th ed., pp. 244-245). St. Louis: Saunders.

---

953. A nurse who is assisting in an ambulatory care clinic takes a client's blood pressure in the left arm and notes that it is 200/118 mm Hg. The first action of the nurse is to:

1 Check the blood pressure in the right arm.
2 Inquire about the presence of kidney disorders.
3 Report the elevation to the registered nurse (RN).
4 Recheck the blood pressure in the same arm within 30 seconds.

Level of Cognitive Ability: Application
Client Needs: Physiological Integrity
Integrated Process: Nursing Process/Implementation
Content Area: Adult Health/Cardiovascular

Answer: 1

Rationale: After obtaining a high initial reading, the nurse takes the blood pressure in the opposite arm to see if the pressure is elevated in one extremity only. The nurse also rechecks the blood pressure in the same arm but waits at least 2 minutes between readings. The nurse inquires about the presence of kidney disorders, which could contribute to elevated blood pressure. The nurse would notify the RN, who would then contact the physician because immediate treatment is necessary. However, this should not be done without obtaining verification of the blood pressure elevation.

Test-Taking Strategy: Use the process of elimination, and note the strategic word *first.* This tells you that more than one or all of the options may be partially or totally correct. In this instance, eliminate option 4 first because it is incorrect. Choose option 1 over the other options because it provides verification of the initial reading. Review the procedures for obtaining a blood pressure reading if you had difficulty with this question.

Reference

Christensen, B., & Kockrow, E. (2006). *Foundations of nursing* (5th ed., pp. 258-260). St. Louis: Mosby.

---

954. A hospitalized client has been diagnosed with thrombophlebitis. The nurse plans to avoid doing which of the following during the care of this client?

1 Applying moist heat to the leg
2 Maintaining the client on bedrest
3 Elevating the feet above heart level
4 Placing a pillow under the client's knees

Level of Cognitive Ability: Application
Client Needs: Physiological Integrity
Integrated Process: Nursing Process/Implementation
Content Area: Adult Health/Cardiovascular

Answer: 4

Rationale: Thrombophlebitis is the inflammation of a vein accompanied by the formation of a clot. The nurse avoids placing a pillow under the knees of a client with thrombophlebitis because it obstructs venous return to the heart and exacerbates the impairment of blood flow. The client is maintained on bedrest as prescribed after a diagnosis of thrombophlebitis is made to prevent the occurrence of pulmonary embolus. The feet are elevated above heart level to help with venous return, and warm, moist heat may be used to provide comfort and reduce venospasm.

Test-Taking Strategy: Use the process of elimination, and note the strategic word *avoid.* This word indicates a negative event query and asks you to select an option that is an incorrect action. Use principles related to gravity and to the relief of inflammation to answer this question; this should direct you to option 4. Review the care of the client with thrombophlebitis if you had difficulty with this question.

Reference

Christensen, B., & Kockrow, E. (2006). *Adult health nursing* (5th ed., p. 390). St. Louis: Mosby.

---

955. A new prenatal client is 6 months pregnant. On the first prenatal visit, the nurse notes that the client is gravida 4, para 0, aborta 3. The client is 5 feet, 6 inches tall; she weighs 130 pounds and is 25 years old. The client states, "I get really tired after working all day and I can't keep up with my housework." Which factor

Answer: 4

Rationale: Gestational diabetes mellitus is characterized by an impaired ability to metabolize carbohydrates that is usually caused by a deficiency of insulin that occurs during pregnancy. Fatigue is a normal occurrence during pregnancy. The client is not obese. To be at high risk for gestational diabetes, the maternal age should be more than 30 years. However, a history of unexplained stillbirths or miscarriages puts the client at high risk for gestational diabetes.

in the preceding data leads the nurse to suspect gestational diabetes mellitus?
1 Fatigue
2 Obesity
3 Maternal age
4 Previous fetal demise

Level of Cognitive Ability: Comprehension
Client Needs: Physiological Integrity
Integrated Process: Nursing Process/Data Collection
Content Area: Maternity/Antepartum

Test-Taking Strategy: Use the process of elimination. Option 1 can be eliminated by recalling that fatigue normally occurs during pregnancy. Options 2, 3, and 4 are all risk factors for gestational diabetes, but options 2 and 3 do not apply to this client. Review the risk factors associated with gestational diabetes if you had difficulty with this question.

Reference

Leifer, G. (2007). *Introduction to maternity and pediatric nursing* (5th ed., p. 97). Philadelphia: Saunders.

---

956. A nurse in the emergency department is caring for a client who is bleeding from a scalp laceration obtained during a fall from a stepladder. The nurse should take which action first to care for the wound?
1 Prepare to suture the area.
2 Administer a prophylactic antibiotic.
3 Cleanse the wound with sterile normal saline.
4 Ask the client about the timing of the last tetanus vaccination.

Level of Cognitive Ability: Application
Client Needs: Physiological Integrity
Integrated Process: Nursing Process/Implementation
Content Area: Adult Health/Integumentary

Answer: 3
Rationale: The first nursing action is to cleanse the wound thoroughly with sterile normal saline. This removes dirt or foreign matter from the wound and allows for the visualization of the size of the wound. Direct pressure is also applied initially, as needed, to control bleeding. If suturing is necessary, the surrounding hair may be shaved. Prophylactic antibiotics are often ordered. The date of the client's last tetanus shot is determined, and prophylaxis is given, if needed, as prescribed.

Test-Taking Strategy: Use the process of elimination, and note the strategic words *care for the wound* and *first*. The first action that focuses on the actual care of the wound is option 3. Review the care of the client with a laceration if you had difficulty with this question.

Reference

Christensen, B., & Kockrow, E. (2006). *Foundations of nursing* (5th ed., p. 768). St. Louis: Mosby.

---

957. A client is admitted to the hospital with a diagnosis of malnutrition and does not understand the results of the various prescribed laboratory tests. The nurse should make which accurate statement to the client?
1 "Elevated albumin levels indicate dehydration."
2 "Elevated creatinine levels indicate respiratory problems."
3 "Normal red blood cell levels indicate adequate vitamin B_6 intake."
4 "Normal hemoglobin levels indicate that iron and protein intake is sufficient."

Level of Cognitive Ability: Comprehension
Client Needs: Physiological Integrity
Integrated Process: Nursing Process/Implementation
Content Area: Fundamental Skills

Answer: 4
Rationale: Malnutrition is a disorder of nutrition that may result from an unbalanced, insufficient diet or from the impaired absorption, assimilation, or use of foods. Normal hemoglobin levels indicate that iron and protein intake are sufficient. Elevated albumin levels do not necessarily indicate dehydration. Elevated creatinine levels indicate kidney problems. Normal red blood cell levels indicate adequate vitamin B_{12} intake.

Test-Taking Strategy: Use the process of elimination, and focus on the subject. Remember that normal hemoglobin levels indicate that iron and protein intake is sufficient. Review the blood tests that indicate malnutrition if you had difficulty with this question.

Reference

Ignatavicius, D., & Workman, M. (2010). *Medical-surgical nursing: Patient-centered collaborative care* (6th ed., pp. 1393-1394). St. Louis: Saunders.

---

958. A licensed practical nurse (LPN) is assisting with the care of a client who has a diagnosis of suspected myocardial infarction. The client has been experiencing chest pain that is unrelieved by nitroglycerin, and the registered nurse administers morphine sulfate 5 mg intravenously as prescribed by the physician. After the administration of the morphine sulfate, the LPN should:

1 Monitor urinary output.
2 Increase the oxygen flow rate.
3 Monitor respirations and blood pressure.
4 Place the client in Trendelenburg's position.

Level of Cognitive Ability: Application
Client Needs: Physiological Integrity
Integrated Process: Nursing Process/Implementation
Content Area: Pharmacology

Answer: 3

Rationale: Morphine sulfate is an opiate analgesic that is administered to control chest pain. The LPN must monitor the client's heart rhythm and vital signs, especially the client's respirations. Signs of morphine sulfate toxicity include respiratory depression and hypotension. Urinary output is not directly related to the administration of this medication. The oxygen flow rate is not increased without a physician's order to do so. The client will be placed in Trendelenburg's position if a sudden drop in blood pressure occurs.

Test-Taking Strategy: Focus on the subject of the question, and recall the side effects associated with the administration of morphine sulfate. Remember that this medication affects the respiratory status to direct you to option 3. Review the side effects of morphine sulfate if you had difficulty with this question.

References

Christensen, B., & Kockrow, E. (2006). *Adult health nursing* (5th ed., p. 356). St. Louis: Mosby.
Hodgson, B., & Kizior, R. (2009). *Saunders nursing drug handbook 2009* (p. 787). St. Louis: Saunders.

---

959. A client has returned to the nursing unit after a gastroscopy procedure. The nurse should take which postprocedural action?

1 Place the client in a supine position for comfort.
2 Monitor the client's vital signs every hour for 4 hours.
3 Check the gag reflex by stroking the back of the client's throat.
4 Provide saline gargles to aid in comfort as soon as the client returns.

Level of Cognitive Ability: Application
Client Needs: Physiological Integrity
Integrated Process: Nursing Process/Implementation
Content Area: Adult Health/Gastrointestinal

Answer: 3

Rationale: A gastroscopy is the visual inspection of the interior of the stomach by means of a gastroscope inserted through the esophagus. Before the procedure, medication is given to provide conscious sedation and prevent gagging. After the procedure, the nurse must check for the return of the gag reflex to prevent aspiration. In addition, the client must be placed in a side-lying or semi-Fowler's position to prevent aspiration. The client's vital signs should be taken every 30 minutes for 2 hours to detect abnormalities. Saline gargles must only be administered when the presence of the gag reflex has been confirmed.

Test-Taking Strategy: Use the process of elimination, and read each option carefully. Use the ABCs—airway, breathing, and circulation—and recall the importance of determining the presence of a gag reflex during the postprocedural period. Review postprocedural care after gastroscopy if you had difficulty with this question.

Reference

Chernecky, C., & Berger, B. (2008). *Laboratory tests and diagnostic procedures* (5th ed., p. 569). Philadelphia: Saunders.

---

960. A client is on a regular diet and is a pesco vegetarian. Which food item on the diet menu will the client be willing to eat?

1 Scrambled eggs
2 Buttered wheat toast
3 Stir-fried vegetables
4 Chocolate milk shake

Answer: 3

Rationale: A pesco vegetarian consumes seafood but excludes meat, poultry, eggs, and dairy products from the diet. Stir-fried vegetables are allowed on a pesco-vegetarian diet. Eggs, butter, and milk shakes are dairy products and thus are not eaten by a strict vegetarian.

Level of Cognitive Ability: Comprehension
Client Needs: Physiological Integrity
Integrated Process: Nursing Process/Data Collection
Content Area: Fundamental Skills

Test-Taking Strategy: Use the process of elimination, and note that options 1, 2, and 4 are comparable or alike in that they are all dairy products. Review the pesco-vegetarian diet if you had difficulty with this question.

Reference

Grodner, M., Long, S., & Walkingshaw, B. (2007). *Foundations and clinical applications of nutrition* (4th ed., pp. 119-120). St. Louis: Mosby.

---

961. An older client has been complaining about suffering from heartburn. Which statement about lessening the symptoms should the nurse provide to the client?

1 "Eat a high-protein, low-fat diet on a daily basis."
2 "Drink at least three fruit juices a day as a main beverage."
3 "After 20 to 30 minutes of eating, lie down to help the food digest."
4 "Try to eat more after you feel full to keep the stomach at full capacity."

Level of Cognitive Ability: Application
Client Needs: Physiological Integrity
Integrated Process: Nursing Process/Implementation
Content Area: Fundamental Skills

Answer: 1
Rationale: Heartburn is usually caused by the reflux of gastric contents into the esophagus, but it may result form hyperacidity or peptic ulcer. A high-protein, low-fat diet is recommended for a client with heartburn. This type of diet allows the stomach valve to close and prevents gastric secretions from upsetting the stomach. Fruit juices should be avoided because their high level of acidity aggravates symptoms. At least 2 hours should pass before the client lies down after eating to allow enough time for the stomach acid to decrease. Clients should not be encouraged to overeat, which increases acid production and causes stomach pressure.

Test-Taking Strategy: Note the strategic words *lessening the symptoms.* Recall the causes of heartburn to direct you to the correct option. Review the causes of heartburn if you had difficulty with this question.

Reference

deWit, S. (2009). *Medical-surgical nursing: Concepts & practice* (p. 691). St. Louis: Saunders.

---

962. A client with unstable angina is returning to the nursing unit after an coronary angioplasty. The nurse observes the client for mental status changes, knowing that a change could indicate which specific complication of this procedure?

1 Cerebral emboli
2 Cerebral hemorrhage
3 Increased intraocular pressure
4 Reactions from the contrast medium

Level of Cognitive Ability: Analysis
Client Needs: Physiological Integrity
Integrated Process: Nursing Process/Data Collection
Content Area: Adult Health/Cardiovascular

Answer: 1
Rationale: Angioplasty involves using a balloon-tipped catheter to displace or flatten the plaque built up along the arterial walls, thereby enlarging the diameter of the vessel. There is a chance for a small piece of the plaque to become dislodged, which could create an embolus. Reactions from the contrast most likely will occur immediately rather than when the client returns to the nursing unit. Cerebral hemorrhage and increased intraocular pressure are not directly related to postangioplasty complications.

Test-Taking Strategy: Note the strategic words *returning to the nursing unit* and *mental status changes.* Recall what is involved in an angioplasty and the associated complications to direct you to option 1. Review the complications of an angioplasty if you had difficulty with this question.

Reference

Ignatavicius, D., & Workman, M. (2010). *Medical-surgical nursing: Patient-centered collaborative care* (6th ed., p. 724). St. Louis: Saunders.

---

963. A nurse administers an antiemetic to a client who has vomited. Three hours later, the client tells the nurse that he is

Answer: 2
Rationale: Room-temperature or cold foods are better tolerated by the client with episodes of nausea and vomiting. Hot items

hungry and would like something to eat. Which food item is best for the nurse to give the client at this time?
1 Hot tea
2 Apple juice
3 Chicken soup
4 Buttered toast

Level of Cognitive Ability: Application
Client Needs: Physiological Integrity
Integrated Process: Nursing Process/Implementation
Content Area: Fundamental Skills

may increase the nausea because of the aromas that they emit. Dry toast (without butter) would be better tolerated by the client.

Test-Taking Strategy: Use the process of elimination. Eliminate options 1 and 3 because they are comparable or alike in that they are both hot items. From the remaining options, recall that clear liquids are best tolerated after episodes of vomiting. Review the care of the client with nausea and vomiting if you had difficulty with this question.

Reference
deWit, S. (2009). *Medical-surgical nursing: Concepts & practice* (p. 41). St. Louis: Saunders.

---

964. A nurse is caring for a client with a diagnosis of malnutrition. Which of the following is the most effective measure for monitoring the client's status?
1 Calorie count
2 Daily weights
3 Intake and output
4 Skin fold measurements

Level of Cognitive Ability: Comprehension
Client Needs: Physiological Integrity
Integrated Process: Nursing Process/Data Collection
Content Area: Fundamental Skills

Answer: 2
Rationale: Malnutrition is a disorder of nutrition that may result from an unbalanced, insufficient diet or from the impaired absorption, assimilation, or use of foods. Daily weights are the most accurate way to monitor the client's progress. It is important to weigh the client at the same time each day and for the client to have the same amount of clothes on, to urinate beforehand, and to use the same scale. It also is recommended that the client be weighed before breakfast. Options 1, 3, and 4 provide data about nutrition but are not the most effective measures.

Test-Taking Strategy: Focus on the client's diagnosis and the subject of the question. Recall that the client's weight accurately provides data about the client's nutritional status. Review nutritional data collection measures if you had difficulty with this question.

Reference
Ignatavicius, D., & Workman, M. (2010). *Medical-surgical nursing: Patient-centered collaborative care* (6th ed., p. 1395). St. Louis: Saunders.

---

965. A nurse plans to apply a moisturizer to an older client's dry skin. For maximum effectiveness, the nurse chooses which of the following?
1 A lotion
2 An oil-based cream
3 An oil for the bath water
4 A petrolatum-based product

Level of Cognitive Ability: Application
Client Needs: Physiological Integrity
Integrated Process: Nursing Process/Implementation
Content Area: Fundamental Skills

Answer: 4
Rationale: Petrolatum provides the most effective moisturizing by forming an occlusive barrier on the skin and reducing water loss. Creams and lotions are mostly water based, less occlusive, and less likely to reduce skin dryness than petrolatum-based products. Bath oils are not the most effective moisturizer.

Test-Taking Strategy: Although all of the options are products that are used for dry skin, note the strategic words *maximum effectiveness*. Knowledge of skin preparation ingredients and how they work will direct you to option 4. Remember that petrolatum provides the most effective moisturization. Review moisturizing products if you had difficulty with this question.

Reference
Wold, G. (2008). *Basic geriatric nursing* (4th ed., pp. 274-275). St. Louis: Mosby.

966. A nurse auscultates bowel sounds in a client and identifies an early sign of intestinal obstruction when which of the following is heard?

1 Resonance
2 Diminished sounds
3 Absent bowel sounds
4 High-pitched tinkling sounds

Level of Cognitive Ability: Comprehension
Client Needs: Physiological Integrity
Integrated Process: Nursing Process/Data Collection
Content Area: Adult Health/Gastrointestinal

Answer: 4

Rationale: An intestinal obstruction is any obstruction that results in the failure of the contents of the intestine to progress through the lumen of the bowel. High-pitched tinkling sounds indicate an intestinal obstruction. Absent or diminished sounds may signify a paralytic ileus or later signs of an obstruction. Resonance is not a finding of auscultation.

Test-Taking Strategy: Use the process of elimination, and note the strategic word *auscultates.* Eliminate option 1 because it does not deal with auscultation. Eliminate options 2 and 3 next because they are comparable or alike. Review the findings associated with an intestinal obstruction if you had difficulty with this question.

Reference

Christensen, B., & Kockrow, E. (2006). *Adult health nursing* (5th ed., p. 240). St. Louis: Mosby.

---

967. A nurse in a long-term care facility documents a client's apical pulse rate as 82 beats/min, strong, and irregular. The nurse notes that the client complains of "feeling tired lately" and that prior baseline data indicate that the client's apical pulse rate ranged from 60 to 90 beats/min and that it was strong and regular. Which of the following is a priority nursing action?

1 Place the client on bedrest.
2 Notify the client's physician.
3 Schedule the client for a cardiac stress test.
4 Initiate a fluid restriction of 1000 mL for 24 hours.

Level of Cognitive Ability: Application
Client Needs: Physiological Integrity
Integrated Process: Nursing Process/Implementation
Content Area: Fundamental Skills

Answer: 2

Rationale: Any change in the rate, quality, or character of the pulse should be reported to the physician because this occurrence could be an indication of developing cardiac problems related to atherosclerosis, medication, or disease. With the data given here, there is no need for bedrest or fluid restriction. A physician's order must be obtained before scheduling the client for a stress test.

Test-Taking Strategy: Use the process of elimination, and note the strategic word *priority.* Options 1, 3, and 4 require a physician's order. Review the nursing interventions when a change of cardiac status occurs if you had difficulty with this question.

Reference

Wold, G. (2008). *Basic geriatric nursing* (4th ed., pp. 136-137). St. Louis: Mosby.

---

968. A client with congestive heart failure has been receiving furosemide (Lasix) daily. Which finding indicates the ineffectiveness of diuretic therapy?

1 Pitting pedal edema
2 Clear lung sounds bilaterally
3 Decreased exertional dyspnea
4 A weight loss of 3 lbs in 24 hours

Level of Cognitive Ability: Analysis
Client Needs: Physiological Integrity
Integrated Process: Nursing Process/Evaluation
Content Area: Pharmacology

Answer: 1

Rationale: Furosemide (Lasix) is a loop diuretic. Pitting pedal edema is a sign of excess fluid volume. Options 2, 3, and 4, are all signs of decreased edema, which is an indication that diuretic therapy has been effective for the excretion of excess fluid.

Test-Taking Strategy: Note the strategic word *ineffectiveness.* Use the process of elimination, and select the option that would indicate the presence of edema. Review the characteristics of furosemide if you had difficulty with this question.

Reference

Hodgson, B., & Kizior, R. (2009). *Saunders nursing drug handbook 2009* (p. 524). St. Louis: Saunders.

969. A nurse is caring for an older client who has been prescribed bedrest and who is concerned about the prevention of pneumonia. To detect early signs of pneumonia, the nurse monitors for which of the following?

1 Poor skin turgor
2 Diminished respiratory rate
3 Copious amounts of blood-tinged sputum
4 A rectal temperature of 100.8° F or higher

Level of Cognitive Ability: Application
Client Needs: Physiological Integrity
Integrated Process: Nursing Process/Data Collection
Content Area: Adult Health/Respiratory

Answer: 4

Rationale: Pneumonia is an acute inflammation of the lung. The older client may not present with the usual signs and symptoms of illness. Because of the lower-than-normal body temperature in an older client, an early sign of pneumonia would be a temperature elevation. Poor skin turgor is a sign of dehydration. In the later stages of pneumonia, the respiratory rate increases in an attempt to compensate for poor oxygen exchange. Blood-tinged sputum may be a sign of congestive heart failure.

Test-Taking Strategy: Note the strategic word *early*, and focus on the subject—pneumonia. Recall the pathophysiology associated with this lung inflammation to direct you to option 4. Review the signs of pneumonia if you had difficulty with this question.

Reference

Wold, G. (2008). *Basic geriatric nursing* (4th ed., pp. 41, 75). St. Louis: Mosby.

---

970. A client is receiving phenobarbital (Luminal) orally for the treatment of a seizure disorder. The nurse monitors for which common side effect that can occur with the administration of this medication?

1 Drowsiness
2 Blurred vision
3 Hypocalcemia
4 Seizure activity

Level of Cognitive Ability: Application
Client Needs: Physiological Integrity
Integrated Process: Nursing Process/Implementation
Content Area: Pharmacology

Answer: 1

Rationale: Phenobarbital (Luminal) is a barbiturate, and drowsiness is a common side effect of this medication. Blurred vision is not an associated side effect. Hypocalcemia is a rare toxic reaction. Seizure activity could occur as a result of the abrupt withdrawal of medication therapy or as a toxic reaction.

Test-Taking Strategy: Note the strategic words *common side effect*. Use the process of elimination and your knowledge of the action of this medication to direct you to option 1. Review phenobarbital if you had difficulty with this question.

Reference

Hodgson, B., & Kizior, R. (2009). *Saunders nursing drug handbook 2009* (p. 921). St. Louis: Saunders.

---

971. A client with a cardiac disorder is placed on complete bedrest. The nurse plans this client's care, knowing that a potential complication related to complete bedrest is:

1 Arthritis
2 Constipation
3 Increased anxiety
4 Increased chest pain.

Level of Cognitive Ability: Comprehension
Client Needs: Physiological Integrity
Integrated Process: Nursing Process/Planning
Content Area: Fundamental Skills

Answer: 2

Rationale: Constipation occurs as a result of inactivity and is an undesirable complication for cardiac clients; straining or bearing down triggers Valsalva's maneuver, which increases cardiac workload. Options 1, 3, and 4 are unrelated to bedrest.

Test-Taking Strategy: Use the process of elimination, and focus on the subject—a complication of complete bedrest. This will direct you to option 2. Review the complications associated with bedrest if you had difficulty with this question.

References

Christensen, B., & Kockrow, E. (2006). *Foundations of nursing* (5th ed., p. 596). St. Louis: Mosby.
Linton, A. (2007). *Introduction to medical-surgical nursing* (4th ed., p. 319). Philadelphia: Saunders.

972. The nurse best identifies that an older client is having a sleep pattern disturbance when which of the following is noted during data collection?

1 Apraxia
2 Occasional nocturia
3 Hypersalivation
4 Verbal complaints of difficulty falling asleep

Level of Cognitive Ability: Comprehension
Client Needs: Physiological Integrity
Integrated Process: Nursing Process/Data Collection
Content Area: Fundamental Skills

Answer: 4

Rationale: Many older clients experience changes in their activity and rest cycles. Apraxia (the inability to perform purposeful movements), nocturia (excessive nighttime urination), and hypersalivation are not indicators of a disturbed sleep pattern.

Test-Taking Strategy: Focus on the subject—sleep pattern disturbance. Note the relationship between this subject and option 4. Review age-related changes if you had difficulty with this question.

Reference

Wold, G. (2008). *Basic geriatric nursing* (4th ed. p. 329-330, 334). St. Louis: Mosby.

---

973. A nurse encourages an older client to perform deep-breathing and coughing exercises. The nurse understands that which normal age-related changes place the older client at higher risk for respiratory infections?

1 The alveolar membrane thins.
2 The alveolar walls are destroyed.
3 The lung tissue becomes less elastic and less rigid.
4 Reduced ciliary movement creates an ineffective cough.

Level of Cognitive Ability: Comprehension
Client Needs: Physiological Integrity
Integrated Process: Nursing Process/Implementation
Content Area: Fundamental Skills

Answer: 4

Rationale: As aging occurs, the lung tissue becomes less elastic and more rigid (not less rigid), the alveolar membranes thicken (not thin), and ciliary movement is reduced. The destruction of alveolar walls is a characteristic of chronic obstructive pulmonary disease (not a normal age-related change).

Test-Taking Strategy: Note the strategic words *normal age-related changes.* Read each option carefully, and use your knowledge of the aging process to answer the question; this will direct you to option 4. Review age-related changes if you had difficulty with this question.

Reference

Wold, G. (2008). *Basic geriatric nursing* (4th ed., pp. 39-40). St. Louis: Mosby.

---

974. A nurse is caring for a hospitalized older client with diabetes mellitus who has been diagnosed with dehydration. The client is alert but disoriented, pale, and slightly diaphoretic, and the nurse suspects that the client is hypoglycemic. The initial nursing intervention is to:

1 Administer oral glucose.
2 Obtain a fingerstick blood sample and test the glucose level.
3 Assist the client to bed, put the side rails up, and call the physician.
4 Seat the client at the nurse's desk while checking the physician's orders.

Level of Cognitive Ability: Application
Client Needs: Physiological Integrity
Integrated Process: Nursing Process/Implementation
Content Area: Adult Health/Endocrine

Answer: 2

Rationale: The nurse should confirm that the client is hypoglycemic by checking the blood glucose level. Option 1 is incorrect because the hypoglycemia has not been determined. More information should be gathered before calling the physician; therefore, option 3 is incorrect. Option 4 does not meet the client's immediate needs.

Test-Taking Strategy: Note strategic word *suspects*. Focus on the information in the question to direct you to option 2. In addition, option 2 is the only option that addresses the first step of the nursing process, which is data collection. Review the nursing actions to take if hypoglycemia is suspected if you had difficulty with this question.

Reference

Wold, G. (2008). *Basic geriatric nursing* (4th ed., p. 69). St. Louis: Mosby.

975. A physician has ordered 10 units of regular insulin with 20 units of NPH insulin to be administered subcutaneously every morning. The nurse should:

1. Shake the NPH insulin vial to distribute the suspension.
2. Administer both the regular insulin and the NPH insulin at 10:00 AM.
3. Draw up the regular insulin first and then add the NPH insulin to the same syringe.
4. Draw up the NPH insulin first and then add the regular insulin to the same syringe.

Level of Cognitive Ability: Application
Client Needs: Physiological Integrity
Integrated Process: Nursing Process/Implementation
Content Area: Pharmacology

Answer: 3

Rationale: Regular insulin is always drawn up before the NPH insulin. Insulin is usually administered 15 to 30 minutes before a meal. To mix the NPH insulin suspension, the vial should be gently rotated. Shaking introduces air bubbles into the solution.

Test-Taking Strategy: Use the process of elimination. Remember "R then N" (RN) when drawing up both types of insulin into the same syringe. Review the technique for administering insulin if you had difficulty with this question.

References

Ignatavicius, D., & Workman, M. (2010). *Medical-surgical nursing: Patient-centered collaborative care* (6th ed., p. 1486). St. Louis: Saunders.

Kee, J., Hayes, E., & McCuistion, L. (2009). *Pharmacology: A nursing process approach* (6th ed., p. 797). St. Louis: Saunders.

---

976. A nurse is assigned to care for a client with a history of coronary artery disease (CAD). The nurse reviews the client's health record, knowing that which data documented in the record is related to CAD?

1. Edema
2. Hyperlipidemia
3. Increased urinary output
4. Decreased urinary output

Level of Cognitive Ability: Comprehension
Client Needs: Physiological Integrity
Integrated Process: Nursing Process/Data Collection
Content Area: Fundamental Skills

Answer: 2

Rationale: CAD occurs as a result of the accumulation of fatty plaque in the coronary arteries or because of other arteriosclerotic changes. Elevated serum cholesterol and triglyceride levels (hyperlipidemia) play a major role in the development of CAD. Edema may be present if the client has congestive heart failure, but edema and changes in urinary output are not significant contributors to the development of CAD.

Test-Taking Strategy: Use the process of elimination. Think about the pathophysiology associated with CAD, and recall that hyperlipidemia is associated with this disease. Review the risk factors for CAD if you had difficulty with this question.

References

Christensen, B., & Kockrow, E. (2006). *Adult health nursing* (5th ed., p. 376). St. Louis: Mosby.

Christensen, B., & Kockrow, E. (2006). *Foundations of nursing* (5th ed., p. 650). St. Louis: Mosby.

---

977. A nurse is assigned to care for a client with a diagnosis of coronary artery disease (CAD). The nurse plans care, knowing that:

1. Activity and stress improve coronary blood flow.
2. Activity and stress are not related to coronary blood flow.
3. Chest pain experienced during exercise indicates necrosis.
4. Chest pain experienced during exercise may indicate ischemia.

Answer: 4

Rationale: CAD may go unrecognized for a period of time in persons with a sedentary lifestyle because adequate blood flow to the myocardium may be maintained despite the CAD. However, during times of emotional stress, increased physical activity, or both, the diseased coronary arteries may not be able to supply the myocardium with adequate blood. The inadequate perfusion of the myocardium, which is referred to as ischemia, causes pain; however, no damage to the heart muscle occurs. Necrosis is a result of prolonged oxygen deprivation of the myocardium and tissue death (myocardial infarction).

Level of Cognitive Ability: Application
Client Needs: Physiological Integrity
Integrated Process: Nursing Process/Planning
Content Area: Adult Health/Cardiovascular

Test-Taking Strategy: Use the process of elimination and your knowledge of CAD to answer the question. Remember that as a result of the pathophysiology associated with CAD, chest pain experienced during exercise may indicate ischemia. Review CAD if you had difficulty with this question.

References

deWit, S. (2009). *Medical-surgical nursing: Concepts & practice* (p. 489). St. Louis: Saunders.

Ignatavicius, D., & Workman, M. (2010). *Medical-surgical nursing: Patient-centered collaborative care* (6th ed., p. 847). St. Louis: Saunders.

---

978. A nurse is reinforcing heath care instructions to a client with coronary artery disease (CAD). Which statement by the client indicates the need for additional instruction?

1 "My diet should be low in salt and fat."
2 "I should conserve my energy and avoid stress."
3 "I must keep these prongs in my nose to get the extra oxygen that the doctor has prescribed."
4 "I can have someone from my office bring over my unfinished work so that I can complete it as long as I do not get out of bed."

Level of Cognitive Ability: Comprehension
Client Needs: Physiological Integrity
Integrated Process: Teaching and Learning
Content Area: Adult Health/Cardiovascular

Answer: 4

Rationale: CAD is an abnormal condition that may affect the heart's arteries and produce pathologic effects, especially the reduced flow of oxygen and nutrients to the myocardium. Reducing the demands on the heart by encouraging rest and relaxation is important for the hospitalized client with CAD. Oxygen therapy frequently is ordered for cardiac clients to provide supplemental oxygen. A diet low in salt and fat is also prescribed.

Test-Taking Strategy: Note the strategic words *need for additional instruction*. These words indicate a negative event query and ask you to select an option that is an incorrect statement. Recall that the goal of the care of this client is reducing the demands placed on the heart; this will direct you to option 4. Review the care of the client with CAD if you had difficulty with this question.

Reference

deWit, S. (2009). *Medical-surgical nursing: Concepts & practice* (pp. 494-495). St. Louis: Saunders.

---

979. A nurse is assigned to care for a client with coronary artery disease who is scheduled for a cardiac catheterization. After the catheterization, the priority nursing action is to monitor the:

1 Urine output
2 Temperature
3 Potassium level
4 Catheter insertion site

Level of Cognitive Ability: Application
Client Needs: Physiological Integrity
Integrated Process: Nursing Process/Implementation
Content Area: Delegating/Prioritizing

Answer: 4

Rationale: Cardiac catheterization is a diagnostic procedure during which a catheter is introduced through an incision into a large blood vessel and threaded through the circulatory system of the heart to visualize the coronary artery vessels. After cardiac catheterization, priorities of nursing care include the frequent monitoring of the blood pressure and pulse. The catheter insertion site is checked frequently for signs of bleeding and swelling, and the distal pulses are also assessed. The potassium level, temperature, and urine output should also be monitored, but they are not the priorities of the items identified in the options.

Test-Taking Strategy: Note the strategic word *priority*, and note the relationship between the word *catheterization* in the question and *catheter* in the correct option. Review nursing care after a cardiac catheterization if you had difficulty with this question.

Reference

Chernecky, C., & Berger, B. (2008). *Laboratory tests and diagnostic procedures* (5th ed., p. 297). Philadelphia: Saunders.

---

980. A client has coronary artery disease, and blood samples are obtained to evaluate the client's serum cholesterol levels. Which result should the nurse consider most desirable?

1 Elevated total lipoprotein levels
2 Decreased total lipoprotein levels
3 Decreased low-density lipoprotein (LDL) levels and increased high-density lipoprotein (HDL) levels
4 Increased LDL levels and decreased HDL levels

Level of Cognitive Ability: Analysis
Client Needs: Physiological Integrity
Integrated Process: Nursing Process/Evaluation
Content Area: Fundamental Skills

Answer: 3
Rationale: HDLs are considered the "good" cholesterol, and LDLs are the "bad" cholesterol. LDLs come mainly from animal fats; therefore, option 3 is correct.

Test-Taking Strategy: Note the strategic words *most desirable.* Remember that LDLs are "bad" and HDLs are "good" to assist you with answering this question. Review these laboratory tests and their significance if you had difficulty with this question.

References

Chernecky, C., & Berger, B. (2008). *Laboratory tests and diagnostic procedures* (5th ed., pp. 714-716). Philadelphia: Saunders.
Christensen, B., & Kockrow, E. (2006). *Adult health nursing* (5th ed., p. 336). St. Louis: Mosby.

---

981. A pregnant client asks the nurse why tetracycline (Sumycin) cannot be prescribed for her acne. The nurse responds by telling the client that the medication:

1 May cause premature labor
2 May cause deafness in the fetus
3 Is more likely to produce an allergic reaction
4 May darken the teeth and disrupt the bone growth of the fetus

Level of Cognitive Ability: Analysis
Client Needs: Physiological Integrity
Integrated Process: Nursing Process/Implementation
Content Area: Pharmacology

Answer: 4
Rationale: Tetracycline is an antibiotic that readily crosses the placenta and that is deposited in the teeth and bones of the fetus. This medication can cause permanent tooth enamel discoloration, and it can depress bone growth. Tetracycline does not induce labor. Option 3 is incorrect because the allergic potential of any medication does not increase during pregnancy. Option 2 is incorrect.

Test-Taking Strategy: Knowledge of the effects of tetracycline on the fetus is necessary to answer this question. Remember that tetracyclines readily cross the placenta and that they are deposited in the teeth and bones of the fetus. Review tetracyclines if you had difficulty with this question.

Reference

Kee, J., Hayes, E., & McCuistion, L. (2009). *Pharmacology: A nursing process approach* (6th ed., p. 445). St. Louis: Saunders.

---

982. A nurse is caring for an older client who is receiving triazolam (Halcion). The nurse monitors the client closely, knowing that this medication can cause:

1 Blood clots
2 Constipation
3 Urinary retention
4 Impaired mobility

Level of Cognitive Ability: Application
Client Needs: Physiological Integrity
Integrated Process: Nursing Process/Implementation
Content Area: Pharmacology

Answer: 4
Rationale: Medications are metabolized and excreted more slowly in older clients; therefore, the risk of adverse effects is increased. Triazolam (Halcion) is a benzodiazepine sedative and hypnotic, and it can cause confusion and dizziness that lead to impaired mobility. Options 1, 2, and 3 are incorrect.

Test-Taking Strategy: Recall that older clients are more likely to experience adverse side effects of any medication to direct you to option 4. Remember that safety is a priority concern with the older client. Review the adverse effects of triazolam if you had difficulty with this question.

Reference

Edmunds, M. (2010). *Introduction to clinical pharmacology* (6th ed., p. 283). St. Louis: Mosby.

---

983. When administering both cimetidine (Tagamet) and sucralfate (Carafate) to a client, the nurse should plan to give these medications:

1 2 hours apart
2 15 minutes apart
3 At the same time
4 Only when the client complains of pain

Level of Cognitive Ability: Application
Client Needs: Physiological Integrity
Integrated Process: Nursing Process/Planning
Content Area: Pharmacology

Answer: 1

Rationale: Cimetidine (Tagamet) is a gastric acid secretion inhibitor. Sucralfate (Carafate) is an antiulcer agent that forms a protective barrier at the stomach mucosal surface and that can prevent other medications from being absorbed. Sucralfate should be given 2 hours before or after other medications. Options 2, 3, and 4 are incorrect.

Test-Taking Strategy: Use the process of elimination. Recall that sucralfate forms a protective barrier at the stomach mucosal surface to direct you to option 1. Review cimetidine and sucralfate if you had difficulty with this question.

Reference

Hodgson, B., & Kizior, R. (2009). *Saunders nursing drug handbook 2009* (pp. 245, 1082). St. Louis: Saunders.

---

984. A nurse is caring for a client receiving furosemide (Lasix). To evaluate the effectiveness of diuretic therapy, the nurse should monitor the client's:

1 Pulse
2 Weight
3 Potassium level
4 Level of consciousness

Level of Cognitive Ability: Analysis
Client Needs: Physiological Integrity
Integrated Process: Nursing Process/Evaluation
Content Area: Pharmacology

Answer: 2

Rationale: Furosemide (Lasix) is a loop diuretic. All diuretic medications result in an increased urinary output, thus reducing body weight. The pulse may be affected as a result of decreased circulating volume, but this is not an expected outcome of diuretic therapy. Potassium levels are monitored with diuretics, but this is for the purpose of monitoring for side effects (not for monitoring the effectiveness of therapy). Option 4 is unrelated to the action of this medication.

Test-Taking Strategy: Note the strategic word *effectiveness*. Recall the action and effects of diuretic therapy to direct you to option 2. Review furosemide if you had difficulty with this question.

Reference

Hodgson, B., & Kizior, R. (2009). *Saunders nursing drug handbook 2009* (p. 524). St. Louis: Saunders.

---

985. A nurse is caring for a client who is taking warfarin sodium (Coumadin). To evaluate the effectiveness of therapy, the nurse monitors the client's:

1 Daily weight
2 Urinary output
3 Blood pressure
4 Prothrombin time (PT)

Level of Cognitive Ability: Analysis
Client Needs: Physiological Integrity
Integrated Process: Nursing Process/Evaluation
Content Area: Pharmacology

Answer: 4

Rationale: Warfarin sodium is an anticoagulant that is given to maintain a PT of 1.5 times the normal level. Therefore, checking blood coagulation tests is an effective measure for determining effectiveness. Options 1, 2, and 3 are not affected by warfarin therapy.

Test-Taking Strategy: Focus on the action of the mediation. Recall that warfarin sodium (Coumadin) is an anticoagulant to direct you to option 4. Review warfarin sodium if you had difficulty with this question.

Reference

Edmunds, M. (2010). *Introduction to clinical pharmacology* (6th ed., p. 325). St. Louis: Mosby.

---

986. A nurse is caring for a client who is taking digoxin (Lanoxin). Before administering the medication, the nurse checks the client's:

Answer: 4

Rationale: Digoxin (Lanoxin) is a cardiotonic and antidysrhythmic medication. One of the adverse effects of digoxin is the slowing of the pulse rate, which occurs as a result of decreased conduction at

1 Temperature
2 Blood pressure
3 Respiratory rate
4 Apical pulse rate

Level of Cognitive Ability: Application
Client Needs: Physiological Integrity
Integrated Process: Nursing Process/Implementation
Content Area: Pharmacology

the atrioventricular node. Therefore, the nurse checks the client's apical pulse rate. In addition, if the pulse is less than 60 beats/min, the medication is held, and the physician is notified. Options 1, 2, and 3 are usually not directly affected by digoxin.

Test-Taking Strategy: Focus on the name of the medication. Recall that digoxin (Lanoxin) is a cardiotonic and antidysrhythmic medication to direct you to option 4. Review the nursing interventions related to digoxin if you had difficulty with this question.

Reference

Hodgson, B., & Kizior, R. (2009). *Saunders nursing drug handbook 2009* (p. 356). St. Louis: Saunders.

---

987. Chlorpromazine (Thorazine) has been prescribed for a client. The client returns to the physician's office for a follow-up examination and complains of restlessness and agitation. The nurse observes the client and collects additional data, knowing that which of the following signs may indicate a potentially serious complication related to this medication?
1 The client is picking at skin sores.
2 The client's lips smack repetitively.
3 The client's weight has gone up 1 lb.
4 The client's blood pressure is slightly elevated.

Level of Cognitive Ability: Analysis
Client Needs: Physiological Integrity
Integrated Process: Nursing Process/Data Collection
Content Area: Pharmacology

Answer: 2
Rationale: Chlorpromazine (Thorazine) is a phenothiazine antipsychotic. The most serious side effect of the phenothiazine antipsychotics is tardive dyskinesia. Early signs of this condition are lip sucking and smacking behaviors, tongue protrusion, facial grimacing, and choreiform movements. Options 1, 3, and 4 are not indicative of a complication related to this medication.

Test-Taking Strategy: Focus on the name of the medication. Recall that chlorpromazine (Thorazine) is a phenothiazine antipsychotic and that the most serious side effect of these medications is tardive dyskinesia. Review the phenothiazine antipsychotics and their adverse reactions if you had difficulty with this question.

Reference

Hodgson, B., & Kizior, R. (2009). *Saunders nursing drug handbook 2009* (pp. 236-237). St. Louis: Saunders.

---

988. A school-age child has history of upper respiratory infection accompanied by sore throat. The physician explains to the nurse that the modified Jones criteria are being used to diagnose rheumatic fever. The nurse understands that the physician is looking for:
1 An elevation in antistreptolysin-O antibodies
2 A significant decrease in the child's sedimentation rate
3 Emotional instability, purposeless movement, and muscular weakness
4 Evidence of streptococcal infection and the presence of two major manifestations or one major and two minor manifestations of rheumatic fever

Answer: 4
Rationale: The Jones criteria are a standardized set of guidelines for the diagnosis of rheumatic fever. Rheumatic fever is a systemic inflammatory disease that often occurs 1 to 5 weeks after recovery from a sore throat. A high probability of rheumatic fever is indicated when there is evidence of at least two of the major or one major and two minor manifestations of the Jones criteria and evidence of a streptococcal infection. The sedimentation rate is normally increased in a client with rheumatic fever. An elevation in antistreptolysin-O antibodies indicates a recent streptococcal infection but does not alone diagnose rheumatic fever. Option 3 identifies clinical manifestations of chorea, which is one major manifestation. However, these alone are not enough to diagnose rheumatic fever, according to the modified Jones criteria.

Test-Taking Strategy: Focus on the data in the question. Note the relationship between the words *rheumatic fever* in the question and the correct option. Review the Jones criteria if you had difficulty with this question.

Level of Cognitive Ability: Analysis
Client Needs: Physiological Integrity
Integrated Process: Nursing Process/Data Collection
Content Area: Child Health

Reference
Leifer, G. (2007). *Introduction to maternity and pediatric nursing* (5th ed., pp. 604-605). Philadelphia: Saunders.

---

989. A school-age child sustains a fracture along the epiphyseal line of the femur after a fall from the garage roof. The nurse plans care, knowing that a potential long-term effect of this type of injury likely is:
1 Osteomyelitis
2 Muscle atrophy
3 Growth disturbance
4 Paresthesias, paralysis, or both

Level of Cognitive Ability: Comprehension
Client Needs: Physiological Integrity
Integrated Process: Nursing Process/Planning
Content Area: Child Health

Answer: 3
Rationale: Growth takes place at the epiphysis of the long bone. A fracture at this level can destroy the layer of germinal cells of the epiphysis and result in a growth disturbance. Osteomyelitis is an infection of the bone that is more likely to occur with a compound (open) fracture rather than with an epiphyseal fracture. Muscle atrophy may result from immobility or casting, but this resolves as activity increases. Paresthesias and paralysis can result from edema and the constriction of a cast but not specifically from a fracture of the epiphysis.

Test-Taking Strategy: Note the strategic words *long-term effect.* Use the process of elimination, and focus on the subject—the epiphyseal line; this will direct you to option 3. Review the complications associated with a fractured femur if you had difficulty with this question.

Reference
McKinney, E., James, S., Murray, S., & Ashwill, J. (2009). *Maternal-child nursing* (3rd ed., p. 1400). St. Louis: Mosby.

---

990. A nurse is reinforcing instructions to an 8-year-old child about measures to take to identify the early signs of an asthma episode. The nurse instructs the child to first:
1 Perform chest percussion and postural drainage immediately.
2 Open the airway passages by using a handheld nebulizer treatment.
3 Use a peak-flow meter to measure for a drop in the expiratory flow rate.
4 Deliver a dose of a bronchodilator with a metered-dose inhaler to see if it helps.

Level of Cognitive Ability: Application
Client Needs: Physiological Integrity
Integrated Process: Teaching and Learning
Content Area: Child Health

Answer: 3
Rationale: An asthmatic child who is more than 4 years old should be able to measure his or her own expiratory flow. A drop in the expiratory flow is the most reliable early sign of an asthma episode. Chest percussion and postural drainage normally are used to clear the air passages of children with cystic fibrosis (not asthma). Medications would be administered with a metered-dose inhaler or a hand-held nebulizer if an asthma attack actually occurs.

Test-Taking Strategy: Note the strategic word *first,* and focus on the subject—measures to take to identify the early signs of an asthma episode. This will direct you to option 3 because it relates to data collection. Review instructions for children with asthma if you had difficulty with this question.

Reference
Price, D., & Gwin, J. (2008). *Pediatric nursing: An introductory text* (10th ed., p. 310). St. Louis: Saunders.

---

991. A nurse is caring for a client with terminal cancer. When planning for the administration of an opioid pain reliever, the nurse understands that:
1 Not all pain is real.
2 Opioid analgesics are highly addictive.

Answer: 4
Rationale: Administering pain medication around the clock provides increased pain relief and decreases the stressors associated with pain (e.g., anxiety, fear). Opioid analgesics may be addictive, but this is not a concern for a client with terminal cancer. Not all opioid analgesics cause tachycardia. Although option 1 may be

3 Opioid analgesics can cause tachycardia.
4 Around-the-clock dosing gives better pain relief than PRN dosing.

Level of Cognitive Ability: Comprehension
Client Needs: Physiological Integrity
Integrated Process: Caring
Content Area: Pharmacology

accurate, this is not a concern in this situation; the client's pain needs to be relieved.

Test-Taking Strategy: Use the process of elimination, your knowledge of the effects of opioid analgesics, and the client's diagnosis to answer the question. This will direct you to option 4. Review pain management and the administration of opioid analgesics if you had difficulty with this question.

Reference
Black, J., & Hawks, J. (2009). *Medical-surgical nursing: Clinical management for positive outcomes* (8th ed., p. 392). St. Louis: Saunders

---

992. A pediatrician is evaluating a school-age child after the teacher reports that the child is not paying attention during class. The teacher reports that the child appears to be daydreaming and staring off into space 40 or 50 times during the day but that the child is alert and participates in classroom activities for the remainder of the day. The nurse who is assisting the pediatrician expects that the pediatrician will note which of the following on physical examination?

1 The child has a school phobia, and the source of the problem needs to be determined.
2 The child has attention-deficit/hyperactivity disorder (ADHD) and needs medication.
3 The child has a behavioral problem, and a referral to a special class may be necessary if things do not improve.
4 The child is probably experiencing absence seizures and will need to have an electroencephalogram (EEG) performed to confirm this diagnosis.

Level of Cognitive Ability: Analysis
Client Needs: Physiological Integrity
Integrated Process: Nursing Process/Data Collection
Content Area: Child Health

Answer: 4
Rationale: Numerous and frequent episodes of a child staring off into space and then quickly returning to conversation or activities is a classic sign of absence seizures that can be confirmed by an EEG. Classic symptoms of ADHD include easy distraction, fidgeting, and problems following directions. School phobia includes physical symptoms that usually occur at home and that may prevent the child from attending school. Severe behavior problems that necessitate placement in a special class involve more overt behavior than that described in the question.

Test-Taking Strategy: Focus on the description provided in the question and use your knowledge of the symptoms associated with absence seizures to direct you to option 4. Remember that numerous and frequent episodes of a child staring off into space and then quickly returning to conversation or activities is a classic sign of absence seizures. Review the indicators of absence seizures if you had difficulty with this question.

Reference
Price, D., & Gwin, J. (2008). *Pediatric nursing: An introductory text* (10th ed., p. 253). St. Louis: Saunders.

---

993. An adolescent female is admitted to the hospital for severe weight loss. During data collection, the nurse notes that the client is suffering from a disturbed body image and amenorrhea and that she appears to be depressed. A primary goal is to improve the client's nutritional status. Which nursing action should the nurse implement first?

Answer: 4
Rationale: Until the client begins to take adequate nutrition and is physiologically stable, the nurse cannot work with the client on other levels. Options 1, 2, and 3 are appropriate interventions that should be instituted after the client's nutrition status has improved.

1 Establish a behavioral contract with the client in which she agrees to adhere to a diet and a realistic exercise program.
2 Weigh the client daily in her gown and without shoes, and observe for any hidden objects that could alter her weight.
3 Involve the client and her parents in family group sessions to work through psychological problems related to anorexia.
4 Observe the client during and after meals to be sure that proper foods are eaten and that the client does not discard the food after apparently consuming it.

Level of Cognitive Ability: Application
Client Needs: Physiological Integrity
Integrated Process: Nursing Process/Implementation
Content Area: Delegating/Prioritizing

Test-Taking Strategy: Note the strategic word *first*. Use Maslow's Hierarchy of Needs theory, and remember that physiological needs are the priority; this will direct you to option 4. In addition, note that option 4 is the only option that relates to data collection, which is the first step of the nursing process. Review interventions for the client with anorexia if you had difficulty with this question.

Reference
Price, D., & Gwin, J. (2008). *Pediatric nursing: An introductory text* (10th ed., p. 344). St. Louis: Saunders.

---

994. A client is placed on a magnesium-containing antacid. The nurse reviews the client's health record and determines that which preexisting condition requires the cautious use of this antacid?
1 Angina
2 Renal failure
3 Hypertension
4 Diabetes mellitus

Level of Cognitive Ability: Analysis
Client Needs: Physiological Integrity
Integrated Process: Nursing Process/Data Collection
Content Area: Pharmacology

Answer: 2
Rationale: Renal failure is the inability of the kidneys to excrete waste, concentrate urine, and conserve electrolytes. The administration of magnesium-containing antacids can cause increased magnesium levels in the client with renal failure. Options 1, 3, and 4 identify disorders with pathophysiologies that are not affected by magnesium.

Test-Taking Strategy: Note the strategic words *requires the cautious use.* Recall the pathophysiology associated with renal failure to direct you to option 2. Review the contraindications for magnesium-containing antacids if you had difficulty with this question.

Reference
Hodgson, B., & Kizior, R. (2009). *Saunders nursing drug handbook 2009* (p. 710). St. Louis: Saunders.

---

995. A nurse is reviewing the health record of a client who is taking a daily dose of digoxin (Lanoxin). Which of the following, if noted in the health record, would place the client at risk for digoxin toxicity?
1 Peptic ulcer disease
2 Hyperthyroidism and hyperthermia
3 Hypothyroidism and loop diuretic use
4 Muscle spasms and ibuprofen (Motrin) use

Level of Cognitive Ability: Analysis
Client Needs: Physiological Integrity

Answer: 3
Rationale: Digoxin (Lanoxin) is a cardiotonic and antidysrhythmic medication. Digoxin must be used cautiously in clients who are taking loop diuretics because electrolyte imbalances such as hypokalemia can occur, thus increasing the risk for toxicity. The risk for toxicity also can occur in clients with an impaired ability to metabolize medication, such as what occurs with hypothyroidism. Options 1, 2, and 4 are not associated with the risk for toxicity.

Test-Taking Strategy: Focus on the subject—the condition that will place the client at risk for digoxin toxicity. Recall the causes and pathophysiology of digoxin toxicity to direct you to option 3. Review the causes of digoxin toxicity if you had difficulty with this question.

Integrated Process: Nursing Process/Data Collection
Content Area: Pharmacology

Reference
Edmunds, M. (2010). *Introduction to clinical pharmacology* (6th ed., p. 228). St. Louis: Mosby.

---

996. A 5-year-old boy has a deficiency of factor VIII. An important goal is to relieve the pain caused by bleeding into the joints. Which interventions does the nurse expect will be prescribed to achieve this goal?

1 Joint immobilization
2 Hot packs for the affected joints
3 Nonsteroidal antiinflammatory drugs (NSAIDs)
4 Physical therapy to help the child through the acute period

Level of Cognitive Ability: Comprehension
Client Needs: Physiological Integrity
Integrated Process: Nursing Process/Planning
Content Area: Child Health

Answer: 1
Rationale: A deficiency in factor VIII places the child at risk for bleeding. Joint immobilization assists with preventing bleeding and pain. Heat application increases blood flow to the area and promotes bleeding. NSAIDs can prolong bleeding time and increase the bleeding and pain caused by the pressure of the confined fluid in the narrow joint space. Physical therapy can be helpful after the bleeding episode is under control, but therapy can increase bleeding during the acute period.

Test-Taking Strategy: Focus on the subject—relieving the pain caused by bleeding into the joints. Use the principles related to the effects of heat and cold to eliminate option 2. Eliminate option 4 because of the word *acute* in this option. Recalling that NSAIDs present the risk of bleeding assists with directing you to option 1. Review the measures to relieve the pain caused by bleeding into the joints if you had difficulty with this question.

Reference
McKinney, E., James, S., Murray, S., & Ashwill, J. (2009). *Maternal-child nursing* (3rd ed., p. 1293). St. Louis: Mosby.

---

997. A 3-year-old child is admitted to the hospital with a diagnosis of acute lymphocytic leukemia (ALL). The nurse assigned to care for the child is concerned because the child is crying and stating, "My knees hurt." Which intervention does the nurse plan for the child?

1 Applying heat to the knees
2 Applying cold packs to the knees
3 Administering 2.5 grains of aspirin
4 Attempting to involve the child in diversional activities so that he or she will forget the discomfort

Level of Cognitive Ability: Application
Client Needs: Physiological Integrity
Integrated Process: Nursing Process/Implementation
Content Area: Child Health

Answer: 2
Rationale: ALL is a hematologic, malignant disease that is characterized by large numbers of immature cells (lymphoblasts) in the bone marrow, circulating blood, lymph nodes, spleen, liver, and other organs. Bleeding into the joints can occur, and cold applications will decrease joint discomfort. Aspirin has anticoagulant properties and should not be prescribed. Heat applications will cause more blood circulation, which increases any pain and bleeding that is present. Diversional activities do not relieve the pain.

Test-Taking Strategy: Focus on the child's diagnosis, and use the process of elimination. Recall that the associated risk of bleeding exists to assist you with eliminating options 1 and 3. In addition, recall the effect of heat to assist you with eliminating option 1. From the remaining options, option 2 is the one that addresses the child's physiological need. Review the care of the child with ALL if you had difficulty with this question.

Reference
McKinney, E., James, S., Murray, S., & Ashwill, J. (2009). *Maternal-child nursing* (3rd ed., p. 1293). St. Louis: Mosby.

---

998. A child is brought to the urgent care clinic. The mother is concerned because the child is difficult to awaken, complains of a "tummy ache," and is irritable. Of the following questions, which one does

Answer: 1
Rationale: Lead poisoning is a toxic condition that is caused by the inhalation or ingestion of lead or lead compounds. Homes that are more than 25 years old may have lead paint and will most likely have lead pipes. A fruity breath odor is a symptom of

the nurse expect the physician to ask the mother if lead poisoning is suspected?
1 "Do you live in a home that is more than 25 years old?"
2 "Does your child's breath have a sweet or fruity odor?"
3 "Does you child chew on pencils or crayons while drawing?"
4 "Has your child been breathing rapidly and sweating profusely?"

Level of Cognitive Ability: Analysis
Client Needs: Physiological Integrity
Integrated Process: Nursing Process/Data Collection
Content Area: Child Health

ketoacidosis. Hyperventilation and diaphoresis are signs of salicylate (not lead) poisoning. Pencil lead is made of graphite, so it does not present a hazard. Crayons are not toxic.

Test-Taking Strategy: Focus on the subject—the contributing factors of lead poisoning. Note the words *home that is more than 25 years old* to direct you to option 1. Review the risk factors for lead poisoning if you had difficulty with this question.

Reference
Hockenberry, M., & Wilson, D. (2009). *Wong's essentials of pediatric nursing* (8th ed., p. 478). St. Louis: Mosby.

---

999. A client with acute inferior myocardial infarction (MI) is receiving heparin therapy. The nurse monitors for which associated complication of this therapy?
1 Bleeding
2 Infection
3 Constipation
4 Decreased urine output

Level of Cognitive Ability: Application
Client Needs: Physiological Integrity
Integrated Process: Nursing Process/Implementation
Content Area: Pharmacology

Answer: 1
Rationale: Heparin is an anticoagulant that prevents clotting. The nurse monitors the client for signs of bleeding, such as bleeding gums, petechiae, hematoma formation, and blood in the stool and urine. Infection, constipation, and decreased urine output are not related to heparin therapy.

Test-Taking Strategy: Focus on the action of the medication. Recall that heparin is an anticoagulant to direct you to option 1. Review the care of a client receiving heparin if you had difficulty with this question.

Reference
Hodgson, B., & Kizior, R. (2009). *Saunders nursing drug handbook 2009* (pp. 563-566). St. Louis: Saunders.

1000. A client is preparing for discharge after coronary artery bypass graft surgery (CABG) and asks the nurse if sexual activity is permitted. The nurse should make which response to the client?
1 "I do not know. Wait and discuss this with your physician."
2 "No. Sexual activity is not recommended after heart surgery."
3 "No. Sexual activity can cause the rupture of your cardiac suture lines."
4 "Sexual activity will be allowed. The physician will tell you when you can resume sexual activity."

Level of Cognitive Ability: Application
Client Needs: Physiological Integrity
Integrated Process: Nursing Process/Implementation
Content Area: Adult Health/Cardiovascular

Answer: 4
Rationale: CABG surgery is a procedure in which a prosthesis or section of a blood vessel is grafted into one of the coronary arteries, thus bypassing a narrowing or blockage in a coronary artery. Activity restrictions are often a concern of clients after CABG. Resuming normal sexual relations will be allowed, but the physician decides when the client can safely resume this activity. Options 1, 2, and 3 are incorrect.

Test-Taking Strategy: Use your knowledge of client instructions after CABG and therapeutic communication techniques to answer this question. Eliminate options 2 and 3 first because they are comparable or alike in that they could cause increased anxiety in the client. Eliminate option 1 next because it places the client's feelings on hold. Review client instructions after CABG if you had difficulty with this question.

Reference
Ignatavicius, D., & Workman, M. (2010). *Medical-surgical nursing: Patient-centered collaborative care* (6th ed., p. 872). St. Louis: Saunders.

1001. A 4-week-old infant is brought to the pediatrician for the first well-baby appointment. The mother is concerned because the child has been vomiting after meals and the vomiting is becoming more frequent and forceful. The physician suspects pyloric stenosis. Which clinical manifestation helps to establish the diagnosis?

1 A previously happy and healthy infant suddenly becomes pale, cries out, and draws up the legs to the chest.
2 Ribbon-like stool, bile-stained emesis, and the absence of peristalsis and abdominal distention are apparent.
3 The infant cries loudly and continuously during the evening hours, appears to be in considerable pain, but otherwise nurses or takes formula well.
4 The vomitus contains sour undigested food, but no bile. The child is constipated, and visible peristaltic waves move from left to right across the child's abdomen.

Level of Cognitive Ability: Analysis
Client Needs: Physiological Integrity
Integrated Process: Nursing Process/Data Collection
Content Area: Child Health

Answer: 4
Rationale: Pyloric stenosis is the narrowing of the pyloric sphincter at the outlet of the stomach, which causes an obstruction that blocks the flow of food into the small intestine. Option 4 identifies the classic symptoms of pyloric stenosis. An infant who suddenly becomes pale, cries out, and draws the legs up to the chest is demonstrating physical signs of intussusception. Ribbon-like stool, bile-stained emesis, with the absence of peristalsis and abdominal distention are symptoms of congenital megacolon (Hirschsprung's disease). Crying during the evening hours, appearing to be in pain, but otherwise eating well are clinical manifestations of colic.

Test-Taking Strategy: Focus on the subject—pyloric stenosis. Recall that pyloric stenosis involves the narrowing of the pyloric sphincter to direct you to the correct option. Review pyloric stenosis if you had difficulty with this question.

References
Leifer, G. (2007). *Introduction to maternity and pediatric nursing* (5th ed., p. 636). Philadelphia: Saunders.
Price, D., & Gwin, J. (2008). *Pediatric nursing: An introductory text* (10th ed., p. 159). St. Louis: Saunders.

1002. A nurse is caring for a child with *Haemophilus influenzae* meningitis. As a part of the nursing care plan, the nurse will monitor the child for nerve deafness. The nurse anticipates that the most likely medication to be prescribed to decrease the incidence of nerve deafness will be:

1 Furosemide (Lasix)
2 Ceftazidime (Fortaz)
3 Hydrocortisone (Solu-Cortef)
4 Ceftriaxone sodium (Rocephin)

Level of Cognitive Ability: Analysis
Client Needs: Physiological Integrity
Integrated Process: Nursing Process/Planning
Content Area: Child Health

Answer: 3
Rationale: Meningitis is an infection or inflammation of the membranes that cover the brain and spinal cord. The administration of an intravenous corticosteroid early during the course of the disease has decreased the incidence of nerve deafness as a complication. Ceftriaxone sodium and ceftazidime are third-generation cephalosporins that are prescribed as the antibiotics of choice for *Haemophilus influenzae* meningitis, but they do not specifically decrease the incidence of nerve deafness. Furosemide is a diuretic.

Test-Taking Strategy: Focus on the subject—decreasing the incidence of nerve deafness. Eliminate options 2 and 4 first because they are comparable or alike in that they are antibiotics. From the remaining options, recall that furosemide is a diuretic to eliminate option 1. Review the care of the child with meningitis if you had difficulty with this question.

Reference
Price, D., & Gwin, J. (2008). *Pediatric nursing: An introductory text* (10th ed., p. 165). St. Louis: Saunders.

1003. A client is hospitalized with chest pain, and a myocardial infarction is suspected. The client tells the nurse that the chest pain has returned, and the nurse administers one 0.4-mg nitroglycerin tablet sublingually as prescribed. If the pain is not relieved, what should the nurse do next?

1 Notify the physician.
2 Increase the oxygen flow rate.
3 Place the client in Trendelenburg's position.
4 Administer another sublingual nitroglycerin tablet in 5 minutes.

Level of Cognitive Ability: Application
Client Needs: Physiological Integrity
Integrated Process: Nursing Process/Implementation
Content Area: Pharmacology

Answer: 4

Rationale: Nitroglycerin is a coronary vasodilator. One tablets is administered every 5 minutes (not exceeding three tablets) for chest pain as long as the client maintains a systolic blood pressure of 100 mm Hg or more. The physician is notified if the chest pain is not relieved after administration of the three tablets. Placing the client in Trendelenburg's (head-lowered) position may be necessary with sudden drops in blood pressure, at which time the physician should be notified. Increasing oxygen flow rates are done with an order from a physician.

Test-Taking Strategy: Knowledge of the administration procedure for nitroglycerin when a client is experiencing chest pain is necessary to answer this question. Remember that one tablet of nitroglycerin is administered every 5 minutes (not exceeding three tablets) for chest pain as long as the client maintains a systolic blood pressure of 100 mm Hg or more. Review the procedure for the administration of nitroglycerin if you had difficulty with this question.

Reference

Christensen, B., & Kockrow, E. (2006). *Adult health nursing* (5th ed., p. 351). St. Louis: Mosby.

1004. A nurse is caring for a client with chest pain who is suspected of having a myocardial infarction (MI). The physician has ordered laboratory studies to evaluate the client's progress. Which laboratory data report is significant to the diagnosis of an MI?

1 Increased hematocrit (HCT) level
2 Decreased white blood cell (WBC) count
3 Increased creatine kinase (CK-MB) level
4 Increased creatine kinase (CK-MM) level

Level of Cognitive Ability: Comprehension
Client Needs: Physiological Integrity
Integrated Process: Nursing Process/Data Collection
Content Area: Adult Health/Cardiovascular

Answer: 3

Rationale: Cardiac enzymes and isoenzymes are used to confirm a myocardial infarction. CK-MB is specific for the heart tissue, CK-MM reflects injury to the general skeletal muscle, and CK-BB reflects brain tissue injury. The WBC count tends to increase during acute myocardial infarction. The HCT level is not specifically related to an MI.

Test-Taking Strategy: Focus on the client's diagnosis. Eliminate option 2 first because of the word *decreased*. Eliminate option 1 next because it is unrelated to the client's diagnosis. From the remaining options, remember that CK-MB is specific to the cardiac muscle. Review the creatine kinase isoenzymes if you had difficulty with this question.

References

Christensen, B., & Kockrow, E. (2006). *Adult health nursing* (5th ed., pp. 352-353). St. Louis: Mosby.
deWit, S. (2009). *Medical-surgical nursing: Concepts & practice* (p. 496). St. Louis: Saunders.

1005. A nurse is caring for a client with angina who requests something to drink. Which of the following beverages should the nurse give to the client?

1 Tea
2 Cola
3 Coffee
4 Lemonade

Answer: 4

Rationale: Clients with angina should not consume caffeinated beverages because of the vasoconstriction effect associated with caffeine. Options 1, 2, and 3 are items that contain caffeine.

Test-Taking Strategy: Use the process of elimination. Note that options 1, 2, and 3 are comparable or alike in that they all contain caffeine. Review the food items that contain caffeine if you had difficulty with this question.

Level of Cognitive Ability: Application
Client Needs: Physiological Integrity
Integrated Process: Nursing Process/Implementation
Content Area: Fundamental Skills

Reference

Ignatavicius, D., & Workman, M. (2010). *Medical-surgical nursing: Patient-centered collaborative care* (6th ed., p. 778). St. Louis: Saunders.

1006. A client has been placed in seclusion. The nurse is responsible for assisting with providing care and documenting the care of the client. Which of the following most completely identifies the components that require documentation?

1 Vital signs, reason for seclusion, date, and time
2 Vital signs, toileting, and checking on the client in accordance with the protocol time frame (e.g., every 15 minutes)
3 Ambulating, toileting, and checking on the client in accordance with the protocol time frame (e.g., every 15 minutes)
4 Vital signs, toileting, feeding or fluid intake, and checking on client in accordance with the protocol time frame (e.g., every 15 minutes)

Level of Cognitive Ability: Comprehension
Client Needs: Physiological Integrity
Integrated Process: Communication and Documentation
Content Area: Mental Health

Answer: 4

Rationale: Seclusion is the isolation of a client in a special room to decrease stimuli that may cause or exacerbate the client's emotional distress. The room is free from objects that the client might use to cause self-harm or harm to others. Option 4 addresses the client's basic needs during seclusion. Option 1 contains data that are documented at the time that seclusion is initiated. Options 2 and 3 are not complete in terms of identifying physiological needs.

Test-Taking Strategy: Use the process of elimination. Eliminate option 1 first because these data are documented at the time that seclusion is initiated. From the remaining options, use Maslow's Hierarchy of Needs theory to prioritize. Option 4 most completely addresses the client's basic needs. Review the care of the client in seclusion if you had difficulty with this question.

Reference

Varcarolis, E., & Halter, M. (2009). *Essentials of psychiatric mental health nursing: A communication approach to evidence-based care* (p. 524). St. Louis: Saunders.

1007. A client with a Sengstaken-Blakemore tube in place is admitted to the hospital from the emergency department. The nurse assigned to assist with caring for the client plans the client's care, understanding that the purpose of this tube is to:

1 Control ascites
2 Control bleeding from gastritis
3 Apply pressure to esophageal varices
4 Remove ammonia-forming bacteria from the gastrointestinal tract

Level of Cognitive Ability: Comprehension
Client Needs: Physiological Integrity
Integrated Process: Nursing Process/Planning
Content Area: Adult Health/Gastrointestinal

Answer: 3

Rationale: A Sengstaken-Blakemore tube is inserted in a client with cirrhosis with ruptured esophageal varices. It has esophageal and gastric balloons. The esophageal balloon exerts pressure on the ruptured esophageal varices and stops the bleeding. The gastric balloon holds the tube in the correct position and prevents the migration of the esophageal balloon, which would harm the client. Options 1, 2, and 4 identify treatment goals for clients with ruptured esophageal varices and do not describe the purpose of this tube.

Test-Taking Strategy: Focus on the subject, and use the process of elimination. Option 3 correctly defines the purpose of the tube. All of the other options identify treatment goals for clients with ruptured esophageal varices. Review the purpose of the Sengstaken-Blakemore tube if you had difficulty with this question.

Reference

Christensen, B., & Kockrow, E. (2006). *Adult health nursing* (5th ed., pp. 260-261). St. Louis: Mosby.

1008. A nurse is instructing a client with chronic obstructive pulmonary disease (COPD) about breathing techniques. The nurse incorporates which of the following modalities?

1 Pursed-lip breathing
2 Inspiratory breathing
3 Chest physical therapy
4 Intercostal chest expansion

Level of Cognitive Ability: Application
Client Needs: Physiological Integrity
Integrated Process: Teaching and Learning
Content Area: Adult Health/Respiratory

Answer: 1

Rationale: COPD is a progressive and irreversible disease that is characterized by the diminished inspiratory and expiratory capacity of the lungs. Pursed-lip breathing allows the client to slowly exhale carbon dioxide while keeping the airways open. Intercostal chest expansion, inspiratory breathing, and chest physical therapy are not breathing techniques.

Test-Taking Strategy: Use the process of elimination. Eliminate options 2, 3, and 4 because they are comparable or alike in that they are not breathing techniques. Remember that pursed-lip breathing is associated with the COPD client to direct you to option 1. Review breathing techniques for the client with COPD if you had difficulty with this question.

Reference

Linton, A. (2007). *Introduction to medical-surgical nursing* (4th ed., p. 557). Philadelphia: Saunders.

1009. A physician has ordered a partial rebreathing face mask for a client who has terminal lung cancer. The nurse plans care knowing that the mask:

1 Delivers an accurate fraction of inspired oxygen (FIO_2) to the client
2 Requires a low liter flow to prevent the rebreathing of carbon dioxide
3 Requires that the reservoir bag be deflated during inspiration to work effectively
4 Conserves oxygen by having the client rebreathe some of his or her own exhaled air

Level of Cognitive Ability: Comprehension
Client Needs: Physiological Integrity
Integrated Process: Nursing Process/Planning
Content Area: Adult Health/Respiratory

Answer: 4

Rationale: Rebreathing masks have a reservoir bag that conserves oxygen and that requires a high liter flow to achieve concentrations of 40% to 60%. It does not deliver accurate FIO_2 to the client. The bag should not deflate during inspiration. A rebreathing bag conserves oxygen by having the client rebreathe his or her own exhaled air.

Test-Taking Strategy: Use the process of elimination. Note the relationship of the words *partial rebreathing* in the question and *rebreathe some of his or her own exhaled air* in the correct option. Review oxygen delivery systems if you had difficulty with this question.

Reference

deWit, S. (2009). *Medical-surgical nursing: Concepts & practice* (p. 353). St. Louis: Saunders.

1010. A 48-year-old man is brought to the emergency department complaining of chest pain. His vital signs are blood pressure (BP), 150/90 mm Hg; pulse (P), 88 beats/min; and respirations (R), 20 breaths/min. The nurse administers nitroglycerin 0.4 mg sublingually. To evaluate the effectiveness of this medication, the nurse should expect which of the following changes in the vital signs?

1 BP, 150/90 mm Hg; P, 70 beats/min; R, 24 breaths/min
2 BP, 100/60 mm Hg; P, 96 beats/min; R, 20 breaths/min

Answer: 2

Rationale: Nitroglycerin dilates both arteries and veins, thereby causing blood to pool in the periphery. This causes a reduced preload and thus a drop in cardiac output. This vasodilation causes the blood pressure to fall. The drop in cardiac output causes the sympathetic nervous system to respond and to attempt to maintain cardiac output by increasing the pulse. Therefore, option 2 is correct.

Test-Taking Strategy: Use the process of elimination. Recall that nitroglycerin is a vasodilator and that it causes the BP to drop to eliminate options 1 and 4. In addition, if chest pain and cardiac workload are reduced, the client will be more comfortable; therefore, a rise in respirations should not be seen. This assists with directing you to option 2. Review the effects of nitroglycerin if you had difficulty with this question.

3 BP, 100/60 mm Hg; P, 70 beats/min; R, 24 breaths/min
4 BP, 160/100 mm Hg; P, 120 beats/min; R, 16 breaths/min

Level of Cognitive Ability: Analysis
Client Needs: Physiological Integrity
Integrated Process: Nursing Process/Evaluation
Content Area: Pharmacology

Reference

Linton, A. (2007). *Introduction to medical-surgical nursing* (4th ed., pp. 633, 642). Philadelphia: Saunders.

1011. A client who had abdominal surgery 1 day ago has a nasogastric tube. The nurse who is assisting with caring for the client notes the absence of bowel sounds. The nurse's best action is to:

1 Feed the client.
2 Remove the nasogastric tube.
3 Continue to monitor for bowel sounds.
4 Contact the registered nurse (RN) immediately.

Level of Cognitive Ability: Application
Client Needs: Physiological Integrity
Integrated Process: Nursing Process/Implementation
Content Area: Adult Health/Gastrointestinal

Answer: 3

Rationale: Bowel sounds may be absent for 2 to 3 days after surgery because of bowel manipulation during surgery. The nurse should continue to monitor the client. If a nasogastric tube is present, it should stay in place, and the client should be kept NPO until after the onset of bowel sounds. In addition, the nurse should not remove the nasogastric tube. There is no need to contact the RN immediately, although the finding should be reported.

Test-Taking Strategy: Use the process of elimination. Note the strategic words *1 day ago* and *best*. Recall that bowel sounds may not return for 2 to 3 days after this type of operation. Review normal postoperative findings after abdominal surgery if you had difficulty with this question.

Reference

deWit, S. (2009). *Medical-surgical nursing: Concepts & practice* (p. 98). St. Louis: Saunders.

1012. Which statement by the mother of a newly circumcised infant indicates knowledge of necessary postcircumcision care?

1 "I should clean his penis every hour with baby wipes."
2 "I should check for bleeding every hour for the first 12 hours."
3 "My baby will not urinate for the next 24 hours because of swelling."
4 "I should wrap his penis completely in dry sterile gauze and make sure that it is dry when I change his diaper."

Level of Cognitive Ability: Comprehension
Client Needs: Physiological Integrity
Integrated Process: Nursing Process/Evaluation
Content Area: Maternity/Postpartum

Answer: 2

Rationale: Circumcision is a surgical procedure in which the prepuce of the penis is excised. The mother should be taught to watch for bleeding, and she should check the site hourly for 8 to 12 hours. Water is used for cleaning because soap or baby wipes may irritate the area and cause discomfort. Voiding should be monitored. The mother should call the physician if the baby has not urinated within 24 hours. Swelling or damage may obstruct urine output. When the diaper is changed, Vaseline gauze should be reapplied, if prescribed. Frequent diaper changes prevent the contamination of the site.

Test-Taking Strategy: Use the process of elimination. Eliminate option 1 because baby wipes cause stinging in the newly circumcised penis. Eliminate option 3 because penile swelling prevents voiding, and this should be reported to the physician. Eliminate option 4 because gauze that is completely dry sticks to the penis. Review postcircumcision care if you had difficulty with this question.

Reference

Leifer, G. (2008). *Maternity nursing: An introductory text* (10th ed., p. 198). Philadelphia: Saunders.

1013. A nurse plans to reinforce which essential discharge instruction to the client with testicular cancer after testicular surgery?

1 "You cannot drive for 6 weeks."
2 "You must refrain from sitting for long periods."
3 "You cannot be fitted for a prosthesis for 6 months."
4 "Report any elevation in temperature to your physician."

Level of Cognitive Ability: Application
Client Needs: Physiological Integrity
Integrated Process: Teaching and Learning
Content Area: Adult Health/Oncology

Answer: 4
Rationale: For the client who has had testicular surgery, the nurse should emphasize the importance of notifying the physician if chills, fever, drainage, redness, or discharge occurs. These symptoms may indicate the presence of an infection. The client may drive 1 week after testicular surgery. A prosthesis is often inserted during surgery. Sitting should be avoided after prostate surgery because of the risk of hemorrhage; however, the risk is not as high with testicular surgery.

Test-Taking Strategy: Use Maslow's Hierarchy of Needs theory. Infection is the priority. An elevation of temperature could signal an infection after any surgical procedure and should be reported. Note the close-ended words *cannot, must,* and *cannot* in options 1, 2, and 3, respectively. Review the care of the client after testicular surgery if you had difficulty with this question.

Reference
Linton, A. (2007). *Introduction to medical-surgical nursing* (4th ed., p. 1100). Philadelphia: Saunders.

1014. A nurse is caring for a client with Parkinson's disease who is taking benztropine mesylate (Cogentin) daily. The nurse understands that the priority nursing action when caring for clients who are taking his medication is to monitor which of the following?

1 Pulse
2 Pupil response
3 Intake and output
4 Respiratory status

Level of Cognitive Ability: Application
Client Needs: Physiological Integrity
Integrated Process: Nursing Process/Data Collection
Content Area: Pharmacology

Answer: 3
Rationale: Benztropine mesylate (Cogentin) is an anticholinergic. Urinary retention is a side effect of this medication. The nurse should observe for dysuria, a distended abdomen, the infrequent voiding of small amounts, and overflow incontinence. Options 1, 2, and 4 are not related to this medication.

Test-Taking Strategy: Use the process of elimination. Remember that urinary retention is a concern with benztropine mesylate to direct you to option 3. Review benztropine mesylate and its side effects if you had difficulty with this question.

Reference
Edmunds, M. (2010). *Introduction to clinical pharmacology.* (6th ed., p. 263). St. Louis: Mosby.

1015. A nurse is teaching a client with chronic obstructive pulmonary disease (COPD) pursed-lip breathing. The nurse tells the client:

1 That exhalation should be twice as long as inhalation
2 That inhalation should be twice as long as exhalation
3 To loosen the abdominal muscles while breathing out
4 To inhale with pursed lips and exhale with the mouth open wide

Level of Cognitive Ability: Application
Client Needs: Physiological Integrity

Answer: 1
Rationale: COPD is a progressive and irreversible condition that is characterized by the diminished inspiratory and expiratory capacity of the lungs. Prolonging the time of exhaling reduces the air trapping caused by airway narrowing or collapse in clients with COPD. Tightening the abdominal muscles helps with the expelling of air. Exhaling through pursed lips increases the intraluminal pressure and prevents the airways from collapsing. Options 2, 3, and 4 are incorrect actions.

Test-Taking Strategy: Use the process of elimination. Recall that the major purpose of pursed-lip breathing is to prevent air trapping during exhalation to direct you to the option 1. Review the principles of pursed-lip breathing if you had difficulty with this question.

Integrated Process: Teaching and Learning
Content Area: Adult Health/Respiratory

Reference
deWit, S. (2009). *Medical-surgical nursing: Concepts & practice* (p. 336). St. Louis: Saunders.

1016. A client is taking lithium carbonate (Lithobid) for the treatment of bipolar disorder. Which question should the nurse ask the client when collecting data to determine signs of early drug toxicity?

1 "Do you frequently have headaches?"
2 "Have you noted excessive urination?"
3 "Have you been experiencing seizures over the past few days?"
4 "Have you been experiencing any nausea, vomiting, or diarrhea?"

Level of Cognitive Ability: Application
Client Needs: Physiological Integrity
Integrated Process: Nursing Process/Data Collection
Content Area: Pharmacology

Answer: 4
Rationale: Lithium carbonate is an antimanic medication. Common early signs of lithium toxicity are gastrointestinal (GI) disturbances such as nausea, vomiting, and diarrhea. The questions identified in options 1, 2, and 3 are unrelated to lithium toxicity.

Test-Taking Strategy: Note the strategic word *early,* and focus on the subject. The question asks for the early signs of lithium toxicity. Recall that GI disturbances occur early during the course of lithium toxicity to direct you to option 4. Review the signs of lithium toxicity if you had difficulty with this question.

Reference
Hodgson, B., & Kizior, R. (2009). *Saunders nursing drug handbook 2009* (p. 693). St. Louis: Saunders.

1017. A client is admitted to the hospital for the repair of an unruptured cerebral aneurysm. The nurse assigned to care for the client monitors the client for signs of aneurysm rupture. Which finding will the nurse note first if the aneurysm ruptures?

1 Widened pulse pressure
2 Unilateral motor weakness
3 Unilateral slowing of pupil response
4 A decline in the level of consciousness

Level of Cognitive Ability: Comprehension
Client Needs: Physiological Integrity
Integrated Process: Nursing Process/Data Collection
Content Area: Adult Health/Neurological

Answer: 4
Rationale: An aneurysm is a localized dilation of the wall of a blood vessel. The rupture of a cerebral aneurysm usually results in increased intracranial pressure. The first sign of increased intracranial pressure is a change in the level of consciousness caused by the compression of the reticular formation. This change in consciousness can be as subtle as drowsiness or restlessness. Because centers that control blood pressure are located lower in the brainstem than those that control consciousness, a pulse pressure alteration is a later sign. Although options 1, 2, and 3 can occur, these are not early signs of increased intracranial pressure.

Test-Taking Strategy: Use the process of elimination, and note the strategic word *first.* Remember that changes in the level of consciousness are the first indication of increased intracranial pressure. Review the clinical manifestations associated with increased intracranial pressure and aneurysm rupture if you had difficulty with this question.

Reference
deWit, S. (2009). *Medical-surgical nursing: Concepts & practice* (p. 572). St. Louis: Saunders.

1018. A client has just undergone an upper gastrointestinal (GI) series. When the client returns to the unit, the nurse plans to implement which of the following, which is an important part of routine postprocedural care?

Answer: 1
Rationale: Barium sulfate, which is used as contrast material during an upper GI series, is a constipating material. If it is not eliminated from the GI tract, it can cause obstruction. Therefore, laxatives or cathartics are administered as part of routine postprocedural care. Options 2 and 4 are unnecessary. Increased fluids are helpful, but a liquid diet is not necessary.

1 Laxative
2 Bland diet
3 Liquid diet
4 NPO status

Level of Cognitive Ability: Application
Client Needs: Physiological Integrity
Integrated Process: Nursing Process/Planning
Content Area: Adult Health/Gastrointestinal

Test-Taking Strategy: Use the process of elimination. Recall that barium is administered during this test and remember its side effects to direct you to option 1. Review postprocedural care after an upper GI series if you had difficulty with this question.

Reference

Chernecky, C., & Berger, B. (2008). *Laboratory tests and diagnostic procedures* (5th ed., p. 1133). Philadelphia: Saunders.

1019. A nurse is administering continuous nasogastric tube feedings to a client. The nurse should take which action as part of the routine care of this client?
1 Check the residual every 4 hours.
2 Change the feeding bag and tubing every 12 hours.
3 Pour additional feeding into the bag when 25 mL is left.
4 Hold the feeding if more than 200 mL of residual is aspirated.

Level of Cognitive Ability: Application
Client Needs: Physiological Integrity
Integrated Process: Nursing Process/Implementation
Content Area: Fundamental Skills

Answer: 1
Rationale: A nasogastric feeding tube is checked at least every 4 hours for residual when administering continuous tube feedings. Placement is checked before each bolus with intermittent feedings and before medications are administered. The bag and tubing are completely changed every 24 hours. The bag should be rinsed before adding new formula to a bag that is already hanging. The feeding should be withheld for 30 to 60 minutes if the residual is more than 100 mL or if it is an amount greater than that prescribed by the physician or designated by agency protocol.

Test-Taking Strategy: Note the strategic words *continuous nasogastric tube feedings.* Use the nursing process to answer the question. Option 1 is the only option that addresses data collection. Review the nursing care associated with continuous nasogastric tube feedings if you had difficulty with this question.

Reference

Christensen, B., & Kockrow, E. (2006). *Foundations of nursing* (5th ed., p. 655). St. Louis: Mosby.

1020. A nurse is asked to obtain dressing supplies for a client who is scheduled to have a chest tube inserted by the physician. The nurse selects which material to be used as the first layer of the dressing at the chest tube insertion site?
1 Petrolatum jelly gauze
2 Sterile 4 × 4 gauze pad
3 Absorbent Kerlix dressing
4 Gauze impregnated with povidone-iodine

Level of Cognitive Ability: Application
Client Needs: Physiological Integrity
Integrated Process: Nursing Process/Implementation
Content Area: Adult Health/Respiratory

Answer: 1
Rationale: The first layer of the chest tube dressing is petrolatum jelly gauze, which allows for an occlusive seal at the chest tube insertion site. Additional layers of gauze cover this layer, and the dressing is secured with a strong adhesive tape or Elastoplast tape. Absorbent Kerlix dressing or gauze impregnated with povidone-iodine is not used.

Test-Taking Strategy: Use the process of elimination, and note the strategic words *first layer.* Recall that it is imperative to have an occlusive seal at the site and remember which dressing material to use to help achieve that occlusive seal to direct you to option 1. Review chest tube dressings if you had difficulty with this question.

Reference

Perry, A. & Potter, P. (2010). *Clinical nursing skills & techniques* (7th ed., p. 704). St. Louis: Mosby.

1021. A client is seen in the ambulatory care clinic with a complaint of feeling something in the eye. The nurse is asked to

Answer: 3
Rationale: Ocular irrigation is performed with sterile normal saline because it is an isotonic solution. Fluorescein is used to visualize a

prepare for ocular irrigation and obtains which solution to be used as an irrigant?
1 Sterile water
2 Fluorescein
3 Sterile normal saline (0.9%)
4 Proparacaine hydrochloride (Ophthaine)

Level of Cognitive Ability: Application
Client Needs: Physiological Integrity
Integrated Process: Nursing Process/Planning
Content Area: Adult Health/Eye

corneal abrasion secondary to injury. Proparacaine hydrochloride is used as a topical anesthetic before irrigation is performed.

Test-Taking Strategy: Use the process of elimination, and note the strategic word *irrigant*. Recall that normal saline is an isotonic solution to direct you to option 3. Review the procedure for eye irrigation if you had difficulty with this question.

Reference

Linton, A. (2007). *Introduction to medical-surgical nursing* (4th ed., p. 1165). Philadelphia: Saunders.

1022. A client who had intracranial surgery has a decreasing pulse rate with an increasing blood pressure. The nurse avoids which activity until the client has stabilized?
1 Suctioning
2 Keeping the neck midline
3 Carefully monitoring fluid intake
4 Elevating the head of the bed to 30 degrees

Level of Cognitive Ability: Application
Client Needs: Physiological Integrity
Integrated Process: Nursing Process/Implementation
Content Area: Adult Health/Neurological

Answer: 1
Rationale: The client is showing signs of increasing intracranial pressure (ICP). The nurse avoids activities that further increase the ICP (e.g., suctioning). The nurse positions the head of the bed at 30 degrees and keeps the client's neck midline to promote venous drainage from the cranium. The nurse carefully monitors fluid intake to prevent fluid overload.

Test-Taking Strategy: Use the process of elimination, and note the strategic word *avoids*. This word indicates a negative event query and asks you to select an option that is an incorrect action. Note that the client is exhibiting signs of increased ICP, and recall the preventive measures. The nurse will avoid suctioning because it would increase intracranial pressure; this directs you to option 1. Review the care of the client after intracranial surgery if you had difficulty with this question.

References

Christensen, B., & Kockrow, E. (2006). *Adult health nursing* (5th ed., p. 705). St. Louis: Mosby.
deWit, S. (2009). *Medical-surgical nursing: Concepts & practice* (p. 549). St. Louis: Saunders.

1023. A nurse is assigned to care for a client with angina pectoris. While the nurse is providing care, the client develops acute anginal chest discomfort. The nurse prepares to immediately administer:
1 Morphine sulfate
2 Propranolol (Inderal)
3 Nifedipine (Procardia)
4 Nitroglycerin (Nitrostat)

Level of Cognitive Ability: Application
Client Needs: Physiological Integrity
Integrated Process: Nursing Process/Implementation
Content Area: Adult Health/Cardiovascular

Answer: 4
Rationale: The relief of pain related to angina usually begins within 1 or 2 minutes after the administration of sublingual nitroglycerin. Morphine sulfate is usually administered if the sublingual route has failed to relieve the pain. Propranolol is used to treat certain cardiac disorders and also may be used to treat hypertension. Nifedipine is often used for the maintenance treatment of angina rather than for acute episodes.

Test-Taking Strategy: Knowledge of the actions to take and the medication that is used to treat an acute episode of angina is necessary to answer this question. Remember that nitroglycerin (Nitrostat) is used to treat anginal pain. Review angina and the use of nitroglycerin if you had difficulty with this question.

Reference

Christensen, B., & Kockrow, E. (2006). *Adult health nursing* (5th ed., p. 346). St. Louis: Mosby.

1024. A nurse is preparing to feed a client who has dysphagia. The nurse plans to do which of the following to assist the client with swallowing?

1 Place the food on the tip of the tongue.
2 Provide foods that have a soft consistency.
3 Place the equivalent of 30 mL of food on the fork.
4 Use water to help the client swallow food that is in the mouth.

Level of Cognitive Ability: Application
Client Needs: Physiological Integrity
Integrated Process: Nursing Process/Planning
Content Area: Adult Health/Neurological

Answer: 2
Rationale: No more than a standard amount of food (approximately 15 mL) should be placed on the feeding utensil. Food should be placed on the posterior part of the tongue to aid with swallowing. Foods with a soft consistency should be provided. Liquids are thickened and are given separately from solid foods to prevent choking.

Test-Taking Strategy: Use the process of elimination. Note the strategic word *dysphagia,* and recall that this term indicates that the client has difficulty swallowing; this will direct you to option 2. Review the care of the client with dysphagia if you had difficulty with this question.

References
deWit, S. (2009). *Medical-surgical nursing: Concepts & practice* (p. 596). St. Louis: Saunders.
Linton, A. (2007). *Introduction to medical-surgical nursing* (4th ed., p. 482). Philadelphia: Saunders.

1025. A client with chronic renal failure did not receive any juice on the breakfast meal tray. The nurse obtains a cup of which of the following juices from the unit kitchen?

1 Grape
2 Prune
3 Orange
4 Grapefruit

Level of Cognitive Ability: Application
Client Needs: Physiological Integrity
Integrated Process: Nursing Process/Implementation
Content Area: Adult Health/Renal

Answer: 1
Rationale: Renal failure is the inability of the kidneys to excrete waste, concentrate urine, and conserve electrolytes properly. Apple and grape juices are low in potassium and are better choices for a client with chronic renal failure. Prune, orange, and grapefruit juices are high in potassium and should be used cautiously or avoided in these clients.

Test-Taking Strategy: Use the process of elimination, and remember that potassium is limited for the client with chronic renal failure. Use basic nutritional principles to recall the potassium content of the various juices listed; this will direct you to option 1. Review dietary measures for the client with renal failure if you had difficulty with this question.

References
Ignatavicius, D., & Workman, M. (2010). *Medical-surgical nursing: Patient-centered collaborative care* (6th ed., p. 1607). St. Louis: Saunders.
Nix, S. (2009). *Williams' basic nutrition and diet therapy* (13th ed., pp. 418-419). St. Louis: Mosby.

1026. A nurse is assisting with preparing a plan of care for a client who is scheduled for an abdominal perineal resection. Which nursing intervention should the nurse suggest be included in the plan?

1 Clamp the Penrose drain.
2 Change the wound dressing.
3 Remove and replace the perineal packing 12 hours after the procedure.
4 Notify the physician if serosanguineous drainage from the wound is present.

Level of Cognitive Ability: Application
Client Needs: Physiological Integrity

Answer: 2
Rationale: Immediately after abdominal perineal resection, profuse serosanguineous drainage from the perineal wound is expected. There is no need to notify the physician at this time. A Penrose drain should not be clamped because this will cause the accumulation of fluid within the tissue. Both Penrose drains and packing are removed gradually over a period of 5 to 7 days. The nurse should not remove the perineal packing.

Test-Taking Strategy: Use the process of elimination. Eliminate options 1 and 3 because these are inappropriate interventions. From the remaining options, recall the normal expectations after this type of surgery to direct you to option 2. Review postoperative expectations after abdominal perineal resection if you had difficulty with this question.

Integrated Process: Nursing Process/Planning
Content Area: Fundamental Skills

Reference
deWit, S. (2009). *Medical-surgical nursing: Concepts & practice* (pp. 725-726). St. Louis: Saunders.

1027. A nurse is assisting with planning care for a client with aldosteronism. The nurse plans to monitor for which of the following in the client?

1 Hypoglycemia
2 Fluid overload
3 Urinary retention
4 Gastrointestinal bleeding

Level of Cognitive Ability: Application
Client Needs: Physiological Integrity
Integrated Process: Nursing Process/Planning
Content Area: Adult Health/Endocrine

Answer: 2
Rationale: Aldosteronism is characterized by the hypersecretion of aldosterone. Aldosterone plays a major role in fluid and electrolyte balance. The hypersecretion of aldosterone leads to sodium and water retention, which can lead to fluid overload. The other options are not part of the clinical picture that occurs with this health problem.

Test-Taking Strategy: Use the process of elimination, and recall the pathophysiology of aldosteronism and its effects on the status of the client. Remember that the hypersecretion of aldosterone leads to sodium and water retention to direct you to option 2. Review aldosteronism if you had difficulty with this question.

Reference
Black, J, & Hawks, J. (2009). *Medical-surgical nursing: Clinical management for positive outcomes* (8th ed., pp. 1050-1051). St. Louis: Saunders.

1028. A client is experiencing a sleep pattern disturbance. The nurse plans to do which of the following to best help the client obtain sufficient rest?

1 Use maximum doses of sedative medication at bedtime.
2 Institute a rigid time frame for the delivery of nursing care.
3 Allow for at least 60 minutes of uninterrupted sleep at a time.
4 Adjust the number of pillows, the lights, and the noise level to the client's preference.

Level of Cognitive Ability: Application
Client Needs: Physiological Integrity
Integrated Process: Nursing Process/Planning
Content Area: Fundamental Skills

Answer: 4
Rationale: An environment that is conducive to sleep is one that simulates the client's natural environment, including the number of pillows; the type of bedcovers; and the light, temperature, and noise levels. The nurse should be flexible with care delivery times to allow the client rest periods as needed. Sedative medications are used as necessary and ideally are limited to three times per week. The client needs at least 90 minutes without interruption to complete one sleep cycle.

Test-Taking Strategy: Use the process of elimination, and note the strategic words *best* and *sufficient rest.* Eliminate options 1 and 2 first because they contain the words *maximum* and *rigid,* respectively. Remember that a full sleep cycle is 90 minutes long to help you choose option 4 over option 3. Review measures to promote sleep if you had difficulty with this question.

Reference
Christensen, B., & Kockrow, E. (2006). *Foundations of nursing* (5th ed., pp. 417-418). St. Louis: Mosby.

1029. A nurse is asked to reinforce teaching with a client with chronic renal failure who has been started on hemodialysis. The nurse includes which of the following pieces of information in discussions with the client?

1 It is all right to eat unlimited protein on the day before hemodialysis.

Answer: 2
Rationale: Many medications are dialyzable, which means that they are removed from the bloodstream during dialysis. Because of this, many medications are withheld on the day of dialysis until after the procedure. It is not typical for double doses of medication to be given because there is no way to be certain how much of each medication is cleared by dialysis. Clients who are receiving hemodialysis are not told that it is acceptable to disregard dietary and fluid restrictions.

2 Most daily medications should be taken after hemodialysis rather than before.
3 Double doses of most daily medications should be given on the day of hemodialysis.
4 It is unnecessary to stay within fluid restriction limits on the day before hemodialysis.

Level of Cognitive Ability: Application
Client Needs: Physiological Integrity
Integrated Process: Nursing Process/Implementation
Content Area: Adult Health/Renal

Test-Taking Strategy: Use the process of elimination. Eliminate options 1 and 4 first because they are comparable or alike. From the remaining options, use general principles related to medication administration to direct you to option 2. Remember that medications should not be double-dosed. Review preprocedural measures for dialysis if you had difficulty with this question.

References

Christensen, B., & Kockrow, E. (2006). *Adult health nursing* (5th ed., p. 506). St. Louis: Mosby.
Linton, A. (2007). *Introduction to medical-surgical nursing* (4th ed., p. 874). Philadelphia: Saunders.

1030. A client with acquired immunodeficiency syndrome (AIDS) is experiencing shortness of breath because of *Pneumocystis jiroveci* pneumonia. The nurse plans to do which of the following to assist the client with performing activities of daily living?
1 Provide supportive care.
2 Provide small, frequent meals.
3 Offer food with a low microbial content.
4 Provide meals and snacks with high protein, calorie, and nutritional values.

Level of Cognitive Ability: Application
Client Needs: Physiological Integrity
Integrated Process: Nursing Process/Planning
Content Area: Adult Health/Respiratory

Answer: 1
Rationale: Providing supportive care as needed reduces the client's physical and emotional energy demands and conserves energy resources for other functions (e.g., breathing). Options 2, 3, and 4 are important interventions for the client with AIDS, but they do not address the subject of the question. Option 2 assists the client with better tolerating meals. Option 3 decreases the client's risk for infection. Option 4 assists the client with maintaining an appropriate weight and proper nutrition.

Test-Taking Strategy: Use the process of elimination, and focus on the subject—shortness of breath. Note that options 2, 3, and 4 are comparable or alike in that they are all dietary interventions; option 1 is the one that is different. Review the care of the client with AIDS if you had difficulty with this question.

Reference

Christensen, B., & Kockrow, E. (2006). *Adult health nursing* (5th ed., pp. 802, 806). St. Louis: Mosby.

1031. A client is admitted to the nursing unit after a fall from a roof. The client has multiple lacerations and a right leg fracture that has been treated with a plaster cast. The nurse positions the right leg in which manner to promote optimal circulation?
1 In a flat or level position
2 Flat for 3 hours and then elevated for 1 hour
3 Elevated for 3 hours and then flat for 1 hour
4 Elevated on pillows continuously for 24 to 48 hours

Level of Cognitive Ability: Application
Client Needs: Physiological Integrity

Answer: 4
Rationale: A casted extremity is elevated continuously for the first 24 to 48 hours to minimize swelling and to promote venous drainage. The other options are not part of the standard positioning of the newly casted extremity.

Test-Taking Strategy: Use the process of elimination. Remember that edema sets in after a fracture and that it can be increased by casting. Use the concepts related to gravity to assist you with eliminating options 1, 2, and 3. Review appropriate positioning after the casting of an extremity if you had difficulty with this question.

Reference

Christensen, B., & Kockrow, E. (2006). *Adult health nursing* (5th ed., p. 172). St. Louis: Mosby.

Integrated Process: Nursing Process/Implementation
Content Area: Adult Health/Musculoskeletal

1032. A client has had a repair of an abdominal aortic aneurysm (AAA). The nurse assigned to assist with caring for the client places the highest priority on which of the following nursing activities immediately after surgery?
1 Checking peripheral pulses
2 Pulmonary hygiene measures
3 Application of pneumatic boots
4 Administration of oral opioid analgesics

Level of Cognitive Ability: Application
Client Needs: Physiological Integrity
Integrated Process: Nursing Process/Implementation
Content Area: Adult Health/Cardiovascular

Answer: 1
Rationale: Checking the peripheral pulses is the highest priority immediately after the repair of an AAA; this indicates whether the graft is patent and perfusing the lower extremities. The client would receive parenteral opioids immediately after surgery. The prevention of respiratory and circulatory complications (options 2 and 3) is also important, but it does not supersede the determination of graft patency.

Test-Taking Strategy: Note the strategic words *highest priority*. Recall that this surgical procedure is vascular in nature, and look for the option that most directly addresses the prevention or treatment of a vascular complication. Use the ABCs—airway, breathing, and circulation—to direct you to option 1. Review the care of the client after the repair of an AAA if you had difficulty with this question.

Reference
Linton, A. (2007). *Introduction to medical-surgical nursing* (4th ed., pp. 691, 705). Philadelphia: Saunders.

1033. A client who is scheduled for annuloplasty asks the nurse to explain again what the surgical procedure entails. When planning a response, the nurse should incorporate which of the following points?
1 The valve is replaced with a biologic valve.
2 The valve is replaced with a mechanical valve.
3 The valve leaflets are repaired, with possible implantation of a prosthetic ring.
4 The stenotic valve leaflets are separated, and any calcium deposits are removed.

Level of Cognitive Ability: Comprehension
Client Needs: Physiological Integrity
Integrated Process: Nursing Process/Planning
Content Area: Adult Health/Cardiovascular

Answer: 3
Rationale: Annuloplasty is used for mitral or tricuspid regurgitation and the involves reconstruction of the annulus and the valve leaflets. Annulus repair may or may not involve the insertion of a prosthetic ring. Option 4 describes commissurotomy, and options 1 and 2 are types of valve replacement.

Test-Taking Strategy: It is necessary to be familiar with the different types of cardiac valvular surgery to answer this question correctly. Remember that during an annuloplasty the valve leaflets are repaired, with possible implantation of a prosthetic ring. Review the various types of valvular repair procedures if you had difficulty with this question.

References
Lewis, S., Heitkemper, M., Dirksen, S., & Bucher, L. (2007). *Medical-surgical nursing: Assessment and management of clinical problems* (7th ed., p. 882). St. Louis: Mosby.
Monahan, F., Sands, J., Marek, J., Neighbors, M., & Green, C. (2007). *Phipps' medical-surgical nursing: Health and illness perspectives* (8th ed., pp. 842-843). St. Louis: Mosby.

1034. A nurse has been assigned to care for a client who is in the diuretic phase of renal failure. The nurse reviews the plan of care and monitors for signs of which of the following?
1 Hyponatremia and hypokalemia
2 Hypocalcemia and hyperkalemia

Answer: 1
Rationale: During the diuretic phase of acute renal failure, the client loses large amounts of fluid. This is accompanied by losses of sodium and potassium because of the kidneys' inability to properly concentrate urine. The nurse monitors the client for these electrolyte imbalances and for signs of dehydration.

3 Hypernatremia and hypokalemia
4 Hypermagnesemia and hyperkalemia

Level of Cognitive Ability: Application
Client Needs: Physiological Integrity
Integrated Process: Nursing Process/Data Collection
Content Area: Adult Health/Renal

Test-Taking Strategy: Use the process of elimination, and note the strategic words *diuretic phase.* During the diuretic phase, you would expect losses of both fluids and electrolytes. The only option that addresses conditions that begin with *hypo-* in the entire option is option 1. Review the clinical manifestations that occur during the diuretic phase of renal failure if you had difficulty with this question.

References

Ignatavicius, D., & Workman, M. (2010). *Medical-surgical nursing: Patient-centered collaborative care* (6th ed., p. 1602) St. Louis: Saunders.
Linton, A. (2007). *Introduction to medical-surgical nursing* (4th ed., p. 868). Philadelphia: Saunders.

1035. A client with chronic renal failure has a protein restriction in the diet. The nurse avoids giving the client which of the following sources of incomplete protein in the diet?
1 Nuts
2 Eggs
3 Milk
4 Fish

Level of Cognitive Ability: Application
Client Needs: Physiological Integrity
Integrated Process: Nursing Process/Implementation
Content Area: Adult Health/Renal

Answer: 1
Rationale: The client whose diet has a protein restriction should be careful to ensure that the proteins that are eaten are complete and that they have the highest biologic value. Foods such as meat, fish, milk, and eggs are complete proteins, which are optimal for the client with chronic renal failure. Nuts are an incomplete protein.

Test-Taking Strategy: Use the process of elimination. Note the strategic word *avoids,* and focus on the subject—an incomplete protein. Use your knowledge of basic nutritional principles and of foods that are complete and incomplete proteins to answer this question. Review these nutritional concepts if you had difficulty with this question.

References

Grodner, M., Long, S., & Walkingshaw, B. (2007). *Foundations and clinical applications of nutrition* (4th ed., p. 117). St. Louis: Mosby.
Ignatavicius, D., & Workman, M. (2010). *Medical-surgical nursing: Patient-centered collaborative care* (6th ed., pp. 1615-1616). St. Louis: Saunders.
Schlenker, E., & Long, S. (2007). *Williams' essentials of nutrition & diet therapy* (9th ed., p. 73). St. Louis: Mosby.

1036. A nurse looks at the clock and notes that a client is due in hydrotherapy for a burn dressing change in 30 minutes. The nurse plans to do which of the following next for the care of this client?
1 Get out a robe and slippers.
2 Immediately place the client on NPO status.
3 Administer an opioid analgesic that was last given 6 hours ago.
4 Gather dressing supplies to send with the client to hydrotherapy.

Level of Cognitive Ability: Application
Client Needs: Physiological Integrity
Integrated Process: Nursing Process/Planning
Content Area: Adult Health/Integumentary

Answer: 3
Rationale: The client should receive pain medication approximately 20 minutes before a burn dressing change; this helps the client to tolerate an otherwise painful procedure. The client does not need to be NPO for this procedure. Dressing supplies are not sent with the client because they are normally available in the hydrotherapy area. A robe and slippers are given to the client for transport but are not indicated 30 minutes ahead of time.

Test-Taking Strategy: Note the strategic word *next.* Use Maslow's Hierarchy of Needs theory and the ability to sequence nursing activities in terms of time to answer this question. Think about the procedure to be done and note the client's diagnosis to direct you to option 3. Review the care of the client who is scheduled for hydrotherapy if you had difficulty with this question.

Reference
Ignatavicius, D., & Workman, M. (2010). *Medical-surgical nursing: Patient-centered collaborative care* (6th ed., p. 539). St. Louis: Saunders.

1037. A client is complaining of skin irritation from the edges of a cast that was applied the previous day. The skin edges are pink and irritated. The nurse plans to do which of the following as a corrective action?

1 Petal the edges of the cast with tape.
2 Massage the skin at the rim of the cast.
3 Shake a small amount of powder under the cast rim.
4 Use a hair dryer set on a cool, high setting to soothe the irritation.

Level of Cognitive Ability: Application
Client Needs: Physiological Integrity
Integrated Process: Nursing Process/Planning
Content Area: Adult Health/Musculoskeletal

Answer: 1
Rationale: The nurse should petal the edges of the cast with tape to minimize skin irritation. A hair dryer is used on a cool, low setting if a nonplaster cast becomes wet or if the client's skin itches under the cast. Massaging the skin does not alleviate the problem. Powder should not be shaken under the cast because it could clump, become moist, and cause skin breakdown.

Test-Taking Strategy: Begin to answer this question by determining the cause of the client's skin irritation. Because the question tells you that the cast edges are the cause, you can then systematically eliminate each of the incorrect options. Note the relationship between the words *skin edges are pink and irritated* in the question and the words in option 1. Review the principles of cast care if you had difficulty with this question.

Reference
deWit, S. (2009). *Medical-surgical nursing: Concepts & practice* (p.793). St. Louis: Saunders.

1038. A client with Guillain-Barré syndrome is being admitted to the hospital. The client's chief complaint is an ascending paralysis that has reached the level of the waist. The nurse plans to have which of the following items available for emergency use?

1 Nebulizer and pulse oximeter
2 Blood pressure cuff and flashlight
3 Flashlight and incentive spirometer
4 Cardiac monitor and intubation tray

Level of Cognitive Ability: Comprehension
Client Needs: Physiological Integrity
Integrated Process: Nursing Process/Planning
Content Area: Adult Health/Neurological

Answer: 4
Rationale: Guillain-Barré syndrome is a peripheral polyneuritis that occurs 1 to 3 weeks after an episode of fever that is associated with a viral infection or an immunization. The client with Guillain-Barré syndrome is at risk for respiratory failure because of ascending paralysis. An intubation tray should be available for use. Another complication of this syndrome is cardiac dysrhythmia, which necessitates the use of cardiac monitoring. Although some of the items in options 1, 2, and 3 may be used during the routine care of the client, they are not needed for emergency use.

Test-Taking Strategy: Use the process of elimination, and note the strategic words *emergency use*. These words tell you that the correct answer is an option that contains equipment that is not routinely used for the provision of care. With this in mind, eliminate options 2 and 3 first. From the remaining options, recall the complications of this syndrome to direct you to option 4. Review nursing care measures for the client with Guillain-Barré syndrome if you had difficulty with this question.

Reference
Christensen, B., & Kockrow, E. (2006). *Adult health nursing* (5th ed., p. 737). St. Louis: Mosby.

1039. A nurse responds to a call bell and finds a client lying on the floor after a fall. The nurse suspects that the client's arm may be broken. Which action is the highest priority of the nurse before moving the client?

Answer: 1
Rationale: When a fracture is suspected, it is imperative that the area be splinted and immobilized before the client is moved. Emergency help should be called for if the client is external to a hospital, and a physician should be called if the client is

1 Immobilizing the arm
2 Taking the client's vital signs
3 Calling the radiology department
4 Telling the client that there will be no permanent damage

Level of Cognitive Ability: Application
Client Needs: Physiological Integrity
Integrated Process: Nursing Process/Implementation
Content Area: Adult Health/Musculoskeletal

hospitalized. The nurse should remain with the client and provide realistic reassurance. The client should not be told that there will be no permanent damage.

Test-Taking Strategy: Use the process of elimination, and note the strategic words *highest priority*. Eliminate option 3 because the physician will order radiology films. Option 4 is eliminated next because the nurse does not make a statement that provides false reassurance. When considering the remaining options, focus on the situation in the question. Immobilizing the limb is imperative for the client's safety, which makes it a better choice than taking the client's vital signs. Review the care of the client with a suspected extremity fracture if you had difficulty with this question.

Reference
Christensen, B., & Kockrow, E. (2006). *Foundations of nursing* (5th ed., p. 764). St. Louis: Mosby.

1040. A nurse is preparing a client for surgery. Which of the following is a component of the plan of care?
1 Be sure that the prescribed preoperative studies are performed.
2 Instruct the client to avoid oral hygiene on the morning of surgery.
3 Verify that the client has remained NPO for 24 hours before surgery.
4 Report any increases in blood pressure on the day of surgery to the physician.

Level of Cognitive Ability: Application
Client Needs: Physiological Integrity
Integrated Process: Nursing Process/Planning
Content Area: Fundamental Skills

Answer: 1
Rationale: The nurse should be sure that any preoperative studies that were prescribed were performed. If any abnormal findings are noted, the nurse should alert the registered nurse, who in turn should notify the physician. Oral hygiene is allowed preoperatively, but the client should not swallow any water. The client usually has a restriction of food and fluids for 8 hours (not 24 hours) before surgery. Some increase in both blood pressure and pulse is common because of client anxiety about the surgery.

Test-Taking Strategy: Read the options carefully, and use the process of elimination. Recall that surgery can produce anxiety in the client to assist you with eliminating option 4. Option 2 can be eliminated next because there is no reason to avoid oral hygiene as long as the client does not swallow any water. Careful reading of option 3 assists you with eliminating this option and directs you to option 1. Review general preoperative care if you had difficulty with this question.

Reference
deWit, S. (2009). *Medical-surgical nursing: Concepts & practice* (pp. 69-72). St. Louis: Saunders.

1041. A nurse has been told to institute aneurysm precautions for a client with a cerebral aneurysm. Which item does the nurse plan for this client?
1 Allow ambulation in the room only.
2 Allow the client to read and watch television.
3 Encourage the client to take his or her own daily bath.
4 Instruct the client to not strain with bowel movements.

Answer: 4
Rationale: Aneurysm precautions include placing the client on bedrest in a quiet setting. The lights are kept dim to minimize environmental stimulation. Any activity that increases the blood pressure (BP) or that impedes venous return from the brain is prohibited (e.g., pushing, pulling, sneezing, coughing, straining). The nurse provides all physical care to minimize increases in BP. For the same reason, visitors, radio, television, and reading materials are prohibited or limited. Stimulants such as caffeine and nicotine are prohibited; decaffeinated coffee or tea may be used.

Level of Cognitive Ability: Application
Client Needs: Physiological Integrity
Integrated Process: Nursing Process/Planning
Content Area: Adult Health/Neurological

Test-Taking Strategy: To answer this question, you must understand that universal principles of aneurysm precautions include limiting the amount of stimulation (in any form) that the client receives and preventing increased intracranial pressure (ICP). With this in mind, eliminate options 1 and 3 first. From the remaining options, recall that straining can increase ICP, so it is appropriate to tell the client not to do so. Review the components of aneurysm precautions if you had difficulty with this question.

Reference
Monahan, F., Sands, J., Marek, J., Neighbors, M., & Green, C. (2007). *Phipps' medical-surgical nursing: Health and illness perspectives* (8th ed., p. 1441). St. Louis: Mosby.

1042. A client with a spinal cord injury is wheelchair bound. The nurse plans to obtain which most effective pressure relief device to place in the seat of the client's wheelchair?
1 Air ring
2 Gel pad
3 Soft pillow
4 Egg crate pad

Level of Cognitive Ability: Application
Client Needs: Physiological Integrity
Integrated Process: Nursing Process/Planning
Content Area: Fundamental Skills

Answer: 2
Rationale: The client who is wheelchair bound is at risk for skin breakdown under bony prominences and benefits greatly from special pressure-relief devices, such as gel pads. The other items listed in the options are useful for some clients in selected situations, but they do not disperse pressure the way that this special device does.

Test-Taking Strategy: Use the process of elimination, and note the strategic words *most effective.* Visualize each of these items and think about how they will relieve pressure to direct you to the correct option. Review the effects and use of pressure-relief devices if you had difficulty with this question.

References
deWit, S. (2009). *Medical-surgical nursing: Concepts & practice* (p. 555). St. Louis: Saunders.
Linton, A. (2007). *Introduction to medical-surgical nursing* (4th ed., p. 497). Philadelphia: Saunders.

1043. A client is admitted to the hospital with unstable angina. For this client, it is imperative that:
1 Large meals are served three times a day.
2 Visitors are permitted liberal visiting hours.
3 The client performs all activities of daily living.
4 Plenty of time is allotted for rest and relaxation.

Level of Cognitive Ability: Application
Client Needs: Physiological Integrity
Integrated Process: Nursing Process/Planning
Content Area: Adult Health/Cardiovascular

Answer: 4
Rationale: The client with unstable angina requires plenty of rest and relaxation to prevent decreased blood supply to the myocardium as a result of increased demands. Large meals are contraindicated because of the increased metabolic requirement for digestion and consumption. Visitors are limited to ensure proper rest. The client needs assistance with activities of daily living because rest is important.

Test-Taking Strategy: Focus on the client's diagnosis, and use the process of elimination. Remember that clients with angina require rest to direct you to option 4. Review the care of the client with angina if you had difficulty with this question.

Reference
Christensen, B., & Kockrow, E. (2006). *Adult health nursing* (5th ed., p. 349). St. Louis: Mosby.

1044. When the nurse is changing the back dressing of a client who has had a lumbar laminectomy, bulging at the incision site is observed. The nurse should take which action?

1 Notify the registered nurse (RN).
2 Apply a clean transparent dressing.
3 Try to express fluid from the incision site.
4 Place a soft, multilayer, absorbent dressing on the site.

Level of Cognitive Ability: Application
Client Needs: Physiological Integrity
Integrated Process: Nursing Process/ Implementation
Content Area: Adult Health/Neurological

Answer: 1

Rationale: After laminectomy or diskectomy, bulging at the incision site could indicate the formation of a hematoma or a cerebrospinal fluid leak. This must be reported to the RN, who then contacts the surgeon. The nurse should not try to express the fluid because this could disrupt the incision and possibly introduce pathogens. A dressing should be replaced as part of routine nursing practice, but the most important action is the notification of the RN regarding this complication.

Test-Taking Strategy: Use the process of elimination. Recall that bulging at the incisional site indicates a complication of surgery to direct you to option 1. Review the complications associated with laminectomy if you had difficulty with this question.

Reference

Christensen, B., & Kockrow, E. (2006). *Adult health nursing* (5th ed., p. 184). St. Louis: Mosby.

1045. A client being seen in the physician's office for follow-up 2 weeks after pneumonectomy complains of numbness and tenderness at the surgical site. The nurse tells the client that this is:

1 Not likely to be permanent but that it may last for some months
2 A severe problem and that the client probably will be rehospitalized
3 Probably caused by permanent nerve damage as a result of the surgery
4 Often the first sign of wound infection and that the client's temperature will need to be checked

Level of Cognitive Ability: Application
Client Needs: Physiological Integrity
Integrated Process: Nursing Process/ Implementation
Content Area: Adult Health/Respiratory

Answer: 1

Rationale: Pneumonectomy is the surgical excision of a lung. Clients who undergo pneumonectomy may experience numbness, altered sensation, or tenderness in the area that surrounds the incision. These sensations may last for months. They are not considered to be a severe problem, and they are not indicative of wound infection.

Test-Taking Strategy: Use the process of elimination. Eliminate option 2 because of the word *severe.* Eliminate option 3 because of the word *permanent.* Eliminate option 4 because numbness and tenderness are not signs of infection. Review the effects of pneumonectomy if you had difficulty with this question.

Reference

Ignatavicius, D., & Workman, M. (2010). *Medical-surgical nursing: Patient-centered collaborative care* (6th ed., pp. 649-650). St. Louis: Saunders.

1046. A nurse inspects a client's right lower extremity and finds an open area that measures 3 cm × 4 cm in size. The area has a deep reddish base, and it is surrounded by skin that is edematous, with a brownish color to it. Pedal pulses are palpable in the right leg. The nurse interprets that the ulcerated area is a result of which of the following predisposing conditions?

1 Atrial fibrillation
2 Venous insufficiency
3 Pulmonary embolism
4 Arterial insufficiency

Answer: 2

Rationale: The wound described in the question has the characteristics of a venous stasis ulcer. These ulcers are caused by conditions that result in chronic venous congestion in the extremities. Examples of such conditions include venous insufficiency (varicose veins) and chronic deep vein thrombosis. Pulmonary embolism is a complication of deep vein thrombosis. Arterial insufficiency is accompanied by pain, and typical findings include pale, cool extremities that have diminished or absent pedal pulses. Atrial fibrillation may cause cardiac thrombi, which could break loose and travel to any area of the body, including the legs. This also would cause an acute onset of the classic symptoms found in clients with arterial insufficiency.

Level of Cognitive Ability: Analysis
Client Needs: Physiological Integrity
Integrated Process: Nursing Process/Data Collection
Content Area: Adult Health/Cardiovascular

Test-Taking Strategy: Focus on the subject—the findings that characterize arterial versus venous disease. Eliminate options 1 and 3 first because they are not directly related to wound development. From the remaining options, focus on the differences between arterial and venous disorders to direct you to option 2. Review these differences if you had difficulty with this question.

Reference

Linton, A. (2007). *Introduction to medical-surgical nursing* (4th ed., p. 710). Philadelphia: Saunders.

1047. A nurse is assisting with delivering nursing care to an adult male client who has received tissue plasminogen activator (Activase). The nurse allows which of the following items to be used by this client at the bedside?

1. Dental floss
2. Electric razor
3. Firm-bristle toothbrush
4. Small nail trimming scissors

Level of Cognitive Ability: Application
Client Needs: Physiological Integrity
Integrated Process: Nursing Process/Implementation
Content Area: Pharmacology

Answer: 2

Rationale: Tissue plasminogen activator is a thrombolytic medication that is used to dissolve thrombi or emboli caused by thrombus. A frequent and potentially severe side effect of therapy is bleeding. The nurse manipulates the client's environment to reduce the hazard of bleeding associated with the use of sharp items at the bedside. The nurse provides a soft toothbrush for mouth care and allows an electric razor for shaving. The nurse does not allow dental floss, a firm-bristle toothbrush, or scissors at the bedside; these items could cause trauma that results in bleeding.

Test-Taking Strategy: Focus on the name of the medication. Recall that bleeding is a side effect of this therapy and remember which common items used in personal care could cause bleeding to direct you to option 2. Review the characteristics of tissue plasminogen activator if you had difficulty with this question.

Reference

Hodgson, B., & Kizior, R. (2009). *Saunders nursing drug handbook 2009* (p. 45). St. Louis: Saunders.

1048. A nurse is planning to teach a client with angina pectoris about the appropriate use of nitroglycerin sublingual tablets. Which item should the nurse include in the plan?

1. Keep the tablets in a shirt pocket.
2. Stop taking the medication if a headache occurs.
3. Replace the medication 6 months after opening the bottle.
4. Take up to five doses 5 minutes apart if chest pain occurs.

Level of Cognitive Ability: Application
Client Needs: Physiological Integrity
Integrated Process: Teaching and Learning
Content Area: Pharmacology

Answer: 3

Rationale: Nitroglycerin is a coronary vasodilator. It is relatively unstable, and the medication should be replaced 6 months after the bottle is opened. The tablets should be kept away from heat, light, and moisture. The client may take up to three doses 5 minutes apart. If chest pain is not relieved at that time, the client should seek emergency care. Headache is an expected side effect of the medication and usually diminishes as the client becomes accustomed to the medication.

Test-Taking Strategy: Focus on the medication, and recall that medication names that contain the letters *nitro* in their names are vasodilators. Recall the proper use and storage of nitroglycerin sublingual tablets to direct you to the correct option. Remember that nitroglycerin is relatively unstable and that the medication should be replaced 6 months after the bottle is opened. Review nitroglycerin guidelines if you had difficulty with this question.

Reference

Ignatavicius, D., & Workman, M. (2010). *Medical-surgical nursing: Patient-centered collaborative care* (6th ed., p. 857). St. Louis: Saunders.

1049. A client is taking labetalol hydrochloride (Normodyne) to treat hypertension. The nurse informs the client that which side effect can occur with the use of this medication?

1 Impotence
2 Tachycardia
3 Night blindness
4 Increased energy level

Level of Cognitive Ability: Application
Client Needs: Physiological Integrity
Integrated Process: Nursing Process/Implementation
Content Area: Pharmacology

Answer: 1
Rationale: Labetalol hydrochloride (Normodyne) is a β-adrenergic blocking agent that is used to treat hypertension. Impotence is a common side effect of labetalol and may be distressing to the client. Other side effects of this medication are bradycardia, weakness, and fatigue. Night blindness is unrelated to this medication, although this medication can cause blurred vision and dry eyes.

Test-Taking Strategy: Use the process of elimination. Recall that medication names that end with *-lol* are β-adrenergic blocking agents. Recall the side effects associated with this classification of medications and that impotence is a side effect that may be distressing to the client to direct you to option 1. Review the side effects of labetalol hydrochloride if you had difficulty with this question.

Reference
Hodgson, B., & Kizior, R. (2009). *Saunders nursing drug handbook 2009* (p. 652). St. Louis: Saunders.

1050. A client has a new prescription for nifedipine (Procardia). The nurse reinforces medication instructions and teaches the client which of the following?

1 Monitor the pulse daily.
2 Limit alcohol to 2 oz per day.
3 Expect urinary retention as a side effect.
4 Cut the dose in half if dizziness or syncope occurs.

Level of Cognitive Ability: Application
Client Needs: Physiological Integrity
Integrated Process: Teaching and Learning
Content Area: Pharmacology

Answer: 1
Rationale: Nifedipine (Procardia) is a calcium-channel blocking agent that can cause bradycardia as a side effect. For this reason, clients taking this medication are taught to monitor the pulse on a daily basis. Urinary frequency is a side effect, but urinary retention is not. Alcohol should not be used at all by a client taking a medication such as nifedipine because it could cause or worsen hypotension. Clients are not instructed to change medication doses on the basis of symptoms.

Test-Taking Strategy: Use the process of elimination. Recall that many of the calcium-channel blocking agents have names that end with the suffix *-dipine*. This may be helpful when trying to remember the classification of this medication. Use general medication guidelines to eliminate option 2. From this point, note the relationship between this cardiac medication and option 1 to direct you to this option. Review nifedipine if you had difficulty with this question.

Reference
Hodgson, B., & Kizior, R. (2009). *Saunders nursing drug handbook 2009* (p. 832). St. Louis: Saunders.

1051. A nurse is told that a client with a history of heart failure who is undergoing peritoneal dialysis has developed crackles in the lower lung fields. The nurse interprets that this finding is most likely related to which of the following?

1 Natural progression of the renal failure
2 Compliance with dietary sodium restriction

Answer: 3
Rationale: Peritoneal dialysis is a dialysis procedure in which the peritoneum is used as a diffusible membrane. Crackles in the lung fields of the peritoneal dialysis client result from overhydration or insufficient fluid removal during dialysis. An intake that is greater than the output of peritoneal dialysis fluid overhydrates the client, thus resulting in lung crackles; adherence to medication and diet therapy should control this sign (not make it worse). If dialysis is effective, there is no connection between the progression of renal failure and the development of signs of overhydration.

3 Intake greater than output on the dialysis record
4 Adherence to digoxin (Lanoxin) therapy schedule

Level of Cognitive Ability: Analysis
Client Needs: Physiological Integrity
Integrated Process: Nursing Process/Data Collection
Content Area: Adult Health/Renal

Test-Taking Strategy: Use the process of elimination. Begin to answer this question by eliminating options 2 and 4. These options are incorrect because adherence to standard therapy should control the signs of heart failure (not make them worse). From the remaining options, remember that crackles are caused by excess fluid in the body to direct you to option 3. Review the care of the client with peritoneal dialysis if you had difficulty with this question.

References

Ignatavicius, D., & Workman, M. (2010). *Medical-surgical nursing: Patient-centered collaborative care* (6th ed., pp. 1614, 1618). St. Louis: Saunders.
Monahan, F., Sands, J., Marek, J., Neighbors, M., & Green, C. (2007). *Phipps' medical-surgical nursing: Health and illness perspectives* (8th ed., p. 1031). St. Louis: Mosby.

1052. The nurse is collecting data from a client who is taking an oral bronchodilator. The nurse notes that which symptom is a common side effect of this type of medication?
1 Diarrhea
2 Bradycardia
3 Nervousness
4 Urinary retention

Level of Cognitive Ability: Application
Client Needs: Physiological Integrity
Integrated Process: Nursing Process/Data Collection
Content Area: Pharmacology

Answer: 3
Rationale: Bronchodilators commonly cause side effects such as nervousness, anxiety, nausea, vomiting, tachycardia, and palpitations. The nurse monitors for these symptoms in clients taking this type of medication. Urinary retention and diarrhea are not side effects of this medication.

Test-Taking Strategy: Focus on the medication classification. Recall the effects of bronchodilators to direct you to option 3. Remember that bronchodilators commonly cause side effects such as nervousness, anxiety, nausea, vomiting, tachycardia, and palpitations. Review the characteristics of bronchodilators if you had difficulty with this question.

References

Ignatavicius, D., & Workman, M. (2010). *Medical-surgical nursing: Patient-centered collaborative care* (6th ed., p. 620). St. Louis: Saunders.
Kee, J., Hayes, E., & McCuistion, L. (2009). *Pharmacology: A nursing process approach* (6th ed, p. 608). St. Louis: Saunders.

1053. A client who is scheduled for pneumonectomy asks the nurse how long the chest tubes will be in place. The nurse responds that:
1 They will be in for 24 to 48 hours.
2 They will be removed after 3 to 4 days.
3 They usually function for a full week after surgery.
4 It is likely that there will be no chest tubes in place after surgery.

Level of Cognitive Ability: Application
Client Needs: Physiological Integrity
Integrated Process: Nursing Process/Implementation
Content Area: Adult Health/Respiratory

Answer: 4
Rationale: Pneumonectomy involves the removal of the entire lung, usually because of extensive disease (e.g., bronchogenic carcinoma, unilateral tuberculosis, lung abscess). Chest tubes are not usually inserted because the cavity is left to fill with serosanguineous fluid, which later solidifies. The phrenic nerve is severed to elevate the diaphragm, thus further decreasing the size of the chest cavity on the operative side. Options 1, 2, and 3 are incorrect.

Test-Taking Strategy: Use the process of elimination. Recall that the entire lung is removed with this procedure. Hence, chest tubes are unnecessary because there is no lung remaining to reinflate to fill the pleural space. Review pneumonectomy if you had difficulty with this question.

Reference

Black, J., & Hawks, J. (2009). *Medical-surgical nursing: Clinical management for positive outcomes* (8th ed., p. 1615). St. Louis: Saunders.

1054. A nurse is assigned to assist with caring for a client with a diagnosis of a dissecting abdominal aortic aneurysm. The nurse avoids doing which of the following while caring for this client?

1 Monitoring the vital signs
2 Performing deep palpation of the abdomen
3 Telling the client to report back, shoulder, or neck pain
4 Turning the client to the side to look for ecchymosis on the lower back

Level of Cognitive Ability: Application
Client Needs: Physiological Integrity
Integrated Process: Nursing Process/Implementation
Content Area: Adult Health/Cardiovascular

Answer: 2

Rationale: An aneurysm is a localized dilation of the wall of a blood vessel. The nurse avoids deep palpation in the client in which a dissecting aneurysm is known or suspected because doing so could place the client at risk for rupture. The nurse looks for ecchymosis on the lower back to determine aneurysm leaking and tells the client to report back, neck, shoulder, or extremity pain. An important nursing action is monitoring for changes in vital signs that may indicate worsening of the condition.

Test-Taking Strategy: Use the process of elimination, and note the strategic word *avoids.* With the diagnosis presented, the only option that could cause harm to the client is the option that addresses deep palpation. Review the care of the client with a dissecting abdominal aortic aneurysm if you had difficulty with this question.

Reference

Ignatavicius, D., & Workman, M. (2010). *Medical-surgical nursing: Patient-centered collaborative care* (6th ed., p. 811). St. Louis: Saunders.

1055. A nurse is assigned to assist with caring for a client who sustained a closed head injury 6 hours previously. After report, the nurse finds that the client has vomited and is confused and that she complains of dizziness and a headache. Which of the following is the first nursing action?

1 Administer an antiemetic.
2 Notify the registered nurse (RN).
3 Reorient the client to her surroundings.
4 Change the client's gown and bed linens.

Level of Cognitive Ability: Application
Client Needs: Physiological Integrity
Integrated Process: Nursing Process/Implementation
Content Area: Adult Health/Neurological

Answer: 2

Rationale: The client with a closed head injury is at risk for developing increased intracranial pressure. This is evidenced by symptoms such as headache, dizziness, confusion, weakness, and vomiting. Because of the implications of the symptoms, the first nursing action is to notify the RN, who then contacts the physician. Other nursing actions that are appropriate include the physical care of the client and reorienting the client to her surroundings.

Test-Taking Strategy: Use the process of elimination, and note the strategic words *first nursing action.* This directs you to prioritize the nursing actions. Considering the closed head injury and the developing signs and symptoms, the nurse should suspect increased intracranial pressure; this should direct you to option 2. Review the care of the client with a closed head injury if you had difficulty with this question.

Reference

Christensen, B., & Kockrow, E. (2006). *Adult health nursing* (5th ed., p. 743). St. Louis: Mosby.

1056. A client is brought into the emergency department after suffering a head injury. The first action by the nurse is to determine the client's:

1 Level of consciousness
2 Pulse and blood pressure
3 Respiratory rate and depth
4 Ability to move extremities

Answer: 3

Rationale: The first action of the nurse is to ensure that the client has an adequate airway and respiratory status. In rapid sequence, the client's circulatory and neurological statuses are evaluated.

Test-Taking Strategy: Use the ABCs—airway, breathing, and circulation. The correct option deals with the client's airway. Respiratory rate and depth support this action. Review the initial care of the client with a head injury if you had difficulty with this question.

Level of Cognitive Ability: Application
Client Needs: Physiological Integrity
Integrated Process: Nursing Process/Implementation
Content Area: Adult Health/Neurological

Reference

Christensen, B., & Kockrow, E. (2006). *Adult health nursing* (5th ed., p. 742). St. Louis: Mosby.

1057. A client has been diagnosed with deep vein thrombosis (DVT) of the left leg. The nurse determines that the client's condition is improving if which of the following outcomes is noted?

1 Edema is resolving.
2 Homans' sign is positive.
3 The skin on the left leg is reddened and warm.
4 The calf circumference is half an inch greater than the baseline measurement.

Answer: 1

Rationale: DVT involves a thrombus in one of the deep veins of the body, most commonly the iliac or femoral vein. Symptoms of DVT include warm, reddened skin over the affected area; edema of the extremity; enlarged calf circumference; and a positive Homans' sign (pain with dorsiflexion of the foot). Indications that the condition is resolving are a reduction in these signs and symptoms.

Test-Taking Strategy: Use the process of elimination, and note the strategic words *condition is improving.* Recall the signs and symptoms of DVT and focus on the strategic words to direct you to option 1. Review DVT if you had difficulty with this question.

Level of Cognitive Ability: Comprehension
Client Needs: Physiological Integrity
Integrated Process: Nursing Process/Evaluation
Content Area: Adult Health/Cardiovascular

Reference

Linton, A. (2007). *Introduction to medical-surgical nursing* (4th ed., p. 709). Philadelphia: Saunders.

1058. A client with a spinal cord injury is at risk for the development of foot drop. The nurse uses which item as the most effective preventive measure?

1 Footboard
2 Heel protectors
3 Posterior splints
4 Pneumatic boots

Answer: 3

Rationale: The most effective means of preventing foot drop are the use of posterior splints or high-top sneakers. A footboard prevents plantar flexion, but it also places the client more at risk for developing pressure ulcers of the feet. Heel protectors protect the skin but do not prevent foot drop. Pneumatic boots prevent deep vein thrombosis but not foot drop.

Test-Taking Strategy: Use the process of elimination, and focus on the subject—the prevention of foot drop. This guides you to select the option that immobilizes the foot in a functional position while protecting the skin of the extremities. Review the purposes of immobilization devices if you had difficulty with this question.

Level of Cognitive Ability: Application
Client Needs: Physiological Integrity
Integrated Process: Nursing Process/Implementation
Content Area: Fundamental Skills

Reference

Black, J., & Hawks, J. (2009). *Medical-surgical nursing: Clinical management for positive outcomes* (8th ed., p. 1962). St. Louis: Saunders.

1059. A client is ambulatory and wearing a halo vest after a cervical spine fracture. The nurse tells the client to avoid which of the following because it will present a risk for injury?

Answer: 2

Rationale: A halo vest is an orthopedic device that is used to help immobilize the neck and head. The client with a halo vest should avoid bending at the waist because the halo vest is heavy, and the client's trunk is limited in flexibility. It is helpful for the client to scan the environment visually because the client's peripheral vision is diminished due to the need to

Level of Cognitive Ability: Application
Client Needs: Physiological Integrity
Integrated Process: Nursing Process/Implementation
Content Area: Pharmacology

Reference
Hodgson, B., & Kizior, R. (2009). *Saunders nursing drug handbook 2009* (p. 46). St. Louis: Saunders.

1064. A client has been placed on medication therapy with amitriptyline. The nurse monitors the client for which common side effect of this medication?
1 Diarrhea
2 Polyuria
3 Hypertension
4 Drowsiness and fatigue

Level of Cognitive Ability: Application
Client Needs: Physiological Integrity
Integrated Process: Nursing Process/Implementation
Content Area: Pharmacology

Answer: 4
Rationale: Amitriptyline is a tricyclic antidepressant. Common side effects of medication therapy with amitriptyline are the central nervous system effects of drowsiness, fatigue, lethargy, and sedation. Other common side effects include dry mouth, dry eyes, blurred vision, hypotension, and constipation.

Test-Taking Strategy: Use the process of elimination. Recall that this medication is an antidepressant to direct you to option 4. Review the side effects of amitriptyline if you had difficulty with this question.

Reference
Hodgson, B., & Kizior, R. (2009). *Saunders nursing drug handbook 2009* (p. 59). St. Louis: Saunders.

1065. A client with a 5-year history of depression has been admitted to the nursing unit on a voluntary basis. When collecting data from the client, which comment by the nurse would best obtain data about the client's recent sleeping patterns?
1 "How did you sleep last night?"
2 "Tell me about your sleeping patterns."
3 "You look as if you could use some sleep."
4 "Have you been having trouble sleeping at home?"

Level of Cognitive Ability: Application
Client Needs: Physiological Integrity
Integrated Process: Nursing Process/Data Collection
Content Area: Mental Health

Answer: 2
Rationale: Option 2 is open-ended and allows the client to say what is most relevant and important at the time. One night of sleep does not tell the nurse how the pattern has been over time. Anyone may or may not sleep well for one night, and that night's sleep or lack of sleep does not indicate a problem. Option 3 could be interpreted by the depressed person as a negative statement and could shut down the further communication that is needed for thorough data collection. Option 4 could lead to a one-word answer, and that is not the desired response for adequate data collection.

Test-Taking Strategy: Use therapeutic communication techniques. Select the option that allows the client to take the lead in the conversation. In addition, note that option 2 is the only open-ended question. Review therapeutic communication techniques if you had difficulty with this question.

Reference
Varcarolis, E., & Halter, M. (2009). *Essenials of psychiatric mental health nursing: A communication approach to evidence-based care* (pp. 95-98, 222). St. Louis: Saunders.

1066. When administering an intramuscular injection in the gluteal muscle, the best position for the client to assume to relax the muscle is:
1 Prone position, with a toe-in position
2 Sims' position, with a toe-in position
3 On the side, with the knee of the upper leg flexed
4 On the side, with the knee of the lower leg flexed

Answer: 1
Rationale: A prone, toe-in position promotes the internal rotation of the hips, which relaxes the muscle and makes the injection less painful. Options 2, 3, and 4 will not relax the muscle.

Test-Taking Strategy: Use the process of elimination, and note the strategic words *best position* and *relax the muscle.* Visualize each position described in the options to direct you to option 1. Review positioning for the administration of intramuscular medications if you had difficulty with this question.

Level of Cognitive Ability: Application
Client Needs: Physiological Integrity
Integrated Process: Nursing Process/Implementation
Content Area: Fundamental Skills

Reference
Christensen, B., & Kockrow, E. (2006). *Foundations of nursing* (5th ed., p. 726). St. Louis: Mosby.

1067. Which nursing intervention is appropriate when caring for a child after a tepid tub bath to treat hyperthermia?
1 Help the child put on a cotton sleep shirt.
2 Leave the child uncovered for 15 minutes.
3 Take the child's axillary temperature in 2 hours.
4 Place the child in bed, and cover the child with a blanket.

Level of Cognitive Ability: Application
Client Needs: Physiological Integrity
Integrated Process: Nursing Process/Implementation
Content Area: Child Health

Answer: 1
Rationale: Cotton is a lightweight material that protects the child from becoming chilled after the bath. Option 2 is incorrect because the child should not be left uncovered. Option 3 is incorrect because the child's temperature should be reassessed half an hour after the bath. Option 4 is incorrect because a blanket is heavy and may increase the child's body temperature and metabolism.

Test-Taking Strategy: Use the process of elimination. Eliminate option 2 because the child should not be left uncovered. Eliminate option 3 because the child's temperature should be reassessed in half an hour. Eliminate option 4 because of the word *blanket.* Review the care of a child with hyperthermia if you had difficulty with this question.

Reference
McKinney, E., James, S., Murray, S., & Ashwill, J. (2009). *Maternal-child nursing* (3rd ed., p. 935). St. Louis: Mosby.

1068. A nurse is caring for an infant with diarrhea. Which clinical manifestation should the nurse recognize as the earliest symptom of dehydration?
1 Cool extremities
2 Gray, mottled skin
3 Capillary refill of 2 seconds
4 Apical pulse rate of 160 beats/min

Level of Cognitive Ability: Comprehension
Client Needs: Physiological Integrity
Integrated Process: Nursing Process/Data Collection
Content Area: Child Health

Answer: 4
Rationale: Dehydration causes interstitial fluid to shift to the vascular compartment in an attempt to maintain fluid volume. Circulatory failure occurs when the body is unable to compensate for fluid that has been lost; the blood pressure decreases, and the pulse increases. This is followed by peripheral symptoms. Options 1, 2, and 3 are incorrect; these findings reflect diminished peripheral circulation.

Test-Taking Strategy: Use the process of elimination, and focus on the strategic word *earliest.* Options 1, 2, and 3 are comparative or alike and relate to diminished perpheral circulation. Review the early signs of dehydration if you had difficulty with this question.

Reference
Price, D., & Gwin, J. (2008). *Pediatric nursing: An introductory text* (10th ed., pp. 32, 90). St. Louis: Saunders.

1069. A nurse administers acetylsalicylic acid (aspirin) as prescribed before a percutaneous transluminal coronary angioplasty (PTCA) for coronary artery disease to:
1 Relieve postprocedural pain
2 Prevent thrombus formation
3 Prevent postprocedural hyperthermia
4 Prevent inflammation of the puncture site

Answer: 2
Rationale: PTCA is used for the treatment of atherosclerotic coronary heart disease and angina pectoris in which some plaques in the arteries of the heart are flattened against the arterial walls, thus resulting in improved circulation. Before PTCA, the client is usually given an anticoagulant (commonly a low dose of aspirin) to reduce the risk of the occlusion of the artery during the procedure. Options 1, 3, and 4 are unrelated to the purpose of administering aspirin to this client.

Level of Cognitive Ability: Application
Client Needs: Physiological Integrity
Integrated Process: Nursing Process/Implementation
Content Area: Adult Health/Cardiovascular

Test-Taking Strategy: Use the process of elimination. Recall the action and properties of aspirin to direct you to option 2. In addition, awareness of the potential complications of PTCA and the nursing measures to use to prevent these complications assists you with answering the question. Review the actions and uses of aspirin and the complications associated with PTCA if you had difficulty with this question.

References

deWit, S. (2009). *Medical-surgical nursing: Concepts & practice* (p. 497). St. Louis: Saunders.
Hodgson, B., & Kizior, R. (2009). *Saunders nursing drug handbook 2009* (p. 94). St. Louis: Saunders.

1070. A nurse plans to administer acetaminophen (Tylenol), as prescribed, before the administration of topical nitrates because:

1 Headache is a common side effect of nitrates.
2 Fever usually accompanies myocardial infarction.
3 Acetaminophen potentiates the therapeutic effects of nitrates.
4 Acetaminophen does not interfere with platelet action the way that aspirin (acetylsalicylic acid) does.

Level of Cognitive Ability: Application
Client Needs: Physiological Integrity
Integrated Process: Nursing Process/Implementation
Content Area: Pharmacology

Answer: 1
Rationale: Nitrates vasodilate. Headache occurs as a side effect of nitrates. Acetaminophen may be given before nitrates to prevent headaches or to minimize the discomfort caused by the headaches. Options 2, 3, and 4 do not identify the purpose for administering acetaminophen.

Test-Taking Strategy: Use the process of elimination. Focus on the subject of the question and recall that headache is a common side effect of nitrates to direct you to option 1. Review the side effects of nitrates and the purpose of administering acetaminophen before these medications if you had difficulty with this question.

Reference

Kee, J., Hayes, E., & McCuistion, L. (2009). *Pharmacology: A nursing process approach* (6th ed., p. 634). St. Louis: Saunders.

1071. A nurse is caring for a male client with urolithiasis. Important care and teaching include which of the following?

1 Weigh the client daily.
2 Restrict physical activities.
3 Strain all urine after each voiding.
4 Turn, cough, and deep breathe every 2 hours

Level of Cognitive Ability: Application
Client Needs: Physiological Integrity
Integrated Process: Nursing Process/Implementation
Content Area: Adult Health/Renal

Answer: 3
Rationale: Urolithiasis is the presence of calculi in the urinary system. The obstruction of the urinary tract is the primary problem associated with urolithiasis. Stones recovered from straining the urine can be analyzed and can provide direction for the prevention of further stone formation. Activities should not be restricted. Options 1 and 4 are not specifically related to the subject of the question.

Test-Taking Strategy: Use the process of elimination, and select the option that is associated most commonly with a client with urolithiasis. In this situation, straining all urine is the most common or typical intervention. Review the care of the client with urolithiasis if you had difficulty with this question.

Reference

Christensen, B., & Kockrow, E. (2006). *Adult health nursing* (5th ed., p. 491). St. Louis: Mosby.

1072. A nurse is assigned to assist with caring for a newly delivered breast-feeding infant. Which intervention performed by the nurse best prevents jaundice in this infant?

1 Placing the infant under phototherapy.
2 Keeping the infant NPO until the second period of reactivity.
3 Requesting that the mother breast-feed the infant every 2 to 3 hours.
4 Encouraging the mother to offer a formula supplement after each breast-feeding session.

Level of Cognitive Ability: Application
Client Needs: Physiological Integrity
Integrated Process: Nursing Process/Implementation
Content Area: Maternity/Postpartum

Answer: 3

Rationale: To help facilitate a decrease in jaundice, the mother should breast-feed the infant frequently during the immediate period after birth, because colostrum is a natural laxative that helps to promote the passage of meconium. Phototherapy requires a physician's order and is not implemented until bilirubin levels are 12 mg/dL or higher in the healthy term infant. Breast-feeding should begin as soon as possible after birth while the infant is in the first period of reactivity. Delaying breast-feeding decreases the production of prolactin, which decreases the mother's milk production. Offering the infant a formula supplement will cause nipple confusion and decrease the amount of milk produced by the mother.

Test-Taking Strategy: Use the process of elimination. Recall the pathophysiology related to jaundice. Remember that to facilitate a decrease in jaundice, the mother should breast-feed the infant frequently during the period immediately after birth. Review these important nursing interventions if you had difficulty with this question.

Reference

McKinney, E., James, S., Murray, S., & Ashwill, J. (2009). *Maternal-child nursing* (3rd ed., pp. 501-502). St. Louis: Mosby.

1073. A nurse is caring for a client who is scheduled for arthroscopy. During the postoperative period, which of the following is the priority nursing action?

1 Monitoring the intake and output
2 Monitoring for numbness or tingling
3 Checking the dressing at the surgical site
4 Checking the complete blood count results

Level of Cognitive Ability: Application
Client Needs: Physiological Integrity
Integrated Process: Nursing Process/Implementation
Content Area: Adult Health/Musculoskeletal

Answer: 2

Rationale: Arthroscopy is the examination of the interior of a joint that is performed by inserting a specially designed endoscope through a small incision. The priority nursing action is monitoring the affected area for numbness or tingling. Options 1, 3, and 4 are components of postoperative care, but, considering the options presented, they are not the priority.

Test-Taking Strategy: Note the strategic word *priority*. Use the ABCs—airway, breathing, and circulation—to answer the question; this will direct you to option 2. Review nursing care after arthroscopy if you had difficulty with this question.

References

Christensen, B., & Kockrow, E. (2006). *Adult health nursing* (5th ed., p. 129). St. Louis: Mosby.
Ignatavicius, D., Workman, M. (2010). *Medical-surgical nursing: Patient-centered collaborative care* (6th ed., pp. 1150-1151). St. Louis: Saunders.

1074. A nurse is caring for a client with active tuberculosis who has started medication therapy that includes rifampin (Rifadin). Which of the following is an expected observation?

1 Bilious urine
2 Yellow sclera
3 Clay-colored stools
4 Orange-colored body secretions

Answer: 4

Rationale: Rifampin (Rifadin) is an antitubercular medication. Secretions are orange in color when the client is taking rifampin. The client should be instructed that the secretions will be orange and that soft contact lenses can be permanently discolored. Options 1, 2, and 3 are not expected observations.

Level of Cognitive Ability: Analysis
Client Needs: Physiological Integrity
Integrated Process: Nursing Process/Data Collection
Content Area: Adult Health/Respiratory

Test-Taking Strategy: Focus on the subject—the expected observations. Options 1, 2, and 3 are not expected observations. In addition, note that these options are comparable or alike in that they are all symptoms of intrahepatic obstruction as seen in clients with viral hepatitis. Review rifampin if you had difficulty with this question.

Reference

Hodgson, B., & Kizior, R. (2009). *Saunders nursing drug handbook 2009* (p. 1017). St. Louis: Saunders.

1075. A nurse sends a sputum specimen from a client with suspected active tuberculosis (TB) to the laboratory for culture. The nurse is told that the results report that *Mycobacterium tuberculosis* has been cultured. The nurse determines that these results are:

1 Positive for active TB
2 Positive for a less virulent strain of TB
3 Inconclusive until a repeat sputum sample is sent
4 Not reliable unless the client has also had a positive Mantoux test

Level of Cognitive Ability: Analysis
Client Needs: Physiological Integrity
Integrated Process: Nursing Process/Data Collection
Content Area: Adult Health/Respiratory

Answer: 1

Rationale: TB is a chronic granulomatous infection caused by an acid-fast bacillus. The culturing of *Mycobacterium tuberculosis* from sputum or other body secretions or tissue is the only method of confirming the diagnosis of TB. Options 2 and 3 are incorrect statements. The Mantoux test is used to support the diagnosis but does not confirm active disease.

Test-Taking Strategy: Recall that *Mycobacterium tuberculosis* is the bacteria that is responsible for TB and that the culturing of the bacteria from sputum confirms the diagnosis to direct you to option 1. Because TB affects the respiratory system, it makes sense that the bacteria will be found in the sputum if the client has active disease. Review the diagnostic tests associated with active TB if you had difficulty with this question.

References

Chernecky, C., & Berger, B. (2008). *Laboratory tests and diagnostic procedures* (5th ed., pp. 955-956). Philadelphia: Saunders.
deWit, S. (2009). *Medical-surgical nursing: Concepts & practice* (p. 325). St. Louis: Saunders.

1076. A nurse is preparing to administer betamethasone (Celestone) by the intramuscular route, as prescribed, to a client who is 30 weeks pregnant and who is in preterm labor. The client asks the nurse why she is receiving steroids, and the nurse responds by telling the client that the betamethasone will:

1 Help stop the labor contractions
2 Help the baby's lungs mature faster
3 Decrease the incidence of fetal infection
4 Prevent the client's membranes from rupturing

Level of Cognitive Ability: Application
Client Needs: Physiological Integrity
Integrated Process: Nursing Process/Implementation
Content Area: Maternity/Intrapartum

Answer: 2

Rationale: Respiratory distress syndrome is the most common cause of morbidity and mortality in preterm infants. Betamethasone, which is a corticosteroid, is given to enhance fetal lung maturity. The medication's optimal benefits begin 24 hours after initial therapy. Options 3 and 4 are incorrect; betamethasone can actually mask signs of infection, and it does not prevent the rupture of the membranes. Although betamethasone may be given during the time that tocolytic agents are administered, it does not inhibit preterm labor.

Test-Taking Strategy: Focus on the name of the medication, and recall that medication names that end with the letters *-sone* are corticosteroids. Note the words *preterm labor* to assist you with recalling that this medication is given to enhance fetal lung maturity. Review the action of betamethasone if you had difficulty with this question.

Reference

Leifer, G. (2008). *Maternity nursing: An introductory text* (10th ed., p. 279). Philadelphia: Saunders.

1077. A nurse is caring for a client with a history of congestive heart failure. The physician has ordered furosemide (Lasix) 40 mg daily to prevent fluid overload. Which laboratory value should be most closely monitored by the nurse?

1 Sodium
2 Glucose
3 Potassium
4 Magnesium

Level of Cognitive Ability: Analysis
Client Needs: Physiological Integrity
Integrated Process: Nursing Process/Data Collection
Content Area: Pharmacology

Answer: 3
Rationale: Furosemide is a potassium-losing diuretic. Insufficient potassium replacement may lead to hypokalemia. Options 1, 2, and 4 are not a concern when administering this medication.

Test-Taking Strategy: Note that the question states that furosemide (Lasix) is ordered to prevent fluid overload. This indicates that this medication is a diuretic. Remember that with a potassium-losing diuretic, the most critical laboratory value to monitor is the potassium level. Review furosemide if you had difficulty with this question.

Reference
Edmunds, M. (2010). *Introduction to clinical pharmacology* (6th ed., p. 37). St. Louis: Mosby.

1078. A nurse is reinforcing teaching to a client who is being discharged and going home with orders for the self-administration of subcutaneous enoxaparin (Lovenox). The nurse plans to tell the client to monitor for which of the following highest priority items?

1 Headaches
2 Constipation
3 Nausea or vomiting
4 Bleeding gums or bruising

Level of Cognitive Ability: Application
Client Needs: Physiological Integrity
Integrated Process: Nursing Process/Planning
Content Area: Pharmacology

Answer: 4
Rationale: Enoxaparin (Lovenox) is an anticoagulant, and a common side effect of anticoagulant therapy is bleeding. Because of this, the nurse instructs the client to monitor for signs that could indicate bleeding, such as bleeding gums, bruising, hematuria, and dark, tarry stools. Options 1, 2, and 3 are not associated with the use of this medication.

Test-Taking Strategy: Use the process of elimination, and note the strategic words *highest priority*. Recall that this medication is an anticoagulant to direct you to option 4. Review enoxaparin if you had difficulty with this question.

Reference
Hodgson, B., & Kizior, R. (2009). *Saunders nursing drug handbook 2009* (p. 914). St. Louis: Saunders.

1079. A client has been given a prescription for sulfasalazine (Azulfidine) for the treatment of ulcerative colitis. When conducting the medication teaching, the nurse asks the client if the client has a history of allergy to:

1 Sulfonamides or salicylates
2 Diuretics or acetaminophen
3 Shellfish or calcium-channel blockers
4 Histamine receptor antagonists or β-blockers

Level of Cognitive Ability: Application
Client Needs: Physiological Integrity
Integrated Process: Nursing Process/Data Collection
Content Area: Pharmacology

Answer: 1
Rationale: Sulfasalazine (Azulfidine) is a sulfonamide and an anti-inflammatory medication. The client who has been prescribed sulfasalazine should be checked for a history of allergy to either sulfonamides or salicylates because of the chemical composition of the medication. The other options are incorrect because they are not a concern when the client is taking this medication.

Test-Taking Strategy: Use the process of elimination. Note the relationship of the words *sulfasalazine* in the question and *sulfonamides* in the correct option. Review the contraindications associated with the use of sulfasalazine if you had difficulty with this question.

Reference
Skidmore-Roth, L. (2008). *2008 Mosby's nursing drug reference* (21st ed., p. 952). St. Louis: Mosby.

1080. A nurse is caring for a client who is experiencing an alteration in the oral mucous membranes. The nurse should avoid using which of the following items when providing mouth care to this client?

1 Lip moistener
2 Soft toothbrush
3 Lemon-glycerin swabs
4 Nonalcoholic mouthwash

Level of Cognitive Ability: Application
Client Needs: Physiological Integrity
Integrated Process: Nursing Process/Implementation
Content Area: Fundamental Skills

Answer: 3

Rationale: The nurse avoids using lemon-glycerin swabs for the client with altered oral mucous membranes because they dry the membranes further and could cause pain. Items that are helpful include a soft toothbrush to prevent trauma; lip moistener to prevent lip cracking; and soothing, cleansing rinses, such as nonalcoholic mouthwash.

Test-Taking Strategy: Use the process of elimination, and note the strategic word *avoid*. This word indicates a negative event query and asks you to select an option that is an incorrect item. Evaluate each of the options in terms of the likelihood of causing trauma to at-risk tissue. Review the principles of mouth care if you had difficulty with this question.

Reference

Potter, P., & Perry, A. (2009) *Fundamentals of nursing* (7th ed., p. 886). St. Louis: Mosby.

1081. A client has asymptomatic hypocalcemia from decreased dietary intake. The nurse who is giving the client an oral calcium supplement should administer this medication with:

1 Water
2 Fruit juice
3 A carbonated beverage
4 Any lactose-free product

Level of Cognitive Ability: Application
Client Needs: Physiological Integrity
Integrated Process: Nursing Process/Implementation
Content Area: Pharmacology

Answer: 1

Rationale: Calcium supplements should be taken with a large glass of water. Administration with or after meals promotes absorption. Options 2, 3, and 4 are incorrect.

Test-Taking Strategy: Use the process of elimination. Recall absorption factors associated with the administration of calcium to direct you to option 1. Remember that it is best to administer calcium supplements with a large glass of water. Review the administration of oral calcium if you had difficulty with this question.

Reference

Hodgson, B., & Kizior, R. (2009). *Saunders nursing drug handbook 2009* (p. 172). St. Louis: Saunders.

1082. A nurse has an order to administer two ophthalmic medications to a client who has undergone eye surgery. The nurse waits how many minutes after administering the first medication before giving the second?

1 1 minute
2 2 minutes
3 5 minutes
4 10 minutes

Level of Cognitive Ability: Application
Client Needs: Physiological Integrity
Integrated Process: Nursing Process/Implementation
Content Area: Adult Health/Eye

Answer: 3

Rationale: The nurse waits for at least 3 to 5 minutes before administering the second of two separate ophthalmic medications. This allows for the adequate ocular absorption of the first medication, and it prevents the second medication from flushing out the first. Options 1, 2, and 4 are incorrect.

Test-Taking Strategy: Specific knowledge of time frames for the administration of ocular medications is needed to answer this question. Remember that the nurse waits for at least 3 to 5 minutes between the administration of two separate ophthalmic medications. Review the principles of ocular medication administration if you had difficulty with this question.

Reference

Linton, A. (2007). *Introduction to medical-surgical nursing* (4th ed., p. 1165). Philadelphia: Saunders.

1083. Serum calcium levels indicate that the client has hypercalcemia. The nurse avoids doing which of the following, which would aggravate the condition?

1 Limit the sodium intake.
2 Limit calcium-containing foods.
3 Encourage increased fluid intake.
4 Withhold calcium carbonate antacids.

Level of Cognitive Ability: Application
Client Needs: Physiological Integrity
Integrated Process: Nursing Process/ Implementation
Content Area: Fundamental Skills

Answer: 1
Rationale: Sodium should not be limited for the client with hypercalcemia, unless sodium is contraindicated (e.g., in the client with heart failure). The retention of sodium promotes a loss of calcium by the kidneys. Fluid intake is increased to help flush calcium from the body, and calcium-containing medications and foods are withheld or limited, respectively.

Test-Taking Strategy: Use the process of elimination, and note the strategic word *avoids*. This word indicates a negative event query and asks you to select an option that is an incorrect action. Focus on the client's diagnosis to assist you with eliminating options 2, 3, and 4. Review the treatment for hypercalcemia if you had difficulty with this question.

References
Christensen, B., & Kockrow, E. (2006). *Foundations of nursing* (5th ed., p. 676). St. Louis: Mosby.
Linton, A. (2007). *Introduction to medical-surgical nursing* (4th ed., p. 393). Philadelphia: Saunders.

1084. A client receiving lithium carbonate (Lithobid) is noted to be drowsy. He has slurred speech, and he is experiencing muscle twitching and impaired coordination. Which action should the nurse take?

1 Hold one dose of lithium.
2 Double the next dose of lithium.
3 Notify the registered nurse (RN).
4 Increase fluids to 2000 mL per day.

Level of Cognitive Ability: Application
Client Needs: Physiological Integrity
Integrated Process: Nursing Process/ Implementation
Content Area: Pharmacology

Answer: 3
Rationale: Lithium carbonate is an antimanic medication. Signs and symptoms of lithium toxicity include vomiting and diarrhea and nervous system changes such as slurred speech, incoordination, drowsiness, muscle weakness, and twitching. The nurse should notify the RN if the client experiences signs of toxicity; the RN will in turn notify the physician before administering any additional doses of the medication. As long as there are no contraindications, the client should routinely take in between 2000 to 3000 mL of fluid per day while taking this medication.

Test-Taking Strategy: Use the process of elimination. Eliminate options 1 and 2 first, recalling that it is not common practice to either hold one dose or double a medication dose without a specific order. From the remaining options, recall the signs of lithium toxicity to direct you to option 3. Review the signs of lithium toxicity if you had difficulty with this question.

Reference
Hodgson, B., & Kizior, R. (2009). *Saunders nursing drug handbook 2009* (p. 693). St. Louis: Saunders.

1085. A client has started medication therapy with metoclopramide (Reglan). The nurse monitors which of the following items to determine the effectiveness of therapy?

1 Urine output
2 Breath sounds
3 Vomiting episodes
4 Complaints of headache

Level of Cognitive Ability: Application
Client Needs: Physiological Integrity

Answer: 3
Rationale: Metoclopramide (Reglan) is an antiemetic. The nurse monitors to see whether the client has experienced a decrease or absence of vomiting to determine the effectiveness of therapy. Options 1, 2, and 4 are not associated with the use of this medication.

Test-Taking Strategy: Focus on the name of the medication. Recall that this medication is an antiemetic to direct you to the correct option. Review metoclopramide if you had difficulty with this question.

Integrated Process: Nursing Process/ Implementation
Content Area: Pharmacology

Reference
Hodgson, B., & Kizior, R. (2009). *Saunders nursing drug handbook 2009* (p. 751). St. Louis: Saunders.

1086. When checking the height of a cane before ambulating a client, the nurse checks to be sure that the top of the cane is parallel to the:
1 Waistline
2 Uppermost level of the thigh
3 Greater trochanter of the femur
4 Midline between the greater trochanter and the waist

Level of Cognitive Ability: Application
Client Needs: Physiological Integrity
Integrated Process: Nursing Process/ Implementation
Content Area: Fundamental Skills

Answer: 3
Rationale: The top of the cane should reach the level of the greater trochanter of the client's femur. Options 1, 2, and 4 are incorrect.

Test-Taking Strategy: Use the process of elimination, and visualize each of the positions described in the options. Eliminate options 1 and 4 because these positions are too high. Conversely, eliminate option 2 because this position is too low. Review safe procedures for ambulation with a cane if you had difficulty with this question.

Reference
Linton, A. (2007). *Introduction to medical-surgical nursing* (4th ed., p. 924). Philadelphia: Saunders.

1087. When ambulating a client, it is best for the nurse to stand:
1 Behind the client
2 In front of the client
3 On the affected side of the client
4 On the unaffected side of the client

Level of Cognitive Ability: Application
Client Needs: Physiological Integrity
Integrated Process: Nursing Process/ Implementation
Content Area: Fundamental Skills

Answer: 3
Rationale: When walking with the client, the nurse should stand on the client's affected side. The nurse should position the free hand at the client's shoulder area so that the client can be pulled toward the nurse in the event that the client falls forward. The client is instructed to look up and outward rather than at his or her feet.

Test-Taking Strategy: Use the process of elimination. Eliminate options 1 and 2 because neither position places the nurse in a strategic position should the client lose balance and begin to fall forward or backward. Recall that support is needed on the affected side to direct you to option 3. Review ambulation procedures if you had difficulty with this question.

Reference
Perry, A., Potter, P. (2010). *Clinical nursing skills and techniques* (7th ed., p. 253). St. Louis: Mosby.

1088. A nurse is preparing to administer an intramuscular injection as prescribed to a 2-year-old child. The nurse selects which best site to administer the medication?
1 Deltoid muscle
2 Dorsal gluteal muscle
3 Ventral gluteal muscle
4 Vastus lateralis muscle

Level of Cognitive Ability: Application
Client Needs: Physiological Integrity
Integrated Process: Nursing Process/ Implementation
Content Area: Child Health

Answer: 4
Rationale: The vastus lateralis muscle is well developed at birth. It is the best choice for all pediatric age groups, but it should always be used for children who are less than 3 years old. This muscle is able to tolerate larger volumes of medication, and it is not located near vital structures such as nerves and blood vessels.

Test-Taking Strategy: The strategic word *best* requires prioritizing. Because options 2 and 3 are comparable or alike anatomical areas, neither are likely to be correct. Remember that the deltoid is a smaller muscle that is near important nerves and that it is generally not a preferred site for an intramuscular injection. Review the procedure for administering intramuscular injections to a 2-year-old child if you had difficulty with this question.

Reference

Price, D., & Gwin, J. (2008). *Pediatric nursing: An introductory text* (10th ed., p. 384). St. Louis: Saunders.

1089. Which statement by an adolescent indicates a need for follow-up data collection and intervention?

1 "I tend to get very moody."
2 "When I get stressed out about school, I just like to be alone."
3 "I don't eat anything with fat in it, and I've lost 8 pounds in 2 weeks!"
4 "I can't seem to wake up in the morning. I would sleep until noon if I could."

Level of Cognitive Ability: Comprehension
Client Needs: Physiological Integrity
Integrated Process: Nursing Process/Data Collection
Content Area: Child Health

Answer: 3

Rationale: Undereating is a common problem in teenagers who have a heightened awareness of body image and who receive peer pressure to try excessively restrictive diets. Omitting all fat and undergoing a major weight loss during a time of growth suggest inadequate nutrition and a possible eating disorder. Options 1, 2, and 4 are common and normal behaviors or feelings during adolescence.

Test-Taking Strategy: Use the process of elimination, and note the words *need for follow-up*. Select the option that indicates a problem or abnormality. Options 1, 2, and 4 are common and normal behaviors or feelings during adolescence. Review the development stage of the adolescent if you had difficulty with this question.

Reference

Price, D., & Gwin, J. (2008). *Pediatric nursing: An introductory text* (10th ed., pp. 334-335). St. Louis: Saunders

---

1090. A nurse is caring for a client who has bipolar disorder and who is having a manic episode. Which of the following would be the best menu choice for this client?

1 Beef stew, fruit salad, and tea
2 Cheeseburger, banana, and milk
3 Macaroni and cheese, apple, and milk
4 Scrambled eggs, orange juice, and coffee with cream and sugar

Level of Cognitive Ability: Application
Client Needs: Physiological Integrity
Integrated Process: Nursing Process/Implementation
Content Area: Mental Health

Answer: 2

Rationale: Bipolar disorder is a mental disorder that is characterized by episodes of mania, depression, or mixed mood. The client in a manic state often has inadequate food and fluid intake because of physical agitation. Foods that the client can eat "on the run" are best because the client is too active to sit at meals and use utensils; thus option 2 is the best menu choice.

Test-Taking Strategy: Use the process of elimination, and focus on the client's diagnosis. Recall that the client in a manic state should not have caffeine-containing products; thus options 1 and 4 can be eliminated. From the remaining options, note that option 2 identifies finger foods; remember the concept of finger foods with regard to these clients. Review the nutritional needs of the client with mania if you had difficulty with this question.

Reference

Varcarolis, E., & Halter, M. (2009). *Essentials of psychiatric mental health nursing: A communication approach to evidence-bared care* (p. 260). St. Louis: Saunders.

1091. A nurse is caring for a client who is receiving lithium carbonate (Lithobid). The nurse is told that the result of the client's lithium level is 2.0 mEq/L. The nurse determines this result to be:

1 Insignificant
2 Within normal limits
3 Lower than normal limits
4 Higher than normal limits, thus indicating toxicity

Answer: 4

Rationale: Lithium carbonate (Lithobid) is an antimanic medication. The therapeutic level for lithium is 0.6 to 1.2 mEq/L. A level of 2.0 mEq/L indicates toxicity and requires that the medication be withheld and the blood work repeated. The physician is also notified.

Level of Cognitive Ability: Comprehension
Client Needs: Physiological Integrity
Integrated Process: Nursing Process/Evaluation
Content Area: Pharmacology

Test-Taking Strategy: Knowledge of the therapeutic lithium level is necessary to answer this question. Recall that the therapeutic level for lithium is 0.6 to 1.2 mEq/L to direct you to option 4. Review this therapeutic level if you had difficulty with this question.

Reference
Hodgson, B., & Kizior, R. (2009). *Saunders nursing drug handbook 2009* (pp. 961-963). St. Louis: Saunders.

1092. A client calls the physician's office and tells the nurse that she found an area that looks like the peel of an orange when performing a breast self-examination but that she found no other changes. The nurse should:

1. Tell the client that there is nothing to worry about.
2. Arrange for the client to be seen by the physician as soon as possible.
3. Tell the client to take her temperature and to call back if she has a fever.
4. Tell the client to point the area out to the physician at her next regularly scheduled appointment.

Level of Cognitive Ability: Application
Client Needs: Physiological Integrity
Integrated Process: Nursing Process/Implementation
Content Area: Adult Health/Oncology

Answer: 2
Rationale: Peau d'orange or an orange-peel appearance of the skin of the breast is associated with late breast cancer. Realizing that this is what the client is describing, the nurse should arrange for the client to be seen by the physician as soon as possible. Peau d'orange is not indicative of an infection, so it is not necessary to have the client take her temperature.

Test-Taking Strategy: Use the process of elimination, and focus on the data in the question. Recall that peau d'orange is a sign of breast cancer to direct you to option 2. Review the signs of breast cancer if you had difficulty with this question.

Reference
Christensen, B., & Kockrow, E. (2006). *Adult health nursing* (5th ed., p. 605). St. Louis: Mosby.

1093. A client with Cushing's syndrome is being instructed by the nurse regarding follow-up care. Which statement by the client indicates the need for further instruction?

1. "I should avoid contact sports."
2. "I should avoid foods rich in potassium."
3. "I should check my ankles for swelling."
4. "I should check my blood sugar regularly."

Level of Cognitive Ability: Comprehension
Client Needs: Physiological Integrity
Integrated Process: Teaching and Learning
Content Area: Adult Health/Endocrine

Answer: 2
Rationale: Cushing's syndrome is a metabolic disorder that results from the chronic and excessive production of cortisol by the adrenal cortex. Hypokalemia is associated with this condition, and the client should consume foods that are high in potassium. Clients experience activity intolerance, osteoporosis, and frequent bruising. Fluid volume excess results from water and sodium retention. Hyperglycemia is caused by an increased cortisol secretion.

Test-Taking Strategy: Use the process of elimination, and note the strategic words *need for further instruction*. These words indicate a negative event query and ask you to select an option that is an incorrect statement. Recall the pathophysiology associated with this disorder to direct you to option 2. Remember that hypokalemia is associated with Cushing's syndrome and that the client should consume foods high in potassium. Review Cushing's syndrome if you had difficulty with this question.

Reference
Christensen, B., & Kockrow, E. (2006). *Adult health nursing* (5th ed., pp. 538-539). St. Louis: Mosby.

1094. A client with aldosteronism is being treated with spironolactone (Aldactone). Which of the following parameters indicates to the nurse that the treatment is effective?

1 A decrease in blood pressure
2 A decrease in sodium excretion
3 A decrease in body metabolism
4 An increase in potassium excretion

Level of Cognitive Ability: Analysis
Client Needs: Physiological Integrity
Integrated Process: Nursing Process/Evaluation
Content Area: Pharmacology

Answer: 1
Rationale: Spironolactone (Aldactone) is a potassium-sparing diuretic that antagonizes the effect of aldosterone and decreases circulating volume by promoting sodium and water excretion. Spironolactone increases potassium retention and it lowers the blood pressure. This medication has no effect on body metabolism.

Test-Taking Strategy: Use the process of elimination, and note the strategic word *effective.* Recall that this medication is also used to treat hypertensive conditions to direct you to option 1. Review the effects of spironolactone if you had difficulty with this question.

Reference
Hodgson, B., & Kizior, R. (2009). *Saunders nursing drug handbook 2009* (p. 1077). St. Louis: Saunders.

1095. A client with cancer tells the nurse that the food on the meal tray "tastes funny." Which intervention by the nurse is appropriate?

1 Keeping the client NPO
2 Providing frequent oral hygiene care
3 Administering an antiemetic as ordered
4 Asking for an order for parenteral nutrition

Level of Cognitive Ability: Application
Client Needs: Physiological Integrity
Integrated Process: Nursing Process/Implementation
Content Area: Adult Health/Oncology

Answer: 2
Rationale: Cancer treatments may cause a distortion of taste. Frequent oral hygiene aids in preserving taste function. Keeping a client NPO increases nutritional risks. Antiemetics are used when nausea and vomiting are a problem. Parenteral nutrition is used when oral intake is not possible.

Test-Taking Strategy: Use the process of elimination, and focus on the subject—taste sensation. Only option 2 addresses this subject. Review the effects of cancer treatments if you had difficulty with this question.

Reference
Christensen, B., & Kockrow, E. (2006). *Adult health nursing* (5th ed., pp. 833, 838). St. Louis: Mosby.

1096. A common finding in the health history of a client with chronic pancreatitis that the nurse may expect to note is:

1 Weight gain
2 Use of alcohol
3 Exposure to occupational chemicals
4 Abdominal pain relieved with food or antacids

Level of Cognitive Ability: Comprehension
Client Needs: Physiological Integrity
Integrated Process: Nursing Process/Data Collection
Content Area: Adult Health/Gastrointestinal

Answer: 2
Rationale: Chronic pancreatitis occurs most often in alcoholics. Abstinence from alcohol is important to prevent the client from developing chronic pancreatitis. Clients usually have malabsorption with weight loss. Chemical exposure is associated with cancer of the pancreas. Pain is not relieved with food or antacids.

Test-Taking Strategy: Use the process of elimination. Focus on the diagnosis of chronic pancreatitis to direct you to option 2. Review the most common causes of pancreatitis if you had difficulty with this question.

Reference
Christensen, B., & Kockrow, E. (2006). *Adult health nursing* (5th ed., p. 277). St. Louis: Mosby.

1097. A client has just been admitted to the hospital with a nonhealing arterial ischemic leg ulcer. The nurse inspects the ulcer for which characteristics?

1 Deep, pale, and painful
2 Deep, ruddy, and painless
3 Shallow, pale, and painful
4 Shallow, ruddy, and painless

Level of Cognitive Ability: Comprehension
Client Needs: Physiological Integrity
Integrated Process: Nursing Process/Data Collection
Content Area: Adult Health/Cardiovascular

Answer: 1
Rationale: Arterial ischemic leg ulcers are characteristically deep, pale, and painful. By contrast, venous stasis ulcers are more shallow, with a ruddy color to the ulcer. Venous ulcers are also painful but less so than arterial ulcers. There is no ulcer that is characteristically painless.

Test-Taking Strategy: Use the process of elimination. Eliminate options 2 and 4 first, knowing that ulcers are painful to clients. From the remaining options, select option 1 by recalling that arterial ulcers are deep because they are caused by tissue malnutrition. Review the characteristics of arterial ulcers if you had difficulty with this question.

Reference
Linton, A. (2007). *Introduction to medical-surgical nursing* (4th ed., pp. 699, 702). Philadelphia: Saunders.

1098. A client has been taking corticosteroids to control rheumatoid arthritis. What laboratory value most likely will be noted as a result of this medication?

1 Increased serum glucose
2 Decreased serum sodium
3 Elevated serum potassium
4 Increased white blood cells

Level of Cognitive Ability: Analysis
Client Needs: Physiological Integrity
Integrated Process: Nursing Process/Data Collection
Content Area: Pharmacology

Answer: 1
Rationale: Glucocorticoid (corticosteroid) medications have three primary uses: replacement therapy for adrenal insufficiency, immunosuppressive therapy, and anti-inflammatory therapy. Exogenous glucocorticoids cause the same effects on cellular activity as the naturally produced glucocorticoids; however, exogenous glucocorticoids may produce undesired clinical outcomes. The glucocorticoids stimulate appetite, increase caloric intake, and increase the availability of glucose for energy. These combined effects cause the blood glucose levels to rise, thus making clients prone to hyperglycemia. Options 2, 3, and 4 are not associated with the use of glucocorticoids.

Test-Taking Strategy: Knowledge of the side effects of glucocorticoids helps you to answer this question. Remember that corticosteroids cause blood glucose levels to rise, thereby making clients prone to hyperglycemia. Review glucocorticoids if you had difficulty with this question.

Reference
Edmunds, M. (2010). *Introduction to clinical pharmacology* (6th ed., p. 345). St. Louis: Mosby.

1099. A nurse is assigned to care for a group of clients in the clinical nursing unit. The nurse determines that which of the following clients is most at risk for the development of a pulmonary embolism?

1 A 25-year-old woman with diabetic ketoacidosis
2 A 65-year-old man out of bed 1 day after prostate resection
3 A 73-year-old woman who has just had a hip fracture pinned
4 A 38-year-old man with pulmonary contusion after an auto accident

Answer: 3
Rationale: Pulmonary embolism is the blockage of a pulmonary artery by fat, air, tumor tissue, or a thrombus that usually has arisen from a peripheral vein. Clients who are most at risk for pulmonary embolism include those who are immobilized, particularly after an operation. Other causes of pulmonary embolism include conditions that are characterized by hypercoagulability, endothelial disease, and advancing age.

Level of Cognitive Ability: Comprehension
Client Needs: Physiological Integrity
Integrated Process: Nursing Process/Data Collection
Content Area: Fundamental Skills

Test-Taking Strategy: Use the process of elimination. The options can be best compared by evaluating the degree of immobility that each client has as well as by considering the age of the client, which is given in each option. The clients in options 1 and 2 have the least long-term anticipated immobility, so they should be eliminated first. From the remaining options, the younger client with the lung contusion is expected to be more mobile than the elderly woman with a hip fracture, so you are directed to option 3. Review the causes of pulmonary embolism if you had difficulty with this question.

Reference

Christensen, B., & Kockrow, E. (2006). *Adult health nursing* (5th ed., p. 446). St. Louis: Mosby.

1100. A physician has inserted a nasoenteric tube for the treatment of an intestinal obstruction. The nurse raises the head of the bed and tells the client to lie in which position to help the tube advance into the duodenum through the pyloric sphincter?

1 On the left side
2 On the right side
3 Supine, with the head of the bed flat
4 Supine, with the head of the bed elevated 30 degrees

Level of Cognitive Ability: Application
Client Needs: Physiological Integrity
Integrated Process: Nursing Process/Implementation
Content Area: Adult Health/Gastrointestinal

Answer: 2

Rationale: After the insertion of a nasoenteric tube for the treatment of an intestinal obstruction, the client is instructed to lie on the right side with the head of the bed elevated to aid in the passage of the tube from the stomach into the duodenum, past the pyloric sphincter. The positions in options 1, 3, and 4 will not help with tube advancement.

Test-Taking Strategy: Use your knowledge of basic anatomy and of the position of the stomach to assist you with answering this question. Knowledge of this position can be applied to the management of a client with any type of nasoenteric tube. Review the anatomy of the gastrointestinal tract if you had difficulty with this question.

References

Ignatavicius, D., Workman, M. (2010). *Medical-surgical nursing: Patient-centered collaborative care* (6th ed., p. 1277). St. Louis: Saunders.
Potter, P., & Perry, A. (2009) *Fundamentals of nursing* (7th ed., p. 1024). St. Louis: Mosby.

1101. A nurse is monitoring the renal function of a client. After directly noting urine volume and characteristics, the nurse checks which item as the best indirect indicator of renal status?

1 Pulse rate
2 Blood pressure
3 Bladder distention
4 Level of consciousness

Level of Cognitive Ability: Application
Client Needs: Physiological Integrity
Integrated Process: Nursing Process/Implementation
Content Area: Adult Health/Renal

Answer: 2

Rationale: The kidneys normally receive 20% to 25% of the cardiac output, even under conditions of rest. Adequate renal perfusion is necessary for kidney function to be optimal. Perfusion can be estimated best by the blood pressure, which is an indirect reflection of the adequacy of the cardiac output. The pulse rate affects the cardiac output, but it can be altered by factors unrelated to kidney function. Bladder distention reflects a problem or obstruction that is most often distal to the kidneys. The level of consciousness is an unrelated item.

Test-Taking Strategy: Use the process of elimination. Eliminate the level of consciousness first as the item that is most unrelated to kidney function. Because bladder distention can be affected by a number of other factors besides renal function, this is eliminated next. To choose between pulse and blood pressure, remember that the cardiac output overall helps to determine the blood pressure and renal perfusion. Thus, blood pressure is the umbrella option and the one that is more directly related to kidney perfusion. Review the factors that affect renal perfusion if you had difficulty with this question.

Reference

Ignatavicius, D., Workman, M. (2010). *Medical-surgical nursing: Patient-centered collaborative care* (6th ed., p. 1535). St. Louis: Saunders.

1102. A client with ascites and slight jaundice is seen in the ambulatory care clinic. The nurse collecting data from the client asks the client about a history of chronic use of which of the following medications?

1 Ibuprofen (Advil)
2 Ranitidine (Zantac)
3 Acetaminophen (Tylenol)
4 Acetylsalicylic acid (Aspirin)

Level of Cognitive Ability: Analysis
Client Needs: Physiological Integrity
Integrated Process: Nursing Process/Data Collection
Content Area: Adult Health/Gastrointestinal

Answer: 3
Rationale: Acetaminophen (Tylenol) is an analgesic and a potentially hepatotoxic medication. The use of this medication and other hepatotoxic agents should be investigated whenever a client presents with symptoms that are compatible with liver disease (e.g., ascites, jaundice). Options 1, 2, and 4 are not as toxic to the liver.

Test-Taking Strategy: To answer this question, it is first necessary to know that the symptoms identified in the question are compatible with liver disease. With this in mind, evaluate each of the options for their relative ability to be toxic to the liver. Remember that acetaminophen (Tylenol) is a potentially hepatotoxic medication. Review the medications that are hepatotoxic if you had difficulty with this question.

Reference

Hodgson, B., & Kizior, R. (2009). *Saunders nursing drug handbook 2009* (pp. 12-13). St. Louis: Saunders.

1103. A nurse is assigned to care for a client who has just undergone eye surgery. The nurse plans to instruct the client that which activity is permitted during the postoperative period?

1 Reading
2 Bending over
3 Lifting objects
4 Watching television

Level of Cognitive Ability: Application
Client Needs: Physiological Integrity
Integrated Process: Nursing Process/Planning
Content Area: Adult Health/Eye

Answer: 4
Rationale: After eye surgery, the client is taught to avoid doing activities that raise intraocular pressure and that could cause complications during the postoperative period. The client is also taught to avoid activities that cause rapid eye movements, which are irritating in the presence of postoperative inflammation. For these reasons, the client is taught to avoid bending over, lifting heavy objects, straining, sneezing, making sudden movements, or reading. Watching television is permissible because the eye does not need to move rapidly with this activity and because this activity does not increase intraocular pressure.

Test-Taking Strategy: Think about the subject of intraocular pressure when answering this question. Eliminate options 2 and 3 first because they obviously increase intraocular pressure. From the remaining options, choose option 4 instead of option 1 because it is less taxing to the eyes. Review the care of the client after eye surgery if you had difficulty with this question.

Reference
Christensen, B., & Kockrow, E. (2006). *Adult health nursing* (5th ed., p. 652). St. Louis: Mosby.

1104. A female client with a history of chronic infection of the urinary system complains of burning and urinary frequency. To determine whether the current problem is of renal origin, the nurse asks the client if she is experiencing pain or discomfort in the:
1 Labium
2 Flank area
3 Urinary meatus
4 Suprapubic area

Level of Cognitive Ability: Application
Client Needs: Physiological Integrity
Integrated Process: Nursing Process/Data Collection
Content Area: Adult Health/Renal

Answer: 2
Rationale: Pain or discomfort from a problem that originates in the kidney is felt at the costovertebral angle (flank area) on the affected side. Ureteral pain is felt in the ipsilateral labium in the female client or the ipsilateral scrotum in the male client. Bladder infection is often accompanied by suprapubic pain and pain or burning at the urinary meatus when voiding.

Test-Taking Strategy: Use the process of elimination, and focus on the subject—renal origin. Recalling that the kidneys sit higher than the level of the bladder and retroperitoneally helps you eliminate the incorrect options. Review the effects of a renal disorder if you had difficulty with this question.

Reference
deWit, S. (2009). *Medical-surgical nursing: Concepts & practice* (p. 845). St. Louis: Saunders.

1105. A nurse is assigned to assist with caring for a client who has just had an insertion of an inferior vena cava (IVC) filter. During the first 24 hours after the procedure, the nurse plans to monitor the insertion site for which of the following?
1 Infection
2 Bleeding
3 Necrosis
4 Poor wound healing

Level of Cognitive Ability: Application
Client Needs: Physiological Integrity
Integrated Process: Nursing Process/Implementation
Content Area: Adult Health/Cardiovascular

Answer: 2
Rationale: The care of the client who has had an insertion of an IVC filter is similar to that of any surgical client. During the first 24 hours after the procedure, the nurse is most concerned with signs of bleeding. Signs of infection or poor wound healing would not be apparent during this time frame. Option 3 is incorrect.

Test-Taking Strategy: Use the process of elimination, and note the strategic words *monitor* and *first 24 hours.* These words tell you that the correct answer is the option that poses the greatest risk to the client immediately after the procedure is completed. This directs you to option 2. Review basic postoperative care if you had difficulty with this question.

Reference
Ignatavicius, D., Workman, M. (2010). *Medical-surgical nursing: Patient-centered collaborative care* (6th ed., p. 682). St. Louis: Saunders.

1106. During a routine visit to the physician's office, an older client with diabetes mellitus complains of vision changes. The client describes vision blurring that has resulted in difficulty with reading and with driving at night. Given the client's history, the nurse interprets that the client is probably developing:
1 Cataracts
2 Glaucoma
3 Papilledema
4 A detached retina

Answer: 1
Rationale: A cataract is an opacity of the lens of the eye that can develop as part of the aging process. Although the incidence of cataracts increases with age, the older client with diabetes mellitus is at greater risk for the development of cataracts. The most frequent complaint is of blurred vision that is not accompanied by pain. The client may also experience difficulty when reading or driving at night, and glare may also be a problem. Glaucoma is characterized by elevated pressure within the eye. Papilledema is a swelling of the optic disc. A detached retina involves the separation of the retina from the retinal pigment epithelium in the back of the eye.

Level of Cognitive Ability: Comprehension
Client Needs: Physiological Integrity
Integrated Process: Nursing Process/Data Collection
Content Area: Adult Health/Eye

Test-Taking Strategy: Use the process of elimination, and focus on the information in the question. Recall the signs and symptoms of cataracts to direct you to option 1. Review the signs and symptoms of cataracts if you had difficulty with this question.

Reference
Christensen, B., & Kockrow, E. (2006). *Adult health nursing* (5th ed., p. 651). St. Louis: Mosby.

1107. A nurse inquires about a smoking history when collecting data from a client with coronary artery disease. The most important item for the nurse to identify is the:
1 Desire to quit smoking
2 Number of pack years
3 Brand of cigarettes used
4 Number of past attempts to quit smoking

Level of Cognitive Ability: Comprehension
Client Needs: Physiological Integrity
Integrated Process: Nursing Process/Data Collection
Content Area: Adult Health/Cardiovascular

Answer: 2
Rationale: The number of cigarettes smoked daily and the duration of the habit are used to calculate the number of pack years, which is the standard method of documenting a client's history of smoking. The brand of cigarettes may give a general indication of tar and nicotine levels, but the information has no immediate clinical use. The desire to quit and the number of past attempts to quit smoking may be useful when the nurse develops a smoking cessation plan with the client.

Test-Taking Strategy: Use the process of elimination, and note the strategic words *most important item*. This indicates that more than one option is correct. The option that most closely predicts the degree of added risk of coronary artery disease is the number of pack years. Review the risks associated with coronary artery disease if you had difficulty with this question.

Reference
Ignatavicius, D., & Workman, M. (2010). *Medical-surgical nursing: Patient-centered collaborative care* (6th ed., p. 558). St. Louis: Saunders.

1108. A client with primary open-angle glaucoma has been prescribed timolol maleate (Timoptic) ophthalmic drops. The client asks the nurse how this medication works. The nurse tells the client that the medication lowers intraocular pressure by:
1 Constricting the pupil
2 Reducing intracranial pressure
3 Reducing the production of aqueous humor
4 Increasing the contractions of the ciliary muscle

Level of Cognitive Ability: Application
Client Needs: Physiological Integrity
Integrated Process: Nursing Process/Implementation
Content Area: Pharmacology

Answer: 3
Rationale: β-Adrenergic–blocking agents such as timolol reduce intraocular pressure by decreasing the production of aqueous humor. Miotic agents (e.g., pilocarpine) increase contractions of the ciliary muscle and constrict the pupil, thereby increasing the outflow of aqueous humor.

Test-Taking Strategy: Use the process of elimination. Eliminate option 2 because this medication is unrelated to intracranial pressure. Eliminate options 1 and 4 next because these are both actions of miotic agents. Review timolol maleate if you had difficulty with this question.

Reference
Hodgson, B., & Kizior, R. (2009). *Saunders nursing drug handbook 2009* (p. 1136). St. Louis: Saunders.

1109. A client is complaining of knee pain. The knee is swollen, red, and warm to the touch. The nurse interprets that the client's signs and symptoms are not associated with which condition?

Answer: 4
Rationale: Redness and heat are associated with musculoskeletal inflammation, infection, or a recent injury. Degenerative disease is accompanied by pain, but there is no redness. Swelling may or may not occur.

1 Infection
2 Recent injury
3 Inflammation
4 Degenerative disease

Level of Cognitive Ability: Comprehension
Client Needs: Physiological Integrity
Integrated Process: Nursing Process/Data Collection
Content Area: Adult Health/Musculoskeletal

Test-Taking Strategy: Use the process of elimination, and note the strategic words *not associated*. Swelling, redness, and warmth are signs of inflammation. The body's inflammatory response is triggered by inflammation, infection, and injury; this should direct you to option 4. Review the signs of inflammation if you had difficulty with this question.

References

Christensen, B., & Kockrow, E. (2006). *Foundations of nursing* (5th ed., p. 278). St. Louis: Mosby.
Linton, A. (2007). *Introduction to medical-surgical nursing* (4th ed., p. 162). Philadelphia: Saunders.

1110. A client seeks treatment in the emergency department for a lower-leg injury. There is a visible deformity of the lower aspect of the leg, and the injured leg appears to be shorter than the other leg. The area is painful, swollen, and beginning to become ecchymotic. The nurse interprets that this client has experienced a:
1 Strain
2 Sprain
3 Fracture
4 Contusion

Level of Cognitive Ability: Comprehension
Client Needs: Physiological Integrity
Integrated Process: Nursing Process/Data Collection
Content Area: Adult Health/Musculoskeletal

Answer: 3
Rationale: Typical signs and symptoms of a fracture include pain, loss of function in the area, deformity, shortening of the extremity, crepitus, swelling, and ecchymosis. Not all fractures lead to the development of every sign. A strain results from a pulling force on the muscle; symptoms include soreness and pain with muscle use. A sprain is an injury to a ligament caused by a wrenching or twisting motion; symptoms include pain, swelling, and an inability to use the joint or to bear weight normally. A contusion results from a blow to the soft tissue and causes pain, swelling, and ecchymosis.

Test-Taking Strategy: Use the process of elimination. Within the list of signs and symptoms in the question, note the one that states that one leg is shorter than the other. Only a fractured bone (which shortens with displacement) could cause this sign. Review the signs of a fracture if you had difficulty with this question.

Reference

Linton, A. (2007). *Introduction to medical-surgical nursing* (4th ed., p. 918). Philadelphia: Saunders.

1111. A client presents to the emergency department with a chemical burn of the left eye. The immediate action of the nurse is to:
1 Apply a cold compress to the injured eye.
2 Apply a nonocclusive bandage to the eye.
3 Determine the nature of the chemical agent.
4 Flush the eye continuously with a sterile solution.

Level of Cognitive Ability: Application
Client Needs: Physiological Integrity
Integrated Process: Nursing Process/Implementation
Content Area: Adult Health/Eye

Answer: 4
Rationale: When the client has suffered a chemical burn of the eye, the nurse immediately flushes the eye with a sterile solution continuously for 15 minutes. If a sterile eye irrigation solution is not available, running water may be used. Applying compresses or bandages is an incorrect action because this does not rid the eye of the damaging chemical. Cold compresses are used for blows to the eye, whereas light bandages may be placed over cuts of the eye or eyelid. Determining the nature of the chemical is helpful but is not the priority action.

Test-Taking Strategy: Use the process of elimination. Focus on the type of eye injury, and note the strategic word *chemical;* this will direct you to option 4. Review emergency care related to chemical burns of the eye if you had difficulty with this question.

Reference

Black, J., & Hawks, J. (2009). *Medical-surgical nursing: Clinical management for positive outcomes* (8th ed., p. 1252). St. Louis: Saunders.

1112. A client tells the nurse about a pattern of getting a strong urge to void that is followed by incontinence before the client can get to the bathroom. The nurse determines that the client is experiencing which problem?

1 Urge incontinence
2 Total incontinence
3 Stress incontinence
4 Reflex incontinence

Level of Cognitive Ability: Comprehension
Client Needs: Physiological Integrity
Integrated Process: Nursing Process/Data Collection
Content Area: Adult Health/Renal

Answer: 1
Rationale: Urge incontinence occurs when the client has urinary incontinence soon after experiencing urgency. Total incontinence occurs when there is an unpredictable and continuous loss of urine. Stress incontinence occurs as a sudden leakage of urine with activities that increase intraabdominal pressure. Reflex incontinence occurs when incontinence occurs at rather predictable times that correspond with the attainment of a certain bladder volume.

Test-Taking Strategy: Use the process of elimination, and focus on the data in the question. Note the relationship of the words *strong urge to void* in the question and the word *urge* in option 1. Review the types of incontinence if you had difficulty with this question.

Reference
deWit, S. (2009). *Medical-surgical nursing: Concepts & practice* (p. 833). St. Louis: Saunders.

1113. A nurse is instilling an otic solution into an adult client's left ear. The nurse avoids doing which of the following as part of this procedure?

1 Pulling the auricle backward and upward
2 Warming the solution to room temperature
3 Placing the tip of the dropper on the edge of the ear canal
4 Placing the client in a side-lying position with the ear facing up

Level of Cognitive Ability: Application
Client Needs: Physiological Integrity
Integrated Process: Nursing Process/Implementation
Content Area: Adult Health/Ear

Answer: 3
Rationale: When instilling eardrops, the dropper is not allowed to touch any object or any part of the client's skin. The solution is warmed before use. The client is placed on the side with the affected ear directed upward. The nurse pulls the auricle backward and upward and instills the medication by holding the dropper about 1 cm above the ear canal.

Test-Taking Strategy: Use the process of elimination, and note the strategic word *avoids.* This word indicates a negative event query and asks you to select an option that is an incorrect action. Visualizing this procedure assists with directing you to option 3. Review this basic nursing procedure if you had difficulty with this question.

Reference
Christensen, B., & Kockrow, E. (2006). *Foundations of nursing* (5th ed., p. 714). St. Louis: Mosby.

1114. Catatonic excitement has been diagnosed in a client who has been rapidly pacing nonstop for several hours and who is not eating or drinking. The nurse recognizes that in this situation:

1 There is an urgent need for restraint.
2 The client will soon become catatonic stuporous.
3 There is a need to encourage verbalization of feelings.
4 There is an urgent need for physical and medical control.

Level of Cognitive Ability: Comprehension
Client Needs: Physiological Integrity

Answer: 4
Rationale: Catatonic excitement is manifested by a state of extreme psychomotor agitation. Clients urgently require physical and medical control because they are often destructive and violent to others, and their excitement can cause them to injure themselves or collapse from complete exhaustion. Options 1, 2, and 3 are incorrect.

Test-Taking Strategy: Focus on the data in the question, and use Maslow's Hierarchy of Needs theory to answer the question. Remember that physiological needs come first. This will direct you to option 4. Review the priority needs for the client with catatonic excitement if you had difficulty with this question.

Integrated Process: Nursing Process/Evaluation
Content Area: Mental Health

References
Fortinash, K., & Holoday-Worret, P. (2008). *Psychiatric mental health nursing* (4th ed., pp. 259-260). St. Louis: Mosby.
Keltner, N., Schwecke, L., & Bostrom, C. (2007) *Psychiatric nursing* (5th ed., pp. 370-371). St. Louis: Mosby.

1115. Which of the following laboratory data indicate a potential complication associated with type 1 diabetes mellitus?
1 Ketonuria
2 Potassium, 4.2 mEq
3 Blood glucose, 112 mg/dL
4 Blood urea nitrogen, 18 mg/dL

Level of Cognitive Ability: Comprehension
Client Needs: Physiological Integrity
Integrated Process: Nursing Process/Data Collection
Content Area: Adult Health/Endocrine

Answer: 1
Rationale: Ketonuria is an abnormal finding in the diabetic client that indicates ketosis. Ketosis is a metabolic effect of fat metabolism that results from a lack of insulin, and it occurs in clients with type 1 diabetes mellitus. It is associated with severe complications of diabetic ketoacidosis (e.g., hyperglycemia, ketosis, acidosis). Option 2, 3, and 4 are all normal laboratory findings.

Test-Taking Strategy: Use the process of elimination, and focus on the client's diagnosis and the subject of the question—a complication. Recall the normal range of the laboratory values listed in the options to direct you to option 1. Remember that ketonuria is an abnormal finding. Review the complications of diabetes mellitus if you had difficulty with this question.

References
Christensen, B., & Kockrow, E. (2006). *Adult health nursing* (5th ed., p. 470). St. Louis: Mosby.
deWit, S. (2009). *Medical-surgical nursing: Concepts & practice* (p. 911). St. Louis: Saunders.

1116. A nurse is collecting data from a male client with diabetes mellitus who has been taking insulin for many years. The client states that he is currently experiencing periods of hypoglycemia followed by periods of hyperglycemia. The nurse determines that the most likely cause for this occurrence is:
1 Eating snacks between meals
2 Initiating the use of the insulin pump
3 Injecting insulin at the site of lipodystrophy
4 Adjusting insulin according to the blood glucose level

Level of Cognitive Ability: Comprehension
Client Needs: Physiological Integrity
Integrated Process: Nursing Process/Data Collection
Content Area: Adult Health/Endocrine

Answer: 3
Rationale: Tissue hypertrophy (lipodystrophy) involves the thickening of the subcutaneous tissue at an injection site. This can interfere with the absorption of insulin and result in erratic blood glucose levels. Because the client has been taking insulin for many years, this is the most likely cause of poor control.

Test-Taking Strategy: Use the process of elimination, and note the strategic words *taking insulin for many years.* These words indicate that you must consider a long-term complication of insulin administration, such as lipodystrophy. Options 1, 2, and 4 are actually appropriate techniques to use to regulate blood glucose levels. Review lipodystrophy if you had difficulty with this question.

References
Christensen, B., & Kockrow, E. (2006). *Adult health nursing* (5th ed., p. 551). St. Louis: Mosby.
Ignatavicius, D., Workman, M. (2010). *Medical-surgical nursing: Patient-centered collaborative care* (6th ed., p. 1486). St. Louis: Saunders.

1117. A nurse is assisting with caring for a client after a suprapubic prostatectomy. The nurse monitors the continuous bladder irrigation to detect which of the following signs of catheter blockage?

Answer: 4
Rationale: Catheter blockage or occlusion by clots after prostatectomy can result in urine backup and leakage around the catheter at the urethral meatus. This is accompanied by a stoppage of outflow through the catheter into the drainage bag. Pale pink

1 Drainage that is pale pink
2 Drainage that is bright red
3 True urine output of 50 mL/hour
4 Urine leakage around the three-way catheter at the meatus

Level of Cognitive Ability: Application
Client Needs: Physiological Integrity
Integrated Process: Nursing Process/Data Collection
Content Area: Adult Health/Renal

drainage indicates sufficient flow; bright red drainage indicates that the irrigant is running too slowly. A true urine output of 50 mL/hour indicates catheter patency.

Test-Taking Strategy: Use the process of elimination, and focus on the subject—catheter blockage. Eliminate options 1 and 2 first because of the word *drainage,* which implies catheter patency. Apply basic principles related to Foley catheter management to select the correct option from those remaining. A leakage around the catheter at the meatus indicates blockage. Review the signs of catheter blockage if you had difficulty with this question.

References
Christensen, B., & Kockrow, E. (2006). *Foundations of nursing* (5th ed., p. 579). St. Louis: Mosby.
Potter, P., & Perry, A. (2009) *Fundamentals of nursing* (7th ed., p. 1167). St. Louis: Mosby.

1118. A nurse is assigned to assist with caring for a client after transurethral prostatectomy. The nurse avoids doing which of the following after this procedure?
1 Reporting signs of confusion
2 Monitoring hourly urine output
3 Removing the traction tape on the three-way catheter
4 Administering belladonna and opium (B&O) suppositories at room temperature as prescribed

Level of Cognitive Ability: Application
Client Needs: Physiological Integrity
Integrated Process: Nursing Process/Implementation
Content Area: Adult Health/Renal

Answer: 3
Rationale: Transurethral prostatectomy involves the resection of the prostate by means of a cystoscope passed through the urethra. The nurse avoids removing the traction tape applied by the surgeon in the operating room. The purposes of this tape are to place pressure on the prostate and to reduce hemorrhage. The nurse monitors for confusion, which could result from hyponatremia secondary to the hypotonic irrigant used during the surgical procedure. The nurse also routinely monitors hourly urine output because the client has a three-way bladder irrigation running. B&O suppositories, which are ordered on a PRN basis for bladder spasm, should be warmed to room temperature before administration.

Test-Taking Strategy: Use the process of elimination, and note the strategic word *avoids.* This word indicates a negative event query and asks you to select an option that is an incorrect action. Eliminate options 1 and 2 first because they are part of routine nursing care and are not contraindicated as part of the care of this client. Knowledge of the use of bladder antispasmodics or of this specific surgical procedure will direct you to option 3. Review transurethral prostatectomy if you had difficulty with this question.

Reference
deWit, S. (2009). *Medical-surgical nursing: Concepts & practice* (pp. 982-983). St. Louis: Saunders.

1119. A client is due for a dose of bumetanide (Bumex). The nurse temporarily withholds the dose and notifies the physician if which laboratory result is noted?
1 Sodium, 137 mEq/L
2 Chloride, 106 mEq/L
3 Potassium, 2.9 mEq/L
4 Magnesium, 2.5 mg/dL

Answer: 3
Rationale: Bumetanide (Bumex) is a loop diuretic, which is not potassium sparing. The value given in the options for potassium is below the therapeutic range of 3.5 to 5.1 mEq/L for this electrolyte. The nurse should notify the physician before giving the dose of medication so that potassium may be ordered. Options 1, 2, and 4 are all normal laboratory values.

Level of Cognitive Ability: Application
Client Needs: Physiological Integrity
Integrated Process: Nursing Process/ Implementation
Content Area: Pharmacology

Test-Taking Strategy: Use the process of elimination, and focus on the subject—withholding a dose of medication and notifying the physician. Eliminate options 1, 2, and 4 because they are normal laboratory values. Review bumetanide and the normal potassium level if you had difficulty with this question.

References

Chernecky, C., & Berger, B. (2008). *Laboratory tests and diagnostic procedures* (5th ed., p. 891). Philadelphia: Saunders.
Hodgson, B., & Kizior, R. (2009). *Saunders nursing drug handbook 2009* (p. 156). St. Louis: Saunders.

1120. A client with heart failure is receiving digoxin (Lanoxin) daily. When the nurse enters the client's room to administer the morning medications, the client complains of anorexia, nausea, and yellow vision. The nurse should plan to do which of the following first?

1 Give the digoxin immediately.
2 Administer all medications.
3 Check the morning serum digoxin level.
4 Check the morning serum potassium level.

Level of Cognitive Ability: Application
Client Needs: Physiological Integrity
Integrated Process: Nursing Process/ Implementation
Content Area: Pharmacology

Answer: 3
Rationale: Digoxin (Lanoxin) is a cardiac glycoside and antidysrhythmic. The nurse should check for the result of the digoxin level that was drawn because the symptoms described by the client are compatible with toxicity. Because a low potassium level may contribute to toxicity, checking the serum potassium level may provide useful additional information, but this is not the first action. The digoxin should be withheld until the level is known, thus making options 1 and 2 incorrect.

Test-Taking Strategy: Use the process of elimination, and note the strategic word *first*. Eliminate options 1 and 2 because it is inappropriate to administer the client's medications without investigating further. From the remaining options, note that the client's complaints indicate toxicity to direct you to option 3. Review the signs of digoxin toxicity if you had difficulty with this question.

Reference

Hodgson, B., & Kizior, R. (2009). *Saunders nursing drug handbook 2009* (p. 356). St. Louis: Saunders.

1121. A nurse is administering an oral dose of erythromycin (Erythrocin) to an assigned client. The nurse understands that it is best to give this medication with a:

1 Full glass of milk
2 Full glass of water
3 Sip of orange juice
4 Any noncitrus beverage

Level of Cognitive Ability: Application
Client Needs: Physiological Integrity
Integrated Process: Nursing Process/ Implementation
Content Area: Pharmacology

Answer: 2
Rationale: Erythromycin is a macrolide antibiotic that should be taken with a full glass of water. Sufficient volume is needed to obtain the maximal effect of the medication. Depending on the specific type of erythromycin, it may need to be administered on an empty stomach, with meals, or regardless of the timing of meals. The nurse should verify the best method of administration for the type of medication ordered.

Test-Taking Strategy: Use the process of elimination, and note the strategic word *best*. Eliminate options 1, 3, and 4 because they are comparable or alike in that they indicate administering the medication with some type of liquid food substance. Review erythromycin if you had difficulty with this question.

Reference

Hodgson, B., & Kizior, R. (2009). *Saunders nursing drug handbook 2009* (p. 436). St. Louis: Saunders.

1122. A client with a fractured femur who has had an open reduction and an internal fixation is receiving ketorolac (Toradol). The nurse evaluates the effectiveness of the medication by monitoring the client's:

1 Pain rating
2 Temperature
3 Serum calcium level
4 White blood cell count

Level of Cognitive Ability: Analysis
Client Needs: Physiological Integrity
Integrated Process: Nursing Process/Evaluation
Content Area: Pharmacology

Answer: 1

Rationale: Ketorolac (Toradol) is a nonopioid analgesic and a nonsteroidal anti-inflammatory drug. It acts by inhibiting prostaglandin synthesis, and it produces analgesia that is peripherally mediated. The nurse evaluates the effectiveness of this medication by using the pain rating scale with the client. Options 2, 3, and 4 are incorrect.

Test-Taking Strategy: Use the process of elimination. Note the client's diagnosis to provide you with a clue that the medication is an analgesic; this will direct you to option 1. Review ketorolac if you had difficulty with this question.

References

Christensen, B., & Kockrow, E. (2006). *Foundations of nursing* (5th ed., pp. 405-406). St. Louis: Mosby.

Hodgson, B., & Kizior, R. (2009). *Saunders nursing drug handbook 2009* (pp. 648-650). St. Louis: Saunders.

1123. A client has an order for beclomethasone (Beconase AQ) to be given via the intranasal route. The client also has an order for a nasal decongestant. Which of the following methods of administration by the nurse is correct?

1 Administer the decongestant 15 minutes before the beclomethasone.
2 Administer the beclomethasone 15 minutes before the decongestant.
3 Administer the beclomethasone immediately before the decongestant.
4 Administer the decongestant immediately before the beclomethasone.

Level of Cognitive Ability: Application
Client Needs: Physiological Integrity
Integrated Process: Nursing Process/Implementation
Content Area: Pharmacology

Answer: 1

Rationale: The nasal decongestant should be administered 15 minutes before the beclomethasone, which is a glucocorticoid, to clear the nasal passages and enhance the absorption of the medication. Options 2, 3, and 4 are incorrect.

Test-Taking Strategy: Use the same principles when answering this question that you would use when administering bronchodilators and corticosteroids together; this will direct you to option 1. Remember that the nasal decongestant should be administered before the beclomethasone. Review these medications and their appropriate methods of administration if you had difficulty with this question.

Reference

Hodgson, B., & Kizior, R. (2009). *Saunders nursing drug handbook 2009* (pp. 120-121). St. Louis: Saunders.

1124. A client is receiving tobramycin (Tobrex). The nurse determines that the client is responding well to the medication therapy if which of the following laboratory results are noted?

1 Sodium, 145 mEq/L; chloride, 106 mEq/L
2 Sodium, 140 mEq/L; potassium, 3.9 mEq/L
3 White blood cell count, 8000/mm^3; creatinine, 0.9 mg/dL
4 White blood cell count, 15,000/mm^3; blood urea nitrogen, 38 mg/dL

Answer: 3

Rationale: Tobramycin is an antibiotic (aminoglycoside) that causes nephrotoxicity and ototoxicity. The medication is effective if the white blood cell count drops back into the normal range and the kidney function remains normal. Option 4 indicates an abnormal white blood cell count and an elevated blood urea nitrogen level. Options 1 and 2 are not related to this medication.

Test-Taking Strategy: Use the process of elimination, and note the strategic words *responding well*. Eliminate options 1 and 2 first because tobramycin is an antibiotic. Recall that aminoglycosides cause nephrotoxicity to direct you to choose option 3 over option 4, using laboratory values as your guide. Review tobramycin and normal laboratory values if you had difficulty with this question.

Level of Cognitive Ability: Analysis
Client Needs: Physiological Integrity
Integrated Process: Nursing Process/Evaluation
Content Area: Pharmacology

Reference

Hodgson, B., & Kizior, R. (2009). *Saunders nursing drug handbook 2009* (p. 1146). St. Louis: Saunders.

1125. Which of the following is a nursing intervention for the client who is taking maintenance dosages of lithium carbonate (Lithobid)?

1 Monitoring intake and output
2 Monitoring daily serum lithium levels
3 Observing for remission of depressive states
4 Performing a weekly electrocardiogram (ECG)

Level of Cognitive Ability: Application
Client Needs: Physiological Integrity
Integrated Process: Nursing Process/Implementation
Content Area: Pharmacology

Answer: 1

Rationale: Lithium carbonate is used to treat manic disorders (not depression). The side effects of lithium are nausea, tremors, polyuria, and polydipsia, and the nurse should monitor intake and output. The serum lithium concentration is checked approximately every 2 to 4 days during initial therapy and at longer intervals thereafter. Toxic levels of lithium may induce ECG changes; however, there is no need to perform weekly ECGs if maintenance levels are maintained.

Test-Taking Strategy: Use the process of elimination. Eliminate options 2 and 4 first because of the words *daily* and *weekly*, respectively. From the remaining options, use your knowledge of the side effects and use of the medication to direct you to option 1. Review nursing interventions related to the administration of lithium if you had difficulty with this question.

Reference

Hodgson, B., & Kizior, R. (2009). *Saunders nursing drug handbook 2009* (p. 693). St. Louis: Saunders.

1126. A nurse is caring for a client who has recently been diagnosed with a spinal cord injury. The nurse reviews the client's record and anticipates that the most likely medication to be prescribed will be which of the following?

1 Morphine sulfate
2 Mannitol (Osmitrol)
3 Propranolol (Inderal)
4 Methylprednisolone (Solu-Medrol)

Level of Cognitive Ability: Analysis
Client Needs: Physiological Integrity
Integrated Process: Nursing Process/Planning
Content Area: Adult Health/Neurological

Answer: 4

Rationale: A spinal cord injury is a traumatic disruption of the spinal cord that is often associated with extensive musculoskeletal involvement. The most likely medication to be ordered for a recently diagnosed spinal cord injury is methylprednisolone. This medication is a glucocorticoid, and it is given to reduce traumatic edema. The use of propranolol (a β-blocker), mannitol (an osmotic diuretic), or morphine sulfate (an opioid analgesic) is not indicated based on the information provided in the question.

Test-Taking Strategy: Use the process of elimination, and note the strategic words *recently been diagnosed with a spinal cord injury*. Recall the association between injury and edema and remember the actions of the medications listed in the options to direct you to option 4. Review the medications listed and the treatment of spinal cord injury if you had difficulty with this question.

References

Hodgson, B., & Kizior, R. (2009). *Saunders nursing drug handbook 2009* (p. 749). St. Louis: Saunders.
Linton, A. (2007). *Introduction to medical-surgical nursing* (4th ed., p. 497). Philadelphia: Saunders.

1127. A nurse is collecting data from a client admitted to the hospital with a diagnosis of Raynaud's disease. The nurse accurately

Answer: 4

Rationale: Raynaud's disease produces closure of the small arteries in the distal extremities in response to cold, vibration, or external

checks for the symptoms associated with Raynaud's disease when the nurse:
1 Checks for a rash on the digits
2 Observes for softening of the nails or nail beds
3 Palpates for a rapid or irregular peripheral pulse
4 Palpates for diminished or absent peripheral pulses

Level of Cognitive Ability: Application
Client Needs: Physiological Integrity
Integrated Process: Nursing Process/Data Collection
Content Area: Adult Health/Cardiovascular

stimuli. Palpation for diminished or absent peripheral pulses checks for the interruption of circulation. The nails grow slowly, become brittle or deformed, and heal poorly around the nail beds when infected. Skin changes include hair loss, thinning or tightening of the skin, and delayed healing of cuts or injuries. Although the palpation of the peripheral pulses is correct, it is incorrect to find a rapid or irregular pulse. The peripheral pulses may be normal, absent, or diminished.

Test-Taking Strategy: Use the ABCs—airway, breathing, and circulation; this will direct you to option 4. Review the manifestations associated with Raynaud's disease if you had difficulty with this question.

Reference

Linton, A. (2007). *Introduction to medical-surgical nursing* (4th ed., p. 704). Philadelphia: Saunders.

1128. A nurse monitors the respiratory status of a client being treated for acute exacerbation of chronic obstructive pulmonary disease (COPD). Which initial finding indicates a deterioration in ventilation?
1 Cyanosis
2 Barrel chest
3 Hyperinflated chest
4 Rapid, shallow respirations

Level of Cognitive Ability: Comprehension
Client Needs: Physiological Integrity
Integrated Process: Nursing Process/Data Collection
Content Area: Adult Health/Respiratory

Answer: 4

Rationale: COPD is a progressive and irreversible condition that is characterized by the diminished inspiratory and expiratory capacity of the lungs. An increase in the rate of respirations and a decrease in the depth of respirations indicates a deterioration in ventilation. Cyanosis is not a good indicator of oxygenation in the client with COPD; it may be present with some but not all clients. A hyperinflated chest (barrel chest) and hypertrophy of the accessory muscles of the upper chest and neck may normally be found in clients with severe COPD.

Test-Taking Strategy: Use the process of elimination. Note the strategic words *initial* and *deterioration in ventilation.* Eliminate options 2 and 3 first because they are comparable or alike. Because cyanosis is not a good indicator of oxygenation in the client with COPD, eliminate option 1. Review the clinical manifestations associated with COPD if you had difficulty with this question.

Reference

Linton, A. (2007). *Introduction to medical-surgical nursing* (4th ed., p. 553). Philadelphia: Saunders.

1129. Which data collection finding indicates the effectiveness of postural drainage and chest physiotherapy (CPT) in the client with chronic obstructive pulmonary disease (COPD)?
1 The client's cough is suppressed.
2 The client expectorates large amounts of sputum.
3 The client's expiration time becomes less prolonged.
4 The client is able to maintain the necessary position for postural drainage and chest physiotherapy.

Answer: 2

Rationale: COPD is a progressive and irreversible condition that is characterized by the diminished inspiratory and expiratory capacity of the lungs. Postural drainage and CPT aid in improving airway clearance by mobilizing secretions to make them easier to expectorate. It is necessary for the client to cough effectively to expectorate secretions. The ability to maintain the necessary position for these respiratory treatments does not demonstrate the effectiveness of the treatment. It is a normal expectation that clients with even stable COPD will demonstrate a prolonged expiration time that exceeds 4 seconds.

Level of Cognitive Ability: Analysis
Client Needs: Physiological Integrity
Integrated Process: Nursing Process/Evaluation
Content Area: Adult Health/Respiratory

Test-Taking Strategy: Use the process of elimination, and note the strategic words *indicates the effectiveness.* Keep this in mind as you remember the purpose of CPT and postural drainage to direct you to option 2. Options 1 and 4 do not determine effectiveness. A prolonged expiration time is a normal expectation in a client with this disorder and has no relationship to these respiratory treatments. Review the purpose of postural drainage and CPT if you had difficulty with this question.

References

Christensen, B., & Kockrow, E. (2006). *Adult health nursing* (5th ed., p. 451). St. Louis: Mosby.
Linton, A. (2007). *Introduction to medical-surgical nursing* (4th ed., p. 559). Philadelphia: Saunders.

1130. Diazepam (Valium) is prescribed for a client. The nurse reinforces instructions to the client and tells the client to expect which side effect?

1 Cough
2 Tinnitus
3 Hypertension
4 Incoordination

Level of Cognitive Ability: Application
Client Needs: Physiological Integrity
Integrated Process: Teaching and Learning
Content Area: Pharmacology

Answer: 4
Rationale: Diazepam, which is a benzodiazepine, can cause motor incoordination and ataxia; safety precautions should be instituted for clients taking this medication. Options 1, 2, and 3 are unrelated to this medication.

Test-Taking Strategy: Use the process of elimination, and focus on the classification of the medication. Recalling that a benzodiazepine can cause incoordination assists you with answering the question. Review the side effects of diazepam if you had difficulty with this question.

Reference

Christensen, B., & Kockrow, E. (2006). *Adult health nursing* (5th ed., p. 40). St. Louis: Mosby.

1131. A nurse is assisting with caring for a client who is receiving oxytocin (Pitocin) to induce labor. During the administration of oxytocin, it is most important for the nurse to monitor the:

1 Urinary output
2 Fetal heart rate
3 Maternal temperature
4 Maternal blood glucose level

Level of Cognitive Ability: Application
Client Needs: Physiological Integrity
Integrated Process: Nursing Process/Data Collection
Content Area: Pharmacology

Answer: 2
Rationale: Oxytocin (Pitocin) is a uterine smooth muscle stimulant that produces uterine contractions. Uterine contractions can cause fetal anoxia; therefore, it is most important to monitor the fetal heart rate. Options 1, 3, and 4 are unrelated to the administration of this medication.

Test-Taking Strategy: Use the ABCs—airway, breathing, and circulation—to answer the question; this will direct you to option 2. Review the action and nursing implications associated with the administration of oxytocin if you had difficulty with this question.

Reference

Hodgson, B., & Kizior, R. (2009). *Saunders nursing drug handbook 2009* (p. 884). St. Louis: Saunders.

1132. A nursing instructor asks a nursing student about the reason for medication toxicity occurring in a neonate. The student understands the reason for this occurrence when the student verbalizes that the neonate's:

Answer: 3
Rationale: The liver is not fully developed in the neonate and thus cannot detoxify many medications. Options 1, 2, and 4 are incorrect.

1 Lungs are immature
2 Kidneys are smaller
3 Liver is not fully developed
4 Cerebral function is not fully developed

Level of Cognitive Ability: Comprehension
Client Needs: Physiological Integrity
Integrated Process: Teaching and Learning
Content Area: Maternity/Postpartum

Test-Taking Strategy: Use the process of elimination and your knowledge of the normal physiological maturity associated with the neonate. Recall that the liver is associated with the detoxification of medications to direct you to option 3. Review the normal physiological findings in the neonate if you had difficulty with this question.

Reference

McKinney, E., James, S., Murray, S., & Ashwill, J. (2009). *Maternal-child nursing* (3rd ed., p. 499). St. Louis: Saunders.

1133. A client is hospitalized for ingesting an overdose of acetaminophen (Tylenol). The nurse prepares to administer which specific antidote as prescribed for this medication overdose?
1 Protamine sulfate
2 Phytonadione (Vitamin K)
3 Acetylcysteine (Mucomyst)
4 Naloxone hydrochloride (Narcan)

Level of Cognitive Ability: Application
Client Needs: Physiological Integrity
Integrated Process: Nursing Process/Planning
Content Area: Pharmacology

Answer: 3
Rationale: Acetylcysteine (Mucomyst) restores the sulfhydryl groups that are depleted by acetaminophen metabolism. Protamine sulfate is the antidote for heparin. Vitamin K is the antidote for warfarin sodium (Coumadin). Naloxone hydrochloride reverses respiratory depression.

Test-Taking Strategy: Use the process of elimination. Recall the specific antidotes for both heparin and warfarin sodium (Coumadin) to eliminate options 1 and 2. Recall that naloxone hydrochloride reverses respiratory depression to eliminate option 4. Review the antidotes listed in the options if you had difficulty with this question.

Reference

Hodgson, B., & Kizior, R. (2009). *Saunders nursing drug handbook 2009* (p. 13). St. Louis: Saunders.

1134. A nurse is observing a client to determine whether the client is correctly using a walker. When evaluating the client's use of a walker, the nurse expects to note which of the following?
1 The client puts weight on the hand pieces, slides the walker forward, and then walks into it.
2 The client puts weight on the hand pieces, moves the walker forward, and then walks into it.
3 The client puts all four points of the walker flat on the floor, puts weight on the hand pieces, and then walks into the walker.
4 The client walks into the walker, puts weight on the hand pieces, and then puts all four points of the walker flat on the floor.

Level of Cognitive Ability: Comprehension
Client Needs: Physiological Integrity
Integrated Process: Nursing Process/Evaluation
Content Area: Fundamental Skills

Answer: 3
Rationale: When the client uses a walker, the nurse stands adjacent to the affected side. The client is instructed to put all four points of the walker 2 feet forward and flat on the floor before putting weight on the hand pieces; this ensures client safety and prevents stress cracks in the walker. The client is then instructed to move the walker forward and to walk into it.

Test-Taking Strategy: Attempt to visualize this procedure. Options 1 and 2 can be eliminated because putting weight on the hand pieces initially will cause an unsafe situation. From the remaining options, recall that the walker is placed on all four points first to direct you to option 3. Review the procedure for walking with a walker if you had difficulty with this question.

Reference

deWit, S. (2009). *Medical-surgical nursing: Concepts & practice* (p. 779). St. Louis: Saunders.

1135. When evaluating a client for the correct height of crutches, the nurse expects to note which of the following?

1 The client is able to rest the axillae on the axillary bars.
2 The nurse is able to place two fingers comfortably between the axillae and the axillary bars.
3 The nurse is able to place four fingers comfortably between the axillae and the axillary bars.
4 The client is able to maintain the arms in a straight position when standing with the crutches.

Level of Cognitive Ability: Comprehension
Client Needs: Physiological Integrity
Integrated Process: Nursing Process/Evaluation
Content Area: Fundamental Skills

Answer: 2

Rationale: With the client's elbows flexed 20 to 30 degrees, the shoulders in a relaxed position, and the crutches placed approximately 15 cm (6 inches) anterolateral from the toes, the nurse should be able to place two fingers comfortably between the axillae and the axillary bars. The crutches are adjusted if there is too much or too little space in the axillary area. The client is advised to never rest the axillae on the axillary bars because this could injure the brachial plexus (the nerve in the axillae that supplies the arm and shoulder area). Ambulation is stopped if the client complains of numbness or tingling in the hands or arms.

Test-Taking Strategy: Use the process of elimination. Visualize each of the options and eliminate those that are not reasonable and that will not provide safety; this will direct you to option 2. Review the procedure for correct crutch placement if you had difficulty with this question.

Reference

Perry, A. & Potter, P. (2010). *Clinical nursing skills & techniques* (7th ed., pp. 252-253). St. Louis: Mosby.

1136. A client with myasthenia gravis is admitted to the hospital. The nurse reviews the health record and notes that the client is taking pyridostigmine (Mestinon). The nurse checks the client for which side effect of this medication?

1 Depression
2 Mouth ulcers
3 Abdominal cramps
4 Unexplained weight gain

Level of Cognitive Ability: Application
Client Needs: Physiological Integrity
Integrated Process: Nursing Process/Data Collection
Content Area: Pharmacology

Answer: 3

Rationale: Pyridostigmine is an acetylcholinesterase inhibitor. Abdominal discomfort and cramps are side effects of the medication. Options 1, 2, and 4 are not specific side effects associated with the use of this medication.

Test-Taking Strategy: Recall that myasthenia gravis is a neuromuscular disorder. Use your knowledge of the side effects of this medication and recall that pyridostigmine is an acetylcholinesterase inhibitor to direct you to option 3. Review the side effects associated with pyridostigmine if you had difficulty with this question.

Reference

Hodgson, B., & Kizior, R. (2009). *Saunders nursing drug handbook 2009* (p. 983). St. Louis: Saunders.

1137. A client with a fractured right ankle has a short leg plaster cast applied. During discharge teaching, the nurse reinforces which of the following information to prevent complications?

1 Trim the rough edges of the cast after it is dry.
2 Bear weight on the right leg only after the cast is dry.
3 Expect burning and tingling sensations under the cast for 3 to 4 days.
4 Keep the right ankle elevated with pillows above the height of the heart for 24 to 48 hours.

Answer: 4

Rationale: Leg elevation is important to increase venous return and to decrease edema; edema can cause compartment syndrome, which is a major complication of fractures and casting. Option 1 is incorrect because any cast modifications should be performed by trained personnel under medical supervision. However, the client, family, or both may be taught how to "petal" the cast to prevent skin irritation and breakdown. Option 2 is incorrect because the bearing of weight on a fractured extremity is determined by the physician during a follow-up examination after radiography. Although the client may feel heat after the cast is applied, a burning or tingling sensation indicates nerve damage and ischemia and is not expected; it should be reported immediately.

Level of Cognitive Ability: Application
Client Needs: Physiological Integrity
Integrated Process: Teaching and Learning
Content Area: Adult Health/Musculoskeletal

Test-Taking Strategy: Remember that skin breakdown, compartment syndrome, cast damage, and venous thrombosis are all potential complications associated with casting. Use the ABCs—airway, breathing, and circulation. Option 4 is associated with the maintenance of circulation. Review client instructions regarding cast care if you had difficulty with this question.

Reference

Christensen, B., & Kockrow, E. (2006). *Adult health nursing* (5th ed., p. 172). St. Louis: Mosby.

1138. An older adult female client with a fractured left tibia has a long leg cast and is using crutches to ambulate. When caring for the client, the nurse should be alert for which sign that indicates a complication associated with crutch walking?

1 Weak biceps brachii
2 Left leg paresthesias
3 Triceps muscle spasms
4 Forearm muscle weakness

Level of Cognitive Ability: Analysis
Client Needs: Physiological Integrity
Integrated Process: Nursing Process/Data Collection
Content Area: Adult Health/Musculoskeletal

Answer: 4

Rationale: Forearm muscle weakness is a sign of radial nerve injury caused by crutch pressure on the axillae. When clients lack upper body strength, especially in the flexor and extensor muscles of the arms, they frequently allow their weight to rest on their axillae instead of their arms while ambulating with crutches. Older adult women tend to have poor upper body strength. Option 1 is a common physical finding in older adults (especially women), and it is not a complication of crutch walking. Option 2 is a sign of compartment syndrome, which is a complication of fractures (not of crutch walking). Option 3 may occur as a result of increased muscle use, but it is not a complication of crutch walking.

Test-Taking Strategy: Use the process of elimination. When asked about a complication of the use of crutches, think about nerve injury caused by crutch pressure on the axillae; this will direct you to option 4. Review the complications of crutch walking if you had difficulty with this question.

Reference

deWit, S. (2009). *Medical-surgical nursing: Concepts & practice* (pp. 781, 813). St. Louis: Saunders.

1139. A client is diagnosed with angina. The nurse reviews the client's diagnostic and laboratory results, knowing that which finding is indicative of myocardial ischemia?

1 Increased serum potassium levels
2 Decreased serum potassium levels
3 Electroencephalogram (EEG) wave increases
4 S-T wave depression on electrocardiogram (ECG)

Level of Cognitive Ability: Analysis
Client Needs: Physiological Integrity
Integrated Process: Nursing Process/Data Collection
Content Area: Adult Health/Cardiovascular

Answer: 4

Rationale: Ischemia represents a decreased amount of oxygen to the myocardium. Ischemia may be detected on an ECG by changes in the S-T wave or by T-wave inversion. EEG and potassium level findings are not directly related to coronary ischemia.

Test-Taking Strategy: Focus on the subject—myocardial ischemia. Note the relationship between the subject and option 4. Review these diagnostic findings if you had difficulty with this question.

Reference

Ignatavicius, D., & Workman, M. (2010). *Medical-surgical nursing: Patient-centered collaborative care* (6th ed., pp. 848-849). St. Louis: Saunders.

1140. A nurse is caring for a client admitted to the hospital with a diagnosis of active tuberculosis (TB). The nurse understands that this diagnosis was confirmed by:

1 A Mantoux test
2 A sputum culture
3 A chest radiograph
4 Clinical manifestations

Level of Cognitive Ability: Comprehension
Client Needs: Physiological Integrity
Integrated Process: Nursing Process/Data Collection
Content Area: Adult Health/Respiratory

Answer: 2
Rationale: TB is a granulomatous infection caused by an acid-fast bacillus. A sputum culture of *Mycobacterium tuberculosis* confirms the diagnosis of TB. Usually three sputum samples are obtained for the acid-fast smear. After the start of therapy, sputum samples are obtained again to determine the effectiveness of therapy. A positive Mantoux test indicates exposure to TB but does not confirm its presence. Clinical manifestations do not confirm the injection. A positive chest radiograph may indicate the presence of TB lesions but again does not confirm active disease.

Test-Taking Strategy: Use the process of elimination, and note the strategic word *confirmed*. Active TB can be confirmed only by the presence of acid-fast bacilli. The sputum culture is the only method of determining the presence of this organism. Review the diagnostic tests for TB if you had difficulty with this question.

Reference
deWit, S. (2009). *Medical-surgical nursing: Concepts & practice* (p. 325). St. Louis: Saunders.

1141. A nurse employed in an obstetrician's office checks the fundal height of a client who is in the second trimester of pregnancy. When measuring this, the nurse most likely expects the measurement:

1 To be less than the gestational age
2 To correlate with the gestational age
3 To be greater than the gestational age
4 To have no correlation with the gestational age

Level of Cognitive Ability: Comprehension
Client Needs: Physiological Integrity
Integrated Process: Nursing Process/Data Collection
Content Area: Maternity/Antepartum

Answer: 2
Rationale: Up to the third trimester, the measurement of the fundal height roughly correlates with the gestational age.

Test-Taking Strategy: Note the strategic words *second trimester*. Use these words and your knowledge of the fundal height and the gestational age to answer the question. Review data collection findings during the prenatal period if you had difficulty with this question.

Reference
Leifer, G. (2008). *Maternity nursing: An introductory text* (10th ed., pp. 62, 86). Philadelphia: Saunders.

1142. A nurse is reviewing the health record of a neonate admitted to the nursery. The nurse notes documentation that the anterior fontanel of the neonate is soft. The nurse interprets this finding as indicative of:

1 Dehydration
2 Normal development
3 Increased intracranial pressure
4 Decreased intracranial pressure

Level of Cognitive Ability: Comprehension
Client Needs: Physiological Integrity
Integrated Process: Nursing Process/Data Collection
Content Area: Maternity/Postpartum

Answer: 2
Rationale: The anterior fontanel is normally 2 to 3 cm wide, 3 to 4 cm long, and in the shape of a diamond. It can be described as soft, which is normal, or as full and bulging, which can indicate increased intracranial pressure. Conversely, a depressed fontanel can mean that the neonate is dehydrated.

Test-Taking Strategy: Knowledge of the normal findings in a neonate is necessary to answer this question. Remember that the anterior fontanel is normally 2 to 3 cm wide, 3 to 4 cm long, in the shape of a diamond, and soft. Review the findings related to neonatal fontanels if you had difficulty with this question.

Reference
Leifer, G. (2008). *Maternity nursing: An introductory text* (10th ed., p. 177). Philadelphia: Saunders.

1143. A nurse is caring for a client who had abdominal surgery. While the nurse is caring for the client, the client complains of pain in the calf. The nurse should:

1 Ask the client to walk and observe the client's gait.
2 Lightly massage the client's calf to relieve muscle pain.
3 Observe the client's calf for temperature, color, and size.
4 Administer PRN meperidine hydrochloride (Demerol) as ordered.

Level of Cognitive Ability: Application
Client Needs: Physiological Integrity
Integrated Process: Nursing Process/Data Collection
Content Area: Fundamental Skills

Answer: 3

Rationale: The nurse monitors for postoperative complications such as deep vein thrombosis (DVT), pulmonary emboli, and wound infection. Pain in the calf may indicate DVT; changes in color, temperature, or size of the calf also may indicate this complication. Options 1 and 2 may result in an embolus if the client does in fact have DVT. Administering pain medication for this client's complaint is not the appropriate nursing action.

Test-Taking Strategy: Use the process of elimination. Remember that data collection is the first step of the nursing process. Only option 3 specifically addresses data collection. Review postoperative complications and appropriate interventions if you had difficulty with this question.

Reference

Christensen, B., & Kockrow, E. (2006). *Adult health nursing* (5th ed., pp. 56, 389). St. Louis: Mosby.

1144. A nurse is checking the patency of a peripheral intravenous (IV) site and suspects an infiltration. The nurse performs which action to determine whether the IV has infiltrated?

1 Checking the surrounding tissue for edema and coolness
2 Stripping the tubing quickly while checking for a rapid blood return
3 Checking the area around the IV site for discomfort, redness, and warmth
4 Increasing the IV flow rate and observing the site for an immediate tightening of tissue

Level of Cognitive Ability: Application
Client Needs: Physiological Integrity
Integrated Process: Nursing Process/Implementation
Content Area: Fundamental Skills

Answer: 1

Rationale: Infiltration occurs when IV fluid seeps into the tissues. When checking an IV site for signs of infiltration, it is important to check the site for edema and coolness. Stripping the tubing does not cause a blood return but instead forces IV fluids into the vein or the surrounding tissues, which could cause more tissue damage. Increasing the flow rate may be damaging to the tissues if the IV has infiltrated. The IV site feels cool if the IV fluid has infiltrated into the surrounding tissues.

Test-Taking Strategy: Use the process of elimination, and focus on the subject—infiltration. Recall that edema and coolness occur with an infiltration to direct you to option 1. Review the signs of infiltration if you had difficulty with this question.

Reference

deWit, S. (2009). *Medical-surgical nursing: Concepts & practice* (p. 59). St. Louis: Saunders.

1145. A client is brought into the emergency department after a motor vehicle accident, and a neck injury is suspected. The client is unresponsive, not breathing, and pulseless. The nurse prepares to open the client's airway with the use of which method?

1 Tilt the head and lift the chin.
2 Use the jaw-thrust maneuver.
3 Keep the client flat and grasp the tongue.
4 Lift the head up, put it on two pillows, and attempt to ventilate.

Answer: 2

Rationale: The appropriate way to open the airway in a client with a suspected neck injury is the jaw-thrust maneuver. This maneuver will prevent further injury if a neck injury is present. Options 1, 3, and 4 are incorrect actions.

Test-Taking Strategy: Use the process of elimination, and note the strategic words *neck injury is suspected.* Knowledge of airway management should assist you with eliminating options 3 and 4. From the remaining options, eliminate option 1 because this method will cause further damage to client with a neck injury. Review basic life support measures if you had difficulty with this question.

Level of Cognitive Ability: Application
Client Needs: Physiological Integrity
Integrated Process: Nursing Process/Implementation
Content Area: Fundamental Skills

References

deWit, S. (2009). *Medical-surgical nursing: Concepts & practice* (p. 93). St. Louis: Saunders.
Proehl, J. (2009). *Emergency nursing procedures* (4th ed., p. 10-12). St. Louis: Saunders.

1146. A nurse is caring for a child with Reye's syndrome. The nurse determines that a major symptom associated with Reye's syndrome is present when which of the following is noted?

1 Persistent vomiting
2 Protein in the urine
3 Symptoms of hyperglycemia
4 A history of a staphylococcal infection

Level of Cognitive Ability: Analysis
Client Needs: Physiological Integrity
Integrated Process: Nursing Process/Data Collection
Content Area: Child Health

Answer: 1

Rationale: Reye's syndrome is a combination of acute encephalopathy and fatty infiltration of the internal organs that may follow acute viral infections. Persistent vomiting is a major symptom associated with increased intracranial pressure (ICP). ICP and encephalopathy are major symptoms of Reye's syndrome. Options 2, 3, and 4 are incorrect. Protein is not present in the urine of clients with this condition. Reye's syndrome is related to a history of viral infections, and hypoglycemia is a symptom of this disease.

Test-Taking Strategy: Use the process of elimination, and recall that increased ICP is associated with Reye's syndrome; this will direct you to option 1. Review the symptoms of Reye's syndrome and the signs of increased ICP if you had difficulty with this question.

Reference

Price, D., & Gwin, J. (2008). *Pediatric nursing: An introductory text* (10th ed., p. 318). St. Louis: Saunders.

1147. A nurse is caring for an adolescent client with conjunctivitis and is planning to reinforce home-care instructions. Which instruction should the nurse include in the plan of care?

1 Replace contact lenses.
2 Apply hot compresses to lessen irritation.
3 Avoid using all eye makeup to prevent possible reinfection.
4 Stay home for 3 days after starting antibiotic eye drops to avoid the spread of infection.

Level of Cognitive Ability: Application
Client Needs: Physiological Integrity
Integrated Process: Teaching and Learning
Content Area: Child Health

Answer: 1

Rationale: Conjunctivitis is an inflammation of the conjunctiva that is caused by bacterial or viral infection, allergy, or environmental factors. All contact lenses should be replaced. Eye makeup should be replaced but can still be worn. Hot compresses are not used and can burn the eye and the surrounding skin. Cool compresses decrease pain and irritation. Isolation for 24 hours after antibiotics are initiated is necessary.

Test-Taking Strategy: Use the process of elimination. Eliminate option 3 because of the close-ended word *all*. Eliminate option 4 because 3 days is a lengthy period to remain isolated, particularly if antibiotics have been initiated. Select option 1 over option 2, knowing that cool (not hot) compresses decrease pain and irritation. Review home-care instructions for the client with conjunctivitis if you had difficulty with this question.

References

Lewis, S., Heitkemper, M., Dirksen, S., & Bucher, L. (2007). *Medical-surgical nursing: Assessment and management of clinical problems* (7th ed., p. 422). St. Louis: Mosby.
McKinney, E., James, S., Murray, S., & Ashwill, J (2009). *Maternal-child nursing* (3rd ed., p. 1563). St. Louis: Mosby.

1148. A child is admitted to the hospital with a suspected diagnosis of pneumococcal pneumonia. The nurse initially prepares:

Answer: 2

Rationale: A complication of pneumococcal pneumonia can be pleural effusion, so the respiratory status of the child should be

1 To start antibiotic therapy immediately
2 To monitor the child's respiratory rate and breath sounds
3 To allow the child to go to the playroom to play with other children
4 For a chest x-ray to be done to determine how much consolidation there is in the lungs

Level of Cognitive Ability: Application
Client Needs: Physiological Integrity
Integrated Process: Nursing Process/Implementation
Content Area: Child Health

monitored. Antibiotic therapy is not started until cultures are obtained. The child should not be allowed in the playroom at this time. Option 4 is part of medical management rather than nursing care.

Test-Taking Strategy: Use the process of elimination, and note the strategic word *initially.* Option 2 addresses data collection, which is the first step of the nursing process. This option addresses the ABCs—airway, breathing, and circulation, and it is also the option that is directly related to the child's diagnosis. Review the care of the client with pneumococcal pneumonia if you had difficulty with this question.

Reference
Leifer, G. (2007). *Introduction to maternity and pediatric nursing* (5th ed., pp. 578-579). Philadelphia: Saunders.

1149. A nurse is assigned to care for a client who is suspected of having bulimia. When collecting data from the client, the nurse is aware that a characteristic of bulimia is that the client:
1 Binge eats, then purges
2 Is accepting of body size
3 Overeats for the enjoyment of food
4 Overeats in response to losing control over a weight-loss diet

Level of Cognitive Ability: Comprehension
Client Needs: Physiological Integrity
Integrated Process: Nursing Process/Data Collection
Content Area: Mental Health

Answer: 1
Rationale: Bulimia is characterized by an insatiable craving for food that often results in episodes of continuous eating that are followed by purging, depression, and self-deprivation. Clients with this condition seldom attempt to diet and have no sense of loss of control. Options 2, 3, and 4 are true of the obese person who may binge eat.

Test-Taking Strategy: Use the process of elimination. Eliminate options 3 and 4 because they are comparable or alike. From the remaining options, recall the definition of bulimia to direct you to option 1. Review the characteristics of bulimia if you had difficulty with this question.

Reference
Varcarolis, E., & Halter, M. (2009). *Essentials of psychiatric mental health nursing: A communication approach to evidence-based care* (p. 199). St. Louis: Saunders.

1150. A nurse is caring for a client with angina who received nitroglycerin sublingually for chest pain. Which vital sign must the nurse monitor closely when administering nitroglycerin?
1 Heart rate
2 Respirations
3 Temperature
4 Blood pressure

Level of Cognitive Ability: Application
Client Needs: Physiological Integrity
Integrated Process: Nursing Process/Implementation
Content Area: Pharmacology

Answer: 4
Rationale: Nitroglycerin is a vasodilator that is used to increase coronary artery blood flow. The side effects of nitroglycerin include postural hypotension, flushing, headache, dizziness, and rash. Monitoring the client's blood pressure is most important at this time. Although the nurse may also monitor the client's heart rate, respirations, and temperature, these items are not directly related to the medication.

Test-Taking Strategy: Use the process of elimination. Recall that nitroglycerin is a vasodilator to direct you to option 4. Review the side effects of nitroglycerin if you had difficulty with this question.

Reference
Hodgson, B., & Kizior, R. (2009). *Saunders nursing drug handbook 2009* (p. 841). St. Louis: Saunders.

1151. A client who has experienced a brain attack (stroke) has partial hemiplegia of the left leg. The straight leg cane formerly used by the client is not quite sufficient now. The nurse determines that the client could benefit from the somewhat greater support and stability provided by a:

1 Quad cane
2 Wheelchair
3 Wooden crutch
4 Lofstrand crutch

Level of Cognitive Ability: Comprehension
Client Needs: Physiological Integrity
Integrated Process: Nursing Process/Planning
Content Area: Adult Health/Neurological

Answer: 1
Rationale: A quad cane may be used by the client who requires more support and stability than what is provided by a straight leg cane. The quad cane provides a four-point base of support and is indicated for use by clients with partial or complete hemiplegia. Crutches and wheelchairs are not indicated for use by a client such as the one described in the question. Lofstrand crutches are useful for clients with bilateral weakness.

Test-Taking Strategy: Use the process of elimination. Giving a wheelchair to a client with partial hemiplegia is excessive and should be eliminated first. Wooden crutches are not indicated because there is no restriction with regard to bearing weight. Lofstrand crutches are useful with bilateral weakness. Review each of these assistive devices if you had difficulty with this question.

Reference
Potter, P., & Perry, A. (2009). *Fundamentals of nursing* (7th ed., p. 803). St. Louis: Mosby.

1152. A nurse is caring for a client who has developed compartment syndrome from a severely fractured arm. The client asks the nurse how this happened. The nurse's response is based on the understanding that:

1 A bone fragment has injured the nerve supply in the area.
2 Bleeding and swelling cause increased pressure in an area that cannot expand.
3 An injured artery caused impaired arterial perfusion throughout the compartment.
4 The fascia expands with injury, thereby causing pressure on underlying nerves and muscles.

Level of Cognitive Ability: Comprehension
Client Needs: Physiological Integrity
Integrated Process: Nursing Process/Implementation
Content Area: Adult Health/Musculoskeletal

Answer: 2
Rationale: Compartment syndrome is caused by bleeding and swelling within a compartment that is lined by fascia and that does not expand. The bleeding and swelling put pressure on the nerves, muscles, and blood vessels in the compartment, which triggers the symptoms. Options 1, 3, and 4 are incorrect.

Test-Taking Strategy: Use the process of elimination. Option 3 should be eliminated first because compartment syndrome is not caused by an arterial injury. Knowing that the fascia itself cannot expand helps you to eliminate option 4. It is necessary to know that bleeding and swelling (not nerve injury) cause the symptoms of compartment syndrome. Review the cause of compartment syndrome if you had difficulty with this question.

Reference
Christensen, B., & Kockrow, E. (2006). *Adult health nursing* (5th ed., pp. 164-165). St. Louis: Mosby.

1153. A client has undergone fasciotomy to treat compartment syndrome of the leg. The nurse plans to provide which type of prescribed wound care to the fasciotomy site?

1 Dry, sterile dressings
2 Hydrocolloid dressings
3 Moist, sterile, saline dressings
4 Half-strength Betadine dressings

Answer: 3
Rationale: A fasciotomy is a surgical incision into an area of fascia. The fasciotomy site is not sutured; it is left open to relieve pressure and edema. The site is covered with moist (not dry), sterile, saline dressings. After 3 to 5 days, when perfusion is adequate and edema subsides, the wound is debrided and closed. A hydrocolloid dressing is not used with clean, open incisions. The incision is clean (not dirty), so there should be no reason to use Betadine.

Level of Cognitive Ability: Application
Client Needs: Physiological Integrity
Integrated Process: Nursing Process/Planning
Content Area: Adult Health/Musculoskeletal

Test-Taking Strategy: Use the process of elimination and your knowledge of the basics of wound care. Recall that with a fasciotomy, the skin is not sutured closed but rather left open for pressure relief. Moist tissue must remain moist, which eliminates option 1. A hydrocolloid dressing is not indicated for use with clean, open incisions, so option 2 can be eliminated. The incision is clean (not dirty), so there should be no reason to use Betadine, which can be irritating to normal tissues. This will direct you to option 3. Review care after a fasciotomy if you had difficulty with this question.

References

Ignatavicius, D., Workman, M. (2010). *Medical-surgical nursing: Patient-centered collaborative care* (6th ed., p. 1181). St. Louis: Saunders.
Linton, A. (2007). *Introduction to medical-surgical nursing* (4th ed., p. 917). Philadelphia: Saunders.

1154. A client has been diagnosed with myocardial infarction. The cardiac catheterization findings reveal 99% occlusion of the left anterior descending (LAD) coronary artery. What parts of the heart does the nurse expect to be affected?

1 Left atrium
2 Right ventricle
3 Left ventricle and septum
4 Right ventricle and septum

Answer: 3
Rationale: The LAD coronary artery perfuses most of the left ventricular muscle mass and the septum. Options 1, 2, and 4 are not affected by the LAD.

Test-Taking Strategy: Note the strategic word *left;* this will help you to eliminate options 2 and 4. For the remaining options, recall that the LAD perfuses the left ventricle. Review the anatomy of the coronary arteries if you had difficulty with this question.

References

Ignatavicius, D., Workman, M. (2010). *Medical-surgical nursing: Patient-centered collaborative care* (6th ed., pp. 706, 850). St. Louis: Saunders.
Linton, A. (2007). *Introduction to medical-surgical nursing* (4th ed., p. 628). Philadelphia: Saunders.

Level of Cognitive Ability: Comprehension
Client Needs: Physiological Integrity
Integrated Process: Nursing Process/Data Collection
Content Area: Fundamental Skills

1155. Which of the following is the appropriate method to use to administer eardrops to an infant?

1 Pull down and back on the auricle and direct the solution onto the eardrum.
2 Pull up and back on the earlobe and direct the solution toward the wall of the canal.
3 Pull down and back on the earlobe and direct the solution toward the wall of the canal.
4 Pull up and back on the auricle and direct the solution toward the wall of the ear canal.

Answer: 3
Rationale: The infant should be turned on his or her side, with the affected ear facing up. With the nondominant hand, the nurse pulls the earlobe down and back. The medication is administered by aiming it at the wall of the canal rather than directly onto the eardrum. The infant should be held or positioned with the affected ear up for 10 to 15 minutes so that the solution is retained. For an adult client, the ear is pulled up and back to straighten the auditory canal.

Test-Taking Strategy: Use the process of elimination, and note that the question addresses an infant. Eliminate option 1 because the solution should not be directed onto the eardrum. Visualize each of the remaining options. Option 4 is eliminated because it is the adult procedure. It would be difficult to pull up and back on an infant's earlobe; therefore option 2 can be eliminated. Review the procedure for administering ear medications to an infant if you had difficulty with this question.

Level of Cognitive Ability: Application
Client Needs: Physiological Integrity
Integrated Process: Nursing Process/Implementation
Content Area: Child Health

Reference
Price, D., & Gwin, J. (2008). *Pediatric nursing: An introductory text* (10th ed., p. 384). St. Louis: Saunders.

1156. A nurse is asked to assist the physician with the removal of a chest tube. The nurse plans to instruct the client to:
1 Hold the breath
2 Breathe in deeply
3 Breathe normally
4 Breathe out forcefully

Level of Cognitive Ability: Application
Client Needs: Physiological Integrity
Integrated Process: Nursing Process/Implementation
Content Area: Adult Health/Respiratory

Answer: 1
Rationale: When preparing for chest tube removal, the client is instructed in how to perform Valsalva's maneuver so that he or she can hold his or her breath and bear down as the physician removes the tube. This increases intrathoracic pressure, thereby lessening the potential for air to enter the pleural space. Options 2, 3, and 4 are incorrect.

Test-Taking Strategy: Use the process of elimination. Eliminate options 2 and 3 because they are comparable or alike in that breathing causes air to enter the pleural space. From the remaining options, eliminate option 4 because of the word *forcefully*. Review the procedure for the removal of a chest tube if you had difficulty with this question.

Reference
Perry, A., & Potter, P. (2010). *Clinical nursing skills & techniques* (7th ed., p. 715). St. Louis: Mosby.

1157. An older client who was recently admitted to the hospital with a hip fracture is placed in Buck's traction. The nurse assigned to care for the client should frequently monitor the client's:
1 Vital signs
2 Mental state
3 Neurovascular status
4 Ability to perform range-of-motion exercises

Level of Cognitive Ability: Application
Client Needs: Physiological Integrity
Integrated Process: Nursing Process/Implementation
Content Area: Adult Health/Musculoskeletal

Answer: 3
Rationale: Buck's traction is a type of skin traction. The neurovascular status of the extremity of the client in Buck's traction must be checked every 2 hours for the first 24 hours. Older clients are especially at risk for neurovascular compromise because many of these clients already have disorders that affect the peripheral vascular system. The client's physiological status (not the presence of Buck's traction) determines the frequency of the monitoring of the vital signs. Although clients in some types of traction do become depressed after a few days or weeks, Buck's traction is usually used preoperatively, typically for a few hours or 1 to 2 days at most. Range-of-motion exercises of the involved leg are contraindicated in clients with hip fractures.

Test-Taking Strategy: Use the process of elimination. Eliminate option 4 first because range-of-motion exercises are contraindicated in a client with hip fracture. From the remaining options, focus on the subject—Buck's traction; visualize this type of device. Although determining vital signs is the umbrella option, neurovascular status is specific to the use of traction and addresses the ABCs—airway, breathing, and circulation. Review nursing care of the client in traction if you had difficulty with this question.

References
deWit, S. (2009). *Medical-surgical nursing: Concepts & practice* (p. 793). St. Louis: Saunders.
Ignatavicius, D., & Workman, M. (2010). *Medical-surgical nursing: Patient-centered collaborative care* (6th ed., p. 1190). St. Louis: Saunders.

1158. A client who has a renal mass asks the nurse why an ultrasound has been scheduled as opposed to other diagnostic tests that may be ordered. The nurse

Answer: 3
Rationale: A significant advantage of an ultrasound is that it can differentiate a solid mass from a fluid-filled mass. It is noninvasive, and it does not require any special aftercare. There are other

formulates a response based on the understanding that:

1 All other tests are more invasive than an ultrasound.
2 All other tests require more elaborate postprocedural care.
3 An ultrasound can differentiate a solid mass from a fluid-filled cyst.
4 An ultrasound is much more cost effective than other diagnostic tests.

Level of Cognitive Ability: Comprehension
Client Needs: Physiological Integrity
Integrated Process: Nursing Process/Implementation
Content Area: Adult Health/Renal

diagnostic tests that are also noninvasive (unless contrast is used) and that also require no special aftercare. However, it is the ultrasound that can most optimally discriminate between solid and fluid-filled masses.

Test-Taking Strategy: Use the process of elimination. Eliminate options 1 and 2 first because of the close-ended word *all.* From the remaining options, recall that ultrasonography uses sound waves that are reflected back from tissues of different densities to direct you to option 3. Review the purpose of ultrasound if you had difficulty with this question.

References

Chernecky, C., & Berger, B. (2008). *Laboratory tests and diagnostic procedures* (5th ed., pp. 693-694). Philadelphia: Saunders.
deWit, S. (2009). *Medical-surgical nursing: Concepts & practice* (p. 823). St. Louis: Saunders.

1159. A client has been admitted to the hospital with acute glomerulonephritis. The nurse plans to collect data and initially asks the client about a recent history of:

1 Hypertension
2 Bleeding ulcer
3 Fungal infection
4 Streptococcal infection

Level of Cognitive Ability: Application
Client Needs: Physiological Integrity
Integrated Process: Nursing Process/Data Collection
Content Area: Adult Health/Renal

Answer: 4
Rationale: Acute glomerulonephritis is an acute inflammation of the glomerulus of the kidney that is characterized by proteinuria, hematuria, decreased urine production, and edema. The predominant cause of acute glomerulonephritis is infection with beta hemolytic streptococcus 3 weeks before the onset of symptoms. Other infectious agents besides bacteria that could trigger the disorder include viruses and parasites. Hypertension and bleeding ulcer are not precipitating causes.

Test-Taking Strategy: Use the process of elimination. Knowing that infection is a common trigger for glomerulonephritis helps you to eliminate options 1 and 2 first. From the remaining options, it is necessary to know that streptococcal infections are a common cause of this problem. Review the causes of glomerulonephritis if you had difficulty with this question.

Reference

Linton, A. (2007). *Introduction to medical-surgical nursing* (4th ed., p. 857). Philadelphia: Saunders.

1160. A nurse is caring for a client who is receiving bolus feedings via a nasogastric tube. As the nurse is finishing the feeding, the client asks for the head of the bed to be positioned flat so that she may sleep. Which position is the appropriate choice for this client at this time?

1 Head of bed flat with the client in the supine position for at least 30 minutes
2 Head of bed flat with the client in the supine position for at least 60 minutes
3 Head of bed in semi-Fowler's position with the client in the left lateral position for at least 60 minutes

Answer: 4
Rationale: Aspiration is a possible complication associated with a nasogastric tube feeding. The head of the bed is elevated 35 to 40 degrees for at least 30 minutes after a bolus tube feeding to prevent vomiting and aspiration. The right lateral position uses gravity to facilitate gastric retention to prevent vomiting. The flat supine position is avoided for the first 30 minutes after a tube feeding.

Test-Taking Strategy: Use the process of elimination. Eliminate options 1 and 2 first because a flat position places the client at risk for aspiration. From the remaining options, think about the anatomy of the gastrointestinal system. Option 3 and 4 indicate the same head elevation, but the right lateral position uses gravity to facilitate gastric retention to prevent vomiting. Review the care of the client after a nasogastric tube feeding if you had difficulty with this question.

4 Head of bed elevated 35 to 40 degrees with the client in the right lateral position for at least 30 minutes

Level of Cognitive Ability: Application
Client Needs: Physiological Integrity
Integrated Process: Nursing Process/Implementation
Content Area: Fundamental Skills

Reference

Linton, A. (2007). *Introduction to medical-surgical nursing* (4th ed., p. 740). Philadelphia: Saunders.

1161. A nurse is caring for a client with acute pancreatitis and a history of alcoholism. Which data would be a sign of paralytic ileus, which is a complication of acute pancreatitis?

1 Inability to pass flatus
2 Loss of anal sphincter control
3 Severe, constant pain with rapid onset
4 Firm, nontender mass palpable at the lower right costal margin

Level of Cognitive Ability: Comprehension
Client Needs: Physiological Integrity
Integrated Process: Nursing Process/Data Collection
Content Area: Adult Health/Gastrointestinal

Answer: 1

Rationale: An inflammatory reaction such as acute pancreatitis can cause paralytic ileus, which is the most common form of nonmechanical obstruction. The inability to pass flatus is a clinical manifestation of paralytic ileus. A loss of sphincter control is not a sign of paralytic ileus. Pain is associated with paralytic ileus, but the pain usually presents as a more constant generalized discomfort. Pain that is severe, constant, and rapid in onset is more likely caused by strangulation of the bowel. Option 4 is the description of the physical finding of liver enlargement. The liver is usually enlarged in cases of cirrhosis or hepatitis. Although this client may have an enlarged liver, that is not a sign of paralytic ileus or intestinal obstruction.

Test-Taking Strategy: Use the process of elimination, and focus on the subject—paralytic ileus. Recall the pathophysiology of this complication and note the word *paralytic* to direct you to option 1. Review the signs of paralytic ileus if you had difficulty with this question.

Reference

Christensen, B., & Kockrow, E. (2006). *Adult health nursing* (5th ed., p. 240). St. Louis: Mosby.

1162. After collecting data from a client with cholelithiasis, the nurse reports that the bowel sounds are normal. The nurse documents which description of normal bowel sounds?

1 Waves of loud gurgles auscultated in all four quadrants
2 Low-pitched swishing auscultated in one or two quadrants
3 Relatively high-pitched clicks or gurgles auscultated in all four quadrants
4 Very high-pitched loud rushes auscultated, especially in one or two quadrants

Level of Cognitive Ability: Application
Client Needs: Physiological Integrity
Integrated Process: Communication and Documentation
Content Area: Adult Health/Gastrointestinal

Answer: 3

Rationale: Although the frequency and intensity of bowel sounds vary depending on the phase of digestion, normal bowel sounds are relatively high-pitched clicks or gurgles. Loud gurgles (borborygmi) indicate hyperperistalsis. Bowel sounds are higher pitched and loud (hyperresonance) when the intestines are under tension (e.g., with intestinal obstruction). A swishing or buzzing sound represents turbulent blood flow that may be associated with a bruit.

Test-Taking Strategy: Use the process of elimination. Normal bowel sounds should be audible in all four quadrants, so options 2 and 4 can be eliminated. Focus on the subject—normal bowel sounds; this will direct you to option 3. Review the characteristics of bowel sounds if you had difficulty with this question.

References

Jarvis, C. (2008) *Physical examination and health assessment* (5th ed, p. 570). Philadelphia: Saunders.
Linton, A. (2007). *Introduction to medical-surgical nursing* (4th ed., p. 734). Philadelphia: Saunders.

1163. A nurse is assigned to care for a client with nephrotic syndrome. The nurse checks which most important parameter on a daily basis?
1 Weight
2 Albumin level
3 Activity tolerance
4 Blood urea nitrogen (BUN) level

Level of Cognitive Ability: Application
Client Needs: Physiological Integrity
Integrated Process: Nursing Process/Data Collection
Content Area: Adult Health/Renal

Answer: 1
Rationale: The client with nephrotic syndrome (an abnormal condition of the kidney) typically presents with edema, hypoalbuminemia, and proteinuria. The nurse carefully checks the fluid balance of the client, which includes the daily monitoring of weight, intake and output, edema, and girth measurements. Albumin, BUN, and creatinine levels are monitored as prescribed. The client's activity level is adjusted according to the amount of edema and water retention; the activity level should be restricted as edema increases.

Test-Taking Strategy: Use the process of elimination. Recall that the activity level is adjusted according to the volume of fluid retention to eliminate option 3. From the remaining options, recall that edema is a significant clinical manifestation, and note the word *daily* in the question; this will direct you to option 1. Review nursing interventions for the client with nephrotic syndrome if you had difficulty with this question.

Reference
Christensen, B., & Kockrow, E. (2006). *Adult health nursing* (5th ed., p. 499). St. Louis: Mosby.

1164. A client is being admitted to the nursing unit with urolithiasis and ureteral colic. The nurse checks the client for pain that is:
1 Dull and aching in the costovertebral area
2 Aching and cramp-like throughout the abdomen
3 Sharp and radiating posteriorly to the spinal column
4 Excruciating, wave-like, and radiating toward the genitalia

Level of Cognitive Ability: Comprehension
Client Needs: Physiological Integrity
Integrated Process: Nursing Process/Data Collection
Content Area: Adult Health/Renal

Answer: 4
Rationale: Urolithiasis is the presence of calculi in the urinary system, and ureteral colic is the pain that is associated with the presence of calculi. The pain of ureteral colic is caused by the movement of a stone through the ureter; it is sharp, excruciating, and wave-like pain that radiates to the genitalia and thigh. The stone causes a reduced flow of urine, and the urine also contains blood because of the stone's abrasive action on the urinary tract mucosa. Stones in the renal pelvis cause deep, aching pain in the costovertebral area. Renal colic is characterized by pain that is acute, with nausea, vomiting, and tenderness over the costovertebral area.

Test-Taking Strategy: Use the process of elimination. Begin to answer this question by eliminating option 2 because this pattern of pain is nonspecific and is the least likely to be the correct option. From the remaining options, recall the anatomical location of the kidneys and ureters. Because the kidneys are located in the posterior abdomen near the rib cage, pain in the costovertebral area is more likely to be associated with stones in the renal pelvis. Alternatively, sharp wave-like pain that radiates toward the genitalia is more consistent with the location of the ureters. Review the characteristics of the pain associated with urolithiasis and ureteral colic if you had difficulty with this question.

References
Christensen, B., & Kockrow, E. (2006). *Adult health nursing* (5th ed., p. 490). St. Louis: Mosby.
Linton, A. (2007). *Introduction to medical-surgical nursing* (4th ed., p. 858). Philadelphia: Saunders.

1165. A nurse is collecting data from a client with left-sided heart failure. The client states that it is necessary to use three pillows under the head and chest at night to be able to breathe comfortably while sleeping. The nurse documents that the client is experiencing:

1 Orthopnea
2 Dyspnea at rest
3 Dyspnea on exertion
4 Paroxysmal nocturnal dyspnea

Level of Cognitive Ability: Comprehension
Client Needs: Physiological Integrity
Integrated Process: Communication and Documentation
Content Area: Adult Health/Cardiovascular

Answer: 1

Rationale: Dyspnea is a subjective problem that can range from an awareness of breathing to physical distress; it does not necessarily correlate with the degree of heart failure. Dyspnea can be exertional, or it may occur when the client is at rest. Orthopnea is a more severe form of dyspnea that requires the client to use pillows to support the head and thorax at night. Paroxysmal nocturnal dyspnea is a severe form of dyspnea that occurs suddenly at night because of rapid fluid reentry into the vasculature from the interstitium during sleep.

Test-Taking Strategy: Use the process of elimination. Eliminate options 3 and 4 because the question mentions nothing about exertion or a sudden (paroxysmal) event. Select option 1 instead of 2 because the client is breathing comfortably with the use of pillows. Review the characteristics associated with orthopnea if you had difficulty with this question.

References

Christensen, B., & Kockrow, E. (2006). *Foundations of nursing* (5th ed., p. 56). St. Louis: Mosby.
deWit, S. (2009). *Medical-surgical nursing: Concepts & practice* (p. 293). St. Louis: Saunders.

1166. A client with renal cancer is being treated preoperatively with radiation therapy. The nurse determines that the client has an understanding of the proper care of the skin over the treatment field if the client states to:

1 Avoid skin exposure to direct sunlight and chlorinated water.
2 Use lanolin-based cream on the affected skin on a daily basis.
3 Use the hottest water possible to wash the treatment site twice daily.
4 Remove the lines or ink marks using a gentle soap after each treatment.

Level of Cognitive Ability: Comprehension
Client Needs: Physiological Integrity
Integrated Process: Nursing Process/Evaluation
Content Area: Adult Health/Oncology

Answer: 1

Rationale: The client undergoing radiation therapy should avoid washing the site until instructed to do so. At that time, the client should wash using mild soap and warm or cool water and then pat the area dry. No lotions, creams, alcohol, or deodorants should be placed on the skin over the treatment site. Lines or ink marks that are placed on the skin to guide the radiation therapy should be left in place. The affected skin should be protected from temperature extremes, direct sunlight, and chlorinated water (e.g., swimming pools).

Test-Taking Strategy: Use the process of elimination. Eliminate options 2 and 3 because of the words *lanolin* and *hottest*, respectively, in these options. Recall that the markings used to guide therapy are to be left in place to help you to choose option 1 instead of option 4. Review skin care for the client who is receiving radiation therapy if you had difficulty with this question.

Reference

deWit, S. (2009). *Medical-surgical nursing: Concepts & practice* (p. 173). St. Louis: Saunders.

1167. Which of the following sites is best for checking the pulse during the cardiopulmonary resuscitation (CPR) of a 6-month-old infant?

1 Radial
2 Carotid
3 Femoral
4 Brachial

Answer: 4

Rationale: The carotid is the most central and accessible artery in children who are older than 1 year. However, the very short and often flat neck of the infant renders the carotid pulse difficult to palpate. In these children, it is preferable to use the brachial pulse, which is located on the inner side of the upper arm midway between the elbow and the shoulder. The radial and femoral pulses are also difficult to palpate in an infant.

Level of Cognitive Ability: Comprehension
Client Needs: Physiological Integrity
Integrated Process: Nursing Process/Data Collection
Content Area: Child Health

Test-Taking Strategy: Use the process of elimination, and focus on the age of the infant. Recall the principles related to CPR, and visualize the anatomical location of the pulses identified in the options; this will direct you to option 4. Review the principles of CPR if you had difficulty with this question.

Reference

Hockenberry, M., & Wilson, D. (2009). *Wrong's essentials of pediatric nursing* (8th ed., p. 806). St. Louis: Mosby.

1168. A client with renal failure is receiving epoetin alfa (Epogen) to support erythropoiesis. The nurse questions the client about compliance with taking which medication, which supports red blood cell (RBC) production?

1 Iron supplement
2 Zinc supplement
3 Calcium supplement
4 Magnesium supplement

Level of Cognitive Ability: Application
Client Needs: Physiological Integrity
Integrated Process: Nursing Process/Data Collection
Content Area: Adult Health/Renal

Answer: 1

Rationale: Epoetin alfa (Epogen) induces erythropoiesis. Iron is needed for RBC production; otherwise, the body cannot produce sufficient erythrocytes. The client is not receiving the full benefit of the therapy with epoetin alfa if iron is not taken. The medications in options 2, 3, and 4 do not support RBC production.

Test-Taking Strategy: Use the process of elimination. Note the relationship of the words *RBC production* in the question with the word *iron* in the correct option. Review the concepts related to epoetin alfa and RBC production if you had difficulty with this question.

Reference

Hodgson, B., & Kizior, R. (2009). *Saunders nursing drug handbook 2009* (pp. 423-425). St. Louis: Saunders.

1169. A client who just underwent tonsillectomy has become restless. The nurse notes an increasing pulse rate, slight pallor, and frequent swallowing. The nurse interprets that:

1 The client needs pain medication.
2 This is an expected postoperative finding.
3 The client most likely has some mild postoperative edema.
4 The client may have postoperative bleeding or hemorrhage.

Level of Cognitive Ability: Analysis
Client Needs: Physiological Integrity
Integrated Process: Nursing Process/Evaluation
Content Area: Adult Health/Respiratory

Answer: 4

Rationale: A tonsillectomy is the surgical excision of the palatine tonsils. Signs of postoperative hemorrhage include pallor, restlessness, frequent swallowing, large amounts of bloody drainage or vomitus, increasing pulse rate, and a falling blood pressure. These signs should be reported to the surgeon. Although some of the signs and symptoms exhibited by the client could also result from pain (e.g., restlessness, increasing pulse), the presence of the others indicates bleeding.

Test-Taking Strategy: Use the process of elimination. Recall the concepts related to hemorrhage and shock and focus on the signs presented in the question to direct you to option 4. Review postoperative complications after tonsillectomy if you had difficulty with this question.

Reference

Linton, A. (2007). *Introduction to medical-surgical nursing* (4th ed., p. 1225). Philadelphia: Saunders.

1170. A nurse is reviewing the results of a sweat test performed on a child with cystic fibrosis (CF). The nurse should expect to note which of the following?

Answer: 3

Rationale: CF is an inherited autosomal-recessive disorder of the exocrine glands that causes these glands to produce abnormally thick secretions of mucus, an elevation of sweat electrolytes, increased organic and enzymatic constituents of saliva, and an

1 A sweat potassium concentration of less than 40 mEq/L
2 A sweat potassium concentration of less than 60 mEq/L
3 A sweat chloride concentration of greater than 60 mEq/L
4 A sweat bicarbonate concentration of less than 40 mEq/L

Level of Cognitive Ability: Comprehension
Client Needs: Physiological Integrity
Integrated Process: Nursing Process/Data Collection
Content Area: Child Health

overactivity of the autonomic nervous system. The consistent finding of abnormally high chloride concentrations in the sweat is a unique characteristic of CF. Normally the sweat chloride concentration is less than 40 mEq/L. A chloride concentration of greater than 60 mEq/L is diagnostic of CF. Bicarbonate and potassium concentrations are unrelated to the sweat test.

Test-Taking Strategy: Use the process of elimination. Eliminate options 1, 2, and 4 because the bicarbonate and potassium levels are unrelated to the sweat test. In addition, note that option 3 is different in that it indicates a "greater than" value. Review the sweat test if you had difficulty with this question.

Reference

Price, D., & Gwin, J. (2008). *Pediatric nursing: An introductory text* (10th ed., p. 153). St. Louis: Saunders.

1171. A nurse performs a neurovascular check on a client with a newly applied cast. Close observation and further evaluation will be necessary if the nurse notes:
1 Capillary refill of 6 seconds
2 Palpable pulses distal to the cast
3 Blanching of the nail bed when depressed
4 Sensation when the area distal to the cast is pinched

Level of Cognitive Ability: Comprehension
Client Needs: Physiological Integrity
Integrated Process: Nursing Process/Data Collection
Content Area: Adult Health/Neurological

Answer: 1

Rationale: To check for adequate circulation (capillary refill), the nail bed of each finger or toe is depressed until it blanches and then the pressure is released. Optimally, the color will change from white to pink rapidly (less than 3 seconds). If this does not occur, the toes or fingers require close observation and further evaluation. Palpable pulses and sensations distal to the cast are expected. However, the physician must be notified if pulses cannot be palpated or the client complains of numbness or tingling.

Test-Taking Strategy: Use the process of elimination, and note the strategic words *close observation and further evaluation.* Eliminate options 2, 3, and 4 because these options identify normal and expected findings. Option 1 identifies an abnormal or unexpected finding. Review the technique for checking capillary refill if you had difficulty with this question.

Reference

Jarvis, C. (2008) *Physical examination and health assessment* (5th ed., pp. 237, 537). Philadelphia: Saunders.

1172. A client undergoes a cholecystectomy and returns from surgery with a T tube in place. The nurse is assigned to assist with caring for the client and is instructed to monitor the drainage from the T tube. During the first 24 hours after surgery, the nurse expects how much bile to drain from the T tube?
1 50 mL
2 100 mL
3 500 mL
4 1500 mL

Level of Cognitive Ability: Comprehension
Client Needs: Physiological Integrity
Integrated Process: Nursing Process/Evaluation
Content Area: Adult Health/Gastrointestinal

Answer: 3

Rationale: A cholecystectomy is the removal of the gall bladder. During the initial postoperative period, bloody drainage is expected; this will then become greenish-brown bile. Bile output is approximately 400 to 500 mL a day, with a gradual decrease in amount. Bile drainage amounts in excess of 1000 mL a day should be reported to the physician.

Test-Taking Strategy: Use the process of elimination, and note the strategic words *during the first 24 hours.* This provides you with a clue that the output will be on the higher side, so options 1 and 2 can be eliminated. Visualize the amounts identified in the remaining options. Option 4 identifies an excessive amount and should be eliminated. Review postoperative expectations after cholecystectomy if you had difficulty with this question.

References

Christensen, B., & Kockrow, E. (2006). *Adult health nursing* (5th ed., p. 276). St. Louis: Mosby.

Linton, A. (2007). *Introduction to medical-surgical nursing* (4th ed., p. 821). Philadelphia: Saunders.

1173. A client with diabetes mellitus receives 8 units of humulin regular insulin subcutaneously at 7:30 AM. The nurse would be most alert for signs of hypoglycemia at what time of the day?

1 1:30 PM to 3:30 PM
2 3:30 PM to 5:30 PM
3 11:30 AM to 1:30 PM
4 9:30 AM to 11:30 AM

Level of Cognitive Ability: Analysis
Client Needs: Physiological Integrity
Integrated Process: Nursing Process/Data Collection
Content Area: Pharmacology

Answer: 4

Rationale: Humulin regular insulin is a short-acting insulin. Its onset of action occurs after half an hour, and it peaks in 2 to 4 hours. Its duration of action is 4 to 6 hours. A hypoglycemic reaction will most likely occur at peak time, which, in this situation, would be between 9:30 AM and 11:30 AM.

Test-Taking Strategy: Use the process of elimination. Recall that regular insulin is a short-acting insulin to direct you to option 4. Review both NPH and regular insulin if you had difficulty with this question.

Reference

Hodgson, B., & Kizior, R. (2009). *Saunders nursing drug handbook 2009* (p. 612). St. Louis: Saunders.

1174. A nurse is assisting with collecting assessment data from a newborn who is suspected of having Down syndrome. When checking the newborn's skin, which of the following does the nurse expect to note if this syndrome is present?

1 A single crease across the palm
2 Two large creases across the palm
3 Several creases noted across the palm
4 The absence of creases across the palm

Level of Cognitive Ability: Comprehension
Client Needs: Physiological Integrity
Integrated Process: Nursing Process/Data Collection
Content Area: Maternity/Postpartum

Answer: 1

Rationale: Down syndrome is a congenital condition characterized by varying degrees of mental retardation and multiple defects. A single crease across the palm (simian crease) is often associated with chromosomal abnormalities, most notably Down syndrome. Options 2, 3, and 4 are not associated with Down syndrome.

Test-Taking Strategy: Knowledge of the characteristics associated with Down syndrome is needed to answer this question. Remember that a single crease across the palm (simian crease) is often associated with chromosomal abnormalities, most notably Down syndrome. Review the characteristics of Down syndrome if you had difficulty with this question.

Reference

Price, D., & Gwin, J. (2008). *Pediatric nursing: An introductory text* (10th ed., p. 110). St. Louis: Saunders.

1175. A nurse is caring for a client who was admitted to the surgical nursing unit after a right modified radical mastectomy. The nurse should include which intervention when caring for this client?

1 Take blood pressures in the right arm only.
2 Have serum laboratory samples drawn from the right arm only.
3 Position the client supine with the right arm elevated on a pillow.

Answer: 4

Rationale: If there is drainage or bleeding from the surgical site after mastectomy, gravity causes the drainage to seep down and soak the posterior axillary portion of the dressing first. The nurse should check this area to detect early bleeding. The client should be positioned with the head in semi-Fowler's position and the arm elevated on pillows to decrease edema. Edema is likely to occur because lymph drainage channels have been resected during the surgical procedure. Blood pressure, venipunctures, and intravenous sites should not involve the use of the operative arm.

4 Check the right posterior axilla area when checking the surgical dressing.

Level of Cognitive Ability: Application
Client Needs: Physiological Integrity
Integrated Process: Nursing Process/Implementation
Content Area: Adult Health/Oncology

Test-Taking Strategy: Use the process of elimination. Eliminate options 1 and 2 first because they are comparable or alike, and note the close-ended word *only* in these options. From the remaining options, use your knowledge of the effects of gravity to direct you to option 4. Review the care of the client after a modified radical mastectomy if you had difficulty with this question.

Reference

Black, J., & Hawks, J. (2009). *Medical-surgical nursing: Clinical management for positive outcomes* (8th ed., pp. 956-957). St. Louis: Saunders.

1176. A client is at risk for infection after a radical vulvectomy. The nurse avoids doing which of the following when providing perineal care to this client?

1 Intermittently exposing the wound to air
2 Providing prescribed sitz baths after the sutures are removed
3 Providing perineal care after each voiding and bowel movement
4 Cleansing the perineum using warm tap water and a bulb syringe

Level of Cognitive Ability: Application
Client Needs: Physiological Integrity
Integrated Process: Nursing Process/Implementation
Content Area: Adult Health/Oncology

Answer: 4

Rationale: A vulvectomy is the surgical removal of part or all of the tissues of the vulva. A sterile solution (e.g., normal saline) should be used for perineal care with the use of an aseptic syringe; this should be done regularly twice a day and after each voiding and bowel movement. The wound is intermittently exposed to air to permit drying and to prevent maceration. After the sutures are removed, sitz baths may be prescribed to stimulate healing and to soothe the area.

Test-Taking Strategy: Use the process of elimination, and note the strategic word *avoids*. This word indicates a negative event query and asks you to select an option that is an incorrect action. Eliminate options 2 and 3 first because these are accepted practices. From the remaining options, note the words *tap water* in option 4. Knowledge of principles of asepsis and of the conditions that cause a wound infection directs you to option 4. Review the principles of asepsis and of the prevention of wound infections if you had difficulty with this question.

References

Ignatavicius, D., Workman, M. (2010). *Medical-surgical nursing: Patient-centered collaborative care* (6th ed., p. 1707-1708). St. Louis: Saunders.
Lewis, S., Heitkemper, M., Dirksen, S., & Bucher, L. (2007). *Medical-surgical nursing: Assessment and management of clinical problems* (7th ed., pp. 1406-1407). St. Louis: Mosby.

1177. A nurse is assisting a client with hepatic encephalopathy with filling out the dietary menu. The nurse advises the client to avoid which entree item, which could aggravate the client's condition?

1 Tomatoes
2 Fresh fruit plate
3 Vegetable lasagna
4 Ground beef patty

Level of Cognitive Ability: Application
Client Needs: Physiological Integrity
Integrated Process: Nursing Process/Implementation
Content Area: Adult Health/Gastrointestinal

Answer: 4

Rationale: Clients with hepatic encephalopathy have an impaired ability to convert ammonia into urea and therefore must limit the intake of protein and ammonia-containing foods in the diet. The client should avoid foods such as chicken, beef, ham, cheese, buttermilk, peanut butter, and gelatin.

Test-Taking Strategy: Use the process of elimination. Recall that clients with hepatic encephalopathy must limit the intake of protein to direct you to option 4. Note that options 1, 2, and 3 are comparable or alike in that they address food items of a fruit or vegetable nature. Option 4 is the option that is different. Review dietary measures for the client with hepatic encephalopathy if you had difficulty with this question.

Reference
Christensen, B., & Kockrow, E. (2006). *Adult health nursing* (5th ed., p. 261). St. Louis: Mosby.

1178. A client with a colostomy is complaining of gas building up in the colostomy bag. The nurse tells the client that which food item is least likely to aggravate this problem?
1 Corn
2 Beans
3 Potatoes
4 Cauliflower

Level of Cognitive Ability: Application
Client Needs: Physiological Integrity
Integrated Process: Nursing Process/ Implementation
Content Area: Adult Health/Gastrointestinal

Answer: 3
Rationale: Gas-forming foods include corn, cauliflower, onions, beans, and cabbage. These should be avoided by the client with a colostomy until tolerance to them is determined. Potatoes are not a gas-forming food.

Test-Taking Strategy: Use the process of elimination, and note the strategic words *least likely to aggravate.* Use your knowledge of the basic principles of nutrition, and focus on the subject—gas-forming foods. This will direct you to option 3. Review gas-forming food items if you had difficulty with this question.

Reference
Black, J., & Hawks, J. (2009). *Medical-surgical nursing: Clinical management for positive outcomes* (8th ed., p. 709). St. Louis: Saunders.

1179. A client admitted to the hospital with a diagnosis of cirrhosis has massive ascites and difficulty breathing. The nurse performs which intervention as a priority measure to assist the client with breathing?
1 Elevating the head of the client's bed
2 Encouraging deep breathing every 2 hours
3 Checking the client's respirations every 4 hours
4 Repositioning the client from one side to the other every 2 hours

Level of Cognitive Ability: Application
Client Needs: Physiological Integrity
Integrated Process: Nursing Process/ Implementation
Content Area: Adult Health/Gastrointestinal

Answer: 1
Rationale: Ascites is the abnormal intraperitoneal accumulation of a fluid that contains large amounts of protein and electrolytes. The client is having difficulty breathing because of upward pressure on the diaphragm from the ascitic fluid. Elevating the head of the bed enlists the aid of gravity in relieving pressure on the diaphragm. The other options are appropriate general measures for the client with ascites, but the priority measure is the one that relieves diaphragmatic pressure.

Test-Taking Strategy: Use the process of elimination, and note the strategic words *priority measure.* These words tells you that more than one or all of the options may be partially or totally correct. In this case, every option is a correct nursing action, but elevating the head of the bed takes highest priority for providing immediate relief of the client's symptoms. Review the care of the client with ascites if you had difficulty with this question.

Reference
Christensen, B., & Kockrow, E. (2006). *Adult health nursing* (5th ed., p. 260). St. Louis: Mosby.

1180. The nurse teaches a client with asymptomatic diverticulitis to consume which type of diet?
1 High in protein
2 Moderate in fat
3 High in carbohydrates
4 Soft foods high in fiber

Level of Cognitive Ability: Application
Client Needs: Physiological Integrity

Answer: 4
Rationale: Diverticulitis is the inflammation of one or more diverticula in the colon. With asymptomatic diverticulitis, the goal is to prevent constipation, and the client is taught to consume soft foods that are high in fiber. The client should avoid foods such as nuts, corn, popcorn, and raw celery because these substance can become trapped in the diverticula and cause pain and inflammation. Although it is acceptable for the client to consume protein, fats, and carbohydrates, it is not necessary that the diet be high in protein or carbohydrates or moderate in fat.

Integrated Process: Nursing Process/Implementation
Content Area: Adult Health/Gastrointestinal

Test-Taking Strategy: Use the process of elimination, and note the word *asymptomatic*. Recalling that preventing constipation is the goal will direct you to option 4. Review the diet prescribed for diverticulitis if you had difficulty with this question.

References

Black, J., & Hawks, J. (2009). *Medical-surgical nursing: Clinical management for positive outcomes* (8th ed., p. 761). St. Louis: Saunders.
deWit, S. (2009). *Medical-surgical nursing: Concepts & practice* (p. 715). St. Louis: Saunders.

1181. A nurse caring for a client with hepatic encephalopathy checks the client for asterixis. To appropriately check for asterixis, the nurse:

1 Checks the stools for clay-colored pigmentation
2 Asks the client to sign something and notes any difficulty with writing
3 Reviews serum levels of bilirubin and alkaline phosphatase for elevation
4 Asks the client to extend an arm, dorsiflex the wrist, and extend the fingers

Level of Cognitive Ability: Application
Client Needs: Physiological Integrity
Integrated Process: Nursing Process/Data Collection
Content Area: Adult Health/Gastrointestinal

Answer: 4
Rationale: Asterixis is an abnormal muscle tremor that is often associated with hepatic encephalopathy. The nurse asks the client to extend an arm, dorsiflex the wrist, and extend the fingers. The nurse then checks for muscle tremors. Asterixis is sometimes also called "liver flap." Options 1, 2, and 3 are associated interventions in the care of a client with hepatitis, but they are not signs of asterixis.

Test-Taking Strategy: Focus on the subject—checking for asterixis. Recall that asterixis is an abnormal muscle tremor to direct you to option 4. Review the technique for testing for asterixis if you had difficulty with this question.

Reference

deWit, S. (2009). *Medical-surgical nursing: Concepts & practice* (p. 757). St. Louis: Saunders.

1182. A nurse instructs a preoperative client regarding the proper use of an incentive spirometer. During the postoperative period, the nurse determines that use of the incentive spirometer was effective if the client exhibits:

1 Coughing
2 Shallow breaths
3 Audible wheezing
4 Unilateral chest expansion

Level of Cognitive Ability: Comprehension
Client Needs: Physiological Integrity
Integrated Process: Nursing Process/Evaluation
Content Area: Fundamental Skills

Answer: 1
Rationale: Incentive devices have many desired and positive effects, such as providing the stimulus for a spontaneous deep breath. With the use of the sustained maximal inspiration concept, spontaneous deep breathing reduces atelectasis, opens airways, stimulates coughing, and actively encourages an individual's participation in recovery. Shallow breaths, wheezing, and unilateral chest expansion indicate that the incentive spirometry was not effective. Wheezing indicates a narrowing or obstruction of the airway, and unilateral chest expansion could indicate atelectasis.

Test-Taking Strategy: Use the process of elimination, and focus on the subject—the effectiveness of the incentive spirometer. Options 2, 3, and 4 indicate abnormal findings and so can be eliminated. Review the purpose of an incentive spirometer if you had difficulty with this question.

Reference

deWit, S. (2009). *Medical-surgical nursing: Concepts & practice* (p. 79). St. Louis: Saunders.

1183. A nurse is caring for a client who was admitted to the hospital with a diagnosis of angina. While the nurse is caring for the client, the client begins to experience chest pain. Which of the following data should be obtained by the nurse immediately?

1 Blood pressure
2 Presence of a fever
3 Symptoms of nausea
4 Location and intensity of pain

Level of Cognitive Ability: Application
Client Needs: Physiological Integrity
Integrated Process: Nursing Process/Data Collection
Content Area: Delegating/Prioritizing

Answer: 4
Rationale: If a client experiences chest pain, the nurse must assess the pain by requesting a description of pain intensity, location, duration, and quality. The assessment of the pain is the priority, although the nurse may check the client's vital signs and for symptoms of nausea.

Test-Taking Strategy: Note the strategic word *immediately.* Focus on the subject of the question, and note the relationship between the subject and option 4. Review the immediate care of the client who is experiencing chest pain if you had difficulty with this question.

References
Christensen, B., & Kockrow, E. (2006). *Adult health nursing* (5th ed., pp. 346-347). St. Louis: Mosby.
Linton, A. (2007). *Introduction to medical-surgical nursing* (4th ed., pp. 653-654). Philadelphia: Saunders.

1184. A client is to be started on prazosin (Minipress), and the client asks the nurse why the first three doses must be taken at bedtime. The nurse's response is based on the understanding that, during early use, prazosin:

1 Results in extreme drowsiness
2 Can cause significant dependent edema
3 Should be taken when the stomach is empty
4 Can cause dizziness, lightheadedness, or possible syncope

Level of Cognitive Ability: Comprehension
Client Needs: Physiological Integrity
Integrated Process: Nursing Process/Implementation
Content Area: Pharmacology

Answer: 4
Rationale: Prazosin (Minipress) is an α-adrenergic blocking agent. First-dose hypotensive reaction may occur during early therapy; this is characterized by dizziness, lightheadedness, and possible syncope, and it can also occur during periods when the dosage is increased. The effect usually disappears with continued use or when the dosage is decreased. Options 1, 2, and 3 are incorrect.

Test-Taking Strategy: Focus on the name of the medication. Recall that prazosin (Minipress) is an antihypertensive agent to direct you to option 4. Remember that orthostatic hypotension, which causes dizziness, lightheadedness, and possible syncope, can occur with the use of antihypertensives. Review prazosin if you had difficulty with this question.

Reference
Hodgson, B., & Kizior, R. (2009). *Saunders nursing drug handbook 2009* (p. 949). St. Louis: Saunders.

1185. A nurse has applied the prescribed dressing to the leg of a client with an ischemic arterial leg ulcer. The nurse uses which of the following methods of covering the dressing?

1 Apply a Kling roll, and tape it to the skin.
2 Apply a sterile pad, and tape it to the skin.
3 Apply small Montgomery straps, and tie the edges together.
4 Apply a Kling roll, and tape the edge of the roll onto the bandage.

Level of Cognitive Ability: Application
Client Needs: Physiological Integrity

Answer: 4
Rationale: With an arterial ulcer, the nurse applies tape only to the bandage itself. Tape is never used directly on the skin because it could cause further tissue damage. For the same reason, Montgomery straps are not applied to the skin (although these are generally intended for use on abdominal wounds). Standard dressing technique includes the use of Kling rolls on circumferential dressings.

Test-Taking Strategy: Use the process of elimination. Recall that tape is not applied to the skin to assist you with eliminating options 1 and 2. For the same reason, eliminate option 3 because the Montgomery straps also must adhere to the skin. Review the care of the client with an arterial ulcer if you had difficulty with this question.

Integrated Process: Nursing Process/Implementation
Content Area: Adult Health/Cardiovascular

References
Black, J., & Hawks, J. (2009). *Medical-surgical nursing: Clinical management for positive outcomes* (8th ed., p. 1325). St. Louis: Saunders.
Ignatavicius, D., & Workman, M. (2010). *Medical-surgical nursing: Patient-centered collaborative care* (6th ed., p. 493). St. Louis: Saunders.

1186. Breathing exercises and postural drainage are ordered for a child with cystic fibrosis (CF). The appropriate plan to implement these procedures includes which of the following?

1 Perform the postural drainage and then the breathing exercises
2 Perform the breathing exercises and then the postural drainage
3 Perform the postural drainage in the morning and the breathing exercises in the evening
4 Plan the breathing exercises and the postural drainage so that they are scheduled 4 hours apart

Level of Cognitive Ability: Application
Client Needs: Physiological Integrity
Integrated Process: Nursing Process/Planning
Content Area: Child Health

Answer: 1
Rationale: CF is an inherited autosomal-recessive disorder of the exocrine glands that causes these glands to produce abnormally thick secretions of mucus, an elevation of sweat electrolytes, increased organic and enzymatic constituents of saliva, and the overactivity of the autonomic nervous system. Breathing exercises are recommended for the majority of children with CF, even for those with minimal pulmonary involvement. The exercises are usually performed twice daily, and they are preceded with postural drainage. The postural drainage mobilizes secretions, and the breathing exercises then assist with expectoration. Exercises to assist with posture and to mobilize the thorax are included (e.g., swinging the arms, bending and twisting the trunk). The ultimate aim of these exercises is to establish a good habitual breathing pattern. Options 2, 3, and 4 are incorrect.

Test-Taking Strategy: Use the process of elimination. Recall that postural drainage and breathing exercises are most effective when performed together to assist you with eliminating options 3 and 4. From the remaining options, consider the effectiveness that each procedure will have on the mobilization of secretions to direct you to option 1. Review the effects of postural drainage and breathing exercises if you had difficulty with this question.

References
Leifer, G. (2007). *Introduction to maternity and pediatric nursing* (5th ed., p. 589). Philadelphia: Saunders.
Price, D., & Gwin, J. (2008). *Pediatric nursing: An introductory text* (10th ed., p. 157). St. Louis: Saunders.

1187. A child is admitted to the pediatric unit with a diagnosis of celiac disease. Based on this diagnosis, the nurse expects that the child's stools will be:

1 Dark in color
2 Unusually hard
3 Abnormally small in amount
4 Particularly offensive in odor

Level of Cognitive Ability: Comprehension
Client Needs: Physiological Integrity
Integrated Process: Nursing Process/Data Collection
Content Area: Child Health

Answer: 4
Rationale: Celiac disease is an inborn error of metabolism that is characterized by the inability to hydrolyze the peptides that are contained in gluten. The stools of a child with celiac disease are characteristically malodorous, pale, large (bulky), and soft (loose). Excessive flatus is common, and bouts of diarrhea may occur. Options 1, 2, and 3 are not characteristics of this disorder.

Test-Taking Strategy: Knowledge of the manifestations of celiac disease is necessary to answer this question. Remember that the stools of a child with celiac disease are characteristically malodorous, pale, large (bulky), and soft (loose). Review these manifestations if you had difficulty with this question.

Reference
Price, D., & Gwin, J. (2008). *Pediatric nursing: An introductory text* (10th ed., p. 250). St. Louis: Saunders.

1188. A nurse is caring for a client who is comatose. The nurse notes in the chart that the client is exhibiting decerebrate posturing. The nurse monitors the client, knowing that decerebrate posturing can best be described as:

1 The flexion of the extremities after a stimulus
2 The extension of the extremities after a stimulus
3 Upper-extremity flexion with lower-extremity extension
4 Upper-extremity extension with lower-extremity flexion

Level of Cognitive Ability: Comprehension
Client Needs: Physiological Integrity
Integrated Process: Nursing Process/Data Collection
Content Area: Adult Health/Neurological

Answer: 2
Rationale: Decerebrate posturing, which can occur with upper brainstem injury, is the extension of the extremities after a stimulus. Options 1, 3, and 4 are incorrect descriptions.

Test-Taking Strategy: Use the process of elimination. Remember that decerebrate also is known as extension to direct you to option 2. Review posturing and its relationship to neurological disorders if you had difficulty with this question.

Reference
Linton, A. (2007). *Introduction to medical-surgical nursing* (4th ed., p. 433). Philadelphia: Saunders.

1189. A client who undergoes a gastric resection is at risk for developing dumping syndrome. The nurse monitors for which of the following that is a symptom of this syndrome?

1 Dizziness
2 Bradycardia
3 Constipation
4 Extreme thirst

Level of Cognitive Ability: Application
Client Needs: Physiological Integrity
Integrated Process: Nursing Process/Data Collection
Content Area: Adult Health/Gastrointestinal

Answer: 1
Rationale: Dumping syndrome is experienced by clients who have undergone a subtotal gastrectomy. The clinical manifestations of dumping syndrome occur 5 to 30 minutes after eating. Symptoms include vasomotor disturbances (e.g., vertigo), tachycardia, syncope, sweating, pallor, palpations, and the desire to lie down. Options 2, 3, and 4 are not associated with dumping syndrome.

Test-Taking Strategy: Use the process of elimination. Recall that the symptoms associated with dumping syndrome are vasomotor in nature to direct you to option 1. Review dumping syndrome and the appropriate treatment measures if you had difficulty with this question.

Reference
Linton, A. (2007). *Introduction to medical-surgical nursing* (4th ed., p. 742). Philadelphia: Saunders.

1190. When assessing a client for the major postoperative complication after a craniotomy, the nurse monitors for:

1 Bleeding
2 Tachycardia
3 Hypotension
4 Restlessness

Level of Cognitive Ability: Analysis
Client Needs: Physiological Integrity
Integrated Process: Nursing Process/Data Collection
Content Area: Adult Health/Neurological

Answer: 4
Rationale: A craniotomy is any surgical opening into the skull. The major postoperative complication after craniotomy is increased intracranial pressure (ICP) from cerebral edema, hemorrhage, or the obstruction of the normal flow of cerebrospinal fluid. Symptoms of increased ICP include severe headache, deteriorating level of consciousness, restlessness, irritability, and dilated or pinpoint pupils that are slow to react or that do not react to light. Although the nurse may monitor for bleeding, hypotension, and tachycardia, these signs do not relate to the presence of increased ICP.

Test-Taking Strategy: Use the process of elimination. Remember to always monitor the neurological client for increased ICP. Recall that a change in the level of consciousness (LOC) is the first indicator of increased ICP. Option 4 is the only option that addresses the LOC. Review the signs of increased ICP and postoperative complications after craniotomy if you had difficulty with this question.

Reference

Christensen, B., & Kockrow, E. (2006). *Adult health nursing* (5th ed., p. 702). St. Louis: Mosby.

1191. Buck's traction is applied to a client after a hip fracture, and the client asks the nurse about this type of traction. The nurse responds that Buck's traction is a:

1 Plaster traction that involves the use of a cast
2 Skeletal traction that involves the use of surgically inserted pins
3 Circumferential traction that involves the use of a belt around the body
4 Skin traction that involves the use of traction attached to the skin and soft tissues

Level of Cognitive Ability: Comprehension
Client Needs: Physiological Integrity
Integrated Process: Nursing Process/Implementation
Content Area: Adult Health/Musculoskeletal

Answer: 4

Rationale: Buck's traction is a form of skin traction that involves the use of a belt or halter that is attached to the skin and soft tissues. The purpose of this type of traction is to decrease painful muscle spasms that accompany fractures. The weight that is used as a pulling force is limited to 5 to 10 lbs to prevent injury to the skin. Pins, a belt around the body, and plaster are not used with this type of traction.

Test-Taking Strategy: Use the process of elimination. Recall that Buck's traction is a skin traction to assist you with eliminating options 1, 2, and 3. Review the purpose and principles related to Buck's traction if you had difficulty with this question.

Reference

deWit, S. (2009). *Medical-surgical nursing: Concepts & practice* (pp. 789-790). St. Louis: Saunders.

1192. A nurse reinforces instructions to a postpartum client about the observation of lochia. The nurse determines that the client understands what to expect when the client states that, on the second day postpartum, the lochia should be:

1 Red
2 Pink
3 White
4 Yellow

Level of Cognitive Ability: Comprehension
Client Needs: Physiological Integrity
Integrated Process: Nursing Process/Evaluation
Content Area: Maternity/Postpartum

Answer: 1

Rationale: The uterus rids itself of the debris that remains after birth through a discharge called lochia, which is classified according to its appearance and contents. Lochia rubra is dark red in color. It occurs for the first 2 to 3 days after delivery, and it contains epithelial cells, erythrocytes, leukocytes, shreds of decidua, and occasionally fetal meconium, lanugo, and vernix caseosa. Lochia should not contain large clots; if it does, the cause should be investigated without delay. Lochia serosa is a brownish-pink discharge that normally occurs from days 4 to 10 postpartum. Lochia alba is the whitish discharge that normally occurs from days 10 to 14 postpartum.

Test-Taking Strategy: Use the process of elimination. Note the strategic words *second day postpartum* to direct you to option 1. Review normal postpartum findings if you had difficulty with this question.

Reference

Leifer, G. (2008). *Maternity nursing: An introductory text* (10th ed., p. 228). Philadelphia: Saunders.

1193. Skin closure with a heterograft is performed on a client with burn injuries. The client asks the nurse about this type of graft. The nurse bases the response on the knowledge that a heterograft can best be described as:

1 Skin from a cadaver
2 Skin from a skin bank
3 Skin from another species
4 Skin from the burned client

Level of Cognitive Ability: Comprehension
Client Needs: Physiological Integrity
Integrated Process: Nursing Process/Implementation
Content Area: Adult Health/Integumentary

Answer: 3

Rationale: Biologic dressings are usually heterograft or homograft material. Heterograft is skin from another species. The most commonly used type of heterograft is pig skin because of its availability and its relative compatibility with human skin. Homograft is skin from another human, which is usually obtained from a cadaver and provided by a skin bank. An autograft is skin from the burned client.

Test-Taking Strategy: Use the process of elimination. Options 1, 2, and 4 are comparable or alike in that they relate to grafts from human skin. Option 3 is the option that is different. Review the various types of skin grafts if you had difficulty with this question.

Reference

Christensen, B., & Kockrow, E. (2006). *Adult health nursing* (5th ed., p. 110). St. Louis: Mosby.

1194. A nurse is assigned to assist with caring for a hospitalized client who sustained a head injury. The nurse positions this client:

1 In left Sims' position
2 In reverse Trendelenburg's position
3 With the client's head elevated on a pillow
4 With the head of the bed elevated 30 to 45 degrees

Level of Cognitive Ability: Application
Client Needs: Physiological Integrity
Integrated Process: Nursing Process/Implementation
Content Area: Adult Health/Neurological

Answer: 4

Rationale: The client who has sustained a head injury is positioned to avoid extreme flexion or extension of the neck and to maintain the head in a midline, neutral position. The client is logrolled when turned to avoid extreme hip flexion. The head of the bed is elevated 30 to 45 degrees. All of these measures are used to enhance venous drainage, which helps to prevent increased intracranial pressure (ICP). Options 1, 2, and 3 are incorrect positions.

Test-Taking Strategy: Use the process of elimination, and focus on the subject—concern about increased ICP. Keep this in mind and consider the principles of gravity to eliminate options 1, 2, and 3. Review the care of the client after a head injury if you had difficulty with this question.

Reference

deWit, S. (2009). *Medical-surgical nursing: Concepts & practice* (p. 544). St. Louis: Saunders.

1195. An infant is admitted to the pediatric unit with a diagnosis of esophageal atresia. The nurse reviews the health history and expects to note which typical finding of this disorder documented in the record?

1 Slowed reflexes
2 Continuous drooling
3 Diaphragmatic breathing
4 Passage of large amounts of frothy stool

Level of Cognitive Ability: Comprehension
Client Needs: Physiological Integrity
Integrated Process: Nursing Process/Data Collection
Content Area: Child Health

Answer: 2

Rationale: Esophageal atresia is an abnormal esophagus that ends in a blind pouch or that narrows to a thin cord and thus does not provide a continuous passage to the stomach. The condition prevents the passage of swallowed mucus and saliva into the stomach. After fluid has accumulated in the pouch, it flows from the mouth, and the infant then drools continuously. Options 1, 3, and 4 are not associated with this disorder.

Test-Taking Strategy: Use the process of elimination. Eliminate options 3 and 4 by considering the anatomical location of the disorder. Focus on the word *atresia* to direct you to the correct option. Review the manifestations associated with esophageal atresia if you had difficulty with this question.

Reference

Leifer, G. (2007). *Introduction to maternity and pediatric nursing* (5th ed., p. 635). Philadelphia: Saunders.

1196. A nurse is monitoring a client with acquired immunodeficiency syndrome (AIDS) for early signs of Kaposi's sarcoma. The nurse observes the client for lesion(s) that are:

1 Unilateral, raised, and bluish-purple in color
2 Bilateral, flat, brownish, and scaly in appearance
3 Unilateral, red, raised, and blister-like in appearance
4 Bilateral, flat, and pink, turning to dark violet or black in color

Level of Cognitive Ability: Application
Client Needs: Physiological Integrity
Integrated Process: Nursing Process/Data Collection
Content Area: Adult Health/Respiratory

Answer: 4
Rationale: Kaposi's sarcoma is a malignant multifocal neoplasm of the reticuloendothelial cells. These lesions generally start with an area that is flat and pink and that changes to a dark violet or black color. The lesions are usually present bilaterally. They may appear in many areas of the body, and they are treated with radiation, chemotherapy, and cryotherapy. Options 1, 2, and 3 are incorrect descriptions.

Test-Taking Strategy: Use the process of elimination. Recall that Kaposi's sarcoma occurs in a bilateral pattern to help you to eliminate options 1 and 3. Knowledge of the character of the lesions is necessary to discriminate between options 2 and 4. Remember that Kaposi's sarcoma generally starts with an area that is flat and pink and that changes to a dark violet or black color. Review the characteristics of Kaposi's sarcoma if you had difficulty with this question.

Reference
Linton, A. (2007). *Introduction to medical-surgical nursing* (4th ed., p. 619). Philadelphia: Saunders.

1197. A nurse is told that a client is suspected of having pleural effusion. The nurse monitors the client for the typical manifestations of this condition, including:

1 Dyspnea at rest and a moist, productive cough
2 Dyspnea at rest and a dry, nonproductive cough
3 Dyspnea on exertion and a moist, productive cough
4 Dyspnea on exertion and a dry, nonproductive cough

Level of Cognitive Ability: Application
Client Needs: Physiological Integrity
Integrated Process: Nursing Process/Data Collection
Content Area: Adult Health/Respiratory

Answer: 4
Rationale: Pleural effusion is the abnormal accumulation of fluid in the pleural spaces of the lungs. Typical findings in a client with a pleural effusion include dyspnea that usually occurs with exertion and a dry, nonproductive cough. The cough is caused by bronchial irritation and possible mediastinal shift. Options 1, 2, and 3 are incorrect descriptions.

Test-Taking Strategy: Use the process of elimination. Recall that a pleural effusion occurs in the pleural space (not the airways) to help you to eliminate options 1 and 3, which mention a productive cough. Remember that dyspnea occurs on exertion before it occurs at rest to help you to choose option 4 over option 3. Review the manifestations associated with pleural effusion if you had difficulty with this question.

References
Christensen, B., & Kockrow, E. (2006). *Adult health nursing* (5th ed., pp. 360, 437). St. Louis: Mosby.
deWit, S. (2009). *Medical-surgical nursing: Concepts & practice* (p. 329). St. Louis: Saunders.

1198. A nurse explains to the mother of a newborn the purpose of giving the vitamin K injection to the newborn. The nurse determines that the mother understands the primary purpose of the injection when the mother states:

1 "The newborn lacks vitamins."
2 "The newborn's blood levels are low."
3 "The newborn lacks intestinal bacteria."
4 "The newborn's liver can't produce vitamin K."

Answer: 3
Rationale: The absence of the normal flora needed to synthesize vitamin K in the normal newborn gut results in low levels of vitamin K and creates a transient blood coagulation deficiency between the second and fifth day of life. From a low point at about 2 to 3 days after birth, these coagulation factors rise slowly, but they do not approach normal adult levels until 9 months of age or later. Increasing levels of these vitamin-K–dependent factors indicate a response to dietary intake and to the bacterial colonization of the intestines. An injection of vitamin K is given prophylactically on the day of birth to combat the deficiency. Options 1, 2, and 4 are incorrect.

Level of Cognitive Ability: Comprehension
Client Needs: Physiological Integrity
Integrated Process: Nursing Process/Evaluation
Content Area: Maternity/Postpartum

Test-Taking Strategy: Knowledge of the synthesis of vitamin K is necessary to answer this question. Remember that the absence of the normal flora needed to synthesize vitamin K in the normal newborn gut results in low levels of vitamin K. Review the purpose of administering vitamin K to the newborn if you had difficulty with this question.

Reference

Leifer, G. (2008). *Maternity nursing: An introductory text* (10th ed., p. 137). Philadelphia: Saunders.

1199. A nurse notes that a client's urinalysis report contains a notation of positive red blood cells (RBCs). The nurse interprets that this finding is unrelated to which of the following items that is part of the client's clinical picture?

1 Diabetes mellitus
2 History of kidney stones
3 Concurrent anticoagulant therapy
4 History of recent blow to the right flank

Level of Cognitive Ability: Comprehension
Client Needs: Physiological Integrity
Integrated Process: Nursing Process/Data Collection
Content Area: Adult Health/Renal

Answer: 1
Rationale: Hematuria can be caused by trauma to the kidney, such as blunt trauma to the lower posterior trunk or flank. Kidney stones can cause hematuria as they scrape the endothelial lining of the urinary system. Anticoagulant therapy can cause hematuria as a side effect. Diabetes mellitus does not cause hematuria.

Test-Taking Strategy: Use the process of elimination, and note the strategic word *unrelated*. Begin to answer this question by eliminating options 3 and 4, which are most obviously likely to cause RBCs to be found in the urine. From the remaining options, recall that the scraping of the stones against the mucosa could cause minor trauma and bleeding to help you to eliminate option 2 as well. Thus diabetes mellitus is unrelated to positive RBCs in the urine. Review the causes of hematuria if you had difficulty with this question.

References

deWit, S. (2009). *Medical-surgical nursing: Concepts & practice* (pp. 826-827). St. Louis: Saunders.
Ignatavicius, D., & Workman, M. (2010). *Medical-surgical nursing: Patient-centered collaborative care* (6th ed., p. 885). St. Louis: Saunders.

1200. A nurse is instructed to ambulate a client with a Foley catheter four times a day in the hall. The nurse understands that the safest way to accomplish this while maintaining the integrity of the catheter is to:

1 Change the drainage bag to a leg-collection bag.
2 Tie the drainage bag to the client's waist while ambulating.
3 Use a walker to hang the drainage bag from while ambulating.
4 Tell the client to hold the drainage bag lower than the level of the bladder.

Level of Cognitive Ability: Comprehension
Client Needs: Physiological Integrity

Answer: 1
Rationale: The safest way to protect the integrity of the catheter with a mobile client is to attach the tube to a leg-collection bag. This allows for greater freedom of movement while alleviating worry about accidental disconnection or dislodgment. The drainage bag should be maintained below the level of the bladder; therefore options 2 and 3 are incorrect. Options 2, 3, and 4 all present the potential risk for tension or for the client to pull on the catheter during ambulation.

Test-Taking Strategy: Use the process of elimination. Recalling that the drainage bag should be maintained below the level of the bladder eliminates options 2 and 3. In addition, note that options 2, 3, and 4 all present the risk for tension or for the client to pull on the catheter during ambulation. Review the care of the client with a Foley catheter if you had difficulty with this question.

Integrated Process: Nursing Process/Implementation
Content Area: Adult Health/Renal

Reference
Christensen, B., & Kockrow, E. (2006). *Foundations of nursing* (5th ed., p. 582). St. Louis: Mosby.

1201. A client who was recently diagnosed with polycystic kidney disease has just finished speaking with the physician about the disorder. The client asks the nurse to explain again what the most serious complication of the disorder might be. When formulating a response, the nurse incorporates the understanding that the most serious complication is:

1 Diabetes insipidus
2 End-stage renal disease (ESRD)
3 Chronic urinary tract infection (UTI)
4 Syndrome of inappropriate antidiuretic hormone (SIADH) secretion

Answer: 2
Rationale: Polycystic kidney disease is an abnormal condition in which the kidneys are enlarged and contain many cysts. The most serious complication of polycystic kidney disease is ESRD, which would be managed with dialysis or transplant. Chronic UTI is the most common complication because of the altered anatomy of the kidney and the development of resistant strains of bacteria. Diabetes insipidus and SIADH secretion are unrelated disorders.

Test-Taking Strategy: Use the process of elimination. Note the relationship between the words *most serious* in the question and the words *end-stage* in option 2. Review the complications of polycystic kidney disease if you had difficulty with this question.

Level of Cognitive Ability: Comprehension
Client Needs: Physiological Integrity
Integrated Process: Nursing Process/Implementation
Content Area: Adult Health/Renal

Reference
Linton, A. (2007). *Introduction to medical-surgical nursing* (4th ed., p. 857). Philadelphia: Saunders.

1202. It has been 12 hours since a postpartum client's delivery of a healthy newborn. The nurse checks the mother's uterus for the process of involution and documents that it is progressing normally when palpation of the client's fundus is noted:

1 At the level of the umbilicus
2 One fingerbreadth below the umbilicus
3 Two fingerbreadths below the umbilicus
4 Midway between the umbilicus and the symphysis pubis

Answer: 1
Rationale: The term involution is used to describe the rapid reduction in size and the return of the uterus to a normal condition that is similar to its nonpregnant state. Immediately after the delivery of the placenta, the uterus contracts to the size of a large grapefruit. The fundus is situated in the midline between the symphysis pubis and the umbilicus. Within 6 to 12 hours after birth, the fundus of the uterus rises to the level of the umbilicus. The top of the fundus remains at the level of the umbilicus for a day or so and then descends into the pelvis by approximately one fingerbreadth on each succeeding day.

Test-Taking Strategy: Knowledge of the normal process of involution is necessary to answer the question. Note the strategic words *12 hours* and visualize the process of involution and the expected findings to direct you to option 1. Review the process of involution if you had difficulty with this question.

Level of Cognitive Ability: Comprehension
Client Needs: Physiological Integrity
Integrated Process: Nursing Process/Data Collection
Content Area: Maternity/Postpartum

Reference
Leifer, G. (2008). *Maternity nursing: An introductory text* (10th ed., p. 227). Philadelphia: Saunders.

1203. A client with a gastric tumor is scheduled for a subtotal gastrectomy (Billroth II procedure) and asks the nurse about the procedure. The nurse explains the procedure, knowing that the best description is that:

Answer: 3
Rationale: During the Billroth II procedure, the lower portion of the stomach is removed, and the remainder is anastomosed to the jejunum. This technique is preferred for the treatment of duodenal ulcer because recurrent ulceration develops less frequently. The duodenal stump is preserved to permit

1 The proximal end of the distal stomach is anastomosed to the duodenum.
2 The entire stomach is removed, and the esophagus is anastomosed to the duodenum.
3 The lower portion of the stomach is removed, and the remainder is anastomosed to the jejunum.
4 The antrum of the stomach is removed, and the remaining portion is anastomosed to the duodenum.

Level of Cognitive Ability: Comprehension
Client Needs: Physiological Integrity
Integrated Process: Nursing Process/Implementation
Content Area: Adult Health/Gastrointestinal

bile flow to the jejunum. Options 1, 2, and 4 are incorrect descriptions.

Test-Taking Strategy: Use the process of elimination. Gastrectomy is the removal of the stomach; this should assist you with eliminating option 1. The fact that this is a subtotal procedure should direct you to option 3. Review the Billroth II procedure if you had difficulty with this question.

Reference

Linton, A. (2007). *Introduction to medical-surgical nursing* (4th ed., pp. 768-769). Philadelphia: Saunders.

1204. A nurse assigned to care for a client with cancer reviews the plan of care and notes that the client has a nursing diagnosis of *Risk for injury* related to thrombocytopenia secondary to the adverse effects of chemotherapy. Based on the plan of care, the nurse plans to monitor the results of which of the following laboratory studies closely?
1 Platelet count
2 White blood cell (WBC) count
3 Antinuclear antibody (ANA) titer
4 Erythrocyte sedimentation rate (ESR)

Level of Cognitive Ability: Analysis
Client Needs: Physiological Integrity
Integrated Process: Nursing Process/Data Collection
Content Area: Adult Health/Oncology

Answer: 1
Rationale: The client with thrombocytopenia has an insufficient number of platelets, which puts the client at risk for bleeding. Other related studies that should be monitored include hemoglobin, hematocrit, and coagulation studies. The WBC count is a test that indicates the risk for or the presence of infection, whereas the ESR is a nonspecific test that indicates inflammation. The ANA titer is a test of immune function that can indicate the presence of certain autoimmune disorders.

Test-Taking Strategy: Use the process of elimination. Recall the definition of thrombocytopenia to direct you to option 1. Review the adverse effects of chemotherapy if you had difficulty with this question.

References

Christensen, B., & Kockrow, E. (2006). *Adult health nursing* (5th ed., p. 834). St. Louis: Mosby.
Linton, A. (2007). *Introduction to medical-surgical nursing* (4th ed., p. 587). Philadelphia: Saunders.

1205. A nurse is assigned to care for a client with bladder cancer who recently received chemotherapy and who has a platelet count of 20,000/mm^3. Based on this laboratory value, the nurse plans to do which of the following?
1 Tell the client to not eat any fresh fruits.
2 Monitor for signs of infection in the client.
3 Monitor the client's skin for the presence of petechiae.
4 Tell the client that if anyone delivers fresh flowers, they should be returned to the florist.

Answer: 3
Rationale: When the platelet count is decreased, the client is at risk for bleeding. A high risk of hemorrhage exists when the platelet count is less than 20,000/mm^3. The client should be monitored for signs of bleeding, and petechiae are such a sign. Options 1, 2, and 4 are specific interventions related to the risk of infection; although they may be components of the plan of care, they are not specific to the risk for bleeding. Option 4 is not a therapeutic statement to make to the client.

Test-Taking Strategy: Use the process of elimination. Recall the normal platelet count and that a low count places the client at risk for bleeding to assist you with eliminating options 1, 2, and 4. Review the normal platelet count and the plan of care for a client with a low count if you had difficulty with this question.

Level of Cognitive Ability: Analysis
Client Needs: Physiological Integrity
Integrated Process: Nursing Process/Planning
Content Area: Adult Health/Oncology

Reference
Ignatavicius, D., & Workman, M. (2010). *Medical-surgical nursing: Patient-centered collaborative care* (6th ed., p. 426). St. Louis: Saunders.

ALTERNATE ITEM FORMAT QUESTIONS

Prioritizing (Ordered Response)

1206. A licensed practical nurse (LPN) witnesses a client going into pulmonary edema. The client exhibits respiratory distress, but the blood pressure is stable at this time. The LPN contacts the registered nurse (RN) immediately and prepares to take the following actions in which order of priority? (Number 1 is the first action.)

____ Recheck the vital signs.
____ Place the client in high-Fowler's position.
____ Call the respiratory therapy department for a ventilator.
____ Begin the client's PRN oxygen at 2 L via nasal cannula.
____ Place the client on a pulse oximeter and a cardiac monitor.
____ Assist the RN with preparing the client for the administration of PRN morphine sulfate intravenous injection.

Level of Cognitive Ability: Application
Client Needs: Physiological Integrity
Integrated Process: Nursing Process/Implementation
Content Area: Delegating/Prioritizing

Answer: 4, 1, 6, 2, 3, 5
Rationale: The client in pulmonary edema is immediately placed in high-Fowler's position, and an oxygen delivery apparatus is applied. The nurse would also place the client on a pulse oximeter and a cardiac monitor to monitor the cardiopulmonary status. The nurse would monitor the client's vital signs closely. Next, the LPN would assist the RN with preparing the client for the administration of PRN morphine sulfate intravenous injection. Because a ventilator may or may not be needed, calling the respiratory therapy department would be the final action of the actions provided. Additional interventions include the administration of diuretics and the insertion of a Foley catheter. The RN should also notify the client's physician when signs of pulmonary edema are initially observed.

Test-Taking Strategy: Remember that in a respiratory emergency situation, client positioning may be the first action because it will alleviate dyspnea. Next, use the ABCs—airway, breathing, and circulation—to determine that the application of a nasal mask or cannula will improve the client's available ambient oxygen supply. Placing the client on a pulse oximeter and a cardiac monitor would be the next action. From the remaining options, the nurse would recheck the vital signs and determine if the client is stable, and then would administer morphine sulfate as ordered. Recall that mechanical ventilation may or may not be needed; this recollection will assist you with determining that this is the final action from the options provided. Review the immediate nursing actions for a client in pulmonary edema if you had difficulty with this question.

References
Christensen, B., & Kockrow, E. (2006). *Adult health nursing* (5th ed., p. 446). St. Louis: Mosby.
Ignatavicius, D., & Workman, M. (2010). *Medical-surgical nursing: Patient-centered collaborative care* (6th ed., pp. 775-776). St. Louis: Saunders.

Fill-in-the-Blank

1207. A nurse is assessing a client's cigarette smoking habit. The client states that he has smoked three fourths of a pack per day for the last 10 years. The nurse calculates that the client has a smoking history of how many pack years?

Answer: _______ pack years

Answer: 7.5 pack years
Rationale: The standard method for quantifying smoking history is to multiply the number of packs smoked per day by the number of years of smoking. This number is recorded as the number of pack years. The number of pack years for the client who has smoked three fourths of a pack per day for 10 years is calculated as follows: 0.75 packs × 10 years = 7.5 pack years.

Level of Cognitive Ability: Application
Client Needs: Physiological Integrity
Integrated Process: Nursing Process/Data Collection
Content Area: Adult Health/Respiratory

Test-Taking Strategy: Focus on the information in the question, and multiply the number of packs of cigarettes smoked per day by the number of years of smoking. Review the calculation of pack years if you had difficulty with this question.

Reference

Ignatavicius, D. & Workman, M. (2010). *Medical-surgical nursing: Patient-centered collaborative care* (6th ed., p. 558). St. Louis: Saunders.

Multiple Response

1208. A client is admitted to the hospital with a diagnosis of acute bacterial pericarditis, and the licensed practical nurse (LPN) reviews the admission assessment performed by the nurse who admitted the client. Which of the following findings, which are associated with this inflammatory heart disease, would the LPN expect to note on the admission assessment form? Select all that apply.

❒ 1 Fever
❒ 2 Leukopenia
❒ 3 Bradycardia
❒ 4 Pericardial friction rub
❒ 5 Decreased erythrocyte sedimentation rate
❒ 6 Severe precordial chest pain that intensifies when in the supine position

Level of Cognitive Ability: Analysis
Client Needs: Physiological Integrity
Integrated Process: Nursing Process/Data Collection
Content Area: Adult Health/Cardiovascular

Answer: 1, 4, 6

Rationale: With acute pericarditis, the membranes that surround the heart become inflamed and rub against each other, thus producing the classic pericardial friction rub. The client complains of severe precordial chest pain that intensifies when lying supine and that decreases when in a sitting position. The pain also intensifies when the client breathes deeply. Fever typically occurs and is accompanied by leukocytosis and an elevated erythrocyte sedimentation rate. Malaise, myalgias, and tachycardia are common.

Test-Taking Strategy: Focus on the diagnosis to assist you with determining that the client would have a fever (option 1); the compensatory response to fever is an increased metabolic rate and tachycardia. Remember that, when the client has an inflammatory disease, the erythrocyte sedimentation rate and the white blood cell count would increase (leukocytosis not leukopenia). Lastly, focus on the diagnosis to assist you with determining that a pericardial friction rub and severe precordial chest pain will be present (options 4 and 6). Review the characteristics associated with acute bacterial pericarditis if you had difficulty with this question.

Reference

Ignatavicius, D. & Workman, M. (2010). *Medical-surgical nursing: Patient-centered collaborative care* (6th ed., p. 786). St. Louis: Saunders.

Prioritizing (Ordered Response)

1209. A client who works as a security guard at night in an industrial building is brought to the emergency department with suspected carbon monoxide poisoning. List in order of priority the actions that the nurse prepares to take when the client arrives. (Number 1 is the first action.)

___ Administer 100% oxygen.
___ Check the blood pressure and pulse.
___ Check the client's airway for patency.
___ Draw blood for carboxyhemoglobin levels.
___ Document the findings, treatment, and client response.

Answer: 2, 3, 1, 4, 5, 6

Rationale: When the client arrives, the nurse immediately checks the client's airway for patency and then quickly prepares to administer 100% oxygen at atmospheric pressure or hyperbaric pressure to speed up the elimination of carbon monoxide from the hemoglobin and to reverse hypoxia. The next most important action is the assessment of the client's vital signs. Blood is then drawn (initially and serially) to monitor carboxyhemoglobin levels; when they drop below 5%, oxygen may be discontinued. After assessment, treatment, and the evaluation of the client's response, the nurse documents the findings. If the episode was unintentional and precipitated by conditions in a dwelling, the health department is notified.

____ Notify the local health department and request an inspection of the industrial building.

Level of Cognitive Ability: Application
Client Needs: Physiological Integrity
Integrated Process: Nursing Process/Implementation
Content Area: Delegating/Prioritizing

Test-Taking Strategy: Note the data in the question. Use the ABCs—airway, breathing, and circulation—to direct you to first check the client's airway and then to administer 100% oxygen. Use the steps of the nursing process to finish collecting data about the client. From the remaining actions listed, use Maslow's Hierarchy of Needs theory, and recall that physiological needs are the priority. This will assist you with determining that drawing blood for carboxyhemoglobin levels is the next action and that this is followed by documentation. Review the care of the client with carbon monoxide poisoning if you had difficulty with this question.

Reference

Chernecky, C., & Berger, B. (2008). *Laboratory tests and diagnostic procedures* (5th ed., pp. 292-293). Philadelphia: Saunders.

Figure/Illustration and Fill-in-the-Blank

1210. A client is to receive 6000 units of heparin subcutaneously. How many milliliters will the nurse prepare for administration? (Refer to the medication label.)

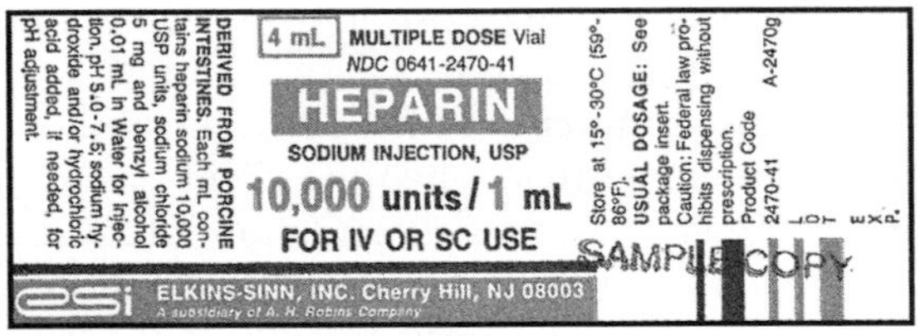

Figure 9-1 From Kee, J., & Marshall, S. (2009). *Clinical calculations: With applications to general and specialty areas* (6th ed., p. 170). Philadelphia: Saunders.

Answer: _______ mL

Level of Cognitive Ability: Application
Client Needs: Physiological Integrity
Integrated Process: Nursing Process/Implementation
Content Area: Fundamental Skills

Answer: 0.6 mL

Rationale: Calculate the dosage by dividing the amount ordered by the amount available. The physician ordered 6000 units of heparin, and there are 10,000 units/mL available; therefore, divide 6000 units by 10,000. Use the formula of dividing what is available by what is desired, and then multiply by 1 mL; this will result in a dose of 0.6 mL.

Test-Taking Strategy: Read carefully to see that there are 10,000 units of heparin in 1 mL, so less than 1 mL of solution is necessary for the prescribed dose. Recheck your calculation with a calculator before documenting your answer, and be sure that the calculated dose makes sense. Review medication calculations if you had difficulty with this question.

References

Kee, J., & Marshall, S. (2009). *Clinical calculations: With applications to general and specialty areas* (6th ed., p. 170). Philadelphia: Saunders.
Potter, P., & Perry, A. (2009) *Fundamentals of nursing* (7th ed., pp. 697-700). St. Louis: Mosby.

Chart/Exhibit

1211. A second-day postpartum client with diabetes mellitus has scant lochia with a foul odor and a temperature of 101.6° F. The physician suspects infection and writes the following orders for the treatment of the client. Which order should the nurse complete first?

Answer: 3

Rationale: A culture and sensitivity should be obtained before any antibiotic therapy is begun to avoid masking the microorganisms identified by the culture. Options 1, 2, and 4 are standard parts of therapy for this type of infection but are not completed first.

Test-Taking Strategy: Use the process of elimination, and note the strategic word *first*. Remember that a culture and sensitivity specimen is always obtained before the initiation of antibiotic therapy. Review the care of the client with a potential postpartum infection if you had difficulty with this question.

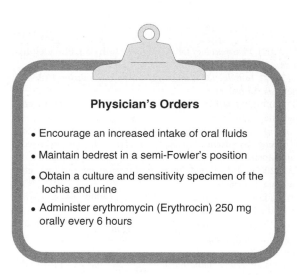

Physician's Orders

- Encourage an increased intake of oral fluids
- Maintain bedrest in a semi-Fowler's position
- Obtain a culture and sensitivity specimen of the lochia and urine
- Administer erythromycin (Erythrocin) 250 mg orally every 6 hours

1 Encourage an increased intake of oral fluids.
2 Maintain bedrest in a semi-Fowlers position
3 Obtain a culture and sensitivity specimen of the lochia and urine.
4 Administer erythromycin (Erythrocin) 250 mg orally every 6 hours.

Level of Cognitive Ability: Application
Client Needs: Physiological Integrity
Integrated Process: Nursing Process/Implementation
Content Area: Maternity/Postpartum

Reference

Leifer, G. (2008). *Maternity nursing: An introductory text* (10th ed., pp. 344-345). Philadelphia: Saunders.

Multiple Response

1212. A client is receiving desmopressin (DDAVP) intranasally. The nurse should use which measurements to determine the effectiveness of this medication? Select all that apply.

❐ 1 Fluid intake
❐ 2 Urine output
❐ 3 Daily weight
❐ 4 Pupillary response
❐ 5 Presence of edema
❐ 6 Ability to perform full range-of-motion exercises

Level of Cognitive Ability: Analysis
Client Needs: Physiological Integrity
Integrated Process: Nursing Process/Evaluation
Content Area: Pharmacology

Answer: 1, 2, 3, 5

Rationale: DDAVP is an analogue of vasopressin (antidiuretic hormone) that is used for the management of diabetes insipidus. The nurse monitors the client's fluid balance to determine the effectiveness of the medication. Fluid status can be evaluated by noting intake and output, daily weight, and the presence of edema.

Test-Taking Strategy: Use the process of elimination. Recall that DDAVP is an antidiuretic hormone to direct you to the options that address fluid balance. Review DDAVP if you had difficulty with this question.

Reference

Hodgson, B., & Kizior, R. (2009). *Saunders nursing drug handbook 2009* (p. 334). St. Louis: Saunders.

REFERENCES

Black, J., & Hawks, J. (2009). *Medical-surgical nursing: Clinical management for positive outcomes* (8th ed.). St. Louis: Saunders.

Chernecky, C., & Berger, B. (2008). *Laboratory tests and diagnostic procedures* (5th ed.). Philadelphia: Saunders.

Christensen, B., & Kockrow, E. (2006). *Adult health nursing* (5th ed.). St. Louis: Mosby.

Christensen, B., & Kockrow, E. (2006). *Foundations of nursing* (5th ed.). St. Louis: Mosby.

Copstead, L., & Bansilk, J. (2010). *Pathophysiology* (4th ed.). St. Louis: Mosby.

deWit, S. (2009). *Medical-surgical nursing: Concepts & practice*. St. Louis: Saunders.

Edmunds, M. (2010). Introduction to clinical pharmacology (6th ed.). St. Louis: Mosby.

Fortinash, K., & Holoday-Worret, P. (2008). *Psychiatric mental health nursing* (4th ed.). St. Louis: Mosby.

Gahart, B., & Nazareno, A. (2009). *Intravenous medications* (25th ed.). St. Louis: Mosby.

Grodner, M., Long, S., & Walkingshaw, B. (2007). *Foundations and clinical applications of nutrition* (4th ed.). St. Louis: Mosby.

Hockenberry, M., & Wilson, D. (2009). *Wong's essentials of pediatric nursing* (8th ed.). St. Louis: Mosby.

Hodgson, B., & Kizior, R. (2009). *Saunders nursing drug handbook 2009*. St. Louis: Saunders.

Ignatavicius, D., & Workman, M. (2010). *Medical-surgical nursing: Patient-centered collaborative care* (6th ed.). St. Louis: Saunders.

Jarvis, C. (2008). *Physical examination and health assessment* (5th ed.). Philadelphia: Saunders.

Kee, J., Hayes, E., & McCuistion, L. (2009). *Pharmacology: A nursing process approach* (6th ed.). Philadelphia: Saunders.

Kee, J., & Marshall, S. (2009). *Clinical calculations: With applications to general and specialty areas* (6th ed.). Philadelphia: Saunders.

Keltner, N., Schwecke, L., & Bostrom, C. (2007). *Psychiatric nursing* (5th ed.). St. Louis: Mosby.

Lehne, R. (2007). *Pharmacology for nursing care* (6th ed.). Philadelphia: Saunders.

Leifer, G. (2007). *Introduction to maternity and pediatric nursing* (5th ed.). Philadelphia: Saunders.

Leifer, G. (2008). *Maternity nursing: An introductory text* (10th ed.). Philadelphia: Saunders.

Lewis, S., Heitkemper, M., Dirksen, S., & Bucher, L. (2007). *Medical-surgical nursing: Assessment and management of clinical problems* (7th ed.). St. Louis: Mosby.

Linton, A. (2007). *Introduction to medical-surgical nursing* (4th ed.). Philadelphia: Saunders.

McKinney, E., James, S., Murray, S., & Ashwill, J (2009). *Maternal-child nursing* (3rd ed.). St. Louis: Mosby.

Monahan, F., Sands, J., Marek, J., Neighbors, M., & Green, C. (2007). *Phipps' medical-surgical nursing: Health and illness perspectives* (8th ed.). St. Louis: Mosby.

Nix, S. (2009). *Williams' basic nutrition and diet therapy* (13th ed.). St. Louis: Mosby.

Perry, A., & Potter, P. (2010). *Clinical nursing skills & techniques* (7th ed.). St. Louis: Mosby.

Potter, P., & Perry, A. (2009). *Fundamentals of nursing* (7th ed.). St. Louis: Mosby.

Price, D., & Gwin, J. (2008). *Pediatric nursing: An introductory text* (10th ed.). St. Louis: Saunders.

Schlenker, E., & Long, S. (2007). *Williams' essentials of nutrition & diet therapy* (9th ed.). St. Louis: Mosby.

Skidmore-Roth, L. (2008). *Mosby's nursing drug reference* (21st ed.). St. Louis: Mosby.

Varcarolis, E., & Halter, M. (2009). *Essentials of psychiatric mental health nursing: A communication approach to evidence-based care.* St. Louis: Saunders.

Wold, G. (2008). *Basic geriatric nursing* (4th ed.). St. Louis: Mosby.

UNIT

III

Integrated Processes

CHAPTER

10

Integrated Processes and the NCLEX-PN® Test Plan

INTEGRATED PROCESSES

In the new test plan that was implemented in April 2008, the National Council of State Boards of Nursing (NCSBN) identified a framework based on client needs. This framework was selected based on the analysis of the findings of a practice analysis study of newly licensed practical and vocational nurses in the United States, NCSBN content experts, and boards of nursing. The NCSBN identified four major Client Needs categories: Safe and Effective Care Environment, Health Promotion and Maintenance, Psychosocial Integrity, and Physiological Integrity. These categories are described in Chapter 5, "Client Needs and the NCLEX-PN® Test Plan." The 2008 test plan also identifies four processes that are fundamental to the practice of nursing and that are known as Integrated Processes: Clinical Problem-Solving Process (Nursing Process), Caring, Communication and Documentation, and Teaching and Learning. These processes are integrated throughout the four major Client Needs categories. They are described in this chapter and listed in Box 10-1.

Box 10-1 ▲ INTEGRATED PROCESSES

Clinical Problem-Solving Process (Nursing Process)
Caring
Communication and Documentation
Teaching and Learning

CLINICAL PROBLEM-SOLVING PROCESS (NURSING PROCESS)

The Clinical Problem-Solving Process (Nursing Process) provides a systematic and organized approach for delivering care to clients. The steps of this process are Data Collection, Planning, Implementation, and Evaluation (Box 10-2).

Box 10-2 ▲ CLINICAL PROBLEM-SOLVING PROCESS (NURSING PROCESS)

Data Collection
Planning
Implementation
Evaluation

Data Collection

Data collection is the first step of the nursing process, when the nurse participates in a systematic method of establishing a database about the client. This step of the nursing process includes gathering information about the client, communicating the information gained during the data collection, and contributing to the formulation of nursing diagnoses. The database provides the foundation for the remaining steps of the nursing process.

Data collection begins with the first contact with the client. During all successive contacts, the nurse continues to collect information that is significant and relevant to the needs of the client. With each contact, the nurse uses all of the senses to gather data about the client.

The nurse collects data about the client from a variety of sources during this process. The client is the primary source of data. Family members or significant others are secondary sources of data, and these sources may supplement or verify the information provided by the client. Data may also be obtained from other health care team members and from the client's current and prior health records.

The information collected by the nurse includes both subjective and objective data. Subjective data include the information that the client states and that is based on the client's opinion. Objective data are the observable, measurable pieces of information about the client. Objective data include measurements (e.g., vital signs, laboratory findings) and information obtained from the observation of the client. Objective data also include clinical manifestations (e.g., the signs and symptoms of an illness or disease).

As part of the process of data collection, the nurse is responsible for recognizing significant findings in the client, determining the need for additional information, reporting findings to the registered nurse (RN) or other relevant health care team members (e.g., the physician), and documenting findings thoroughly and accurately.

The nurse contributes to the formulation of nursing diagnoses by assisting with organizing relevant health care data and determining significant relationships between the data and client needs, problems, or both.

On the NCLEX-PN, remember that data collection is the first step of the nursing process. When answering these type of questions, focus on the data in the question, and select the option that addresses a data collection action. The exception to this guideline is if the question identifies an emergency situation; in an emergency situation, a nursing action may be the priority. In addition, use skills of prioritizing (e.g., Maslow's Hierarchy of Needs theory, the ABCs—airway, breathing, and circulation) to answer the question (Box 10-3).

Planning

Planning is the second step of the nursing process. In this step, the nurse provides input into plan development, participates in setting goals for meeting the client's needs, and helps to design strategies to achieve these goals.

During the planning phase, the nurse assists with the formulation of the goals of care by participating in the identification of nursing interventions to achieve goals and by communicating client needs that may require the alteration of the goals of care. The nurse takes the nursing diagnosis written by the RN and states it as a nursing problem in objective, specific terms. The nurse then sets goals and lists interventions. When evidence of a new client problem emerges, the nurse collects data about the problem and collaborates with the RN, and then the RN formulates a new nursing diagnosis. Setting priorities assists the nurse with organizing and planning care that solves the most urgent problems. The client should be included in discussions when identifying the priorities of care. Priorities may change as the client's level of wellness changes. The most important problems—those that are potentially life threatening—must be taken care of immediately.

After priorities are established, the client and the nurse mutually decide on the expected goals. A goal must be set for each priority or client need. The selected goals serve as a guide for individualizing the care of the client. The goals must be client centered, measurable, realistic, time referenced, and determined by the client and nurse together. Unless criteria for the goals have been predetermined, it is difficult to know whether the goal is achieved and if the problem has been resolved.

The nurse assists with the development of the plan of care by collaborating with the client and health care team members to select nursing interventions that will achieve the goals and by planning for client safety, comfort, and the maintenance of optimal functioning. The nurse participates in the identification of health and social resources available to the client and family and collaborates with other health care team members when planning the delivery of care. The nurse should communicate client needs, review the plan of care with the RN, and document the plan of care thoroughly and accurately.

When answering questions on the NCLEX-PN, remember that this is a nursing examination. The answer to the question most likely will involve something that is included in the nursing care plan rather than the medical plan, unless the question asks what the nurse anticipates that the physician will prescribe. In addition, remember that actual problems are usually more important than potential or at-risk problems and that physiological needs are usually the priority (Box 10-4).

Box 10-3 ▲ NURSING PROCESS: DATA COLLECTION

QUESTION

A nurse assigned to care for a client with a tracheostomy tube is asked to check the client for subcutaneous emphysema, which is a complication of a tracheostomy. The nurse checks the client for which of the following?

1. Signs of respiratory distress
2. Crackling sounds heard in the lungs
3. Abnormal skin and mucous membrane color
4. A puffy and crackling sensation on palpation of the tissues surrounding the tracheostomy site

ANSWER: 4

Rationale: Subcutaneous emphysema, which is also known as crepitus, occurs when air escapes from the tracheostomy incision into the tissues, dissects fascial planes under the skin, and accumulates around the face, neck, and upper chest. These areas appear puffy, and slight finger pressure will produce a crackling sound and sensation. This is not generally a serious condition because the air will eventually be absorbed. Options 1, 2, and 3 are not characteristics of subcutaneous emphysema.

Box 10-4 ▲ NURSING PROCESS: PLANNING

QUESTION

In a client's nursing care plan, a nurse notes a nursing diagnosis of *Ineffective coping* related to decreased activity tolerance and respiratory disease. The nurse determines that the client is showing an adaptive response if which behavior is observed?

1. Secluding himself to decrease fatigue
2. Stating that his appetite has decreased
3. Trying to increase ambulation each day
4. Increasing the use of medication to help with sleep

ANSWER: 3

Rationale: The client with respiratory disease may experience ineffective coping related to the inability to tolerate activity and as a result of social isolation. The client demonstrates adaptive responses by increasing activity to the highest level possible before respiratory symptoms are triggered, using relaxation or other learned coping skills, and participating in a pulmonary rehabilitation program. Enhancing one's own seclusion, anorexia, and insomnia are not adaptive responses.

Implementation

Implementation is the third step of the nursing process, and it includes initiating and completing the nursing actions that are required to accomplish the defined goals. This step is the action phase, and it involves assisting with organizing and managing client care, providing care to achieve established goals of care, and communicating nursing interventions.

The nurse assists with organizing and managing the client's care by implementing the established plan of care and by participating in client care conferences. The nurse is responsible for using safe and appropriate techniques and precautionary and preventive interventions when providing care to a client. The nurse is also responsible for instituting nursing interventions if adverse responses occur, initiating life-saving interventions for emergency situations, and providing an environment that is conducive to the attainment of the goals of care.

This step of the nursing process also includes providing care based on the client's needs, preferences, or both; encouraging the client to follow the prescribed treatment plan; and assisting the client with maintaining optimal functioning. In addition, the process of implementation includes monitoring the client care administered by unlicensed nursing personnel and reinforcing teaching about the principles, procedures, and techniques required for the maintenance and promotion of health.

The implementation step concludes when the nurse's actions are completed and when these actions, including their effects and the client's response, are communicated to the relevant members of the health care team and documented.

The NCLEX-PN is an examination about nursing, so focus on the nursing action rather than the medical action unless the question is asking what prescribed medical action is anticipated (Box 10-5).

Box 10-5 ▲ NURSING PROCESS: IMPLEMENTATION

QUESTION

A nurse is changing a dressing on a hospitalized client who had abdominal surgery. When the nurse removes the abdominal dressing, the nurse notes the protrusion of the bowel through the incision. List in order of priority the actions that the nurse will take. Number 1 is the first action, and number 6 is the last action.

____ Notify the registered nurse.
____ Check the client's vital signs.
____ Prepare the client for surgery.
____ Document the findings, the actions taken, and the client response.
____ Place the client in semi-Fowler's position, with the knees slightly flexed.
____ Cover the protruding bowel with a sterile dressing that has been moistened with sterile normal saline solution.

ANSWER: 1, 4, 5, 6, 2, 3

Rationale: Evisceration is the protrusion of an internal organ (e.g., a bowel loop) through an incision. Wound eviscerations are emergencies, and, if an evisceration occurs, the registered nurse is immediately notified and will then contact the surgeon. The client is placed in a supine (on the back) and semi-Fowler's position, with the knees slightly flexed. This position eases pressure on the wound, prevents further tearing of the wound edges, and reduces the risk of further evisceration. The nurse next covers the protruding bowel with a sterile dressing that has been moistened with sterile normal saline solution to help prevent wound contamination and to keep the abdominal contents moist. After these immediate interventions have been performed, the nurse checks the client's vital signs and pulse oximetry for abnormalities and signs of shock. An intravenous device will be inserted if one is not in place, and the client will be placed on NPO status because surgery will most likely be needed to repair the wound. Finally, the nurse documents the findings, the actions taken, and the client's response.

Evaluation

Evaluation is the fourth step of the nursing process, and it is a way of measuring client progress toward the meeting of established goals. Although evaluation is the final step of the nursing process, it is an ongoing and integral component of each step. The process of data collection is reviewed to determine whether sufficient information was obtained and whether the information obtained was specific and appropriate. The plan and expected outcomes are examined to determine if they are realistic, achievable, time referenced, measurable, and effective. Interventions are examined to determine their effectiveness for achieving the expected outcomes.

Because evaluation is an ongoing process, it is vital to all steps of the nursing process. Evaluation is the continuous process of comparing actual outcomes with the expected outcomes of care, and it provides the means for determining the need to modify the plan of care. Inherent in this step of the nursing process are the communication of evaluation findings; the process of documenting and reporting the client's response to treatment and care; and the determination of the effectiveness of teaching to relevant members of the health care team.

Evaluation questions on the NCLEX-PN may be written to address a client's response to treatment measures or to determine a client's understanding of the prescribed treatment measures (Box 10-6).

CARING

Caring is the essence of nursing, and it is basic to any helping relationship; it is central to every encounter that the nurse has with a client. Through caring, the

Box 10-6 ▲ NURSING PROCESS: EVALUATION

QUESTION

A nurse administers hydralazine hydrochloride (Apresoline) to a client with autonomic dysreflexia. Which finding indicates that the medication is effective?

1. Muscle spasms subside.
2. The blood pressure declines.
3. The client says that he feels better.
4. The intensity of seizure activity declines.

ANSWER: 2

Rationale: Hydralazine hydrochloride is an antihypertensive agent that decreases the blood pressure by providing vasodilation. Options 1, 3, and 4 do not indicate a specific response and are unrelated to the action of the medication.

nurse humanizes the client. Treating the client with respect and dignity is a true expression of caring. In the technological environment of health care, emphasizing the client's individuality counteracts any potential process of depersonalization. Caring is an Integrated Process of the test plan of the NCLEX-PN, so this concept is central to all Client Needs categories of the plan. The NCSBN describes caring as the interaction of the nurse and client in an atmosphere of mutual respect and trust; in this collaborative environment, the nurse provides support and compassion to help achieve the desired outcomes.

In the NCLEX-PN, the concept of caring is primary. It is easy to become involved with looking at a question from a technological viewpoint. However, the concept of caring should be addressed when reading a test question and when selecting an option. Always address the client's feelings and provide support. Remember that this examination is all about nursing and that nursing is caring (Box 10-7).

Box 10-7 ▲ CARING

QUESTION

A client and her infant have undergone testing for human immunodeficiency virus (HIV), and both clients were found to be positive. The news is devastating, and the mother is crying. The appropriate intervention at this time is to:

1. Examine with the mother how she got HIV.
2. Listen quietly while the mother talks and cries.
3. Describe the progressive stages and treatments of HIV.
4. Call an HIV counselor and make an appointment for them.

ANSWER: 2

Rationale: HIV is a retrovirus that causes acquired immunodeficiency syndrome. The client has just received devastating news and should have someone present with her as she begins to cope with this issue. The nurse should sit and actively listen while the mother talks and cries. Calling an HIV counselor may be helpful, but it is not what the client needs at this time. The other options are not appropriate for this stage of coping with the news that both the mother and the infant are HIV-positive. Remember to address the client's feelings and to support the client. The nurse should sit, listen, and provide support because this is the most caring response.

COMMUNICATION AND DOCUMENTATION

The process of communication occurs as the nurse interacts either verbally or nonverbally with a client. Therapeutic communication techniques are key to an effective nurse–client relationship. Communication questions are integrated throughout the NCLEX-PN test plan, and they may address a client situation in any health care setting. The NCSBN describes communication and documentation as both the verbal and nonverbal interactions between the client, the significant others, and the members of the health care team, as well as the events and activities associated with client care as validated through a written or electronic record that reflects standards of practice and accountability into the provision of care.

When answering a question on the NCLEX-PN, the use of an effective communication technique indicates a correct option, and the use of an ineffective communication technique indicates an incorrect option. In addition, some communication questions may focus on psychosocial issues or issues related to client anxiety, fears, and concerns. With these types of questions, always focus on the client's feelings, concerns, and anxieties first. If an option reflects the client's feelings, concerns, or anxieties, select that option.

Documentation is a critical component of a nurse's responsibilities. The process of documentation serves many purposes and provides a comprehensive representation of the client's health status and of the care provided by all members of the health care team. There are many methods of documentation, but the responsibilities surrounding this practice remain the same.

When answering a question on the NCLEX-PN that is related to documentation, consider the associated ethical and legal responsibilities and the specific guidelines that are related to both narrative and computerized documentation systems (Box 10-8).

TEACHING AND LEARNING

Client and family education are primary nursing responsibilities. The NCSBN describes teaching and learning as facilitating the acquisition of knowledge, skills, and attitudes that lead to a change in behavior.

Box 10-8 ▲ COMMUNICATION AND DOCUMENTATION

COMMUNICATION

QUESTION

A client with depression tells a nurse that he is going to "put an end to my misery." The nurse should provide which response to the client?

1. "We all feel like that at times."
2. "Why do you feel like you need to say that?"
3. "Can you tell me more about what you plan to do?"
4. "You feel like that now, but soon you'll regain your will to live."

ANSWER: 3

Rationale: All suicidal threats must be taken seriously, and their meaning must be thoroughly explored. Options 1 and 4 devalue and ignore the client's feelings. Option 2 is incorrect because "why" questions are demeaning and belittling, and they will make the client feel guilty.

DOCUMENTATION

QUESTION

A nurse hears a client calling out for help. The nurse hurries down the hallway to the client's room and finds the client lying on the floor. The nurse checks the client thoroughly and assists the client back to bed. The nurse notifies the registered nurse of the incident and completes an incident report. Which of the following should the nurse document in the incident report?

1. The client fell out of bed.
2. The client climbed over the side rails.
3. The client was found lying on the floor.
4. The client became restless and tried to get out of bed.

ANSWER: 3

Rationale: The incident report should contain the client's name, age, and diagnosis. It should contain a factual description of the incident, any injuries experienced by those involved, and the outcome of the situation. Option 3 is the only option that describes the facts as observed by the nurse. Options 1, 2, and 4 are interpretations of the situation and are not factual data as observed by the nurse. Remember to focus on factual information when documenting and to avoid including interpretations.

Box 10-9 ▲ TEACHING AND LEARNING

QUESTION

Digoxin (Lanoxin) and hydrochlorothiazide (HydroDIURIL) are prescribed for a client with congestive heart failure, and the nurse provides instructions to the client about the medications. Which client statement indicates the need for further instruction?

1. "These medications cause an increase in urine output."
2. "I should take my radial pulse before taking these medications."
3. "I should decrease my intake of foods high in potassium, such as bananas."
4. "These medications should be taken in the morning rather than in the evening."

ANSWER: 3

Rationale: Digoxin (Lanoxin) is a cardiac glycoside, and hydrochlorothiazide (HydroDIURIL) is a diuretic. Clients who are taking digoxin have an increased risk of toxicity from the potassium-depleting effect of the hydrochlorothiazide. Therefore, the diet should be high in potassium. The client should take his or her pulse before taking cardiac glycosides. For best therapeutic effects, these medications should be taken at the same time in the morning. A combined therapeutic effect of these medications is to increase urine output. The increased blood flow to the kidneys as a result of enhanced cardiac contractility caused by the digoxin promotes urinary output. Hydrochlorothiazide increases the urine excretion of sodium and water by inhibiting sodium reabsorption in the nephron.

The principles related to the teaching and learning process are used when the nurse functions in the role of a teacher. The nurse should remember that determining the client's readiness and motivation to learn is the initial step of the teaching and learning process.

When answering a question on the NCLEX-PN that is related to the teaching and learning process, use the principles related to teaching and learning theory. If a test question addresses client education, remember that client motivation and readiness to learn are the first priorities (Box 10-9).

REFERENCES

Black, J., & Hawks, J. (2009). *Medical-surgical nursing: Clinical management for positive outcomes* (8th ed.). Philadelphia: Saunders.

Christensen, B., & Kockrow, E. (2006). *Foundations of nursing* (5th ed.). St. Louis: Mosby.

deWit, S. (2009). *Medical-surgical nursing: Concepts & practice.* St. Louis: Saunders.

Hill, S., & Howlett, H. (2009). *Success in practical/vocational nursing: From student to leader* (6th ed.). Philadelphia: Saunders.

Hodgson, B., & Kizior, R. (2009). *Saunders nursing drug handbook 2009.* St. Louis: Saunders.

Lehne, R. (2010). *Pharmacology for nursing care* (7th ed.). St. Louis: Saunders.

Lilley, L., Harrington, S., & Snyder, J. (2007). *Pharmacology and the nursing process* (5th ed.). St. Louis: Mosby.

Linton, A., & Maebius, N. (2007). *Introduction to medical-surgical nursing* (4th ed.). Philadelphia: Saunders.

National Council of State Boards of Nursing (Eds.) (2008). *2008 Detailed Test Plan for the NCLEX-PN® Examination.* Chicago: Author.

National Council of State Boards of Nursing, Inc. Web site: www.ncsbn.org. Accessed August 30, 2009.

Stuart, G. (2009). *Principles and practices of psychiatric nursing* (9th ed.). St. Louis: Mosby.

CHAPTER

11

Integrated Processes

CLINICAL PROBLEM-SOLVING PROCESS (NURSING PROCESS)

Nursing Process: Data Collection

1213. A nurse is assisting with collecting data from a pregnant client with a history of cardiac disease and checking the client for venous congestion. The nurse checks which of the following body areas, knowing that venous congestion is most commonly noted in this area?

1 Vulva
2 Around the eyes
3 Fingers
4 Around the abdomen

Level of Cognitive Ability: Application
Client Needs: Health Promotion and Maintenance
Integrated Process: Nursing Process/Data Collection
Content Area: Maternity/Antepartum

Answer: 1

Rationale: The assessment of the cardiovascular system includes observation for venous congestion that can develop into varicosities. Venous congestion is most commonly noted in the legs, vulva, and rectum. It would be difficult to check for the presence of edema in the abdominal area of a client who is pregnant. Although edema may be noted in the fingers and around the eyes, edema in these areas would not be directly associated with venous congestion.

Test-Taking Strategy: Use the process of elimination. Focus on the strategic words *venous congestion* to direct you to option 1. Review data collection techniques for the cardiovascular system of a pregnant client if you had difficulty with this question.

Reference

Leifer, G. (2007). *Introduction to maternity and pediatric nursing* (5th ed., pp. 102-103). Philadelphia: Saunders.

1214. A client who has been receiving long-term diuretic therapy is admitted to the hospital with a diagnosis of dehydration (fluid volume deficit). The nurse should check the client for which sign or symptom that correlates with this fluid imbalance?

1 Decreased pulse
2 Bibasilar crackles
3 Dry mucous membranes
4 Increased blood pressure

Level of Cognitive Ability: Comprehension
Client Needs: Physiological Integrity
Integrated Process: Nursing Process/Data Collection
Content Area: Fundamental Skills

Answer: 3

Rationale: Dehydration is an excessive loss of water from the body tissues. Findings that occur with fluid volume deficit (dehydration) are increased pulse and respirations, weight loss, poor skin turgor, dry mucous membranes, decreased urine output, concentrated urine with increased specific gravity, increased hematocrit level, and altered level of consciousness. The signs in options 1, 2, and 4 occur with fluid volume excess.

Test-Taking Strategy: Use the process of elimination, and focus on the client's diagnosis. Note the relationship between the client's diagnosis and the word *dry* in option 3. Review the signs and symptoms of fluid volume deficit if you had difficulty with this question.

Reference

Linton, A. (2007). *Introduction to medical-surgical nursing* (4th ed., p. 192). Philadelphia: Saunders.

1215. A nurse is monitoring the level of consciousness of a child with a head injury and documents that the child is obtunded. Based on this documentation, which of the following observations did the nurse make?

1 The child is unable to think clearly and rapidly.
2 The child is unable to recognize place or person.
3 The child requires considerable stimulation for arousal.
4 The child sleeps unless aroused and, once aroused, has limited interaction with the environment.

Level of Cognitive Ability: Comprehension
Client Needs: Physiological Integrity
Integrated Process: Nursing Process/Data Collection
Content Area: Child Health

Answer: 4
Rationale: If a child is obtunded, he or she sleeps unless aroused and, once aroused, has limited interaction with the environment. Option 1 describes confusion. Option 2 describes disorientation. Option 3 describes stupor.

Test-Taking Strategy: Use the process of elimination, and note the strategic word *obtunded.* Knowledge of the standard terms used to identify levels of consciousness will direct you to option 4. Remember that, if the child is obtunded, the child sleeps unless aroused and, once aroused, has limited interaction with the environment. Review the monitoring of the level of consciousness if you had difficulty with this question.

References
Wong, D., Hockenberry, M., Perry, S., Lowdermilk, D., & Wilson, D. (2006). *Maternal-child nursing care* (3rd ed., p. 1672). St. Louis: Mosby.
Hockenberry, M., & Wilson, D. (2009). *Wong's essentials of pediatric care* (8th ed., p. 976). St. Louis: Mosby.

1216. An Hispanic-American mother brings her child to the clinic for an examination. Which of the following would be most important during data collection about the child?

1 Avoiding eye contact
2 Using body language only
3 Avoiding speaking to the child
4 Touching the child during the examination

Level of Cognitive Ability: Application
Client Needs: Psychosocial Integrity
Integrated Process: Nursing Process/Data Collection
Content Area: Fundamental Skills

Answer: 4
Rationale: In the Hispanic-American culture, eye behavior is significant. The "evil eye" can be given to a child if a person looks at and admires a child without touching the child, so touching the child during the examination is very important. Although avoiding eye contact indicates respect and attentiveness, this is not the most important intervention during data collection. Avoiding speaking to the child and using body language only are not therapeutic interventions.

Test-Taking Strategy: Use the process of elimination, and note the strategic words *most important.* Eliminate options 2 and 3 first because they are comparable or alike. From the remaining options, select the intervention that is the most therapeutic, which is touch. Review the characteristics associated with Hispanic Americans if you had difficulty with this question.

Reference
Christensen, B., & Kockrow, E. (2006). *Foundations of nursing* (5th ed., p. 143). St. Louis: Mosby.

1217. A nurse is obtaining a history from a client admitted to the hospital with a cerebral thrombotic stroke. The nurse collects data from the client, knowing that, before this type of stroke, the client likely experienced:

1 No symptoms at all
2 Throbbing headaches
3 Transient hemiplegia and loss of speech
4 Unexplained episodes of loss of consciousness

Answer: 3
Rationale: Cerebral thrombosis does not occur suddenly. During the few hours or days that precede a thrombotic stroke, the client may experience a transient loss of speech, hemiplegia, or paresthesias on one side of the body. Other signs and symptoms of thrombotic stroke vary but may include dizziness, cognitive changes, and seizures. Headache is rare, and a loss of consciousness is not likely to occur.

Level of Cognitive Ability: Analysis
Client Needs: Physiological Integrity
Integrated Process: Nursing Process/Data Collection
Content Area: Adult Health/Neurological

Test-Taking Strategy: Use the process of elimination. Option 1 is eliminated first. From the remaining options, focus on the type of stroke addressed in the question to direct you to option 3. Review the signs and symptoms of a thrombotic stroke if you had difficulty with this question.

Reference

Linton, A. (2007). *Introduction to medical-surgical nursing* (4th ed., pp. 467-468). Philadelphia: Saunders.

1218. A client in a long-term care facility has had a series of gastrointestinal (GI) diagnostic tests, including an upper GI series and endoscopies. When the client returns to the long-term care facility, the priority nursing assessment should focus on the client's:
1 Comfort level
2 Activity tolerance
3 Level of consciousness
4 Hydration and nutrition status

Level of Cognitive Ability: Application
Client Needs: Physiological Integrity
Integrated Process: Nursing Process/Data Collection
Content Area: Adult Health/Gastrointestinal

Answer: 4
Rationale: Many of the diagnostic studies used to identify GI disorders require that the GI tract be cleaned (usually with laxatives and enemas) before testing. In addition, the client most often takes nothing by mouth before and during the testing period. Because the studies may be performed over a period of 24 hours or more, the client may become dehydrated, malnourished, or both. Although options 1, 2, and 3 may be components of an assessment, option 4 is the priority.

Test-Taking Strategy: Note the strategic words *priority nursing assessment.* Use Maslow's Hierarchy of Needs theory to direct you to option 4. Review the care to the client after diagnostic GI tests if you had difficulty with this question.

Reference

Chernecky, C., & Berger, B. (2008). *Laboratory tests and diagnostic procedures* (5th ed., p. 1133). Philadelphia: Saunders.

1219. A nurse is monitoring a client for the vegetative signs of depression. The nurse checks for these signs by determining the client's:
1 Level of self-esteem
2 Level of suicidal ideation
3 Ability to think, concentrate, and make decisions
4 Appetite, weight, sleep patterns, and psychomotor activity

Level of Cognitive Ability: Application
Client Needs: Physiological Integrity
Integrated Process: Nursing Process/Data Collection
Content Area: Mental Health

Answer: 4
Rationale: The vegetative signs of depression are changes in physiological functioning that occur during depression. These include changes in appetite, weight, sleep patterns, and psychomotor activity. Options 1, 2, and 3 represent psychological assessment categories.

Test-Taking Strategy: Use the process of elimination. Recall that the vegetative signs of depression refer to physiological changes to direct you to option 4. Review the characteristics of depression if you had difficulty with this question.

References

Keltner, N., Schwecke, L., & Bostrom, C. (2007). *Psychiatric nursing* (5th ed., pp. 372-373) St. Louis: Mosby.
Varcarolis, E., & Halter, M. (2009). *Essentials of psychiatric mental health nursing: A communication approach to evidence-based care* (p. 222). St. Louis: Saunders.

1220. A nurse is caring for a client with cirrhosis of the liver. The client is receiving spironolactone (Aldactone) daily. Which of the following would indicate to the nurse that the client is experiencing a side effect related to the medication?

Answer: 4
Rationale: Spironolactone is a potassium-sparing diuretic. Side effects include hyperkalemia, dehydration, hyponatremia, and lethargy. Although the concern with most diuretics is hypokalemia, this medication is potassium sparing, which means that the concern with the administration of this medication is hyperkalemia.

1 Edema
2 Dry skin
3 Constipation
4 Hyperkalemia

Level of Cognitive Ability: Analysis
Client Needs: Physiological Integrity
Integrated Process: Nursing Process/Data Collection
Content Area: Pharmacology

Additional side effects include nausea, vomiting, cramping, diarrhea, headache, ataxia, drowsiness, confusion, and fever.

Test-Taking Strategy: Use the process of elimination. Recall that this medication is potassium sparing to direct you to option 4. Review those medications in the classification of potassium-sparing diuretics if you had difficulty with this question.

Reference

Hodgson, B., & Kizior, R. (2009). *Saunders nursing drug handbook 2009* (p. 1076). St. Louis: Saunders.

1221. A nurse is gathering admission data from an African-American client scheduled for a cataract removal and an intraocular lens implant. Which question would be inappropriate for the nurse to ask initially?
1 "Do you ever experience chest pain?"
2 "Do you have any difficulty breathing?"
3 "Do you have a close family relationship?"
4 "Do you frequently have episodes of headache?"

Level of Cognitive Ability: Application
Client Needs: Psychosocial Integrity
Integrated Process: Nursing Process/Data Collection
Content Area: Fundamental Skills

Answer: 3
Rationale: In the African-American culture, it is considered to be intrusive to ask personal questions during the initial contact or meeting. African Americans are highly verbal and express feelings openly to their family and friends, but what transpires within the family is viewed as private. The psychosocial assessment would be of the least priority during the initial admission assessment. In addition, respiratory, cardiovascular, and neurological data are physiological and thus are the priority.

Test-Taking Strategy: Use Maslow's Hierarchy of Needs theory to answer the question. Note the strategic words *inappropriate* and *initially.* Options 1, 2, and 4 address physiological needs. Option 3 addresses a psychosocial need. Review the cultural beliefs of the African-American culture if you had difficulty with this question.

Reference

Christensen, B., & Kockrow, E. (2006). *Foundations of nursing* (5th ed., p. 143). St. Louis: Mosby.

1222. A nurse is preparing a woman in labor for an amniotomy. The nurse should check which priority data before the procedure?
1 Fetal heart rate
2 Maternal heart rate
3 Fetal scalp sampling
4 Maternal blood pressure

Level of Cognitive Ability: Application
Client Needs: Physiological Integrity
Integrated Process: Nursing Process/Data Collection
Content Area: Maternity/Intrapartum

Answer: 1
Rationale: Amniotomy is the artificial rupture of the fetal membranes. Fetal well-being must be confirmed before and after amniotomy. The fetal heart rate should be checked by Doppler or by the application of an external fetal monitor. Although the maternal vital signs may be assessed, the fetal heart rate is the priority. A fetal scalp sampling cannot be done when the membranes are intact.

Test-Taking Strategy: Use the process of elimination, and note the strategic word *priority.* Eliminate option 3 first because a fetal scalp sampling cannot be performed before an amniotomy. Eliminate options 2 and 4 next because they are comparable or alike in that they address maternal vital signs. Option 1 addresses fetal well-being. Review preprocedure care for amniotomy if you had difficulty with this question.

Reference

Christensen, B., & Kockrow, E. (2006). *Foundations of nursing* (5th ed., p. 842). St. Louis: Mosby.

1223. A nurse is assisting with monitoring a client who is receiving an oxytocin (Pitocin) infusion for the induction of labor. The nurse should suspect water intoxication if which of the following is noted?

1 Fatigue
2 Lethargy
3 Tachycardia
4 Bradycardia

Level of Cognitive Ability: Analysis
Client Needs: Physiological Integrity
Integrated Process: Nursing Process/Data Collection
Content Area: Maternity/Intrapartum

Answer: 3
Rationale: During an oxytocin infusion, the woman is monitored closely for water intoxication. Signs of water intoxication include tachycardia, cardiac dysrhythmias, shortness of breath, nausea, and vomiting.

Test-Taking Strategy: Use the process of elimination, and focus on the subject—water intoxication. Think about the physiological response that occurs when fluid overload exists to direct you to option 3. Review the signs of water intoxication if you had difficulty with this question.

Reference

Christensen, B., & Kockrow, E. (2006). *Foundations of nursing* (5th ed., p. 843). St. Louis: Mosby.

1224. A nurse plans to reinforce dietary instructions regarding caloric intake after discharge to a postpartum client. Before the nurse can adequately advise the client, which of the following data need to be collected first?

1 Cultural preferences
2 Concerns about weight gain
3 Information about the presence of fluoride in drinking water
4 The method of infant feeding that the mother has chosen

Level of Cognitive Ability: Comprehension
Client Needs: Psychosocial Integrity
Integrated Process: Nursing Process/Data Collection
Content Area: Maternity/Postpartum

Answer: 4
Rationale: Before the nurse can adequately advise the client, the method of infant feeding that the mother has chosen should be determined. Nonlactating women require a balanced diet of approximately 300 calories a day less than that consumed during pregnancy. The lactating woman will require an increase of 500 calories a day above prepregnancy needs. Good nutrition—not weight loss or gain—is the focus of the postpartum diet. Cultural preferences are important but do not influence the amount of caloric intake required.

Test-Taking Strategy: Focus on the subject of the question and your knowledge of the differences in nutritional requirements between the lactating and nonlactating mother. Note the strategic word *first* to direct you to option 4. Review dietary requirements during the postpartum period if you had difficulty with this question.

Reference

Leifer, G. (2007). *Introduction to maternity and pediatric nursing* (5th ed., p. 233). Philadelphia: Saunders.

1225. A nurse observes that a hospitalized client's daughter is threatening to place the client in a nursing home if the client continues to refuse to take the prescribed medications. The nurse is concerned that the client is a victim of which form of victimization?

1 Neglect
2 Sexual abuse
3 Emotional abuse
4 Economic maltreatment

Level of Cognitive Ability: Comprehension
Client Needs: Psychosocial Integrity
Integrated Process: Nursing Process/Data Collection
Content Area: Mental Health

Answer: 3
Rationale: Emotional abuse is the infliction of mental anguish and includes threatening an individual with abandonment or institutionalization (e.g., a nursing home). Neglect is the failure to provide care, and it can be physical, developmental, or educational. Sexual abuse is any form of sexual contact or exposure without the individual's consent. Economic maltreatment is the illegal or improper exploitation of an individual's funds.

Test-Taking Strategy: Use the process of elimination. Note the relationship between the word *threatening* in the question and option 3. Review the signs of emotional abuse if you had difficulty with this question.

Reference

Varcarolis, E., & Halter, M. (2009). *Essentials of psychiatric mental health nursing: A communication approach to evidence-based care* (pp. 395-396). St. Louis: Saunders.

1226. A woman is admitted to the mental health unit. When asked her name, she responds, "I am our President's wife, the First Lady." The nurse recognizes this response as:

1 A visual illusion
2 A loose association
3 A grandiose delusion
4 An auditory hallucination

Level of Cognitive Ability: Comprehension
Client Needs: Psychosocial Integrity
Integrated Process: Nursing Process/Data Collection
Content Area: Mental Health

Answer: 3

Rationale: Delusion is an important personal belief that is almost certainly not true and that resists modification. An illusion is a misperception or misinterpretation of externally real stimuli. Loose association is thinking that is characterized by speech in which unrelated ideas shift from one subject to another. A hallucination is a false perception.

Test-Taking Strategy: Use the process of elimination. Eliminate options 1 and 4 because the client is not having any visual or auditory disturbances. Eliminate option 2 because there is no indication of shifting from one subject to another. Making a reference to being the First Lady is a grandiose assumption. Review the characteristics of delusions if you had difficulty with this question.

Reference

Christensen, B., & Kockrow, E. (2006). *Foundations of nursing* (5th ed., p. 1145). St. Louis: Mosby.

1227. A nurse is monitoring a client with Addison's disease for signs of hyperkalemia. The nurse expects to note which of the following if hyperkalemia is present?

1 Polyuria
2 Cardiac dysrhythmias
3 Dry mucous membranes
4 Prolonged bleeding time

Level of Cognitive Ability: Comprehension
Client Needs: Physiological Integrity
Integrated Process: Nursing Process/Data Collection
Content Area: Adult Health/Endocrine

Answer: 2

Rationale: Addison's disease is caused by the partial or complete failure of adrenocortical function. The inadequate production of aldosterone in a client with Addison's disease causes the inadequate excretion of potassium and results in hyperkalemia. The clinical manifestations of hyperkalemia are the result of altered nerve transmission. The most harmful consequence of hyperkalemia is its effect on cardiac function. Options 1, 3, and 4 are not associated with Addison's disease or hyperkalemia.

Test-Taking Strategy: Use the process of elimination. Recall the effects of hyperkalemia to direct you to option 2. Remember that the most harmful consequence of hyperkalemia is its effect on cardiac function. Review the pathophysiology associated with Addison's disease and the effects of hyperkalemia if you had difficulty with this question.

Reference

Linton, A. (2007). *Introduction to medical-surgical nursing* (4th ed., pp. 972-973). Philadelphia: Saunders.

1228. A client goes into respiratory distress, and arterial blood gases (ABGs) are drawn from the radial artery. The nurse assists with performing Allen's test before the ABGs are drawn to determine the adequacy of the:

1 Ulnar circulation
2 Carotid circulation
3 Femoral circulation
4 Brachial circulation

Level of Cognitive Ability: Application
Client Needs: Physiological Integrity

Answer: 1

Rationale: Before radial puncture is performed to obtain an arterial specimen for ABGs, Allen's test should be performed to determine adequate ulnar circulation. The failure to assess the collateral circulation could result in severe ischemic injury to the hand should damage to the radial artery occur with arterial puncture. The other options are incorrect.

Test-Taking Strategy: Use the process of elimination, and note the strategic words *radial artery*. Use your knowledge of the anatomy of the cardiovascular system to eliminate options 2, 3, and 4. Review the purpose and procedure of Allen's test if you had difficulty with this question.

Integrated Process: Nursing Process/Data Collection
Content Area: Fundamental Skills

Reference

Linton, A. (2007). *Introduction to medical-surgical nursing* (4th ed., p. 518). Philadelphia: Saunders.

1229. A nurse is checking a client's functional abilities and his ability to perform activities of daily living (ADLs). The nurse focuses data collection on which of the following?

1 The client's ability to drive a car
2 The client's normal everyday routine in the home
3 The client's self-care needs, such as toileting, feeding, and ambulating
4 The client's ability to do light and heavy housework and to pay the bills

Level of Cognitive Ability: Application
Client Needs: Physiological Integrity
Integrated Process: Nursing Process/Data Collection
Content Area: Fundamental Skills

Answer: 3

Rationale: ADLs are activities such as bathing, toileting, ambulating, dressing, and feeding oneself. The abilities to do housework, pay bills, and drive a car are considered instrumental ADLs. The normal routine in the home is not a component of a functional assessment.

Test-Taking Strategy: Use the process of elimination, and focus on the subject—the ability to perform ADLs. Recall that ADLs involve self-care needs to direct you to option 3. Review the concepts of ADLs if you had difficulty with this question.

References

Christensen, B., & Kockrow, E. (2006). *Foundations of nursing* (5th ed., pp. 1201-1202). St. Louis: Mosby.
deWit, S. (2009). *Medical-surgical nursing: Concepts & practice* (p. 773). St. Louis: Saunders.

1230. A client is to undergo renal arteriography (angiography) to rule out renal pathology. As an essential element of care, the nurse asks the client about a history of:

1 Frequent antibiotic use
2 Long-term diuretic therapy
3 Allergy to shellfish or iodine
4 Allergy to peanuts or bananas

Level of Cognitive Ability: Application
Client Needs: Physiological Integrity
Integrated Process: Nursing Process/Data Collection
Content Area: Adult Health/Renal

Answer: 3

Rationale: Arteriography is a method of radiologically visualizing the arteries that is performed after a radiopaque contrast medium is introduced into the bloodstream or into a specific vessel by injection or through a catheter. The client undergoing any type of arteriography should be questioned about allergies to shellfish, seafood, or iodine; this is essential to identify a potential allergic reaction to the contrast dye that may be used in some diagnostic tests. The other items are also useful as part of data collection, but they are not as critical as the allergy determination.

Test-Taking Strategy: Use the process of elimination, and note the strategic word *essential*. This word implies that more than one or all of the options may be correct but that one of them is of highest priority. Option 4 can be eliminated first as the least pertinent to current care. Because the question indicates that arteriography is planned, the items are evaluated with regard to their potential connection to this test. Thus, all of the options except option 3 should be eliminated because option 3 is directly related to the test. Review preprocedural care for arteriography if you had difficulty with this question.

Reference

Linton, A. (2007). *Introduction to medical-surgical nursing* (4th ed., pp. 692, 844). Philadelphia: Saunders.

1231. A client has a cuffed tracheostomy tube and is being weaned from its use. The nurse who is assisting with caring for

Answer: 1

Rationale: The cuff must be deflated before a cuffed tracheostomy tube is plugged; the client cannot ventilate around the tube

the client checks for which critical occurrence before plugging the client's tracheostomy?

1 The cuff is fully deflated.
2 The oxygen saturation is at least 99%.
3 The airway is totally free of secretions.
4 The respiratory rate is 16 breaths/min.

Level of Cognitive Ability: Analysis
Client Needs: Physiological Integrity
Integrated Process: Nursing Process/Data Collection
Content Area: Adult Health/Respiratory

and could suffer respiratory arrest. Other correct nursing actions include suctioning the airway to promote ventilation and monitoring the adequacy of the client's oxygen saturation. (Baseline oxygen saturation may vary slightly, depending on the client, and may not be 99%.) The nurse cannot expect that the airway will be totally free of secretions. A respiratory rate of 16 breaths/min is within the normal range and is not a critical observation in this situation.

Test-Taking Strategy: Use the process of elimination. The question asks for a critical observation before plugging the tracheostomy. Options 2 and 4 indicate good respiratory status, but these values or results may not be realistic for every client and are not critical. Likewise, it is hard to ensure that the airway is completely free of secretions. The best option to address is that the tracheostomy cuff be deflated. Also, note that the correct option relates to the ABCs—airway, breathing, and circulation. If the tracheostomy tube is plugged with the cuff inflated, the client cannot ventilate around the tube and could suffer respiratory arrest. Review the care of the client with a tracheostomy if you had difficulty with this question.

Reference

Potter, P., & Perry, A. (2009). *Fundamentals of nursing* (7th ed., p. 943). St. Louis: Mosby.

1232. A nurse is assigned to collect admission data from a Mexican-American client. During the initial meeting with the client, the nurse should:

1 Avoid touching the client
2 Greet the client with a handshake
3 Smile and use humor throughout the entire admission assessment
4 Avoid any affirmative nods during the conversations with the client

Level of Cognitive Ability: Application
Client Needs: Psychosocial Integrity
Integrated Process: Nursing Process/Data Collection
Content Area: Fundamental Skills

Answer: 2
Rationale: To demonstrate respect, compassion, and understanding, health care providers should greet Mexican-American clients with a handshake. After establishing rapport, care providers may further demonstrate approval and respect through touch, smiling, and affirmative nods of the head. Given the diversity of dialects and the nuances of language, the culturally congruent use of humor is difficult to accomplish and therefore should be avoided.

Test-Taking Strategy: Use the process of elimination. Recall the cultural communication patterns of the Mexican American to direct you to option 2. Remember that to demonstrate respect, compassion, and understanding, health care providers should greet Mexican-American clients with a handshake. Review the characteristics of Mexican Americans if you had difficulty with this question.

Reference

Christensen, B., & Kockrow, E. (2006). *Foundations of nursing* (5th ed., p. 143). St. Louis: Mosby.

1233. A nurse reviews the record of a client receiving external radiation therapy and notes the documentation of a skin finding as moist desquamation. The nurse expects to note which of the following during data collection regarding the client's skin?

Answer: 4
Rationale: Moist desquamation occurs when the basal cells of the skin are destroyed. The dermal level is exposed, which results in the leakage of serum. Reddened skin, a rash, and dermatitis may occur with external radiation but are not described as moist desquamation.

1 A rash
2 Dermatitis
3 Reddened skin
4 Weeping skin

Level of Cognitive Ability: Comprehension
Client Needs: Physiological Integrity
Integrated Process: Nursing Process/Data Collection
Content Area: Adult Health/Oncology

Test-Taking Strategy: Use the process of elimination. Note the strategic word *moist* to direct you to option 4. Options 1, 2, and 3 are eliminated because they are comparable or alike in that they describe a dry rather than a moist skin alteration. Review the signs associated with moist desquamation if you had difficulty with this question.

Reference
Black, J., & Hawks, J. (2009). *Medical-surgical nursing: Clinical management for positive outcomes* (8th ed., p. 276). St. Louis: Saunders.

1234. A nurse is assisting with caring for a child with Reye's syndrome. The nurse monitors the client for:
1 Signs of hyperglycemia
2 Signs of a bacterial infection
3 The presence of protein in the urine
4 Signs of increased intracranial pressure (ICP)

Level of Cognitive Ability: Application
Client Needs: Physiological Integrity
Integrated Process: Nursing Process/Data Collection
Content Area: Child Health

Answer: 4
Rationale: Reye's syndrome is a combination of acute encephalopathy and the fatty infiltration of the internal organs that may follow acute viral infections. Increased ICP, encephalopathy, and hepatic dysfunction can occur in clients with Reye's syndrome. Protein is not present in the urine. Reye's syndrome is related to a history of viral infections. Hypoglycemia is a manifestation of this disease.

Test-Taking Strategy: Use the process of elimination, and focus on the diagnosis. Recall that increased ICP is a major concern in a client with Reye's syndrome to direct you to option 4. Review the care of the child with Reye's syndrome if you had difficulty with this question.

Reference
Price, D., & Gwin, J. (2008). *Pediatric nursing: An introductory text* (10th ed., p. 318). St. Louis: Saunders.

1235. A nurse reads the chart of a client who has stage III Lyme disease. When collecting data from the client, which of the following clinical manifestations should the nurse expect to note?
1 Palpitations
2 Cardiac dysrhythmia
3 Generalized skin rash
4 Enlarged and inflamed joints

Level of Cognitive Ability: Comprehension
Client Needs: Physiological Integrity
Integrated Process: Nursing Process/Data Collection
Content Area: Adult Health/Integumentary

Answer: 4
Rationale: Lyme disease is an infection that is caused by a spirochete transmitted by the bite of an infected tick. Stage III disease develops within a month to several months after the initial infection, and it is characterized by arthritic symptoms (e.g., arthralgias) and enlarged or inflamed joints, which can persist for several years after the initial infection. Cardiac and neurological dysfunction occur in stage II. A rash occurs in stage I.

Test-Taking Strategy: Use the process of elimination. Eliminate options 1 and 2 first because they are both cardiac in nature. Recalling that a rash occurs in stage I will direct you to option 4. Review the clinical manifestations associated with Lyme disease if you had difficulty with this question.

Reference
Copstead, L., & Banasik, J. (2010). *Pathophysiology* (4th ed., pp. 1212-1213). St. Louis: Mosby.

1236. A female client with narcolepsy has been prescribed dextroamphetamine (Dextro-Stat). The client complains to the nurse

Answer: 4
Rationale: Dextroamphetamine is a central nervous system (CNS) stimulant that acts by releasing norepinephrine from the nerve

that she cannot sleep well anymore at night and that she does not want to take the medication any longer. The nurse collects data and asks the client if the medication is taken at which of the following appropriate times?

1 2 hours before bedtime
2 Before a bedtime snack
3 Just before going to sleep
4 At least 6 hours before bedtime

Level of Cognitive Ability: Application
Client Needs: Physiological Integrity
Integrated Process: Nursing Process/Data Collection
Content Area: Pharmacology

endings. The client should take the medication at least 6 hours before going to bed at night to prevent disturbances with sleep. Options 1, 2, and 3 are incorrect.

Test-Taking Strategy: Use the process of elimination. Evaluate each of the options in terms of how far removed the scheduled dose is from the client's bedtime. Recalling that this medication causes CNS stimulation and interferes with sleep will direct you to option 4. Review dextroamphetamine if you had difficulty with this question.

Reference

Lehne, R. (2010). *Pharmacology for nursing care* (7th ed., pp. 399-402). St. Louis: Saunders.

1237. A pregnant client with diabetes mellitus arrives at the health care clinic for a follow-up visit. The nurse most importantly monitors which of the following with this client?

1 Urine for specific gravity
2 For the presence of edema
3 Urine for glucose and ketones
4 Blood pressure, pulse, and respirations

Level of Cognitive Ability: Application
Client Needs: Health Promotion and Maintenance
Integrated Process: Nursing Process/Data Collection
Content Area: Maternity/Antepartum

Answer: 3

Rationale: The nurse monitors the pregnant client with diabetes mellitus for glucose and ketones in the urine at each prenatal visit because the physiological changes of pregnancy can drastically alter insulin requirements. The assessment of the blood pressure, pulse, respirations, and urine for specific gravity as well as looking for the presence of edema are more related to the client with gestational hypertension.

Test-Taking Strategy: Use the process of elimination, and focus on the client's diagnosis. The only option that specifically addresses diabetes mellitus is option 3. Review the prenatal care of the client with diabetes mellitus if you had difficulty with this question.

Reference

Leifer, G. (2008). *Maternity nursing: An introductory text* (10th ed., p. 266). Philadelphia: Saunders.

1238. A nurse is caring for a Hispanic-American client admitted to the hospital with diabetic ketoacidosis. Several family members are present. Which of the following behaviors, if displayed by the family members, would the nurse interpret as being characteristic of this cultural group?

1 Dramatic body language
2 Consistently expressing negative feelings
3 Consistently confronting the nurse directly
4 Maintaining consistent eye contact with the nurse

Level of Cognitive Ability: Comprehension
Client Needs: Psychosocial Integrity

Answer: 1

Rationale: Characteristics of the Hispanic-American culture include the use of dramatic body language (e.g., gestures, facial expressions) to express emotion or pain. This group believes that direct confrontation is disrespectful and that the expression of negative feelings is impolite. In addition, in this culture, avoiding direct eye contact indicates respect and attentiveness.

Test-Taking Strategy: Use the process of elimination, and focus on the Hispanic-American culture. Recall that dramatic body language is a characteristic of this culture to direct you to option 1. Review the beliefs of the Hispanic-American culture if you had difficulty with this question.

Reference

Giger, J., & Davidhizar, R. (2008). *Transcultural nursing assessment & intervention* (5th ed., pp. 673-674). St. Louis: Mosby.

Integrated Process: Nursing Process/Data Collection
Content Area: Fundamental Skills

1239. A nurse is caring for a client at home who is in a body cast. The nurse is collecting data from the client about the psychosocial adjustment of the client to the cast. During data collection, the nurse should check:

1 The need for sensory stimulation
2 The amount of home-care support available
3 The ability to perform activities of daily living
4 The type of transportation available for follow-up care

Level of Cognitive Ability: Analysis
Client Needs: Psychosocial Integrity
Integrated Process: Nursing Process/Data Collection
Content Area: Adult Health/Musculoskeletal

Answer: 1

Rationale: A psychosocial assessment of the client who is immobilized should include the need for sensory stimulation. This assessment should also include such factors as body image, past and present coping skills, and the coping methods used during the period of immobilization. Although home-care support, the ability to perform activities of daily living, and transportation are components of an assessment, they are not as specifically related to psychosocial adjustment as is the need for sensory stimulation.

Test-Taking Strategy: Use the process of elimination, and focus on the strategic word *psychosocial.* Option 3 can be eliminated first because it relates to physiological integrity rather than psychosocial integrity. Eliminate options 2 and 4 next because they are more closely related to physical supports than to the psychosocial needs of the client. Review the components of a psychosocial assessment if you had difficulty with this question.

Reference
deWit, S. (2009). *Medical-surgical nursing: Concepts & practice* (p. 194). St. Louis: Saunders.

1240. A nurse is caring for a client with acquired immunodeficiency syndrome (AIDS). Which finding noted in the client indicates the presence of an opportunistic respiratory infection?

1 Colitis and ulcerated perirectal lesions
2 White plaques on the oral mucosa
3 Ophthalmic nerve involvement causing blindness
4 Fever, exertional dyspnea, and nonproductive cough

Level of Cognitive Ability: Analysis
Client Needs: Physiological Integrity
Integrated Process: Nursing Process/Data Collection
Content Area: Adult Health/Immune

Answer: 4

Rationale: AIDS involves a defect in cell-mediated immunity. Fever, exertional dyspnea, and a nonproductive cough are signs of *Pneumocystis jiroveci* pneumonia, which is a common, life-threatening opportunistic infection among clients with AIDS. Options 1, 2, and 3 are not associated with respiratory infection. Option 1 describes herpes simplex. Option 2 describes the fungal infection oral candidiasis *(Candida albicans)*, which is also called thrush. Option 3 describes the viral infection herpes zoster (shingles) when it has spread to involve the ophthalmic nerve.

Test-Taking Strategy: Use the process of elimination, and focus on the subject—respiratory infection. Option 4 is the only option that identifies symptoms related to the respiratory system. Review the signs of respiratory infection if you had difficulty with this question.

Reference
Linton, A. (2007). *Introduction to medical-surgical nursing* (4th ed., p. 617). Philadelphia: Saunders.

1241. An adult client seeks treatment in a clinic for complaints of a left earache, nausea, and a full feeling in the left ear. The client also has an elevated temperature.

Answer: 4

Rationale: Otitis media in the adult is typically one sided, and it often presents as an acute process with earache, nausea, and possible vomiting, fever, and fullness in the ear. The client may

The nurse first questions the client about:
1 A history of a recent brain abscess
2 Whether hearing is magnified in that ear
3 Whether acetaminophen (Tylenol) relieves the pain
4 A history of a recent upper respiratory infection (URI)

Level of Cognitive Ability: Analysis
Client Needs: Physiological Integrity
Integrated Process: Nursing Process/Data Collection
Content Area: Adult Health/Ear

complain of diminished hearing in the affected ear. The nurse takes a client history first to determine whether the client has had a recent URI. It is unnecessary to question the client about a brain abscess. The nurse may ask the client if anything relieves the pain, but ear infection pain is usually not relieved until antibiotic therapy is initiated.

Test-Taking Strategy: Use the process of elimination, and note the strategic word *first*. Recall the relationship between a URI and otitis media to direct you to option 4. Review otitis media if you had difficulty with this question.

Reference
deWit, S. (2009). *Medical-surgical nursing: Concepts & practice* (p. 657). St. Louis: Saunders.

1242. A nurse is caring for an older client at home who has urinary incontinence and who is very disturbed by the incontinent episodes. The nurse checks the client's home situation to determine environmental barriers to normal voiding. The nurse determines that which item may be contributing to the client's problem?
1 Having a handrail in the bathroom
2 Having one bathroom on each floor of the home
3 Having the bathroom on the second floor and the bedroom on the first floor
4 Having a nightlight present in the hall between the bedroom and bathroom

Level of Cognitive Ability: Comprehension
Client Needs: Safe and Effective Care Environment
Integrated Process: Nursing Process/Data Collection
Content Area: Fundamental Skills

Answer: 3
Rationale: Having the bathroom on the second floor and the bedroom on the first floor may pose a problem for an older client with incontinence. The need to negotiate the stairs and the distance may interfere with reaching the bathroom in a timely fashion. It is more helpful to the incontinent client to have the bathroom on the same floor as the bedroom or to obtain a commode for use. The presence of nightlights and handrails helps the client to reach the bathroom quickly and safely.

Test-Taking Strategy: Use the process of elimination, and focus on the subject—an environmental barrier to normal voiding. Note that options 1, 2, and 4 are comparable or alike in that they all are helpful and safe. Review the measures that promote normal voiding if you had difficulty with this question.

Reference
Christensen, B., & Kockrow, E. (2006). *Foundations of nursing* (5th ed., p. 1100). St. Louis: Mosby.

1243. A nurse is assisting with preparing to administer continuous intravenous (IV) fluid replacement to a client with dehydration. Which of the following is essential for the nurse to check before initiating the IV fluid?
1 Body weight
2 Intake and output
3 Ability to ambulate
4 Usual sleep patterns

Level of Cognitive Ability: Application
Client Needs: Physiological Integrity

Answer: 1
Rationale: Body weight is an accurate indicator of fluid status. As a client is hydrated with IV fluids, the nurse monitors for increasing body weight. Body weight provides a better measurement of gains and losses than intake and output records. An IV should not greatly alter sleep patterns, and clients will still be able to ambulate with an IV in place.

Test-Taking Strategy: Use the process of elimination and focus on the client's diagnosis to direct you to option 1. Remember that body weight is an accurate measurement of gains and losses. Review the care of the dehydrated client if you had difficulty with this question.

Integrated Process: Nursing Process/Data Collection
Content Area: Fundamental Skills

Reference
Linton, A. (2007). *Introduction to medical-surgical nursing* (4th ed., p. 188). Philadelphia: Saunders.

1244. A nurse is monitoring the respiratory status of a client who has expressive aphasia. The nurse uses a visual analog scale to measure which respiratory sign and symptom?
1 Cough
2 Dyspnea
3 Wheezing
4 Hemoptysis

Level of Cognitive Ability: Application
Client Needs: Health Promotion and Maintenance
Integrated Process: Nursing Process/Data Collection
Content Area: Adult Health/Respiratory

Answer: 2
Rationale: Dyspnea is difficult to measure because it tends to be subjective in nature. The client using a visual analog scale points to the description of dyspnea felt when questioned about breathlessness experienced with certain activities. Cough, hemoptysis, and wheezing are all measurable by the nurse without a need for further description by the client.

Test-Taking Strategy: Recall that a visual analog scale is useful for helping to quantify something experienced by the client. This is usually an item that is subjective in nature and that is not readily or directly measurable by the nurse. (Pain is the other symptom that commonly involves use of an analog scale.) It is unnecessary to use an analog scale to rate coughing, wheezing, or hemoptysis because the nurse can directly collect data related to these items using his or her own vision and hearing. Review the visual analog scale if you had difficulty with this question.

Reference
Linton, A. (2007). *Introduction to medical-surgical nursing* (4th ed., p. 210). Philadelphia: Saunders.

1245. A nurse is assisting with performing a cardiovascular assessment on a client with heart failure. Which of the following items should the nurse check to obtain the best information about the client's left-sided heart function?
1 Status of breath sounds
2 Presence of peripheral edema
3 Presence of hepatojugular reflux
4 Presence of jugular vein distention

Level of Cognitive Ability: Analysis
Client Needs: Physiological Integrity
Integrated Process: Nursing Process/Data Collection
Content Area: Adult Health/Cardiovascular

Answer: 1
Rationale: The client with heart failure may present different symptoms depending on whether the right or left side of the heart is failing. Peripheral edema, jugular vein distention, and hepatojugular reflux are all signs of right-sided heart function. The status of breath sounds provides information about left-sided heart function.

Test-Taking Strategy: Use the process of elimination, and focus on the subject—the status of left-sided heart function. Remember to associate the words *left* and *lungs*. Options 2, 3, and 4 reflect right-sided heart failure. Review the signs of right- and left-sided heart failure if you had difficulty with this question.

Reference
Christensen, B., & Kockrow, E. (2006). *Adult health nursing* (5th ed., pp. 361, 366). St. Louis: Mosby.

Nursing Process: Planning

1246. A nurse is preparing to care for an infant with pertussis. When planning care, the nurse addresses which most critical problem first?
1 Fluid volume excess
2 High risk for infection
3 Sleep-pattern disturbance
4 Ineffective airway clearance

Answer: 4
Rationale: Pertussis is an acute, highly contagious respiratory disease that is characterized by paroxysmal coughing that ends in a loud whooping inspiration. The most important problem relates to adequate air exchange. Because of the copious, thick secretions that occur with pertussis and the small airways of an infant, air exchange is critical. A fluid volume deficit is more likely to occur in this infant because of the thick secretions and vomiting. Infection is an important consideration, but the airway is the priority. Sleep

Level of Cognitive Ability: Application
Client Needs: Physiological Integrity
Integrated Process: Nursing Process/Planning
Content Area: Child Health

patterns may be disturbed because of the coughing, but they are not the most critical issue.

Test-Taking Strategy: Use the process of elimination and the ABCs—airway, breathing, and circulation. The airway is always the most critical concern; this should direct you to option 4. Review the care of the infant with pertussis if you had difficulty with this question.

Reference

Christensen, B., & Kockrow, E. (2006). *Foundations of nursing* (5th ed., p. 1068). St. Louis: Mosby.

1247. A nurse receives a telephone call from the emergency department about a 7-month-old infant with febrile seizures who will be admitted to the pediatric unit. When planning care for this infant, the nurse should anticipate the need for which of the following?

1 Restraints at the bedside
2 A code cart at the bedside
3 Suction equipment at the bedside
4 A padded tongue blade taped to the head of the bed

Level of Cognitive Ability: Application
Client Needs: Physiological Integrity
Integrated Process: Nursing Process/Planning
Content Area: Child Health

Answer: 3
Rationale: During a seizure, the infant should be placed in a side-lying position but should not be restrained. Suctioning may be necessary during a seizure to remove secretions that obstruct the airway. A padded tongue blade should never be used; in fact, nothing should be placed in a client's mouth during a seizure. It is not necessary to place a code cart at the bedside, but a cart should be readily available in the nursing unit.

Test-Taking Strategy: Use the process of elimination and the ABCs—airway, breathing, and circulation—to answer the question. Option 3 is the only option that specifically relates to airway. Review nursing interventions for an infant with seizures if you had difficulty with this question.

Reference

Hockenberry, M., & Wilson, D. (2009). *Wong's essentials of pediatric care* (8th ed., p. 1015). St. Louis: Mosby.

1248. A client with a brain attack (stroke) is prepared for discharge from the hospital. The physician has prescribed range-of-motion (ROM) exercises for the client's right side. When planning for the client's care, the nurse:

1 Implements ROM exercises to the point of pain for the client
2 Considers the use of active, passive, or active-assisted exercises in the home
3 Develops a schedule of ROM exercises for every 2 hours while awake, even if the client is fatigued
4 Encourages the client to be dependent on a home health care nurse to complete the exercise program

Level of Cognitive Ability: Application
Client Needs: Health Promotion and Maintenance
Integrated Process: Nursing Process/Planning
Content Area: Adult Health/Neurological

Answer: 2
Rationale: The nurse must consider all forms of ROM exercise for the client. Even if the client has right hemiplegia, the client can assist in some of his or her own rehabilitative care. In addition, the goal is for the client to assume as much self-care and independence as possible. The nurse needs to plan care so that the client becomes self-reliant. Options 1 and 3 are incorrect from a physiological perspective.

Test-Taking Strategy: Use the process of elimination. Options 1 and 3 can be eliminated first because these actions can be harmful to the client. From the remaining options, recall that dependency is not in the best interest of a client's sense of health promotion, which eliminates option 4. Note that option 2 is the umbrella option. Review ROM exercises and self-care if you had difficulty with this question.

References

Christensen, B., & Kockrow, E. (2006). *Foundations of nursing* (5th ed., pp. 385-388). St. Louis: Mosby.
deWit, S. (2009). *Medical-surgical nursing: Concepts & practice* (p. 577). St. Louis: Saunders.

1249. A nurse assists with developing a plan of care for a client with a spica cast that covers a lower extremity. When planning for bowel elimination needs, the nurse includes which of the following in the plan?

1 Administer an enema daily.
2 Use a fracture pan for bowel elimination.
3 Use a bedside commode for all elimination needs.
4 Use a regular bedpan to prevent the spilling of contents in the bed.

Level of Cognitive Ability: Application
Client Needs: Physiological Integrity
Integrated Process: Nursing Process/Planning
Content Area: Fundamental Skills

Answer: 2
Rationale: A fracture pan is designed for use with clients with body or leg casts. A client with a spica cast (body cast) that covers a lower extremity cannot bend at the hips to sit up, so a regular bedpan or a commode would be inappropriate. Daily enemas are not a part of routine care.

Test-Taking Strategy: Focus on the strategic words *covers a lower extremity.* Use the process of elimination, and note the strategic word *fracture* in the correct option. Review the care of the client with a spica cast if you had difficulty with this question.

Reference
Christensen, B., & Kockrow, E. (2006). *Foundations of nursing* (5th ed., pp. 472-473). St. Louis: Mosby.

1250. A nurse is developing a plan of care for a hospitalized Asian-American client. The nurse avoids including which of the following in the plan of care?

1 Limiting eye contact
2 Clarifying responses to questions
3 Maintaining physical space with the client
4 Providing light touch to the head for comfort

Level of Cognitive Ability: Application
Client Needs: Psychosocial Integrity
Integrated Process: Nursing Process/Planning
Content Area: Fundamental Skills

Answer: 4
Rationale: Avoiding physical closeness, limiting eye contact, avoiding hand gestures, and clarifying responses to questions are all components of the plan of care for an Asian-American client. In the Asian-American culture, the head is considered to be sacred; touching someone on the head is thought to be disrespectful. When working with clients from this culture, remember to touch the client's head only when necessary and to inform the client before doing so.

Test-Taking Strategy: Use the process of elimination, and note the strategic word *avoids.* This word indicates a negative event query and asks you to select an option that is an incorrect action. Eliminate options 1 and 3 because they are comparable or alike in that they both address avoiding contact. Eliminate option 2 because it is a therapeutic communication technique. Review the beliefs associated with the Asian-American culture if you had difficulty with this question.

Reference
Giger, J., & Davidhizar, R. (2008). *Transcultural nursing assessment & intervention* (5th ed., p. 446). St. Louis: Mosby.

1251. A nurse is caring for a client who is receiving parenteral nutrition. The nurse plans which nursing intervention to prevent infection in the client?

1 Weighing the client daily
2 Encouraging increased fluid intake
3 Monitoring the serum blood urea nitrogen daily
4 Using strict aseptic technique for intravenous site dressing changes

Answer: 4
Rationale: Strict aseptic technique is vital during dressing changes because the intravenous catheter can serve as a direct entry point for microorganisms. Options 1, 2, and 3 are not measures that will prevent infection.

Test-Taking Strategy: Use the process of elimination. Note the relationship between the word *infection* in the question and *aseptic* in the correct option. The only option that will prevent infection is option 4. Review the care of a client receiving parenteral nutrition if you had difficulty with this question.

Level of Cognitive Ability: Application
Client Needs: Safe and Effective Care Environment
Integrated Process: Nursing Process/Planning
Content Area: Fundamental Skills

Reference

Linton, A. (2007). *Introduction to medical-surgical nursing* (4th ed., p. 744). Philadelphia: Saunders.

1252. A nurse is preparing to give a client a dose of iron dextran (InFeD) via the intramuscular route. The nurse should plan to:

1 Inject the medication deeply using a Z-track technique.
2 Administer the medication into the deltoid muscle of the arm.
3 Use a 5/8-inch, 25-gauge needle to administer the medication.
4 Avoid changing the needle between the drawing up of the medication and the injection.

Level of Cognitive Ability: Application
Client Needs: Physiological Integrity
Integrated Process: Nursing Process/Planning
Content Area: Pharmacology

Answer: 1
Rationale: Iron dextran may permanently stain subcutaneous tissue. For this reason, the medication is administered using the Z-track technique deep into the upper outer quadrant of the buttock. It is never given in the arm or in other exposed areas. An intramuscular 2- to 3-inch, 19- or 20-gauge needle is used. The needle is changed after drawing up the medication and before administration to minimize subcutaneous staining.

Test-Taking Strategy: Use the process of elimination, and note the strategic words *intramuscular route.* This will assist you with eliminating options 2 and 3. Remember that iron stains to assist you with eliminating option 4. Review the procedure for administering iron dextran if you had difficulty with this question.

Reference

Linton, A. (2007). *Introduction to medical-surgical nursing* (4th ed., p. 582). Philadelphia: Saunders.

1253. A nurse is planning to implement a bladder retraining program for a client with incontinence. Which intervention is contraindicated as the nurse develops this plan?

1 Ensure the accessibility of a toilet.
2 Limit the oral fluid intake of the client.
3 Strictly adhere to scheduled toileting times.
4 Teach pelvic-muscle–strengthening exercises.

Level of Cognitive Ability: Application
Client Needs: Physiological Integrity
Integrated Process: Nursing Process/Planning
Content Area: Adult Health/Renal

Answer: 2
Rationale: For a bladder retraining program to be successful, several components must be in place. The client should learn and practice pelvic-muscle–strengthening exercises to promote bladder emptying. The nurse should ensure the accessibility of bathroom facilities and strictly adhere to the toileting schedule. Limiting fluid intake is contraindicated; adequate fluid intake is necessary to produce enough urine to stimulate micturition.

Test-Taking Strategy: Use the process of elimination, and note the strategic word *contraindicated.* This word indicates a negative event query and asks you to select an option that is an incorrect action. Because options 1 and 3 are most obviously correct, they are eliminated in accordance with the wording of the question. From the remaining options, it is necessary to know that sufficient fluid is necessary to cause bladder filling and the proper stimulation of the micturition reflex; this will help you to select option 2 as the intervention that is contraindicated. Review the components of a bladder retraining program if you had difficulty with this question.

Reference

Linton, A. (2007). *Introduction to medical-surgical nursing* (4th ed., pp. 333, 342). Philadelphia: Saunders.

1254. A nurse is planning a menu with the hospital dietitian for a Chinese client. The meal plan is designed to include

Answer: 2
Rationale: The Chinese diet is generally vegetarian. Native Chinese clients generally do not drink milk or eat milk products

which food that is generally included in the diet of members of this cultural group?
1 Milk
2 Vegetables
3 Large portions of meat
4 A dessert high in sugar content

Level of Cognitive Ability: Application
Client Needs: Psychosocial Integrity
Integrated Process: Nursing Process/Planning
Content Area: Fundamental Skills

because of a genetic tendency toward lactose intolerance. Most Chinese clients do not eat large portions of meat or desserts high in sugar content.

Test-Taking Strategy: Use the process of elimination. Recall the food rituals related to the Chinese culture to direct you to option 2. Remember that the Chinese diet is generally vegetarian. Review the dietary characteristics of the Chinese culture if you had difficulty with this question.

References
Giger, J., & Davidhizar, R. (2008). *Transcultural nursing assessment & intervention* (5th ed., p. 460). St. Louis: Mosby.
Nix, S. (2009). *Williams' basic nutrition and diet therapy* (13th ed., pp. 262-263, 520). St. Louis: Mosby.

1255. A male client who initially denied that he drank 12 beers per day is being discharged from the hospital. He is now willing to admit that he has a problem with drinking, and he states that he will "get some help" to live a healthier lifestyle. The nurse plans for a meeting with a representative from which of the following groups to meet with the client before discharge?
1 Al-Anon
2 Fresh Start
3 Families Anonymous
4 Alcoholics Anonymous

Level of Cognitive Ability: Application
Client Needs: Psychosocial Integrity
Integrated Process: Nursing Process/Planning
Content Area: Mental Health

Answer: 4
Rationale: Alcoholics Anonymous is a major self-help organization for the treatment of alcoholism. Option 1 is a group for families of alcoholics. Option 2 is for nicotine addicts. Option 3 is for parents of children who abuse substances.

Test-Taking Strategy: Use the process of elimination. Note the relationship between the word *drinking* in the question and *Alcoholics* in the correct option. Review the purposes of specific support groups if you had difficulty with this question.

Reference
deWit, S. (2009). *Medical-surgical nursing: Concepts & practice* (pp. 1124-1125). St. Louis: Saunders.

1256. A nurse is assisting with admitting a client who recently had a bilateral adrenalectomy. Which intervention is essential for the nurse to suggest to include in the client's plan of care?
1 Preventing social isolation
2 Considering occupational therapy
3 Discussing changes in body image
4 Avoiding stress-producing situations and procedures

Level of Cognitive Ability: Application
Client Needs: Physiological Integrity
Integrated Process: Nursing Process/Planning
Content Area: Adult Health/Endocrine

Answer: 4
Rationale: A bilateral adrenalectomy involves the removal of the adrenal glands. This surgical procedure can lead to adrenal insufficiency. Adrenal hormones are essential for maintaining homeostasis in response to stressors. Options 1, 2, and 3 are not essential interventions specific to this client's problem.

Test-Taking Strategy: Note the strategic word *essential* in the question; this words indicates the need to prioritize. Remember that, according to Maslow's Hierarchy of Needs theory, physiological needs come first. The stress reaction involves physiological processes. Options 1, 2, and 3 relate to psychosocial needs. Review the postoperative effects after an adrenalectomy if you had difficulty with this question.

Reference
deWit, S. (2009). *Medical-surgical nursing: Concepts & practice* (p. 902). St. Louis: Saunders.

1257. A perinatal client is admitted to the obstetric unit during an exacerbation of a heart condition. When planning for the nutritional requirements of the client, the nurse should consult with the dietitian to ensure which of the following?

1 A low-calorie diet to ensure an absence of weight gain
2 A diet low in fluids and fiber to decrease blood volume
3 A diet adequate in fluids and fiber to decrease constipation
4 Unlimited sodium intake to increase the circulating blood volume

Level of Cognitive Ability: Application
Client Needs: Physiological Integrity
Integrated Process: Nursing Process/Planning
Content Area: Maternity/Antepartum

Answer: 3
Rationale: Constipation can cause the client to use Valsalva's maneuver, which can cause blood to rush to the heart and overload the cardiac system. A low-calorie diet is not recommended during pregnancy. Diets low in fluid and fiber can cause a decrease in blood volume that can deprive the fetus of nutrients, so adequate fluid intake and high-fiber foods are important. Sodium should be restricted to some degree, as prescribed by the physician, because sodium can cause an overload to the circulating blood volume and contribute to cardiac complications.

Test-Taking Strategy: Use the process of elimination. Think about the physiology of the cardiac system, maternal and fetal needs, and the factors that increase the workload of the heart to answer the question; this will direct you to option 3. Review nursing measures for the pregnant client with cardiac disease if you had difficulty with this question.

Reference
McKinney, E., James, S., Murray, S., & Ashwill, J. (2009). *Maternal-child nursing* (3rd ed., pp. 306, 646). St. Louis: Mosby.

1258. A nurse is assisting with preparing a plan of care for a client with Ménière's disease who is experiencing severe vertigo. Which nursing intervention should the nurse suggest to include in the plan of care to assist the client with this condition?

1 Instructing the client to increase the sodium in the diet
2 Encouraging the client to increase the daily fluid intake
3 Instructing the client to cut down on cigarette smoking
4 Encouraging the client to avoid sudden head movements

Level of Cognitive Ability: Application
Client Needs: Safe and Effective Care Environment
Integrated Process: Nursing Process/Planning
Content Area: Adult Health/Ear

Answer: 4
Rationale: Vertigo is a sensation of instability or disequilibrium that can result in the risk for injury. The nurse instructs the client to make slow head movements to prevent the worsening of the vertigo. Dietary changes that reduce the amount of endolymphatic fluid (e.g., salt and fluid restrictions) are sometimes prescribed. Clients are advised to stop smoking because of the vasoconstrictive effects.

Test-Taking Strategy: Use the process of elimination, and focus on the subject—severe vertigo. Note the relationship between the words *vertigo* in the question and *to avoid sudden head movements* in the correct option. Recall that salt and fluid restrictions are sometimes prescribed to assist you with eliminating options 1 and 2. Note the words *cut down* to eliminate option 3. Review the measures that will reduce vertigo in the client with Ménière's disease if you had difficulty with this question.

References
deWit, S. (2009). *Medical-surgical nursing: Concepts & practice* (p. 633). St. Louis: Saunders.
Linton, A. (2007). *Introduction to medical-surgical nursing* (4th ed., p. 1203). Philadelphia: Saunders.

1259. An 18-year-old woman is admitted to a mental health unit with a diagnosis of anorexia nervosa. The nurse assists with planning this client's care, knowing that health promotion should focus on:

1 Providing a supportive environment
2 Examining intrapsychic conflicts and past issues

Answer: 4
Rationale: Anorexia nervosa is characterized by a prolonged refusal to eat adequately that results in emaciation, amenorrhea, emotional disturbances involving the body image, and a fear of becoming obese. Health promotion focuses on helping clients to identify and examine both dysfunctional thoughts and the values and beliefs that maintain these thoughts. Providing a supportive environment is important but is not as primary as option 4 for

3 Emphasizing social interaction with clients who are withdrawn
4 Helping the client to identify and examine dysfunctional thoughts and beliefs

Level of Cognitive Ability: Application
Client Needs: Health Promotion and Maintenance
Integrated Process: Nursing Process/Planning
Content Area: Mental Health

this client. Emphasizing social interaction is not appropriate at this time. Examining intrapsychic conflicts and past issues is not directly related to the client's problem.

Test-Taking Strategy: Use the process of elimination, and focus on the subject—health promotion. Option 4 is the only option that is specifically client centered. This option also focuses on data collection, which is the first step of the nursing process. Review the care of the client with anorexia nervosa if you had difficulty with this question.

Reference
deWit, S. (2009). *Medical-surgical nursing: Concepts & practice* (p. 1114). St. Louis: Saunders.

1260. A nurse is assisting with preparing discharge plans for a client who has attempted suicide. The nurse suggests including which of the following in the plan?
1 Weekly follow-up appointments
2 Contracts and immediately available crisis resources
3 Encouraging family and friends to always be present
4 Providing phone numbers for the hospital and physician

Level of Cognitive Ability: Application
Client Needs: Psychosocial Integrity
Integrated Process: Nursing Process/Planning
Content Area: Mental Health

Answer: 2
Rationale: Crisis times may occur between appointments. Contracts facilitate clients feeling responsible for keeping a promise, which gives the client control. Family and friends cannot always be present. Providing phone numbers will not ensure available and immediate crisis resources.

Test-Taking Strategy: Use the process of elimination, and focus on the subject—the availability of immediate resources for the client. Eliminate option 3 first because this is unrealistic. Options 1 and 4 will not necessarily provide immediate resources. In addition, note the word *immediately* in option 2. Review discharge plans for a client who has attempted suicide if you had difficulty with this question.

Reference
deWit, S. (2009). *Medical-surgical nursing: Concepts & practice* (p. 1114). St. Louis: Saunders.

1261. A nurse is planning to instruct a Mexican-American client about nutrition and dietary restrictions. When developing the plan, the nurse is aware that this ethnic group:
1 Primarily eats raw fish
2 Primarily enjoys eating red meat
3 Views food as a primary form of socialization
4 Eats only food that lacks color, flavor, and texture

Level of Cognitive Ability: Comprehension
Client Needs: Psychosocial Integrity
Integrated Process: Nursing Process/Planning
Content Area: Fundamental Skills

Answer: 3
Rationale: Mexican foods are rich in color, flavor, texture, and spiciness. In the Mexican-American culture, any occasion is seen as a time to celebrate with food and to enjoy the companionship of family and friends. Because food is a primary form of socialization in the Mexican culture, Mexican Americans may have difficulty adhering to a prescribed diet. Asian Americans eat raw fish, rice, and soy sauce. European Americans prefer carbohydrates and red meat.

Test-Taking Strategy: Use the process of elimination. Recall the food practices and preferences and the meaning of food in the Mexican-American culture to direct you to option 3. Review the food preferences associated with the Mexican-American culture if you had difficulty with this question.

Reference
Giger, J., & Davidhizar, R. (2008). *Transcultural nursing: Assessment & intervention* (5th ed., p. 250). St. Louis: Mosby.

1262. A nurse is assisting with developing a plan of care for a newborn infant diagnosed with bilateral clubfeet. The nurse includes instructions in the plan to tell the parents that:

1 The regimen of manipulation and casting is effective in all cases of bilateral clubfeet.
2 Genetic testing is wise for future pregnancies because other children born to this couple may also be affected.
3 If casting is needed, it will begin at birth and continue for 12 weeks, at which point the condition will be reevaluated.
4 Surgery performed immediately after birth has been found to be most effective for achieving a complete recovery.

Level of Cognitive Ability: Application
Client Needs: Physiological Integrity
Integrated Process: Nursing Process/Planning
Content Area: Child Health

Answer: 3
Rationale: Clubfoot is a congenital deformity of the foot that is characterized by the unilateral or bilateral deviation of the metatarsal bones of the forefoot. Casting should begin at birth and continue for at least 12 weeks or until maximum correction is achieved. At this time, corrective shoes may provide support to maintain alignment, or surgery can be performed. Surgery is usually delayed until the age of 4 to 12 months. Options 1 and 4 are inaccurate. Option 2 does not address the subject of the question.

Test-Taking Strategy: Use the process of elimination, and focus on the subject—parental instructions for the child with bilateral clubfeet. Eliminate option 2 because this is not the time to discuss the future. Eliminate option 4 because of the word *immediately*. From the remaining options, note that option 3 provides accurate information and that option 1 contains the close-ended word *all*. Review the treatment plan for bilateral clubfeet if you had difficulty with this question.

Reference
Price, D., & Gwin, J. (2008). *Pediatric nursing: An introductory text* (10th ed., p. 106). St. Louis: Saunders.

1263. A nurse is planning to assist with obtaining a set of arterial blood gases on a client. In addition to sending the specimen to the laboratory immediately, the nurse plans to provide which item to obtain the specimen and to optimally maintain the integrity of the specimen?

1 A syringe that contains a preservative
2 A heparinized syringe and a bag of ice
3 A heparinized syringe and a preservative
4 A syringe that contains a preservative and a bag of ice

Level of Cognitive Ability: Application
Client Needs: Physiological Integrity
Integrated Process: Nursing Process/Planning
Content Area: Adult Health/Respiratory

Answer: 2
Rationale: The arterial blood gas sample is obtained with the use of a heparinized syringe. The sample of blood is placed on ice and sent to the laboratory immediately. A preservative is not used.

Test-Taking Strategy: Use the process of elimination. Note that options 1, 3, and 4 are comparable and alike in that they indicate the use of a preservative. Review the method for obtaining an arterial blood gas sample if you had difficulty with this question.

Reference
Linton, A. (2007). *Introduction to medical-surgical nursing* (4th ed., p. 518). Philadelphia: Saunders.

1264. A client is experiencing diabetes insipidus secondary to cranial surgery. The nurse who is assisting with caring for the client plans to implement which of the following anticipated prescribed therapies?

1 Fluid restriction
2 Administering diuretics
3 Increased sodium intake
4 Intravenous (IV) replacement of fluid losses

Answer: 4
Rationale: Diabetes insipidus is a metabolic disorder caused by injury of the neurohypophyseal system. The client with diabetes insipidus excretes large amounts of extremely dilute urine. This usually occurs as a result of decreased synthesis or release of antidiuretic hormone with conditions such as head injury, surgery near the hypothalamus, and increased intracranial pressure. Corrective measures include allowing ample oral fluid intake, administering IV fluid as needed to replace sensible and insensible losses, and administering vasopressin (Pitressin). Sodium is not

Level of Cognitive Ability: Analysis
Client Needs: Physiological Integrity
Integrated Process: Nursing Process/Planning
Content Area: Adult Health/Neurological

administered because the serum sodium level is usually high, as is the serum osmolality. Diuretics will exacerbate the fluid loss.

Test-Taking Strategy: Use the process of elimination, and focus on the client's diagnosis. Recall that a large fluid loss is the problem in this client; this will assist you with eliminating options 1 and 2. From the remaining options, recall that the serum sodium level is already elevated in a client with this disorder. Remember that fluid replacement is the most direct form of therapy for fluid loss to direct you to option 4. Review the treatment for diabetes insipidus if you had difficulty with this question.

Reference

Christensen, B., & Kockrow, E. (2006). *Adult health nursing* (5th ed., pp. 524-525). St. Louis: Mosby.

1265. A nurse is assisting with planning care for a child with an infectious communicable disease. The nurse determines that which of the following is the primary goal?

1 The public health department will be notified.
2 The child will experience only mild discomfort.
3 The child will not spread the infection to others.
4 The child will experience only minor complications.

Level of Cognitive Ability: Analysis
Client Needs: Safe and Effective Care Environment
Integrated Process: Nursing Process/Planning
Content Area: Child Health

Answer: 3

Rationale: The primary goal is to prevent the spread of the disease to others. Although the health department may need to be notified at some point, it is not the most important primary goal. It is also important to prevent client discomfort as much as possible. The child should experience no complications.

Test-Taking Strategy: Use the process of elimination, and note the strategic words *primary goal*. In addition, note the relationship between the words *infectious communicable disease* in the question and *infection* in the correct option. Review the goals of care for the child with an infectious communicable disease if you had difficulty with this question.

Reference

Leifer, G. (2007). *Introduction to maternity and pediatric nursing* (5th ed., p. 717). Philadelphia: Saunders.

1266. A nurse is assisting with planning care for an infant who has pyloric stenosis. To most effectively meet the infant's preoperative needs, the nurse includes which of the following in the plan of care?

1 Administering enemas until returns are clear
2 Providing the mother with privacy to breast-feed every 2 hours
3 Providing small, frequent feedings of glucose, water, and electrolytes
4 Monitoring the intravenous (IV) infusion, intake and output, and weight

Level of Cognitive Ability: Application
Client Needs: Physiological Integrity
Integrated Process: Nursing Process/Planning
Content Area: Child Health

Answer: 4

Rationale: Pyloric stenosis is a narrowing of the pyloric sphincter at the outlet of the stomach, which causes an obstruction that blocks the flow of food into the small intestine. Important preoperative nursing responsibilities include monitoring the IV infusion, intake and output, and weight and obtaining urine specific gravity measurements. In addition, weighing the infant's diapers provides information about output. The infant is kept NPO preoperatively unless the physician prescribes a thickened formula. Enemas until returns are clear would further compromise the fluid volume status.

Test-Taking Strategy: Use the process of elimination, and note the strategic word *preoperative*. Eliminate option 1 because enemas would further compromise the fluid balance status. Eliminate options 2 and 3 because the infant should be NPO during the preoperative period. Review the preoperative care of an infant with pyloric stenosis if you had difficulty with this question.

Reference
Christensen, B., & Kockrow, E. (2006). *Foundations of nursing* (5th ed., p. 1029). St. Louis: Mosby.

1267. A nurse plans to call the dietary department to obtain a dinner meal for an Italian-American client who was admitted to the hospital at 4:00 PM. The physician prescribed a diet "as tolerated." Considering the practices and preferences of the Italian-American culture, which of the following should the nurse plan to request for the meal?
1 Rice
2 Kosher foods
3 Blue cornmeal
4 Bread and pasta

Level of Cognitive Ability: Application
Client Needs: Psychosocial Integrity
Integrated Process: Nursing Process/Planning
Content Area: Fundamental Skills

Answer: 4
Rationale: Food preferences of Italian Americans include bread, pasta, cheese, meats, poultry, and fish. Asian Americans prefer rice and raw fish. Dietary kosher laws are adhered to by members of the Jewish community. Native-American preferences include blue cornmeal, fish, game, fruits, and berries.

Test-Taking Strategy: Use the process of elimination. Remember that kosher foods are important to the Jewish population, that blue cornmeal is associated with Native Americans, and that Asian Americans prefer rice. Review the food preferences of the various cultures if you had difficulty with this question.

Reference
Nix, S. (2009). *Williams' basic nutrition and diet therapy* (13th ed., p. 263). St. Louis: Mosby.

1268. A client who was a victim of a gunshot incident states, "I feel like I am losing my mind. I keep hearing the gunshots and seeing my friend lying on the ground." The nurse plans strategies to formulate a therapeutic relationship that will include:
1 Teaching the client relaxation techniques
2 Asking the psychiatrist to order an antianxiety medication
3 Encouraging the client to think about how lucky he or she is to be alive
4 Encouraging the client to talk about the incident and the feelings related to it

Level of Cognitive Ability: Application
Client Needs: Psychosocial Integrity
Integrated Process: Nursing Process/Planning
Content Area: Mental Health

Answer: 4
Rationale: When developing a therapeutic relationship, it is important to acknowledge and validate the client's feelings. Although teaching the client relaxation techniques may be helpful at some point, this process is not related to the subject of the question. Options 2 and 3 are nontherapeutic techniques and do not promote a therapeutic relationship.

Test-Taking Strategy: Use therapeutic communication techniques. Eliminate options 2 and 3 because they do not encourage further discussion about the client's feelings. Teaching the client how to relax may be helpful at some point but not at the beginning of the therapeutic relationship. Remember to address the client's feelings. Review therapeutic communication techniques if you had difficulty with this question.

References
Fortinash, K., & Holoday-Worret, P. (2008). *Psychiatric mental health nursing* (4th ed., pp. 278-279). St. Louis: Mosby.
Varcarolis, E., & Halter, M. (2009). *Essentials of psychiatric mental health nursing: A communication approach to evidence-based care* (pp. 91-95). St. Louis: Saunders.

1269. A nurse is caring for a hospitalized child with a diagnosis of rheumatic fever who has developed carditis. The mother asks the nurse to explain the meaning of carditis. The nurse plans to respond that

Answer: 1
Rationale: Carditis is the inflammation of the heart (primarily the mitral valve), and it is a complication of rheumatic fever. Option 2 describes chorea. Option 3 describes polyarthritis. Option 4 describes erythema marginatum.

carditis is a complication of rheumatic fever that results in:
1 The inflammation of the heart (primarily the mitral valve)
2 Involuntary movements that affect the legs, arms, and face
3 Tender, painful joints (especially the elbows, knees, ankles, and wrists)
4 Red skin lesions that start as flat or slightly raised macules, usually over the trunk, that spread peripherally

Level of Cognitive Ability: Application
Client Needs: Physiological Integrity
Integrated Process: Nursing Process/Planning
Content Area: Child Health

Test-Taking Strategy: Use the process of elimination. Note the relationship between the word *carditis* in the question and *heart* in the correct option. Review carditis if you had difficulty with this question.

Reference
Leifer, G. (2007). *Introduction to maternity and pediatric nursing* (5th ed., p. 604). Philadelphia: Saunders.

1270. A nurse is told that a child with Reye's syndrome is being admitted to the hospital. The nurse assists with developing a plan of care for the child and suggests including which priority nursing action in the plan?
1 Monitoring for hearing loss
2 Positioning the child supine
3 Monitoring intake and output (I&O)
4 Providing a quiet environment with low lighting

Level of Cognitive Ability: Application
Client Needs: Physiological Integrity
Integrated Process: Nursing Process/Planning
Content Area: Child Health

Answer: 4
Rationale: Reye's syndrome is a combination of acute encephalopathy and fatty infiltration of the internal organs that may follow an acute viral infection. Cerebral edema is a progressive part of the disease process in Reye's syndrome. A major component of the care of a child with Reye's syndrome is maintaining effective cerebral perfusion and controlling intracranial pressure. Decreasing stimuli in the environment decreases the stress on the cerebral tissue and the neuron responses. Hearing loss does not occur with this disorder. The child should be in a head-elevated position to decrease the progression of cerebral edema and to promote the drainage of cerebrospinal fluid. Although monitoring I&O may be a component of the plan, it is not the priority.

Test-Taking Strategy: Use the process of elimination, and note the strategic words *priority nursing action*. Recall that increased intracranial pressure is a concern to direct you to option 4. Review the priorities in the plan of care for the child with Reye's syndrome if you had difficulty with this question.

Reference
Leifer, G. (2007). *Introduction to maternity and pediatric nursing* (5th ed., pp. 529-530). Philadelphia: Saunders.

1271. A nurse who is caring for an Orthodox Jewish client plans a diet that adheres to the practices of Judaism. The nurse avoids including which of the following in the diet plan?
1 Well-cooked meats
2 Fish with scales and fins
3 Meat and milk together
4 Unleavened bread during Passover week

Answer: 3
Rationale: Dietary kosher laws must be adhered to by Orthodox Jews. Rare meats are prohibited. Fish that have scales and fins are allowed; however, any combination of meat and milk is prohibited. During Passover week, only unleavened bread is eaten.

Test-Taking Strategy: Use the process of elimination, and note the strategic word *avoids*. This word indicates a negative event query and asks you to select an option that is an incorrect dietary plan. Recall the dietary practices of Judaism to direct you to option 3. Review the dietary practices of this cultural group if you had difficulty with this question.

Level of Cognitive Ability: Application
Client Needs: Psychosocial Integrity
Integrated Process: Nursing Process/Planning
Content Area: Fundamental Skills

Reference

Nix, S. (2009). *Williams' basic nutrition and diet therapy* (13th ed., p. 256). St. Louis: Mosby.

1272. A nursing student is asked to conduct a clinical conference about autism. The student plans to include in the discussion that the primary characteristic associated with autism is:

1 Normal social play
2 Normal verbal communication
3 Lack of social interaction and awareness
4 The consistent imitation of others' actions

Level of Cognitive Ability: Application
Client Needs: Psychosocial Integrity
Integrated Process: Nursing Process/Planning
Content Area: Child Health

Answer: 3

Rationale: Autism is a severe developmental disorder that begins during infancy or toddlerhood. A primary characteristic is a lack of social interaction and awareness. Social behaviors in autism include a lack of or abnormal imitations of others' actions and a lack of or abnormal social play. Additional characteristics include a lack of or impaired verbal communication and marked abnormal nonverbal communication.

Test-Taking Strategy: Use the process of elimination. Eliminate options 1 and 2 first because they address normal behaviors. From the remaining options, recall that the autistic child lacks social interaction and awareness to direct you to option 3. Review the characteristics associated with autism if you had difficulty with this question.

Reference

Christensen, B., & Kockrow, E. (2006). *Foundations of nursing* (5th ed., p. 1076). St. Louis: Mosby.

1273. A nurse is assisting with developing a plan of care for a child returning from the recovery room after a tonsillectomy. The nurse avoids placing which intervention in the plan of care?

1 Suctioning whenever necessary
2 Offering clear, cool liquids when awake
3 Monitoring for bleeding from the surgical site
4 Eliminating milk and milk products from the diet

Level of Cognitive Ability: Application
Client Needs: Physiological Integrity
Integrated Process: Nursing Process/Planning
Content Area: Child Health

Answer: 1

Rationale: After tonsillectomy, suction equipment should be available. However, suctioning is not performed unless there is an airway obstruction because of the risk of traumatizing the tissue in the surgical area. If suctioning must be performed, it needs to be performed carefully to avoid trauma. Clear, cool liquids are encouraged. Milk and milk products are avoided initially because they coat the throat and cause the child to clear the throat, thus increasing the risk of bleeding. Monitoring for bleeding is an important intervention after any type of surgery.

Test-Taking Strategy: Use the process of elimination, and note the strategic word *avoids*. This word indicates a negative event query and asks you to select an option that is an incorrect action. Eliminate option 3 first because this is an expected general nursing procedure. From the remaining options, think about the anatomical location of the surgery to direct you to option 1. Suctioning after tonsillectomy will disrupt the integrity of the surgical site and can cause bleeding. Review postoperative care after tonsillectomy if you had difficulty with this question.

Reference

McKinney, E., James, S., Murray, S., & Ashwill, J. (2009). *Maternal-child nursing* (3rd ed., p. 1184). St. Louis: Mosby.

1274. A nurse is assisting with preparing a plan of care for a child being admitted to the hospital with a diagnosis of congestive

Answer: 4

Rationale: CHF is an abnormal condition that reflects impaired cardiac pumping. Measures that will decrease the workload on the

heart failure (CHF). The nurse avoids including which of the following in the plan?

1 Elevating the head of the bed
2 Providing oxygen during stressful periods
3 Limiting the time that the child is allowed to bottle-feed
4 Waking the child for feeding to ensure adequate nutrition

Level of Cognitive Ability: Application
Client Needs: Physiological Integrity
Integrated Process: Nursing Process/Planning
Content Area: Child Health

heart include limiting the time that the child is allowed to bottle- or breast-feed, elevating the head of the bed, allowing for uninterrupted rest periods, and providing oxygen during stressful periods.

Test-Taking Strategy: Use the process of elimination, and note the strategic word *avoids.* This word indicates a negative event query and asks you to select an option that is an incorrect statement. Review each option carefully, and recall that the goal for a child with CHF is decreasing the workload on the heart. Option 4 is the only option that will not provide this measure. Review the measures associated with caring for a child with CHF if you had difficulty with this question.

Reference

Leifer, G. (2007). *Introduction to maternity and pediatric nursing* (5th ed., p. 602). Philadelphia: Saunders.

1275. A 10-month-old infant is hospitalized for respiratory syncytial virus (RSV), and the nurse assists with developing a plan of care for the infant. Based on the developmental stage of the infant, the nurse suggests including which of the following in the plan of care?

1 Restraining the infant with a total body restraint to prevent any tubes from being dislodged
2 Following the home feeding schedule and allowing the infant to be held only when the parents visit
3 Washing hands, wearing a mask when caring for the child, and keeping the child as quiet as possible
4 Providing a consistent routine and touching, rocking, and cuddling the infant throughout the hospitalization

Level of Cognitive Ability: Application
Client Needs: Physiological Integrity
Integrated Process: Nursing Process/Planning
Content Area: Child Health

Answer: 4
Rationale: A 10-month-old infant is in the trust versus mistrust stage of psychosocial development (Erikson) and in the sensorimotor period of cognitive development (Piaget). Hospitalization may have an adverse effect. A consistent routine accompanied by touching, rocking, and cuddling will help the child to develop trust and provide sensory stimulation. Total body restraint is unnecessary and an incorrect action. RSV is not airborne (a mask is not required); it is usually transmitted by the hands. Touching and holding the infant only when the parents visit will not provide adequate stimulation and interpersonal contact for the infant.

Test-Taking Strategy: Note the age and diagnosis of the infant. Focus on the strategic words *developmental stage of the infant* to direct you to option 4. Review the psychosocial needs of a 10-month-old infant if you had difficulty with this question.

Reference

Christensen, B., & Kockrow, E. (2006). *Foundations of nursing* (5th ed., pp. 156, 1017). St. Louis: Mosby.

1276. A nurse is planning activities for a client who is severely depressed. Which of the following activities would be appropriate for this client?

1 Dance therapy
2 Playing cards with the nurse
3 Ping-Pong with another client
4 Role-playing during a group activity

Level of Cognitive Ability: Comprehension
Client Needs: Psychosocial Integrity
Integrated Process: Nursing Process/Planning
Content Area: Mental Health

Answer: 2
Rationale: When a client is severely depressed, he or she should be involved in quiet, one-on-one activities. Because concentration is impaired when the client is severely depressed, this strategy maximizes the potential for interacting and may minimize anxiety levels. Options 1, 3, and 4 are incorrect.

Test-Taking Strategy: Use the process of elimination, and note the strategic words *severely depressed.* In addition, note the words *with the nurse* in the correct option. The activities identified in options 1, 3, and 4 indicate interaction with individuals other than the nurse. Review the care of the client who is severely depressed if you had difficulty with this question.

References
Stuart, G. (2009). *Principles and practices of psychiatric nursing* (9th ed., p. 307). St. Louis: Mosby.
Swearingen, P. (2008). *All-in-one care planning resource: Medical-surgical, pediatric, maternity & psychiatric nursing care plans* (2nd ed., p. 766). St. Louis: Mosby.

1277. A licensed practical nurse (LPN) is assisting a forensic psychiatric nurse with conducting a group session for female offender clients. Which of the following should the LPN identify as a priority and plan to suggest to include in the group session with these clients?

1 Psychodrama
2 Self-defense skills
3 Medication education
4 Coping skills and stress management

Level of Cognitive Ability: Analysis
Client Needs: Psychosocial Integrity
Integrated Process: Nursing Process/Planning
Content Area: Mental Health

Answer: 4
Rationale: The most useful survival skills for female offender clients in a group session would include effective problem-solving and coping skills to enhance the ability to manage stress. Option 1 may be used to assist clients to express their feelings more appropriately, but this would not be a priority. Option 2 is incorrect, although self-defense skills used to channel the aggressive drive appropriately may be useful. Option 3 is incorrect because these clients do not normally receive medication.

Test-Taking Strategy: Note the data in the question, and focus on the subject—female offender clients; this will direct you to option 4. Review the therapies described in the options and their uses if you had difficulty with this question.

Reference
Newell, R., & Gournay, K. (2009). *Mental health nursing: An evidence-based approach* (2nd ed., p. 387). St. Louis: Churchill Livingstone.

Nursing Process: Implementation

1278. A nurse is collecting data from a client who is in the second trimester of pregnancy. If the nurse notes that the fetal heart rate (FHR) is 100 beats/min, what action should be taken?

1 Document the findings.
2 Notify the registered nurse (RN).
3 Inform the mother that the FHR is normal and that everything is fine.
4 Instruct the mother to return to the clinic in 1 week for reevaluation of the FHR.

Level of Cognitive Ability: Application
Client Needs: Physiological Integrity
Integrated Process: Nursing Process/Implementation
Content Area: Maternity/Antepartum

Answer: 2
Rationale: The FHR should be between 120 and 160 beats/min during pregnancy. An FHR of 100 beats/min would require that the RN be notified and the client be further evaluated. Options 1, 3, and 4 are inaccurate nursing actions.

Test-Taking Strategy: Use the process of elimination. Knowing that the limits for the FHR are between 120 and 160 beats/min will direct you to option 2. Review the normal findings of the pregnant client if you had difficulty with this question.

Reference
Christensen, B., & Kockrow, E. (2006). *Foundations of nursing* (5th ed., p. 814). St. Louis: Mosby.

1279. A client with a closed head injury has fluid leaking from the ear. The nurse should first:

1 Notify the physician.
2 Test the drainage's pH level.
3 Irrigate the ear canal gently.
4 Test the drainage for glucose.

Answer: 4
Rationale: The client with a closed head injury may have leakage of cerebrospinal fluid (CSF) from the nose or ear. The nurse first determines whether the fluid tests positive for glucose, which indicates that it is indeed CSF. The nurse then notifies the registered nurse, who then notifies the physician. Testing of pH is not indicated. The ear is not irrigated because of the risk of infection.

Level of Cognitive Ability: Application
Client Needs: Physiological Integrity
Integrated Process: Nursing Process/Implementation
Content Area: Adult Health/Neurological

Test-Taking Strategy: Note the strategic words *closed head injury*. Recall that this client is at risk for CSF leakage, and remember the appropriate method of determining the presence of CSF. With this in mind, eliminate options 2 and 3. From the remaining options, note the strategic word *first* to direct you to option 4. Review the care of the client with a closed head injury if you had difficulty with this question.

References

Christensen, B., & Kockrow, E. (2006). *Adult health nursing* (5th ed., p. 742). St. Louis: Mosby.
deWit, S. (2009). *Medical-surgical nursing: Concepts & practice* (p. 543). St. Louis: Saunders.

1280. A nurse is assigned to care for a client with a history of asthma. In the event that the client experiences an asthma attack, the nurse should do which of the following first?
1 Obtain a set of vital signs.
2 Prepare to administer oxygen at 21%.
3 Place the client in a high-Fowler's position.
4 Obtain an intravenous (IV) cannula for starting an IV line.

Answer: 3
Rationale: Asthma is a respiratory disorder that is characterized by recurring episodes of paroxysmal dyspnea; wheezing on expiration or inspiration caused by the constriction of the bronchi; coughing; and viscous, mucoid bronchial secretions. The initial nursing action is to place the client in a position that is helpful for breathing, such as sitting bolt upright or in a high-Fowler's position. Other nursing actions follow in rapid sequence and include monitoring the vital signs and administering bronchodilators and oxygen (but at levels of 2 to 5 L/min or 24% to 28% by Venti-mask). The insertion of an IV line and the ongoing monitoring of the respiratory status are also indicated.

Level of Cognitive Ability: Application
Client Needs: Physiological Integrity
Integrated Process: Nursing Process/Implementation
Content Area: Delegating/Prioritizing

Test-Taking Strategy: Use the process of elimination, and note the strategic word *first*. Eliminate option 2 first because oxygen at 21% is ambient air (not supplemental oxygen). Option 1 is not the best first choice when a client is in respiratory distress, so this option can be eliminated. The correct option protects the client's airway; this will guide you to choose option 3 instead of option 4. Review the care of the client experiencing an asthma attack if you had difficulty with this question.

Reference

Christensen, B., & Kockrow, E. (2006). *Adult health nursing* (5th ed., p. 458). St. Louis: Mosby.

1281. A client has a compulsive bed-making ritual in which the client makes and remakes a bed numerous times. The client often misses breakfast and some morning activities because of the ritual. Which nursing action is most helpful?
1 Discuss the ridiculousness of the behavior.
2 Verbalize tactful, mild disapproval of the behavior.
3 Help the client to make the bed so that the task can be finished quicker.
4 Offer reflective feedback, such as "I see you have made your bed several times."

Answer: 4
Rationale: Reflective feedback acknowledges the client's behavior. The client is usually aware of the irrationality (or ridiculousness) of the behavior. Verbalizing disapproval would increase the client's anxiety and reinforce the need to perform the ritual. Helping with the ritual is nontherapeutic and also reinforces the behavior.

Test-Taking Strategy: Use the process of elimination. Recall that the purpose of the ritual is to relieve anxiety to assist you with eliminating options 1 and 2 because these actions would increase the anxiety. Eliminate option 3 because there is no therapeutic value in participating in the ritual. Review the appropriate interventions for the client with compulsive behaviors if you had difficulty with this question.

Level of Cognitive Ability: Application
Client Needs: Psychosocial Integrity
Integrated Process: Nursing Process/ Implementation
Content Area: Mental Health

Reference

Fortinash, K., & Holoday-Worret, P. (2008). *Psychiatric mental health nursing* (4th ed., pp. 185-186). St. Louis: Mosby.

1282. When collecting data about a child, a nurse notes that the child's genitals are swollen. The nurse suspects that the child is being sexually abused. The nurse should take which action?

1 Document the child's physical findings.
2 Refer the family to appropriate support groups.
3 Report the case in which the abuse is suspected.
4 Assist the family with identifying resources and support systems.

Level of Cognitive Ability: Application
Client Needs: Psychosocial Integrity
Integrated Process: Nursing Process/ Implementation
Content Area: Child Health

Answer: 3
Rationale: The primary legal responsibility of the nurse when child abuse is suspected is to report the case. All 50 states require health care professionals to report all cases of suspected abuse. Although documenting findings, assisting the family, and referring the family to appropriate resources and support groups are important, the primary legal responsibility is to report the case.

Test-Taking Strategy: Focus on the subject—that the child is being sexually abused. In addition to the many implications associated with child abuse, recall that abuse is a crime; this will direct you to option 3. Review the responsibilities of the nurse when child abuse is suspected if you had difficulty with this question.

Reference

Christensen, B., & Kockrow, E. (2006). *Foundations of nursing* (5th ed., pp. 25, 27). St. Louis: Mosby.

1283. A nurse is caring for a child with a head injury. When reviewing the record, the nurse notes that the physician has documented decorticate posturing. During care of the child, the nurse notes extension of the upper extremities and internal rotation of the upper arm and wrist. The nurse also notes that the lower extremities are extended, with some internal rotation noted at the knees and feet. Based on these findings, the nurse should take which action?

1 Document the findings.
2 Notify the registered nurse (RN).
3 Attempt to flex the child's lower extremities.
4 Continue to monitor for posturing of the child.

Level of Cognitive Ability: Application
Client Needs: Physiological Integrity
Integrated Process: Nursing Process/ Implementation
Content Area: Child Health

Answer: 2
Rationale: Decorticate posturing refers to the flexion of the upper extremities and the extension of the lower extremities. Plantarflexion of the feet may also be observed. Decerebrate posturing involves the extension of the upper extremities with the internal rotation of the upper arms and wrists. The lower extremities will extend, with some internal rotation noted at the knees and feet. The progression from decorticate to decerebrate posturing usually indicates deteriorating neurological function and warrants the notification of the RN; the RN will then contact the physician. Options 1, 3, and 4 are incorrect.

Test-Taking Strategy: Focus on the data in the question, and use your knowledge of the findings associated with decerebrate and decorticate positioning. Note that a change in the client's condition has occurred and that the neurological findings indicate deterioration of the client's condition to direct you to the correct option. Review the different types of posturing if you had difficulty with this question.

Reference

Price, D., & Gwin, J. (2008). *Pediatric nursing: An introductory text* (10th ed., pp. 211, 213). St. Louis: Saunders.

1284. An older client who has undergone internal fixation after fracturing a left hip has developed a reddened left heel. The nurse obtains which priority item to manage this problem?

1 Trapeze
2 Sheepskin
3 Bed cradle
4 Draw sheet

Level of Cognitive Ability: Application
Client Needs: Physiological Integrity
Integrated Process: Nursing Process/ Implementation
Content Area: Adult Health/Musculoskeletal

Answer: 2

Rationale: The reddened heel results from the pressure of the foot against the mattress. The nurse obtains a sheepskin, heel protectors, or an alternating pressure mattress. The bed cradle is unnecessary for managing this problem. A draw sheet and trapeze are of general use for this client but are not specific for dealing with the reddened heel.

Test-Taking Strategy: Use the process of elimination, and focus on the subject—a reddened left heel. Eliminate option 3 first as an unnecessary measure. Eliminate options 1 and 4 next because, although they are generally helpful for the client's mobility, they are not related to the subject of the question. Option 2 addresses the problem stated in the question. Review the measures that prevent skin breakdown in the immobile client if you had difficulty with this question.

Reference

Linton, A. (2007). *Introduction to medical-surgical nursing* (4th ed., pp. 315-316). Philadelphia: Saunders.

1285. A nurse is caring for an African-American client. The nurse enters the room and, after greeting and introducing herself to the client, begins to describe the angiography procedure scheduled for the next day. The client turns away from the nurse. Which of the following nursing actions is appropriate?

1 Continue with the explanation.
2 Ask the client if he or she can hear the nurse.
3 Walk around to the other side of the client so that the nurse faces the client.
4 Leave the room and return later to continue with the explanation.

Level of Cognitive Ability: Application
Client Needs: Psychosocial Integrity
Integrated Process: Nursing Process/ Implementation
Content Area: Fundamental Skills

Answer: 1

Rationale: In the African-American culture, direct eye contact is often viewed as being rude. If the client turns away from the nurse during a conversation, the appropriate action is to continue with the conversation. Walking around to the other side of the client so that the nurse faces the client is in direct conflict with this cultural practice. Asking the client if he or she can hear the nurse or leaving the room and returning later to continue with the explanation may be viewed as rude by the client.

Test-Taking Strategy: Use the process of elimination and therapeutic communication techniques. Eliminate options 2 and 4 first because these are nontherapeutic actions. From the remaining options, option 1 is the most therapeutic. Review the communication practices of the African-American cultural group if you had difficulty with this question.

Reference

Christensen, B., & Kockrow, E. (2006). *Foundations of nursing* (5th ed., p. 143). St. Louis: Mosby.

1286. A nurse teaches a client with a rib fracture to cough and deep breathe. The client resists directions by the nurse because of the pain. The nurse should take which action?

1 Request that a nerve block be performed to deaden the pain.
2 Continue to give the client gentle encouragement to cough and deep breathe.

Answer: 4

Rationale: The shallow respirations that occur with rib fracture predispose the client to developing atelectasis and pneumonia. It is essential that the client perform coughing and deep breathing to prevent these complications. The nurse accomplishes this most effectively by premedicating the client with pain medication and assisting the client with splinting during the exercises. Continuing to give the client gentle encouragement to cough and deep breathe and explaining in detail the potential complications of a lack of coughing and deep breathing do not address the client's

3 Explain in detail the potential complications of a lack of coughing and deep breathing.
4 Premedicate the client and assist the client to splint the area during these exercises.

Level of Cognitive Ability: Application
Client Needs: Physiological Integrity
Integrated Process: Nursing Process/Implementation
Content Area: Adult Health/Respiratory

pain. Requesting that a nerve block be performed to deaden the pain is extreme and unrealistic.

Test-Taking Strategy: Use the process of elimination. Eliminate option 1 because it is an extreme and unrealistic action. Options 2 and 3 can be eliminated because they do not address the subject of the client's pain. Review the care of the client with a rib fracture if you had difficulty with this question.

Reference

deWit, S. (2009). *Medical-surgical nursing: Concepts & practice* (p. 342). St. Louis: Saunders.

1287. An older client who has been in traction for several days is becoming disoriented. The best intervention to deal with the disorientation is to:

1 Let the family reorient the client.
2 Order laboratory tests to check for imbalances.
3 Go along with the disorientation to not upset the client.
4 Use environmental clues (e.g., calendars, clocks) and gentle corrective reminders to reorient the client.

Level of Cognitive Ability: Application
Client Needs: Psychosocial Integrity
Integrated Process: Nursing Process/Implementation
Content Area: Fundamental Skills

Answer: 4

Rationale: An inactive older person may become disoriented because of a lack of sensory stimulation. The family can help with orientation, but it is the nurse's responsibility to help reorient the client. This client is in traction, so the client's understanding and cooperation are essential to the treatment; therefore the disorientation cannot be ignored. Ordering laboratory tests is outside of the scope of practice of a nurse.

Test-Taking Strategy: Note the strategic word *best,* and use the process of elimination. Options 2 and 3 can be eliminated first because they do not directly deal with the subject of disorientation. From the remaining options, select option 4 because it is the nurse's responsibility to care for the client. Review nursing measures for the disoriented client if you had difficulty with this question.

References

Linton, A. (2007). *Introduction to medical-surgical nursing* (4th ed., p. 325). Philadelphia: Saunders.
Wold, G. (2008). *Basic geriatric nursing* (4th ed., p. 178). St. Louis: Mosby

---

1288. A nurse is caring for a 14-year-old child who is hospitalized and placed in Crutchfield traction. The child is having difficulty adjusting to the length of the hospital confinement. The nurse should take which action to meet the child's needs?

1 Let the child wear his or her own clothing when friends visit.
2 Allow the child to play loud music in the hospital room.
3 Allow the child to have his or her hair dyed if the parent agrees.
4 Allow the child to keep the shades closed and the room darkened at all times

Level of Cognitive Ability: Application
Client Needs: Psychosocial Integrity

Answer: 1

Rationale: Crutchfield traction involves the use of skeletal pins, and the client is immobilized. Adolescents need to identify with peers and belong to a group; they like to dress like the group and wear similar hairstyles. The hospitalized child should be allowed to wear his or her own clothing to feel a sense of belonging to the group. Because Crutchfield traction involves skeletal pins, hair dye is not appropriate. Loud music may disturb others in the hospital. The child's request for a darkened room is indicative of a possible problem with depression that may require further evaluation and intervention.

Test-Taking Strategy: Use the process of elimination, and focus on the subjects—Crutchfield traction and a 14-year-old child. Knowledge of Crutchfield traction and its limitations as well as of growth and development concepts will direct you to option 1. Review growth and development and the care of the child in traction if you had difficulty with this question.

Integrated Process: Nursing Process/Implementation
Content Area: Child Health

Reference
McKinney, E., James, S., Murray, S., & Ashwill, J. (2009). *Maternal-child nursing* (3rd ed., p. 891). St. Louis: Mosby.

1289. A nurse is told that a client in leg traction will be admitted to the nursing unit. The nurse prepares for the arrival and obtains which item that will be essential for helping the client to move in bed while in the leg traction?
1 A footboard
2 Extra pillows
3 A bed trapeze
4 An electric bed

Level of Cognitive Ability: Application
Client Needs: Physiological Integrity
Integrated Process: Nursing Process/Implementation
Content Area: Adult Health/Musculoskeletal

Answer: 3
Rationale: A trapeze is a device that will allow the client to lift straight up while being moved so that the amount of pull exerted on the limb in traction is not altered. A footboard and extra pillows do not facilitate moving. An electric bed or a manual bed can be used for traction, but neither one specifically assists the client with moving in bed.

Test-Taking Strategy: Note the strategic words *essential* and *move in bed*. Visualize the items in the options, and focus on the subject—helping the client to move in bed. This will direct you to option 3. Review the care of the client in traction if you had difficulty with this question.

Reference
Christensen, B., & Kockrow, E. (2006). *Adult health nursing* (5th ed., p. 175). St. Louis: Mosby.

1290. A nurse is assisting with caring for a client after a craniectomy. The nurse is told that the client's incision is supratentorial. How should the nurse position the client?
1 Head of the bed flat
2 Lying on the operative side
3 Head of the bed elevated 30 degrees
4 Head of the bed elevated 90 degrees

Level of Cognitive Ability: Application
Client Needs: Physiological Integrity
Integrated Process: Nursing Process/Implementation
Content Area: Adult Health/Neurological

Answer: 3
Rationale: Craniectomy involves the removal of a portion of the client's cranium; therefore, lying on the operative side is contraindicated because the bony protection of the skull has been removed. The head of the bed should be elevated 30 degrees to promote optimal venous drainage while maintaining arterial perfusion to the brain.

Test-Taking Strategy: Use the process of elimination. Recall the impact of craniectomy on client positioning and the concepts related to the general positioning of the client with a neurological problem. Note the strategic word *supratentorial*, and remember that *supra-* means *up*. This will assist you with eliminating options 1 and 2. Visualize the positions described in the remaining two options. Option 3 provides more client comfort than option 4 and does not potentially interfere with arterial circulation to the brain. Review the care of the client after craniectomy if you had difficulty with this question.

Reference
deWit, S. (2009). *Medical-surgical nursing: Concepts & practice* (p. 544). St. Louis: Saunders.

1291. A client is admitted to the hospital with a leaking cerebral aneurysm and scheduled for surgery. The nurse implements which of the following during the preoperative period?
1 Placing the client on bedrest
2 Allowing the client to ambulate to the bathroom

Answer: 1
Rationale: A cerebral aneurysm is an abnormal localized dilation of a cerebral artery. The client's activity is kept at a minimum to prevent Valsalva's maneuver. Clients often hold their breath and strain while pulling up to get out of bed; this exertion may cause a rise in blood pressure, which increases bleeding. Clients who have bleeding aneurysms in any vessel will have their activity curtailed.

3 Obtaining a bedside commode for the client's use
4 Encouraging the client to be up at least twice a day

Level of Cognitive Ability: Application
Client Needs: Physiological Integrity
Integrated Process: Nursing Process/ Implementation
Content Area: Adult Health/Neurological

Test-Taking Strategy: Use the process of elimination, and focus on the client's diagnosis and the strategic words *preoperative period*. Eliminate options 2, 3, and 4 because they are comparable or alike in that they all involve out-of-bed activity. Review aneurysm precautions if you had difficulty with this question.

Reference
Black, J., & Hawks, J. (2009). *Medical-surgical nursing: Clinical management for positive outcomes* (8th ed., p. 1330). St. Louis: Saunders.

1292. A physician calls a nurse to obtain the daily laboratory results of a client receiving parenteral nutrition. The nurse obtains which laboratory result because it would provide the most valuable information about the client's status related to the parenteral nutrition?
1 Serum electrolyte levels
2 Arterial blood gas levels
3 White blood cell (WBC) count
4 Complete blood cell count (CBC)

Level of Cognitive Ability: Application
Client Needs: Physiological Integrity
Integrated Process: Nursing Process/ Implementation
Content Area: Fundamental Skills

Answer: 1
Rationale: Parenteral nutrition solutions contain amino acid and dextrose solutions with electrolytes and trace elements added. The physician uses the electrolyte values to determine whether changes are needed in the composition of the parenteral nutrition solutions that will be administered during the next 24 hours; this prevents the client from developing an electrolyte imbalance. Options 2, 3, and 4 are not directly related to the client's status relative to parenteral nutrition.

Test-Taking Strategy: Use the process of elimination. Eliminate options 3 and 4 first because a CBC includes a WBC count. From the remaining options, focus on the subject and consider the composition of parenteral nutrition solutions to direct you to option 1. Review the composition of parenteral nutrition if you had difficulty with this question.

Reference
deWit, S. (2009). *Medical-surgical nursing: Concepts & practice* (p. 706). St. Louis: Saunders.

1293. A nurse is caring for an infant after pyloromyotomy performed to treat hypertrophic pyloric stenosis. The nurse should place the infant in which position after surgery?
1 Flat on the operative side
2 Flat on the unoperative side
3 Prone, with the head of the bed elevated
4 Supine, with the head of the bed elevated

Level of Cognitive Ability: Application
Client Needs: Physiological Integrity
Integrated Process: Nursing Process/ Implementation
Content Area: Child Health

Answer: 3
Rationale: A pyloromyotomy involves the incision of the longitudinal and circular muscle of the pylorus, which leaves the mucosa intact but separates the incised muscle fibers. After pyloromyotomy, the head of the bed is elevated, and the infant is placed prone to reduce the risk of aspiration. Options 1, 2, and 4 are incorrect positions after this type of surgery.

Test-Taking Strategy: Consider the anatomical location of the surgical procedure and the risks associated with the procedure to answer the question. Visualize each of the positions identified in the options. Keep in mind that aspiration is a major concern to direct you to option 3. Review nursing care measures after pyloromyotomy if you had difficulty with this question.

References
Leifer, G. (2007). *Introduction to maternity and pediatric nursing* (5th ed., p. 636). Philadelphia: Saunders.
Price, D., & Gwin, J. (2008). *Pediatric nursing: An introductory text* (10th ed., p. 160). St. Louis: Saunders.

1294. The mother of a child with mumps calls the health care clinic to tell the nurse that the child has been very lethargic and has been vomiting. The nurse should tell the mother:

1 To continue to monitor the child
2 To bring the child to the clinic to be seen by the physician
3 That lethargy and vomiting are normal manifestations of mumps
4 That as long as there is no fever there is nothing to be concerned about

Level of Cognitive Ability: Application
Client Needs: Physiological Integrity
Integrated Process: Nursing Process/ Implementation
Content Area: Child Health

Answer: 2

Rationale: Mumps generally affect the salivary glands, but they can also affect multiple organs. The most common complication of mumps is septic meningitis, with the virus being identified in the cerebrospinal fluid. Common signs include nuchal rigidity, lethargy, and vomiting. The child described in the question should be seen by the physician. Options 1, 3, and 4 are incorrect and delay necessary intervention.

Test-Taking Strategy: Use the process of elimination. Focus on the signs and symptoms presented in the question and recall that meningitis is a complication of mumps to direct you to option 2. Review the complications of mumps and the associated clinical manifestations if you had difficulty with this question.

Reference

Christensen, B., & Kockrow, E. (2006). *Foundations of nursing* (5th ed., p. 1067). St. Louis: Mosby.

1295. A nurse is reviewing the physician's orders for a child admitted to the hospital with vaso-occlusive pain crisis as a result of sickle cell anemia. The nurse should question the registered nurse about which prescribed order?

1 Bedrest
2 Intravenous fluids
3 Supplemental oxygen
4 Meperidine hydrochloride (Demerol) for pain

Level of Cognitive Ability: Application
Client Needs: Physiological Integrity
Integrated Process: Nursing Process/ Implementation
Content Area: Child Health

Answer: 4

Rationale: During a vaso-occlusive crisis, clumps of sickled erythrocytes obstruct blood vessels, which results in occlusion, ischemia, and the infarction of adjacent tissue. Meperidine hydrochloride is contraindicated for ongoing pain management because of the increased risk for seizures associated with the use of the medication. The management of severe pain generally includes the use of strong opioid analgesics (e.g., morphine sulfate, hydromorphone [Dilaudid]). These medications are usually most effective when given as a continuous infusion or at regular intervals around the clock. Options 1, 2, and 3 are appropriate prescriptions for the treatment of vaso-occlusive pain crisis.

Test-Taking Strategy: Use the process of elimination, and focus on the subject—questioning an order. Recall that oxygen, fluids, and bedrest are components of care for this condition to direct you to option 4. Review the care of a child with sickle cell anemia if you had difficulty with this question.

Reference

Price, D., & Gwin, J. (2008). *Pediatric nursing: An introductory text* (10th ed., pp. 147-148). St. Louis: Saunders.

1296. A nurse is caring for an infant with laryngomalacia (congenital laryngeal stridor). In which position should the nurse place the infant to decrease the incidence of stridor?

1 Prone
2 Supine
3 Supine, with the neck flexed
4 Prone, with the neck hyperextended

Level of Cognitive Ability: Application
Client Needs: Physiological Integrity

Answer: 4

Rationale: To decrease the incidence of stridor and improve the child's breathing, the child is placed in a prone position with the neck hyperextended. Options 1, 2, and 3 are not appropriate positions.

Test-Taking Strategy: Use the process of elimination, and note the strategic words *decrease the incidence of stridor.* Visualize each of the positions identified in the options to direct you to option 4. Review the care of the infant with stridor if you had difficulty with this question.

Integrated Process: Nursing Process/ Implementation
Content Area: Child Health

Reference

McKinney, E., James, S., Murray, S., & Ashwill, J. (2009). *Maternal-child nursing* (3rd ed., p. 1191). St. Louis: Mosby.

1297. A nurse in the newborn nursery prepares to admit a newborn infant with spina bifida, myelomeningocele type. Which nursing action is the priority?

1 Monitor the temperature.
2 Monitor the blood pressure.
3 Monitor the specific gravity of the urine.
4 Inspect the anterior fontanel for bulging.

Level of Cognitive Ability: Application
Client Needs: Physiological Integrity
Integrated Process: Nursing Process/ Implementation
Content Area: Child Health

Answer: 4

Rationale: Spina bifida is a congenital neural tube defect in which there is a developmental anomaly in the posterior vertebral arch. Increased intracranial pressure is a complication associated with this condition. A sign of increased intracranial pressure in the newborn infant with spina bifida is a bulging or tough anterior fontanel. The newborn infant is at risk for infection before the surgical procedure and the closure of the gibbus, and monitoring the temperature is an important intervention; however, inspecting the anterior fontanel for bulging is the immediate priority. A normal saline dressing is placed over the affected site to maintain the moisture of the gibbus and its contents; this prevents tearing or the breakdown of skin integrity at the site. The blood pressure is difficult to check during the newborn period, and it is not the best indicator of infection or a potential complication. Urine concentration is not well developed during the newborn stage of development.

> ***Test-Taking Strategy***: Use the process of elimination. Eliminate options 2 and 3 first because blood pressure and specific gravity are not as reliable as indicators of changes in the newborn status as they are for older children. From the remaining options, focus on the strategic word *priority* to direct you to option 4. Review the care of the infant with spina bifida if you had difficulty with this question.

Reference

Price, D., & Gwin, J. (2008). *Pediatric nursing: An introductory text* (10th ed., pp. 113-115). St. Louis: Saunders.

1298. A child with hepatitis B is being cared for at home. The mother of the child calls the health care clinic and tells the nurse that the jaundice seems to be worsening. The nurse should make which response to the mother?

1 "The hepatitis may be spreading."
2 "It is necessary to isolate the child from the others."
3 "The jaundice may appear to get worse before it resolves."
4 "You should bring the child to the health care clinic to see the physician."

Level of Cognitive Ability: Application
Client Needs: Physiological Integrity
Integrated Process: Nursing Process/ Implementation
Content Area: Child Health

Answer: 3

Rationale: Hepatitis is an inflammatory condition of the liver that is characterized by jaundice, hepatomegaly, anorexia, abdominal and gastric discomfort, abnormal liver function, clay-colored stools, and tea-colored urine. The parents should be instructed that jaundice may appear to get worse before it resolves. The parents of a child with hepatitis should also be taught the danger signs that could indicate a worsening of the child's condition, specifically changes in neurological status, bleeding, and fluid retention. Jaundice does not indicate that the condition is worsening or that the child requires isolation or needs to be seen by the physician.

> ***Test-Taking Strategy***: Use the process of elimination and your knowledge of the physiology associated with hepatitis to answer this question. Remember that jaundice worsens before it resolves. Review the instructions for the parents of a child with hepatitis if you had difficulty with this question.

Reference

McKinney, E., James, S., Murray, S., & Ashwill, J. (2009). *Maternal-child nursing* (3rd ed., p. 1132). St. Louis: Mosby.

1299. A nurse is preparing to suction an infant's tracheotomy. The nurse obtains the equipment for the procedure and turns the suction to which setting?

1 40 mm Hg
2 90 mm Hg
3 110 mm Hg
4 120 mm Hg

Level of Cognitive Ability: Application
Client Needs: Physiological Integrity
Integrated Process: Nursing Process/Implementation
Content Area: Child Health

Answer: 2

Rationale: The suctioning procedure for pediatric clients varies from that used for adults; suctioning in infants and children requires the use of a smaller suction catheter and lower suction settings. Suction settings should range from 60 to 100 mm Hg for infants and children and from 40 to 60 mm Hg for preterm infants.

Test-Taking Strategy: Use the process of elimination, and note the strategic word *infant.* Recall the procedure that is used in an adult to direct you to option 2. Remember that suction settings should range from 60 to 100 mm Hg for infants. Review infant suctioning if you had difficulty with this question.

Reference

Christensen, B., & Kockrow, E. (2006). *Foundations of nursing* (5th ed., p. 981). St. Louis: Mosby.

1300. A nurse is caring for a client who is at risk for aspiration who begins to experience seizure activity while in bed. Which action by the nurse will prevent aspiration from occurring?

1 Raising the head of the bed
2 Loosening the client's restrictive clothing
3 Removing the pillow and raising the padded side rails
4 Positioning the client on the side, if possible, with the head flexed forward

Level of Cognitive Ability: Application
Client Needs: Physiological Integrity
Integrated Process: Nursing Process/Implementation
Content Area: Adult Health/Neurological

Answer: 4

Rationale: Positioning the client on one side with the head flexed forward allows the tongue to fall forward and facilitates the drainage of secretions, which could help prevent aspiration. The nurse should also loosen or remove the client's restrictive clothing, remove the bed pillow, and raise the padded side rails. These actions would not decrease the risk of aspiration, but they are general safety measures to use during seizure activity. The nurse should not raise the head of the bed.

Test-Taking Strategy: Use the process of elimination, and note the strategic words *prevent aspiration.* Visualizing the effect that each of the options would have on airway and aspiration will direct you to option 4. Review the care of the client with seizures who is at risk for aspiration if you had difficulty with this question.

References

deWit, S. (2009). *Medical-surgical nursing: Concepts & practice* (p. 567). St. Louis: Saunders.

Linton, A. (2007). *Introduction to medical-surgical nursing* (4th ed., p. 437). Philadelphia: Saunders.

1301. A client with a brain attack (stroke) has episodes of coughing while swallowing liquids. The client has a temperature of 101° F, an oxygen saturation of 91% (down from 98% previously), slight confusion, and noticeable dyspnea. Which action should the nurse take?

1 Notify the registered nurse (RN).
2 Encourage the client to cough and deep breathe.
3 Administer an acetaminophen (Tylenol) suppository.
4 Administer a bronchodilator ordered on a PRN basis.

Answer: 1

Rationale: The client is exhibiting clinical signs and symptoms of aspiration, which include fever, dyspnea, decreased arterial oxygen levels, and confusion. Other symptoms that occur with this complication are difficulty with managing saliva and coughing or choking while eating. Because the client has developed a complication that requires medical intervention, the nurse should notify the RN, who will then intervene.

Test-Taking Strategy: Use the process of elimination. Focus on the data in the question, which will indicate that aspiration has most likely occurred. Eliminate options 2, 3, and 4 because these actions will not assist with alleviating this life-threatening condition. Review the findings in the client who is aspirating and the appropriate nursing interventions if you had difficulty with this question.

Level of Cognitive Ability: Application
Client Needs: Physiological Integrity
Integrated Process: Nursing Process/ Implementation
Content Area: Adult Health/Neurological

References
Christensen, B., & Kockrow, E. (2006). *Foundations of nursing* (5th ed., p. 1103-1104). St. Louis: Mosby.
Linton, A. (2007). *Introduction to medical-surgical nursing* (4th ed., pp. 468, 474). Philadelphia: Saunders.

1302. A nurse is caring for a client with depression who also has a problem with consuming adequate nutrition. Which initial nursing measure should the nurse implement?

1 Asking the client to identify preferred foods and drinks
2 Allowing the client to eat alone if the client prefers to do so
3 Offering high-protein, low-calorie fluids frequently throughout the day and evening
4 Offering low-calorie, high-protein snacks frequently throughout the day and evening

Level of Cognitive Ability: Application
Client Needs: Psychosocial Integrity
Integrated Process: Nursing Process/ Implementation
Content Area: Mental Health

Answer: 1
Rationale: It is important to ask the client to identify preferred foods and drinks and to offer choices when possible. The client is more likely to eat the foods provided if choices are offered. The client should be offered high-calorie, high-protein fluids and snacks frequently throughout the day and evening. When possible, the nurse should remain with the client during meals. This strategy reinforces the idea that someone cares, which can raise the client's self-esteem and serve as an incentive to eat.

Test-Taking Strategy: Use the process of elimination, and note the strategic word *initial.* Recall the basic principles related to nutrition and the importance of offering the client choices to direct you to option 1. Review effective measures related to the client with a problem with nutrition if you had difficulty with this question.

Reference
Linton, A. (2007). *Introduction to medical-surgical nursing* (4th ed., p. 1259). Philadelphia: Saunders.

1303. A client with urolithiasis is being evaluated to determine the type of stone that is being formed. The nurse should provide the client with which item to assist with this process?

1 A strainer
2 A calorie-count sheet
3 A vital signs graphic sheet
4 An intake-and-output record

Level of Cognitive Ability: Application
Client Needs: Physiological Integrity
Integrated Process: Nursing Process/ Implementation
Content Area: Adult Health/Renal

Answer: 1
Rationale: Urolithiasis is the presence of calculi in the urinary tract. The urine is strained to catch small stones that can be sent to the laboratory for analysis. After the type of stone has been determined, an individualized plan of care and prevention is developed. Options 2, 3, and 4 will not assist with determining the stone type.

Test-Taking Strategy: Use the process of elimination, and note that the question asks for an item that will help with the determination of the type of stone. Therefore, even if several of the options may be appropriate for use with the client with urolithiasis, you must select the one that is specific for this purpose. Begin by eliminating options 3 and 4; these items provide information about vital signs and fluid balance, but they do not provide data that will help to determine the type of stone. From the remaining options, select option 1, knowing that straining the urine would allow for the possible capture of small stones that could then be sent to the laboratory for analysis. Review the care of the client with urolithiasis if you had difficulty with this question.

Reference
Christensen, B., & Kockrow, E. (2006). *Adult health nursing* (5th ed., p. 491). St. Louis: Mosby.

1304. A nurse is providing care to a client after a bone biopsy. Which action should the nurse take as part of the aftercare for this procedure?

1 Monitor the vitals signs once per day.
2 Keep the area in a dependent position.
3 Administer intramuscular opioid analgesics.
4 Monitor the site for swelling, bleeding, and hematoma formation.

Level of Cognitive Ability: Application
Client Needs: Physiological Integrity
Integrated Process: Nursing Process/Implementation
Content Area: Adult Health/Musculoskeletal

Answer: 4

Rationale: Nursing care after bone biopsy includes monitoring the site for swelling, bleeding, and hematoma formation. The vital signs are monitored every 4 hours for 24 hours. The biopsy site is elevated for 24 hours to reduce edema. The client usually requires mild analgesics; more severe pain usually indicates that complications are arising.

Test-Taking Strategy: Use the process of elimination. Remember that the client must have periodic assessments after this procedure. With this in mind, eliminate option 1 because the time frame is too infrequent. Remember that the procedure is done with the client under local anesthesia to eliminate option 3 next. From the remaining options, recall the principles related to circulation and positioning to direct you to option 4. Review the care of a client after bone biopsy if you had difficulty with this question.

Reference

deWit, S. (2009). *Medical-surgical nursing: Concepts & practice* (p. 771). St. Louis: Saunders.

1305. A newborn infant is diagnosed with respiratory distress syndrome (RDS). Which nursing intervention is most effective for keeping the infant's oxygen needs as low as possible?

1 Monitoring the heart rate
2 Reviewing the blood gas reports
3 Maintaining a neutral thermal environment
4 Performing heelsticks for blood glucose screening

Level of Cognitive Ability: Application
Client Needs: Physiological Integrity
Integrated Process: Nursing Process/Implementation
Content Area: Maternity/Postpartum

Answer: 3

Rationale: RDS is an acute lung disease of the newborn that is characterized by airless alveoli, inelastic lungs, a respiration rate of more than 60 breaths/min, nasal flaring, retractions, grunting on expiration, and peripheral edema. Every effort should be made to maintain the infant in a neutral thermal environment. Oxygen needs will increase rapidly if the infant's body temperature is above or below the neutral thermal range. Handling the newborn, which includes monitoring the heart rate and performing heelsticks, stimulates movement and oxygen consumption. The interpretation of blood gases is diagnostic and indicates the effectiveness of employed interventions.

Test-Taking Strategy: Use the process of elimination, and focus on the subject—keeping the infant's oxygen needs as low as possible. Visualizing the actions described in each option will direct you to option 3. Review the measures that prevent an increase in oxygen needs if you had difficulty with this question.

Reference

Christensen, B., & Kockrow, E. (2006). *Foundations of nursing* (5th ed., p. 1010). St. Louis: Mosby.

1306. A nurse in the postpartum unit checks the temperature of a client who delivered a healthy newborn infant 4 hours previously. The mother's temperature is 100.8° F. The nurse provides oral hydration to the mother and encourages fluid intake. Four hours later, the nurse rechecks the temperature and notes that

Answer: 2

Rationale: A temperature of more than 100.4° F for two consecutive readings is considered febrile, and the RN should be notified. The RN will then contact the physician. Options 1, 3, and 4 are incorrect actions based on the data in the question. In addition, a nurse should not increase IV fluids without an order to do so.

it is still 100.8° F. The nurse should take which action?
1 Document the temperature.
2 Notify the registered nurse (RN).
3 Increase the intravenous (IV) fluids.
4 Continue hydration and recheck the temperature 4 hours later.

Level of Cognitive Ability: Application
Client Needs: Physiological Integrity
Integrated Process: Nursing Process/Implementation
Content Area: Maternity/Postpartum

Test-Taking Strategy: Use the process of elimination. Option 3 can be eliminated first because this action requires a physician order. From the remaining options, note that the temperature has remained unchanged after nursing intervention to provide you with the clue that further intervention is necessary; this will direct you to option 2. Review normal and abnormal findings during the postpartum period if you had difficulty with this question.

Reference
Leifer, G. (2008). *Maternity nursing: An introductory text* (10th ed., p. 344). Philadelphia: Saunders.

1307. A nurse is checking the fundus of a postpartum woman and notes that the uterus is soft and spongy. The nurse should take which action initially?
1 Notify the registered nurse (RN).
2 Encourage the mother to ambulate.
3 Massage the fundus gently until it becomes firm.
4 Document fundal position, consistency, and height.

Level of Cognitive Ability: Application
Client Needs: Physiological Integrity
Integrated Process: Nursing Process/Implementation
Content Area: Maternity/Postpartum

Answer: 3
Rationale: If the fundus is boggy (soft and spongy), it should be massaged gently until firm by the nurse, who observes for increased bleeding or clots. The RN is notified and will contact the physician if uterine massage is not helpful. Option 2 is an inappropriate action at this time. The nurse should document fundal position, consistency, and height; the need to perform fundal massage; and the client's response to the intervention. The initial action, however, is stated in option 3.

Test-Taking Strategy: Use the process of elimination, and note the strategic word *initially*. Note the relationship between the words *soft and spongy* in the question and *until it becomes firm* in option 3. Review nursing interventions related to a soft and spongy fundus if you had difficulty with this question.

Reference
Leifer, G. (2008). *Maternity nursing: An introductory text* (10th ed., p. 227). Philadelphia: Saunders.

1308. A nurse is assisting with caring for a client 3 hours after an upper right lung lobectomy. The client has a closed chest drainage system that has 150 mL of bloody drainage in the collection chamber. The client's vital signs are as follows: blood pressure, 100/50 mm Hg; heart rate, 100 beats/min; and respiratory rate, 26 breaths/min. There is intermittent bubbling in the water-seal chamber. One hour later, the nurse notes that the bubbling is now constant and that the client appears dyspneic. The nurse should first check the:
1 Client's vital signs
2 Client's lung sounds
3 Chest tube connections
4 Amount of drainage in the collection chamber

Answer: 3
Rationale: Constant bubbling in the water-seal chamber of a closed chest drainage system indicates an air leak. In addition, the change in the client's status is most likely related to an air leak caused by a loose connection. Other possible causes of the change in the client's status include a tear or incision in the pulmonary pleura. Although the other options are correct, they should be pursued after initial attempts to locate and correct the air leak. It takes only a moment to check the connections; if a leak is found and corrected, the client's symptoms should resolve. The registered nurse should be notified of the change in the client's condition.

Test-Taking Strategy: Use the process of elimination, and note the strategic word *first*. Recall that a constant bubbling in the water-seal chamber could indicate a leak to direct you to option 3. Review basic knowledge of closed chest drainage systems if you had difficulty with this question.

Level of Cognitive Ability: Application
Client Needs: Physiological Integrity
Integrated Process: Nursing Process/Implementation
Content Area: Adult Health/Respiratory

References

Christensen, B., & Kockrow, E. (2006). *Adult health nursing* (5th ed., p. 439). St. Louis: Mosby.
deWit, S. (2009). *Medical-surgical nursing: Concepts & practice* (p. 348). St. Louis: Saunders.

1309. A client is admitted to the emergency department with complaints of severe, radiating chest pain. The client is extremely restless, frightened, and dyspneic. Immediate admission orders include oxygen by nasal cannula at 4 L/min, creatine phosphokinase and isoenzymes, a chest radiograph, and a 12-lead electrocardiogram (ECG). The nurse should take which initial action?

1 Obtain the 12-lead ECG.
2 Apply the oxygen to the client.
3 Call radiology to order the chest radiograph.
4 Call the laboratory to order the blood work.

Level of Cognitive Ability: Application
Client Needs: Physiological Integrity
Integrated Process: Nursing Process/Implementation
Content Area: Adult Health/Cardiovascular

Answer: 2

Rationale: The initial action for a client who is experiencing chest pain is to apply oxygen because the client may be experiencing myocardial ischemia. The ECG can provide evidence of cardiac damage and the location of myocardial ischemia. However, oxygen is the priority to prevent further cardiac damage. The blood work is not a priority. Cardiac isoenzymes can help with determining the choice of treatment; however, they do not begin to rise until 1 to 2 hours after the onset of a myocardial infarction. Although the chest radiograph can show cardiac enlargement, it does not influence the immediate treatment.

Test-Taking Strategy: Use the process of elimination, and note the strategic word *initial*. Remember that the immediate goal of therapy is to prevent myocardial ischemia; only option 2 achieves that goal. In addition, use the ABCs—airway, breathing, and circulation—to direct you to the correct option. Review the care of the client with a myocardial infarction if you had difficulty with this question.

Reference

Linton, A. (2007). *Introduction to medical-surgical nursing* (4th ed., p. 658). Philadelphia: Saunders.

Nursing Process: Evaluation

1310. A nurse has been encouraging the intake of oral fluids in a laboring woman to improve hydration. Which of the following indicates a successful outcome of this action?

1 Ketones in the urine
2 A urine specific gravity of 1.020
3 A blood pressure of 150/90 mm Hg
4 Continued leaking of amniotic fluid

Level of Cognitive Ability: Comprehension
Client Needs: Health Promotion and Maintenance
Integrated Process: Nursing Process/Evaluation
Content Area: Maternity/Intrapartum

Answer: 2

Rationale: Urine specific gravity measures the concentration of the urine, and the normal range is from 1.015 to 1.025. During the first stage of labor, the renal system has a tendency to concentrate urine. Labor and birth require hydration and caloric intake to replenish energy expenditure and to promote efficient uterine function. An elevated blood pressure and ketones in the urine are not expected outcomes related to labor and hydration. After the membranes have ruptured, it is expected that amniotic fluid may continue to leak.

Test-Taking Strategy: Use the process of elimination, and focus on the subject—a successful outcome related to oral intake. Recall the relationship of oral intake to urine concentration to direct you to option 2. Review the importance of hydration for the woman in labor if you had difficulty with this question.

Reference

McKinney, E., James, S., Murray, S., & Ashwill, J. (2009). *Maternal-child nursing* (3rd ed., pp. 363, 365). St. Louis: Mosby.

1311. A postpartum client has a nursing diagnosis of *Risk for infection*. A goal has been developed that states, "The client will not develop an infection during her hospital stay." Which data would support that the goal has been met?

1 Loss of appetite
2 Absence of fever
3 Presence of chills
4 Abdominal tenderness

Level of Cognitive Ability: Comprehension
Client Needs: Physiological Integrity
Integrated Process: Nursing Process/Evaluation
Content Area: Maternity/Postpartum

Answer: 2

Rationale: Fever is the first indication of an infection. Chills, abdominal tenderness, and loss of appetite also indicate the presence of an infection. Therefore, the absence of a fever indicates that an infection is not present.

Test-Taking Strategy: Use the process of elimination, and note the strategic words *that the goal has been met.* The question is asking for a means of evaluating the effectiveness of a goal that relates to infection. Options 1, 3, and 4 would indicate that the goal had not been met. Review the signs of postpartum infection if you had difficulty with this question.

Reference

Leifer, G. (2008). *Maternity nursing: An introductory text* (10th ed., pp. 129, 344). Philadelphia: Saunders.

1312. A nurse is monitoring the nutritional status of the client who is receiving enteral nutrition as a result of dysphagia caused by a head injury. The nurse monitors which of the following to best determine the effectiveness of the tube feedings for this client?

1 Daily weight
2 Calorie count
3 Serum protein level
4 Daily intake and output

Level of Cognitive Ability: Comprehension
Client Needs: Physiological Integrity
Integrated Process: Nursing Process/Evaluation
Content Area: Fundamental Skills

Answer: 1

Rationale: The most accurate measurement of the effectiveness of the nutritional management of the client is the monitoring of the daily weight. This should be done at the same time each day (preferably early morning), with the client wearing the same clothes and using the same scale. Options 2, 3, and 4 assist with the measurement of the nutrition and hydration status. However, the effectiveness of the diet is measured by the maintenance of the body weight.

Test-Taking Strategy: Use the process of elimination, and note the strategic word *effectiveness.* This tells you that the correct option is an outcome. With this in mind, eliminate options 2 and 4 first because these are tools that the nurse uses to measure nutrition and fluid status. Eliminate option 3 next because it reflects only one component of the diet—protein. Review the methods of monitoring nutritional status if you had difficulty with this question.

Reference

Christensen, B., & Kockrow, E. (2006). *Foundations of nursing* (5th ed., p. 656). St. Louis: Mosby.

1313. An adult client with a critically high potassium level has received sodium polystyrene sulfonate (Kayexalate). The nurse determines that the medication was most effective if the client's repeat serum potassium level is:

1 4.9 mEq/L
2 5.4 mEq/L
3 5.8 mEq/L
4 6.2 mEq/L

Level of Cognitive Ability: Comprehension
Client Needs: Physiological Integrity
Integrated Process: Nursing Process/Evaluation
Content Area: Fundamental Skills

Answer: 1

Rationale: The normal serum potassium level in the adult is 3.5 to 5.1 mEq/L. Option 1 is the only option that reflects a value that has dropped down into the normal range. Options 2, 3, and 4 identify elevated potassium levels.

Test-Taking Strategy: Use the process of elimination, and note the strategic words *critically high.* Recall the normal serum potassium level to direct you to option 1. Review the expected effects of sodium polystyrene sulfonate and the normal potassium level if you had difficulty with this question.

References

deWit, S. (2009). *Medical-surgical nursing: Concepts & practice* (p. 45). St. Louis: Saunders.
Linton, A. (2007). *Introduction to medical-surgical nursing* (4th ed., pp. 184, 196). Philadelphia: Saunders.

1314. A client with a history of hypertension has been prescribed triamterene (Dyrenium). The nurse determines that the client understands the impact of this medication on the diet if the client states the need to avoid which of the following fruits?

1 Pears
2 Apples
3 Bananas
4 Cranberries

Level of Cognitive Ability: Analysis
Client Needs: Physiological Integrity
Integrated Process: Nursing Process/Evaluation
Content Area: Adult Health/Cardiovascular

Answer: 3
Rationale: Triamterene is a potassium-sparing diuretic, so the client should avoid foods high in potassium. Fruits that are naturally higher in potassium include avocados, bananas, fresh oranges, mangoes, nectarines, papayas, and dried prunes.

Test-Taking Strategy: Use the process of elimination, and note the strategic word *avoid.* This word indicates a negative event query and asks you to select an option that is an incorrect food. Recall that triamterene is a potassium-sparing diuretic, and then identify the high-potassium food. Review triamterene and those food items that are high in potassium if you had difficulty with this question.

Reference
deWit, S. (2009). *Medical-surgical nursing: Concepts & practice* (p. 747). St. Louis: Saunders.

1315. A perinatal client has been instructed about the prevention of genital tract infections. Which statement by the client indicates an understanding of these preventive measures?

1 "I can douche anytime I want."
2 "I can wear my tight-fitting jeans."
3 "I should avoid the use of condoms."
4 "I should wear underwear with a cotton panel liner."

Level of Cognitive Ability: Comprehension
Client Needs: Health Promotion and Maintenance
Integrated Process: Nursing Process/Evaluation
Content Area: Maternity/Antepartum

Answer: 4
Rationale: Wearing items with cotton panel liners allows for air movement in and around the genital area and assists with the prevention of genital tract infections. Douching is to be avoided. Wearing tight clothes irritates the genital area and does not allow for air circulation. Condoms should be used to minimize the spread of genital tract infections.

Test-Taking Strategy: Use the process of elimination, and note the strategic words *indicates an understanding.* Options 1, 2, and 3 are all incorrect statements about client self-care. Review prevention measures associated with genital tract infections if you had difficulty with this question.

Reference
deWit, S. (2009). *Medical-surgical nursing: Concepts & practice* (p. 943). St. Louis: Saunders.

1316. The registered nurse (RN) has documented a nursing diagnosis of *Ineffective airway clearance.* The licensed practical nurse (LPN) uses which of the following indicators as the best guide to determine when the client needs suctioning?

1 Respiratory rate
2 Arterial blood gas results
3 Inability to expectorate mucus
4 Oxygen saturation measurement

Level of Cognitive Ability: Analysis
Client Needs: Physiological Integrity
Integrated Process: Nursing Process/Evaluation
Content Area: Fundamental Skills

Answer: 3
Rationale: Suctioning is indicated when the client cannot expectorate mucus after a variety of other assistive methods have been used. The need for suctioning is best determined by listening for coarse gurgling or bubbling respirations or by hearing abnormal breath sounds with auscultation. The other options could be affected by factors other than the accumulation of secretions.

Test-Taking Strategy: Use the process of elimination, and focus on the subject—the need for suctioning; this will direct you to option 3. Remember that arterial blood gas results, oxygen saturation, and the respiratory rate may change as a result of mucus accumulation. However, the client's inability to expectorate mucus and the presence of noisy respirations or abnormal breath sounds indicate the presence of secretions that require removal. Review suctioning procedures and indications of the need for suctioning if you had difficulty with this question.

References
deWit, S. (2009). *Medical-surgical nursing: Concepts & practice* (pp. 310, 312). St. Louis: Saunders.
Linton, A. (2007). *Introduction to medical-surgical nursing* (4th ed., p. 1214). Philadelphia: Saunders.

1317. A nurse is reviewing a plan of care for a client who is in traction and notes a nursing diagnosis of *Self-care deficit.* The nurse evaluates the plan of care and determines that which observation indicates a successful outcome?

1 The client refuses care.
2 The client allows the family to assist with care.
3 The client assists with self-care as much as possible.
4 The client allows the nurse to complete the care on a daily basis.

Level of Cognitive Ability: Analysis
Client Needs: Physiological Integrity
Integrated Process: Nursing Process/Evaluation
Content Area: Adult Health/Musculoskeletal

Answer: 3
Rationale: A successful outcome for the nursing diagnosis of *Self-care deficit* is for the client to do as much of the self-care as possible. The nurse should promote the client's independence and allow the client to perform as much self-care as is optimal, considering the client's condition. The nurse would determine that the outcome is unsuccessful if the client refused care or allows others to handle the care.

Test-Taking Strategy: Use the process of elimination, and focus on the strategic words *successful outcome.* Option 1 can be eliminated first because of the words *refuses care.* Note that options 2 and 4 are comparable or alike in that they indicate that the client relies on others to perform care. Review successful outcomes related to the nursing diagnosis of *Self-care deficit* if you had difficulty with this question.

References
deWit, S. (2009). *Medical-surgical nursing: Concepts & practice* (p. 776). St. Louis: Saunders.
Linton, A. (2007). *Introduction to medical-surgical nursing* (4th ed., p. 311). Philadelphia: Saunders.

1318. A nurse instructs a parent about the appropriate actions to take when the toddler has a temper tantrum. Which statement by the parent indicates an understanding of the instructions?

1 "I will ignore the tantrums as long as there is no physical danger."
2 "I will give frequent reminders that only bad children have tantrums."
3 "I will send my child to a room alone for 10 minutes after every tantrum."
4 "I will reward my child with candy at the end of each day without a tantrum."

Level of Cognitive Ability: Comprehension
Client Needs: Health Promotion and Maintenance
Integrated Process: Nursing Process/Evaluation
Content Area: Child Health

Answer: 1
Rationale: Ignoring a negative attention-seeking behavior is considered the best way to extinguish it, provided that the child is safe from injury. Option 2 is untrue and negative. Option 3 gives attention to the tantrum. Providing candy for rewards is unhealthy and unlikely to be effective at the end of the day.

Test-Taking Strategy: Use the process of elimination, and focus on the subject—appropriate actions to take when a toddler has a temper tantrum. Recall that ignoring a tantrum is the best way to extinguish it to direct you to option 1. Review the interventions for a child who has temper tantrums if you had difficulty with this question.

Reference
Christensen, B., & Kockrow, E. (2006). *Foundations of nursing* (5th ed., p. 164). St. Louis: Mosby.

1319. A nurse who is caring for a client in seclusion determines that it is safe for the client to come out of seclusion when the nurse hears the client say which of the following?

Answer: 2
Rationale: Option 2 indicates that the client may be safely removed from seclusion. The client in seclusion must be assessed at regular intervals (usually every 15 to 30 minutes) for physical needs, safety, and comfort. Option 1 indicates a physical need that

1 "I need to use the restroom right away."
2 "I no longer want to hurt myself or others."
3 "I can't breathe in here. The walls are closing in on me."
4 "I'd like to go back to my room and be alone for a while."

Level of Cognitive Ability: Comprehension
Client Needs: Psychosocial Integrity
Integrated Process: Nursing Process/Evaluation
Content Area: Mental Health

could be met with a urinal, bedpan, or commode; it does not indicate that the client has calmed down enough to leave the seclusion room. Option 3 could be handled by supportive communication or a PRN medication, if indicated; it does not necessitate discontinuing seclusion. Option 4 could be an attempt to manipulate the nurse; it gives no indication that the client will control himself or herself when alone in the room.

Test-Taking Strategy: Use the process of elimination, and focus on the subject—removing a client from seclusion. Recall the purpose and the use of seclusion to direct you to option 2. Review seclusion procedure if you had difficulty with this question.

Reference
Varcarolis, E., & Halter, M. (2009). *Essentials of psychiatric mental health nursing: A communication approach to evidence-based care* (p. 524). St. Louis: Saunders.

1320. A client has had a laryngectomy for throat cancer and has started oral intake. The nurse determines that the client has tolerated the first stage of dietary advancement if the client takes which of the following types of diet without aspiration or choking?
1 Bland
2 Full liquids
3 Clear liquids
4 Semisolid foods

Level of Cognitive Ability: Analysis
Client Needs: Physiological Integrity
Integrated Process: Nursing Process/Evaluation
Content Area: Adult Health/Oncology

Answer: 4
Rationale: Oral intake after laryngectomy is started with semisolid foods. When the client can manage this type of food, liquids may be introduced. Thin liquids are not given until the risk of aspiration is negligible. A bland diet is not appropriate because the client may not be able to tolerate the texture of some of the solid foods that would be included in a bland diet.

Test-Taking Strategy: Use the process of elimination. Eliminate options 2 and 3 first because a client with swallowing difficulty will be unable to manage liquids. From the remaining options, recall that a bland diet provides no control over the consistency or texture of the food. Review dietary measures for a client after laryngectomy if you had difficulty with this question.

Reference
Linton, A. (2007). *Introduction to medical-surgical nursing* (4th ed., p. 1233). Philadelphia: Saunders.

1321. An older client who is a victim of elder abuse and his family have been seen in the counseling center weekly for the past month. Which statement, if made by the abusive family member, indicates that he or she has learned more positive coping skills?
1 "I will be more careful to make sure that my father's needs are 100% met."
2 "I am so sorry and embarrassed that the abusive event occurred. It won't happen again."
3 "Now that my father is moving into my home, I will have to stop drinking alcohol."
4 "I feel better equipped to care for my father now that I know where to turn if I need assistance."

Answer: 4
Rationale: Elder abuse sometimes results when family members are expected to care for their aging parents. This care can cause the family to become overextended, frustrated, or financially depleted. Knowing where to turn in the community for assistance with caring for an aging family member can bring much-needed relief. Using these alternatives is a positive coping skill for many families. Options 1, 2, and 3 are statements of good faith or promises that may or may not be kept in the future.

Test-Taking Strategy: Use the process of elimination, and focus on the subject—a positive coping skill. Only option 4 identifies a means of coping that outlines a definitive plan for handling the pressure associated with the older client's care. Review the concepts related to elder abuse if you had difficulty with this question.

Level of Cognitive Ability: Analysis
Client Needs: Psychosocial Integrity
Integrated Process: Nursing Process/Evaluation
Content Area: Mental Health

Reference

Christensen, B., & Kockrow, E. (2006). *Foundations of nursing* (5th ed., pp. 27, 155). St. Louis: Mosby.

1322. A nurse is caring for a 24-hour-old term infant who had a confirmed episode of hypoglycemia at 1 hour old. Which observation by the nurse would indicate the need for further evaluation?

1 Weight loss of 4 ounces and dry, peeling skin
2 Breast-feeding for 20 minutes or more, with strong sucking
3 Blood glucose level of 40 mg/dL before the last feeding
4 High-pitched cry and eating 10 to 15 mL of formula per feeding

Level of Cognitive Ability: Analysis
Client Needs: Physiological Integrity
Integrated Process: Nursing Process/Evaluation
Content Area: Maternity/Postpartum

Answer: 4

Rationale: At 24 hours old, a term infant should be able to consume at least 1 oz of formula per feeding. A high-pitched cry is indicative of neurological involvement. Hypoglycemia causes central nervous system symptoms (high-pitched cry) and weakness, which makes the infant unable to eat enough for growth. Weight loss during the first few days of life and dry, peeling skin are normal findings for term infants. Breast-feeding for 20 minutes with a strong suck is an excellent finding. Blood glucose levels are acceptable at 40 mg/dL during the first few days of life.

Test-Taking Strategy: Use the process of elimination, and note the strategic words *need for further evaluation*. These words indicate a negative event query and ask you to select an option that is an abnormal finding. Eliminate options 1, 2, and 3 because these are normal findings. In addition, the words *high-pitched cry* should direct you to option 4. Review normal newborn findings and the indications of hypoglycemia if you had difficulty with this question.

References

Leifer, G. (2008). *Maternity nursing: An introductory text* (10th ed., p. 323). Philadelphia: Saunders.
Price, D., & Gwin, J. (2008). *Pediatric nursing: An introductory text* (10th ed., p. 77). St. Louis: Saunders.

1323. A nurse is caring for a client with tuberculosis who is receiving rifampin (Rifadin) daily. Which of the following indicates to the nurse that the client is experiencing an adverse reaction?

1 A total bilirubin level of 0.5 mg/dL
2 A sedimentation rate of 15 mm/hr
3 A white blood cell count of 6000 cells/mm^3
4 An alkaline phosphatase level of 25 units/dL

Level of Cognitive Ability: Analysis
Client Needs: Physiological Integrity
Integrated Process: Nursing Process/Evaluation
Content Area: Pharmacology

Answer: 4

Rationale: Rifampin (Rifadin) is an antitubercular medication. Adverse reactions or toxic effects of rifampin include hepatotoxicity, hepatitis, blood dyscrasias, Stevens-Johnson syndrome, and antibiotic-related colitis. The nurse monitors for increased liver enzymes, bilirubin, blood urea nitrogen, and uric acid because elevations indicate an adverse reaction. The normal alkaline phosphatase level is 4.5 to 13 King-Armstrong units/dL. The normal total bilirubin level is less than 1.5 mg/dL. A normal white blood cell count is 4500 to 11,000 cells/mm^3. The normal sedimentation rate is 0 to 30 mm/hr.

Test-Taking Strategy: Use the process of elimination. Remember that the medication is metabolized in the liver to assist you with eliminating options 2 and 3; these laboratory studies are not directly related to the assessment of liver function. From the remaining options, knowledge of normal laboratory values will direct you to option 4. Review rifampin and the associated laboratory values if you had difficulty with this question.

Reference

Kee, J., Hayes, E., & McCuistion, L. (2009). *Pharmacology: A nursing process approach* (6th ed., p. 463). St. Louis: Saunders.

1324. A client being discharged from the mental health unit has a history of anxiety and command hallucinations to harm self or others. The nurse teaches the client about interventions for hallucinations and anxiety. The nurse determines that the client understands these measures when the client says:

1 "If I take my medication, I won't be anxious."
2 "I can go to a support group and talk about my feelings."
3 "If I get enough sleep and eat well, I won't get anxious and hear things."
4 "I can call my clinical specialist when I'm hallucinating so that I can talk about my feelings and plans and not hurt anyone."

Level of Cognitive Ability: Comprehension
Client Needs: Psychosocial Integrity
Integrated Process: Nursing Process/Evaluation
Content Area: Mental Health

Answer: 4
Rationale: There may be an increased risk for impulsive behavior, aggressive behavior, or both if a client is receiving command hallucinations to harm self or others. Talking about auditory hallucinations can interfere with the subvocal muscular activity associated with a hallucination. Options 1, 2, and 3 are general interventions that are not specific to anxiety and hallucinations.

Test-Taking Strategy: Focus on the subject—anxiety and hallucinations. Options 1, 2, and 3 are all interventions that a client can do to help maintain wellness. However, option 4 is specific to the subject and indicates self-responsible commitment and control over personal behavior. In addition, note the relationship between the words *hallucinations* in the question and *hallucinating* in option 4. Review the interventions for anxiety and hallucinations if you had difficulty with this question.

Reference
deWit, S. (2009). *Medical-surgical nursing: Concepts & practice* (p. 1160). St. Louis: Saunders.

1325. A nurse is assigned to care for a preschooler who has a diagnosis of scarlet fever and who is on bedrest. What data obtained by the nurse would indicate that the child is coping with the illness and bedrest?

1 The child insists that the mother stay in the room.
2 The child is coloring and drawing pictures in a notebook.
3 The mother keeps providing new activities for the child to do.
4 The child sucks the thumb whenever he or she does not get what is asked for.

Level of Cognitive Ability: Comprehension
Client Needs: Psychosocial Integrity
Integrated Process: Nursing Process/Evaluation
Content Area: Child Health

Answer: 2
Rationale: According to Piaget, play is the best way for preschoolers to understand and adjust to life's experiences. They are able to use pencils and crayons at this age, and they can draw stick figures and other rudimentary things. A child with scarlet fever needs quiet play, and drawing will provide that. Options 1, 3, and 4 do not address positive coping mechanisms.

Test-Taking Strategy: Think about the developmental level of preschoolers, and focus on the subject—determining whether the child is coping with the disease and bedrest. Option 2 is a positive coping mechanism for preschoolers. Options 1, 3, and 4 do not address positive coping mechanisms. Review the expected developmental level of a preschooler and the effects of bedrest on a child if you had difficulty with this question.

Reference
Christensen, B., & Kockrow, E. (2006). *Foundations of nursing* (5th ed., p. 1067). St. Louis: Mosby.

1326. A European-American client maintains eye contact with the nurse during a conversation about the preoperative teaching plan. The nurse interprets this nonverbal communication as:

1 Rudeness
2 Arrogance
3 Indicating uneasiness
4 Indicating trustworthiness

Answer: 4
Rationale: In the European-American culture, eye contact is viewed as indicating trustworthiness. Alternatively, eye contact is considered rude in Asian-American culture. Arrogance and uneasiness are incorrect interpretations of this nonverbal communication from the European-American client.

Level of Cognitive Ability: Comprehension
Client Needs: Psychosocial Integrity
Integrated Process: Nursing Process/Evaluation
Content Area: Fundamental Skills

Test-Taking Strategy: Use the process of elimination, and note that options 1, 2, and 3 are comparable or alike in that they indicate a negative response. Option 4 is the only option that is positive. Review the communication practices of the European-American culture if you had difficulty with this question.

References

Giger, J., & Davidhizar, R. (2008) *Transcultural nursing assessment & intervention* (5th ed., p. 32). St. Louis: Mosby.
Jarvis, C. (2008). *Physical examination and health assessment* (5th ed., p. 73). Philadelphia: Saunders.

1327. A client has just taken a dose of trimethobenzamide (Tigan). The nurse determines that the medication has been effective if the client states relief of:

1 Heartburn
2 Constipation
3 Abdominal pain
4 Nausea and vomiting

Level of Cognitive Ability: Analysis
Client Needs: Physiological Integrity
Integrated Process: Nursing Process/Evaluation
Content Area: Pharmacology

Answer: 4
Rationale: Trimethobenzamide (Tigan) is an antiemetic agent that is used for the treatment of nausea and vomiting. The medication is not used to treat heartburn, constipation, or abdominal pain.

Test-Taking Strategy: Use the process of elimination, and focus on the medication. Recall that this medication is an antiemetic to direct you to option 4. Review the action of trimethobenzamide if you had difficulty with this question.

Reference

Hodgson, B., & Kizior, R. (2009). *Saunders nursing drug handbook 2009* (p. 1175). Philadelphia: Saunders.

1328. A client with a short-leg plaster cast complains of an intense itching under the cast, and the nurse provides instructions to the client about relief measures for the itching. Which statement by the client indicates an understanding of the measures to use to relieve the itching?

1 "I can use the blunt part of a ruler to scratch the area."
2 "I can trickle small amounts of water down inside the cast."
3 "I can use a hair dryer on a cool setting and allow the air to blow into the cast."
4 "I need to obtain assistance when placing an object into the cast for the itching."

Level of Cognitive Ability: Comprehension
Client Needs: Safe and Effective Care Environment
Integrated Process: Nursing Process/Evaluation
Content Area: Adult Health/Musculoskeletal

Answer: 3
Rationale: Itching is a common complaint of clients with casts. Objects should not be put inside a cast because of the risk of scratching the skin and providing a point of entry for bacteria. A plaster cast can break down when wet. The best way to relieve itching is by blowing cool air inside the cast with a hair dryer.

Test-Taking Strategy: Use the process of elimination. Eliminate options 1 and 4 first because they both involve the use of an object being placed inside the cast. Recall that water can soften a plaster cast and cause maceration of the skin to direct you to option 3. Review client education about cast care if you had difficulty with this question.

Reference

Christensen, B., & Kockrow, E. (2006). *Adult health nursing* (5th ed., p. 171). St. Louis: Mosby.

1329. A nurse is reinforcing instructions to the mother of a child with strabismus of the left eye and reviews the procedure

Answer: 3
Rationale: Patching may be used for the treatment of strabismus to strengthen the weak eye. With this treatment, the good eye is

for patching the child. The nurse determines that the mother understands the procedure if the mother makes which statement?

1 "I will place patches on both eyes."
2 "I will place the patch on the left eye."
3 "I will place the patch on the right eye."
4 "I will alternate the patch from the right eye to the left eye every hour."

Level of Cognitive Ability: Comprehension
Client Needs: Physiological Integrity
Integrated Process: Nursing Process/Evaluation
Content Area: Child Health

patched; this encourages the child to use the weaker eye. This type of treatment is most successful when it is performed during the preschool years. The schedule for patching is individualized and prescribed by the ophthalmologist. Options 1, 2, and 4 are incorrect.

Test-Taking Strategy: Use the process of elimination. Remember that strabismus is a lazy eye to direct you to the correct option. It makes sense to patch the unaffected eye to strengthen the muscles in the affected eye. Review the procedure for patching for strabismus if you had difficulty with this question.

Reference

Price, D., & Gwin, J. (2008). *Pediatric nursing: An introductory text* (10th ed., p. 241). St. Louis: Saunders.

1330. A nurse has taught a client who is taking a xanthine bronchodilator about beverages to avoid. The nurse determines that the client understands the information if the client chooses which beverage from the dietary menu?

1 Cola
2 Coffee
3 Cranberry juice
4 Chocolate milk

Level of Cognitive Ability: Analysis
Client Needs: Physiological Integrity
Integrated Process: Nursing Process/Evaluation
Content Area: Pharmacology

Answer: 3

Rationale: Cola, coffee, and chocolate contain xanthine and should be avoided by the client who is taking a xanthine bronchodilator. These substances could lead to an increased incidence of the cardiovascular and central nervous system side effects that can occur with the use of this type of bronchodilator. The beverages in options 1, 2, and 4 are not acceptable to consume.

Test-Taking Strategy: Use the process of elimination. Note that options 1, 2, and 4 are comparable or alike in that they contain some form of stimulant. Review the dietary measures for a client taking a xanthine bronchodilator if you had difficulty with this question.

Reference

Lehne, R. (2010). *Pharmacology for nursing care* (7th ed., pp. 394, 906). St. Louis: Saunders.

1331. A client is started on tolbutamide (Orinase) once daily. The nurse observes for which intended effect of this medication?

1 Weight loss
2 Resolution of infection
3 Decreased blood glucose level
4 Decreased blood pressure

Level of Cognitive Ability: Analysis
Client Needs: Physiological Integrity
Integrated Process: Nursing Process/Evaluation
Content Area: Pharmacology

Answer: 3

Rationale: Tolbutamide is an oral hypoglycemic agent that is taken in the morning. It is not used to enhance weight loss, treat infection, or decrease blood pressure.

Test-Taking Strategy: Use the process of elimination, and note the strategic words *intended effects.* Focus on the name of the medication and recall that this medication is an oral hypoglycemic to direct you to option 3. Review the action of this medication if you had difficulty with this question.

Reference

Lehne, R. (2010). *Pharmacology for nursing care* (7th ed., p. 687). St. Louis: Saunders.

1332. A nurse is assigned to care for a client with acquired immunodeficiency syndrome (AIDS) who is receiving amphotericin B (Fungizone) to treat a fungal

Answer: 1

Rationale: Amphotericin B (Fungizone) is an antifungal and antiprotozoal medication. Clients taking amphotericin B may develop hypokalemia, which can be severe and lead to extreme muscle

respiratory infection. Which of the following indicates an adverse reaction to the medication?
1 Hypokalemia
2 Hyperkalemia
3 Hypocalcemia
4 Hypercalcemia

Level of Cognitive Ability: Analysis
Client Needs: Physiological Integrity
Integrated Process: Nursing Process/Evaluation
Content Area: Pharmacology

weakness and electrocardiogram changes. Distal renal tubular acidosis commonly occurs and contributes to the development of hypokalemia. High potassium levels do not occur. The medication does not cause calcium levels to fluctuate.

Test-Taking Strategy: Focus on the client's diagnosis and the name of the medication to determine that it is an antifungal medication. With this in mind, use your knowledge of the medication and remember that hypokalemia is an adverse reaction to amphotericin B. Review amphotericin B if you had difficulty with this question.

Reference
Hodgson, B., & Kizior, R. (2009). *Saunders nursing drug handbook 2009* (p. 67). Philadelphia: Saunders.

1333. A client has received a dose of a PRN medication called loperamide (Imodium). The nurse monitors the client after administration to see if the client has relief of:
1 Diarrhea
2 Tarry stools
3 Constipation
4 Abdominal pain

Level of Cognitive Ability: Analysis
Client Needs: Physiological Integrity
Integrated Process: Nursing Process/Evaluation
Content Area: Pharmacology

Answer: 1
Rationale: Loperamide is an antidiarrheal agent that is commonly administered after loose stools. It is used for the management of both acute and chronic (e.g., with inflammatory bowel disease) diarrhea. It can also be used to reduce the volume of drainage from an ileostomy. It is not used to treat tarry stools, constipation, or abdominal pain.

Test-Taking Strategy: Use the process of elimination, and focus on the name of the medication. Recall that this medication is an antidiarrheal agent to direct you to option 1. Review the purpose of loperamide if you had difficulty with this question.

Reference
Hodgson, B., & Kizior, R. (2009). *Saunders nursing drug handbook 2009* (p. 695). St. Louis: Saunders.

1334. A client is using diphenhydramine hydrochloride (Benadryl) 1% as a topical agent for allergic dermatosis. The medication is having the intended effect if which of the following is observed?
1 Nighttime sedation
2 Decrease in urticaria
3 Healing of burned tissue
4 Resolution of ecchymoses

Level of Cognitive Ability: Analysis
Client Needs: Physiological Integrity
Integrated Process: Nursing Process/Evaluation
Content Area: Pharmacology

Answer: 2
Rationale: The antihistamine medication diphenhydramine has many uses. It reduces the symptoms of allergic reaction (e.g., itching, urticaria) when used as a topical agent. It is not used to treat burns or ecchymoses. Mild nighttime sedation is a side effect but not an intended effect.

Test-Taking Strategy: Use the process of elimination and focus on the diagnosis to direct you to option 2. Review diphenhydramine if you had difficulty with this question.

Reference
Linton, A. (2007). *Introduction to medical-surgical nursing* (4th ed., p. 1215). Philadelphia: Saunders.

1335. A client has begun medication therapy with colchicine. The nurse monitors for which expected effect of this medication?
1 Joint pain reduction
2 Urine output increase

Answer: 1
Rationale: Colchicine is classified as an antigout agent. Its expected effects include reduced joint swelling and pain and the prevention of acute gouty attacks. It is not an antipyretic, antihypertensive, or diuretic medication.

3 Temperature reduction
4 Blood pressure increase

Level of Cognitive Ability: Analysis
Client Needs: Physiological Integrity
Integrated Process: Nursing Process/Evaluation
Content Area: Pharmacology

Test-Taking Strategy: Note the strategic words *expected effects.* Recall that this medication is an antigout agent to direct you to option 1. Review the actions and uses of colchicine if you had difficulty with this question.

Reference

Lehne, R. (2010). *Pharmacology for nursing care* (7th ed., p. 867). St. Louis: Saunders.

1336. A nurse has instructed a client about a low-sodium diet. The nurse determines that the client understands the information if the client selects which of the following dairy products as appropriate for use?
1 Yogurt
2 Whole milk
3 Powdered milk
4 American cheese

Level of Cognitive Ability: Comprehension
Client Needs: Health Promotion and Maintenance
Integrated Process: Nursing Process/Evaluation
Content Area: Adult Health/Cardiovascular

Answer: 3
Rationale: The client on a low-sodium diet should be taught that any foods that are derived from animal sources contain physiological saline and are therefore higher in sodium than many foods from plant sources. Powdered milk is often manufactured to be lower in sodium, so it is the best dairy choice of those presented in the options for clients on a low-sodium diet.

Test-Taking Strategy: Use the process of elimination. Note that options 1, 2, and 4 are comparable or alike in that they are directly derived from animal sources. Review sodium-restricted diets if you had difficulty with this question.

References

Christensen, B., & Kockrow, E. (2006). *Foundations of nursing* (5th ed., pp. 648-649). St. Louis: Mosby.
deWit, S. (2009). *Medical-surgical nursing: Concepts & practice* (p. 484). St. Louis: Saunders.
Linton, A. (2007). *Introduction to medical-surgical nursing* (4th ed., p. 107). Philadelphia: Saunders.

1337. In the care plan of a client with Graves' disease, the nurse notes a nursing diagnosis of *Imbalanced nutrition, less than body requirements* related to the effects of the hypercatabolic state. Which of the following indicates a successful outcome for this diagnosis?
1 The client verbalizes the need to avoid snacking between meals.
2 The client discusses the relationship between meal time and the blood glucose level.
3 The client maintains his or her normal weight or gradually gains weight if it is below normal.
4 The client demonstrates knowledge of the need to consume a diet that is high in fat and low in protein.

Level of Cognitive Ability: Analysis
Client Needs: Physiological Integrity
Integrated Process: Nursing Process/Evaluation
Content Area: Adult Health/Endocrine

Answer: 3
Rationale: Graves' disease is characterized by hyperthyroidism. It causes a state of chronic nutritional and caloric deficiency as a result of the metabolic effects of excessive T3 and T4. Clinical manifestations include weight loss and increased appetite, so it is therefore a nutritional goal that the client will not lose additional weight and will gradually return to the ideal body weight, if necessary. To accomplish this, the client must be encouraged to eat frequent high-calorie, high-protein, and high-carbohydrate meals and snacks. The relationship between mealtime and the blood glucose level is unrelated to the subject of the question.

Test-Taking Strategy: Use the process of elimination, and focus on the strategic words *hypercatabolic state.* Options 1 and 4 would not be beneficial for a client in a hypercatabolic state. Option 2 can be eliminated because discussing the fluctuation in the blood glucose level will not assist a client who is hypercatabolic. Review altered nutrition and Graves' disease if you had difficulty with this question.

Reference

Christensen, B., & Kockrow, E. (2006). *Adult health nursing* (5th ed., p. 530). St. Louis: Mosby.

1338. A nurse is assisting with caring for a woman in labor who is receiving oxytocin (Pitocin) by intravenous infusion. The nurse monitors the client, knowing that which of the following indicates an adequate contraction pattern?

1 One contraction per minute, with resultant cervical dilation
2 Four contractions every 5 minutes, with resultant cervical dilation
3 One contraction every 10 minutes, without resultant cervical dilation
4 Three to five contractions in 10 minutes, with resultant cervical dilation

Level of Cognitive Ability: Analysis
Client Needs: Physiological Integrity
Integrated Process: Nursing Process/Evaluation
Content Area: Maternity/Intrapartum

Answer: 4
Rationale: The preferred oxytocin dosage is the minimal amount necessary to maintain an adequate contraction pattern, which is characterized by three to five contractions in a 10-minute period, with resultant cervical dilation. If contractions are more frequent than every 2 minutes, contraction quality may be decreased.

Test-Taking Strategy: Use the process of elimination, and focus on the subject—an adequate contraction pattern; this will assist you with eliminating option 3. Eliminate options 1 and 2 next because they are comparable or alike. Review the expected effects of oxytocin if you had difficulty with this question.

Reference

Leifer, G. (2008). *Maternity nursing: An introductory text* (10th ed., pp. 288-289). Philadelphia: Saunders.

1339. A client has been given a prescription for a course of azithromycin (Zithromax). The nurse determines that the medication is having the intended effect if which of the following is noted?

1 Pain is relieved.
2 Blood pressure is lower.
3 Joint discomfort is reduced.
4 Signs and symptoms of infection are relieved

Level of Cognitive Ability: Analysis
Client Needs: Physiological Integrity
Integrated Process: Nursing Process/Evaluation
Content Area: Pharmacology

Answer: 4
Rationale: Azithromycin is a macrolide antibiotic that is used to treat infection. It is not ordered for the treatment of pain, blood pressure, or joint discomfort.

Test-Taking Strategy: Use the process of elimination. Eliminate options 1 and 3 first because they are comparable or alike. From the remaining options, focus on the name of the medication, and recall that many antibiotic names end with the letters *-mycin;* this will direct you to option 4. Review the action and purpose of azithromycin if you had difficulty with this question.

Reference

Hodgson, B., & Kizior, R. (2009). *Saunders nursing drug handbook 2009* (pp. 111-114). St. Louis: Saunders.

1340. A client has begun medication therapy with betaxolol (Kerlone). The nurse determines that the client is experiencing the intended effects of therapy if which of the following is noted?

1 Edema present at +3
2 Weight gain of 5 lbs
3 Pulse rate increased from 58 to 74 beats/min
4 Blood pressure decreased from 142/94 to 128/82 mm Hg

Level of Cognitive Ability: Analysis
Client Needs: Physiological Integrity
Integrated Process: Nursing Process/Evaluation
Content Area: Pharmacology

Answer: 4
Rationale: Betaxolol is a β-adrenergic–blocking agent used to lower blood pressure, relieve angina, or eliminate dysrhythmias. Side effects include bradycardia and symptoms of congestive heart failure (e.g., weight gain, increased edema).

Test-Taking Strategy: Use the process of elimination, and note that the question asks for the intended effect of the medication. Remember that β-adrenergic–blocking agents medication names end with *-olol.* Recall the action of the medication to direct you to option 4. Review the intended effects of betaxolol if you had difficulty with this question.

Reference

Hodgson, B., & Kizior, R. (2009). *Saunders nursing drug handbook 2009* (pp. 129-130). St. Louis: Saunders.

1341. A nurse is caring for a client who has a nasogastric tube (NG) in place that has been connected to suction after abdominal surgery. Which observation by the nurse indicates that the tube is functioning properly?

1 The suction gauge reads low intermittent suction.
2 The client indicates that pain is a 3 on a 1-to-10 scale.
3 The distal end of the NG tube is pinned to the client's gown.
4 The client denies nausea and has 250 mL of fluid in the suction collection container.

Level of Cognitive Ability: Comprehension
Client Needs: Physiological Integrity
Integrated Process: Nursing Process/Evaluation
Content Area: Adult Health/Gastrointestinal

Answer: 4

Rationale: An NG tube connected to suction is used postoperatively to decompress and rest the bowel because the gastrointestinal tract lacks peristaltic activity as a result of manipulation during surgery. Although the nurse makes pertinent observations of the tube to ensure that it is secure and properly connected to suction, the client is assessed for the effect. The client should not experience symptoms of ileus (nausea and vomiting) if the tube is functioning properly. A pain indicator of 3 is an expected finding in a postoperative client.

Test-Taking Strategy: Use the process of elimination, and focus on the subject—the proper functioning of the NG tube. Recall the purpose of the NG tube in a postoperative client to direct you to option 4. Review the care of the client with an NG tube if you had difficulty with this question.

Reference

Christensen, B., & Kockrow, E. (2006). *Foundations of nursing* (5th ed., p. 654). St. Louis: Mosby.

Caring

1342. A 39-year-old man just learned that his 36-year-old wife has an incurable cancer and that she is expected to live for only a few more weeks. The nurse explores the client's feelings and identifies which of the following responses by the husband as indicative of effective individual coping?

1 He states that he will not allow his wife to come home to die.
2 He refuses to visit his wife in the hospital or to discuss her illness.
3 He expresses his anger at God and the physicians for allowing this to happen.
4 He immediately arranges for their three teenaged children to live with relatives in another state.

Level of Cognitive Ability: Analysis
Client Needs: Psychosocial Integrity
Integrated Process: Caring
Content Area: Fundamental Skills

Answer: 3

Rationale: The expression of anger is known to be a normal response to impending loss, and it may be directed toward the self, the dying person, God or another spiritual being, or the caregivers. Options 1 and 4 indicate possibly rash and unilateral decisions made by the husband without taking into consideration anyone else's feelings. There is evidence of denial in option 2 because the husband refuses to visit or discuss his wife's illness. The only option that indicates effective individual coping by the husband is option 3.

Test-Taking Strategy: Use the process of elimination, and note the strategic words *effective individual coping.* Knowledge of the stages of grief associated with loss will direct you to option 3. Review effective coping mechanisms if you had difficulty with this question.

References

Christensen, B., & Kockrow, E. (2006). *Foundations of nursing* (5th ed., p. 1135). St. Louis: Mosby.
Linton, A. (2007). *Introduction to medical-surgical nursing* (4th ed., p. 360). Philadelphia: Saunders.

1343. A nurse has been caring for a terminally ill client whose death is imminent. The nurse has developed a close relationship with the family of the client. Which of the following nursing interventions will the nurse avoid when dealing with the family during this difficult time?

Answer: 4

Rationale: Maintaining effective and open communication among family members affected by death and grief is of utmost importance. The nurse should maintain and enhance communication and preserve the family's sense of self-direction and control. Option 1 is likely to enhance communication. Option 2 is also an effective technique, and the family needs to know that

1 Encouraging family discussion of feelings
2 Accepting the family's expressions of anger
3 Facilitating the use of spiritual practices identified by the family
4 Making the decisions for the family during the difficult moments

Level of Cognitive Ability: Application
Client Needs: Psychosocial Integrity
Integrated Process: Caring
Content Area: Fundamental Skills

someone will be there who is supportive and nonjudgmental. Option 3 is also an effective intervention because spiritual practices give meaning to life and have an impact on how people react to crisis. Option 4 removes autonomy and decision making from the family at a time when they are already experiencing feelings of loss of control. This is an ineffective intervention that can impair communication.

Test-Taking Strategy: Note the strategic word *avoid*. This word indicates a negative event query and asks you to select an option that is an incorrect nursing action. Use the process of elimination, and focus on therapeutic communication techniques; this will direct you to option 4. Review therapeutic techniques for individuals in crisis if you had difficulty with this question.

References
deWit, S. (2009). *Medical-surgical nursing: Concepts & practice* (pp. 1174-1175). St. Louis: Saunders.
Linton, A. (2007). *Introduction to medical-surgical nursing* (4th ed., p. 75). Philadelphia: Saunders.

1344. A client brought to the emergency department is dead on arrival (DOA). The family of the client tells the physician that the client had terminal cancer. The emergency department physician examines the client and asks the nurse to contact the medical examiner about an autopsy. The family of the client tells the nurse that they do not want an autopsy performed. Which response to the family is appropriate?
1 "The decision is made by the medical examiner."
2 "An autopsy is mandatory for any client who is DOA."
3 "I will contact the medical examiner regarding your request."
4 "It is required by federal law. Why don't we talk about it, and why don't you tell me how you feel?"

Level of Cognitive Ability: Application
Client Needs: Safe and Effective Care Environment
Integrated Process: Caring
Content Area: Fundamental Skills

Answer: 3
Rationale: An autopsy may be required by state law in certain circumstances, including the sudden death of a client and a death that occurs under suspicious circumstances. It is not a requirement by federal law, and it is not mandatory that every client who is DOA undergo an autopsy. If a family requests to not have an autopsy performed on a family member, then the nurse should contact the medical examiner about the request.

Test-Taking Strategy: Use the process of elimination, your knowledge of the laws and issues surrounding autopsy, and therapeutic communication techniques to answer the question. Eliminate options 2 and 4 first because these statements are not accurate. From the remaining options, option 3 is the most therapeutic and caring response to make to the family. Review the issues and laws that surround autopsy if you had difficulty with this question.

Reference
Linton, A. (2007). *Introduction to medical-surgical nursing* (4th ed., p. 361). Philadelphia: Saunders.

1345. An older client with coronary artery disease is scheduled for hospital discharge and lives alone. The client states, "I don't know how I'll be able to remember all these instructions and take care of myself when I get home." The nurse should plan which action to assist the client?

Answer: 4
Rationale: With earlier hospital discharge, clients are returning home with more acute problems than before, and they may require support from a home health agency until they can function independently. Option 3 does nothing to actively assist the client, and option 2 is not realistic in the current health care environment. Although option 1 is a viable option, it does not ensure

1 Ask an out-of-town relative to stay with the client for a day or so.
2 Ask the physician to delay the discharge until the client is better able to manage self-care.
3 Suggest that the social worker follow up with a telephone call after discharge to ensure that the client is progressing.
4 Suggest that the physician be asked for a referral to a home health agency for nursing and home health aide support.

Level of Cognitive Ability: Application
Client Needs: Safe and Effective Care Environment
Integrated Process: Caring
Content Area: Fundamental Skills

that the client has continued care until he or she is able to independently manage his or her own care.

Test-Taking Strategy: Use the process of elimination, and focus on the subject and the client's concern. Note that option 4 is the only action that will ensure that the client has the necessary assistance until independence is achieved. Review the concepts related to home care support if you had difficulty with this question.

Reference

Linton, A. (2007). *Introduction to medical-surgical nursing* (4th ed., p. 8). Philadelphia: Saunders.

1346. A nurse had been caring for a client who died a few minutes ago, and the nurse reflects on the care given to the client. Which statement supports the nurse's belief that the client died with dignity?
1 A new nurse states that it is difficult to give that kind of care to a dying client.
2 The nurse gave increasing doses of pain medication to keep the client well sedated.
3 The physician recognizes that all the orders were carried out and that there were no questions.
4 The family thanks the nurse and states that the client was not in pain and was peaceful at the end.

Level of Cognitive Ability: Comprehension
Client Needs: Psychosocial Integrity
Integrated Process: Caring
Content Area: Fundamental Skills

Answer: 4

Rationale: The family response is an external perception, and it is extremely important. Families derive a great deal of comfort knowing that their loved one received the best care possible. Option 4 provides external validation that the client received comprehensive, quality care. Option 1 focuses on the feelings of a new nurse who may be expressing his or her own anxiety. Option 2 reflects on only one aspect of caring for a dying client. Option 3 focuses on physician orders rather than client care.

Test-Taking Strategy: Use the process of elimination, and focus on the subject—the client dying with dignity. The only option that addresses this subject is option 4. Review the concepts related to death and dying if you had difficulty with this question.

References

Christensen, B., & Kockrow, E. (2006). *Foundations of nursing* (5th ed., p. 200). St. Louis: Mosby.
Linton, A. (2007). *Introduction to medical-surgical nursing* (4th ed., pp. 87-88). Philadelphia: Saunders.

1347. While talking to a prenatal client about her dietary and alcohol-drinking habits, the nurse observes that the client has difficulty concentrating and appears agitated. The nurse should proceed with the conversation using which guideline?
1 A nonjudgmental approach may help to gain maternal trust.
2 Provoking maternal guilt may help a woman recognize her problem and seek support services.

Answer: 1

Rationale: The potential effects of alcohol use during pregnancy for both the mother and the fetus have been well documented. The nurse who expresses genuine concern with suspected abusers and who displays a nonjudgmental approach may motivate positive behavioral changes during the prenatal period. The maternal behaviors of lack of concentration and agitation are frequently seen in childbearing women who are abusing alcohol. Options 2, 3, and 4 are inappropriate guidelines for the nurse to follow in this situation, and they do not address a caring approach.

3 A discussion of the possible consequences of drinking alcohol during pregnancy should be avoided.
4 Women respond negatively to the hopeful message of the potential benefits of drinking cessation during pregnancy.

Level of Cognitive Ability: Application
Client Needs: Psychosocial Integrity
Integrated Process: Caring
Content Area: Maternity/Antepartum

Test-Taking Strategy: Use therapeutic caring techniques and the process of elimination. Remember that it is important to display a caring and nonjudgmental approach to the client. Review therapeutic caring techniques if you had difficulty with this question.

Reference

Christensen, B., & Kockrow, E. (2006). *Foundations of nursing* (5th ed., p. 792). St. Louis: Mosby.

1348. A woman who was drinking alcohol fell asleep while driving and was injured in an automobile accident. The client's only daughter, who was a passenger in the car, was killed instantly. During report, the nurse is told that the client is upset and withdrawn. When caring for the client, what is the appropriate initial nursing action?

1 Reflect back to the client that she appears upset.
2 Let the client have some time alone to grieve over the loss.
3 Request medication to assist the client with coping with the loss.
4 Tell the client that the injury and her daughter's death were the result of alcohol abuse, and refer the client for counseling.

Level of Cognitive Ability: Application
Client Needs: Psychosocial Integrity
Integrated Process: Caring
Content Area: Mental Health

Answer: 1

Rationale: The nurse should encourage the client to express her feelings. Reflection statements tend to elicit a deeper awareness of feelings. In addition, option 1 validates the perception that the client is upset. Options 2 and 3 address interventions before assessing the situation. Option 4 is inappropriate and is a block to communication.

Test-Taking Strategy: Note the strategic words *appropriate initial nursing action*. Use therapeutic communication techniques and the process of elimination. Select the option that encourages the client to express her feelings and to talk more. Remember to always address the client's feelings. Review therapeutic communication and caring techniques if you had difficulty with this question.

Reference

Christensen, B., & Kockrow, E. (2006). *Foundations of nursing* (5th ed., p. 42). St. Louis: Mosby.

1349. A nurse is collecting data from a client being admitted to the hospital. The client has right-sided weakness, aphasia, and urinary incontinence. One of the client's children states, "If this is a stroke, it's the kiss of death." The nurse should make which response to the family member?

1 "A stroke is not the kiss of death."
2 "You feel as if your parent is dying?"
3 "These symptoms may be reversible."
4 "Wait until the doctor gets here to think like that."

Answer: 2

Rationale: Option 2 allows the family member to verbalize and to begin to cope and adapt to what is happening. By restating what was said, the nurse is able to clarify the family member's feelings and to begin to offer information that will help to ease some of the fears that the family member may face at the moment. Options 1 and 4 offer disapproval and put the family member's feelings on hold. Option 3 provides false hope at this point.

Test-Taking Strategy: Use therapeutic communication techniques. Option 2 is the only option that addresses the family member's feelings. Review therapeutic caring and communication techniques if you had difficulty with this question.

Level of Cognitive Level: Application
Client Needs: Psychosocial Integrity
Integrated Process: Caring
Content Area: Fundamental Skills

Reference
deWit, S. (2009). *Medical-surgical nursing: Concepts & practice* (p. 576). St. Louis: Saunders.

1350. A nurse is assisting with planning care for a suicidal client. To provide a caring, therapeutic environment, which of the following is included in the nursing care plan?

1 Placing the client in a private room to ensure privacy and confidentiality
2 Establishing a therapeutic relationship and conveying unconditional positive regard
3 Maintaining a distance of 12 inches at all times to ensure the client that control will be provided
4 Placing the client in charge of a meaningful unit activity, such as the morning chess tournament

Level of Cognitive Ability: Application
Client Needs: Safe and Effective Care Environment
Integrated Process: Caring
Content Area: Mental Health

Answer: 2
Rationale: The establishment of a therapeutic relationship with the suicidal client increases feelings of acceptance. Although the suicidal behavior and thinking of the client are unacceptable, the use of unconditional positive regard acknowledges the client in a human-to-human context and increases the client's sense of self-worth. The client would not be placed in a private room because this is an unsafe action and may intensify the client's feelings of worthlessness. Distances of 18 inches or less between two individuals constitute intimate space; the invasion of this space may be misinterpreted by the client and increase the client's tension and feelings of helplessness. Placing the client in charge of the morning chess game is a premature intervention that can overwhelm the client and cause him or her to fail, which can reinforce the client's feelings of worthlessness.

Test-Taking Strategy: Use the process of elimination. Eliminate option 1 because isolation (i.e., a private room) is not a safe and therapeutic intervention. Option 4 may produce feelings of worthlessness. Eliminate option 3 because a distance of 12 inches is restrictive. Option 2 is the only option that addresses a caring and therapeutic environment. Review the care of the suicidal client if you had difficulty with this question.

Reference
deWit, S. (2009). *Medical-surgical nursing: Concepts & practice* (p. 1114). St. Louis: Saunders.

1351. A client has died, and the nurse asks one of the client's family members about the funeral arrangements. The family member refuses to discuss the subject. The nurse should take which appropriate action at this time?

1 Provide the information needed for decision making.
2 Demonstrate acceptance of the family member's feelings.
3 Remain with the family member without discussing funeral arrangements.
4 Assess the risk of self-harm, and refer the family member to a mental health professional.

Level of Cognitive Ability: Application
Client Needs: Psychosocial Integrity
Integrated Process: Caring
Content Area: Fundamental Skills

Answer: 3
Rationale: The family member is exhibiting the first stage of grief, which is denial. Option 1 may be an appropriate intervention during the bargaining stage. Option 2 is an appropriate intervention for the acceptance or reorganization and restitution stage. Option 4 may be an appropriate intervention for depression.

Test-Taking Strategy: Note the strategic words *appropriate action*, and use therapeutic caring and communication techniques. Eliminate options 1 and 4 because they do not address the subject of the question. From the remaining options, note the strategic words *refuses to discuss the subject* to direct you to option 3. The acceptance of feelings is important, but, in this situation, remaining with the family member is most appropriate. Review the grieving process and therapeutic caring and communication techniques if you had difficulty with this question.

Reference
Linton, A. (2007). *Introduction to medical-surgical nursing* (4th ed., p. 75). Philadelphia: Saunders.

1352. A nurse employed in the emergency department is assigned to care for an older client who has been identified as a victim of physical abuse. When planning care for this client, which of the following is the nurse's priority?

1. Adhering to the mandatory abuse reporting laws
2. Referring the abusing family member for treatment
3. Determining if the client is in any immediate danger
4. Encouraging the client to file charges against the abuser

Level of Cognitive Ability: Application
Client Needs: Safe and Effective Care Environment
Integrated Process: Caring
Content Area: Mental Health

Answer: 3

Rationale: Whenever the abused client remains in the abusive environment, priority must be placed on determining if the person is in any immediate danger. If so, emergency action must be taken to remove the client from the abusive situation. Options 1 and 2 may be appropriate interventions, but they are not the priority. Option 4 is not an appropriate intervention at this time and may produce increased fear and anxiety in the client.

Test-Taking Strategy: Use the process of elimination. Eliminate option 4 first because this action may produce increased fear and anxiety in the client. Use Maslow's Hierarchy of Needs theory to select from the remaining options. Remember that if a physiological need is not present, safety is the priority; this should direct you to option 3. The correct option also addresses the first step of the nursing process, which is data collection. Review the principles related to caring for the abused client if you had difficulty with this question.

Reference

Fortinash, K., & Holoday-Worret, P. (2008). *Psychiatric mental health nursing* (4th ed., p. 504). St. Louis: Mosby.

1353. A woman comes into the emergency department in a severe state of anxiety after a car accident. The important nursing intervention at this time would be to:

1. Remain with the client.
2. Put the client in a quiet room.
3. Teach the client deep breathing.
4. Encourage the client to talk about her feelings and concerns.

Level of Cognitive Ability: Application
Client Needs: Psychosocial Integrity
Integrated Process: Caring
Content Area: Mental Health

Answer: 1

Rationale: If the client with severe anxiety is left alone, she may feel abandoned and become overwhelmed. Placing the client in a quiet room is indicated, but the nurse must stay with the client. It is not possible to teach the client deep breathing or relaxation exercises until the anxiety decreases. Encouraging the client to discuss feelings and concerns would not take place until the anxiety has decreased.

Test-Taking Strategy: Use the process of elimination, and note the strategic words *severe state of anxiety.* Because the anxiety state is severe, eliminate options 3 and 4. From the remaining options, consider the word *important* in the question; this should direct you to option 1. Review the care of the client with severe anxiety if you had difficulty with this question.

Reference

deWit, S. (2009). *Medical-surgical nursing: Concepts & practice* (p. 1104). St. Louis: Saunders.

1354. During the transition period of labor, the nurse notes that a client is having difficulty concentrating on her breathing technique. The client's coach anxiously states that he does not know how to help her. The appropriate intervention is to:

1. Tell them that, during transition, no interventions are effective.
2. Keep them informed about the labor process and events using positive terms.

Answer: 2

Rationale: During the transition period of active labor, the client and her support system must be kept informed with appropriate information so that they can better take part in the labor process and remain in control. Option 1 is incorrect. Options 3 and 4 are inappropriate.

Test-Taking Strategy: Use the process of elimination, and note the strategic word *appropriate.* Use therapeutic communication techniques and note the word *positive* in option 2 to direct you to this option. Review the care of the client during the transition period of labor if you had difficulty with this question.

3 Relieve the coach of the responsibilities because he does not know how to help.
4 Provide pharmacological interventions so that the client does not have to concentrate.

Level of Cognitive Ability: Application
Client Needs: Psychosocial Integrity
Integrated Process: Caring
Content Area: Maternity/Intrapartum

Reference

Christensen, B., & Kockrow, E. (2006). *Foundations of nursing* (5th ed., p. 828). St. Louis: Mosby.

1355. The family of a client with Parkinson's disease tells the nurse that the client is having difficulty adjusting to the disorder and that they do not know what to do to help. The nurse advises the family that which of the following would be therapeutic to assist the client with coping with the disease?

1 Plan only a few activities for the client during the day.
2 Cluster activities at the end of the day, when the client is restless and bored.
3 Assist the client with activities of daily living (ADLs) as much as possible.
4 Encourage and praise client efforts to exercise and perform ADLs.

Level of Cognitive Ability: Application
Client Needs: Psychosocial Integrity
Integrated Process: Caring
Content Area: Adult Health/Neurological

Answer: 4

Rationale: Parkinson's disease is a slowly progressing degenerative neurological disorder. The client with Parkinson's disease has a tendency to become withdrawn and depressed, which can be limited by encouraging the client to be an active participant in his or her own care. The family should also give the client encouragement and praise for perseverance in these efforts. The family should plan activities intermittently throughout the day to inhibit daytime sleeping and boredom. Options 1, 2, and 3 are incorrect.

Test-Taking Strategy: Use the process of elimination. Eliminate option 1 first because of the close-ended word *only.* Eliminate option 2 next because clustering activities at one time will tire the client. From the remaining options, recall that the client should be an active participant in his or her own care to direct you to option 4. Review therapeutic techniques for the client with Parkinson's disease to assist with adjustment to the disease if you had difficulty with this question.

Reference

Linton, A. (2007). *Introduction to medical-surgical nursing* (4th ed., p. 448). Philadelphia: Saunders.

1356. A nurse is assisting with caring for a group of homeless people in a certain area of a city. When planning for the potential needs of this group, what is the most immediate concern?

1 Peer support through structured groups
2 Finding affordable housing for the group
3 Setting up a 24-hour crisis center and hotline
4 Meeting the basic needs to ensure that adequate food, shelter, and clothing are available

Level of Cognitive Ability: Analysis
Client Needs: Physiological Integrity
Integrated Process: Caring
Content Area: Delegating/Prioritizing

Answer: 4

Rationale: The question asks about the most immediate concern, which is always attending to the basic needs of food, shelter, and clothing. Options 1, 2, and 3 are other activities that may be carried out at a later time.

Test-Taking Strategy: Use Maslow's Hierarchy of Needs theory to answer the question. Option 4 addresses basic physiological needs. Although options 1, 2, and 3 are also appropriate actions, option 4 is the immediate concern. Review the needs of the homeless population if you had difficulty with this question.

References

Fortinash, K., & Holoday-Worret, P. (2008). *Psychiatric mental health nursing* (4th ed., p. 636). St. Louis: Mosby.
Mauer, F., & Smith, C. (2009). *Community/public health nursing practices: Health for families and populations.* (4th ed., pp. 541-542). St. Louis: Saunders.

1357. A nurse is providing care to a Cuban-American client who is terminally ill. Numerous family members are present most of the time, and many of the family members are very emotional. The appropriate nursing action is to:

1 Restrict the number of family members visiting at one time.
2 Inform the family that emotional outbursts are to be avoided.
3 Contact the physician to speak to the family members about their behaviors.
4 Request permission to move the client to a private room, and allow the family members to visit.

Level of Cognitive Ability: Application
Client Needs: Psychosocial Integrity
Integrated Process: Caring
Content Area: Fundamental Skills

Answer: 4

Rationale: In the Cuban-American culture, loud crying and other physical manifestations of grief are considered socially acceptable. Of the options provided, option 4 is the only option that identifies a culturally sensitive and caring approach on the part of the nurse. Options 1, 2, and 3 are inappropriate nursing interventions.

Test-Taking Strategy: Focus on the clients of the question, who are the family members of a Cuban-American client. Use the process of elimination, and recall the characteristics of this culture and the importance of cultural sensitivity; this will direct you to option 4. Review the characteristics of the Cuban-American culture if you had difficulty with this question.

Reference

Potter, P., & Perry, A. (2009) *Fundamentals of nursing* (7th ed., p. 316). St. Louis: Mosby.

1358. A nurse is caring for an older client who has been recently admitted from home to a long-term care facility. The client has a diagnosis of end-stage renal cancer, and the nurse recognizes that the client is coping with many losses. The best way to address the client's psychosocial needs is to:

1 Provide total care to the client.
2 Sit with the client and allow the client to verbalize feelings.
3 Medicate the client for pain every 4 hours as prescribed.
4 Encourage the client to participate in daily social activities.

Level of Cognitive Ability: Application
Client Needs: Psychosocial Integrity
Integrated Process: Caring
Content Area: Fundamental Skills

Answer: 2

Rationale: Clients admitted from home into a long-term care facility are dealing with losses in control over their environment, independence, and privacy. Sitting with the client and allowing the client to express feelings is the best way to address the client's psychosocial needs. Providing total care does not facilitate independence. Medicating for pain will keep the client comfortable, but this does not address the client's psychosocial needs. Participation in daily social activities will not meet the special psychosocial needs of this client.

Test-Taking Strategy: Use the process of elimination, and focus on the strategic words *psychosocial needs.* Eliminate options 1 and 3 first because these options deal with physiological needs. From the remaining options, recall that the client's feelings should be addressed first to direct you to option 2. Review the care of the client experiencing loss if you had difficulty with this question.

References

deWit, S. (2009). *Medical-surgical nursing: Concepts & practice* (pp. 205-206). St. Louis: Saunders.
Linton, A. (2007). *Introduction to medical-surgical nursing* (4th ed., p. 1243). Philadelphia: Saunders.

1359. A client with diabetes mellitus is told that amputation of the leg is necessary to sustain her life. The client is very upset and says to the nurse, "This is all the doctor's fault! I did everything that the doctor asked me to do!" The nurse interprets the client's statement as:

1 An expected coping mechanism
2 An ineffective coping mechanism

Answer: 1

Rationale: The expression of anger is known to be a normal response to impending loss, and the anger may be directed toward self, God or another spiritual being, or a caregiver. The nurse should be aware of the effective and ineffective coping mechanisms that can occur in a client when loss is anticipated. Notifying the hospital lawyer is inappropriate. Guilt may or may not be a component of the client's feelings, but the information in the question does not provide an indication that guilt is present.

3 A need to notify the hospital lawyer
4 An expression of guilt on the part of the client

Level of Cognitive Ability: Analysis
Client Needs: Psychosocial Integrity
Integrated Process: Caring
Content Area: Fundamental Skills

Test-Taking Strategy: Focus on the data provided in the question. Note that options 1 and 2 address coping mechanisms; this may provide you with a clue that one of these may be the correct option. Note that the client is blaming the doctor. Use your knowledge of the stages of grief associated with loss to direct you to option 1. Review the stages of grief and expected client expressions of grief if you had difficulty with this question.

References

Christensen, B., & Kockrow, E. (2006). *Adult health nursing* (5th ed., p. 556). St. Louis: Mosby.
Christensen, B., & Kockrow, E. (2006). *Foundations of nursing* (5th ed., p. 1134). St. Louis: Mosby.
Linton, A. (2007). *Introduction to medical-surgical nursing* (4th ed., pp. 1237-1240). Philadelphia: Saunders.

1360. A nurse is interacting with the family of a client who is unconscious as a result of a head injury. Which approach should the nurse use to help the family cope with this situation?
1 Discourage the family from touching the client.
2 Explain equipment and procedures on an ongoing basis.
3 Enforce adherence to visiting hours to ensure the client's rest.
4 Encourage the family to not give in to their feelings of grief.

Level of Cognitive Ability: Application
Client Needs: Psychosocial Integrity
Integrated Process: Caring
Content Area: Adult Health/Neurological

Answer: 2
Rationale: Families often need assistance with coping with the sudden severe illness of a loved one. The nurse should explain all equipment, treatments, and procedures and supplement or reinforce the information given by the physician. Family members should be encouraged to touch and speak to the client and to become involved in the client's care in some way if they are comfortable doing so. The nurse should allow the family to stay with the client whenever possible. The nurse also encourages the family members to eat properly and to obtain enough sleep to maintain their strength.

Test-Taking Strategy: Use the process of elimination and therapeutic caring and communication techniques to answer this question. Each of the incorrect options places distance between the family and the client. Review the techniques that assist family members with dealing with a sudden illness if you had difficulty with this question.

Reference

deWit, S. (2009). *Medical-surgical nursing: Concepts & practice* (p. 546). St. Louis: Saunders.

Communication and Documentation

1361. A client with myasthenia gravis is having difficulty with the motor aspects of speech. He has difficulty forming words, and his voice has a nasal tone. The nurse should use which communication strategy when working with this client?
1 Encourage the client to speak quickly.
2 Nod continuously while the client is speaking.
3 Repeat what the client said to verify the message.
4 Engage the client in lengthy discussions to strengthen his voice.

Answer: 3
Rationale: Myasthenia gravis is an abnormal condition that is characterized by chronic fatigability and muscle weakness, especially in the face and throat, as a result of a defect in the conduction of the nerve impulses at the neuromuscular junction. The client has speech that is nasal in tone and dysarthric as a result of cranial nerve involvement of the muscles that govern speech. The nurse listens attentively and verbally verifies what the client has said. Other helpful techniques are to ask questions that require a yes or no response and to develop alternative communication methods (e.g., letter board, picture board, pen and paper, flash cards). Encouraging the client to speak quickly is inappropriate and counterproductive. Continuous nodding may be distracting

Level of Cognitive Ability: Application
Client Needs: Physiological Integrity
Integrated Process: Communication and Documentation
Content Area: Adult Health/Neurological

and is unnecessary. Lengthy discussions will tire the client rather than strengthen his voice.

Test-Taking Strategy: Use the process of elimination and basic principles of communication to answer this question; this will direct you to option 3. Review myasthenia gravis and effective communication strategies if you had difficulty with this question.

References

deWit, S. (2009). *Medical-surgical nursing: Concepts & practice* (pp. 606-607). St. Louis: Saunders.
Linton, A. (2007). *Introduction to medical-surgical nursing* (4th ed., pp. 454-456). Philadelphia: Saunders.

1362. A nurse has an order to institute aneurysm precautions for a client with a cerebral aneurysm. Which item should the nurse document on the plan of care for this client?

1 Limit out-of-bed activities to twice daily.
2 Allow the client to read and watch television.
3 Encourage the client to take his or her own daily bath.
4 Instruct the client to not strain with bowel movements.

Level of Cognitive Ability: Application
Client Needs: Physiological Integrity
Integrated Process: Communication and Documentation
Content Area: Adult Health/Neurological

Answer: 4
Rationale: Aneurysm precautions include placing the client on bedrest in a quiet setting. The lights are kept dim to minimize environmental stimulation. Any activity that increases the blood pressure or that impedes venous return from the brain is prohibited (e.g., pushing, pulling, sneezing, coughing, straining). The nurse provides all physical care to minimize increases in blood pressure. For the same reason, visitors, radio, television, and reading materials are prohibited or limited. Stimulants such as caffeine and nicotine are prohibited. The nurse documents that the client is instructed to avoid straining with bowel movements.

Test-Taking Strategy: Use the process of elimination. Recall that the components of aneurysm precautions are to limit the amount of stimulation (in any form) that the client receives and to prevent increased intracranial pressure (ICP). With this in mind, eliminate options 1 and 3 first. From the remaining options, recall that straining can increase ICP, so it is appropriate to tell the client not to do so. Review the components of aneurysm precautions if you had difficulty with this question.

Reference

Monahan, F., Sands, J., Marek, J., Neighbors, M., & Green, C. (2007). *Phipps' medical-surgical nursing: Health and illness perspectives* (8th ed., p. 1441). St. Louis: Mosby.

1363. A nurse is trying to determine the client's adjustment to a new diagnosis of coronary heart disease before discharging the client from the hospital. Of the following questions, which one should the nurse ask to elicit the most useful response to determine the client's adjustment?

1 "Do you understand the use of your new medications?"
2 "Are you going to book your follow-up physician visit?"
3 "Do you have anyone at home to help with housework and shopping?"
4 "How do you feel about the lifestyle changes you are planning to make?"

Answer: 4
Rationale: All of these questions relate to aspects of care after discharge, but only option 4 explores the client's feelings about adjustment to the disease. Options 1, 2, and 3 do not address these feelings.

Test-Taking Strategy: Use therapeutic communication techniques. Open-ended questions explore the client's reactions or feelings to a particular situation, whereas closed-ended responses generally elicit a response of "yes" or "no." All of the incorrect options are closed-ended questions. Review therapeutic communication techniques if you had difficulty with this question.

Level of Cognitive Ability: Application
Client Needs: Health Promotion and Maintenance
Integrated Process: Communication and Documentation
Content Area: Fundamental Skills

References
Christensen, B., & Kockrow, E. (2006). *Adult health nursing* (5th ed., p. 345). St. Louis: Mosby.
Christensen, B., & Kockrow, E. (2006). *Foundations of nursing* (5th ed., pp. 39-42). St. Louis: Mosby.

1364. A female client who is experiencing disordered thinking about food being poisoned is admitted to the mental health unit. The nurse uses which communication technique to encourage the client to eat dinner?
1 Open-ended questions and silence
2 Offering opinions about the need to eat
3 Focusing on self-disclosure of personal food preferences
4 Verbalizing reasons that the client may choose not to eat

Level of Cognitive Ability: Application
Client Needs: Physiological Integrity
Integrated Process: Communication and Documentation
Content Area: Mental Health

Answer: 1
Rationale: Open-ended questions and silence are strategies that encourage a client to discuss the problem in a descriptive manner. Options 2 and 4 are not helpful because they do not encourage the client to express her feelings. Option 3 is not a client-centered intervention.

Test-Taking Strategy: Use the process of elimination and therapeutic communication techniques. Eliminate options 2 and 4 first because they do not support client expression of feelings. Eliminate option 3 next because it is not a client-centered response. Review therapeutic communication techniques if you had difficulty with this question.

Reference
Christensen, B., & Kockrow, E. (2006). *Foundations of nursing* (5th ed., pp. 39-42). St. Louis: Mosby.

1365. A pregnant client reports that the prescribed iron supplement is causing nausea, constipation, and heartburn and that she plans to stop taking the medication. The nurse should make which response to the client?
1 "You will get used to the side effects in time."
2 "Your baby needs that iron, you can't stop taking it."
3 "Do not stop taking your medication without talking to the doctor."
4 "These gastric reactions are most intense during initial therapy. They become less bothersome with continued use."

Level of Cognitive Ability: Application
Client Needs: Psychosocial Integrity
Integrated Process: Communication and Documentation
Content Area: Fundamental Skills

Answer: 4
Rationale: It is most important that pregnant clients receive iron supplements because of the extra demands placed on maternal circulation by the fetus. Option 4 offers needed information to the client and addresses the issues that are bothersome. Options 2 and 3 show disapproval of the client's feelings. Option 1 places the client's issue on hold.

Test-Taking Strategy: Use therapeutic communication techniques. Remember to focus on the client's feelings and concerns to direct you to option 4. Review therapeutic communication techniques if you had difficulty with this question.

Reference
Christensen, B., & Kockrow, E. (2006). *Adult health nursing* (5th ed., p. 302). St. Louis: Mosby.

1366. A client with type 2 diabetes mellitus was recently hospitalized for hyperglycemic hyperosmolar nonketotic syndrome

Answer: 4
Rationale: The nurse should provide time and listen to the client's concerns. In option 4, the nurse is attempting to clarify the

(HHNS). Upon discharge from the hospital, the client expresses concern about the recurrence of HHNS. Which statement by the nurse is therapeutic?

1 "I'm sure this won't happen again."
2 "Don't worry, your family will help you."
3 "I think you might need to go to a nursing home."
4 "You have concerns about the treatment of your condition?"

Level of Cognitive Ability: Application
Client Needs: Psychosocial Integrity
Integrated Process: Communication and Documentation
Content Area: Adult Health/Endocrine

client's feelings. Options 1 and 2 provide inappropriate false reassurance. In addition, the nurse would not tell the client not to worry. Option 3 is not an appropriate nursing response because it disregards the client's concerns and gives advice.

> ***Test-Taking Strategy***: Use therapeutic communication techniques. Remember to always address the client's feelings to direct you to option 4. Review therapeutic communication techniques if you had difficulty with this question.

References

Christensen, B., & Kockrow, E. (2006). *Adult health nursing* (5th ed., p. 557). St. Louis: Mosby.
deWit, S. (2009). *Medical-surgical nursing: Concepts & practice* (p. 8). St. Louis: Saunders.

1367. The husband of a client who has a Sengstaken-Blakemore tube states to the nurse, "I thought having this tube down her nose the first time would convince my wife to quit drinking." The nurse should make which response to the client's husband?

1 "I think you are a good person to stay with your wife."
2 "Alcoholism is a disease that affects the whole family."
3 "Have you discussed this subject at the support group meetings?"
4 "You sound frustrated with dealing with your wife's drinking problem."

Level of Cognitive Ability: Application
Client Needs: Psychosocial Integrity
Integrated Process: Communication and Documentation
Content Area: Adult Health/Gastrointestinal

Answer: 4

Rationale: In option 4, the nurse uses the therapeutic communication techniques of clarifying and focusing to assist the client (the spouse) with expressing his feelings about his wife's chronic illness. Showing approval (option 1), stereotyping (option 2), and changing the subject (option 3) are nontherapeutic techniques that block communication.

> ***Test-Taking Strategy***: Use therapeutic communication techniques. Remember to always address the client's feelings to direct you to option 4. Review therapeutic communication techniques if you had difficulty with this question.

References

Christensen, B., & Kockrow, E. (2006). *Foundations of nursing* (5th ed., pp. 39-42). St. Louis: Mosby.
Linton, A. (2007). *Introduction to medical-surgical nursing* (4th ed., pp. 740, 813-814). Philadelphia: Saunders.

1368. A nurse is assigned to care for a client who is in a state of catatonic stupor. When the nurse enters the client's room, the client is found lying on the bed with his body pulled into a fetal position. The nurse should take which action?

1 Ask the client direct questions to encourage talking.
2 Take the client into the dayroom to be with other clients.
3 Leave the client alone and continue with providing care to other clients.
4 Sit beside the client in silence and occasionally ask open-ended questions.

Answer: 4

Rationale: Clients who are withdrawn may be immobile and mute, and they require consistent, repeated approaches. Intervention includes the establishment of interpersonal contact. Communication with withdrawn clients requires much patience from the nurse. The nurse facilitates communication with the client by sitting in silence, asking open-ended questions, and pausing to provide opportunities for the client to respond. The client would not be left alone. It is not appropriate at this time to place the client in a public place (e.g., the dayroom). Asking direct questions to the client is not therapeutic.

Level of Cognitive Ability: Application
Client Needs: Psychosocial Integrity
Integrated Process: Communication and Documentation
Content Area: Mental Health

Test-Taking Strategy: Use the process of elimination. Eliminate option 1 because asking direct questions of this client is not therapeutic. Eliminate option 2 because it is not appropriate to place the client in a public place. Eliminate option 3 because you would not leave the client alone. Option 4 is the best action because it provides both client supervision and communication with the client. Review the care of the client with catatonic stupor if you had difficulty with this question.

Reference

deWit, S. (2009). *Medical-surgical nursing: Concepts & practice* (p. 1157). St. Louis: Saunders.

1369. A nurse is developing a plan of care for an older client and includes strategies that will facilitate effective communication. The nurse should include which strategy to accomplish this goal?

1 Use active listening.
2 Use an authoritarian approach.
3 React only to the facts during conversation.
4 React enthusiastically during the conversation.

Level of Cognitive Ability: Application
Client Needs: Psychosocial Integrity
Integrated Process: Communication and Documentation
Content Area: Fundamental Skills

Answer: 1

Rationale: For effective communication, the nurse uses active listening and creates an environment in which the client feels comfortable expressing feelings. An authoritarian approach is directive rather than permissive and will not create an environment for verbal exchange. Reacting only to the facts is an example of inactive listening. Reacting enthusiastically is not the most effective strategy.

Test-Taking Strategy: Use the process of elimination and therapeutic communication techniques; this will direct you to option 1. Review therapeutic communication techniques if you had difficulty with this question.

Reference

Christensen, B., & Kockrow, E. (2006). *Foundations of nursing* (5th ed., pp. 39-42). St. Louis: Mosby.

1370. A female client with a long-leg cast has been using crutches to ambulate for 1 week. She comes to the clinic with complaints of pain, fatigue, and frustration with crutch walking. She says, "I feel like I have a crippled leg." The nurse should make which response to the client?

1 "Tell me what is bothersome for you."
2 "Why don't you take a couple of days off work and rest."
3 "I know how you feel, I had to use crutches before, too."
4 "Just remember, you'll be done with the crutches in another month."

Level of Cognitive Ability: Application
Client Needs: Psychosocial Integrity
Integrated Process: Communication and Documentation
Content Area: Adult Health/Musculoskeletal

Answer: 1

Rationale: Option 1 involves the therapeutic communication technique of clarification and validation and indicates that the nurse is dealing with the client's problem from the client's perspective. Option 2 gives advice and is a communication block. Option 3 devalues the client's feelings and thus blocks communication. Option 4 provides false reassurance because the client may not be finished using the crutches in another month. In addition, option 4 does not focus on the present problem.

Test-Taking Strategy: Use therapeutic communication techniques. Option 1 is the only response that encourages communication. Review therapeutic communication techniques if you had difficulty with this question.

References

Christensen, B., & Kockrow, E. (2006). *Foundations of nursing* (5th ed., pp. 39-42). St. Louis: Mosby.
Linton, A. (2007). *Introduction to medical-surgical nursing* (4th ed., pp. 923-924). Philadelphia: Saunders.

1371. An 18-year-old client is being discharged from the hospital after surgery and will need to ambulate with a cane for the next 6 months. The nurse asks the client which question that will provide data about the psychosocial status of the client regarding the use of the cane?

1 "Time will pass quickly, don't you think?"
2 "You are not worried about what your friends will think, are you?"
3 "Do you have any questions about how to ambulate with the cane?"
4 "How do you feel about having to ambulate with a cane for the next 6 months?"

Level of Cognitive Ability: Application
Client Needs: Psychosocial Integrity
Integrated Process: Communication and Documentation
Content Area: Fundamental Skills

Answer: 4
Rationale: How a client feels is an important part of the psychosocial assessment. Option 1 gives an opinion. Option 2 can be intimidating to the client. Option 3 deals with a physical issue. In addition, options 1, 2, and 3 are closed-ended questions and thus barriers to effective communication.

Test-Taking Strategy: Use therapeutic communication techniques. Avoid responses that include communication blocks. Eliminate options 1, 2, and 3 because they are closed-ended questions that are blocks to communication. Remember to address the client's feelings first. Review therapeutic communication techniques if you had difficulty with this question.

References
Christensen, B., & Kockrow, E. (2006). *Foundations of nursing* (5th ed., pp. 39-42). St. Louis: Mosby.
Linton, A. (2007). *Introduction to medical-surgical nursing* (4th ed., p. 924). Philadelphia: Saunders.

1372. A client will be self-administering an anticoagulant subcutaneously at home and says to the nurse, "I'm not sure I will be able to take this medication at home." The nurse should make which response to the client?

1 "Maybe your wife can give you your shot."
2 "Don't worry. Your doctor knows what's best for you."
3 "You'll be fine once you get used to giving your own shots."
4 "What are your concerns about taking this medication at home?"

Level of Cognitive Ability: Application
Client Needs: Psychosocial Integrity
Integrated Process: Communication and Documentation
Content Area: Fundamental Skills

Answer: 4
Rationale: Option 4 restates the client's concern and provides the client with the opportunity to verbalize. Option 1 offers advice without knowing what the client's concerns really are. Options 2 and 3 provide false reassurance, which invalidates the client's concern.

Test-Taking Strategy: Use therapeutic communication techniques to answer this question. Remember to focus on the client's feelings to direct you to option 4. Review therapeutic communication techniques if you had difficulty with this question.

References
Christensen, B., & Kockrow, E. (2006). *Foundations of nursing* (5th ed., pp. 39-42). St. Louis: Mosby.
deWit, S. (2009). *Medical-surgical nursing: Concepts & practice* (p. 154). St. Louis: Saunders.

1373. A nurse has made an error when documenting the vital signs of a client and obtains the client's record to correct the error. The nurse corrects the error by:

1 Using whiteout
2 Erasing the error
3 Documenting a late entry
4 Drawing one line through the error and initialing and dating the line

Answer: 4
Rationale: If a nurse makes an error when documenting in the client's record, the nurse should follow agency policies to correct the error. This includes drawing one line through the error, initialing and dating the line, and then providing the correct information. Erasing data from the client's record and the use of whiteout are prohibited. A late entry is used to document additional information that was not remembered at the initial time of documentation.

Level of Cognitive Ability: Application
Client Needs: Safe and Effective Care Environment
Integrated Process: Communication and Documentation
Content Area: Fundamental Skills

Test-Taking Strategy: Use the process of elimination and principles related to documentation. Recall that alterations to a client's record are avoided to eliminate options 1 and 2. From the remaining options, focus on the subject to direct you to option 4. Review the principles related to documentation if you had difficulty with this question.

Reference

Linton, A. (2007). *Introduction to medical-surgical nursing* (4th ed., p. 155). Philadelphia: Saunders.

1374. A client with hyperparathyroidism talks to the nurse about the dietary changes prescribed by the physician. The client states, "I guess I'll never be able to eat ice cream and yogurt again." The nurse should make which response to the client?

1 "Why do you say that?"
2 "There are lots of other foods that you can eat."
3 "Ice cream has too much fat content anyway."
4 "You don't think you will be able to eat them at all?"

Level of Cognitive Ability: Application
Client Needs: Psychosocial Integrity
Integrated Process: Communication and Documentation
Content Area: Fundamental Skills

Answer: 4

Rationale: Treatment for clients with hyperparathyroidism includes a low-calcium diet. Ice cream and yogurt are high in calcium and should be restricted. The nurse should respond by rephrasing the client's statement. Options 1, 2, and 3 are examples of communication blocks (e.g., giving advice, requesting an explanation).

Test-Taking Strategy: Use therapeutic communication techniques to answer the question. Options 1, 2, and 3 are communication blocks. Option 4 seeks to validate what the nurse heard to determine whether additional instruction is needed. Review therapeutic communication techniques if you had difficulty with this question.

References

Christensen, B., & Kockrow, E. (2006). *Adult health nursing* (5th ed., p. 536). St. Louis: Mosby.
deWit, S. (2009). *Medical-surgical nursing: Concepts & practice* (pp. 900-901). St. Louis: Saunders.

1375. A client with angina pectoris appears to be very anxious and states, " So I had a heart attack, right?" The nurse should make which response to the client?

1 "Yes, that is why you are here."
2 "Yes, but there is minimal damage to your heart."
3 "No, and we will see to it that you do not have a heart attack."
4 "No, but the doctor wants to monitor you and control or eliminate your pain."

Level of Cognitive Ability: Application
Client Needs: Psychosocial Integrity
Integrated Process: Communication and Documentation
Content Area: Adult Health/Cardiovascular

Answer: 4

Rationale: Angina pectoris occurs as a result of an inadequate blood supply to the myocardium. Neither the nurse nor the physician can guarantee that a heart attack will not occur. A myocardial infarction is a heart attack. Option 3 provides false reassurance. Option 4 is the only option that is accurate and that describes the plan of care to the client.

Test-Taking Strategy: Use therapeutic communication techniques and your knowledge of the definition of angina pectoris to eliminate options 1 and 2. From the remaining options, eliminate option 3 because it provides false reassurance. Review therapeutic communication techniques and the pathophysiology associated with angina pectoris if you had difficulty with this question.

References

Christensen, B., & Kockrow, E. (2006). *Foundations of nursing* (5th ed., pp. 39-42). St. Louis: Mosby.
deWit, S. (2009). *Medical-surgical nursing: Concepts & practice* (p. 493). St. Louis: Saunders.

1376. A nurse is caring for a hospitalized client with depression who is silent and not communicating. The nurse develops a plan of care and incorporates strategies for communicating with the client. Which statement is appropriate for the nurse to make when caring for the client?

1 "Do you feel like talking today?"
2 "You are wearing your new shoes."
3 "Can you tell me how you slept last night?"
4 "Can you tell me how you are feeling today?"

Level of Cognitive Ability: Application
Client Needs: Psychosocial Integrity
Integrated Process: Communication and Documentation
Content Area: Mental Health

Answer: 2

Rationale: When a depressed client is mute or silent, the nurse should use the communication technique of making observations. A statement such as that given in option 2 is appropriate to make to the client. When the client is not ready to talk, direct questions (options 1, 3, and 4) can cause anxiety. Pointing to commonalties in the environment draws the client into and reinforces reality.

Test-Taking Strategy: Use therapeutic communication techniques, and note the client's diagnosis. Eliminate options 1, 3, and 4 because they are comparable or alike in that these options are direct questions that require a response from the client. Review communication techniques for the depressed client if you had difficulty with this question.

References

Christensen, B., & Kockrow, E. (2006). *Foundations of nursing* (5th ed., pp. 39-42). St. Louis: Mosby.
deWit, S. (2009). *Medical-surgical nursing: Concepts & practice* (pp. 10-11). St. Louis: Saunders.

1377. A nurse is caring for a client with delirium who states, "Look at the spiders on the wall." The nurse should make which response to the client?

1 "Would you like me to kill the spiders for you?"
2 "I know you are frightened, but I do not see spiders on the wall."
3 "I can see the spiders on the wall, but they are not going to hurt you."
4 "You're having an hallucination; there are no spiders in this room at all."

Level of Cognitive Ability: Application
Client Needs: Psychosocial Integrity
Integrated Process: Communication and Documentation
Content Area: Mental Health

Answer: 2

Rationale: When hallucinations are present, the nurse should reinforce reality with the client. In option 2, the nurse addresses the client's feelings and reinforces reality. Options 1 and 3 do not reinforce reality. Option 4 reinforces reality but does not address the client's feelings.

Test-Taking Strategy: Use therapeutic communication techniques. Eliminate options 1 and 3 because they reinforce the client's hallucination. Option 4 can be eliminated because, although it reinforces reality, it diminishes the importance of the client's feelings. Review therapeutic communication techniques for the client who is experiencing altered thought processes if you had difficulty with this question.

References

Christensen, B., & Kockrow, E. (2006). *Foundations of nursing* (5th ed., pp. 39-42). St. Louis: Mosby.
deWit, S. (2009). *Medical-surgical nursing: Concepts & practice* (pp. 1137-1138). St. Louis: Saunders.

1378. A nurse is planning a dietary regimen with an anemic client. The client states, "My iron pills will have to do. I can't afford to buy any of that fancy food." The nurse should make which response to the client?

1 "This is very important, so pay attention."
2 "Why don't you ask your family for help?"
3 "Ground beef is not very expensive right now."
4 "Would you like for me to check into some other options for you?"

Answer: 4

Rationale: Option 4 validates the concern that the client has with income. The nurse offers help in a nonthreatening manner that will allow the client to accept or decline. Options 1 and 3 block further communication by placing the client's issues on hold. Option 2 is requesting an explanation by using the word *why.*

Test-Taking Strategy: Use therapeutic communication techniques to answer the question. Note that option 4 is the only option that addresses the client's concern. Remember to always focus on the client's concerns. Review therapeutic communication techniques if you had difficulty with this question.

Level of Cognitive Ability: Application
Client Needs: Psychosocial Integrity
Integrated Process: Communication and Documentation
Content Area: Fundamental Skills

References

Christensen, B., & Kockrow, E. (2006). *Foundations of nursing* (5th ed., pp. 39-42). St. Louis: Mosby.

deWit, S. (2009). *Medical-surgical nursing: Concepts & practice* (pp. 379, 382). St. Louis: Saunders.

1379. A nurse is observing a nursing assistant talking to a client who is hearing impaired. The nurse should intervene if which of the following is done by the nursing assistant during communication with the client?

1 The nursing assistant is speaking clearly to the client.
2 The nursing assistant is facing the client when speaking.
3 The nursing assistant is speaking in a normal tone of voice.
4 The nursing assistant is speaking directly into the client's impaired ear.

Level of Cognitive Ability: Comprehension
Client Needs: Safe and Effective Care Environment
Integrated Process: Communication and Documentation
Content Area: Leadership/Management

Answer: 4

Rationale: When communicating with a hearing-impaired client, the nurse should speak in a normal tone to the client and should not shout. The nurse should talk directly to the client while facing the client and speak clearly. If the client does not seem to understand what is said, the nurse should express the statement differently. Moving closer to the client and toward the better ear may facilitate communication, but the nurse should avoid talking directly into the impaired ear.

Test-Taking Strategy: Use the process of elimination, and note the strategic words *the nurse should intervene.* These words indicate a negative event query and ask you to select an option that is an incorrect action by the nursing assistant. Knowledge of effective communication techniques for the hearing-impaired client will direct you to option 4. Review these therapeutic communication techniques if you had difficulty with this question.

Reference

Linton, A. (2007). *Introduction to medical-surgical nursing* (4th ed., p. 1198). Philadelphia: Saunders.

Teaching and Learning

1380. A nurse has given instructions about site care to a hemodialysis client who had an implantation of an arteriovenous (AV) fistula in the right arm. The nurse determines that the client requires further instruction if the client states to:

1 Sleep on the right side.
2 Avoid carrying heavy objects with the right arm.
3 Report an increased temperature, redness, or drainage at the site.
4 Perform range-of-motion exercises routinely with the right arm.

Level of Cognitive Ability: Comprehension
Client Needs: Physiological Integrity
Integrated Process: Teaching and Learning
Content Area: Adult Health/Renal

Answer: 1

Rationale: Routine instructions to the client with an AV fistula, graft, or shunt include reporting signs and symptoms of infection, performing routine range-of-motion exercises with the affected extremity, avoiding sleeping with the body weight on the extremity with the access site, and avoiding carrying heavy objects with or compressing the extremity that has the access site.

Test-Taking Strategy: Use the process of elimination, and note the strategic words *requires further instruction.* These words indicate a negative event query and ask you to select an option that is an incorrect statement. Recall the importance of maintaining the patency of the AV fistula to direct you to option 1. Review the home-care instructions for a client with an AV fistula if you had difficulty with this question.

References

deWit, S. (2009). *Medical-surgical nursing: Concepts & practice* (pp. 858-859). St. Louis: Saunders.

Linton, A. (2007). *Introduction to medical-surgical nursing* (4th ed., pp. 873-874). Philadelphia: Saunders.

1381. A client is being discharged home but requires ongoing chest pulmonary therapy (CPT). The nurse is asked to reinforce instructions about this procedure. The nurse incorporates which item when reinforcing the instructions to the family about how to correctly perform this procedure?

1 Perform the procedure within 1 hour after a meal.
2 Position the client so that the head and chest are elevated.
3 Continue the therapy up to the prescribed ideal time, if tolerated.
4 Expect that the respiratory status will worsen during the procedure.

Level of Cognitive Ability: Application
Client Needs: Physiological Integrity
Integrated Process: Teaching and Learning
Content Area: Adult Health/Respiratory

Answer: 3
Rationale: CPT should be avoided for 2 hours after meals and for 1 hour after a liquid meal to prevent vomiting. The head and chest are placed in the proper position prescribed for the client; this position incorporates having the head and chest lower than the rest of the body, if tolerated. The client's respiratory status should be monitored and the procedure modified if the respiratory status worsens. The therapy is performed to the ideal time, which is usually 15 minutes, as long as it is tolerated by the client.

Test-Taking Strategy: Use the process of elimination. Recall that CPT makes use of the principles of gravity to assist you with eliminating options 1 and 2. Option 4 does not offer protection for the client's airway and is therefore also eliminated. Review the procedure for CPT if you had difficulty with this question.

References
Linton, A. (2007). *Introduction to medical-surgical nursing* (4th ed., p. 523). Philadelphia: Saunders.
Potter, P., & Perry, A. (2009). *Fundamentals of nursing* (7th ed., pp. 930-931). St. Louis: Mosby.

1382. A nurse has provided instructions to a client about testicular self-examination (TSE). Which statement by the client indicates that the client requires further teaching about TSE?

1 "I will examine myself every 2 months."
2 "I know to report any small lumps."
3 "I should check one testicle at a time."
4 "I will examine myself after I take a warm shower."

Level of Cognitive Ability: Comprehension
Client Needs: Health Promotion and Maintenance
Integrated Process: Teaching and Learning
Content Area: Adult Health/Oncology

Answer: 1
Rationale: TSE should be performed every month, and small lumps or abnormalities should be reported. After a warm bath or shower, the scrotum is relaxed, which makes it easier to perform TSE. The client should check one testicle at a time.

Test-Taking Strategy: Use the process of elimination, and note the strategic words *requires further teaching*. These words indicate a negative event query and ask you to select an option that is an incorrect statement. Remember that breast self-examination needs to be performed monthly to assist you with recalling that TSE is also performed monthly. Review the procedure for TSE if you had difficulty with this question.

Reference
Christensen, B., & Kockrow, E. (2006). *Adult health nursing* (5th ed., p. 619). St. Louis: Mosby.

1383. A client has been prescribed a clonidine patch (Catapres TTS), and the nurse has reinforced instructions with the client regarding the use of the patch. The nurse determines that further instruction is needed if the nurse notes that the client:

1 Verbalized the need to change the patch every 7 days
2 Trimmed the patch because one edge was loose
3 Selected a hairless site on the torso for application

Answer: 2
Rationale: The clonidine patch (Catapres TTS) is an antihypertensive medication. It should be applied to a hairless site on the torso or the upper arm. It is changed every 7 days and left in place when bathing or showering. The patch should not be trimmed because the medication dose will be altered. If the patch becomes slightly loose, it should be covered with an adhesive overlay from the medication package. If it becomes very loose or falls off, it should be replaced. To discard the patch, fold it in half with the adhesive sides together.

4 Verbalized the need to leave the patch in place during bathing or showering

Level of Cognitive Ability: Analysis
Client Needs: Physiological Integrity
Integrated Process: Teaching and Learning
Content Area: Pharmacology

Test-Taking Strategy: Use the process of elimination, and note the strategic words *further instruction is needed.* These words indicate a negative event query and ask you to select an option that is an incorrect statement. The words *trimmed the patch* will direct you to option 2 because this client action would alter the medication dose. Review the clonidine patch if you had difficulty with this question.

Reference

Hodgson, B., & Kizior, R. (2009). *Saunders nursing drug handbook 2009* (p. 268). Philadelphia: Saunders.

1384. A client is being discharged home from the hospital and will be taking cholestyramine (Questran). The nurse determines that further teaching is needed if the client makes which of the following statements?

1 "I should take this medication with meals."
2 "I should mix the Questran with juice or applesauce."
3 "I should call my doctor immediately if I develop diarrhea."
4 "I should increase my fluid intake while taking this medication."

Level of Cognitive Ability: Analysis
Client Needs: Physiological Integrity
Integrated Process: Teaching and Learning
Content Area: Pharmacology

Answer: 3

Rationale: Cholestyramine (Questran) is a cholesterol-lowering (antihyperlipidemic) medication. This medication should not be taken dry; it can be mixed with water, juice, a carbonated beverage, applesauce, or soup. Common side effects include constipation, nausea, indigestion, and flatulence. Increasing fluids will minimize the constipating effects of the medication. Questran must be administered with food to be effective. Diarrhea is not a concern, but severe constipation is.

Test-Taking Strategy: Use the process of elimination, and note the strategic words *further teaching is needed.* These words indicate a negative event query and ask you to select an option that is an incorrect statement. Select option 3 because there are normally measures that can be taken for diarrhea rather than immediately calling the physician. Review cholestyramine if you had difficulty with this question.

Reference

Hodgson, B., & Kizior, R. (2009). *Saunders nursing drug handbook 2009* (p. 238). St. Louis: Saunders.

1385. A nurse is preparing written medication instructions for a client taking colestipol hydrochloride (Colestid). The nurse plans to include instructions about the need for the client to take which of the following to counteract unintended medication effects?

1 Vitamin C
2 Vitamin B
3 B-complex vitamins
4 Fat-soluble vitamins

Level of Cognitive Ability: Application
Client Needs: Physiological Integrity
Integrated Process: Teaching and Learning
Content Area: Pharmacology

Answer: 4

Rationale: Colestipol, which is a bile-sequestering agent, is used to lower blood cholesterol levels. However, the bile salts, which are rich in cholesterol, interfere with the absorption of the fat-soluble vitamins A, D, E, and K, as well as folic acid. With ongoing therapy, the client is at risk for a deficiency of these vitamins and is counseled to take them as supplements.

Test-Taking Strategy: Use the process of elimination. Eliminate options 2 and 3 first because they are comparable or alike. Recall that bile-sequestering agents interfere with the absorption of fat-soluble vitamins and note that option 4 is the umbrella option to assist you with answering the question. Review client teaching points about colestipol hydrochloride if you had difficulty with this question.

Reference

Lehne, R. (2010). *Pharmacology for nursing care* (7th ed., p. 578). St. Louis: Saunders.

1386. A client with tuberculosis (TB) is preparing for discharge from the hospital. Which client statement indicates that further teaching is necessary?

1. "I will not need respiratory isolation when I am home."
2. "I need to place used tissues in a plastic bag when I am home."
3. "I need to eat foods that are high in iron, protein, and vitamin C."
4. "If I miss a dose of medication because of nausea, I just skip that dose and resume my regular schedule."

Level of Cognitive Ability: Analysis
Client Needs: Physiological Integrity
Integrated Process: Teaching and Learning
Content Area: Pharmacology

Answer: 4
Rationale: TB is a chronic granulomatous infection caused by *Mycobacterium tuberculosis.* Because of the resistant strains of TB, the nurse must emphasize that noncompliance with medication requirements could lead to an infection that is difficult to treat and that may cause total drug resistance. Clients may prevent nausea related to the medications by taking the daily dose at bedtime; antinausea medications may also prevent this symptom. Medication doses should not be skipped. Options 1, 2, and 3 are correct statements.

Test-Taking Strategy: Use the process of elimination, and note the strategic words *further teaching is necessary*. These words indicate a negative event query and ask you to select an option that is an incorrect statement. General principles related to medication administration will direct you to option 4. Review medication therapy and its importance in clients with TB if you had difficulty with this question.

Reference
Linton, A. (2007). *Introduction to medical-surgical nursing* (4th ed., p. 563). Philadelphia: Saunders.

1387. A nurse is planning to teach a client who has recently been diagnosed with tuberculosis (TB) about how to prevent the spread of the infection. Which instruction would be least effective to prevent the spread of TB?

1. Teach the client to sterilize dishes at home.
2. Teach the client to properly dispose of Kleenex.
3. Teach the client to cover the mouth when coughing.
4. Teach the client that close contacts should be tested for TB.

Level of Cognitive Ability: Application
Client Needs: Safe and Effective Care Environment
Integrated Process: Teaching and Learning
Content Area: Adult Health/Respiratory

Answer: 1
Rationale: TB is a chronic granulomatous infection caused by *Mycobacterium tuberculosis.* Options 2, 3, and 4 would assist with breaking the chain of infection. Option 1 would not only be impractical, but there is no evidence to suggest that sterilizing dishes would break the chain of infection for a client with TB.

Test-Taking Strategy: Focus on the subject—preventing the spread of TB. Use the process of elimination, and note the strategic words *least effective.* Recall the methods of transmission of TB to direct you to option 1. Review the home-care principles related to TB if you had difficulty with this question.

References
Christensen, B., & Kockrow, E. (2006). *Adult health nursing* (5th ed., p. 429). St. Louis: Mosby.
Linton, A. (2007). *Introduction to medical-surgical nursing* (4th ed., p. 564). Philadelphia: Saunders.

1388. A client is being discharged home after abdominal surgery with a heparin lock (intermittent intravenous catheter) to receive a week of antibiotic intravenous (IV) therapy at home, and the nurse reinforces home-care instructions to the client. Which statement by the client indicates the need for further instruction?

1. "I'll examine the IV site frequently."
2. "If the IV site becomes wet or moist, it can air dry."

Answer: 2
Rationale: Clients who will be at home with an IV site should be instructed about site assessment and about the complications to report to the physician. Clients should also know how to treat complications such as bleeding at the IV site. Clients should be aware that if the dressing is wet or soiled, it needs to be changed immediately to prevent infection.

3 "Pain, redness, and swelling should be reported to the physician."
4 "If the lock or catheter accidentally comes out, I'll apply pressure to the site."

Level of Cognitive Ability: Comprehension
Client Needs: Safe and Effective Care Environment
Integrated Process: Teaching and Learning
Content Area: Fundamental Skills

Test-Taking Strategy: Use the process of elimination, and note the strategic words *need for further instruction*. These words indicate a negative event query and ask you to select an option that is an incorrect statement. Use principles related to asepsis to direct you to option 2. Review these principles if you had difficulty with this question.

References

Christensen, B., & Kockrow, E. (2006). *Foundations of nursing* (5th ed., p. 547). St. Louis: Mosby.
deWit, S. (2009). *Medical-surgical nursing: Concepts & practice* (p. 64). St. Louis: Saunders.

1389. A nurse reinforces instructions to a client who has jaundice and is experiencing pruritus. The nurse avoids telling the client about which incorrect measure to alleviate the discomfort?
1 Wear loose cotton clothing.
2 Use tepid water for bathing.
3 Maintain a warm house temperature.
4 Take the prescribed antihistamines to relieve the itch.

Level of Cognitive Ability: Application
Client Needs: Health Promotion and Maintenance
Integrated Process: Teaching and Learning
Content Area: Adult Health/Gastrointestinal

Answer: 3
Rationale: Pruritus is caused by the accumulation of bile salts in the skin and results from obstructed biliary excretion. The client is instructed to keep the house temperature cool. The client should avoid the use of alkaline soap and wear loose, soft, cotton clothing. Antihistamines, tepid water, and emollient baths may relieve the itching.

Test-Taking Strategy: Use the process of elimination, and note the strategic word *avoids.* This word indicates a negative event query and asks you to select an option that is an incorrect measure. Recall that heat causes vasodilation to direct you to option 3. Review the measures that assist with the alleviation of pruritus if you had difficulty with this question.

References

Christensen, B., & Kockrow, E. (2006). *Adult health nursing* (5th ed., p. 87). St. Louis: Mosby.
Linton, A. (2007). *Introduction to medical-surgical nursing* (4th ed., p. 1132). Philadelphia: Saunders.

1390. A nurse has reinforced instructions to the parents of a child with glomerulonephritis. Which statement by a parent indicates the need for further instruction?
1 "I should monitor the weight of my child."
2 "I should limit play activities to short periods."
3 "I should keep my child on a low-sodium diet."
4 "I should encourage an increased intake of fluids."

Level of Cognitive Ability: Comprehension
Client Needs: Physiological Integrity
Integrated Process: Teaching and Learning
Content Area: Child Health

Answer: 4
Rationale: Glomerulonephritis is an inflammation of the glomerulus of the kidney that is characterized by proteinuria, hematuria, decreased urine production, and edema. In the child with glomerulonephritis, fluid intake should be limited as prescribed. Children with fluid excess may develop pulmonary edema. A low-sodium diet is followed as prescribed because excessive sodium will increase fluid retention. The weight should be monitored to determine fluctuations in fluid status. The child may tire easily, so playtime should be limited to short periods and extended as the condition improves.

Test-Taking Strategy: Use the process of elimination, and note the strategic words *need for further instruction*. These words indicate a negative event query and ask you to select an option that is an incorrect statement. Recall that this disorder relates to an alteration in renal function to direct you to option 4. Review the interventions for glomerulonephritis if you had difficulty with this question.

Reference

Christensen, B., & Kockrow, E. (2006). *Foundations of nursing* (5th ed., p. 1034). St. Louis: Mosby.

1391. A nurse is reinforcing medication instructions to a client receiving furosemide (Lasix). The nurse determines that further teaching is necessary if the client makes which statement?

1 "I should change positions slowly."
2 "I should avoid the use of salt substitutes."
3 "I should talk to my physician about the use of alcohol."
4 "I should be careful not to get overheated in warm weather."

Level of Cognitive Ability: Analysis
Client Needs: Physiological Integrity
Integrated Process: Teaching and Learning
Content Area: Pharmacology

Answer: 2

Rationale: Furosemide is a potassium-losing diuretic, so there is no need to avoid high-potassium products (e.g., salt substitute). Orthostatic hypotension is a risk, and the client must use caution when changing positions and with exposure to warm weather. The client should discuss the use of alcohol with the physician.

Test-Taking Strategy: Use the process of elimination, and note the strategic words *further teaching is necessary.* These words indicate a negative event query and ask you to select an option that is an incorrect statement. Recall that furosemide is a potassium-losing diuretic and that diuretic therapy can induce hypokalemia to direct you to option 2. Review furosemide if you had difficulty with this question.

Reference

Christensen, B., & Kockrow, E. (2006). *Foundations of nursing* (5th ed., p. 672). St. Louis: Mosby.

1392. A client asks the nurse for a recommendation about how to prevent fires and burn injuries. The nurse tells the client that an important intervention to decrease the risk of dying in a residential fire is:

1 The use of operable smoke detectors
2 The installation of a sprinkler system
3 The installation of fire-resistant drywall panels throughout the house
4 Fire extinguishers placed in key areas such as the kitchen, near the furnace, and near the hot water heater

Level of Cognitive Ability: Application
Client Needs: Safe and Effective Care Environment
Integrated Process: Teaching and Learning
Content Area: Fundamental Skills

Answer: 1

Rationale: The early detection of smoke and the subsequent immediate evacuation from the house will significantly impact mortality. The installation of a sprinkler system is expensive and not usually required in residential situations. Although fire-resistant products may help to slow down a blaze, fire-resistant products can eventually catch on fire. Fire extinguishers are important to have in the kitchen for small fires, but they are unrealistic and dangerous to use to attempt to extinguish large fires.

Test-Taking Strategy: Use the process of elimination, and focus on the subject—decreasing the risk of dying in a residential fire. Look for the health prevention measure that is simple to implement and that will alert individuals of the need to evacuate a residence; this will direct you to option 1. Review fire safety if you had difficulty with this question.

Reference

Christensen, B., & Kockrow, E. (2006). *Foundations of nursing* (5th ed., pp. 363, 365). St. Louis: Mosby.

1393. A client has had same-day surgery to insert a ventilating tube in the tympanic membrane. The nurse teaches the client to implement which postoperative measure?

1 Use a shower cap when taking a shower.
2 Swim only with the head above water.
3 Avoid taking any medication for pain.
4 Wash the hair quickly (in 2 minutes or less).

Level of Cognitive Ability: Comprehension
Client Needs: Health Promotion and Maintenance

Answer: 1

Rationale: After the insertion of tubes in the tympanic membrane, it is important to avoid getting water in the ears. For this reason, swimming, showering, and washing the hair are avoided after surgery until the time frame designated for each is identified by the surgeon. A shower cap or earplug may be used when showering, if allowed by the physician. The client should take medication as advised for postoperative discomfort.

Test-Taking Strategy: Use the process of elimination. Eliminate option 2 because of the close-ended word *only* and option 4 because of the word *quickly.* From the remaining options, focus on the anatomical location of the surgery to direct you to option 1. Review client instructions after this type of surgery if you had difficulty with this question.

Integrated Process: Teaching and Learning
Content Area: Adult Health/Ear

Reference
Christensen, B., & Kockrow, E. (2006). *Adult health nursing* (5th ed., p. 679). St. Louis: Mosby.

1394. A nurse is asked to teach a hypertensive client about strategies to prevent episodes of lightheadedness after taking antihypertensive medication. The nurse includes which of the following points in the discussion?

1 Take warm baths to enhance medication effects.
2 Avoid alcohol intake after taking the medication.
3 Move quickly when rising from a sitting to a standing position.
4 Stand motionless during the first hour after the dose is given.

Level of Cognitive Ability: Application
Client Needs: Physiological Integrity
Integrated Process: Teaching and Learning
Content Area: Adult Health/Cardiovascular

Answer: 2
Rationale: The client taking antihypertensive medications should be told to avoid situations that promote lightheadedness and dizziness. These include taking warm baths, drinking alcohol, and standing motionless for long periods of time. The client should rise slowly from a sitting to a standing position, and he or she should wiggle the toes or do leg-muscle setting exercises when standing to avoid lightheadedness.

Test-Taking Strategy: Use the process of elimination, and focus on the subject—preventing lightheadedness. Recall that lightheadedness results from a drop in blood pressure, and select the option that does not aggravate or trigger vasodilatation. Remember that it is best for clients to avoid alcohol when they are taking medications. Review the measures related to preventing the complications associated with antihypertensive medication if you had difficulty with this question.

Reference
deWit, S. (2009). *Medical-surgical nursing: Concepts & practice* (p. 439). St. Louis: Saunders.

1395. A client with acquired immunodeficiency syndrome (AIDS) has a nursing diagnosis of *Fatigue.* The nurse plans to teach the client which of the following strategies to conserve energy after discharge from the hospital?

1 Bathe before eating breakfast.
2 Sit for as many activities as possible.
3 Stand in the shower instead of taking a bath.
4 Group all tasks to be performed early in the morning.

Level of Cognitive Ability: Application
Client Needs: Health Promotion and Maintenance
Integrated Process: Teaching and Learning
Content Area: Adult Health/Immune

Answer: 2
Rationale: AIDS involves a defect in cell-mediated immunity. The client is taught to conserve energy by sitting for as many activities as possible, including dressing, shaving, preparing food, and ironing. The client should also sit in a shower chair instead of standing while bathing. The client should prioritize activities such as eating breakfast before bathing and should alternate major activities with periods of rest.

Test-Taking Strategy: Focus on the subject—conserving energy. Think about the amount of exertion required by the client to perform each of the activities described in the options. Options 3 and 4 are obviously taxing for the client and are thus eliminated first. From the remaining options, recall that bathing may take away energy that could be used for eating; this will direct you to option 2. Review measures that conserve energy if you had difficulty with this question.

Reference
deWit, S. (2009). *Medical-surgical nursing: Concepts & practice* (p. 253). St. Louis: Saunders.

1396. A nurse has reinforced self-care activity instructions to a client after the insertion of an automatic internal cardioverter-defibrillator (AICD). The nurse determines that further instruction is needed

Answer: 2
Rationale: An AICD is implanted in the chest or abdominal area to provide a shock if the client experiences a dysrhythmia (e.g., ventricular fibrillation). Discharge instructions typically include avoiding the following: tight clothing or belts over the

if the client makes which of the following statements?

1 "I need to avoid doing anything where there would be rough contact with the AICD insertion site."
2 "I can perform activities such as swimming, driving, or operating heavy equipment as I need to."
3 "I should try to avoid doing strenuous things that would make my heart rate go up to or above the rate cutoff of the AICD."
4 "I should keep away from electromagnetic sources such as transformers, large electrical generators, and metal detectors, and I should not lean over running motors."

Level of Cognitive Ability: Comprehension
Client Needs: Physiological Integrity
Integrated Process: Teaching and Learning
Content Area: Adult Health/Cardiovascular

AICD insertion sites; rough contact with the AICD insertion site; electromagnetic fields from sources such as electrical transformers and radio, television, or radar transmitters and metal detectors; and close proximity to the running motors of cars or boats. Clients must also alert physicians or dentists to the presence of the device because certain procedures (e.g., diathermy, electrocautery, magnetic resonance imaging) may need to be avoided to prevent device malfunction. Clients should follow the specific advice of a physician regarding activities that are potentially hazardous to the self or others (e.g., swimming, driving, operating heavy equipment).

Test-Taking Strategy: Use the process of elimination, and note the strategic words *further instruction is needed.* These words indicate a negative event query and ask you to select an option that is an incorrect statement. Options 1 and 4 can be eliminated first because they are comparable or alike and are standard instructions after pacemaker insertion. From the remaining options, note the words *heavy equipment* to direct you to option 2. Review client teaching points for AICD if you had difficulty with this question.

References

Ignatavicius, D., & Workman, M. (2010). *Medical-surgical nursing: Patient-centered collaborative care* (6th ed., p. 761). St. Louis: Saunders.

Monahan, F., Sands, J., Marek, J., Neighbors, M., & Green, C. (2007). *Phipps' medical-surgical nursing: Health and illness perspectives* (8th ed., p. 799). St. Louis: Mosby.

1397. A nurse has provided instructions to a client who is receiving external radiation therapy. Which of the following, if stated by the client, would indicate the need for further instruction about self-care related to the radiation therapy?

1 "I should eat a high-protein diet."
2 "I should avoid exposure to sunlight."
3 "I should wash my skin with a mild soap and pat it dry."
4 "I should place pressure on the radiated area to prevent bleeding."

Level of Cognitive Ability: Comprehension
Client Needs: Physiological Integrity
Integrated Process: Teaching and Learning
Content Area: Adult Health/Oncology

Answer: 4

Rationale: The client should avoid pressure on the radiated area and wear loose-fitting clothing. Options 1, 2, and 3 are accurate statements about radiation therapy.

Test-Taking Strategy: Use the process of elimination, and note the strategic words *need for further instruction*. These words indicate a negative event query and ask you to select an option that is an incorrect statement. The word *pressure* in option 4 is an indication that this is an inappropriate measure. Review client teaching points related to skin care and radiation therapy if you had difficulty with this question.

References

Ignatavicius, D., & Workman, M. (2010). *Medical-surgical nursing: Patient-centered collaborative care* (6th ed., p. 420). St. Louis: Saunders.

Monahan, F., Sands, J., Marek, J., Neighbors, M., & Green, C. (2007). *Phipps' medical-surgical nursing: Health and illness perspectives* (8th ed., p. 541). St. Louis: Mosby.

1398. A nurse reinforces home-care instructions to a client who has been hospitalized for a transurethral resection of the prostate (TURP). Which statement by the client indicates the need for further instruction?

Answer: 3

Rationale: After TURP, the client should be advised to avoid strenuous activity for 4 to 6 weeks and to avoid lifting items that weigh more than 20 pounds. Straining during defecation is avoided to prevent bleeding. Prune juice is a satisfactory bowel stimulant to prevent the complication of constipation and straining. The client

1 "I should include prune juice in my diet."
2 "I should avoid strenuous activity for 4 to 6 weeks."
3 "I can lift and push objects up to 30 or 40 pounds in weight."
4 "I should maintain a daily intake of 6 to 8 glasses of water daily."

Level of Cognitive Ability: Comprehension
Client Needs: Physiological Integrity
Integrated Process: Teaching and Learning
Content Area: Adult Health/Renal

should consume a daily intake of at least 6 to 8 glasses of nonalcoholic fluids to minimize clot formation.

Test-Taking Strategy: Use the process of elimination, and note the strategic words *need for further instruction*. These words indicate a negative event query and ask you to select an option that is an incorrect statement. Options 2 and 4 can be eliminated first. Because of the anatomical location of the surgical procedure, it would be reasonable to think that constipation should be avoided, so option 1 can be eliminated as well. Items that weigh 30 or 40 pounds are excessive for these clients to lift or push at this time. Review TURP discharge teaching points if you had difficulty with this question.

Reference
deWit, S. (2009). *Medical-surgical nursing: Concepts & practice* (p. 984). St. Louis: Saunders.

1399. A nurse is reinforcing home-care instructions to a client who will be receiving intravenous (IV) therapy at home. The nurse teaches the client that the most important action to prevent an infection from the IV site is to:
1 Change the IV tubing and fluid containers daily.
2 Redress the IV site daily and cleanse it with alcohol.
3 Check the IV site carefully every day for redness and edema.
4 Carefully wash the hands with antibacterial soap before working with the IV site or equipment.

Level of Cognitive Ability: Application
Client Needs: Safe and Effective Care Environment
Integrated Process: Teaching and Learning
Content Area: Fundamental Skills

Answer: 4
Rationale: It is extremely important for the client to understand the absolute necessity of handwashing before working with IV fluids. IV containers should be changed daily, but the tubing should only be changed every 48 to 72 hours or per agency policy. Although the assessment of the IV site is important, it will not actively prevent an infection. IV sites do not need to be redressed daily unless the dressing becomes soiled, wet, or loose.

Test-Taking Strategy: Use the process of elimination. Note the strategic words *most important*, and focus on the subject—preventing infection. Remember that the priority for infection prevention always includes proper handwashing technique. Review standard precautions and their role in preventing infection if you had difficulty with this question.

Reference
deWit, S. (2009). *Medical-surgical nursing: Concepts & practice* (pp. 64, 120, 1189). St. Louis: Saunders.

1400. A client asks a nurse about the electrocardiographic (ECG) rhythm displayed on the monitor. When planning to discuss basic information about the ECG rhythm, which of the following should the nurse ask the client first?
1 "Are you concerned about the ECG rhythm?"
2 "What do you understand about the ECG rhythm?"
3 "Do you think that there is a problem with your heart?"
4 "Do you know how to interpret an ECG rhythm strip?"

Answer: 2
Rationale: Client-initiated teaching sessions begin with what the client already knows. Options 1 and 3 focus on a problem with the client's heart. Option 4 is not an appropriate question and may devalue the client because it is unlikely that the client will be able to interpret the rhythm strip.

Test-Taking Strategy: Use the process of elimination, and note the strategic word *first*. Eliminate options 1 and 3 because they are comparable or alike. Recall that teaching sessions begin with what the client already knows to direct you to option 2. Review teaching and learning principles if you had difficulty with this question.

Level of Cognitive Ability: Application
Client Needs: Health Promotion and Maintenance
Integrated Process: Teaching and Learning
Content Area: Fundamental Skills

References
deWit, S. (2009). *Medical-surgical nursing: Concepts & practice* (pp. 2-3). St. Louis: Saunders.
Linton, A. (2007). *Introduction to medical-surgical nursing* (4th ed., pp. 673-674). Philadelphia: Saunders.

1401. A nurse reinforces home-care instructions to the parents of a child with generalized tonic-clonic seizures who is being treated with oral phenytoin (Dilantin). The nurse includes instructions about:

1 Monitoring the child's intake and output daily
2 Providing oral hygiene, especially care of the gums
3 Administering the medication 1 hour before food intake
4 Checking the child's blood pressure before the administration of the medication

Level of Cognitive Ability: Application
Client Needs: Physiological Integrity
Integrated Process: Teaching and Learning
Content Area: Pharmacology

Answer: 2
Rationale: Phenytoin (Dilantin) is an anticonvulsant medication. It causes bleeding gums and hyperplasia, so the use of a soft toothbrush and gum massage should be instituted to diminish these complications and prevent trauma. Options 1 and 4 are incorrect because the intake, output, and blood pressure are not affected by this medication. Option 3 is incorrect because the instructions for the administration of this medication include taking it with food to minimize gastrointestinal upset.

Test-Taking Strategy: Use the process of elimination, and focus on the medication. Remember that phenytoin causes gum bleeding and hyperplasia. In addition, note the word *oral* in both the question and the correct option. Review the side effects and the method of administration of phenytoin if you had difficulty with this question.

Reference
Linton, A. (2007). *Introduction to medical-surgical nursing* (4th ed., p. 431). Philadelphia: Saunders.

1402. A nurse notes that a pregnant client is at risk for toxoplasmosis. The nurse should teach the client which of the following to prevent exposure to this disease?

1 Eat raw meats.
2 Wash the hands only before meals.
3 Avoid exposure to litter boxes used by cats.
4 Use topical corticosteroid treatments prophylactically.

Level of Cognitive Ability: Application
Client Needs: Safe and Effective Care Environment
Integrated Process: Teaching and Learning
Content Area: Maternity/Antepartum

Answer: 3
Rationale: Toxoplasmosis is an infection caused by the protozoan parasite *Toxoplasma gondii*. Infected cats transmit toxoplasmosis through the feces, so handling a litter box can transmit the disease to the pregnant client. Meats that are undercooked can harbor microorganisms that can cause infection. The hands should be washed frequently throughout the day. The use of topical corticosteroids will not prevent exposure to the disease.

Test-Taking Strategy: Use the process of elimination. Eliminate option 2 because of the close-ended word *only*. Option 1 represents an extreme statement and thus can also be eliminated. Focus on the strategic words *prevent exposure* to direct you to option 3. Review the causes of toxoplasmosis if you had difficulty with this question.

Reference
Christensen, B., & Kockrow, E. (2006). *Foundations of nursing* (5th ed., p. 914). St. Louis: Mosby.

1403. A nurse plans to instruct a client with candidiasis (thrush) of the oral cavity about care for the disorder. The nurse teaches the client that which action will worsen the disorder?

Answer: 4
Rationale: Candidiasis (thrush) is characterized by the appearance of creamy white patches of exudate on an inflamed tongue or on the buccal mucosa. Clients with thrush cannot tolerate commercial mouthwashes because the high alcohol concentration of these products can cause pain and discomfort of the lesions. A solution

1 Eating foods that are liquid or pureed
2 Eliminating spicy foods from the diet
3 Eliminating citrus juices and hot liquids from the diet
4 Rinsing the mouth four times daily with a commercial mouthwash

Level of Cognitive Ability: Application
Client Needs: Physiological Integrity
Integrated Process: Teaching and Learning
Content Area: Adult Health/Immune

of warm water or a mouthwash formula without alcohol is better tolerated and may promote healing. A change in diet to liquid or pureed food often eases the discomfort of eating. The client should avoid spicy foods, citrus juice, and hot liquids.

Test-Taking Strategy: Use the process of elimination, and note the strategic words *worsen the disorder*. These words indicate a negative event query and ask you to select an option that is an incorrect action. Note the words *commercial mouthwash* in option 4 to direct you to this option. Review the client teaching points related to candidiasis (thrush) if you had difficulty with this question.

Reference

Ignatavicius, D., & Workman, M. (2010). *Medical-surgical nursing: Patient-centered collaborative care* (6th ed., p. 428). St. Louis: Saunders.

1404. A nurse in the ambulatory care unit is reviewing the surgical instructions with a client who will be admitted for knee-replacement surgery. The nurse informs the client that crutches will be needed for ambulation after surgery and that the client will be instructed in the use of the crutches:
1 Before surgery
2 On the first postoperative day
3 On the second postoperative day
4 At the time of discharge after surgery

Level of Cognitive Ability: Application
Client Needs: Physiological Integrity
Integrated Process: Teaching and Learning
Content Area: Adult Health/Musculoskeletal

Answer: 1
Rationale: It is best to determine crutch-walking ability and to instruct the client regarding the use of crutches before surgery because this task can be difficult to learn when the client is in pain postoperatively. Options 2, 3, and 4 are incorrect.

Test-Taking Strategy: Use the process of elimination. Note that options 2, 3, and 4 are comparable or alike in that they all address the postoperative period. Review preoperative teaching principles if you had difficulty with this question.

Reference

deWit, S. (2009). *Medical-surgical nursing: Concepts & practice* (pp. 779-780). St. Louis: Saunders.

1405. A nurse is instructing a client with chronic vertigo about safety measures to prevent the exacerbation of symptoms or injury. The nurse teaches the client that it is important to:
1 Turn the head slowly when spoken to.
2 Remove throw rugs and clutter in the home.
3 Drive at times when the client does not feel dizzy.
4 Go to the bedroom and lie down when vertigo is experienced.

Level of Cognitive Ability: Application
Client Needs: Safe and Effective Care Environment
Integrated Process: Teaching and Learning
Content Area: Adult Health/Ear

Answer: 2
Rationale: Vertigo is a sensation of instability or loss of equilibrium that places the client at risk for injury. The client with chronic vertigo should avoid driving and using public transportation because the sudden movements involved in both methods of transportation could precipitate an attack. To further prevent vertigo attacks, the client should change positions slowly, and he or she should turn the entire body (not just the head) when spoken to. If vertigo does occur, the client should immediately sit down or grasp the nearest piece of furniture. The client should remove clutter and throw rugs from the home because trying to regain balance after slipping could trigger the onset of vertigo.

Test-Taking Strategy: Use the process of elimination, and focus on the subject—safety. Eliminate options 3 and 4 first because they put the client at greatest risk of injury secondary to vertigo. Choose option 2 instead of option 1 because it is the safer intervention of the remaining options. Review safety measures for the client with vertigo if you had difficulty with this question.

Reference

Monahan, F., Sands, J., Marek, J., Neighbors, M., & Green, C. (2007). *Phipps' medical-surgical nursing: Health and illness perspectives* (8th ed., p. 1856). St. Louis: Mosby.

1406. A nurse is instructing the mother of a child with cystic fibrosis about appropriate dietary measures. The nurse tells the mother that the child should consume a:

1 Low-calorie, low-fat diet
2 Low-calorie, restricted fat diet
3 Low-calorie, low-protein diet
4 High-calorie, high-protein diet

Level of Cognitive Ability: Application
Client Needs: Physiological Integrity
Integrated Process: Teaching and Learning
Content Area: Child Health

Answer: 4

Rationale: Cystic fibrosis is a disorder of the exocrine glands that causes those glands to produce abnormally thick secretions of mucus, an elevation of sweat electrolytes, increased organic and enzymatic constituents of saliva, and the overactivity of the autonomic nervous system. Children with cystic fibrosis are managed with a high-calorie, high-protein diet. Pancreatic enzyme replacement therapy and fat-soluble vitamin supplements are administered. Fat restriction is not necessary.

Test-Taking Strategy: Use the process of elimination. Eliminate options 1 and 2 first because they are comparable or alike. Remember the pathophysiology related to cystic fibrosis to direct you to option 4. Review the diet plan for the child with cystic fibrosis if you had difficulty with this question.

Reference

deWit, S. (2009). *Medical-surgical nursing: Concepts & practice* (p. 329). St. Louis: Saunders.

1407. A client is going to have a plaster cast applied, and the nurse explains the procedure to the client. The nurse determines that the client requires further teaching about the procedure if the client states that:

1 The cast will give off heat as it dries.
2 The cast edges may be trimmed with a cast knife.
3 The client may bear weight on the cast after half an hour.
4 A stockinette will be placed over the leg area to be casted.

Level of Cognitive Ability: Comprehension
Client Needs: Physiological Integrity
Integrated Process: Teaching and Learning
Content Area: Adult Health/Musculoskeletal

Answer: 3

Rationale: The procedure for casting involves washing and drying the skin and placing a stockinette material over the area to be casted. A roll of padding is then applied smoothly and evenly. The plaster is rolled onto the padding, and the edges are trimmed or smoothed as needed with a cast knife. A plaster cast gives off heat as it dries. A plaster cast can tolerate weight bearing after it is dry, which may take from 24 to 72 hours, depending on the thickness of the cast.

Test-Taking Strategy: Use the process of elimination, and note the strategic words *requires further teaching*. These words indicate a negative event query and ask you to select an option that is an incorrect statement. Note the word *plaster* in the question, and recall that a plaster cast takes 24 to 72 hours to dry to direct you to option 3. Review the care of the client with a plaster cast if you had difficulty with this question.

Reference

Christensen, B., & Kockrow, E. (2006). *Adult health nursing* (5th ed., p. 172). St. Louis: Mosby.

1408. A nurse has completed diet teaching for a client on a low-sodium diet for the treatment of hypertension. The nurse determines that further teaching is necessary if the client makes which of the following statements?

Answer: 1

Rationale: A low-sodium diet is used as an adjunct to antihypertensive medications for the treatment of hypertension. Sodium retains fluid, which leads to hypertension secondary to increased fluid volume. Frozen foods use salt as a preservative and should not be encouraged as part of a low-sodium diet.

1 "Frozen foods are lowest in sodium."
2 "This diet will help to lower my blood pressure."
3 "This diet is not a replacement for my antihypertensive medications."
4 "The reason I need to lower my salt intake is to reduce fluid retention."

Level of Cognitive Ability: Comprehension
Client Needs: Physiological Integrity
Integrated Process: Teaching and Learning
Content Area: Adult Health/Cardiovascular

Test-Taking Strategy: Note the strategic words *further teaching is necessary*. These words indicate a negative event query and ask you to select an option that is an incorrect statement. Use the process of elimination, and eliminate options 2, 3, and 4 because these are accurate statements related to hypertension. Remember that frozen foods use salt as a preservative. Review the treatment of hypertension and foods that are high in sodium if you had difficulty with this question.

Reference

deWit, S. (2009). *Medical-surgical nursing: Concepts & practice* (p. 48). St. Louis: Saunders.

1409. A client with Parkinson's disease dislikes having muscle tremors and asks the nurse what can be done to make them less noticeable. The nurse should offer which suggestion to the client?

1 "Focus on relaxing your arms as much as possible."
2 "Let your hands rest on your lap or a low table while you are sitting."
3 "Try holding onto the arm of a chair or grasping coins that are in your pocket."
4 "After your medication begins working, the tremors will stop completely on their own."

Level of Cognitive Ability: Application
Client Needs: Physiological Integrity
Integrated Process: Teaching and Learning
Content Area: Adult Health/Neurological

Answer: 3

Rationale: Clients with Parkinson's disease typically have resting tremors that diminish with voluntary activity, thus making option 3 the correct choice. Tremors are worse at rest, so options 1 and 2 incorrect. Medication therapy reduces the severity of tremors but does not stop them completely.

Test-Taking Strategy: Use the process of elimination. Eliminate options 1 and 2 first because they are comparable or alike. Eliminate option 4 next because it contains the close-ended word *completely*. Recall that tremors diminish with voluntary activity to direct you to option 3. Review the care of the client with Parkinson's disease if you had difficulty with this question.

Reference

Swearingen, P. (2008). *All-in-one planning resource: Medical, surgical, pediatric, maternity, & pyschiatric nursing care plan* (2nd ed., p. 316). St. Louis: Mosby.

ALTERNATE ITEM FORMAT QUESTIONS

Fill-in-the-Blank

1410. The physician's order reads as follows: tobramycin sulfate (Nebcin), 7.5 mg intramuscularly twice daily. The medication label reads as follows: 10 mg/mL. The nurse prepares how many milliliters to administer one dose?

Answer: _____ mL

Level of Cognitive Ability: Application
Client Needs: Physiological Integrity
Integrated Process: Nursing Process/Implementation
Content Area: Fundamental Skills

Answer: 0.75 mL

Rationale: Use the formula for calculating a medication dose.
Formula

$$\frac{\text{Desired}}{\text{Available}} \times \text{Volume} = \text{mL per dose}$$

$$\frac{7.5\text{ mg}}{10\text{ mg}} \times 1.0\text{ mL} = 0.75\text{ mL}$$

Test-Taking Strategy: Identify what the question is asking. In this case, the question asks for the number of milliliters per dose. Use the formula to determine the correct dosage, and use a calculator to verify your answer. Review the formula for calculating a medication dose if you had difficulty with this question.

Reference
Potter, P., & Perry, A. (2009) *Fundamentals of nursing* (7th ed., pp. 695-699). St. Louis: Mosby.

Figure/Illustration

1411. A nurse is monitoring a client with a head injury and notes that the client is assuming this posture. The nurse notifies the registered nurse immediately to report that the client is exhibiting:

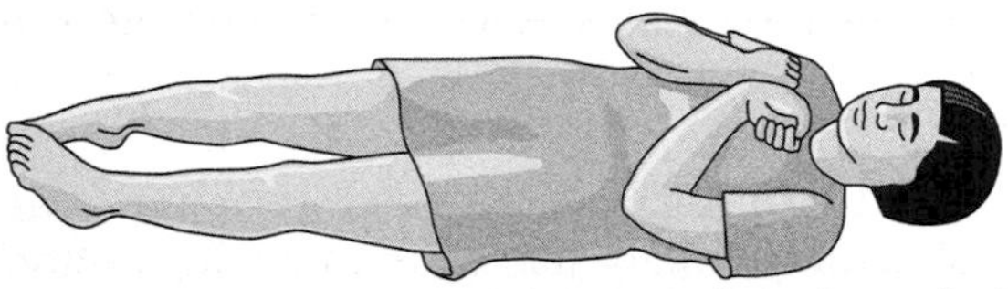

From Ignatavicius, D., & Workman, M. (2006). *Medical surgical nursing: Critical thinking for collaborative care* (5th ed., p. 939). Philadelphia: Saunders.

1 Opisthotonos
2 Decorticate rigidity
3 Decerebrate rigidity
4 Flaccid quadriplegia

Level of Cognitive Ability: Analysis
Client Needs: Physiological Integrity
Integrated Process: Nursing Process/Data Collection
Content Area: Adult Health/Neurological

Answer: 2
Rationale: In decorticate rigidity, the upper extremities (arms, wrists, and fingers) are flexed, with adduction of the arms. The lower extremities are extended, with internal rotation and plantarflexion. Decorticate rigidity indicates a hemispheric lesion of the cerebral cortex. In decerebrate rigidity, the upper extremities are stiffly extended and adducted, with internal rotation and pronation of the palms. The lower extremities are stiffly extended, with plantar flexion. The teeth are clenched, and the back is hyperextended. Decerebrate rigidity indicates a lesion in the brainstem at the midbrain or the upper pons. Flaccid quadriplegia is a complete loss of muscle tone and the paralysis of all four extremities that indicates a completely nonfunctional brainstem. Opisthotonos is prolonged arching of the back, with the head and heels bent backward. Opisthotonos indicates meningeal irritation.

Test-Taking Strategy: Note the position of the client's arms and legs. Remember that in de*cor*ticate rigidity, flexion of the upper extremities toward the *core* of the body occurs; this will direct you to option 2. Review abnormal postures if you had difficulty with this question.

Reference
Ignatavicius, D., & Workman, M. (2010). *Medical-surgical nursing: Patient-centered collaborative care* (6th ed., pp. 941-942). St. Louis: Saunders.

Prioritizing (Ordered Response)

1412. A client arrives in the postanesthesia care unit after colectomy. After listening to a verbal report from the anesthesia care provider, the nurse collects initial data about the client. List, in order of priority, the initial data collection actions. (Number 1 is the first action, and number 6 is the last action.)

___ Checks the blood pressure
___ Checks for airway patency
___ Checks the level of consciousness
___ Documents the initial data collection findings
___ Counts the heart rate and determines the rhythm
___ Counts the respiratory rate and determines the quality of respirations

Answer: 4, 1, 5, 6, 3, 2
Rationale: Postoperative data collection should begin with an evaluation of the ABCs—airway, breathing, and circulation. Airway patency is always checked first to ensure the adequate oxygenation of the body organs and tissues. Next, the rate and quality of the client's respirations are determined, and the breath sounds are auscultated throughout all of the lung fields to ensure adequate respiratory status. The client's heart rate and rhythm are determined, and the client's blood pressure is checked. A neurological assessment is then performed, along with other assessments, such as checking the urinary status, dressings, drains, and tubes and performing a pain assessment as needed. Finally, the nurse documents the initial data collection findings.

Test-Taking Strategy: Note the strategic words *order of priority,* and use the ABCs—airway, breathing, and circulation. The blood pressure is then checked, and this is followed by the assessment of the level of consciousness. Documenting is the last action. Review the initial care of the postoperative client if you had difficulty with this question.

Level of Cognitive Ability: Application
Client Needs: Physiological Integrity
Integrated Process: Nursing Process/Data Collection
Content Area: Fundamental Skills

Reference

Linton, A. (2007). *Introduction to medical-surgical nursing* (4th ed., pp. 264, 267). Philadelphia: Saunders.

Multiple Response

1413. A nurse is monitoring a hospitalized client with diabetes mellitus for signs of hyperglycemia. Select all of the signs of hyperglycemia.

- ❒ 1 Hunger
- ❒ 2 Sweating
- ❒ 3 Diaphoresis
- ❒ 4 Excessive thirst
- ❒ 5 Increased urine output
- ❒ 6 Kussmaul's respirations

Level of Cognitive Ability: Application
Client Needs: Physiological Integrity
Integrated Process: Nursing Process/Data Collection
Content Area: Adult Health/Endocrine

Answer: 1, 4, 5, 6
Rationale: Signs of hyperglycemia include excessive thirst, hunger, fatigue, restlessness, confusion, weakness, Kussmaul's respirations, diuresis, and coma, when severe. If the client presents with these symptoms, the blood glucose level should be checked immediately. Sweating and diaphoresis are signs of hypoglycemia. Hunger can occur with hyperglycemia or hypoglycemia.

> *Test-Taking Strategy*: Focus on the subject—signs of hyperglycemia. Remember the 3 Ps associated with hyperglycemia: polyuria, polydipsia, and polyphagia. Recall that in the client with hyperglycemia, the rate and depth of respirations increase (i.e., Kussmaul's respirations). Review the signs of hyperglycemia if you had difficulty with this question.

Reference

Christensen, B., & Kockrow, E. (2006). *Foundations of nursing* (5th ed., p. 917). St. Louis: Mosby.

Multiple Response

1414. A nurse is providing home-care instructions to the spouse of a client who is confused and who will be cared for at home. Choose the instructions that the nurse provides to the spouse. Check all that apply.

- ❒ 1 Turn the lights off at dusk.
- ❒ 2 Maintain a predictable routine.
- ❒ 3 Use simple, clear communication.
- ❒ 4 Limit the number of choices given to the client.
- ❒ 5 Encourage frequent visits from family and friends.
- ❒ 6 Display a calendar and a clock in the client's room.

Level of Cognitive Ability: Application
Client Needs: Psychosocial Integrity
Integrated Process: Teaching and Learning
Content Area: Mental Health

Answer: 2, 3, 4, 6
Rationale: The caregiver of a confused client is taught measures and techniques that will keep the client oriented and calm. Sensory overload and tasks and activities that are overwhelming for the client will cause disorientation and additional confusion. Therefore, any measures or activities that will increase sensory overload are avoided. Some helpful techniques include displaying a calendar and a clock in the house and in the client's room; maintaining a predictable routine; limiting the number of visitors who come to visit the client; limiting the number of choices given to the client; using simple, clear communication; and turning the lights on at dusk to avoid the sundown syndrome of increased confusion and combative behavior.

> *Test-Taking Strategy*: Focus on the subject—measures that will keep the client oriented and calm. Think about each listed intervention, and remember that measures and activities that will increase sensory overload and that are overwhelming for the client are avoided. This principle will assist you with selecting the correct measures. Review the care of the confused client if you had difficulty with this question.

Reference

Linton, A. (2007). *Introduction to medical-surgical nursing* (4th ed., pp. 325-326). Philadelphia: Saunders.

Fill-in-the-Blank

1415. A nurse tells a client that the physician prescribed 0.4 gram of ibuprofen (Advil) for mild pain. The client tells the nurse that the medication bottle contains 200-mg tablets and asks the nurse about the number of tablets to take. How many tablet(s) will the nurse tell the client to take?

Answer: _____ tablet(s)

Level of Cognitive Ability: Application
Client Needs: Physiological Integrity
Integrated Process: Teaching and Learning
Content Area: Fundamental Skills

Answer: 2

Rationale: Convert 0.4 gram to mg. In the metric system, to convert a larger denomination to smaller one, multiply by 1000 or move the decimal 3 places to the right. Then, use the following formula.

$$0.4 \text{ gram} = 400 \text{ mg}$$

$$\frac{\text{Desired}}{\text{Available}} \times \text{Quantity} = \text{Number of tablets}$$

$$\frac{400 \text{ mg}}{200 \text{ mg}} \times 1 \text{ tablet} = 2 \text{ tablets}$$

Test-Taking Strategy: Knowledge of the formula for the calculation of a medication dosage is required to answer this question. Remember to convert grams to milligrams. Follow the formula, and make sure that the calculated dose makes sense. Use a calculator to verify the answer. Review medication conversions and calculations if you had difficulty with this question.

Reference

Potter, P., & Perry, A. (2009) *Fundamentals of nursing* (7th ed., pp. 695-699). St. Louis: Mosby.

REFERENCES

Black, J., & Hawks, J. (2009). *Medical-surgical nursing: Clinical management for positive outcomes* (8th ed.). St. Louis: Saunders.

Chernecky, C., & Berger, B. (2008). *Laboratory tests and diagnostic procedures* (5th ed.). Philadelphia: Saunders.

Copstead, L., & Banasik, J. (2010). *Pathophysiology* (4th ed.). St. Louis: Mosby.

Christensen, B., & Kockrow, E. (2006). *Adult health nursing* (5th ed.). St. Louis: Mosby.

Christensen, B., & Kockrow, E. (2006). *Foundations of nursing* (5th ed.). St. Louis: Mosby.

deWit, S (2009). *Medical-surgical nursing: Concepts & practice*. St. Louis: Saunders.

Fortinash, K., & Holoday-Worret, P. (2008). *Psychiatric mental health nursing* (4th ed.). St. Louis: Mosby.

Giger, J., & Davidhizar, R. (2008). *Transcultural nursing: Assessment & intervention* (5th ed.). St. Louis: Mosby.

Hockenberry, M., & Wilson, D. (2009). *Wong's essentials of pediatric care* (8th ed.). St. Louis: Mosby.

Hodgson, B., & Kizior, R. (2008). *Saunders nursing drug handbook 2008*. Philadelphia: Saunders.

Ignatavicius, D., & Workman, M. (2010). *Medical-surgical nursing: Patient-centered collaborative care* (6th ed.). St. Louis: Saunders.

Jarvis, C. (2008). *Physical examination and health assessment* (5th ed.). Philadelphia: Saunders.

Kee, J., Hayes, E., & McCuistion, L. (2009). *Pharmacology: A nursing process approach* (6th ed.). St. Louis: Saunders.

Keltner, N., Schwecke, L., & Bostrom, C. (2007). *Psychiatric nursing* (5th ed.). St. Louis: Mosby.

Leifer, G. (2007). *Introduction to maternity and pediatric nursing* (5th ed.). Philadelphia: Saunders.

Leifer, G. (2008). *Maternity nursing: An introductory text* (10th ed.). Philadelphia: Saunders.

Lehne, R. (2010). *Pharmacology for nursing care* (7th ed.). Philadelphia: Saunders.

Linton, A. (2007). *Introduction to medical-surgical nursing* (4th ed). Philadelphia: Saunders.

Maurer, F., & Smith, C. (2009). *Community/public health nursing practices: Health for families and populations.* (4th ed.). St. Louis: Saunders.

McKinney, E., James, S., Murray, S., & Ashwill, J. (2009). *Maternal-child nursing* (3rd ed.). St. Louis: Mosby.

Monahan, F., Sands, J., Marek, J., Neighbors, M., & Green, C. (2007). *Phipps' medical-surgical nursing: Health and illness perspectives* (8th ed.). St. Louis: Mosby.

Mosby. (2008). *2008 Mosby's nursing drug reference* (21st ed.). St. Louis: Mosby.

Newell, R., & Gournay, K. (2009). *Mental health nursing: An evidence-based approach* (2nd ed.). St. Louis: Churchill livingstone.

Nix, S. (2009). *Williams' basic nutrition and diet therapy* (13th ed.). St. Louis: Mosby.

Price, D., & Gwin, J. (2008). *Pediatric nursing: An introductory text* (10th ed.). St. Louis: Saunders.

Potter, P., & Perry, A. (2009). *Fundamentals of nursing* (7th ed). St. Louis: Mosby.

Stuart, G. (2009). *Principles and practices of psychiatric nursing* (9th ed.). St. Louis: Mosby.

Swearingen, P. (2008). *All-in-one care planning resource: Medical-surgical, pediatric, maternity & psychiatric nursing care plans* (2nd ed.). St. Louis: Mosby.

Varcarolis, E., & Halter, M. (2009). *Essentials of psychiatric mental health nursing: A communication approach to evidence-based care*. St. Louis: Saunders.

Wold, G. (2008). *Basic geriatric nursing* (4th ed.). St. Louis: Mosby.

UNIT
IV

Comprehensive Test

Comprehensive Test

1416. A nurse is assisting with developing a plan of care for a client who is at risk for seizures. Select all of the interventions to include in the plan if the client experiences a seizure.

- ❒ 1 Restrain the client's extremities.
- ❒ 2 Place the client in a supine position.
- ❒ 3 Monitor and document the post-seizure status.
- ❒ 4 Place an oral airway between the client's teeth.
- ❒ 5 Note the time that the seizure began and how it progressed.
- ❒ 6 Remove any objects that could cause harm and place them away from the client.

Level of Cognitive Ability: Application
Client Needs: Physiological Integrity
Integrated Process: Nursing Process/Planning
Content Area: Adult Health/Neurological

Answer: 3, 5, 6
Rationale: In the event of a seizure, the nurse would remove any objects that could cause harm and place them away from the client. The nurse would turn the client to his or her side and note the time that the seizure began and how it progressed. The client's extremities are not restrained, and the nurse would not place anything between the client's teeth.

Test-Taking Strategy: Use the process of elimination, and focus on the subject—a client experiencing a seizure. Recall the importance of maintaining a patent airway and that the client should be protected from injury to assist you with identifying the interventions to use to manage a seizure. Remember that documentation is an important component of care. Review the listed interventions if you had difficulty with this question.

References

Christensen, B., & Kockrow, E. (2006). *Adult health nursing* (5th ed., p. 713). St. Louis: Mosby.
Christensen, B., & Kockrow, E. (2006). *Foundations of nursing* (5th ed., p. 362). St. Louis: Mosby.

1417. A nurse is caring for a client with acute cancer pain. The nurse best collects data about the client's pain by:

1 Recognizing nonverbal clues from the client
2 Asking the client about pain using a pain rating scale
3 Reviewing nursing documentation of the client's pain
4 Determining the amount of pain relief after appropriate nursing intervention

Level of Cognitive Ability: Application
Client Needs: Physiological Integrity
Integrated Process: Nursing Process/Data Collection
Content Area: Adult Health/Oncology

Answer: 2
Rationale: The client's perception of pain is the priority of pain data collection. The client is asked to identify the level of pain by a rating scale of 1 to 10, with 10 being the most severe. Nonverbal clues are subjective data. Options 1, 3, and 4 do not provide the best pain assessment method.

Test-Taking Strategy: Focus on the subject—data about the client's pain. Note the strategic word *best.* Use the process of elimination, and note that option 2 is a client-focused answer. Review data collection about pain if you had difficulty with this question.

References

deWit, S. (2009). *Medical-surgical nursing: Concepts & practice* (pp. 141, 183). St. Louis: Saunders.
Linton, A. (2007). *Introduction to medical-surgical nursing* (4th ed., p. 210). Philadelphia: Saunders.

1418. A nurse is caring for a client who received an allogeneic liver transplant and who is receiving tacrolimus (Prograf) daily. The nurse recognizes that the client is experiencing an adverse reaction to the medication if which of the following is noted?

1 Photophobia
2 Hypotension
3 Profuse sweating
4 Decrease in urine output

Answer: 4

Rationale: Tacrolimus is an immunosuppressant medication used for the prophylaxis of organ rejection in clients who are undergoing allogeneic liver transplants. Frequent side effects include headache, tremor, insomnia, paresthesia, diarrhea, nausea, constipation, vomiting, abdominal pain, and hypertension. Adverse reactions and toxic effects include nephrotoxicity, neurotoxicity, and pleural effusion. Nephrotoxicity is characterized by an increasing serum creatinine level and a decrease in urine output. Neurotoxicity—including tremor, headache, and mental status changes—commonly occurs. Photophobia and profuse sweating are unrelated to this medication.

Test-Taking Strategy: Use the process of elimination, and use medical terminology to identify the medication. Look at the medication name, Prograf. Note that *Pro* means *for* and *graf* means *graft.* This assists you with identifying the action of the medication (preventing transplant rejection) and classifying it as an immunosuppressant (which may in turn assist you with remembering its side and adverse effects). Review tacrolimus if you had difficulty with this question.

Level of Cognitive Ability: Analysis
Client Needs: Physiological Integrity
Integrated Process: Nursing Process/Data Collection
Content Area: Pharmacology

Reference

Lehne, R. (2010). *Pharmacology for nursing care* (7th ed., p. 820). St. Louis: Saunders.

1419. A prenatal client is suspected of having iron deficiency anemia. During data collection, the nurse expects to note which of the following?

1 Fluid volume excess
2 Fluid volume deficit
3 Low hemoglobin and hematocrit levels
4 High hemoglobin and hematocrit levels

Answer: 3

Rationale: Iron deficiency is suspected when the hemoglobin level is less than 11 mg/dL. Pathological anemia of pregnancy is primarily caused by iron deficiency. Without iron therapy, even pregnant women who have excellent nutrition end pregnancy with an iron deficit. Iron for the fetus comes from the maternal serum. Options 1, 2, and 4 are not associated with iron deficiency.

Test-Taking Strategy: Use the process of elimination. The words *deficiency* in the question and *low* in option 3 are comparable or alike words that can assist you with selecting the correct option. Review iron deficiency anemia if you had difficulty with this question.

Level of Cognitive Ability: Comprehension
Client Needs: Physiological Integrity
Integrated Process: Nursing Process/Data Collection
Content Area: Maternity/Antepartum

Reference

Leifer, G. (2008). *Maternity nursing: An introductory text* (10th ed., p. 265). Philadelphia: Saunders.

1420. A nurse is assisting with preparing a plan of care for a child with leukemia who is scheduled to receive chemotherapy. Which nursing intervention should be included in the plan of care?

1 Monitor the rectal temperature every 4 hours.
2 Monitor the mouth and anus each shift for signs of breakdown.

Answer: 2

Rationale: When the child is receiving chemotherapy, the nurse should avoid taking rectal temperatures. Oral temperatures are also avoided if mouth ulcers are present. Axillary temperatures should be taken or a tympanic thermometer should be used to prevent alterations in skin integrity. Meticulous mouth care should be performed; the nurse should use a soft-bristled toothbrush and avoid use of alcohol-based mouthwash. The nurse should assess the mouth and anus each shift for ulcers, erythema, or breakdown. Bland, nonirritating foods and liquids should be provided to the

3 Encourage the child to consume fresh fruits and vegetables to maintain the nutritional status.
4 Provide meticulous mouth care several times a day using an alcohol-based mouthwash and a toothbrush.

Level of Cognitive Ability: Application
Client Needs: Physiological Integrity
Integrated Process: Nursing Process/Planning
Content Area: Child Health

child. Fresh fruits and vegetables should be avoided because they can harbor organisms. Chemotherapy can cause neutropenia, and the child should be maintained on a low-bacteria diet if the white blood cell count is low.

Test-Taking Strategy: Use the process of elimination, and read each option carefully. Think about the side effects that can occur with chemotherapy to direct you to option 2. Remember that neutropenia and thrombocytopenia can occur as a result of chemotherapy. Review the nursing plan of care for a client receiving chemotherapy if you had difficulty with this question.

Reference

Christensen, B., & Kockrow, E. (2006). *Foundations of nursing* (5th ed., pp. 1005-1006). St. Louis: Mosby.

1421. A client with Guillain-Barré syndrome is being transferred from the emergency department. The client's chief complaint is an ascending paralysis that has reached the level of the waist. The nurse plans to have which essential item available for emergency use?
1 Flashlight
2 Nebulizer
3 Intubation tray
4 Incentive spirometer

Level of Cognitive Ability: Application
Client Needs: Physiological Integrity
Integrated Process: Nursing Process/Planning
Content Area: Adult Health/Neurological

Answer: 3
Rationale: Guillain-Barré syndrome is a peripheral polyneuritis that is associated with a viral infection or immunizations. The client with Guillain-Barré syndrome is at risk for respiratory failure because of ascending paralysis. An intubation tray should be available for emergency use. Another complication of this syndrome is cardiac dysrhythmias, which necessitate the need for cardiac monitoring. A flashlight, a nebulizer, and an incentive spirometer are not essential items.

Test-Taking Strategy: Use the process of elimination, and note the strategic words *emergency use.* These words tell you that the correct answer will be the option that lists the piece of equipment that is not routinely used to provide care. With this in mind, eliminate options 1, 2, and 4. Review the nursing care measures for the client with Guillain-Barré syndrome if you had difficulty with this question.

References

Christensen, B., & Kockrow, E. (2006). *Adult health nursing* (5th ed., p. 737). St. Louis: Mosby.
Linton, A. (2007). *Introduction to medical-surgical nursing* (4th ed., p. 445). Philadelphia: Saunders.

1422. A nurse is admitting a child with irritable bowel syndrome (IBS) to the hospital. Which information should the nurse expect to obtain when collecting data about the child?
1 Reports of frothy diarrhea
2 Reports of foul-smelling, ribbon-like stools
3 Reports of profuse, watery diarrhea and vomiting
4 Reports of diffuse abdominal pain unrelated to meals or activity

Level of Cognitive Ability: Comprehension
Client Needs: Physiological Integrity

Answer: 4
Rationale: IBS causes diffuse abdominal pain unrelated to meals or activity. Alternating constipation and diarrhea with the presence of undigested food and mucus in the stools may also be noted. Option 1 is a clinical manifestation of lactose intolerance. Option 2 is a clinical manifestation of Hirschsprung's disease. Option 3 is a clinical manifestation of celiac disease.

Test-Taking Strategy: Use the process of elimination, and focus on the child's diagnosis. Note the name of the syndrome to direct you to option 4 because you would expect abdominal pain with such a disorder. Review the clinical manifestations associated with IBS if you had difficulty with this question.

Integrated Process: Nursing Process/Data Collection
Content Area: Child Health

Reference
Hockenberry, M., & Wilson, D. (2009). *Wong's essentials of pediatric care* (8th ed., p. 829). St. Louis: Mosby.

1423. A nurse caring for a child with rubeola (measles) notes that the physician has documented the presence Koplik spots. Based on this documentation, what should the nurse expect to note in the child?

1 Pinpoint petechiae on both legs
2 Whitish vesicles across the chest
3 Reddish pinpoint petechiae on the soft palate
4 Small, bluish-white spots with red bases on the buccal mucosa

Level of Cognitive Ability: Comprehension
Client Needs: Physiological Integrity
Integrated Process: Nursing Process/Data Collection
Content Area: Child Health

Answer: 4
Rationale: Koplik spots appear approximately 2 days before the appearance of the rubeola rash. Koplik spots are small, bluish-white spots with red bases that are found on the buccal mucosa. They last approximately 3 days, after which time they slough off. Options 1, 2, and 3 are incorrect.

Test-Taking Strategy: Knowledge of the characteristics associated with rubeola and Koplik spots is necessary to answer this question. Remember that Koplik spots are small, bluish-white spots with red bases that are found on the buccal mucosa. Review Koplik spots if you had difficulty with this question.

Reference
Christensen, B., & Kockrow, E. (2006). *Foundations of nursing* (5th ed., p. 1065). St. Louis: Mosby.

1424. A child is hospitalized with nephrotic syndrome. Which finding should the nurse expect to note in the child?

1 Weight loss
2 Excitability
3 Constipation
4 Abdominal pain

Level of Cognitive Ability: Comprehension
Client Needs: Physiological Integrity
Integrated Process: Nursing Process/Data Collection
Content Area: Child Health

Answer: 4
Rationale: Nephrotic syndrome is an abnormal condition of the kidney that is characterized by marked proteinuria, hypoalbuminemia, and edema. Clinical manifestations include edema, anorexia, fatigue, and abdominal pain from the presence of extra fluid in the peritoneal cavity. Diarrhea caused by the edema of the bowel occurs and may cause the decreased absorption of nutrients. Increased weight and normal blood pressure are most likely noted.

Test-Taking Strategy: Use the process of elimination. Recall that edema is a clinical manifestation that is associated with nephrotic syndrome to direct you to option 4. Review the clinical manifestations associated with nephrotic syndrome if you had difficulty with this question.

Reference
Christensen, B., & Kockrow, E. (2006). *Foundations of nursing* (5th ed., p. 1033). St. Louis: Mosby.

1425. A nurse is assigned to care for a child with a basilar skull fracture. The nurse reviews the child's record and notes that the physician has documented the presence of Battle's sign. Which of the following should the nurse expect to note in this child?

1 Epistaxis
2 Bruising behind the ear

Answer: 2
Rationale: The most serious type of skull fracture is a basilar skull fracture. Two classic findings associated with this type of fracture are Battle's sign and raccoon eyes. Battle's sign is the presence of bruising or ecchymosis behind the ear that is caused by leaking of blood into the mastoid sinuses. Raccoon eyes occur as a result of blood leaking into the frontal sinus and causing an edematous and bruised periorbital area.

3 Bruised periorbital area
4 Edematous periorbital area

Level of Cognitive Ability: Comprehension
Client Needs: Physiological Integrity
Integrated Process: Nursing Process/Data Collection
Content Area: Child Health

Test-Taking Strategy: Use the process of elimination. Eliminate options 3 and 4 first because they are comparable or alike. From the remaining options, recall the description of Battle's sign to direct you to option 2. Review Battle's sign if you had difficulty with this question.

Reference

McKinney, E., James, S., Murray, S., Ashwill, J. (2009). *Maternal-child nursing* (3rd ed., pp. 1458, 1483). St. Louis: Mosby.

1426. A client has been prescribed phenazopyridine hydrochloride (Pyridium) after a urological procedure. Which of the following should the nurse plan to include when providing medication instructions to the client?

1 The medication exerts an antimicrobial effect.
2 The medication provides an antibacterial effect.
3 The medication must be taken on an empty stomach.
4 The urine may have a reddish-orange discoloration that may stain clothing.

Level of Cognitive Ability: Application
Client Needs: Physiological Integrity
Integrated Process: Nursing Process/Planning
Content Area: Pharmacology

Answer: 4

Rationale: Phenazopyridine is a urinary tract analgesic with no antimicrobial or antibacterial properties. It is used to relieve the frequency, burning, or dysuria that follows urological procedures or that accompanies infection. The medication is usually taken for 2 days or until symptoms have resolved, and then it is discontinued. Any accompanying antibiotics are continued until finished. Phenazopyridine stains clothing and bedclothes an orange-red color that is permanent. For this reason, clients are advised to wear sanitary napkins to protect their undergarments. The medication should be taken with food to avoid gastrointestinal upset.

Test-Taking Strategy: Use the process of elimination. Eliminate options 1 and 2 first because they are comparable or alike. From the remaining options, eliminate option 3 because of the close-ended word *must*. Review phenazopyridine if you had difficulty with this question.

Reference

Christensen, B., & Kockrow, E. (2006). *Adult health nursing* (5th ed., p. 476). St. Louis: Mosby.

1427. A nurse is reviewing the records of several hospitalized clients to identify the clients who are candidates for receiving parenteral nutrition. Select all of the clients who would be candidates.

❒ 1 A client with a severe burn injury
❒ 2 A client with congestive heart failure
❒ 3 A client with severe anorexia nervosa
❒ 4 A client with malabsorption syndrome
❒ 5 A client with uncomplicated gastroenteritis
❒ 6 A client receiving chemotherapy who has severe vomiting and diarrhea

Level of Cognitive Ability: Analysis
Client Needs: Physiological Integrity
Integrated Process: Nursing Process/Data Collection
Content Area: Adult Health/Gastrointestinal

Answers: 1, 3, 4, 6

Rationale: Parenteral nutrition is indicated when the gastrointestinal (GI) tract is severely dysfunctional or nonfunctional; if the client has had multiple GI surgeries, GI trauma, severe intolerance to enteral feedings, or intestinal obstructions; or when the bowel needs to rest for healing. Conditions to consider include acquired immunodeficiency syndrome, cancer, malnutrition, burns, chronic vomiting and diarrhea, diverticulitis hypermetabolic states (e.g., sepsis), inflammatory bowel disease, pancreatitis, and severe anorexia nervosa.

Test-Taking Strategy: Think about the purpose and the components of parenteral nutrition to assist you with identifying the clients who are candidates for this form of nutrition. Note the strategic words *severe* and *malabsorption* in the correct options. Review the indications for parenteral nutrition if you had difficulty with this question.

Reference

Christensen, B., & Kockrow, E. (2006). *Foundations of nursing* (5th ed., p. 718). St. Louis: Mosby.

1428. A nurse is preparing to care for a client with Ménière's disease. The nurse reviews the physician orders and expects to note that which of the following dietary measures is prescribed?

1 Low-fiber diet with decreased fluids
2 Low-sodium diet and fluid restriction
3 Low-fat diet and restriction of citrus fruits
4 Low-carbohydrate diet and the elimination of red meats

Level of Cognitive Ability: Analysis
Client Needs: Physiological Integrity
Integrated Process: Nursing Process/Planning
Content Area: Adult Health/Ear

Answer: 2

Rationale: Ménière's disease is a chronic disease of the inner ear that is characterized by recurrent episodes of vertigo, progressive sensorineural hearing loss that may be bilateral, and tinnitus. Dietary changes that reduce the amount of endolymphatic fluid (e.g., salt and fluid restrictions) are sometimes prescribed for clients with this condition. Options 1, 3, and 4 are not prescribed for this disorder.

Test-Taking Strategy: Use the process of elimination, and focus on the client's diagnosis. Recall that salt and fluid restrictions are sometimes necessary to reduce the amount of endolymphatic fluid to direct you to option 2. Review the pathophysiology and treatment of Ménière's disease if you had difficulty with this question.

Reference

Christensen, B., & Kockrow, E. (2006). *Adult health nursing* (5th ed., p. 676). St. Louis: Mosby.

1429. A nurse consults with a nutritionist about the dietary preferences of an Asian-American client. Which food item should be included in the dietary plan?

1 Rice
2 Chili
3 Red meat
4 Fried foods

Level of Cognitive Ability: Application
Client Needs: Psychosocial Integrity
Integrated Process: Nursing Process/Planning
Content Area: Fundamental Skills

Answer: 1

Rationale: Asian-American food preferences include raw fish, rice, and soy sauce. Hispanic Americans prefer beans, fried foods, spicy foods, chili, and carbonated beverages. European Americans prefer carbohydrates and red meat. African-American food preferences include pork, greens, rice, and fried foods.

Test-Taking Strategy: Use the process of elimination, and correlate rice with Asian Americans. Review the food preferences associated with the Asian-American culture if you had difficulty with this question.

Reference

Christensen, B., & Kockrow, E. (2006). *Foundations of nursing* (5th ed., p. 146). St. Louis: Mosby.

1430. A previously healthy client with a long-leg cast is on prescribed bedrest. The nurse plans to institute which general measure of client care?

1 Request a low-fiber diet.
2 Increase fluids to 3 L per day.
3 Reposition the client every 4 to 6 hours.
4 Check the neurovascular status daily.

Level of Cognitive Ability: Application
Client Needs: Physiological Integrity
Integrated Process: Nursing Process/Planning
Content Area: Adult Health/Musculoskeletal

Answer: 2

Rationale: Routine measures for the immobile client who has had the application of a long-leg cast include checking the neurovascular status every 1 to 4 hours (depending on the time since application), repositioning every 2 to 4 hours, and providing a diet that is high in fiber and fluids (to prevent constipation).

Test-Taking Strategy: Use the process of elimination, and note the strategic words *previously healthy, cast,* and *bedrest.* Knowledge of basic care measures for the immobile client assists you with eliminating options 1 and 3. Recall the concepts related to cast care, data collection, and time frames to assist you with eliminating option 4. Review nursing measures for cast care if you had difficulty with this question.

Reference

Linton, A. (2007). *Introduction to medical-surgical nursing* (4th ed., p. 926). Philadelphia: Saunders.

1431. A client with a long-leg cast is afraid of wetting the top of the cast while urinating. The nurse plans to keep the cast dry by doing which of the following?

1 Petaling the edges of the cast
2 Requesting an order for a Foley catheter
3 Using a trapeze when placing the client on a bedpan
4 Tucking a plastic material (e.g., food wrap) around the area before toileting

Level of Cognitive Ability: Application
Client Needs: Physiological Integrity
Integrated Process: Nursing Process/Planning
Content Area: Adult Health/Musculoskeletal

Answer: 4
Rationale: A waterproof material such as plastic food wrap is very useful for preventing casting material from becoming wet during urination. Petaling the cast edges prevents skin irritation but does not affect the possible wetting of the cast. Foley catheter insertion carries a risk of infection and is not recommended unless it is required for other reasons. Using a trapeze aids in proper positioning but does not necessarily prevent spillage or wetting during urination.

Test-Taking Strategy: Use the process of elimination, and focus on the subject—preventing the wetting of the cast during urination. Eliminate option 2 first using principles of infection control. Eliminate option 1 next because it does not address the subject. From the remaining options, select option 4 because it most directly prevents the problem of getting the cast wet. Review the care of the client with a cast if you had difficulty with this question.

References
Christensen, B., & Kockrow, E. (2006). *Adult health nursing* (5th ed., pp. 171-172). St. Louis: Mosby.
Linton, A. (2007). *Introduction to medical-surgical nursing* (4th ed., p. 920). Philadelphia: Saunders.

1432. A nurse is developing a postoperative plan of care for a 40-year-old male Filipino client scheduled for an appendectomy. The nurse appropriately includes which of the following in the plan of care?

1 Offering pain medication on a regular basis as prescribed
2 Offering pain medication when nonverbal signs of discomfort are identified
3 Informing the client the he will need to ask for pain medication when needed
4 Allowing the client to maintain control and to request pain medication on his own

Level of Cognitive Ability: Application
Client Needs: Psychosocial Integrity
Integrated Process: Nursing Process/Planning
Content Area: Fundamental Skills

Answer: 1
Rationale: Filipinos view pain as part of living an honorable life. The client may appear stoic and may be tolerant of a high degree of pain. The nurse should offer pain medication on a regular basis and in fact encourage pain relief interventions for the Filipino client who does not complain of pain despite physiological indicators. Option 1 is the most appropriate intervention to include in the plan of care.

Test-Taking Strategy: Use the process of elimination. Eliminate options 3 and 4 first because they are comparable or alike. From the remaining options, recall the cultural response to pain in the Filipino client to direct you to option 1. Review the characteristics of the Filipino cultural group if you had difficulty with this question.

Reference
Giger, J., & Davidhizar, R. (2008). *Transcultural nursing assessment & intervention* (5th ed., p. 481). St. Louis: Mosby.

1433. A client with advanced cirrhosis of the liver is not tolerating protein well as evidenced by abnormal laboratory values. The nurse anticipates that which of the following medications will be prescribed for the client?

1 Folic acid (Folvite)
2 Lactulose (Chronulac)

Answer: 2
Rationale: Cirrhosis is a chronic degenerative disease of the liver in which the lobes are covered with fibrous tissue, the parenchyma degenerates, and the lobules are infiltrated with fat. The client with cirrhosis has an impaired ability to metabolize protein as a result of liver dysfunction. The administration of lactulose (Chronulac) aids in the clearance of ammonia via the gastrointestinal tract. Folic acid and thiamine are vitamins that may be used in clients with liver disease as supplemental therapy. Ethacrynic acid is a diuretic.

3 Thiamine (Vitamin B_1)
4 Ethacrynic acid (Edecrin)

Level of Cognitive Ability: Analysis
Client Needs: Physiological Integrity
Integrated Process: Nursing Process/Planning
Content Area: Pharmacology

Test-Taking Strategy: Use the process of elimination. Recall that ammonia levels are elevated with advanced liver disease and that lactulose is a standard form of medication therapy for this condition. Review cirrhosis and the purpose of lactulose if you had difficulty with this question.

Reference

deWit, S. (2009). *Medical-surgical nursing: Concepts & practice* (p. 747). St. Louis: Saunders.

1434. A nurse is caring for a child with renal disease. When analyzing the laboratory results, the nurse notes a sodium level of 148 mEq/L. Based on this finding, which clinical manifestation should the nurse expect to note in this child?
1 Lethargy
2 Cold, clammy skin
3 Increased heart rate
4 Dry, sticky mucous membranes

Level of Cognitive Ability: Analysis
Client Needs: Physiological Integrity
Integrated Process: Nursing Process/Data Collection
Content Area: Child Health

Answer: 4
Rationale: Hypernatremia occurs when the sodium level is more than 145 mEq/L. Clinical manifestations include intense thirst; oliguria; agitation and restlessness; flushed skin; peripheral and pulmonary edema; dry, sticky mucous membranes; and nausea and vomiting. Options 1, 2, and 3 are not associated with the clinical manifestations of hypernatremia.

Test-Taking Strategy: Use the process of elimination. First, determine that the sodium level is elevated and that the child is experiencing hypernatremia. Next, recall the clinical manifestations associated with hypernatremia to direct you to option 4. Review the normal sodium level and the clinical manifestations associated with an imbalance if you had difficulty with this question.

Reference

Christensen, B., & Kockrow, E. (2006). *Foundations of nursing* (5th ed., pp. 671-672). St. Louis: Mosby.

1435. A client is scheduled for a cardiac catheterization. Which data, if noted in the client's health record, must the nurse report to the physician before the catheterization?
1 Allergy to shellfish
2 History of hypertension
3 History of coronary artery disease
4 Allergy to meperidine hydrochloride (Demerol)

Level of Cognitive Ability: Application
Client Needs: Safe and Effective Care Environment
Integrated Process: Nursing Process/Implementation
Content Area: Fundamental Skills

Answer: 1
Rationale: The dye used during the catheterization may contain iodine, so any allergies to shellfish or iodine should be reported immediately to prevent allergic reactions. Coronary artery disease may be the reason for performing the cardiac catheterization, and hypertension is normally associated with coronary artery disease. An allergy to meperidine hydrochloride is not specifically related to a cardiac catheterization, although it must be noted on the client's record.

Test-Taking Strategy: Use the process of elimination. Recall that an allergy to shellfish is significant with any procedure that requires the instillation of a dye to direct you to option 1. Review preprocedure care for a cardiac catheterization if you had difficulty with this question.

Reference

Christensen, B., & Kockrow, E. (2006). *Foundations of nursing* (5th ed., pp. 486, 489). St. Louis: Mosby.

1436. A child was diagnosed with acute poststreptococcal glomerulonephritis, and renal insufficiency is suspected. Which

Answer: 4
Rationale: With poststreptococcal glomerulonephritis, a urinalysis reveals hematuria with red cell casts. Proteinuria is also present.

of the following laboratory results will the nurse expect to note?

1 Negative protein in the urinalysis
2 Negative red blood cells in the urinalysis
3 An elevated white blood cell (WBC) count
4 Elevated blood urea nitrogen (BUN) and creatinine levels

Level of Cognitive Ability: Analysis
Client Needs: Physiological Integrity
Integrated Process: Nursing Process/Data Collection
Content Area: Child Health

If renal insufficiency occurs, the BUN and creatinine levels are elevated. The WBC is usually within normal limits, and mild anemia is common.

Test-Taking Strategy: Use the process of elimination, and focus on the child's diagnosis. Recall that the BUN and creatinine levels are laboratory studies that relate to the renal system to direct you to option 4. Review the clinical manifestations associated with poststreptococcal glomerulonephritis if you had difficulty with this question.

Reference

Christensen, B., & Kockrow, E. (2006). *Foundations of nursing* (5th ed., p. 1034). St. Louis: Mosby.

1437. An infant is brought to the health care clinic, and the mother tells the nurse that her infant has been vomiting after meals, that the vomiting is now becoming more frequent and forceful, and that the infant seems to be constipated. During data collection, the nurse notes visible peristaltic waves moving from left to right across the infant's abdomen. Based on this finding, the nurse should suspect which of the following?

1 Colic
2 Intussusception
3 Pyloric stenosis
4 Congenital megacolon

Level of Cognitive Ability: Analysis
Client Needs: Physiological Integrity
Integrated Process: Nursing Process/Data Collection
Content Area: Child Health

Answer: 3

Rationale: Pyloric stenosis is a narrowing of the pyloric sphincter at the outlet of the stomach; this causes an obstruction that blocks the flow of food into the small intestine. With pyloric stenosis, the vomitus contains sour, undigested food but no bile; the child is constipated, and visible peristaltic waves move from left to right across the abdomen. A movable, palpable, firm, olive-shaped mass in the right upper quadrant may be noted. Crying during the evening hours, appearing to be in pain, but eating well and gaining weight are clinical manifestations of colic. An infant who suddenly becomes pale, cries out, and draws the legs up to the chest is demonstrating the physical signs of intussusception. Ribbon-like stool, bile-stained emesis, the absence of peristalsis, and abdominal distention are symptoms of congenital megacolon (Hirschsprung's disease).

Test-Taking Strategy: Use the process of elimination, and focus on the data provided in the question. Consider each condition presented in the options, and think about the clinical manifestations of each. Recall the manifestations of pyloric stenosis to direct you to option 3. Review the clinical manifestations of pyloric stenosis if you had difficulty with this question.

Reference

Christensen, B., & Kockrow, E. (2006). *Foundations of nursing* (5th ed., p. 1028). St. Louis: Mosby.

1438. A nurse reviews the nursing care plan of a hospitalized child who is immobilized because of skeletal traction. The nurse notes a nursing diagnosis of *Risk for delayed growth and development* related to immobilization and hospitalization. Which evaluative statement indicates a positive outcome for the child?

1 The fracture heals without complications.
2 The caregivers verbalize safe and effective home care.

Answer: 4

Rationale: Regression and inappropriate developmental behaviors may be displayed in response to immobilization and hospitalization. With individualized care planning, a positive outcome of age-appropriate behavior can be achieved. Options 1, 2, and 3 are appropriate evaluative statements for an immobilized child but do not directly address the nursing diagnosis of *Risk for delayed growth and development*.

3 The child maintains normal joint and muscle integrity.
4 The child displays age-appropriate developmental behaviors.

Level of Cognitive Ability: Analysis
Client Needs: Health Promotion and Maintenance
Integrated Process: Nursing Process/Evaluation
Content Area: Child Health

Test-Taking Strategy: Focus on the subject—a nursing diagnosis of *Risk for delayed growth and development*. Use the process of elimination. Recall that delayed growth and development is the state in which an individual is not performing age-appropriate tasks to direct you to option 4. All of the options are evaluative statements, but only option 4 addresses the relevant nursing diagnosis. Review the defining characteristics and the appropriate outcomes for a nursing diagnosis of *Risk for delayed growth and development* if you had difficulty with this question.

References

Christensen, B., & Kockrow, E. (2006). *Foundations of nursing* (5th ed., p. 1133). St. Louis: Mosby.
Hockenberry, M., & Wilson, D. (2009). *Wong's essentials of pediatric* (8th ed., p. 422). St. Louis: Mosby.

1439. A client with a history of self-managed peptic ulcer disease has frequently used excessive amounts of oral antacids. The nurse determines that this client is at risk for which acid-base disturbance?
1 Metabolic acidosis
2 Metabolic alkalosis
3 Respiratory acidosis
4 Respiratory alkalosis

Level of Cognitive Ability: Analysis
Client Needs: Physiological Integrity
Integrated Process: Nursing Process/Data Collection
Content Area: Fundamental Skills

Answer: 2
Rationale: Oral antacids commonly contain bicarbonate or other alkaline components; these bind onto the hydrochloric acid in the stomach to neutralize the acid. The excessive use of oral antacids that contain bicarbonate can cause a metabolic alkalosis over time. Options 1, 3, and 4 are incorrect.

Test-Taking Strategy: Use the process of elimination. Note that the question indicates that the problem is not respiratory in nature. With this in mind, eliminate options 3 and 4 first. Choose correctly from the remaining options knowing that the word *antacid* must work against acids. Review the causes of metabolic alkalosis if you had difficulty with the question.

References

Christensen, B., & Kockrow, E. (2006). *Adult health nursing* (5th ed., p. 214). St. Louis: Mosby.
deWit, S. (2009). *Medical-surgical nursing: Concepts & practice* (p. 54). St. Louis: Saunders.

1440. A nurse is collecting data from a 39-year-old Caucasian female client. The client has a blood pressure of 152/92 mm Hg at rest, a total cholesterol level of 190 mg/dL, and a fasting blood glucose level of 114 mg/dL. The nurse would place priority on which risk factor for coronary artery disease in this client?
1 Age
2 Hypertension
3 Hyperlipidemia
4 Glucose intolerance

Level of Cognitive Ability: Analysis
Client Needs: Health Promotion and Maintenance
Integrated Process: Nursing Process/Data Collection
Content Area: Adult Health/Cardiovascular

Answer: 2
Rationale: Coronary artery disease affects the heart's arteries and results in a reduced flow of oxygen and nutrients to the myocardium. Hypertension, cigarette smoking, and hyperlipidemia are major risk factors for coronary artery disease. Glucose intolerance, obesity, and response to stress are also contributing factors. An age of more than 40 years is a nonmodifiable risk factor. The cholesterol level of 190 mg/dL and the blood glucose level of 114 mg/dL are within the normal range. The nurse places priority on major risk factors that require modification.

Test-Taking Strategy: Use the process of elimination. Focus on the data in the question, and note the strategic word *priority*. Note that the only abnormal value is the blood pressure; this will direct you to option 2. Review the risk factors associated with coronary artery disease if you had difficulty with this question.

References
deWit, S. (2009). *Medical-surgical nursing: Concepts & practice* (pp. 435-436). St. Louis: Saunders.
Linton, A. (2007). *Introduction to medical-surgical nursing* (4th ed., p. 653). Philadelphia: Saunders.

1441. A nurse is caring for a client who has just returned to the nursing unit after an intravenous pyelogram (IVP). The nurse determines that which of the following is a priority for the postprocedure care of this client?

1 Maintaining the client on bedrest
2 Ambulating the client in the hallway
3 Encouraging the increased intake of oral fluids
4 Encouraging the client to try to void frequently

Level of Cognitive Ability: Comprehension
Client Needs: Physiological Integrity
Integrated Process: Nursing Process/Planning
Content Area: Adult Health/Renal

Answer: 3
Rationale: IVP is a radiographic technique for examining the structure and function of the urinary system. After IVP, the client should increase fluid intake to help with the clearance of the dye used for the procedure. The client is usually allowed activity as tolerated, without any specific activity guidelines. It is unnecessary to void frequently after the procedure.

Test-Taking Strategy: Use the process of elimination, and note the strategic word *priority.* Option 4 has no useful purpose and is eliminated first. From the remaining options, recall that there are no specific activity guidelines after IVP. In addition, recall that fluids are necessary to promote the clearance of the dye from the client's system. Review IVP if you had difficulty with this question.

Reference
Christensen, B., & Kockrow, E. (2006). *Foundations of nursing* (5th ed., p. 494). St. Louis: Mosby.

1442. A client with thrombotic brain attack (stroke) experiences periods of emotional lability. The client alternately laughs and cries and intermittently becomes irritable and demanding. The nurse determines that this behavior indicates that:

1 The client is not adapting well to the disability.
2 The problem is likely to get worse before it gets better.
3 The client is experiencing the usual sequelae of a stroke.
4 The client is experiencing side effects of prescribed anticoagulants.

Level of Cognitive Ability: Analysis
Client Needs: Psychosocial Integrity
Integrated Process: Nursing Process/Data Collection
Content Area: Adult Health/Neurological

Answer: 3
Rationale: After a brain attack (stroke), the client often experiences periods of emotional lability that are characterized by sudden bouts of laughing or crying or by irritability, depression, confusion, or being demanding. This is a normal part of the clinical picture for the client with this health problem, although it may be difficult for health care personnel and family members to tolerate. The other options are incorrect.

Test-Taking Strategy: Use the process of elimination. Eliminate options 2 and 4 first; anticoagulants do not cause emotional lability, and there is no information in the question to support option 2. From the remaining options, recall the emotional changes that accompany a stroke to direct you to option 3. Review the effects of a brain attack (stroke) if you had difficulty with this question.

Reference
Linton, A. (2007). *Introduction to medical-surgical nursing* (4th ed., pp. 481-482). Philadelphia: Saunders.

1443. The nurse checks the height of the fundus in a client who is 12 hours postpartum and expects to note that it is at approximately which level? (Refer to the figure to answer the question.)

Answer: 1
Rationale: The location of the fundus helps to determine whether involution is progressing normally. Immediately after delivery, the fundus can be palpated midway between the symphysis pubis and the umbilicus. Within a few hours, the fundus rises to the level of

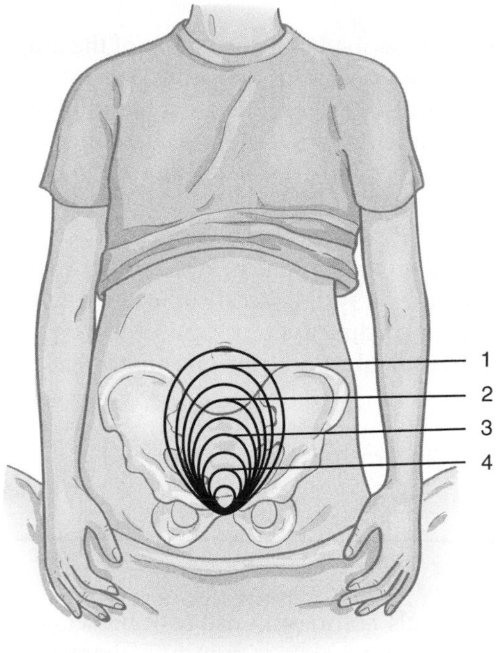

From McKinney, E., James, S., Murray, S., & Ashwill, J. (2005). *Maternal-child nursing* (2nd ed., p. 467). St. Louis: Saunders.

Answer: _____

Level of Cognitive Ability: Comprehension
Client Needs: Health Promotion and Maintenance
Integrated Process: Nursing Process/Data Collection
Content Area: Maternity/Postpartum

the umbilicus and should remain at this level for about 24 hours. After 24 hours, the fundus begins to descend by approximately 1 cm (1 fingerbreadth) per day.

Test-Taking Strategy: Focus on the subject—the height of the fundus in a client who is 12 hours postpartum. Recall that within a few hours of delivery, the fundus rises to the level of the umbilicus and remains at that level for about 24 hours to assist you with answering this question. Review normal postpartum findings if you had difficulty with this question.

References

Christensen, B., & Kockrow, E. (2006). *Foundations of nursing* (5th ed., p. 856). St. Louis: Mosby.

Leifer, G. (2008). *Maternity nursing: An introductory text* (10th ed., p. 227). Philadelphia: Saunders.

1444. A nurse is caring for a client with myasthenia gravis. The client is vomiting and complaining of abdominal cramps and diarrhea. The nurse also notes that the client is hypotensive and experiencing facial muscle twitching. The nurse determines that these symptoms are compatible with:

1 Cholinergic crisis
2 Myasthenic crisis
3 Systemic infection
4 A reaction to plasmapheresis

Level of Cognitive Ability: Analysis
Client Needs: Physiological Integrity
Integrated Process: Nursing Process/Data Collection
Content Area: Adult Health/Neurological

Answer: 1

Rationale: Cholinergic crisis is a pronounced muscular weakness and respiratory paralysis caused by excessive acetylcholine that occurs in clients with myasthenia gravis. Signs and symptoms of cholinergic crisis include nausea, vomiting, abdominal cramping, diarrhea, blurred vision, pallor, facial muscle twitching, pupillary miosis, and hypotension. Cholinergic crisis is a result of overmedication with cholinergic (anticholinesterase) medications, and it is treated by withholding medications. Myasthenic crisis is an exacerbation of myasthenic symptoms caused by undermedication with anticholinesterase medications. There is no information in the question to support options 2, 3, and 4.

Test-Taking Strategy: Use the process of elimination. Note the client's diagnosis, and think about the treatment of this disorder. Recall the effects of cholinergic medications, and focus on the data in the question; this will direct you to option 1. Review the clinical manifestations associated with cholinergic crisis if you had difficulty with this question.

Reference

Linton, A. (2007). *Introduction to medical-surgical nursing* (4th ed., p. 455). Philadelphia: Saunders.

1445. A nurse determines that health teaching regarding arteriosclerosis has been successful when the client describes the condition as:

1 Hardening of the arteries
2 Increased elasticity of the veins
3 Fatty plaques lining the arteries
4 Loss of muscle mass around the heart

Level of Cognitive Ability: Comprehension
Client Needs: Health Promotion and Maintenance
Integrated Process: Teaching and Learning
Content Area: Fundamental Skills

Answer: 1

Rationale: Arteriosclerosis is described as a hardening of the arteries, and it is characterized by thickening, loss of elasticity, and calcification of the arterial walls. The condition can develop as a result of hyperlipidemia or other causes. Option 3 describes atherosclerosis, and option 4 is a normal age-related change in older individuals.

Test-Taking Strategy: Focus on the word *arteriosclerosis* to assist you with eliminating options 2 and 4. Recall that atherosclerosis relates to fatty plaques to direct you to option 1. Review these disorders if you had difficulty with this question.

Reference

deWit, S. (2009). *Medical-surgical nursing: Concepts & practice* (p. 441). St. Louis: Saunders.

1446. A nurse is collecting data from an Hispanic client regarding medication history. The nurse understands that people from this cultural group:

1 Do not permit blood transfusions
2 Often defer all questions to the male members of the family
3 Are offended if direct eye contact is made by the interviewer
4 Often use home remedies in addition to prescription medications

Level of Cognitive Ability: Comprehension
Client Needs: Psychosocial Integrity
Integrated Process: Nursing Process/Data Collection
Content Area: Fundamental Skills

Answer: 4

Rationale: Hispanic individuals commonly use folk healers and home remedies. Options 1, 2, and 3 are not common characteristics of this culture.

Test-Taking Strategy: Knowledge of the cultural practices of the Hispanic population is required to answer this question. Remember that Hispanic individuals commonly use folk healers and home remedies. Review Hispanic cultural practices if you had difficulty with this question.

Reference

Linton, A. (2007). *Introduction to medical-surgical nursing* (4th ed., p. 67). Philadelphia: Saunders.

1447. A client is seen in the health care clinic and diagnosed with conjunctivitis. The nurse provides the client with instructions about care of the disorder while at home. Which statement by the client indicates the need for further instruction?

1 "I do not need to be concerned about spreading this infection to others in my family."
2 "I can use an ophthalmic analgesic ointment at night as prescribed if I have eye discomfort."
3 "I should apply a warm compress before instilling antibiotic drops if purulent discharge is present in my eye."
4 "I should perform a saline eye irrigation before instilling the antibiotic drops into my eye if purulent discharge is present."

Answer: 1

Rationale: Conjunctivitis is an inflammation or infection of the conjunctiva of the eye, and it is highly contagious. Ophthalmic analgesic ointment or drops may be instilled, especially at bedtime, because discomfort becomes more noticeable when the eyelids are closed. Antibiotic drops are usually administered four times a day. When purulent discharge is present, saline eye irrigations or warm compresses to the eye may be necessary before instilling the medication.

Test-Taking Strategy: Use the process of elimination, and note the strategic words *need for further instruction.* These words indicate a negative event query and ask you to select an option that is an incorrect statement. Knowing that this disorder is considered to be highly contagious will direct you to option 1. Review the management of the client with conjunctivitis if you had difficulty with this question.

Level of Cognitive Ability: Comprehension
Client Needs: Safe and Effective Care Environment
Integrated Process: Nursing Process/Evaluation
Content Area: Adult Health/Eye

Reference

Linton, A. (2007). *Introduction to medical-surgical nursing* (4th ed., p. 1172). Philadelphia: Saunders.

1448. A nurse notes documentation of a stage 3 pressure ulcer in a client's record. Which of the following does the nurse expect to note during data collection for this client?

1 A deep ulcer that extends into the muscle and bone
2 An area in which the top layer of skin is missing
3 A deep ulcer that extends into the dermis and the subcutaneous tissue
4 A reddened area that returns to normal skin color after 15 to 20 minutes of pressure relief

Level of Cognitive Ability: Comprehension
Client Needs: Physiological Integrity
Integrated Process: Nursing Process/Data Collection
Content Area: Adult Health/Integumentary

Answer: 3

Rationale: A stage 3 pressure ulcer is a deep ulcer that extends into the dermis and the subcutaneous tissue. White, gray, or yellow eschar is usually present at the bottom of the ulcer, and the ulcer crater may have a lip or an edge. Purulent drainage is common. A stage 2 pressure ulcer is an area in which the top layer of skin is missing. A stage 1 pressure ulcer is a reddened area that returns to normal skin color after 15 to 20 minutes of pressure relief. A stage 4 pressure ulcer is a deep ulcer that extends into the muscle and bone.

Test-Taking Strategy: Use the process of elimination. Note the strategic words *stage 3 pressure ulcer,* and recall that there are four stages of pressure ulcers. Think about the description of each stage. Eliminate option 4 first because it is indicative of a stage 1 pressure ulcer, which is identified by the absence of a break in the skin. Focus on the words *top layer of skin is missing* to help you to eliminate option 2; this is a description of a stage 2 pressure ulcer. From the remaining options, select option 3 over option 1 because option 1 describes the most extensive degree of altered skin integrity and therefore identifies a stage 4 pressure ulcer. Review pressure ulcer stages if you had difficulty with this question.

Reference

Linton, A. (2007). *Introduction to medical-surgical nursing* (4th ed., pp. 316-317). Philadelphia: Saunders.

1449. A client with diabetes mellitus is brought to the urgent care center by the family. The client is lethargic and complains of a dry mouth and thirst. The skin is warm and dry, the skin turgor is poor, and the client has deep respirations and a fruity odor to the breath. Laboratory findings indicate the presence of serum ketones. The nurse concludes that the client is experiencing which complication of diabetes mellitus?

1 Hypoglycemia
2 Diabetic ketoacidosis
3 Stress-induced hypoglycemia
4 Hyperglycemic hyperosmolar nonketotic coma

Level of Cognitive Ability: Analysis
Client Needs: Physiological Integrity

Answer: 2

Rationale: Diabetic ketoacidosis is a complication of uncontrolled diabetes mellitus that is characterized by signs of dehydration (e.g., dry mouth, thirst, poor skin turgor). The client's neurological status declines as the serum glucose level rises. The pulse becomes rapid and weak, and the respirations become deep. The breath has a fruity or acetone odor to it. The client may also complain of abdominal pain, nausea, and vomiting. The presence of serum ketones is noted. Serum ketones are not present in hyperglycemic hyperosmolar nonketotic coma. The serum glucose level is lower than normal in hypoglycemia.

Test-Taking Strategy: Use the process of elimination. Eliminate options 1 and 3 first because they are comparable or alike. In addition, option 3 is not a clinical condition. From the remaining options, recall that a fruity odor to the breath and the presence of serum ketones characterize ketoacidosis to direct you to option 2. Review the signs of diabetic ketoacidosis if you had difficulty with this question.

Integrated Process: Nursing Process/Data Collection
Content Area: Adult Health/Endocrine

Reference

Christensen, B., & Kockrow, E. (2006). *Adult health nursing* (5th ed., p. 558). St. Louis: Mosby.

1450. A client with a head injury and a feeding tube continuously tries to pull out the tube. After receiving an order for restraints from the physician, which method should the nurse use to restrain the client?

1 Vest restraint
2 Mitten splints
3 Waist restraint
4 Wrist restraints

Level of Cognitive Ability: Application
Client Needs: Safe and Effective Care Environment
Integrated Process: Nursing Process/Implementation
Content Area: Adult Health/Neurological

Answer: 2

Rationale: Mitten splints are useful for this client because the client cannot pull against them and create resistance, which could lead to increased intracranial pressure. Vest and waist restraints prevent the client from getting up or falling out of bed but do nothing to limit hand movement. The client can pull against wrist restraints, thereby creating resistance.

Test-Taking Strategy: Use the process of elimination, and look for the option that safely limits hand movement. Eliminate options 1 and 3 first because they do not address the problem stated in the question. Recall the mechanisms and danger of increased intracranial pressure in a client with a head injury to direct you to option 2. Review the care of the client with a head injury if you had difficulty with this question.

References

Christensen, B., & Kockrow, E. (2006). *Adult health nursing* (5th ed., pp. 741-743). St. Louis: Mosby.
deWit, S. (2009). *Medical-surgical nursing: Concepts & practice* (p. 1149). St. Louis: Saunders.

1451. A licensed practical nurse (LPN) is preparing to assist a registered nurse (RN) with the insertion of an oropharyngeal airway into a client. The LPN understands that which of the following is the correct insertion procedure?

1 Flex the client's neck.
2 Leave any dentures in place.
3 Insert the airway with the tip pointed upward.
4 Suction the client's mouth once per shift after insertion.

Level of Cognitive Ability: Application
Client Needs: Physiological Integrity
Integrated Process: Nursing Process/Implementation
Content Area: Adult Health/Respiratory

Answer: 3

Rationale: An oropharyngeal airway of the appropriate size should be selected. The client should be positioned supine, with the neck hyperextended if possible. The airway is inserted with the tip facing upward and then rotated downward after the flange has reached the client's teeth. Any dentures or partial plates should be removed from the client's mouth before the insertion of an oropharyngeal airway. The client's mouth is suctioned every hour or as necessary after insertion.

Test-Taking Strategy: Use the process of elimination, and focus on the subject—the correct insertion procedure. Eliminate option 4 because this is not part of the insertion procedure. Eliminate option 1 next because the neck is hyperextended (unless contraindicated) to open the airway. Finally, recall that dentures should be removed because they are a potential source of airway obstruction. Review airway insertion if you had difficulty with this question.

Reference

Potter, P., & Perry, A. (2009) *Fundamentals of nursing* (7th ed., p. 942). St. Louis: Mosby.

1452. A nurse is caring for a client with a peptic ulcer. When assessing the client for gastrointestinal perforation, the nurse should monitor for which of the following?

Answer: 4

Rationale: Sudden severe abdominal pain is the sign that is most indicative of perforation. The pulse will most likely be weak and rapid when perforation occurs. Positive guaiac tests are not specific

1 Slow, strong pulses
2 Positive guaiac tests
3 Increased bowel sounds
4 Sudden severe abdominal pain

Level of Cognitive Ability: Comprehension
Client Needs: Physiological Integrity
Integrated Process: Nursing Process/Data Collection
Content Area: Adult Health/Gastrointestinal

to perforation and may be obtained from clients with other disorders. The nurse may be unable to hear bowel sounds when perforation of an ulcer occurs.

Test-Taking Strategy: Use the process of elimination and your knowledge of the signs of perforation. Correlate perforation with sudden severe abdominal pain. Note the words *sudden severe* to direct you to option 4. Review the signs of perforation if you had difficulty with this question.

Reference

Linton, A. (2007). *Introduction to medical-surgical nursing* (4th ed., p. 767). Philadelphia: Saunders.

1453. A nurse is caring for a client with a chest tube attached to closed chest drainage. The nurse determines that the client's lung has completely expanded if:
1 Pleuritic chest pain has resolved.
2 The oxygen saturation is more than 92%.
3 Fluctuation in the water-seal chamber has ceased.
4 Suction in the chest drainage system is no longer needed.

Level of Cognitive Ability: Analysis
Client Needs: Physiological Integrity
Integrated Process: Nursing Process/Evaluation
Content Area: Adult Health/Respiratory

Answer: 3
Rationale: When the lung has completely expanded, there is no longer air or fluid in the pleural space to be drained into the water-seal chamber. Thus, an indication that a chest tube is ready for removal is when fluctuation in the water-seal chamber and the drainage of fluid into the collection chamber have ceased. Although air is known to be an irritant to pleural tissue, the cessation of pleuritic pain may not occur when the lung is expanded. The chest tube acts as an irritant; therefore, it contributes to pain. Adequate oxygen saturation does not imply that the lung has fully reexpanded. The use or nonuse of suction in the chest drainage system is not necessarily governed by the degree of lung expansion. Suction is indicated when gravity is not sufficient to drain air and pleural fluid or if the client has a poor respiratory effort and cough. Suction increases the speed at which air and fluid are removed from the pleural space.

Test-Taking Strategy: Use the process of elimination, and note the strategic words *completely expanded*. These words and your knowledge of the functioning of chest tubes should direct you to the correct option. Remember that when the lung has completely expanded, there is no longer air or fluid in the pleural space to be drained into the water-seal chamber and fluctuation ceases. Review chest tube drainage systems if you had difficulty with this question.

Reference

Christensen, B., & Kockrow, E. (2006). *Adult health nursing* (5th ed., p. 439). St. Louis: Mosby.

1454. A client is admitted to the hospital with a tentative diagnosis of pernicious anemia. The nurse checks the client for which of the following symptoms of the disorder?
1 Constipation
2 Shortness of breath
3 Dusky mucous membranes
4 Red tongue that is smooth and sore

Answer: 4
Rationale: Pernicious anemia results from the lack of intrinsic factor, which is essential for the absorption of cyanocobalamin (vitamin B_{12}). Classic signs of pernicious anemia include weakness, mild diarrhea, and a smooth, sore, red tongue. The client may also have nervous system symptoms (e.g., paresthesias, difficulty with balance, occasional confusion). The mucous membranes do not become dusky, and the client does not exhibit shortness of breath.

Level of Cognitive Ability: Application
Client Needs: Physiological Integrity
Integrated Process: Nursing Process/Data Collection
Content Area: Fundamental Skills

Test-Taking Strategy: Focus on the client's diagnosis, and recall the pathophysiology associated with pernicious anemia. Remember that the classic signs of pernicious anemia include weakness, mild diarrhea, and a smooth, sore, red tongue. Review the signs and symptoms associated with pernicious anemia if you had difficulty with the question.

References

Christensen, B., & Kockrow, E. (2006). *Adult health nursing* (5th ed., p. 297). St. Louis: Mosby.
deWit, S. (2009). *Medical-surgical nursing: Concepts & practice* (p. 379). St. Louis: Saunders.

1455. One unit of packed red blood cells has been prescribed for a client postoperatively because the client's hemoglobin level is low. The physician prescribes diphenhydramine hydrochloride (Benadryl) to be dispensed before the administration of the transfusion. The nurse determines that this medication has been prescribed to:

1 Prevent a fever
2 Prevent an urticaria reaction
3 Assist with the absorption of the blood product
4 Promote the movement of the red blood cells into the bone marrow

Level of Cognitive Ability: Analysis
Client Needs: Physiological Integrity
Integrated Process: Nursing Process/Planning
Content Area: Pharmacology

Answer: 2
Rationale: An urticaria reaction is characterized by a rash accompanied by pruritus. This type of transfusion reaction is prevented by pretreating the client with an antihistamine (e.g., diphenhydramine). Options 1, 3, and 4 are incorrect. However, acetaminophen (Tylenol) may be prescribed before the administration of blood to assist with the prevention of an elevated temperature.

Test-Taking Strategy: Use the process of elimination, and eliminate options 3 and 4 first. Blood does not absorb or move into the bone marrow. Recall the classification of diphenhydramine to assist you with eliminating option 1. Review blood transfusion reactions and their management if you had difficulty with this question.

References

Christensen, B., & Kockrow, E. (2006). *Adult health nursing* (5th ed., p. 764). St. Louis: Mosby.
deWit, S. (2009). *Medical-surgical nursing: Concepts & practice* (p. 395). St. Louis: Saunders.

1456. A nurse is providing instructions to a female client about the procedure for collecting a midstream urine sample. Which client statement indicates an understanding of the procedure?

1 "I should douche before collecting the specimen."
2 "I should cleanse the perineum from front to back."
3 "I should collect the urine in the cup as soon as I begin to urinate."
4 "I can collect the specimen tonight and drop it off at the clinic in the morning."

Level of Cognitive Ability: Comprehension
Client Needs: Physiological Integrity
Integrated Process: Nursing Process/Evaluation
Content Area: Fundamental Skills

Answer: 2
Rationale: As part of the correct procedure, the client should cleanse the perineum from front to back with the antiseptic swabs that are packaged with the specimen kit. The client should begin the flow of urine and then collect the sample after starting the flow of urine. The specimen should be sent to the laboratory as soon as possible and not allowed to stand. Improper specimen handling can yield inaccurate test results. It is not normal procedure to douche before collecting the specimen.

Test-Taking Strategy: Use the process of elimination. Note the word *midstream* to assist you with eliminating option 3. Recall that the specimen should be brought to the laboratory after collection to assist you with eliminating option 4. Use basic principles related to hygiene to direct you to option 2 from the remaining options. Review the collection of a midstream urine sample if you had difficulty with this question.

Reference

Christensen, B., & Kockrow, E. (2006). *Foundations of nursing* (5th ed., pp. 503-504). St. Louis: Mosby.

1457. A client scheduled for bone marrow aspiration asks the nurse about possible sites that could be used for the procedure. The nurse tells the client that, in addition to the iliac crest, the test may be performed in which of the following areas?

1 The ribs
2 The femur
3 The scapula
4 The sternum

Level of Cognitive Ability: Application
Client Needs: Physiological Integrity
Integrated Process: Nursing Process/Implementation
Content Area: Fundamental Skills

Answer: 4

Rationale: The most common sites for bone marrow aspiration in the adult are the iliac crest and the sternum. These areas are rich in marrow and easily accessible for aspiration. The ribs, femur, and scapula are incorrect options.

> ***Test-Taking Strategy***: Focus on the diagnostic test. Recall the principles of anatomy and the concepts related to this test to direct you to option 4. Review bone marrow aspiration if you had difficulty with this question.

Reference

deWit, S. (2009). *Medical-surgical nursing: Concepts & practice* (p. 368). St. Louis: Saunders.

1458. The mother of a 3-year-old child calls a neighbor who is a nurse and tells the nurse that the child just ate mouse poison that was stored in a cabinet. The nurse instructs the mother to immediately:

1 Induce vomiting.
2 Call the child's physician.
3 Call the poison control center.
4 Call an ambulance to bring the child to the emergency department.

Level of Cognitive Ability: Application
Client Needs: Physiological Integrity
Integrated Process: Nursing Process/Implementation
Content Area: Child Health

Answer: 3

Rationale: The poison control center should be contacted immediately if a poisoning occurs. Vomiting should not be induced if the victim is unconscious or if the substance ingested was a strong corrosive or a petroleum product. Calling an ambulance or the physician should not be the immediate action because this will delay treatment. If the physician is called, he or she will immediately make a referral to the poison control center. The poison control center may advise the mother to bring the child to the emergency department; the mother should call an ambulance if this is the case.

> ***Test-Taking Strategy***: Use the process of elimination, and note the strategic word *immediately.* Options 2 and 4 delay treatment and are eliminated first. Recall that vomiting should not be induced without appropriate advice to do so to assist you with eliminating option 1. Review poison control measures if you had difficulty with this question.

Reference

Christensen, B., & Kockrow, E. (2006). *Foundations of nursing* (5th ed., pp. 367-368). St. Louis: Mosby.

1459. A client is admitted to the hospital with sickle cell crisis. The nurse monitors the client for which most frequent symptom of the disorder?

1 Pain
2 Diarrhea
3 Bradycardia
4 Blurred vision

Answer: 1

Rationale: Sickle cell crisis is an acute episodic condition that occurs with sickle cell anemia. Sickle cell crisis often causes pain in the bones and joints that is accompanied by joint swelling. Pain is a classic symptom of the disease. Severe pain may require large doses of opioid analgesics. The symptoms listed in options 2, 3, and 4 are not symptoms of sickle cell crisis.

Level of Cognitive Ability: Application
Client Needs: Physiological Integrity
Integrated Process: Nursing Process/Data Collection
Content Area: Fundamental Skills

Test-Taking Strategy: Use the process of elimination. Recall that the primary treatment of sickle cell crisis focuses on the administration of fluids and the management of pain to eliminate the incorrect options. Review the manifestations associated with sickle cell crisis if you had difficulty with this question.

Reference
Christensen, B., & Kockrow, E. (2006). *Adult health nursing* (5th ed., p. 303). St. Louis: Mosby.

1460. A nurse is caring for a client with a brain attack (stroke) who has unilateral neglect, and the nurse provides instructions to the family regarding home care. Which of the following would be included in the nurse's instructions?

1 Assist the client from the affected side.
2 Assist the client from the unaffected side.
3 Place personal items directly in front of the client.
4 Discourage the client from scanning the environment.

Level of Cognitive Ability: Application
Client Needs: Safe and Effective Care Environment
Integrated Process: Teaching and Learning
Content Area: Adult Health/Neurological

Answer: 1
Rationale: Unilateral neglect is a pattern of a lack of awareness of body parts, such as paralyzed arms or legs. Personal items are placed on the unaffected side initially, but thereafter the client's attention is focused to the affected side. The client is assisted from the affected side. The client is also cued to scan the entire environment.

Test-Taking Strategy: Use the process of elimination, and focus on the strategic words *unilateral neglect.* Remember the physiological alteration that occurs with unilateral neglect to direct you to option 1. Review the interventions associated with unilateral neglect if you had difficulty with this question.

Reference
Christensen, B., & Kockrow, E. (2006). *Adult health nursing* (5th ed., p. 733). St. Louis: Mosby.

1461. A nurse has provided discharge instructions to a client who has had surgery for lung cancer. The nurse determines that the client has not understood all of the essential elements of home management if the client verbalizes the need to:

1 Avoid exposure to crowds.
2 Deal with any increases in pain independently.
3 Sit up and lean forward to breathe more easily.
4 Call the physician if increased temperature or shortness of breath occurs.

Level of Cognitive Ability: Comprehension
Client Needs: Physiological Integrity
Integrated Process: Teaching and Learning
Content Area: Adult Health/Oncology

Answer: 2
Rationale: Health teaching includes using positions that facilitate respiration (e.g., sitting up, leaning forward), avoiding exposure to crowds or persons with respiratory infections, and reporting signs and symptoms of respiratory infection or an increase in pain. The client should not deal with any increases in pain independently.

Test-Taking Strategy: Use the process of elimination, and note the strategic words *client has not understood.* These words indicate a negative event query and ask you to select an option that is an incorrect statement. Recall that the client should report signs of infection, difficulty breathing, and increased pain to direct you to option 2. Review client teaching points after lung surgery if you had difficulty with this question.

Reference
deWit, S. (2009). *Medical-surgical nursing: Concepts & practice* (p. 340). St. Louis: Saunders.

1462. A nurse has assisted with providing an educational session about breast self-examination (BSE) to members of the

Answer: 2
Rationale: The best time to perform the BSE is 7 to 10 days after menses, when the breasts are not tender and swollen.

local community. Which client statement indicates the need for further instruction?

1 "I should perform the BSE every month."
2 "I should perform the BSE when I have my period."
3 "It is easiest to perform the BSE when I am in the shower and my hands are soapy."
4 "I'll use the finger pads of my three middle fingers to feel for lumps and thickening."

Level of Cognitive Ability: Comprehension
Client Needs: Health Promotion and Maintenance
Integrated Process: Teaching and Learning
Content Area: Adult Health/Oncology

Options 1, 3, and 4 identify accurate information regarding this important examination.

Test-Taking Strategy: Use the process of elimination, and note the strategic words *need for further instruction*. These words indicate a negative event query and ask you to select an option that is an incorrect statement. Recall that the breasts are tender and swollen during menses to direct you to option 2. Review the BSE if you had difficulty with this question.

References

deWit, S. (2009). *Medical-surgical nursing: Concepts & practice* (pp. 949-950). St. Louis: Saunders.

Linton, A. (2007). *Introduction to medical-surgical nursing* (4th ed., pp. 1038-1039). Philadelphia: Saunders.

1463. A nurse has given the client with a nonplaster (fiberglass) leg cast instructions regarding cast care at home. The nurse determines that the client requires further instruction if the client makes which of the following statements?

1 "I should avoid walking on wet, slippery floors."
2 "I'm not supposed to scratch the skin underneath the cast."
3 "It's OK to wipe dirt off the top of the cast with a damp cloth."
4 "If the cast gets wet, I can dry it with a hair dryer turned to a hot setting."

Level of Cognitive Ability: Comprehension
Client Needs: Safe and Effective Care Environment
Integrated Process: Teaching and Learning
Content Area: Adult Health/Musculoskeletal

Answer: 4

Rationale: Client instructions should include avoiding walking on wet, slippery floors to prevent falls. Surface soil on a cast may be removed with a damp cloth. If the cast gets wet, it can be dried with a hair dryer set to a cool setting to prevent skin breakdown. If the skin under the cast itches, cool air from a hair dryer may be used for relief. The client should never scratch under a cast because of the risk of skin breakdown and ulcer formation.

Test-Taking Strategy: Use the process of elimination, and note the strategic words *requires further instruction*. These words indicate a negative event query and ask you to select an option that is an incorrect statement. Noting the word *hot* in option 4 will direct you to this option. The client should never use a hair dryer on a cast or on the skin under the cast with the dryer set on the hot setting. Only cool settings are used to prevent burns. Review the care of the client with a cast if you had difficulty with this question.

References

Christensen, B., & Kockrow, E. (2006). *Adult health nursing* (5th ed., pp. 171-172). St. Louis: Mosby.

Linton, A. (2007). *Introduction to medical-surgical nursing* (4th ed., p. 922). Philadelphia: Saunders.

1464. A nurse has provided instructions about diet and fluid restriction to a client with chronic renal failure. The nurse determines that the client best understands the information presented if the client selects which of the following desserts from the dietary menu?

1 Jell-O
2 Sherbet

Answer: 4

Rationale: Dietary fluids include anything that is liquid at room temperature (e.g., ice cream, sherbet, Jell-O). When clients are on a fluid-restricted diet, it is helpful to avoid "hidden" fluids to whatever extent possible. This allows the client to drink more fluid, which can alleviate thirst.

3 Ice cream
4 Angel food cake

Level of Cognitive Ability: Comprehension
Client Needs: Physiological Integrity
Integrated Process: Nursing Process/Evaluation
Content Area: Adult Health/Renal

Test-Taking Strategy: Use the process of elimination, and remember that options that are comparable or alike are not likely to be correct. Evaluate each of the options, knowing that there is a greater amount of fluid in options 1, 2, and 3. In addition, these items are fluid at room temperature and therefore must be counted as fluid in the daily allotment. Review diet and fluid restrictions for the client with renal failure if you had difficulty with this question.

Reference

Linton, A. (2007). *Introduction to medical-surgical nursing* (4th ed., p. 876). Philadelphia: Saunders.

1465. A nurse is planning to teach a client with a leg cast how to stand on crutches. The nurse plans to tell the client to place the crutches:

1 3 inches to the front and side of the client's toes
2 8 inches to the front and side of the client's toes
3 15 inches to the front and side of the client's toes
4 20 inches to the front and side of the client's toes

Level of Cognitive Ability: Application
Client Needs: Physiological Integrity
Integrated Process: Teaching and Learning
Content Area: Adult Health/Musculoskeletal

Answer: 2

Rationale: The classic tripod position is taught to the client before instructions about gait are given. The crutches are placed anywhere from 6 to 10 inches in front and to the side of the client, depending on the client's body size. This provides a wide enough base of support to the client and improves balance. Options 1, 3, and 4 are incorrect.

Test-Taking Strategy: Use the process of elimination. Three inches (option 1) and 20 inches (option 4) seem excessively short and long, respectively, so these two options should be eliminated first. From the remaining options, 8 inches seems more in keeping with the normal length of a stride for someone wearing a cast than does 15 inches. Review the procedure for standing with crutches if you had difficulty with this question.

Reference

deWit, S. (2009). *Medical-surgical nursing: Concepts & practice* (pp. 779-781). St. Louis: Saunders.

1466. A nurse is providing instructions to a client who is beginning therapy with digoxin (Lanoxin). The nurse would teach the client to:

1 Take the pulse daily.
2 Monitor the blood pressure once a week.
3 Have electrolyte levels drawn weekly.
4 Measure the weight each morning before breakfast.

Level of Cognitive Ability: Application
Client Needs: Physiological Integrity
Integrated Process: Teaching and Learning
Content Area: Pharmacology

Answer: 1

Rationale: Digoxin (Lanoxin) is a cardiac glycoside and an antidysrhythmic medication. Clients taking digoxin should take the pulse each day and notify the physician if the heart rate drops below 60 beats/min or exceeds 100 beats/min. Options 2, 3, and 4 are not necessary.

Test-Taking Strategy: Use the process of elimination. Digoxin is not an antihypertensive medication, so eliminate option 2 first. The client may need to weigh daily for the condition that requires the digoxin therapy, but it is not absolutely necessary for the safe use of the medication. Weekly electrolyte levels are excessive, which leaves option 1. In addition, this is a "golden rule" of digoxin therapy. Review digoxin if you had difficulty with this question.

Reference

deWit, S. (2009). *Medical-surgical nursing: Concepts & practice* (p. 474). St. Louis: Saunders.

1467. Cyclophosphamide (Cytoxan, Neosar) is prescribed for a client with breast cancer, and the nurse provides instructions to the client about the medication. Which client statement indicates the need for further instruction?

1 "If I lose my hair, it will grow back."
2 "If I develop a sore throat, I should notify the physician."
3 "I should limit my fluid intake while taking this medication."
4 "I should avoid contact with anyone who recently had a live virus vaccine."

Level of Cognitive Ability: Analysis
Client Needs: Physiological Integrity
Integrated Process: Teaching and Learning
Content Area: Pharmacology

Answer: 3

Rationale: Cyclophosphamide is an antineoplastic medication. Hemorrhagic cystitis is an adverse reaction that is associated with this medication. The client should be instructed to consume copious amounts of fluid during therapy. The client's hair will grow back, although it may have a different color and texture. A sore throat may be an indication of an infection and should be reported to the physician. Avoiding contact with persons who recently had a live virus vaccine is important because cyclophosphamide produces immunosuppression, thus placing the client at risk for infection.

Test-Taking Strategy: Use the process of elimination, and note the strategic words *need for further instruction.* These words indicate a negative event query and ask you to select an option that is an incorrect statement. Recall that this medication causes hemorrhagic cystitis and that fluids are important with this therapy to direct you to option 3. Review the adverse effects of cyclophosphamide if you had difficulty with this question.

Reference

Hodgson, B., & Kizior, R. (2009). *Saunders nursing drug handbook 2009* (p. 297). Philadelphia: Saunders.

1468. A nurse has taught the principles of foot care to a client with diabetes mellitus. The nurse determines that the client understood the information if the client states the need to:

1 Cut the toenails down to the cuticle.
2 Wear shoes that are closed at the heel and toe.
3 Put a hot water bottle on the feet if they become cold.
4 Apply lotion to areas of dry skin between the toes.

Level of Cognitive Ability: Comprehension
Client Needs: Physiological Integrity
Integrated Process: Nursing Process/Evaluation
Content Area: Adult Health/Endocrine

Answer: 2

Rationale: The client should wear shoes that are closed at the heel and toe to prevent injury to the feet. The client should avoid other potential sources of injury to the feet. The application of direct heat to the feet could cause burns, and the application of lotion between the toes could cause skin breakdown. The toenails should be cut straight across at the level of the contour of the toe. Other general foot care measures include inspecting the feet daily, cleaning them with mild soap, rinsing and drying them well, and using lanolin-based lotions (except between the toes).

Test-Taking Strategy: Use the process of elimination. Recall concerns related to skin integrity in a client with diabetes mellitus to direct you to option 2. Review diabetic foot care if you had difficulty with this question.

References

deWit, S. (2009). *Medical-surgical nursing: Concepts & practice* (p. 927). St. Louis: Saunders.
Linton, A. (2007). *Introduction to medical-surgical nursing* (4th ed., p. 1006). Philadelphia: Saunders.

1469. A nurse is planning to teach a client with a below-the-knee amputation about skin care to prevent breakdown. Which of the following points would the nurse include in the teaching plan?

1 The residual limb is washed gently and dried every other day.
2 The socket of the prosthesis must be dried carefully before use.

Answer: 2

Rationale: A residual limb sock must be worn at all times to absorb perspiration, and it is changed daily. The residual limb is washed, dried, and inspected for breakdown twice each day. The socket of the prosthesis is cleansed with a mild soap and rinsed and dried carefully each day. A bactericidal agent would not be used.

3 The socket of the prosthesis is washed with a bactericidal agent daily.
4 A residual limb sock must be worn at all times and changed twice a week.

Level of Cognitive Ability: Application
Client Needs: Physiological Integrity
Integrated Process: Teaching and Learning
Content Area: Adult Health/Musculoskeletal

Test-Taking Strategy: Use the process of elimination. Recall that the residual limb is cared for twice a day. With this in mind, eliminate options 1 and 4. From the remaining options, recall that a mild soap is used to wash the prosthesis to direct you to option 2. Review the teaching points for a client after a below-the-knee amputation if you had difficulty with this question.

References

deWit, S. (2009). *Medical-surgical nursing: Concepts & practice* (p. 812). St. Louis: Saunders.
Linton, A. (2007). *Introduction to medical-surgical nursing* (4th ed., p. 944). Philadelphia: Saunders.

1470. A nurse is teaching a client with cholecystitis about foods that must be eliminated from the diet. The nurse tells the client that which food is acceptable to eat?
1 Donuts
2 Baked fish
3 French fries
4 Fried chicken

Level of Cognitive Ability: Application
Client Needs: Physiological Integrity
Integrated Process: Nursing Process/Implementation
Content Area: Adult Health/Gastrointestinal

Answer: 2
Rationale: Cholecystitis is an acute or chronic inflammation of the gallbladder. The client with cholecystitis should decrease the overall intake of dietary fat. Foods that should be avoided include sauces, gravies, fatty meats, fried foods, products made with cream, and heavy desserts. The correct answer is baked fish, which is low in fat.

Test-Taking Strategy: Use the process of elimination, and recall that clients with cholecystitis should decrease their fat intake; this will direct you to option 2. Review food items that are high in fat if you had difficulty with this question.

References

Linton, A. (2007). *Introduction to medical-surgical nursing* (4th ed., pp. 822-823). Philadelphia: Saunders.
Nix, S. (2009). *Williams' basic nutrition and diet therapy* (13th ed., p. 360). St. Louis: Mosby.

1471. The nurse has taught a client who has been newly diagnosed with diabetes mellitus about blood glucose monitoring. The nurse determines that the client understands the information if the client states the need to report blood glucose levels that exceed:
1 350 mg/dL
2 250 mg/dL
3 200 mg/dL
4 150 mg/dL

Level of Cognitive Ability: Comprehension
Client Needs: Physiological Integrity
Integrated Process: Nursing Process/Evaluation
Content Area: Adult Health/Endocrine

Answer: 2
Rationale: It is standard practice to teach the client to report blood glucose levels that exceed 250 mg/dL unless otherwise instructed by the physician. The values in options 3 and 4 are too low to require reporting, and the value in option 1 is too high.

Test-Taking Strategy: Knowledge of the aspects of client teaching for blood glucose monitoring is needed to answer this question correctly. Remember that it is standard practice to teach the client to report blood glucose levels that exceed 250 mg/dL unless otherwise instructed by the physician. Review teaching points for the client with diabetes mellitus if you had difficulty with this question.

Reference

deWit, S. (2009). *Medical-surgical nursing: Concepts & practice* (p. 927). St. Louis: Saunders.

1472. A client with hyperaldosteronism has undergone unilateral adrenalectomy. The nurse includes which of the following items in the postoperative teaching?

Answer: 2
Rationale: The client who has undergone unilateral adrenalectomy must take replacement corticosteroids for up to 2 years after surgery. This allows the remaining gland to resume

1 Diuretics must be taken for life.
2 Glucocorticoids will be needed temporarily.
3 The client is likely to experience hypertension.
4 The client needs to strictly adhere to a low-sodium diet.

Level of Cognitive Ability: Application
Client Needs: Physiological Integrity
Integrated Process: Teaching and Learning
Content Area: Adult Health/Endocrine

function after being suppressed by the excessive hormone production of the diseased gland. Diuretics and a low-sodium diet are used during the preoperative period to manage hypertension; after surgery has been performed, these measures are no longer required.

Test-Taking Strategy: Use the process of elimination, and focus on the anatomical location of the surgery. Note the strategic word *unilateral* to direct you to option 2. Glucocorticoids are only needed temporarily with unilateral adrenalectomy. Review postoperative care after unilateral adrenalectomy if you had difficulty with this question.

Reference

Linton, A. (2007). *Introduction to medical-surgical nursing* (4th ed., p. 976). Philadelphia: Saunders.

1473. The nurse reviews an adult client's laboratory results and reports which abnormal value to the physician?

CLIENT'S CHART

Laboratory	Medications	Progress Notes
Calcium 9 mg/dL		
Potassium 4.0 mEq/L		
Magnesium 2.0 mg/dL		
Blood urea nitrogen 45 mg/dL		

1 Calcium
2 Potassium
3 Magnesium
4 Blood urea nitrogen

Level of Cognitive Ability: Application
Client Needs: Physiological Integrity
Integrated Process: Nursing Process/Implementation
Content Area: Adult Health/Endocrine

Answer: 4
Rationale: The normal calcium level is 8.6 to 10 mg/dL. The normal magnesium level is 1.8 to 3.0 mg/dL. The normal potassium level is 3.5 to 5.1 mEq/L. The normal blood urea nitrogen level is 5 to 20 mg/dL.

Test-Taking Strategy: Focus on the subject—the abnormal laboratory value. Remember that the normal blood urea nitrogen level is 5 to 20 mg/dL. Review these normal laboratory values if you had difficulty with this question.

Reference

Christensen, B., & Kockrow, E. (2006). *Adult health nursing* (5th ed., p. 472). St. Louis: Mosby.

1474. A client is being discharged home after subtotal gastrectomy. The nurse teaches the client to do which of the following to minimize the risk of dumping syndrome?
1 Sit up for 2 hours after eating.
2 Eat only two large meals a day.
3 Avoid drinking liquids during a meal.
4 Eat highly concentrated carbohydrate foods.

Level of Cognitive Ability: Application
Client Needs: Physiological Integrity

Answer: 3
Rationale: Dumping syndrome is experienced by clients who have had a subtotal gastrectomy. Symptoms include profuse sweating, nausea, dizziness, and weakness. To minimize the risk for the condition, the client should avoid taking liquids with meals and should not consume high-carbohydrate food sources. The client should lie down for at least 30 minutes after eating; eat small, frequent meals; and sit semirecumbent while eating. Antispasmodic medications may be prescribed as needed to delay gastric emptying.

Integrated Process: Teaching and Learning
Content Area: Adult Health/Gastrointestinal

Test-Taking Strategy: Use the process of elimination. Note the name of the disorder, and recall the pathophysiology associated with dumping syndrome; this will direct you to option 3. Review the client teaching points related to dumping syndrome if you had difficulty with this question.

Reference
Christensen, B., & Kockrow, E. (2006). *Adult health nursing* (5th ed., p. 218). St. Louis: Mosby.

1475. A physician's order for an adult client reads: Acetaminophen (Tylenol) liquid, 450 mg orally every 4 hours PRN for pain. The medication label reads: 160 mg/5 mL. The nurse prepares how many milliliters to administer one dose?

Answer: _____ mL

Level of Cognitive Ability: Application
Client Needs: Physiological Integrity
Integrated Process: Nursing Process/Implementation
Content Area: Fundamental Skills

Answer: 14 mL
Rationale: Use the formula for calculating medication dosages.
Formula:

$$\frac{\text{Desired}}{\text{Available}} \times \text{Volume} = \text{mL per dose}$$

$$\frac{450\text{mg}}{160\text{mg}} \times 5\text{ mL} = 14\text{ mL}$$

Test-Taking Strategy: Identify the strategic components of the question and what the question is asking. In this case, the question asks for the number of milliliters per one dose. Set up the formula, knowing that the desired dose is 450 mg and that the medication that is available contains 160 mg per 5 mL. Verify the answer with a calculator. Review medication calculations if you had difficulty with this question.

Reference
Kee, J., & Marshall, S. (2009). *Clinical calculations: With applications to general and specialty areas* (6th ed., p. 86). Philadelphia: Saunders.

1476. A client is being discharged home from the hospital after an episode of acute pancreatitis. The nurse would teach the client to call the physician if pain returns in which of the following areas?
1 Epigastric area and radiating to the back
2 Left lower quadrant and radiating to the hip
3 Epigastric area and radiating to the umbilicus
4 Left lower quadrant and radiating to the groin

Level of Cognitive Ability: Application
Client Needs: Physiological Integrity
Integrated Process: Teaching and Learning
Content Area: Adult Health/Gastrointestinal

Answer: 1
Rationale: Pancreatitis is an inflammatory condition of the pancreas that may be acute or chronic. The nurse teaches the client to report the recurrence of pain experienced with pancreatitis. This pain is often severe and unrelenting; it is located in the epigastric region, and it radiates to the back. Options 2, 3, and 4 are incorrect.

Test-Taking Strategy: Use the process of elimination. Because the pain of pancreatitis radiates to the back, it is a little easier to distinguish this pain from other gastrointestinal disorders. Consider the anatomical location of the pancreas to direct you to option 1. Review the signs and symptoms of acute pancreatitis if you had difficulty with this question.

Reference
Christensen, B., & Kockrow, E. (2006). *Adult health nursing* (5th ed., p. 278). St. Louis: Mosby.

1477. A nurse assigned to a client with a stroke who has left homonymous hemianopsia is planning measures to help the client overcome the deficit. The nurse should plan to do which of the following to assist the client with rehabilitation?

1 Place objects in the client's left field of vision.
2 Approach the client from the left field of vision.
3 Remind the client to turn the head to scan the left visual field.
4 Discourage the client from wearing his or her own eyeglasses.

Level of Cognitive Ability: Application
Client Needs: Physiological Integrity
Integrated Process: Nursing Process/Planning
Content Area: Adult Health/Neurological

Answer: 3

Rationale: Homonymous hemianopsia is the loss of one half of the visual field. The client with homonymous hemianopsia should have objects placed in the intact field of vision, and the nurse should also approach the client from the intact side. The nurse instructs the client to scan the environment to overcome the visual deficit and performs client teaching from within the intact field of vision. The nurse encourages the use of personal eyeglasses, if they are available.

Test-Taking Strategy: Use the process of elimination. To answer this question accurately, you must be able to distinguish between homonymous hemianopsia and unilateral neglect. Clients are approached differently with these two deficits. However, the similarity is that the client must be taught to scan the environment; this will direct you to option 3. Review the care of the client with homonymous hemianopsia and review the differences between homonymous hemianopsia and unilateral neglect if you had difficulty with this question.

References

Christensen, B., & Kockrow, E. (2006). *Adult health nursing* (5th ed., p. 730). St. Louis: Mosby.
Ignatavicius, D., & Workman, M. (2010). *Medical-surgical nursing: Patient-centered collaborative care* (6th ed., p. 1035). St. Louis: Saunders.

1478. A nurse is reviewing the laboratory analysis of cerebrospinal fluid (CSF) obtained during a lumbar puncture from a child who is suspected of having bacterial meningitis. Which of the following results would most likely confirm this diagnosis?

1 Clear CSF with low protein and low glucose
2 Cloudy CSF with low protein and low glucose
3 Cloudy CSF with high protein and low glucose
4 Decreased pressure and cloudy CSF with high protein

Level of Cognitive Ability: Analysis
Client Needs: Physiological Integrity
Integrated Process: Nursing Process/Data Collection
Content Area: Child Health

Answer: 3

Rationale: A diagnosis of meningitis is made after testing CSF obtained by lumbar puncture. In the case of bacterial meningitis, the findings usually include increased pressure, cloudy CSF, high protein, and low glucose. Options 1, 2, and 4 are incorrect.

Test-Taking Strategy: Use the process of elimination. Eliminate options 1 and 4 first because clear CSF and decreased pressure are not likely to be found with an infectious process such as meningitis. From the remaining options, recall that high protein indicates a possible diagnosis of meningitis to direct you to option 3. Review the analysis of CSF from lumbar puncture if you had difficulty with this question.

Reference

Christensen, B., & Kockrow, E. (2006). *Foundations of nursing* (5th ed., p. 1047). St. Louis: Mosby.

1479. A mother brings her child to the health care clinic for a routine exam. The mother tells the nurse that the teacher has reported that the child appears to be daydreaming and staring off into space and that this occurs numerous times throughout the day. The nurse reports

Answer: 2

Rationale: Absence seizures are a type of generalized seizure. They consist of a sudden, brief arrest (no longer than 30 seconds) of the child's motor activities that is accompanied by a blank stare and a loss of awareness. The child returns to activity that was in process as though nothing happened. School phobia includes physical symptoms that usually occur at home and that may prevent the

the findings to the registered nurse and suspects that which of the following is occurring with this child?
1 The child probably has school phobia.
2 The child is experiencing absence seizures.
3 The child is showing signs of a behavioral problem.
4 The child has attention-deficit/hyperactivity disorder (ADHD) and is in need of medication.

Level of Cognitive Ability: Application
Client Needs: Physiological Integrity
Integrated Process: Nursing Process/Implementation
Content Area: Child Health

child from attending school. Behavior problems would be noted by more overt symptoms than described in this question. A child with ADHD becomes easily distracted, is fidgety, and has difficulty following instructions.

Test-Taking Strategy: Use the process of elimination, and focus on the information in the question. Note the words *daydreaming and staring off into space* to direct you to option 2. Review the characteristics associated with absence seizures if you had difficulty with this question.

Reference
Price, D., & Gwin, J. (2008). *Pediatric nursing: An introductory text* (10th ed., p. 253). St. Louis: Saunders.

1480. The nurse is sending an arterial blood gas (ABG) specimen to the laboratory for analysis. Which of the following pieces of information should the nurse write on the laboratory requisition? Select all that apply.
❒ 1 Ventilator settings
❒ 2 Client allergies
❒ 3 Client temperature
❒ 4 Date and time the specimen was drawn
❒ 5 Details about any supplemental oxygen that the client is receiving
❒ 6 Extremity from which the specimen was obtained

Level of Cognitive Ability: Application
Client Needs: Physiological Integrity
Integrated Process: Communication and Documentation
Content Area: Adult Health/Respiratory

Answer: 1, 3, 4, 5
Rationale: An ABG requisition usually contains information about the date and time that the specimen was drawn, the client's temperature, whether the specimen was drawn on room air or with the client using supplemental oxygen, and the ventilator settings if the client is on a mechanical ventilator. The client's allergies and the extremity from which the specimen was drawn do not have a direct bearing on the laboratory results.

Test-Taking Strategy: Review the pieces of information from the viewpoint of the relevance of the item to the client's airway status or oxygen use. The only pieces of information that do not relate to airway status or oxygen use are the client's allergies and the extremity from which the specimen was drawn. Review the procedure related to drawing ABGs if you had difficulty with this question.

Reference
Chernecky, C., & Berger, B. (2008). *Laboratory tests and diagnostic procedures* (5th ed., pp. 210-214). Philadelphia: Saunders.

1481. A postoperative client is anemic from blood loss that occurred during the procedure. The nurse determines that which of the following exhibited by the client is most likely attributable to the anemia?
1 Fatigue
2 Bradycardia
3 Muscle cramps
4 Increased respiratory rate

Level of Cognitive Ability: Comprehension
Client Needs: Physiological Integrity
Integrated Process: Nursing Process/Data Collection
Content Area: Fundamental Skills

Answer: 1
Rationale: The client with anemia is likely to complain of fatigue caused by the decreased ability of the body to carry oxygen to tissues to meet metabolic demands. The client is likely to have tachycardia (not bradycardia) because of the body's efforts to compensate for the effects of the anemia. Muscle cramps and increased respiratory rate are not associated findings, although some clients may have shortness of breath.

Test-Taking Strategy: Use the process of elimination. Recall that anemia causes a reduction in oxygen-carrying capacity to direct you to option 1. Review the manifestations of anemia if you had difficulty with this question.

Reference

Christensen, B., & Kockrow, E. (2006). *Adult health nursing* (5th ed., p. 295). St. Louis: Mosby.

1482. A nurse is collecting data from a client who is taking prazosin (Minipress). Which client statement supports the nursing diagnosis of *Noncompliance* related to medication therapy?

1 "If I feel dizzy, I'll skip my dose for a few days."
2 "I can't see the numbers on the label to know how much salt is in food."
3 "I don't understand why I have to keep taking the pills when my blood pressure is normal."
4 "If I have a cold, I shouldn't take any over-the-counter remedies without consulting my doctor."

Level of Cognitive Ability: Analysis
Client Needs: Physiological Integrity
Integrated Process: Nursing Process/Evaluation
Content Area: Pharmacology

Answer: 1

Rationale: Prazosin (Minipress) is an antihypertensive medication. Side effects of prazosin are dizziness and impotence, and the client should be instructed to call the physician if these side effects occur. Holding (skipping) medication causes an abrupt rise in blood pressure. Option 2 indicates a self-care deficit. Option 3 indicates a knowledge deficit. Option 4 indicates client understanding of the medication.

Test-Taking Strategy: Use the process of elimination and focus on the nursing diagnosis to select the correct option. Noting the strategic words *I'll skip my dose* should direct you to option 1. Review the defining characteristics of *Noncompliance* if you had difficulty with this question.

Reference

Hodgson, B., & Kizior, R. (2009). *Saunders nursing drug handbook 2009* (p. 949). Philadelphia: Saunders.

1483. A client is admitted to the hospital with chest pain, and a myocardial infarction is suspected. The nurse informs the client about the importance of notifying a staff member immediately if pain occurs, knowing that the most common psychosocial reaction exhibited by clients with initial chest pain is:

1 Anger
2 Denial
3 Hostility
4 Depression

Level of Cognitive Ability: Comprehension
Client Needs: Psychosocial Integrity
Integrated Process: Nursing Process/Implementation
Content Area: Adult Health/Cardiovascular

Answer: 2

Rationale: Most clients who experience chest discomfort use rationalization and deny that they are experiencing pain. Anger, depression, and hostility may occur, but denial and rationalization are the most common reactions.

Test-Taking Strategy: Focus on the subject—the most common psychosocial reaction exhibited by clients with initial chest pain. Remember that denial is the most common defense mechanism exhibited by clients with chest pain. Review the psychosocial impact of chest pain and cardiac disease if you had difficulty with this question.

Reference

Linton, A. (2007). *Introduction to medical-surgical nursing* (4th ed., pp. 1240, 1242). Philadelphia: Saunders.

1484. A nurse is monitoring a client who is receiving a blood transfusion. The client begins to complain of a sweaty and warm feeling and a backache. The nurse notes that the client's skin is flushed and suspects that the client is having a transfusion reaction. The nurse understands that the immediate

Answer: 4

Rationale: If a transfusion reaction is suspected, the transfusion is stopped, and then normal saline is infused pending further physician orders. This maintains a patent IV access line and aids in maintaining the client's intravascular volume. The IV line is not removed because IV access is needed. Normal saline is the solution of choice instead of solutions that contain dextrose because saline does not cause the red blood cells to clump.

action is to stop the blood transfusion and then:
1 Remove the intravenous (IV) line.
2 Hang an IV bag of 5% dextrose in water.
3 Change the continuous IV to an intermittent needle device.
4 Hang an IV bag of normal saline and infuse it to keep the vein open.

Level of Cognitive Ability: Application
Client Needs: Physiological Integrity
Integrated Process: Nursing Process/Implementation
Content Area: Fundamental Skills

Test-Taking Strategy: Use the process of elimination and your knowledge of blood transfusions to answer the question. Eliminate options 1 and 3 first, knowing that the client requires fluid to maintain intravascular volume. To select from the remaining options, remember that normal saline is used when administering blood. Review blood transfusion reactions if you had difficulty with this question.

Reference

Linton, A. (2007). *Introduction to medical-surgical nursing* (4th ed., p. 581). Philadelphia: Saunders.

1485. A nurse is assigned to assist with caring for a client who is at risk for self-harm. The client says, "You won't have to worry about me much longer." The nurse interprets this statement as:
1 The intention of suicide
2 An expression of depression
3 The expression of hopelessness
4 The intention of self-mutilation

Level of Cognitive Ability: Comprehension
Client Needs: Psychosocial Integrity
Integrated Process: Nursing Process/Evaluation
Content Area: Mental Health

Answer: 1
Rationale: The client at risk for self-harm who says he or she will not be around much longer is expressing suicidal intent. An individual who is depressed is frequently suicidal. The individual with suicidal tendencies frequently performs self-mutilating acts. However, the client's statement is a direct comment about the act. Although hopelessness is associated with a risk for self-harm, the client's statement clearly indicates the intention of suicide.

Test-Taking Strategy: Use the process of elimination. Focus on the client's statement to direct you to option 1. Review the signs of suicide if you had difficulty with this question.

Reference

Linton, A. (2007). *Introduction to medical-surgical nursing* (4th ed., pp. 162-163). Philadelphia: Saunders.

1486. A nurse reviews home-care management instructions with a client who was recently diagnosed with cirrhosis. Which client statement indicates the need for further instruction?
1 "I will obtain adequate rest."
2 "I can include some fat in my diet."
3 "I will take Tylenol if I get a headache."
4 "I should monitor my weight on a regular basis."

Level of Cognitive Ability: Comprehension
Client Needs: Physiological Integrity
Integrated Process: Teaching and Learning
Content Area: Adult Health/Gastrointestinal

Answer: 3
Rationale: Acetaminophen (Tylenol) is avoided because it can cause fatal liver damage in the client with cirrhosis. Adequate rest and nutrition are important. Fat restriction is not necessary, and the diet should supply sufficient carbohydrates, with a total daily intake of 2000 to 3000 calories. The client's weight should be monitored on a regular basis.

Test-Taking Strategy: Note the strategic words *need for further instruction*. These words indicate a negative event query and ask you to select an option that is an incorrect statement. Options 1 and 4 can be easily eliminated. Recall that acetaminophen is hepatotoxic to direct you to option 3. Review the medications that are restricted or avoided in clients with cirrhosis if you had difficulty with this question.

Reference

Christensen, B., & Kockrow, E. (2006). *Adult health nursing* (5th ed., pp. 258-259). St. Louis: Mosby.

1487. A client with a history of gout is also diagnosed with urolithiasis, and the stones are determined to be of the uric acid type. The nurse gives the client instructions to limit the intake of which food item?

1 Milk
2 Liver
3 Apples
4 Carrots

Level of Cognitive Ability: Application
Client Needs: Physiological Integrity
Integrated Process: Teaching and Learning
Content Area: Fundamental Skills

Answer: 2

Rationale: Foods that contain high amounts of purines should be limited or avoided in the client with uric acid stones. This includes limiting or avoiding organ meats, such as liver, brain, heart, kidney, and sweetbreads. Other foods to avoid include herring, sardines, anchovies, meat extracts, consommés, and gravies. Foods that are low in purines include all fruits, many vegetables, milk, cheese, eggs, refined cereals, sugars and sweets, coffee, tea, chocolate, and carbonated beverages.

Test-Taking Strategy: Note the strategic word *limit.* To answer this question, begin by examining the options and classifying the types of food sources that they represent. Options 3 and 4 represent foods that are grown, whereas options 1 and 2 represent foods that are derived from animal sources. Because purines are end products of protein metabolism, eliminate options 3 and 4 first. From the remaining options, you would need to know that organ meats (e.g., liver) provide a greater quantity of protein than milk does. With this in mind, choose option 2 as the food to limit. Review foods that are high in purine if you had difficulty with this question.

References

Christensen, B., & Kockrow, E. (2006). *Adult health nursing* (5th ed., p. 490). St. Louis: Mosby.

Linton, A. (2007). *Introduction to medical-surgical nursing* (4th ed., p. 908). Philadelphia: Saunders.

1488. A client tells the nurse that the client gets dizzy and lightheaded with each use of the incentive spirometer. The nurse asks the client to demonstrate the use of the device, expecting that the client is:

1 Inhaling too slowly
2 Rebreathing exhaled air
3 Not resting adequately between breaths
4 Not forming a tight seal around the mouthpiece

Level of Cognitive Ability: Comprehension
Client Needs: Physiological Integrity
Integrated Process: Nursing Process/Evaluation
Content Area: Adult Health/Respiratory
Answer: 3

Rationale: If the client does not breathe normally between incentive spirometer breaths, hyperventilation and fatigue can result. Hyperventilation is the most common cause of respiratory alkalosis, which is characterized by lightheadedness and dizziness. Options 1, 2, and 4 are not actions that would result in dizziness or lightheadedness. Options 1 and 4 would result in ineffective use, and option 2 would result in confusion.

Test-Taking Strategy: Focus on the subject—the cause of the lightheadedness and dizziness. To answer this question, evaluate each of the possible options to see if they would be expected to cause dizziness or lightheadedness in the client. Only option 3 would result in hyperventilation and subsequent dizziness or lightheadedness. Review the appropriate use of an incentive spirometer if you had difficulty with this question.

References

Christensen, B., & Kockrow, E. (2006). *Adult health nursing* (5th ed., pp. 32-33). St. Louis: Mosby.

deWit, S. (2009). *Medical-surgical nursing: Concepts & practice* (p. 79). St. Louis: Saunders.

1489. A physician orders 0.05 g of pentobarbital (Nembutal) orally at the hour of sleep. The medication label reads: pentobarbital 50-mg capsules. How many

Answer: 1 capsule

Rationale: Convert 0.05 g to milligrams. In the metric system, to convert larger to smaller, multiply by 1000 or move the decimal three places to the right. Then, use the following formula.

capsule(s) should the nurse administer to the client?

Answer: _____ capsule(s)

Level of Cognitive Ability: Application
Client Needs: Physiological Integrity
Integrated Process: Nursing Process/Implementation
Content Area: Fundamental Skills

0.05 g = 50 mg

$$\frac{\text{Desired}}{\text{Available}} \times \text{Quantity} = \text{Capsule(s)}$$

$$\frac{50\text{mg}}{50\text{mg}} \times 1\text{ Capsule} = 1\text{ Capsule}$$

Test-Taking Strategy: Use the formula for the calculation of a medication. Remember to convert grams to milligrams. Follow the formula, and ensure that the calculated dose makes sense. Recheck your answer with a calculator. Review medication conversions and calculations if you had difficulty with this question.

Reference

Potter, P., & Perry, A. (2009) *Fundamentals of nursing* (7th ed., pp. 697-700). St. Louis: Mosby.

1490. A nurse is participating in a health screening clinic. The nurse interprets that which of the following clients has the greatest need for instruction to lower the risk of developing respiratory disease?

1 A 36-year-old who works with pesticides
2 A 40-year-old smoker who works in a hospital
3 A 25-year-old who does woodworking as a hobby
4 A 50-year-old smoker with cracked asbestos lining of the basement pipes in the home

Level of Cognitive Ability: Analysis
Client Needs: Health Promotion and Maintenance
Integrated Process: Nursing Process/Data Collection
Content Area: Adult Health/Respiratory

Answer: 4
Rationale: Smoking greatly enhances the client's risk of developing some form of respiratory disease. Other risk factors include exposure to harmful chemicals, airborne toxins, dust, and fumes. Although all of the clients identified in the options require instruction to lower the risk of developing respiratory disease, the client at greatest risk has two identified risk factors, one of which is smoking.

Test-Taking Strategy: Begin to answer this question by eliminating options 1 and 3 because the most harmful risk factor for the respiratory system is smoking. Select option 4 instead of option 2 because asbestos is toxic to the lungs if particles are inhaled. In addition, option 4 identifies two risk factors, whereas the other options identify only one risk factor. Review the risk factors associated with respiratory disease if you had difficulty with this question.

Reference

Linton, A. (2007). *Introduction to medical-surgical nursing* (4th ed., p. 557). Philadelphia: Saunders.

1491. A female client is being discharged home with an indwelling urinary catheter after the surgical repair of a bladder that was injured as a result of trauma. The nurse concludes that the client understands the principles of catheter management if the client states the need to:

1 Cleanse the perineal area with soap and water once a day.
2 Keep the drainage bag lower than the level of the bladder.

Answer: 2
Rationale: The perineal area should be cleansed with soap and water twice a day and after each bowel movement. The drainage bag should be lower than the level of the bladder, and the tubing should be free of kinks and compression. Adequate fluid intake is necessary to prevent infection and to provide the natural irrigation of the catheter from increased urine flow.

3 Limit fluid intake so that the bag will not become full so quickly.
4 Coil the tubing and place it under the thigh when sitting to avoid tugging on the bladder.

Level of Cognitive Ability: Comprehension
Client Needs: Physiological Integrity
Integrated Process: Nursing Process/Evaluation
Content Area: Fundamental Skills

Test-Taking Strategy: Use the process of elimination. Option 4 is eliminated first because sitting on coiled tubing could cause compression and obstruct drainage. Eliminate option 3 next, knowing that increasing fluids is important. From the remaining options, note that option 1 is insufficient in frequency. Option 2 is correct because this action is consistent with the principles of catheter management. Review these principles if you had difficulty with this question.

Reference
Linton, A. (2007). *Introduction to medical-surgical nursing* (4th ed., p. 848). Philadelphia: Saunders.

1492. A nurse is planning to provide instructions to a client about caring for an ileal conduit. The nurse plans to include which item about ostomy care in discussions with the client?
1 Plan to do appliance changes during the late evening hours.
2 Cleanse the skin around the stoma, use mild soap and water, and rinse and dry the area well.
3 Limit fluids to minimize appliance odor caused by urine breakdown to ammonia.
4 Cut an opening in the faceplate of the appliance that is slightly smaller than the stoma.

Level of Cognitive Ability: Application
Client Needs: Health Promotion and Maintenance
Integrated Process: Teaching and Learning
Content Area: Adult Health/Renal

Answer: 2
Rationale: The skin around the stoma is cleansed at each appliance change using water and a mild, nonresidue soap. The skin is rinsed and then dried thoroughly. The appliance should be changed early in the morning, when urine production is slowest because there is no fluid intake during sleep. Drinking fluids is encouraged to dilute the urine, thereby decreasing the incidence of odor. The appliance is cut so that the opening is not more than 3 mm larger than the stoma. An opening smaller than the stoma will not fit over the stoma.

Test-Taking Strategy: Use the process of elimination. Eliminate option 3 first because limiting fluid intake will not limit ammonia odor; in fact, decreasing fluids will increase the concentration of the urine, thus making it stronger. Option 4 is eliminated next because an appliance cut in this way will be too small to fit over the stoma. From the remaining options, recall that urine flow is slowest in the early morning as a result of decreased intake during the night to direct you to option 2. Review the client teaching points related to an ostomy if you had difficulty with this question.

Reference
Linton, A. (2007). *Introduction to medical-surgical nursing* (4th ed., pp. 409, 411). Philadelphia: Saunders.

1493. A 24-year-old female with a family history of heart disease presents to the physician's office asking to begin oral contraceptive therapy for birth control. The nurse would next inquire whether the client:
1 Exercises regularly
2 Is currently a smoker
3 Eats a low-cholesterol diet
4 Has taken oral contraceptives before

Level of Cognitive Ability: Analysis
Client Needs: Health Promotion and Maintenance

Answer: 2
Rationale: Oral contraceptive use is a risk factor for heart disease, particularly when it is combined with cigarette smoking. Regular exercise and keeping the total cholesterol level under 200 mg/dL are general measures that decrease cardiovascular risk.

Test-Taking Strategy: Use the process of elimination. All of the options are partially correct because they relate either to cardiovascular disease risk factors or medication history. The question asks you to prioritize which option is most important by including the word *next*. The use of oral contraceptives in combination with smoking increases the risk for cardiovascular disease. Review the risks for cardiovascular disease if you had difficulty with this question.

Integrated Process: Nursing Process/Data Collection
Content Area: Pharmacology

Reference
Linton, A. (2007). *Introduction to medical-surgical nursing* (4th ed., p. 1043). Philadelphia: Saunders.

1494. A nurse is implementing measures to maintain adequate peripheral tissue perfusion in a postcardiac surgery client. The nurse avoids which of the following while providing care to this client?

1 Using a knee gatch
2 Elevating the leg while sitting in chair
3 Applying compression stockings
4 Performing range-of-motion (ROM) exercises with the feet

Level of Cognitive Ability: Application
Client Needs: Physiological Integrity
Integrated Process: Nursing Process/Implementation
Content Area: Adult Health/Cardiovascular

Answer: 1
Rationale: After surgery, measures taken to prevent venous stasis include applying elastic stockings or leg wraps, using pneumatic compression boots, discouraging leg crossing, avoiding the use of a knee gatch or placing pillows in the popliteal area, and performing passive and active ROM exercises. Leg elevation while sitting promotes venous drainage and helps to prevent postoperative edema.

Test-Taking Strategy: Note the strategic word *avoids*, and focus on the subject—maintaining adequate tissue perfusion. The use of a knee gatch is contraindicated because it puts pressure on blood vessels in the popliteal area, thus impeding venous return. Review these basic postoperative measures if you had difficulty with this question.

Reference
Christensen, B., & Kockrow, E. (2006). *Adult health nursing* (5th ed., p. 56). St. Louis: Mosby.

1495. A nurse is instructing a client who is in the third trimester of pregnancy about measures to relieve heartburn. Which instruction should the nurse provide to the client?

1 Avoid hot tea.
2 Take frequent sips of milk.
3 Use antacids that contain sodium.
4 Eat fatty foods only once a day in the morning.

Level of Cognitive Ability: Application
Client Needs: Health Promotion and Maintenance
Integrated Process: Teaching and Learning
Content Area: Maternity/Antepartum

Answer: 2
Rationale: Measures to relieve heartburn include small, frequent meals and avoiding fatty fried foods, coffee, and cigarettes. Mild antacids can be used if prescribed and if they do not contain aspirin or sodium. Frequent sips of milk, hot tea, or water are helpful. Gum is also helpful for the relief of heartburn.

Test-Taking Strategy: Use the process of elimination. Eliminate option 3 first because sodium leads to edema and should be avoided. Eliminate option 4 next because fatty and fried foods should be avoided. Knowledge that milk and hot tea can be soothing to the gastrointestinal tract will assist you with eliminating option 1 and direct you to option 2. Review the measures that will reduce heartburn if you had difficulty with this question.

Reference
Christensen, B., & Kockrow, E. (2006). *Foundations of nursing* (5th ed., p. 794). St. Louis: Mosby.

1496. A nurse is providing instructions about home care to the parents of a 3-year-old child with hemophilia. Which statement by the parent indicates the need for further instruction?

1 "My child shouldn't be left unattended."
2 "I need to pad table corners in my home."

Answer: 4
Rationale: The nurse should stress the importance of immunizations, dental hygiene, and routine well-child care. Options 1, 2, and 3 are appropriate. The parents are also instructed in measures to implement in the event of blunt trauma (especially trauma involving the joints), and they are told to apply prolonged pressure to superficial wounds until bleeding has stopped.

3 "I need to remove household items that can tip over."
4 "I need to avoid immunizations and dental hygiene in my child."

Level of Cognitive Ability: Comprehension
Client Needs: Physiological Integrity
Integrated Process: Teaching and Learning
Content Area: Child Health

Test-Taking Strategy: Note the strategic words *need for further instruction.* These words indicate a negative event query and ask you to select an option that is an incorrect statement. Recall that bleeding is a concern in clients with this disorder to assist you with eliminating options 1, 2, and 3, which include measures of protection and safety for the child. Review the care of the child with hemophilia if you had difficulty with this question.

Reference
Price, D., & Gwin, J. (2008). *Pediatric nursing: An introductory text* (10th ed., p. 247). St. Louis: Saunders.

1497. A nurse provides instructions to a client who is taking clorazepate (Tranxene) for the management of an anxiety disorder. Which instruction should the nurse provide to the client?
1 If dizziness occurs, call the physician.
2 Smoking increases the effectiveness of the medication.
3 If gastrointestinal (GI) disturbances occur, discontinue the medication.
4 Drowsiness is a side effect that usually disappears with continued therapy.

Level of Cognitive Ability: Application
Client Needs: Physiological Integrity
Integrated Process: Teaching and Learning
Content Area: Pharmacology

Answer: 4
Rationale: Clorazepate (Tranxene) is a benzodiazepine anxiolytic. The medication can cause drowsiness as a side effect that usually disappears with continued therapy. The client should be instructed to change positions slowly (i.e., from lying to sitting and before standing) to prevent dizziness. Smoking reduces medication effectiveness. GI disturbance is an occasional side effect, and the medication can be given with food if this occurs.

Test-Taking Strategy: Use the process of elimination. Eliminate option 3 first because the client should not be instructed to discontinue the medication. Eliminate option 1 next because episodes of dizziness commonly occur with antianxiety medications, and the client should be told about interventions to alleviate the dizziness. From the remaining options, select option 4 because drowsiness is commonly associated with antianxiety medications and normally disappears with continued therapy. Review clorazepate if you had difficulty with this question.

Reference
Hodgson, B., & Kizior, R. (2009). *Saunders nursing drug handbook 2009* (p. 272). Philadelphia: Saunders.

1498. A client with chlamydial infection has received instructions regarding self-care and the prevention of further infection. The nurse determines that the client requires further instruction if the client states the need to:
1 Use latex condoms to prevent disease transmission.
2 Return to the clinic as requested for a follow-up culture.
3 Use antibiotics prophylactically to prevent symptoms of chlamydia.
4 Reduce the chance of reinfection by limiting the number of sexual partners.

Answer: 3
Rationale: Antibiotics are not taken prophylactically to prevent chlamydia. The risk of reinfection can be reduced by limiting the number of sexual partners and with the use of condoms. In some instances, follow-up culture is requested in 4 to 7 days to confirm a cure.

Test-Taking Strategy: Note the strategic words *requires further instruction.* These words indicate a negative event query and ask you to select an option that is an incorrect action. Options 1 and 4 are correct and are therefore eliminated first. Recall the basic principles of antibiotic therapy to direct you to option 3 because antibiotics are not used intermittently at will for prophylaxis for this infection. Review the measures to prevent chlamydial infection if you had difficulty with this question.

Level of Cognitive Ability: Comprehension
Client Needs: Health Promotion and Maintenance
Integrated Process: Teaching and Learning
Content Area: Fundamental Skills

Reference
Christensen, B., & Kockrow, E. (2006). *Adult health nursing* (5th ed., p. 625). St. Louis: Mosby.

1499. A nurse in the physician's office is reviewing the results of a client's phenytoin (Dilantin) level that was drawn that morning. The nurse determines that the client had a therapeutic drug level if the client's result was:

1 3 mcg/mL
2 8 mcg/mL
3 15 mcg/mL
4 24 mcg/mL

Level of Cognitive Ability: Comprehension
Client Needs: Physiological Integrity
Integrated Process: Nursing Process/Evaluation
Content Area: Pharmacology

Answer: 3
Rationale: Phenytoin is an antiseizure medication. The therapeutic range for serum phenytoin levels is 10 to 20 mcg/mL in clients with normal serum albumin levels and renal function. A level below this range indicates that the client is not receiving sufficient medication and is at risk for seizure activity; the medication dose should be adjusted upward. A level above this range indicates that the client is entering the toxic range and is at risk for toxic side effects of the medication; in this case, the dose should be decreased.

Test-Taking Strategy: To answer this question accurately, you should know the therapeutic drug level for phenytoin. Remember that the therapeutic range for the serum phenytoin level is 10 to 20 mcg/mL in clients with normal serum albumin levels and renal function. Review phenytoin if you had difficulty with this question.

Reference
Hodgson, B., & Kizior, R. (2009). *Saunders nursing drug handbook 2009* (p. 927). St. Louis: Saunders.

1500. A nurse is planning to teach dietary measures to promote fracture healing to a client with a fractured leg in a long-leg cast. Which suggestion would be least helpful to the client?

1 Increase dietary fiber.
2 Follow a high-fat diet.
3 Follow a well-balanced diet.
4 Drink extra fluids.

Level of Cognitive Ability: Application
Client Needs: Physiological Integrity
Integrated Process: Teaching and Learning
Content Area: Adult Health/Musculoskeletal

Answer: 2
Rationale: Clients who are casted have some degree of decreased mobility and should optimize their nutrition to aid in healing. This can be accomplished by increasing the intake of dietary fiber, drinking extra fluids, and following a well-balanced diet.

Test-Taking Strategy: Note the strategic words *least helpful.* Concepts that are useful for answering this question relate to wound healing and decreased mobility. Knowing that wound healing requires balanced nutrition helps you to eliminate option 3. With decreased mobility, there is a risk for constipation, so the client needs increased fluids and dietary fiber. Remember that the question asks for the item that will be least helpful; this will direct you to option 2. Review dietary measures to promote healing if you had difficulty with this question.

Reference
Ignatavicius, D., & Workman, M. (2010). *Medical-surgical nursing: Patient-centered collaborative care* (6th ed., p. 1194). St. Louis: Saunders.

REFERENCES

Christensen, B., & Kockrow, E. (2006). *Adult health nursing* (5th ed.). St. Louis: Mosby.
Christensen, B., & Kockrow, E. (2006). *Foundations of nursing* (5th ed.). St. Louis: Mosby.
deWit, S (2009). *Medical-surgical nursing: Concepts & practice.* St. Louis: Saunders.
Giger, J., & Davidhizar, R. (2008). *Transcultural nursing assessment & intervention* (5th ed.). St. Louis: Mosby.
Hockenberry, M., & Wilson, D. (2009). *Wong's essentials of pediatric care* (8th ed.). St. Louis: Mosby.
Hodgson, B., & Kizior, R. (2009). *Saunders nursing drug handbook 2009.* St. Louis: Saunders.